Dr Ian Morton graduated with a First Class Honours B.Sc. in Pharmacology from Chelsea College, University of London. He gained a Ph.D. from University College London, where he was appointed Lecturer in Pharmacology in 1965. He then moved to King's College London where he became Senior Lecturer in Pharmacology until his retirement. He is now a consultant editor and writer in pharmacology. He is the author of more than one hundred research papers, books and monographs.

Dr Judith Hall graduated with a First Class Honours B.Sc. in Pharmacology from King's College London where she went on to obtain a Ph.D. She has occupied positions in biomedical science at King's College London and the University of Surrey since 1988. In 1995 she was awarded a Wellcome Trust Medical Research Fellowship. She is the author of more than fifty research papers, reviews, books and monographs, and has been an Editor of the *British Journal of Pharmacology*.

Drs Morton and Hall have a keen interest in explaining about drugs and how they work to the non-specialist, and since 1988 have worked together both in writing and editing more than a dozen books as well as contributing to numerous encyclopaedias and medical dictionaries aimed at the general public in both the UK and abroad. They now devote their energies entirely to popular and specialist medical writing.

BY THE SAME AUTHORS

Antibiotics

Medicines for Children

Tranquillizers

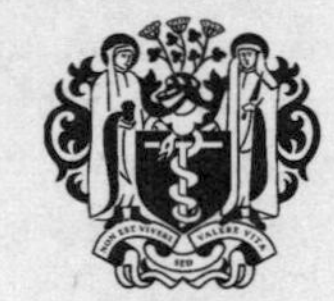

The ROYAL SOCIETY *of* MEDICINE

MEDICINES
THE COMPREHENSIVE GUIDE
SIXTH EDITION

Dr Ian Morton and Dr Judith Hall

BLOOMSBURY

While the creators of this work have made every effort to be as accurate and up to date as possible, medical and pharmacological knowledge is constantly changing and the application of it in particular circumstances depends on many factors. Therefore readers are urged always to consult a qualified medical specialist for individual advice. The writers, researchers, editors and publishers of this book and the Royal Society of Medicine can not be held liable for any errors and omissions, or actions that may be taken as a consequence of using it, nor can they be held responsible for the recommendations of manufacturers regarding uses of proprietary medicines.

All rights reserved; no part of this publication may be reproduced, stored in a retrieval system, or transmitted in any form or by any means, mechanical, photocopying, electronic or otherwise, without the prior written permission of the publishers.

This completely revised edition published in 2002 by
Bloomsbury Publishing Plc
38 Soho Square
London W1D 3HB

www.bloomsburymagazine.com

Text and database copyright © 1995, 1997, 2000, 2002
The Medicines Guide Ltd, London, representing Dr J M Hall and
Dr I K M Morton

Dr I K M Morton and Dr J M Hall assert their moral rights
to be identified as the authors of this work.

British Library Cataloguing in Publication Data

A CIP catalogue for this book is available
from the British Library

ISBN 0 7475 5928 7

This book was produced using Librios®
authoring and content management technology.

www.librios.com

Printed and bound in Great Britain by
Clays Ltd, St Ives plc

CONTENTS

PREFACE

This is the sixth edition of *Medicines: The Comprehensive Guide* – the most popular and best-selling dictionary-style reference source-book for the range of medicines, along with possible side-effects, that is available in the UK today. Previous editions of this book have sold almost two million copies. The text has been extensively revised – to take account of the many new drugs, both generic and proprietary, as well as entire new drug groups, that have been developed and marketed since publication of the fifth edition in 2000. Changes in details of those medicines that remain on the market are also included. Requests from the public have led to the inclusion in this edition of expanded warnings about possible interactions between drugs with other medicines – especially those that can be obtained without a prescription – herbal remedies and nutritional supplements. There is also an expanded glossary of medical terms, which hopefully readers will find useful in understanding some of the more technical terms.

This edition gives international spelling of generic drug names (recommended International Non-proprietary Name; rINN). This changeover from British Approved Names (BAN) reflects the fact that drugs are increasingly often licensed for use in all member states of the European Union (EU) through the European Medicines Evaluation Agency (based in London). But all main generic drug entries in this book give both names (and some US versions), and all names listed A–Z are cross-indexed to the main entries.

The purpose of the book is to give straightforward information on constituent drug components of medicines, describing their uses, explaining in an easy-to-access A–Z format how they work, what side-effects they may have and special conditions or warnings there may be relating to their use. It has been our aim to provide as full and useful a list as is possible and practical, in such a changeable market, of the drug classes (eg antibiotics), non-proprietary (generic) drugs (eg amoxicillin) and most of the proprietary preparations (eg Amoxil) that are available.

There are some categories of preparations we have not felt it was either possible or appropriate to include, however. In particular: [1] preparations of vitamins and minerals that are part of a normal balanced diet are not included, although there are entries on medicines where vitamins and minerals are used medically to correct clinical deficiencies (for example, iron preparations for anaemia, folic acid vitamin supplements in pregnancy); [2] homeopathic or herbal remedies do not fall within the scope of the book, but nevertheless there are many entries on drugs of plant and natural origin, and standardized plant extracts that are part of everyday medicine; [3] the 'social' and non-medical use of drugs is also not covered, although some medicines used to treat drug-overdose and drug-dependence (addiction) are included.

Finally, it is important to note that this book is not intended to be a guide to the prescription or administration of drugs, and it gives neither doses nor recommendations regarding which drugs to use in particular circumstances. A qualified practitioner should always be consulted before any medicine is taken, and the person taking the drug should always read the Patient Information Leaflet (PIL) that now comes with every prescription dispensed.

We hope we have achieved our aim – to help in the public's understanding of the medicines that we all at some time have to take.

IKMM
JMH

HOW TO USE THIS BOOK

The layout of this book was designed to be sufficiently clear for it to be used without further instructions, but some words of explanation may be helpful.

The main section of this book contains entries on the medical drugs (ie medicines) available in the UK, listed A–Z. Drugs are listed under their non-proprietary (generic) and proprietary (brand) names (both will normally appear on packaging of the latter). There are also entries covering the major drug groups that explain in more detail how they work and what they are used for. These are indicated by an ▣ after the name. The A–Z is cross-referenced within the text of one entry to further related entries. These cross-references are indicated when the drug name is printed in the text in SMALL CAPITALS. The side-effects and warnings to be borne in mind when taking a drug are indicated by symbols – ✚ for side-effects and ▲ for warnings – in generic drugs entries. At the end of these articles there is a list of related entries – indicated by a ✪ – which are the proprietary preparations that contain that drug.

At the end of the A–Z section of drugs, there is a Glossary containing explanations of many of the medical and technical terms used in the text, which may be referred to if the reader wants clarification.

Following common practice, drugs are listed in two ways:

The generic name, without an initial capital letter, is the official internationally agreed simplified chemical name of a drug, which unambiguously describes an active constituent of a medicine. For instance, paracetamol is the generic name of an established and familiar drug. In the case of a particular generic formulation, such as paracetamol tablets, even details concerning purity, the time taken for the tablets to dissolve and accuracy of doses are subject to strict control as laid out in the British Pharmacopoeia or other official standards. The generic name is now routinely used in everyday medicine because this is less likely to be misunderstood.

Doctors will often prescribe the generic form of a drug because it costs the NHS less than using a particular proprietary named drug: the active ingredient is identical.

The proprietary name, always with an initial capital letter, is a brand (or trade) name which is a preparation of a drug, or a mixture of drugs, that represents a particular formulation from a particular manufacturer. Manufacturers' names are given in brackets (these are the names that will be found on the packaging and Patient Information Leaflet, or are the companies who can be contacted for more information).

A doctor may prescribe paracetamol simply as 'paracetamol'. In practice, however, common non-prescription drugs such as paracetamol are available not just under their generic name, but also as proprietary preparations under a variety of brand names (Disprol, Panadol etc.). Drugs for many purposes may be prescribed or sold in a variety of forms (capsules, tablets, effervescent tablets, modified-release tablets, powders for solution, suppositories etc.) and sometimes in different strengths (the stronger ones usually have distinguishing names like Forte, Extra or Ultra), and often in varieties that work over longer periods called modified-release preparations (sustained-release preparations or continuous-release preparations; commonly with names containing the terms Continus, CR, MR, SR).

Drugs such as paracetamol are also readily available for non-prescription (over-the-counter; OTC) sale in a combination with other drugs, ie as a 'compound preparation'. For example, there are compound analgesic preparations that contain two or more analgesics (such as paracetamol and codeine), or compound 'cold-cures' (such as paracetamol with a decongestant or a cough suppressant – to treat quite different co-existing symptoms).

Drug class names are used in medicine to group drugs together in various ways, depending on need and emphasis. This can cause confusion even to experts, but in this book there are explanatory entries with cross-referencing between all relevant entries, so navigation between families is straightforward. There are three main ways of grouping drugs. First, and most obvious, is by the purpose of their use (eg antidepressants, contraceptives, antimigraine drugs, HRT, anticancer drugs, vaccines and so on). Second, drugs may be grouped by how they work (eg antihistamines, beta-blockers, calcium-channel blockers etc.). Third, they may be grouped by chemical type (eg barbiturates, benzodiazepines, steroids). The usefulness of these groupings depends on the circumstances, and often one drug may belong to two or more groups.

STEP BY STEP

The following examples highlight the most common points where confusion can arise and serve to illustrate how this book can help. For example, you have bought a proprietary medicine – Nurofen – and want to learn more about its constituents, their other uses, possible side-effects and when such a drug should not be used. Take the following steps:

1. Discover the generic name(s) of the constituent(s)

This information can be obtained by reading the label or packet, or by looking the proprietary (brand) name up in this book. A proprietary entry will list the generic(s) it contains, the drug group the generic(s) belong to (eg analgesics or antibiotics), the form it is available in (eg tablets or nasal spray) and a word or two about its uses. It also provides the manufacturer's name in brackets at the beginning of the entry, which is a useful cross-check of the identity of the preparation. Major pharmaceutical companies, however, may label particular medicines either under their own familiar name or that of a subsidiary. The latter is especially common with OTC (over-the-counter) 'healthcare' products. (Occasionally there may be an unfamiliar name, with some foreign name on the packaging; in which case this may be a 'parallel import' from a country in Europe where the drug is cheaper, therefore look up the generic name – which will use international spelling – and proceed to step 2.)

2. Turn to the generic names or names

Generic entries contain substantially more detail; eg '... is a non-narcotic analgesic with antipyretic properties which is used to treat ...' It also has further information about the drug's main side-effects (✚) and warnings (▲) relating to its administration.

The list of possible side-effects can be extensive, starting with the common and most frequently experienced ones, followed by relatively infrequent reactions and finishing with rarely reported effects. But note, if it is a hospital drug or one used under specialist supervision, then it was not thought appropriate to list all the (often technical) details.

The 'warning' information describes the circumstances when the drug may be unsafe to use or should be used with extreme caution. Two common examples would be during pregnancy or when breast-feeding (where the drug could harm the baby or reduce milk production). Other circumstances may relate to certain diseases, such as kidney or liver disorders which could prevent the drug from being metabolized and excreted normally, or rare but important inherited disorders, such as porphyria, which may cause adverse reactions. These warnings are not exhaustive and do not necessarily apply to all, but they do emphasize the importance of seeking professional medical advice, and explaining all existing medical and other conditions (eg pregnancy). It is always best to check things with your doctor or pharmacist before accepting any sort of medication.

3. For more information read the cross-references

Certain terms or names in SMALL CAPITALS indicate that related or further information can be found at that term's entry. For example, antihypertensives leads to an article that discusses a number of drug types used in treating high blood pressure (eg beta-blockers, diuretics, ACE inhibitors) and its causes (eg lipid-regulating drugs), and can take the reader on to drugs for related conditions (eg anti-angina drugs, heart failure treatment, vasodilators). Some drugs interact with other drugs, herbal remedies or nutritional supplements (such as vitamin tablets) and this can change the effect of the drug or cause adverse reactions. Warnings about interactions are given in these sections. If any technical terms related are not clear, then consult the Glossary at the end of the book which contains explanations of nearly 400 such terms.

4. Going from generic drug names to proprietary preparations

At the end of every generic entry there is a related entry/entries subheading which lists all the proprietaries ('brands') in this book that contain the generic drug in question. Using the A–Z in this way is particularly useful when you are familiar with the generic drug and want to go and buy an appropriate brand.

If you are concerned whether the generic constituents included in, for example, a cold cure have adverse effects in your particular situation, then a glance at the entries would remind you that, say, a sympathomimetic vasoconstrictor should under no circumstances be taken on top of a course of a prescribed monoamine-oxidase inhibitor (MAOI) antidepressant; or that an antihistamine can cause drowsiness to the extent that it would be advisable not to operate machinery or drive a car, and is best taken last thing at night. These examples illustrate, we hope, that gaining an understanding of how prescribed drugs work is not necessarily difficult, and that such an understanding can greatly assist you in getting the most out of the modern healthcare system.

INTRODUCTION

The pharmaceutical industry is one of the UK's most successful industries. There are now about 2,000 prescription-only and 2,000 non-prescription medicines available in the UK alone. Correspondingly, people are increasingly interested in their own health and wellbeing, and particularly in the medicines they take. The medicines available change almost daily, which has meant that this sixth edition of this book is substantially different to the last edition. What are these changes and why have they occurred? And most significantly, what do they mean for those of us who buy and use these medicines?

HOW ARE DRUGS DISCOVERED?

The drug industry

The pharmaceutical industry is one of the most rapidly expanding areas of commerce. Although pharmaceutical companies are increasingly international in their organization, many (whether British or foreign-owned) have a strong base in the UK. In research and development, scientists in the UK have an enviable record of innovation. Also, in the later stages of drug development involving clinical trials, and ultimately the approval and continuing licensing of drugs for use in patients, our Committee on Safety of Medicines and other groups associated with the Medicines Control Agency set world standards for authoritative assessment of safety and efficacy of drugs. In the UK, currently we have one of the most restrictive legislation policies in the world which limits the majority of drugs to prescription-only use.

One outcome of the last couple of decades – the most dynamic period in the history of the pharmaceutical industry – has been the emergence of many new generic drugs, including some entirely new classes of drugs. Some of these have now become famous, such as the beta-blocker 'heart-drugs' and the ulcer-healing H_2-antagonist drugs, which are both British inventions. So extensive has been development work within the pharmaceutical industry, that in this sixth edition, the properties and individual uses of 20 generic beta-blockers (and 68 proprietary formulations) are explained, and they can be used to treat some eight different disease states.

Indeed this edition also sees the introduction or establishment of several promising new drugs or types of drug, including impotence treatment (sildenafil/Viagra), asthma treatment (leukotriene receptor antagonists), potassium-channel activators (to treat angina), new sorts of antidepressants (SNRIs), dementia treatments (donepezil/Aricept) and new types of immunosuppressants for use in organ transplantation (basiliximab, daclizumab, mycophenolate mofetil, alemtuzumab and trastuzumab).

Genetic engineering is proving invaluable in the synthesis of new drugs, sometimes of whole new classes. Drugs that previously required difficult extraction from materials of animal or human origin can now be manufactured by these techniques, including such vital drugs as insulin, hepatitis B vaccine, somatropin (human growth hormone), erythropoietin and interferons. It can confidently be predicted that this trend is set to continue. In some cases literally life-prolonging therapy – for instance, for cancer, AIDS, bleeding and hormone-deficiency diseases – may well become economically as well as theoretically possible. A bonus of these biosynthetically manufactured drugs is their enhanced safety, especially in preventing infection, immune reactions and other biological complications. For example, human growth hormone, used to treat short stature (dwarfism) in children, was at one time isolated from the pituitary glands of cadavers and so brought with it the risk of acquiring Creutzfeldt-Jakob disease due to infecting contamination; however, it has now been replaced in the UK by somatropin, which is a biosynthetic human form that has no risk of contamination.

Nature herself continues to give us new drugs. Pharmacology and medicinal chemistry have a long history of discovering lead compounds in plant and other organisms. In the second half of the twentieth century, hundreds of valuable antibiotics were developed from ferments of fungal moulds. These are used not only for infections by micro-organisms but also in cancer treatment, and as leads in discovery of novel chemicals for a variety of purposes. This edition sees a number of new drugs developed from natural compounds, notably additional and important uses for the taxanes, which are anticancer compounds derived from a complex substance in the yew tree, purified and modified in the laboratory to yield a reliable and safer drug. Herbal medicine is having something of a renaissance, with evidence-based research leading to a better understanding of its risks and benefits.

Future developments

Will this rapid progress continue? Some people within the industry are not optimistic because of escalating costs of drug development; to produce just one new drug can take years and cost millions. However, new research strategies, many involving the emerging science of molecular biology (including genetic engineering), may prove cheaper and more effective, and certainly allow the increased emergence of new sorts of drugs that previously could only be dreamt of. Our new-found ability to manufacture the human form of protein hormones was touched on above. Also a new form of drug called monoclonal antibodies can now be manufactured. These are pure protein molecules of human form, which in principle might work as a sort of specific 'magic bullet' targeting only certain sites in the body so as to deliberately modify function. So far for fairly preliminary indications, they have been harnessed for diverse tasks, including as immunosuppressants for use in organ transplantation, to inhibit platelet aggregation and thrombus formation in heart operations, as antiviral agents, and to destroy certain white blood cells in anticancer treatment for people with lymphoma. Many future applications for such drugs can be envisaged.

Progress in the chemotherapy of infection in the past few decades has gone in fits and starts. In the fight against bacterial and other infections there were several decades of enormous optimism and progress, and we now have about 70 generic antibiotics in the UK alone which can work against a very wide range of infections. But, at the same time there has been worldwide over-use of antibiotics, and strains of bacteria resistant to all but a few 'reserve' antibiotics (eg infections by MRSA; methoxycillin-resistant *Staphylococcus aureus*) are becoming all too common. So the pharmaceutical industry has to look again for sources of new antibacterial drugs. In the search for drugs active against viruses, initial progress was slow. However, the spread of AIDS infection has proved a catalyst in terms of research expenditure, and there are now about 30 antiviral agents available in the UK. In terms of the development of resistance by pathogen organisms, the moral from treatment of TB and other very serious infections has been that multi-drug therapy often proves better in the long run. The concurrent use of two or three different classes of antiviral drugs in the treatment of AIDS (eg protease inhibitors together with reverse transcriptase inhibitors) has proved to be of great benefit to the patient (and the newborn infant).

The next revolutionary advance is expected to be the development of 'individualized' medications tailored to the particular patient being treated. This may be one of the spin-offs of the Human Genome Project and the recent sequencing of the entire human genetic code. It is now technically possible to examine the genome of an individual (eventually with a microchip chemical device in the 'doctor's surgery') that will identify areas within the chromosomes that make that person or their children genetically susceptible to particular diseases (eg sickle-cell anaemia) or to the effects of certain drugs, foodstuffs or environmental chemicals (eg porphyria and G6PD deficiency). Early attempts are already being made to delete, replace or prevent expression of defective genetic material (eg by transfer of DNA in gene therapy for cystic fibrosis).

How are drugs prescribed and used?

Successful medical therapy has always depended on a partnership between the patient and medical professionals – pharmacists, doctors and nursing staff.

Every patient is different and requires individual treatment – a truth that is often easy to forget in a world where the mass production and standardization of products and practice is regarded as the norm. Medicines are prepared and tested according to the most rigorous criteria of standardization, for the sake of safety as well as for economic efficiency. But because people are all likely to be different to some degree, either in their basic genetic make-up or in the circumstances surrounding the condition they are seeking to treat, an individual's response to a certain drug must therefore be taken into account.

Where prescribed medicines are concerned, the doctor has the information and knowledge to allow him or her to help interpret specific needs and situations, and prescribe accordingly. But an increasing number of medicines are now becoming available without prescription and can be bought directly from a pharmacy.

Associated with this is a growing trend to give an increasing share of the advisory role to the pharmacist. However, the doctor will know important details of a patient's history and present condition, which is privileged information that the pharmacist will not have access to. Consequently, this trend towards making more medicines available without prescription places a substantial responsibility for choosing the correct medication on the patient, or on carers in the case of children, the elderly and those who are too ill to co-operate. This book contains much of the information necessary for making sensible choices.

The move to non-prescription drugs

The number of drugs switched each year from prescription-only to an OTC, over-the-counter (non-prescription), status has markedly increased of late. About 50 have moved over in the last couple of decades. This switch has had a great effect on the marketing of proprietary medicines. For example, the analgesic ibuprofen was one of the 11 prescription drugs that changed status in this period, and now there are nearly 50 proprietary preparations of it listed in this book alone.

Members of several major drug groups have quite recently had their status changed from prescription-only to over-the-counter. For example, three members of the ulcer-healing H_2-antagonist group (eg ranitidine/Zantac) are now available OTC (although only for the treatment of dyspepsia rather than ulcers), a number of OTC corticosteroid preparations (for topical use for certain skin conditions) and antifungal treatments (for thrush infections) have all become available without prescription. However, whereas the common analgesics (paracetamol, aspirin and ibuprofen) are on the 'GSL' (General Sales List), and so are available from outlets such as supermarkets and petrol station shops, these latter drugs are on the 'P' list which indicates that they can only be obtained from a qualified pharmacist (normally in a pharmacy).

As more medicines become readily available without prescription, authorities in the UK expect patients to become more skilled at knowing when they should seek expert advice. For much the same reasons, the list of drugs that may be prescribed by nurses and dentists has also been extended, and it is likely that various healthcare workers will be empowered in future either to prescribe or to recommend medication.

Cost considerations

In part, these changes from prescription-only to OTC medicines are motivated by financial objectives. On the one hand, the cost of drugs is the biggest single item of the National Health Service annual bill, so the government is looking to shed some of this load. On the other hand, nearly half of all prescriptions actually cost less than the standard prescription charge, so there are obvious savings in encouraging patients to seek the pharmacist's help over remedies for minor conditions.

Some medicines are so expensive that the NHS has insufficient funds to allow their widespread prescription. Most people will be already aware of the impact of 'post-code prescribing' where the likelihood of a patient receiving one of these very expensive medicines depends on the fund allocations of the district in which they live.

In order to appraise new and existing therapies, and to assess their efficacy and cost-effectiveness, an independent national body, the National Institute for Clinical Excellence (NICE, which was founded in 1999) issues guidance around their use, mainly with respect to their prescription or otherwise within the NHS. Its recommendations have sought to define those types of patients who show the best chance of benefiting from expensive treatments. For example, recommendations have included guidance for taxane anticancer drug therapy for ovarian and breast cancer, and for the prescribing of beta-interferon in the treatment of multiple sclerosis (MS). In March 2002 new guidelines were issued regarding the use of two anticancer drugs, oxaliplatin and irinotecan, for certain types of advanced colorectal cancer.

The move to European practices

Some of the changes in prescribing practice are part of a gradual evolution towards a common standard in Europe. Currently, the UK has one of the most restrictive pharmaceutical legislations in the world, and those who travel widely may already be aware that a very high proportion of the drugs listed in this book as prescription-only are available over-the-counter in much of the rest of Europe (and to an even greater extent in the Americas and in the East). In fact the increasing unification of Europe is having important consequences on medicines legislation. Drugs are increasingly often licensed for use in all member states of the European Union (EU) through the European Medicines Evaluation Agency (EMEA). British legislators have been central to this process, and the EMEA is situated in London. It is the intention of the UK to entirely change over, for generic names, from British Approved Names (BAN) to recommended International Non-proprietary Names (rINN). This book gives both names in all generic drug entries (along with other common names, including some US versions), with all cross-referenced to the main entries (listed by rINN).

Drugs and the traveller

The traveller should note that the generic names of drugs differ little between countries. Since this book lists generic drugs under the new European standard names (as well as major American ones), it should be valuable for use when travelling.

Proprietary names used by a manufacturer for the same generic drug are today less likely to be totally different according to the country in which it is marketed, although there may be minor variations in spelling to accommodate local requirements. It is important to note that some medicines available abroad, both OTC and prescription, may not have been rigorously tested or approved in the UK. A pharmacist should always be consulted in cases of doubt.

Drugs and the Internet

There is now quite wide availability of medicines (and medical advice) on the Internet, and much of this is essentially unregulated and unverified. Some of the medicines apparently freely available for sale (eg Viagra) are actually prescription-only in the UK. Clearly this is yet another set of circumstances where the individual needs access to impartial and accurate information of the type that this book can offer.

USING MEDICINES

How are medicines administered?

Medicines have to able to get to the place where they are to work. How they are given to do this is called the route of administration. They can be applied directly to the site of action (topically), by mouth (orally), by injection (parenterally), by rectum (rectally), via the lungs (by inhalation) and through the skin (transdermally). There are good reasons why different routes of administration are chosen for different purposes.

For example, when a medicine is being used to treat a skin, vaginal, ear, nose, mouth or eye condition, the best way to achieve this is by preparing (formulating) the medicine in a form that can be applied directly (eg as a cream, pessary or drops). When a medicine is applied directly to the site at which it acts, it is called a topical medicine; and because, in general, very little of the medicine enters the body, systemic side-effects are likely to be minimal. Inhalation is another way of delivering a medicine to the site where it is to have its therapeutic effect (the bronchioles of the lungs), and again this route of administration limits side-effects if it is a drug that is little absorbed from there into the bloodstream. However, some drugs are inevitably absorbed in small amounts and so act systemically (eg corticosteroids when inhaled in asthma prophylaxis).

Often, however, medicines need to be inside the body in order to reach the tissue of an organ that needs to be treated (eg kidney, heart, blood vessels). This is mainly achieved by allowing the drug to travel to the relevant tissue or organ in the bloodstream. So when a medicine is taken by mouth (orally), it is absorbed from the stomach or intestine, enters the bloodstream of the body in much the same way as nutrients do from food, and is then transported to its site of action. After transdermal application, the medicine enters the body through the skin (eg HRT therapy, nicotine patches for smoking habituation treatment). Injection is another way of introducing a medicine into the body, and is a useful route of administration when a drug needs to act quickly (and avoids the drug getting broken down by the gastrointestinal tract). Sometimes 'depot' injections are used where the medicine is released slowly into the blood from a 'pool' injected under the skin. These systemic routes of administration, where the medicine is conveyed in the bloodstream, have the consequence that the drug reaches most tissues and organs in the body, in addition to the ones it is being used to treat, and for this reason drugs taken systemically may have quite extensive side-effects.

Sometimes a medicine may have to be taken rectally, in the form of an enema, suppository or solution. This may be because the patient is too ill to take the medicine by mouth (or is vomiting), or because the medicine would be broken down by the stomach.

Using medicines properly

It is important to know why you are taking a medicine, and how to use your medicine properly. Medicines are used to prevent (eg vaccines), cure (eg antibacterials) or control (eg antihypertensives) medical conditions, or to alleviate symptoms (eg painkillers) whilst the condition gets better on its own. Some important things that you should know before taking your medicine are listed below. Each medicine has special instructions unique to itself – therefore if you are at all unsure of any of these points, or they are not clearly explained in the Patient Information Leaflet, it is imperative that you check with either your doctor or pharmacist (often the quickest and easiest approach is to contact your pharmacist first).

What you should know before taking your medicine:

- Are there any important side-effects that should be looked out for or reported?
- Do you have a pre-existing condition or allergy you should have told your doctor or pharmacist about?
- What other medications should not be taken at the same time?
- Did you tell your doctor or pharmacist about any herbal or complementary medicines or supplements you are taking?
- Should it be taken before, during or after food or drink?
- If you miss a dose, should you take two the next time?
- Does 'four times a day' mean at night too?
- Will the medicine make you drowsy so that driving may be dangerous?
- Can you drink alcohol when taking the medicine?
- Should the whole course of medicine be taken even if you get better?
- How should the medicine be stored/discarded?

What are side-effects and why do they occur?

One of the biggest problems associated with taking medicines relates to the side-effects they may have. Drugs act by having specific effects on the body, usually to attack the cause or relieve the symptoms of an illness. However, while dealing with the conditions they were designed to treat, many drugs also affect the body in other, undesirable ways that are incidental to their primary purpose. These adverse reactions, or side-effects, may be so mild as to be barely noticeable, or so severe as to be life-threatening, depending on the drug and the person taking it.

Adverse reactions that result in side-effects can be categorized into one of two main kinds:

'Type A' reactions are inherent in the way the drug acts pharmacologically, and are largely inevitable and very difficult to circumvent. For instance, the side-effects of drowsiness and sedation (due to actions on the brain) are so common with antihistamines that they are accepted by most sufferers as inevitable. However, the pharmaceutical industry is well aware of the inconvenience of side-effects and attempts are continually being made to minimize them. For example, newer antihistamines are altered chemically to restrict the drug's access to the brain. It is important to be aware that such developments are occurring so that, where undesirable side-effects are experienced, discussion with a physician may result in finding a more individually acceptable treatment.

'Type B' reactions are less predictable, and are often referred to as 'idiosyncratic'. A major cause of these idiosyncratic reactions is a true allergic reaction to a drug by the body's immune system. A sensitivity reaction of this kind can present a serious threat to the patient, and the dangers can only be minimized if the patient is aware of the danger because of an earlier reaction to a drug of that class. Physicians routinely ask whether the patient is allergic to antibiotics or local anaesthetics before prescribing them – and each individual must know his or her own idiosyncratic (allergic) responses. After immunizations with vaccines such as those using egg products in their manufacture, the patient is asked to stay afterwards for at least twenty minutes in the waiting-room because of possible allergic reactions. However, some antibiotics, local anaesthetics and other drugs that cause allergic reactions are now available over-the-counter for non-prescription use, so it is vitally important to read the Patient Information Leaflet (PIL) that comes with the medicine, and be aware of the warning signs of reaction. In particular, some medicines contain arachis oil (peanut oil) to which many people are now allergic.

Doctors have a well-tested procedure in the UK whereby they report all suspected adverse drug reactions directly to the Committee on Safety of Medicines (CSM) using so-called 'Yellow Cards' that are issued to them. This has resulted in the amassing of much useful statistical data about the incidence of rarer side-effects. In particular, new medications are listed in a special way, and doctors are asked to be particularly vigilant in reporting unexpected reactions with these – and this has been especially valuable in dealing with this type of danger, leading to specific warnings being issued about the type of patient for whom the drug should not be prescribed (and sometimes resulting in early withdrawal of that drug from the market).

Are drugs really safe?

Questions about drug safety only make sense on a risk-to-benefit basis. In other words, does the severity of the condition warrant risking certain known side-effects? At one end of the scale, for example, is a certain individual's headache sufficiently severe that it is worth risking the known side-effects of aspirin? If the individual is in good health with no history of intolerance to NSAID drugs, and no form of stomach upset, then the answer may well be Yes. On the other hand if the individual is a child, or a person who has a predisposition towards gastric ulcers or asthma, then the answer will be No.

At the other end of the risks-to-benefit scale is the patient who has a life-threatening infection, or cancer. Then the physician may discuss with the patient whether to prescribe treatment with drugs that would be too toxic to use for less-serious conditions.

In terms of risks-to-benefit, vaccination is an extremely valuable precaution. It can, by treating the most vulnerable sectors of the population, completely eliminate some infectious diseases. Smallpox infection no longer exists in the world population, and poliomyelitis may soon be eliminated; both as a result of global vaccination programmes. In the UK, MMR vaccination of children has been introduced with the intention of eliminating mumps, measles and rubella (German measles). Although there may be very rare incidences of serious adverse reactions, most people accept that these risks are far outweighed by the considerable threat to children of contracting the infections themselves. And in any vaccination programme, it is important that all children, rather than just a selection, are vaccinated, or the diseases may regenerate in the unvaccinated group and so become re-established in the population.

When interpreting the side-effects of individual drugs listed in this book, it is important to understand that the longer the period a drug has been in use, the longer the list of possible side-effects is likely to be. Conversely, new drugs may appear to be free of side-effects because less is known about them as they are still going through the reporting processes. In the listings provided in this book, generally the most frequently experienced side-effects appear first, while those at the end of the list are likely to be seen less often.

Similarly, the 'warnings' are based on experience that doctors accumulate in using that drug, and some drugs may not be used by certain people (they are 'contraindicated'), so an alternative drug may be tried.

It can also be seen that the majority of the drugs in this book should be avoided by women who are pregnant or breast-feeding, because, although it is not always known that they are dangerous to the baby, the lessons of the thalidomide disaster have not been forgotten.

Individuals at risk of adverse reaction

People suffering from the following conditions are particularly susceptible to certain drugs or forms of drug therapy. Although the conditions are generally rare, it is very important to be aware of them, and reminders to this effect appear throughout this book under the lists of 'warnings'.

Inherited conditions

Porphyria appears as a 'should not use' warning in many entries. This fairly rare inherited condition, which causes abnormal metabolism of blood pigments, is serious in its own right, but is potentially lethal in combination with a wide range of drugs – some of which are commonly available and otherwise harmless. Normally, individuals who have porphyria know so, but the condition is sufficiently serious that relatives of patients should also be screened.

G6PD deficiency (glucose 6-phosphate dehydrogenase enzyme deficiency) is a genetically inherited condition, and is relatively common in African, Indian and some Mediterranean peoples. Serious adverse reactions occur in those affected when they take any of a range of drugs; for instance, the antimalarial drug primaquine causes red blood cell haemolysis in 5–10% of black males, leading to severe anaemia.

Slow acetylators are people in a similar situation to G6PD deficiency. This describes an inherited condition where an enzyme that breaks down drugs within the body has low activity, and so it is therefore important that lower doses of such drugs (eg isoniazid) are taken by people with this disorder.

Non-inherited conditions

Age needs to be taken into account as a factor in drug doses. The elderly metabolize drugs slowly so lower doses usually need to be used; the elderly are also more likely to become confused with many drugs that act on the brain. Children are especially at risk, and doctors have special ways of working out appropriate doses when it is necessary to prescribe for the young. The manufacturers of OTC medicines always take care to indicate the age-groups and doses for those of their products appropriate for children, and the labelling should be read carefully. It is important to remember that only the current labelling on these OTC products is definitive.

Kidney disorders slow down the excretion of drugs and so active constituents may remain in the body for longer than is intended, therefore doses should be adjusted.

Liver disorders slow down the body's metabolism of drugs, so lower doses may be needed.

Alcoholism is likely to have caused damage to the liver, so the same considerations apply as liver disorders – the slowing down of the body's metabolism of drugs and so lower doses may be required.

Heart disease requires special care when drugs are prescribed, and more usually patients need special advice on the safe use of medicines.

Pregnancy requires special care and, as mentioned already, it is probably best to avoid taking any drugs during pregnancy if this is possible. Even before becoming pregnant it is a good idea to discontinue use of some drugs as well as alcohol to avoid any residual effects. Not all drugs are damaging in pregnancy, and indeed some may be beneficial. The Department of Health now agrees that supplements of the vitamin folic acid help prevent neural tube defects (eg spina bifida) when taken before and during the first three months of pregnancy.

Breast-feeding. Specific information is available on which drugs are of concern because they pass to the baby in the mother's milk or affect milk production. Here, too, as a general rule it is best to avoid all drugs if possible (including smoking and using illicit drugs). If this is not possible then, of course, a doctor should be consulted in every case.

People taking other medications. When buying, or being prescribed a medicine, always tell your doctor or pharmacist if you are taking any other medication – including herbal or homeopathic remedies, because of possible interactions.

Taking more than one drug a time

One of the greatest inherent dangers in the use of either prescription or non-prescription drugs lies in the unpredictability of the interaction between two or more different drugs, or even in the interaction between drugs and foodstuffs or environmental factors.

The risk of serious interactions between monoamine-oxidase inhibitor (MAOI) antidepressants and certain foodstuffs and decongestants is well known. Most people will be aware of the additive or potentiating action that alcohol has on the sedative or sleep-enhancing effects of many drugs, such as benzodiazepine anxiolytics, antihistamines and components of 'cold cures'. It is a legal requirement that medicines are labelled in standard ways to warn the user of such hazards.

There is a widely held belief that antibiotics and alcohol 'do not mix'. This is true for some but not for all. For example, certain antibiotics (eg azole antimicrobials such as metronidazole) interfere with the metabolism of alcohol so that it produces a toxic metabolite, called acetaldehyde, in the body, and this may make the subject feel very ill indeed (see the entry on disulfiram).

Details of some of the more worrying drug interactions are given in the individual generic entries. However, by no means all interactions are detrimental, and two drugs may be specifically prescribed to be taken together for a variety of reasons. For example, one of a pair of drugs may inhibit the break down or excretion of the other drug, so prolonging its beneficial effects (eg clavulanic acid prolongs the duration of action of antibiotics such as amoxycillin by inhibiting bacterial penicillinase enzymes which break down many penicillin antibiotics). Another reason for taking two drugs simultaneously is where one drug counteracts the adverse effects of the other; this can occur in the treatment of Parkinson's disease and other diseases of the central nervous system.

Note that important interactions can occur between conventional drugs, alternative remedies or supplements where either the therapeutic effect of the drugs taken can be changed or there may be adverse reactions. Any prescription, over-the-counter medicines, supplements, herbal remedies or other alternative therapies that you are using, have recently used or plan to use should be discussed with your doctor or pharmacist before you take or are administered any medicine. Important interactions will be detailed in the Patient Information Leaflet that comes with your medication.

In general, however, drug interactions are complex and sometimes difficult to predict, and depend on individual circumstances; and thus full details of all possible interactions are not included in this book. The doctor or pharmacist will have detailed charts of known interactions which in all cases should be consulted, and expert opinion should always be taken if more than one drug is to be used at a time.

In summary

Good medical therapy depends on a partnership between the patient and medical professionals, but deregulation is lowering the protective shield afforded by the prescription-only approach to drug therapy, and as a result greater responsibility is being thrown on the individual. We must therefore become conversant with some facts about our own individual reactions to the basic types of drugs. We must know when it is essential to seek advice from the healthcare professionals and what to ask them. This book is emphatically not a guide to self-medication, but it is intended to help in this process by providing a comprehensive source of understandable information about the medicines themselves.

Other publications

Healthcare professionals use a number of similar guides. The British National Formulary (BNF) – issued twice a year by the British Medical Association and the Royal Pharmaceutical Society of Great Britain – is the standard, impartial and authoritative guide. Along with MIMS (Monthly Index of Medical Specialities, a commercial compendium), the BNF is circulated to prescribing medical practitioners. Over-the-counter drugs are covered by the *OTC Directory*, published by PAGB (Proprietary Association of Great Britain) and issued to healthcare professionals, and can also be obtained by the public.

Detailed information on proprietary drugs is also available to professionals from manufacturers, and is published annually in the ABPI Handbook (Association of British Pharmaceutical Industry). Independent comment on drug-related matters is available to everyone in the *Drug and Therapeutics Bulletin* published by the Consumers' Association.

The *Guide to Drugs and Medicines*, published by the British Medical Association (BMA), and *Which Medicine?*, from the Consumers' Association, deal with drugs under disease-related headings, and this book can act as a complementary reference source to these.

Some useful web sites include: www.nhsdirect.nhs.uk; www.abpi.org.uk (the official site of the Association of the British Pharmaceutical Industry); www.bmjbookshop.com (the online bookshop of the British Medical Association); www.pharmpress.com (the Pharmaceutical Press web site, which is the publications division of the Royal Pharmaceutical Society of Great Britain); and www.netdoctor.co.uk (which provides information on all aspects of health and healthcare). The Royal Society of Medicine's *The Patient's Internet Handbook* (www.patient-handbook.co.uk) is an indispensable guide to finding health information on the Internet.

Readers' letters

The authors welcome any comments, suggestions or criticisms regarding the scope, structure and ease of use of this book, as it is their aim to constantly review and improve the guide during the compiling and revision of each new edition. If you do wish to contact them, please write to Medicines Guide Ltd, 21 Catherine Street, London, WC2B 5JS. Unfortunately, the authors are unable to comment on an individual's course of treatment.

IKMM
JMH
June 2002

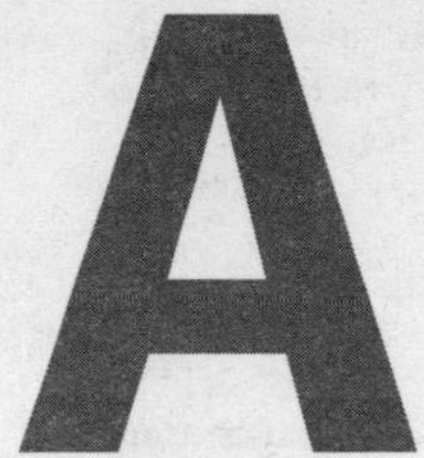

AAA Mouth and Throat Spray

(Manx) is a proprietary, non-prescription preparation of the LOCAL ANAESTHETIC benzocaine, and can be used for the short-term, symptomatic relief of pain associated with sore throat and mouth infections. It is available as a spray, and is not normally given to children under six years, except on medical advice.
✚▲ Side-effects/warnings: See BENZOCAINE.

abacavir

is a (*reverse transcriptase*) ANTIVIRAL drug which can be used in the treatment of HIV infection, in combination with other antivirals. Administration is oral.
✚ Side-effects: Serious hypersensitivity reactions; nausea and vomiting, diarrhoea, abdominal pain; anorexia, fatigue, lethargy, fever, blood changes.
▲ Warnings: It is a specialist drug, and there will be full assessment and patient monitoring throughout treatment.
✪ **Related entries: Trizivir; Ziagen.**

abciximab

is an ANTIPLATELET drug, a monoclonal antibody (a form of pure antibody produced by a type of molecular engineering) which inhibits platelet aggregation and thrombus formation. It is used by specialist doctors as an adjunct to heparin and aspirin for the prevention of complications due to clot formation in high-risk patients undergoing certain types of coronary angioplasty operations. It is administered by intravenous injection or infusion.
✚▲ Side-effects/warnings: It has widespread toxicity, and is used only under close supervision of a hospital specialist.
✪ **Related entry: ReoPro.**

Abelcet

(Elan) is a proprietary, prescription-only preparation of the ANTIFUNGAL and ANTIBIOTIC amphotericin, which has an unusual formulation as a lipid colloidal dispersion (with L-α-dimyristoylphosphatidylcholine and L-α-dimyristoylphosphatidylglycerol) that is intended to minimize toxicity, and can be used for severe systemic fungal infections. It is available in a form for intravenous infusion.
✚▲ Side-effects/warnings: See AMPHOTERICIN.

abortifacient

drugs are used to induce abortion or miscarriage, as a medical alternative to surgical termination. A number of types of drug have been used to procure therapeutic abortion, but commonly the progestogen HORMONE ANTAGONIST drug MIFEPRISTONE is used (given orally) and/or a prostaglandin (eg GEMEPROST, or sometimes DINOPROSTONE), by pessary. A variety of other synthetic or natural agents, and certain microbial toxins, may cause abortion (depending on dose and route of administration).

acamprosate calcium

is a drug used to treat alcoholic patients when they are being withdrawn from alcohol. It is thought to work by affecting the actions of amino acid neurotransmitters in the brain. Administration is oral.
✚ Side-effects: There may be nausea, vomiting, diarrhoea, abdominal pain, itching and other skin reactions; variations in sex drive.
▲ Warnings: It is a specialist drug. It is not used in kidney and severe liver impairment; nor in pregnancy or breast-feeding. It is essential that the patient does not continue alcohol abuse, or the treatment will fail.
✪ **Related entry: Campral EC.**

acarbose

is an ENZYME INHIBITOR that delays the conversion in the intestine of starch and sucrose (sugar) to glucose, and subsequent absorption, and is used in DIABETIC TREATMENT. It has recently been introduced for the treatment of Type II diabetes (non-insulin-dependent diabetes mellitus; NIDDM; maturity-onset diabetes), sometimes in combination with other drugs. It may be of value in patients where other drugs, or diet control, have not been successful, so is useful in obese patients. It is available as tablets to be taken immediately before food.

A

✚ Side-effects: Gastrointestinal disturbances, including diarrhoea, flatulence, bloating, distension and abdominal pain (which become less with time).
▲ Warnings: Because of side-effects it should not be used if there are certain types of intestinal disease. It is not used in pregnancy or when breast-feeding, or when there are certain kidney or liver disorders. Blood glucose and liver enzymes will be monitored. Patients who are also taking INSULIN, or a SULPHONYLUREA-class oral hypoglycaemic drug, in addition to acarbose, need to carry glucose (to counteract hypoglycaemia) rather than sucrose, since acarbose interferes with the conversion and absorption of sucrose.
✪ **Related entry: Glucobay.**

Accolate

(Zeneca; AstraZeneca) is a proprietary, prescription-only preparation of the ANTI-ALLERGIC and ANTI-ASTHMATIC drug zafirlukast, a LEUKOTRIENE-RECEPTOR ANTAGONIST. It is used for the prevention (prophylaxis) of asthma, and is available as tablets.
✚▲ Side-effects/warnings: See ZAFIRLUKAST.

Accupro

(Parke-Davis; Pfizer) is a proprietary, prescription-only preparation of the ACE INHIBITOR quinapril. It can be used as an ANTIHYPERTENSIVE and in HEART FAILURE TREATMENT, and is available as tablets.
✚▲ Side-effects/warnings: See QUINAPRIL.

Accuretic

(Parke-Davis; Pfizer) is a proprietary, prescription-only compound preparation of the ACE INHIBITOR quinapril and the (THIAZIDE) DIURETIC hydrochlorothiazide. It can be used as an ANTIHYPERTENSIVE, and is available as tablets.
✚▲ Side-effects/warnings: See HYDROCHLOROTHIAZIDE; QUINAPRIL.

acebutolol

is a BETA-BLOCKER. It can be used as an ANTIHYPERTENSIVE for raised blood pressure, as an ANTI-ANGINA to relieve symptoms and to improve exercise tolerance and as an ANTI-ARRHYTHMIC to regularize heartbeat and to treat myocardial infarction (damage to heart muscle, usually due to a heart attack). Administration is oral. It is also available, as an antihypertensive, in the form of compound preparations with a DIURETIC.
✚▲ Side-effects/warnings: See PROPRANOLOL HYDROCHLORIDE.
✪ **Related entries: Secadrex; Sectral.**

aceclofenac

is a (NSAID) NON-NARCOTIC ANALGESIC and ANTIRHEUMATIC drug which is used to treat pain and inflammation in rheumatoid arthritis and ankylosing spondylitis, and for short-term treatment of osteoarthritis. Administration is oral.
✚▲ Side-effects/warnings: See NSAID. It should be avoided by those with porphyria.
✪ **Related entry: Preservex.**

ACE inhibitor 🅱

(angiotensin-converting enzyme inhibitor) drugs are used as ANTIHYPERTENSIVE drugs and in HEART FAILURE TREATMENT. They work as ENZYME INHIBITOR drugs by inhibiting the conversion of the natural circulating HORMONE angiotensin I to angiotensin II; and because the latter is a potent VASOCONSTRICTOR, the overall effect is vasodilation (see VASODILATOR) with a HYPOTENSIVE action. This action is of value when the blood pressure is raised (as in hypertension) and also in the treatment of heart failure. There has been a considerable increase recently in the use of ACE inhibitors in moderate hypertension and in severe hypertension when other treatments are not suitable or successful. They are also useful when used as an antihypertensive in insulin-dependent diabetes to protect the kidneys. They are usually used in conjunction with other antihypertensive treatments, especially DIURETIC and sometimes CALCIUM-CHANNEL BLOCKER drugs, and with digoxin in HEART FAILURE TREATMENT. See CAPTOPRIL; CILAZAPRIL; ENALAPRIL MALEATE; FOSINOPRIL; IMIDAPRIL HYDROCHLORIDE; LISINOPRIL; MOEXIPRIL HYDROCHLORIDE; PERINDOPRIL; QUINAPRIL; RAMIPRIL; TRANDOLAPRIL.
✚ Side-effects: ACE inhibitors can cause very marked hypotension (especially when instigating treatment) and also kidney impairment. They may also cause persistent dry cough, angioedema, rash (sometimes with itching and urticaria), pancreatitis, respiratory tract symptoms (eg sinusitis, rhinitis); gastrointestinal effects include

nausea and vomiting, dyspepsia, diarrhoea or constipation. There may be altered liver function, jaundice, hepatitis; changes in blood counts; occasionally headache, dizziness, fatigue and malaise, taste disturbance, tingling in the extremities and bronchospasm.
▲ Warnings: ACE inhibitors should not be used in patients with hypersensitivity to ACE inhibitors, in renovascular disease and certain heart defects, or in pregnancy. They should be used with caution in patients with peripheral vascular disease or severe atherosclerosis. When put on ACE inhibitors, the first doses may cause profound hypotension, especially in people taking diuretics, who are on a low-sodium diet, have heart failure or who are dehydrated. Potassium supplements should be avoided when taking ACE inhibitors or there is a risk of hyperkalemia (high blood potassium levels) developing.

acemetacin

is a (NSAID) NON-NARCOTIC ANALGESIC and ANTIRHEUMATIC. It is used to treat serious rheumatic and arthritic complaints, musculoskeletal pain and postoperative pain. Chemically, it is closely related to indometacin (it is its glycolic acid ester), and is administered orally.
✚▲ Side-effects/warnings: See INDOMETACIN; NSAID. It should not be administered to patients who are breast-feeding.
✪ Related entry: Emflex.

acenocoumarol

(nicoumalone) is a synthetic ANTICOAGULANT which can be used to prevent the formation of clots in heart disease, after heart surgery (especially following implantation of prosthetic heart valves) and to prevent venous thrombosis and pulmonary embolism. Administration is oral.
✚▲ Side-effects/warnings: See WARFARIN SODIUM.
✪ Related entry: Sinthrome.

Acepril

(Squibb; Bristol-Myers Squibb) is a proprietary, prescription-only preparation of the ACE INHIBITOR captopril. It can be used as an ANTIHYPERTENSIVE and in HEART FAILURE TREATMENT, usually in conjunction with other classes of drug. It is available as tablets.
✚▲ Side-effects/warnings: See CAPTOPRIL.

acetaminophen

is the standard name used in the USA for PARACETAMOL.

acetazolamide

is a CARBONIC-ANHYDRASE INHIBITOR with quite wide-ranging actions in the body. It is mainly used in GLAUCOMA TREATMENT to treat several forms of the disorder, because it reduces the formation of aqueous humour in the eye. It acts as a DIURETIC and is sometimes used to treat oedema. It has also been used as an ANTI-EPILEPTIC to assist in the prevention of certain types of epileptic seizures, especially in children. Additionally, it is sometimes used to treat the symptoms of premenstrual syndrome and to prevent mountain sickness. Administration is either oral or by injection.
✚ Side-effects: There may be nausea and vomiting, diarrhoea, taste disturbance; loss of appetite, tingling in the extremities, flushing, headache, dizziness, fatigue, depression, irritability; thirst, increased urine production; reduced libido; changes in blood counts; various other side-effects have been reported.
▲ Warnings: It should be administered with caution to patients who are pregnant or breast-feeding; and avoid its use in patients with severe kidney or liver impairment, certain salt-imbalance states, or who have SULPHONAMIDE sensitivity.
✪ Related entry: Diamox.

acetylcholine

is a neurotransmitter in the body. It has a number of important roles in both the central and peripheral nervous systems, relaying messages between nerves or from nerves to innervated organs. In medicine, it is rarely used as a drug because it is rapidly broken down in the body by widely distributed cholinesterase ENZYMES.

However, in the form of ACETYLCHOLINE CHLORIDE it can be administered in solution to the eyes for cataract surgery and other ophthalmic procedures requiring rapid constriction of the pupil. Although acetylcholine itself is little used therapeutically, a considerable number of drugs work by blocking, mimicking, or exaggerating its actions within the body.

PARASYMPATHOMIMETIC drugs are a class of drugs with effects similar to those of the parasympathetic nervous system and work by mimicking the actions of acetylcholine. Important parasympathomimetic actions include slowing of the heart, vasodilation, constriction of the pupil and altered focusing of the eye. *Direct-acting* parasympathomimetics act at *muscarinic* RECEPTORS for acetylcholine (eg CARBACHOL and PILOCARPINE). *Indirect-acting* parasympathomimetic ANTICHOLINESTERASE drugs prolong the duration of action of naturally released acetylcholine by inhibiting cholinesterase enzymes (eg NEOSTIGMINE).

Certain SKELETAL MUSCLE RELAXANT drugs act by interfering with neurotransmission by acetylcholine at so-called *nicotinic* receptors, which lie at the junction between nerves and voluntary (skeletal) muscles and are called *neuromuscular blocking drugs.* They are used in surgical operations to paralyse skeletal muscles that are normally under voluntary control and so allow maintenance of lighter levels of anaesthesia. These drugs are of one of two sorts: *non-depolarizing* skeletal muscle relaxants (eg GALLAMINE TRIETHIODIDE and tubocurarine); or *depolarizing* skeletal muscle relaxants (eg SUXAMETHONIUM CHLORIDE). The action of the non-depolarizing blocking drugs can be reversed at the end of an operation by administering an anticholinesterase drug.

GANGLION-BLOCKER drugs block the transmission of acetylcholine in the peripheral autonomic nervous system at the junctions called ganglia. The ganglion-blockers are now rarely used in medicine because they have very widespread actions. However, TRIMETAPHAN CAMSYLATE is used as a HYPOTENSIVE to control blood pressure during some types of surgery.

Drugs that mimic acetylcholine through the stimulation of nicotinic receptors also have only a limited use in medicine, because their actions have unacceptable side-effects and are too widespread. Indeed, NICOTINE, as adsorbed into the body by the use of tobacco products, causes widespread and generally undesirable effects, such as an increase in blood pressure, heart rate and blood sugar levels and also a release of adrenaline (which contributes to many of these effects).

In the brain, nicotine acts at nicotinic receptors and causes further stimulation and euphoria, which are all factors in making it such a powerfully habituating (addictive) drug.

Although some ANTICHOLINERGIC drugs act at nicotinic receptors, there is an important group that work by blocking the actions of acetylcholine at muscarinic receptors. The ANTIMUSCARINIC drugs have extensive uses in medicine and it is because they are used so extensively that the term *antimuscarinic* is often used synonymously for *anticholinergic* (even though this is technically inaccurate). Antimuscarinics tend to relax smooth muscle, reduce the secretion of saliva, digestive juices and sweat, and dilate the pupils of the eyes. They can also be used as ANTISPASMODIC and ANTIPARKINSONISM drugs (in the treatment of some of the symptoms of Parkinson's disease), or as ANTINAUSEANT, or ANTI-EMETIC, drugs in the treatment of motion sickness, peptic ulcers, in ophthalmic examinations and in antagonizing adverse effects of anticholinesterases (in medicine, agricultural accidental poisoning or warfare). Examples of antimuscarinic (anticholinergic) drugs include ATROPINE SULPHATE, BENZHEXOL HYDROCHLORIDE and HYOSCINE HYDROBROMIDE.

acetylcholine chloride

is a PARASYMPATHOMIMETIC which is rarely used therapeutically because it is rapidly broken down in the body. However, it can be applied in solution to the eye for cataract surgery, iridectomy and other types of surgery requiring rapid miosis (constriction of the pupil). Administration is by topical application as a solution. (ACETYLCHOLINE is the natural neurotransmitter released from cholinergic nerves in the body.)

✚▲ Side-effects/warnings: See PILOCARPINE.

✪ **Related entry: Miochol-E.**

acetylcysteine

is a drug that is used in two distinct ways. First, it can be used by virtue of its MUCOLYTIC properties applied topically to the eye to increase lacrimation (production of tears) and help treat abnormal or impaired mucus secretion.

Second, it is used as an ANTIDOTE to treat overdose poisoning by the NON-NARCOTIC ANALGESIC paracetamol. The initial symptoms of poisoning, nausea and vomiting, usually settle within 24 hours, but give way to a serious toxic effect on the liver which takes some days to develop. It is to prevent these latter effects that treatment is directed and is required as soon as possible after overdose, normally in hospital.

Administration as an antidote is by intravenous infusion and for other purposes it is topical.

✚▲ Side-effects/warnings: Administer with caution to patients who are asthmatics. Injected there may be rashes and anaphylaxis. As eye-drops, there are minimal side-effects.

✪ Related entries: Ilube; Parvolex.

Acezide

(Squibb; Bristol-Myers Squibb) is a proprietary, prescription-only compound preparation of the ACE INHIBITOR captopril and the DIURETIC hydrochlorothiazide, a combination called *co-zidocapt*. It can be used as an ANTIHYPERTENSIVE, and is available as tablets (in two strengths, one called *LS Tablets*).

✚▲ Side-effects/warnings: See CAPTOPRIL; HYDROCHLOROTHIAZIDE.

Achromycin

(Lederle; Wyeth) is a proprietary, prescription-only preparation of the broad-spectrum ANTIBACTERIAL and (TETRACYCLINES) ANTIBIOTIC tetracycline (as hydrochloride). It can be used to treat many types of infection, and is available as capsules.

✚▲ Side-effects/warnings: See TETRACYCLINE.

aciclovir

(acyclovir) is an ANTIVIRAL which is used specifically to treat infection by the herpes viruses (eg shingles, chickenpox, cold sores, genital herpes and herpes infections of the eye and mouth). It works by inhibiting the action of enzymes in human cells that are used by the virus to replicate itself. To be effective, however, treatment must begin early. It can be valuable in immunocompromised patients. The drug can also be used prophylactically to prevent individuals at risk from contracting a herpes disease. Administration can be oral, as a variety of topical preparations (ointments and creams) or by injection or intravenous infusion.

✚ Side-effects: When applied topically, there may be a temporary burning or stinging sensation; some patients experience a localized drying of the skin. When taken orally, it may give rise to gastrointestinal disturbance and various blood-cell deficiencies. There may also be fatigue, rash, headache, tremor and effects on mood. When injected there may be hallucinations, sleepiness, and severe local inflammation at the injection site.

▲ Warnings: Administer with caution to patients who are pregnant or breast-feeding; or who have impaired kidney function. Adequate fluid intake must be maintained. When given topically, avoid contact with eyes and mucous membranes.

✪ Related entries: Soothelip; Virasorb Cold Sore Cream; Zovirax; Zovirax Cold Sore Cream.

acipimox

is used as a LIPID-REGULATING DRUG in hyperlipidaemia to reduce the levels, or beneficially change the proportions, of various lipids in the bloodstream. It is thought to act in a similar way to NICOTINIC ACID, by inhibiting synthesis of lipids in the liver. Generally, it is administered only to patients in whom a strict and regular dietary regime, alone, is not having the desired effect. Administration is oral.

✚ Side-effects: There may be flushing, itching, rashes and reddening of the skin, nausea and abdominal pain; diarrhoea, malaise, headache, and dry eyes. High doses may cause disorders of liver function, gout, and glucose intolerance.

▲ Warnings: It should not be administered to patients who are pregnant or breast-feeding, or have peptic ulcers; and should be administered with caution to those with impaired kidney function.

✪ Related entry: Olbetam.

Acitak

(Opus; Trinity) is a proprietary, prescription-only preparation of the H_2-ANTAGONIST cimetidine. It can be used as an ULCER-HEALING DRUG for benign peptic ulcers (in the stomach or duodenum), gastro-oesophageal reflux, dyspepsia and associated conditions. It is available as tablets.

✚▲ Side-effects/warnings: See CIMETIDINE.

acitretin

is chemically a RETINOID (it is a metabolite of etretinate, which is a derivative of RETINOL or vitamin A) and has a marked effect on the cells that make up the skin epithelium. It can be taken over a period of weeks to relieve severe psoriasis that is resistant to other treatments and for other

skin conditions (including severe Darier's disease). Treatment is under strict medical supervision. Administration is oral.
✚ Side-effects: These include dryness of skin, conjunctiva and mucous membrane, muscle and joint ache, hair loss, reversible visual disturbances, nausea, headache, sweating, changes in liver function, blood upsets, mood changes, drowsiness, and others.
▲ Warnings: This is a specialist drug and full assessment of patient suitability for treatment will be made. There will be monitoring (eg liver function and blood glucose). Patients must not donate blood during treatment or for one year after. It is not used in patients who are pregnant (and exclude pregnancy before starting and after treatment) or breast-feeding, or who have certain liver or kidney disorders. Avoid excessive exposure to sunlight.
✪ Related entry: Neotigason.

aclarubicin
is a CYTOTOXIC drug (an ANTIBIOTIC in origin) with properties similar to doxorubicin. It is used as an ANTICANCER drug, particularly to treat acute non-lymphocytic leukaemia in patients who have not responded to, or who have relapsed from, other forms of chemotherapy. Administration is by injection.
✚▲ Side-effects/warnings: See CYTOTOXIC.

Acnecide
(Galderma) is a proprietary, non-prescription preparation of the KERATOLYTIC and ANTIMICROBIAL benzoyl peroxide. It can be used to treat acne, and is available as a gel.
✚▲ Side-effects/warnings: See BENZOYL PEROXIDE.

Acnisal
(DermaPharm) is a proprietary, non-prescription preparation of the KERATOLYTIC agent salicylic acid. It can be used to treat acne, and is available as a solution for topical application.
✚▲ Side-effects/warnings: See SALICYLIC ACID.

Acoflam
(Goldshield) is a prescription-only, proprietary version of the (NSAID) NON-NARCOTIC ANALGESIC and ANTIRHEUMATIC diclofenac sodium. It can be used to treat arthritic and rheumatic pain and inflammation and other musculoskeletal disorders. It is available as tablets and modified-release tablets *Acoflam 75 SR* and *Acoflam Retard*.
✚▲ Side-effects/warnings: See DICLOFENAC SODIUM.

Acriflex Cream
(SSL) is a proprietary, non-prescription preparation of the ANTISEPTIC chlorhexidine (as gluconate). It can be used to treat minor wounds and burns on the skin, and is available as a cream.
✚▲ Side-effects/warnings: See CHLORHEXIDINE.

acrivastine
is an ANTIHISTAMINE which has only recently been developed and has fewer sedative side-effects than some of the older antihistamines. It can be used for the symptomatic relief of allergic conditions, such as hay fever and urticaria. Administration is oral.
✚▲ Side-effects/warnings: See ANTIHISTAMINE; but the incidence of sedative and anticholinergic effects is low. Avoid its use in patients with kidney impairment.
✪ Related entries: Benadryl Allergy Relief; Semprex.

Actal Pastils
(Merck Consumer Health; Seven Seas) is a proprietary, non-prescription preparation of the ANTACID hydrotalcite. It can be used to relieve heartburn and acid indigestion, and is available as oral gum. It is not normally given to children, except on medical advice.
✚▲ Side-effects/warnings: See HYDROTALCITE.

Actal Tablets
(Merck Consumer Health; Seven Seas) is a proprietary, non-prescription preparation of the ANTACID alexitol sodium. It can be used to relieve hyperacidity, dyspepsia and indigestion. It is available as tablets and is not normally given to children, except on medical advice.
✚▲ Side-effects/warnings: See ALEXITOL SODIUM.

Act-HIB
(Aventis Pasteur) is a proprietary, prescription-only VACCINE preparation for (*Haemophilus influenzae*) infection, and is available in a form for injection.
✚▲ Side-effects/warnings: See HAEMOPHILUS INFLUENZAE TYPE B VACCINE.

ACT-HIB DTP dc

(Aventis Pasteur) is a non-proprietary, prescription-only preparation of the quadruple VACCINE used to prevent *Haemophilus influenzae* infection, diphtheria, tetanus and pertussis, and may be used as part of childhood immunization. It is available in a form for injection.
✚▲ Side-effects/warnings: See DIPHTHERIA VACCINE; HAEMOPHILUS INFLUENZAE TYPE B VACCINE; PERTUSSIS VACCINE; TETANUS VACCINE.

Acticin

(Strakan) is a proprietary, prescription-only preparation of the (RETINOID) tretinoin. It can be used to treat severe acne, and is available as a cream and a gel.
✚▲ Side-effects/warnings: See TRETINOIN.

Actidose-Aqua Advance

(Cambridge) is a proprietary, non-prescription preparation of activated charcoal. It can be used to treat patients suffering from poisoning or a drug overdose. It is available as an oral suspension.
✚▲ Side-effects/warnings: See ACTIVATED CHARCOAL.

Actifed Compound Linctus

(Warner Lambert Consumer Healthcare; Pfizer) is a proprietary, non-prescription compound preparation of the ANTIHISTAMINE triprolidine hydrochloride, the SYMPATHOMIMETIC and DECONGESTANT pseudoephedrine hydrochloride and the (OPIOID) ANTITUSSIVE dextromethorphan hydrobromide. It can be used for the symptomatic relief of unproductive cough and upper respiratory tract disorders. It is available as a liquid, and is not normally given to children under two years, except on medical advice.
✚▲ Side-effects/warnings: See DEXTROMETHORPHAN HYDROBROMIDE; PSEUDOEPHEDRINE HYDROCHLORIDE; TRIPROLIDINE HYDROCHLORIDE.

Actifed Expectorant

(Warner Lambert Consumer Healthcare; Pfizer) is a proprietary, non-prescription compound preparation of the ANTIHISTAMINE triprolidine hydrochloride, the SYMPATHOMIMETIC and DECONGESTANT pseudoephedrine hydrochloride and the EXPECTORANT agent guaifenesin (guaiphenesin). It can be used for the symptomatic relief of upper respiratory tract disorders accompanied by productive cough. It is available as a liquid, and is not normally given to children under two years, except on medical advice.
✚▲ Side-effects/warnings: See GUAIFENESIN; PSEUDOEPHEDRINE HYDROCHLORIDE; TRIPROLIDINE HYDROCHLORIDE.

Actifed Syrup

(Warner Lambert Consumer Healthcare; Pfizer) is a proprietary, non-prescription compound preparation of the ANTIHISTAMINE triprolidine hydrochloride and the SYMPATHOMIMETIC and DECONGESTANT pseudoephedrine hydrochloride. It can be used for congestion of the upper airways and sinuses, and for the symptomatic treatment of colds, hay fever and rhinitis. It is available as a liquid, and is not normally given to children under two years, except on medical advice.
✚▲ Side-effects/warnings: See PSEUDOEPHEDRINE HYDROCHLORIDE; TRIPROLIDINE HYDROCHLORIDE.

Actifed Tablets

(Warner Lambert Consumer Healthcare; Pfizer) is a proprietary, non-prescription compound preparation of the ANTIHISTAMINE triprolidine hydrochloride and the SYMPATHOMIMETIC and DECONGESTANT pseudoephedrine hydrochloride. It can be used for congestion of the upper airways and sinuses, and for the symptomatic treatment of colds, flu, hay fever and rhinitis. It is available as a liquid, and is not normally given to children under 12 years, except on medical advice.
✚▲ Side-effects/warnings: See PSEUDOEPHEDRINE HYDROCHLORIDE; TRIPROLIDINE HYDROCHLORIDE.

Actilyse

(Boehringer Ingelheim) is a proprietary, prescription-only preparation of the FIBRINOLYTIC alteplase. It can be used to treat myocardial infarction and pulmonary embolism, and is available in a form for injection.
✚▲ Side-effects/warnings: See ALTEPLASE.

Actinac

(Peckforton) is a proprietary, prescription-only compound preparation of the broad-spectrum

A

ANTIBACTERIAL and ANTIBIOTIC chloramphenicol and the ANTI-INFLAMMATORY and CORTICOSTEROID hydrocortisone (as acetate) (also with allantoin, butoxyethyl nicotinate and sulphur). It can be used by topical application to treat acne, and is available as a lotion.
✚▲ Side-effects/warnings: See CHLORAMPHENICOL; HYDROCORTISONE.

actinomycin D
see DACTINOMYCIN.

Actiq
(Elan) is a proprietary, prescription-only preparation of the (OPIOID) NARCOTIC ANALGESIC fentanyl (as citrate), and is on the Controlled Drugs list. It can be used to treat breakthrough pain in patients already receiving opioid therapy for chronic pain. It is available in the form of lozenges for dissolving in the mouth.
✚▲ Side-effects/warnings: See FENTANYL.

activated charcoal
is an adsorbent material. Its primary use is for soaking up poisons in the stomach or small intestine, especially drug overdoses in cases where only a small quantity of the drug may be extremely toxic (eg some ANTIDEPRESSANT drugs). It can help prevent the effects of drug overdose by increasing the elimination of certain drugs even after they have been absorbed (eg PHENOBARBITALand THEOPHYLLINE). It is available as a powder to be taken in solution as often as necessary. It can also be used in ANTIDIARRHOEAL preparations – it is effective in binding together faecal matter – and can relieve flatulence.
✚▲ Side-effects/warnings: As an antidote, the sooner it is given, the more effective it is. It is regarded as safe in normal use. However, when used regularly to treat wind or diarrhoea, it may reduce the absorption of other drugs (eg aspirin, carbamazepine, quinine, and theophylline).
✪ Related entries: Actidose-Aqua Advance; Carbomix; Charcodote; Liqui-Char; Medicoal.

Actonel
(Procter & Gamble Pharm.) is a recently introduced, proprietary, prescription-only preparation of the CALCIUM METABOLISM MODIFIER drug risedronate sodium. It is used in the treatment and prevention of osteoporosis (including corticosteroid-induced osteoporosis) in postmenopausal women, and (at a different dose) for Paget's disease of the bone. It is available in the form of tablets.
✚▲ Side-effects/warnings: See RISEDRONATE SODIUM.

Actonorm Gel
(Wallace) is a proprietary, non-prescription compound preparation of the ANTACID agents magnesium hydroxide and aluminium hydroxide, together with the ANTIFOAMING AGENT dimeticone. It is used for the symptomatic relief of dyspepsia, indigestion, flatulence and gastrointestinal disorders due to overeating. It is available as an oral suspension.
✚▲ Side-effects/warnings: See ALUMINIUM HYDROXIDE; DIMETICONE; MAGNESIUM HYDROXIDE.

Actonorm Powder
(Wallace) is a proprietary, non-prescription compound preparation of the ANTACID agents calcium carbonate, sodium bicarbonate, magnesium carbonate, and aluminium hydroxide, together with the (ANTIMUSCARINIC) ANTICHOLINERGIC atropine sulphate and the ANTISPASMODIC peppermint oil. It can be used for the symptomatic relief of dyspepsia and gastrointestinal disorders due to smooth muscle spasm. It is available as a powder. It is not normally given to children, except on medical advice.
✚▲ Side-effects/warnings: See ALUMINIUM HYDROXIDE; ATROPINE SULPHATE; CALCIUM CARBONATE; MAGNESIUM CARBONATE; PEPPERMINT OIL; SODIUM BICARBONATE.

Actos
(Takeda) is a recently introduced proprietary, prescription-only preparation of PIOGLITAZONE (as hydrochloride). It can be used in combination with other drugs, in DIABETIC TREATMENT of Type II diabetes (non-insulin-dependent diabetes mellitus; NIDDM; maturity-onset diabetes), and is available as tablets.
✚▲ Side-effects/warnings: See PIOGLITAZONE.

Acular
(Allergan) is a proprietary, prescription-only preparation of the (NSAID) NON-NARCOTIC ANALGESIC ketorolac trometamol. It can be used to prevent and reduce inflammation following

eye surgery, and is available as eye-drops.
✚▲ Side-effects/warnings: See KETOROLAC TROMETAMOL.

Acupan

(3M) is a proprietary, prescription-only preparation of the NON-NARCOTIC ANALGESIC nefopam hydrochloride. It can be used to treat moderate pain, and is available as tablets and in a form for injection.
✚▲ Side-effects/warnings: See NEFOPAM HYDROCHLORIDE.

AC Vax

(SmithKline Beecham; GSK) is a proprietary, prescription-only VACCINE preparation. It can be used to give protection against the organism meningococcus (*Neisseria meningitidis* groups A and C), which can cause serious infections such as meningitis. It is available in a form for injection.
✚▲ Side-effects/warnings: See MENINGOCOCCAL POLYSACCHARIDE VACCINE.

ACWY Vax

(SmithKlineBeecham) is a proprietary, prescription-only VACCINE preparation. It can be used to give protection against the organism meningococcus (*Neisseria meningitidis* groups A and C), which can cause serious infections, such as meningitis. It is available in a form for injection.
✚▲ Side-effects/warnings: See MENINGOCOCCAL POLYSACCHARIDE VACCINE.

acyclovir

see ACICLOVIR.

Adalat

(Bayer) is a proprietary, prescription-only preparation of the CALCIUM-CHANNEL BLOCKER nifedipine. It can be used as an ANTI-ANGINA treatment in the prevention of attacks and in peripheral vascular disease (Raynaud's phenomenon). It is available as capsules.
✚▲ Side-effects/warnings: See NIFEDIPINE.

Adalat LA

(Bayer) is a proprietary, prescription-only preparation of the CALCIUM-CHANNEL BLOCKER nifedipine. It can be used as an ANTIHYPERTENSIVE and in ANTI-ANGINA treatment to prevent attacks. Available as modified-release tablets in the doses: *Adalat LA 20, Adalat LA 30*, and *Adalat LA 60*.
✚▲ Side-effects/warnings: See NIFEDIPINE.

Adalat Retard

(Bayer) is a proprietary, prescription-only preparation of the CALCIUM-CHANNEL BLOCKER nifedipine. It can be used as an ANTIHYPERTENSIVE and an ANTI-ANGINA treatment in the prevention of attacks. It is available as modified-release tablets in two doses: *Adalat Retard 10* and *Adalat Retard 20*.
✚▲ Side-effects/warnings: See NIFEDIPINE.

adapalene

is chemically a RETINOID (a derivative of RETINOL, or vitamin A) and can be used to treat mild to moderate acne. Administration is topical as a gel.
✚ Side-effects: There may be skin irritation and other skin reactions.
▲ Warnings: Should not be used in pregnancy, breast-feeding, in cases of eczematous or broken skin, mucous membranes; avoid in severe acne over large areas. Avoid ultraviolet light.
✪ **Related entry: Differin.**

Adcal-D3

(Strakan) is a proprietary, non-prescription compound preparation of the vitamin colecalciferol (cholecalciferol; vitamin D_3) and calcium (in the form of calcium carbonate). It can be used as a MINERAL SUPPLEMENT in the treatment of osteoporosis, supplementation in malnutrition and prevention and treatment of calcium and vitamin D deficiency. It is available in the form of chewable tablets.
✚▲ Side-effects/warnings: See CALCIUM CARBONATE; COLECALCIFEROL.

Adcortyl in Orabase

(Squibb; Bristol-Myers Squibb) is a proprietary, prescription-only preparation of the CORTICOSTEROID and ANTI-INFLAMMATORY triamcinolone (in the form of acetonide). (A version called *Adcortyl in Orabase for Mouth Ulcers* is available without prescription). It can be used to treat mouth ulcers and inflammation, and is available as an oral paste.
✚▲ Side-effects/warnings: See TRIAMCINOLONE.

Adcortyl Intra-articular/ Intradermal

(Squibb; Bristol-Myers Squibb) is a proprietary, prescription-only preparation of the

CORTICOSTEROID and ANTI-INFLAMMATORY triamcinolone (in the form of acetonide). It can be administered by injection to relieve joint and soft tissue pain, swelling and stiffness.
✚▲ Side-effects/warnings: See TRIAMCINOLONE.

Adenocor
(Sanofi-Synthelabo) is a proprietary, prescription-only preparation of the ANTI-ARRHYTHMIC adenosine. It can be used to correct heartbeat irregularities, and is available as tablets and in a form for injection.
✚▲ Side-effects/warnings: See ADENOSINE.

Adenoscan
(Sanofi Winthrop; Sanofi-Synthelabo) is a proprietary, prescription-only preparation of the ANTI-ARRHYTHMIC adenosine. It can be used in conjunction with radionuclide myocardial perfusion imaging in patients who cannot exercise adequately, as a diagnostic procedure. Administration is by injection.
✚▲ Side-effects/warnings: See ADENOSINE.

adenosine
is a specialist drug that can be used as an ANTI-ARRHYTHMIC to correct certain abnormal heart rhythms (eg Wolff-Parkinson-White syndrome) and help in the diagnosis of certain arrhythmias (complex supraventricular tachycardias). Administration is by injection.
✚ Side-effects: Flushes of the face; shortness of breath, feeling of choking and bronchospasm; nausea and light-headedness; extreme slowing of the heart and chest pain.
▲ Warnings: It should be administered with caution in certain heart conditions and is not to be given to patients with asthma.
✪ Related entries: Adenocor; Adenoscan.

Adgyn Combi
(Strakan) is a proprietary, prescription-only compound preparation of the female SEX HORMONES estradiol (an OESTROGEN) and norethisterone (a PROGESTOGEN). It can be used to treat menopausal symptoms in HRT (hormone replacement therapy), and is available as tablets.
✚▲ Side-effects/warnings: See ESTRADIOL; NORETHISTERONE.

Adgyn Estro
Adgyn Estro (Strakan) is a proprietary, prescription-only preparation of the OESTROGEN estradiol. It can be used to treat menopausal symptoms in HRT (hormone replacement therapy), and is available as tablets.
✚▲ Side-effects/warnings: See ESTRADIOL.

Adgyn Medro
(Strakan) is a proprietary, prescription-only preparation of the sex hormone (see SEX HORMONES) medroxyprogesterone acetate (a synthetic PROGESTOGEN). In women it can be used for dysfunctional uterine bleeding, endometriosis and in HRT. Available as tablets.
✚▲ Side-effects/warnings: See MEDROXYPROGESTERONE ACETATE.

ADH (antidiuretic hormone)
see VASOPRESSIN.

Adipine MR
(Trinity) is a proprietary, prescription-only preparation of the CALCIUM-CHANNEL BLOCKER nifedipine. It can be used as an ANTI-ANGINA treatment in the prevention of attacks, and as an ANTIHYPERTENSIVE. It is available as modified-release tablets.
✚▲ Side-effects/warnings: See NIFEDIPINE.

Adizem-SR
(Napp) is a proprietary, prescription-only preparation of the CALCIUM-CHANNEL BLOCKER diltiazem hydrochloride. It can be used as an ANTIHYPERTENSIVE and as an ANTI-ANGINA drug. It is available as modified-release tablets and capsules.
✚▲ Side-effects/warnings: See DILTIAZEM HYDROCHLORIDE.

Adizem-XL
(Napp) is a proprietary, prescription-only preparation of the CALCIUM-CHANNEL BLOCKER diltiazem hydrochloride. It can be used as an ANTIHYPERTENSIVE and as an ANTI-ANGINA drug. It is available as modified-release capsules.
✚▲ Side-effects/warnings: See DILTIAZEM HYDROCHLORIDE.

adrenaline
(epinephrine) is chemically called a *catecholamine*. It is secreted into the bloodstream (along with the closely related substance NORADRENALINE) as an endocrine HORMONE by

the adrenal glands, from the region called the medulla (the central core; hence *adrenomedullary hormone*).

The adrenal glands constitute an important part of the sympathetic nervous system. Together with noradrenaline (which also acts as a neurotransmitter, being released from nerve-endings by electrical signals travelling from the central nervous system via nerves in the body), adrenaline activates or inhibits a wide variety of muscles, exocrine glands, and metabolic processes in the body.

The responses of the body to stimulation of the sympathetic nervous system are primarily concerned with reactions to stress. In the face of stress, or the need for exertion, the body uses adrenaline and noradrenaline to cause constriction of some blood vessels while dilating others, with the net effect that the two catecholamines increase blood flow to the skeletal muscles and heart. The heart rate is raised and there is relaxation of the smooth muscles of the intestine and bronchioles.

There is also a rise in concentration of energy-supplying glucose and free fatty-acids in the bloodstream. The actions of noradrenaline and adrenaline are similar. Adrenaline itself is not greatly used therapeutically because its actions are so widespread. However, in the form of ADRENALINE ACID TARTRATE it may be injected to treat cardiac arrest, bronchoconstriction of anaphylactic shock, and in angioedema. Commonly, it is included in several LOCAL ANAESTHETIC preparations to constrict the blood vessels and help prolong the effect of the local anaesthetic by slowing the rate at which it is 'washed away'; also, it is administered in solution in eye-drops to treat glaucoma.

adrenaline acid tartrate

(epinephrine bitartrate) is the main form of ADRENALINE used clinically. It has both ALPHA-ADRENOCEPTOR STIMULANT and BETA-ADRENOCEPTOR STIMULANT activity, and is not very greatly used therapeutically because its actions are so widespread. In emergencies, however, it may be injected in cardiac arrest, to treat the circulatory collapse and bronchoconstriction of anaphylactic shock, and in angioedema. More commonly, adrenaline is included in several LOCAL ANAESTHETIC preparations, because its pronounced VASOCONSTRICTOR actions considerably prolong anaesthesia by preventing the local anaesthetic from being removed in the bloodstream. Also, it is administered in solution in eye-drops to treat glaucoma. Administration of adrenaline is by injection (as well as various specialized methods with local anaesthetics), by inhalation or as eye-drops.

✚ Side-effects: Depending on the method of administration, there may be an increase in heart rate and irregular rhythms; muscle tremor, dry mouth, anxiety or fear, and coldness in the fingertips and toes. High dosage may lead to tremor, the accumulation of fluid in the lungs and cerebral haemorrhage and other effects. Adrenaline in eye-drops may cause redness and smarting of the eye.

▲ Warnings: Depending on methods of administration and dose, it should be administered with caution to patients who suffer from ischaemic heart disease or hypertension, diabetes or over-activity of the thyroid gland (hyperthyroidism). There may be severe drug interactions in those already taking a number of other drugs, especially antidepressants and beta-blockers.

✪ Related entries: Anapen; EpiPen; Eppy; Ganda; Marcain with Adrenaline; Min-I-Jet Adrenaline.

adrenergic-neurone blocker

drugs act to prevent the release of NORADRENALINE (epinephrine) from the nerves of the sympathetic nervous system, which is involved in controlling involuntary functions such as blood pressure, heart rate and the activity of muscles of internal organs (eg blood vessels, intestines and glandular secretions).

Noradrenaline (norepinephrine) is the main neurotransmitter of the sympathetic nervous system and therefore adrenergic-neurone blockers cause an overall ANTISYMPATHETIC action with a fall in blood pressure. Consequently, the main use of such drugs is as ANTIHYPERTENSIVE agents. However, because of quite marked side-effects, they are not drugs-of-choice in the treatment of moderate to severe high blood pressure. See DEBRISOQUINE; GUANETHIDINE MONOSULPHATE.

▲ Warnings: Some drugs, including NSAIDS and SYMPATHOMIMETIC drugs (eg EPHEDRINE HYDROCHLORIDE in some cold and cough cure preparations) can interfere with the effects of adrenergic-neurone blockers.

A

adrenocorticotrophic hormone (ACTH)
see CORTICOTROPIN.

Adsorbed Diphtheria, Tetanus and [whole-cell] Pertussis Vaccine
(District Health Authorities; Aventis Pasteur; Farillon) (DTPer/Vac/Ads, [DTwP]) is a non-proprietary, prescription-only VACCINE preparation which combines vaccines for IMMUNIZATION against diphtheria and tetanus and pertussis, adsorbed onto a mineral carrier. It is available in a form for injection.

✚▲ Side-effects/warnings: See DIPHTHERIA VACCINE; PERTUSSIS VACCINE; TETANUS VACCINE.

Adsorbed Diphtheria, Tetanus and Pertussis Vaccine
(District Health Authorities) (DTPer/Vac/Ads) is a non-proprietary, prescription-only VACCINE preparation, commonly referred to as *triple vaccine*, which combines (toxoid) vaccines for diphtheria and pertussis (whooping cough) with TETANUS VACCINE adsorbed onto a mineral carrier. It is available in a form for injection (as part of childhood immunization programme, from Health Authorities).

✚▲ Side-effects/warnings: See DIPHTHERIA VACCINE; PERTUSSIS VACCINE; TETANUS VACCINE.

adsorbed diphtheria, tetanus and pertussis vaccine
(DTPer/Vac/Ads) is a VACCINE used for IMMUNIZATION against diphtheria, tetanus and pertussis (whooping cough). It consists of diphtheria vaccine, TETANUS VACCINE and PERTUSSIS VACCINE adsorbed onto a mineral carrier. This *triple vaccine* is used for the primary immunization of children (during first year of life), and is administered by injection.

✚▲ Side-effects/warnings: See DIPHTHERIA VACCINE; PERTUSSIS VACCINE; TETANUS VACCINE.

✪ **Related entries: Adsorbed Diphtheria, Tetanus and Pertussis Vaccine; Infanrix.**

Adsorbed Diphtheria and Tetanus Vaccine
(District Health Authorities; Farillon; Evans; Aventis Pasteur) (DT/Vac/Ads (Child)) is a non-proprietary, prescription-only VACCINE preparation that combines (toxoid) vaccines for diphtheria vaccine and TETANUS VACCINE adsorbed onto a mineral carrier. It is available in a form for injection for adults. (Children over ten years are given ADSORBED DIPHTHERIA AND TETANUS VACCINE FOR ADOLESCENTS AND ADULTS.)

✚▲ Side-effects/warnings: See DIPHTHERIA VACCINE; TETANUS VACCINE.

adsorbed diphtheria and tetanus vaccine
(DT/Vac/Ads) is a VACCINE used for IMMUNIZATION against diphtheria and tetanus and is adsorbed onto a mineral carrier. This combination of diphtheria vaccines and TETANUS VACCINE is used for the primary immunization of children (in a series of administrations including a booster before nursery school entry) and as an alternative to ADSORBED DIPHTHERIA, TETANUS AND PERTUSSIS VACCINE (DTPer/Vac/Ads), for children who can not be given the pertussis vaccine. Subsequently, a similar, but different form is used for adolescents and adults before leaving school or on going to employment or further education. Administration is by injection.

✚▲ Side-effects/warnings: See DIPHTHERIA VACCINE; TETANUS VACCINE.

✪ **Related entries: Adsorbed Diphtheria and Tetanus Vaccine; Adsorbed Diphtheria and Tetanus Vaccine for Adolescents and Adults; Diftavax.**

Adsorbed Diphtheria and Tetanus Vaccine for Adolescents and Adults
(District Health Authorities) (DT/Vac/Ads (Adults) is a non-proprietary, prescription-only VACCINE preparation which combines (toxoid) vaccines for diphtheria and TETANUS VACCINE adsorbed onto a mineral carrier. It is available in a form for injection for children over ten years and adults.

✚▲ Side-effects/warnings: See DIPHTHERIA VACCINE; TETANUS VACCINE.

Adsorbed Diphtheria Vaccine
(District Health Authorities; Farillon) (DT/Vac/Ads (Child)) is a non-proprietary, prescription-only VACCINE preparation that combines (toxoid) vaccine for diphtheria adsorbed onto a mineral carrier. It is available in a form for

injection. (Children over ten years and adults are given Adsorbed Diphtheria and Tetanus Vaccine for Adolescents and Adults.)
✚▲ Side-effects/warnings: See DIPHTHERIA VACCINE.

adsorbed diphtheria vaccine

(Dip/Vac/Ads) is a VACCINE used for IMMUNIZATION against diphtheria and is adsorbed onto a mineral carrier. This form of diphtheria vaccine is administered to those who come into contact with a diphtheria case or a carrier. Administration is by injection.
✚▲ Side-effects/warnings: See DIPHTHERIA VACCINE.
✪ **Related entries: Adsorbed Diphtheria Vaccine; Adsorbed Diphtheria Vaccine for Adults and Adolescents.**

Adsorbed Diphtheria Vaccine for Adults and Adolescents

(District Health Authorities; Farillon) (Dip/Vac/Ads (adult)) is a non-proprietary, prescription-only VACCINE preparation of (toxoid) vaccines for diphtheria adsorbed onto a mineral carrier. It is available in a form for injection..(This preparation is given to children over ten years.)
✚▲ Side-effects/warnings: See DIPHTHERIA VACCINE.

Adsorbed Tetanus Vaccine

(Celltech; Pasteur Mérieux) (Tet/Vac/Ads) is a non-proprietary, prescription-only VACCINE preparation of adsorbed tetanus vaccine. It can be used for active IMMUNIZATION against tetanus, and is available in a form for injection.
✚▲ Side-effects/warnings: See ADSORBED TETANUS VACCINE.

adsorbed tetanus vaccine

(Tet/Vac/Ads) is a VACCINE used for IMMUNIZATION against tetanus and is adsorbed onto a mineral carrier. This form of TETANUS VACCINE is used where a combined vaccine such as *triple vaccine* has not been given or as a booster in later life. Administration is by injection.
✪ **Related entries: Adsorbed Tetanus Vaccine; Clostet.**

Adult Meltus Expectorant for Chesty Coughs and Catarrh

(SSL) is a proprietary, non-prescription compound preparation of the EXPECTORANT agent guaifenesin (guaiphenesin), the ANTISEPTIC agent CETYLPYRIDINIUM CHLORIDE, sucrose and honey. It can be used for the symptomatic relief of coughs and catarrh associated with flu, mild throat infections and colds. It is available as a linctus and is not normally given to children, except on medical advice.
✚▲ Side-effects/warnings: See CETYLPYRIDINIUM CHLORIDE; GUAIFENESIN.

Adult Meltus Expectorant with Decongestant

(SSL) is a proprietary, non-prescription compound preparation of the EXPECTORANT agent guaifenesin (guaiphenesin) and the DECONGESTANT pseudoephedrine hydrochloride. It can be used for the symptomatic relief of chesty coughs and congestion associated with flu and colds. It is available as a linctus and is not normally given to children under one year, except on medical advice.
✚▲ Side-effects/warnings: See GUAIFENESIN; PSEUDOEPHEDRINE HYDROCHLORIDE.

Adult Meltus for Dry Tickly Coughs and Catarrh

(SSL) is a proprietary, non-prescription compound preparation of the SYMPATHOMIMETIC and DECONGESTANT pseudoephedrine hydrochloride and the OPIOID and ANTITUSSIVE dextromethorphan hydrobromide. It can be used for the symptomatic relief of tickly, dry, painful coughs and catarrh. It is available as a liquid, and not normally given to children except on medical advice.
✚▲ Side-effects/warnings: See DEXTROMETHORPHAN HYDROBROMIDE; PSEUDOEPHEDRINE HYDROCHLORIDE.

Adult Meltus Night Time

(SSL) is a proprietary, non-prescription preparation of the ANTIHISTAMINE diphenhydramine hydrochloride with the EXPECTORANT ammonium chloride and sodium citrate. It can be used for the symptomatic relief of deep chesty coughs and colds. It is available as a syrup and is not normally given to children under six years, except on medical advice.
✚▲ Side-effects/warnings: See AMMONIUM CHLORIDE; DIPHENHYDRAMINE HYDROCHLORIDE.

Advil Tablets

(Whitehall Laboratories) is a proprietary, non-prescription preparation of the (NSAID) NON-

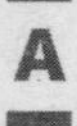

NARCOTIC ANALGESIC and ANTIRHEUMATIC ibuprofen. It can be used for mild to moderate pain, such as dental, period and muscle pain, and also for symptoms of flu and colds (eg fever). It is not normally given to children except on medical advice.
✚▲ Side-effects/warnings: See IBUPROFEN.

Advil Tablets Extra Strength

(Whitehall Laboratories) is a proprietary, non-prescription preparation of the (NSAID) NON-NARCOTIC ANALGESIC and ANTIRHEUMATIC ibuprofen. It can be used for mild to moderate pain, such as dental, period and muscle pain, and also for symptoms of flu and colds (eg fever). Not normally given to children except on medical advice.
✚▲ Side-effects/warnings: See IBUPROFEN.

AeroBec

(3M) is a proprietary, prescription-only preparation of the CORTICOSTEROID and ANTI-ASTHMATIC beclometasone dipropionate. It can be used to prevent asthmatic attacks, and is available in aerosols for inhalation as *AeroBec 50 Autohaler, AeroBec 100 Autohaler*, and a stronger version called *AeroBec Forte*.
✚▲ Side-effects/warnings: See BECLOMETASONE DIPROPIONATE.

Aerocrom

(Castlemead) is a proprietary, prescription-only compound preparation of the ANTI-ALLERGIC sodium cromoglicate and the BETA-RECEPTOR STIMULANT salbutamol (as salbutamol sulphate), which is used as an ANTI-ASTHMATIC. It is important that it is used for the prevention (prophylaxis) of asthma symptoms rather than the acute treatment of asthma attacks. It is available as an aerosol.
✚▲ Side-effects/warnings: See SALBUTAMOL; SODIUM CROMOGLICATE.

Aerodiol

(Servier) is a proprietary, prescription-only preparation of the OESTROGEN estradiol. It can be used in HRT (hormone replacement therapy), and is available as a nasal spray.
✚▲ Side-effects/warnings: See ESTRADIOL. This form of estradiol can also be taken by directing the spray between the cheek and gum above the upper teeth in women who have a severely blocked nose.

Aerolin Autohaler

(3M) is a proprietary, prescription-only preparation of the BETA-RECEPTOR STIMULANT salbutamol (as salbutamol sulphate). It can be used as a BRONCHODILATOR in reversible obstructive airways disease such as as an ANTI-ASTHMATIC, for which it is available as a breath-actuated metered aerosol inhalant.
✚▲ Side-effects/warnings: See SALBUTAMOL.

Afrazine Nasal Spray

(Schering-Plough Consumer Health) is a proprietary, non-prescription preparation of the NASAL DECONGESTANT oxymetazoline hydrochloride. It can be used to relieve nasal congestion associated with a wide variety of upper respiratory tract disorders. It is available as a nasal spray and is not normally given to children under five years, except on medical advice.
✚▲ Side-effects/warnings: See OXYMETAZOLINE HYDROCHLORIDE.

Agenerase

(SmithKlineGlaxo; GSK) is a proprietary, prescription-only preparation of the (*protease inhibitor*) ANTIVIRAL drug AMPRENAVIR. It can be used in the treatment of HIV infection in combination with other antiretroviral drugs, and is available as an oral solution and capsules.
✚▲ Side-effects/warnings: See AMPRENAVIR.

Aggrastat

(MSD) is a proprietary, prescription-only preparation of the ANTIPLATELET drug tirofiban. It can be used, in conjunction with other drugs, to prevent thrombosis in myocardial infarction (under hospital specialist supervision). It is available in a form for intravenous infusion.
✚▲ Side-effects/warnings: See TIROFIBAN.

Agrippal

(Wyeth) is a proprietary, prescription-only preparation of influenza VACCINE (surface antigen vaccine; Flu/Vac/SA). It can be used as immunization for the prevention of influenza, and is available in a form for injection.
✚▲ Side-effects/warnings: INFLUENZA VACCINE.

Ailax

(Galen) is a proprietary, prescription-only preparation of CO-DANTHRAMER 25/200, which is

a (*stimulant*) LAXATIVE based on dantron and poloxamer '188'. It can be used to treat constipation and to prepare patients for abdominal procedures, and is available as an oral suspension.
✚▲ Side-effects/warnings: See DANTRON; POLOXAMER '188'.

Airomir

(3M) is a proprietary, prescription-only preparation of the BETA-RECEPTOR STIMULANT salbutamol. It can be used as a BRONCHODILATOR in reversible obstructive airways disease including as an ANTI-ASTHMATIC treatment. It is available in an aerosol inhalant.
✚▲ Side-effects/warnings: See SALBUTAMOL.

Akineton

(Knoll) is a proprietary, prescription-only preparation of the ANTICHOLINERGIC (ANTIMUSCARINIC) biperiden. It can be used in the treatment of parkinsonism, and is available as tablets and in a form for injection.
✚▲ Side-effects/warnings: See BIPERIDEN.

Aknemin

(Crookes) is a proprietary, prescription-only preparation of the ANTIBACTERIAL and (TETRACYCLINES) ANTIBIOTIC minocycline. It can be used to treat a wide range of infections, and is available as capsules.
✚▲ Side-effects/warnings: See MINOCYCLINE.

Aknemycin Plus

(Crookes) is a proprietary, prescription-only compound preparation of the (RETINOID) tretinoin and the ANTIBACTERIAL and (MACROLIDE) ANTIBIOTIC erythromycin. It can be used to treat acne, and is available as an alcoholic solution.
✚▲ Side-effects/warnings: See ERYTHROMYCIN; TRETINOIN.

albendazole

is an ANTHELMINTIC which is used to provide cover during surgery for the removal of cysts caused by the tapeworm *Echinococcus* and as treatment when surgery is not possible, and to treat strongyloidiasis. Administration is oral.
✚ Side-effects: There may be headache, dizziness, gastrointestinal disturbances, hair loss, rash, and fever. Blood disorders have been reported.
▲ Warnings: It is not to be given to anyone who is pregnant, and administer with care to those who are breast-feeding. Blood and liver function tests will be made.
✪ **Related entry: Zentel.**

alclometasone dipropionate

is a CORTICOSTEROID with ANTI-INFLAMMATORY properties. It is used in the treatment of inflammatory skin disorders, particularly eczema. Administration is by topical application.
✚▲ Side-effects/warnings: See HYDROCORTISONE.
✪ **Related entry: Modrasone.**

Alcoderm

(Galderma) is a proprietary, non-prescription preparation of the SURFACTANT sodium lauryl sulphate with liquid paraffin and a number of other EMOLLIENT agents. It can be used for dry skin conditions, and is available as a cream.
✚▲ Side-effects/warnings: See LIQUID PARAFFIN; SODIUM LAURYL SULPHATE.

alcohol

see ETHANOL; ETHYL ALCOHOL.

alcohols

constitute a large class of chemical compounds, and a number of these are used in medicine or are important toxicologically. *Ethyl alcohol* (ethanol), commonly referred to simply as *alcohol*, is the most familiar and has a number or uses and misuses (it is referred to in a separate article, ETHYL ALCOHOL). *Glycerol* (glycerin(e)) is also an alcohol, and is used in a variety of EMOLLIENT skin preparations, in LAXATIVE suppository preparations, in ear drops, for dry tickly coughs, as a sweetening agent for medications, and as a constituent in many preparations. POLYVINYL ALCOHOL is a constituent in several topical preparations that are used as artificial tears to treat dryness of the eye.

Toxic alcohols notably include *methyl alcohol* (methanol; wood alcohol), which is found both as a contaminant of illicit spirits (through inexpert distillation), and a deliberate additive to ethanol in *methylated spirits* (together with a bitter substances and colouring matter) to discourage its misuse as an alcoholic intoxicant. Ingestion of even small amount of methyl alcohol have a very serious effects due to its metabolism in the body

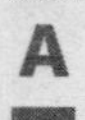

to the much more active chemical, formic acid, which kills nerve cells and the optic nerve, so blinding its victims (as well as having other serious actions). Treatment of ingestion of methanol is touched on in the ANTIDOTE article. Treatment of poisoning after ingestion of another misused alcohol, *ethylene glycol* (antifreeze), may be with the antidote FOMEPIZOLE.

Aldactide 50

(Searle; Pharmacia) is a proprietary, prescription-only compound preparation of the (*aldosterone-antagonist* and *potassium-sparing*) DIURETIC spironolactone and the (THIAZIDE-type) diuretic hydroflumethiazide (a combination called co-flumactone 50/50). It can be used for HEART FAILURE TREATMENT, and is available as tablets.

✚▲ Side-effects/warnings: See HYDROFLUMETHIAZIDE; SPIRONOLACTONE.

Aldactide 25

(Searle; Pharmacia) is a proprietary, prescription-only compound preparation of the (*aldosterone-antagonist* and *potassium-sparing*) DIURETIC spironolactone and the (THIAZIDE) diuretic hydroflumethiazide (a combination called co-flumactone 25/25). It can be used for HEART FAILURE TREATMENT, and is available as tablets.

✚▲ Side-effects/warnings: See HYDROFLUMETHIAZIDE; SPIRONOLACTONE.

Aldactone

(Searle; Pharmacia) is a proprietary, prescription-only preparation of the (*aldosterone-antagonist* and *potassium-sparing*) DIURETIC spironolactone, which can be used in conjunction with other types of diuretic, such as the THIAZIDE, that cause loss of potassium. It can be used to treat oedema associated with aldosteronism, for HEART FAILURE TREATMENT, kidney disease and fluid retention, and ascites caused by cirrhosis of the liver. Available as tablets.

✚▲ Side-effects/warnings: See SPIRONOLACTONE.

Aldara

(3M) is a proprietary, prescription-only preparation of the KERATOLYTIC agent imiquimod. It can be used to remove external genital and perianal warts, and is available as a cream.

✚▲ Side-effects/warnings: See IMIQUIMOD.

aldesleukin

(recombinant interleukin-2), is a one of the cytokine inflammatory mediators called interleukins, produced naturally by cells called macrophages in response to infection or antigenic challenge, being involved in inflammatory reactions, especially fever, in the body. Synthetic (recombinant; rbe) versions can be used as IMMUNOMODULATOR (or IMMUNOSTIMULANT) drugs. Aldesleukin is used as an ANTICANCER drug, mainly for treating metastatic renal cell carcinoma. Administration is by subcutaneous injection.

✚ Side-effects: Toxicity is universal and often severe. A common problem is development of a capillary leak syndrome which causes pulmonary oedema and hypotension. Bone marrow, kidney and liver, thyroid, and CNS toxicity are also common.

▲ Warnings: Aldesleukin is used in specialist units only. It is a very toxic drug, and although it can shrink tumours in a small proportion of patients, there is an insignificant increase in survival.

✪ Related entry: Proleukin.

Aldomet

(MSD) is a proprietary, prescription-only preparation of the ANTISYMPATHETIC methyldopa. It can be used as an ANTIHYPERTENSIVE, and is available as tablets.

✚▲ Side-effects/warnings: See METHYLDOPA.

alemtuzumab

represents a new type of specialist drug. It is a monoclonal antibody (a form of pure antibody produced by a type of molecular engineering) which causes lysis (destruction) of B lymphocytes, so effectively it can be regarded as a specific CYTOTOXIC agent with defined IMMUNOSUPPRESSANT actions. It has recently been introduced for ANTICANCER treatment in those who have chronic lymphocytic leukaemia. Administration is by intravenous infusion.

✚▲ Side-effects/warnings: Alemtuzumab has widespread toxicity and is used only under close supervision of a hospital specialist.

✪ Related entry: MabCampath.

alendronate sodium

see ALENDRONIC ACID.

alendronic acid

is a CALCIUM METABOLISM MODIFIER, a

BISPHOSPHONATE used (as alendronate sodium) to treat disorders of bone metabolism due to HORMONE imbalance. It can be used for treating postmenopausal osteoporosis and corticosteroid-induced osteoporosis. Administration is oral.
✚ Side-effects: Effects on the oesophagus (characterized by oesophagitis, erosions and ulcers), abdominal pain, distension and flatulence, diarrhoea or constipation, muscle pain, headache; rash and skin redness; nausea and vomiting.
▲ Warnings: Not to be administered to patients with certain abnormalities of the oesophagus or other structures, low blood calcium or renal impairment. It is not for use in pregnancy or when breast-feeding. Used with care in kidney impairment and certain gastrointestinal disorders. If there are oesophagus symptoms, such as heartburn, pain on swallowing, medical attention should be sought and the treatment stopped. It is important to follow the instructions on how to take preparations of alendronic acid carefully.
✪ **Related entries: Fosamax; Fosamax Once Weekly.**

alexitol sodium

is an aluminium-containing salt which is used as an ANTACID to relieve hyperacidity, dyspepsia, and indigestion. Administration is oral.
✚ Side-effects: Aluminium salts may cause constipation and sometimes nausea and vomiting.
▲ Warnings: It reduces absorption of phosphates and therefore should not be administered to patients with hypophosphataemia; use with caution in those with porphyria and kidney impairment. It may decrease absorption of a number of other drugs, including ANTIBIOTIC (particularly TETRACYCLINES), ANTIFUNGAL and ACE INHIBITOR drugs.
✪ **Related entry: Actal Tablets.**

alfacalcidol

(1α-hydroxycolecalciferol; 1α-hydroxycholecalciferol) is a synthesized form of CALCIFEROL (VITAMIN D). It is used to make up vitamin D deficiency, particularly in the treatment of types of hypoparathyroidism and prevention of rickets. Administration is oral or by injection.
✪ **Related entries: AlfaD; One-Alpha.**

AlfaD

(Berk; APS) is a proprietary, prescription-only preparation of the VITAMIN D analogue alfacalcidol. It can be used to treat a deficiency of vitamin D, and is available as capsules.
✚▲ Side-effects/warnings: See ALFACALCIDOL.

alfentanil

is an (OPIOID) NARCOTIC ANALGESIC which is used for short surgical operations, outpatient surgery, for pain relief and to enhance the effect of GENERAL ANAESTHETIC and to suppress breathing in patients on artificial ventilation. Administration is by injection. Its proprietary form is on the Controlled Drugs list.
✚▲ Side-effects/warnings: See OPIOID.
✪ **Related entry: Rapifen.**

alfuzosin

is a selective ALPHA-ADRENOCEPTOR BLOCKER which can be used to treat urinary retention in benign prostatic hyperplasia (BPH). Administration is oral.
✚▲ Side-effects/warnings: See ALPHA-ADRENOCEPTOR BLOCKER. Avoid in severe liver impairment.
✪ **Related entries: Xatral; Xatral XL.**

Algesal

(Solvay) is a proprietary, non-prescription preparation of diethylamine salicylate, which has a COUNTER-IRRITANT, OR RUBEFACIENT, action. It can be applied to the skin for the symptomatic relief of musculoskeletal rheumatic conditions. Available as a cream, it is not normally given to children, except on medical advice.
✚▲ Side-effects/warnings: See DIETHYLAMINE SALICYLATE.

Algicon

(Rhône-Poulenc Rorer; Aventis Pharma) is a proprietary, non-prescription compound preparation of the ANTACID agents aluminium hydroxide, magnesium carbonate, potassium bicarbonate, and alginic acid (as magnesium alginate). It can be used to relieve hyperacidity and dyspepsia, and is available as tablets. It is not normally given to children under 12 years, except on medical advice.
✚▲ Side-effects/warnings: See ALGINIC ACID; ALUMINIUM HYDROXIDE; MAGNESIUM CARBONATE; POTASSIUM BICARBONATE.

A

alginic acid

is extracted from seaweed, usually in the form of alginate (magnesium alginate or sodium alginate). It has a viscous, sticky consistency and is used as a DEMULCENT in certain ANTACID preparations to protect against reflux oesophagitis. It is also incorporated in some mouthwashes or gargles to protect and soothe the mouth.
✚▲ Side-effects/warnings: It is regarded as safe in normal use.
✪ **Related entries: Algicon; Asilone Heartburn Liquid; Bisodol Heartburn Relief; Gastrocote Liquid; Gastrocote Tablets; Gaviscon 250; Gaviscon 500 Lemon Flavour Tablets; Gaviscon Advance; Gaviscon Infant; Liquid Gaviscon; Peptac Liquid; Pyrogastrone; Rennie Duo; Setlers Heartburn and Indigestion Liquid; Topal.**

Algipan Rub

(Whitehall Laboratories) is a proprietary, non-prescription compound preparation of capsicum oleoresin and glycol salicylate, which all have COUNTER-IRRITANT, or RUBEFACIENT, actions and the VASODILATOR methyl nicotinate. It can be applied to the skin for the symptomatic relief of muscle pain and stiffness in backache, lumbago, sciatica, rheumatic pain and fibrositis. It is available as a cream and is not normally used for children, except on medical advice.
✚▲ Side-effects/warnings: See CAPSICUM OLEORESIN; GLYCOL SALICYLATE; METHYL NICOTINATE.

alimemazine tartrate

(trimeprazine tartrate) is an ANTIHISTAMINE which is chemically a PHENOTHIAZINE derivative. It can be used to treat the symptoms of allergic disorders, particularly urticaria and pruritus. It also has SEDATIVE properties and is used as a pre-med prior to surgery. Administration is oral.
✚▲ Side-effects/warnings: See ANTIHISTAMINE and CHLORPROMAZINE HYDROCHLORIDE. Because of its sedative property, the performance of skilled tasks, such as driving, may be impaired. It should not be used in pregnancy or breast-feeding.
✪ **Related entry: Vallergan.**

alkaloid 🄴

agents are a group of chemically similar compounds that are used as drugs. The majority of alkaloids were originally extracted from plants and are chemically heterocyclic, often complex, organic compounds with basic (alkali) properties, and in medicine they are usually administered in the form of their salts. Actually, many synthetic drugs are of a similar chemical structure and so also are technically alkaloids. Examples of *plant* alkaloids in medical use include: the BELLADONNA ALKALOID group from the *Atropa belladonna* plant and related species (eg ATROPINE SULPHATE and HYOSCINE HYDROBROMIDE); the alkaloids of opium from the poppy *Papaver somniferum* (eg CODEINE PHOSPHATE, MORPHINE SULPHATE and PAPAVERINE); the ERGOT ALKALOID group (eg ERGOMETRINE MALEATE and ERGOTAMINE TARTRATE); the CINCHONA ALKALOID drugs (QUINIDINE and QUININE) from the bark of the cinchona tree; the vinca alkaloids (eg VINBLASTINE SULPHATE, VINCRISTINE SULPHATE and VINDESINE SULPHATE); EPHEDRINE HYDROCHLORIDE from Chinese plants of the *Ephedra* species; NICOTINE from *Nicotiana tabacum*; tubocurarine, originally a South American arrow-poison from *Chondrodendron tomentosum* and other species; PILOCARPINE from a South American *Pilocarpus* shrub; and IPECACUANHA, which contains emetine and cephaeline from ipecac ('Brazil root').

Alka-Seltzer Original

(Bayer) is a proprietary, non-prescription compound preparation of the (NSAID) NON-NARCOTIC ANALGESIC and ANTIRHEUMATIC aspirin, citric acid, and the ANTACID sodium bicarbonate. It can be used for general aches and pains and for headache with upset stomach. It is available as effervescent tablets and also as *Alka-Seltzer Lemon Flavour*. It is not normally given to children, except on medical advice.
✚▲ Side-effects/warnings: See ASPIRIN; SODIUM BICARBONATE.

Alka-Seltzer XS

(Bayer) is a proprietary, non-prescription compound preparation of the (NSAID) NON-NARCOTIC ANALGESIC and ANTIPYRETIC aspirin, the non-narcotic analgesic and antipyretic paracetamol, and the STIMULANT caffeine (together with citric acid) and the ANTACID sodium bicarbonate. It can be used for general pain relief, headache and upset stomach, for the symptoms of hangover, for the symptoms of flu and also to relieve migraine, toothache and

period pain, as well as muscular aches. It is available as effervescent tablets, and is not normally given to children, except on medical advice.
✚▲ Side-effects/warnings: See ASPIRIN; CAFFEINE; PARACETAMOL; SODIUM BICARBONATE.

Alka XS Go

(Bayer) is a proprietary, non-prescription compound preparation of the (NSAID) NON-NARCOTIC ANALGESIC, ANTIPYRETIC and ANTIRHEUMATIC agents aspirin and paracetamol and the STIMULANT caffeine. It can be used for the relief of headache, migraine, period pain, sore throat, joint swelling and stiffness and the symptoms of colds and flu such as feverishness. It is not normally given to children, except on medical advice.
✚▲ Side-effects/warnings: See ASPIRIN; CAFFEINE; PARACETAMOL.

Alkeran

(GlaxoWellcome; GSK) is a proprietary, prescription-only preparation of the ANTICANCER drug melphalan. It can be used in the treatment of myelomas, and is available as tablets and in a form for injection.
✚▲ Side-effects/warnings: See MELPHALAN.

Allegron

(Dista; Lilly) is a proprietary, prescription-only preparation of the (TRICYCLIC) ANTIDEPRESSANT nortriptyline hydochloride. It can be used to treat depressive illness and to stop children bed-wetting. Available as tablets.
✚▲ Side-effects/warnings: See NORTRIPTYLINE HYDROCHLORIDE.

allopurinol

is a XANTHINE-OXIDASE INHIBITOR that blocks the action of the enzyme xanthine-oxidase, which produces uric acid and so can be used to treat excess uric acid in the blood (hyperuricaemia). It is used to prevent attacks of gout and to treat uric acid and calcium oxalate stones in the urinary tract (renal stones). Administration is oral.
✚ Side-effects: A rash (which may mean that treatment should be stopped), gastrointestinal disorders, fever, skin reactions; rarely, malaise, headache, vertigo, drowsiness, hypertension, taste disturbance, hair loss, liver toxicity and peripheral nerve disorders, and blood disorders.
▲ Warnings: It is not to be used in patients with an acute gout attack (but if an acute attack occurs during treatment, treatment should be continued); concurrent treatment is required with other drugs (eg colchicine and a NSAID, but not aspirin) and an adequate fluid intake must be maintained.
✪ **Related entries: Caplenal; Cosuric; Rimapurinol; Xanthomax; Zyloric.**

Almodan

(Berk; APS) is a proprietary, prescription-only preparation of the broad-spectrum ANTIBACTERIAL and (PENICILLIN) ANTIBIOTIC amoxicillin. It can be used to treat systemic bacterial infections, and is available as capsules and as an oral suspension.
✚▲ Side-effects/warnings: See AMOXICILLIN.

Almogran

(Lundbeck) is a recently introduced proprietary, prescription-only preparation of the (TRIPTAN) ANTIMIGRAINE drug almotriptan. It can be used to treat acute migraine attacks. Available as tablets.
✚▲ Side-effects/warnings: See ALMOTRIPTAN.

almotriptan

is a recently introduced (TRIPTAN) ANTIMIGRAINE drug, which is used to treat acute migraine attacks but not to prevent attacks. It works as a VASOCONSTRICTOR (through acting as a serotonin receptor stimulant selective for serotonin 5-HT_1 receptors), producing a rapid constriction of blood vessels surrounding the brain. Administration is oral.
✚ Side-effects: See SUMATRIPTAN for general side-effects of drugs of this class. Almotriptan may cause a short-lasting increase in blood pressure, drowsiness, dyspepsia and diarrhoea, dry mouth, muscle pains, headache, tinnitus and paraesthesia.
▲ Warnings: See SUMATRIPTAN for general warnings for drugs of this class. It is not to be given to people with peripheral vascular disease, who have had a previous cerebrovascular accident or a transient ischaemic attack. It should be given with caution to people with impaired liver function.
✪ **Related entry: Almogran.**

Alomide

(Alcon) is a proprietary, prescription-only

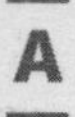

preparation of the ANTI-INFLAMMATORY drug lodoxamide which can be used for seasonal allergic conjunctivitis. It is available as eye-drops.
+▲ Side-effects/warnings: See LODOXAMIDE.

aloxiprin

is a (NSAID) NON-NARCOTIC ANALGESIC and ANTIRHEUMATIC which is incorporated into some proprietary compound analgesic preparations. It is administered orally.
✪ Related entry: Askit Powders.

alpha-adrenoceptor antagonist

see ALPHA-ADRENOCEPTOR BLOCKER.

alpha-adrenoceptor blocker

(alpha-blocker; alpha-adrenoceptor antagonist) drugs inhibit some actions of alpha receptor-stimulant drugs, such as the hormone ADRENALINE (epinephrine; released from the adrenal gland) and the neurotransmitter NORADRENALINE (norepinephrine; which is released from sympathetic nerves). They also inhibit some actions of the SYMPATHOMIMETIC drugs that are used therapeutically. Selective alpha-adrenoceptor blocking drugs work by blocking the receptor sites called alpha-adrenoceptors, thereby preventing the action of adrenaline-like agents. A major use of alpha-blockers is as ANTIHYPERTENSIVE drugs (often in conjunction with other drugs), because they lower blood pressure by preventing VASOCONSTRICTOR actions of noradrenaline and adrenaline (including in the treatment of phaeochromocytoma). They are also used to treat urinary retention in benign prostatic hyperplasia (through an action on the blood circulation within the prostate), also to increase blood flow in Raynaud's syndrome (peripheral vascular disease), for erectile dysfunction (impotence), and sometimes in dementia. See ALFUZOSIN; INDORAMIN; MOXISYLYTE; PHENOXYBENZAMINE HYDROCHLORIDE; PHENTOLAMINE MESILATE; PRAZOSIN HYDROCHLORIDE; TAMSULOSIN HYDROCHLORIDE; TERAZOSIN.
✚ Side-effects: Selective alpha-blockers have a number of side-effects in common. These include sedation, dizziness, hypotension (notably initial postural hypotension); also drowsiness, lack of energy, weakness, depression, headache, dry mouth, nausea, urinary incontinence or increased frequency, speeding of the heart and palpitations.
▲ Warnings: Avoided in those with a history of orthostatic hypotension and micturition difficulties; particular care will be taken at the start of treatment in the elderly, and in kidney and liver impairment. When using these drugs for prostatic hyperplasia, allowance must be made for their antihypertensive actions (with specialist supervision) in people undergoing antihypertensive therapy or for those with cardiac disorders. Selective alpha-blockers may cause drowsiness and so affect ability to drive or operate machinery. Because of possible initial postural hypotension with certain alpha-adrenoceptor blockers, the first dose should be taken on retiring to bed, and if there is dizziness, sweating or fatigue, the individual should remain lying down until these symptoms have passed off. There is a somewhat different prominence of side-effects according to the particular member of this class (and the dose used).

alpha-adrenoceptor stimulant

(alpha-agonist) agents are a class of drugs that act at alpha-receptors, which, along with beta-adrenoceptors, are the sites that recognize and respond to the natural hormones and neurotransmitters (adrenaline and noradrenaline) of the sympathetic nervous system. Drugs that activate this system, by whatever mechanism, are called sympathomimetics (see SYMPATHOMIMETIC).

There are two types of alpha-adrenoceptors. Stimulants acting at the alpha$_1$subtype of receptor are VASOCONSTRICTOR drugs and are widely used as NASAL DECONGESTANT drugs (eg PHENYLEPHRINE HYDROCHLORIDE, OXYMETAZOLINE HYDROCHLORIDE) and also sometimes in ANTIMIGRAINE treatment, or to treat cases of acute hypotension or circulatory shock (eg NORADRENALINE, METHOXAMINE HYDROCHLORIDE and PHENYLEPHRINE HYDROCHLORIDE), locally to facilitate ophthalmological examination (eg phenylephrine hydrochloride) and together with LOCAL ANAESTHETIC drugs to prolong the duration of action of the local anaesthetics. Stimulants acting at the alpha$_2$subtype of receptor are not yet extensively used therapeutically, but recently such agents have been introduced into GLAUCOMA TREATMENT (eg APRACLONIDINE, BRIMONIDINE TARTRATE).

alpha-blocker

see ALPHA-ADRENOCEPTOR BLOCKER.

Alphaderm

(Procter & Gamble Pharm.) is a proprietary, prescription-only compound preparation of the CORTICOSTEROID and ANTI-INFLAMMATORY hydrocortisone and the HYDRATING AGENT urea. Used to treat mild inflammation of the skin, such as eczema. Available as a cream for topical application.

✚▲ Side-effects/warnings: See HYDROCORTISONE; UREA.

Alphagan

(Allergan) is a proprietary, prescription-only preparation of the ALPHA-ADRENOCEPTOR STIMULANT drug brimonidine tartrate that is selective for the $alpha_2$subtype of receptor. It can be used in GLAUCOMA TREATMENT (for open-angle glaucoma and ocular hypertension, particularly when other drugs are not suitable). Available as eye-drops.

✚▲ Side-effects/warnings: See BRIMONIDINE TARTRATE.

Alphanate

(Alpha) is a proprietary, prescription-only preparation of dried human factor VIII fraction, which acts as a HAEMOSTATIC drug to reduce or stop bleeding in the treatment of disorders in which bleeding is prolonged and potentially dangerous (mainly haemophilia A). It is available in a form for intravenous injection or infusion.

✚▲ Side-effects/warnings: See FACTOR VIII FRACTION (DRIED).

AlphaNine

(Alpha) is a proprietary, prescription-only preparation of factor IX fraction, dried, which is prepared from human blood plasma. It can be used in treating patients with a deficiency in factor IX (haemophilia B), and is available in a form for intravenous infusion.

✚▲ Side-effects/warnings: See FACTOR IX FRACTION, DRIED.

Alphaparin

(Grifols) is a proprietary, prescription-only preparation of the ANTICOAGULANT certoparin sodium, a low molecular weight version of heparin. It can be used for prophylaxis of deep-vein thrombosis, and is available in a form for injection.

✚▲ Side-effects/warnings: See CERTOPARIN.

alpha tocopheryl acetate

(tocopherol) is a form of VITAMIN E. It is used in therapeutics to treat deficiency due to malabsorption, such as in abetalipoproteinaemia in young children with congenital cholestasis or cystic fibrosis and as a vitamin supplement. Some people take it in higher doses as a free-radical scavenger in the expectation of protection against a number of disease states. Administration is oral.

✚ Side-effects: Diarrhoea and abdominal pain if used at high doses.

▲ Warnings: It is used with care if there is a predisposition to thrombosis (clot formation). In premature infants there is an increased risk of the disorder known as necrotising enterocolitis.

✪ **Related entry: Ephynal.**

Alphavase

(Ashbourne) is a proprietary, prescription-only preparation of the ALPHA-ADRENOCEPTOR BLOCKER prazosin hydrochloride. It can be used as an ANTIHYPERTENSIVE and in the treatment of urinary retention (eg in benign prostatic hyperplasia; BPH). It is available as tablets.

✚▲ Side-effects/warnings: See PRAZOSIN HYDROCHLORIDE.

Alphosyl 2 in 1 Shampoo

(Stafford-Miller; GSK) is a proprietary, non-prescription preparation of coal tar. It can be used for the treatment of scalp disorders, psoriasis, seborrhoeic dermatitis, scaling, dandruff, and itching.

✚▲ Side-effects/warnings: See COAL TAR.

Alphosyl HC

(Stafford-Miller; GSK) is a proprietary, prescription-only compound preparation of the CORTICOSTEROID and ANTI-INFLAMMATORY hydrocortisone and coal tar (with allantoin). It can be used to treat eczema and psoriasis, and is available as a cream.

✚▲ Side-effects/warnings: See COAL TAR; HYDROCORTISONE.

alprazolam

is a BENZODIAZEPINE which is used as an ANXIOLYTIC in the short-term treatment of anxiety. Administration is oral.

✚▲ Side-effects/warnings: See BENZODIAZEPINE.

✪ **Related entry: Xanax.**

alprostadil

is a PROSTAGLANDIN (PGE_1) which is used to

maintain babies born with congenital heart defects (to maintain patency of ductus arteriosus), while emergency preparations are being made for corrective surgery and intensive care; administration is by intravenous infusion. In men, it is used in IMPOTENCE TREATMENT to treat erectile dysfunction, when it is given by intracavernosal injection into the penis or by direct urethral application.
✚ Side-effects: In babies, it is used under specialist supervision, and there will be careful control and constant monitoring to minimize side-effects and other difficulties. In men, there are many possible side-effects including prolonged erection, painful penis, testicular pain, and swelling during erection. Others side-effects reported include dizziness, headache, effects on the cardiovascular system, fainting, dry mouth, weakness, and many other reactions such as rash, swelling, warmth, burning sensation, and effects on urination.
▲ Warnings: In men it should not be given when there is a predisposition to prolonged erection (myeloma, sickle-cell anaemia, leukaemia); it is given with care to men who have deformed penises.
✪ Related entries: Caverject; MUSE; Prostin VR; Viridal.

Altacite Plus

(Peckforton) is a proprietary, non-prescription compound preparation of the ANTACID hydrotalcite and the ANTIFOAMING AGENT dimeticone. It can be used to relieve hyperacidity, flatulence, gastritis and dyspepsia, and is available as a sugar-free suspension and tablets. It is not normally given to children under eight years, except on medical advice.
✚▲ Side-effects/warnings: See DIMETICONE; HYDROTALCITE.

alteplase

(tissue-type plasminogen activator; rt-PA) has enzyme (see ENZYMES) activity and is used therapeutically as a FIBRINOLYTIC, because it has the property of breaking up blood clots. It is used in serious conditions such as myocardial infarction and pulmonary embolism. Administration is by injection.
✚▲ Side-effects/warnings: See FIBRINOLYTIC.
✪ Related entry: Actilyse.

altretamine

is a CYTOTOXIC drug, which is used as an ANTICANCER drug in the treatment of advanced ovarian cancer. Administration is oral.
✚▲ Side-effects/warnings: See CYTOTOXIC. There will be neurological examinations.
✪ Related entry: Hexalen.

Alu-Cap

(3M) is a proprietary, non-prescription preparation of the ANTACID aluminium hydroxide. It is used to relieve hyperacidity and dyspepsia; also, it can be used as a phosphate-binding agent, as an ANTIDOTE for hyperphosphataemia. It is available as capsules. It is not normally given to children, except on medical advice.
✚▲ Side-effects/warnings: See ALUMINIUM HYDROXIDE.

Aludrox Liquid

(Warner Lambert Consumer Healthcare; Pfizer) is a proprietary, non-prescription preparation of the ANTACID aluminium hydroxide and alumina. It can be used to relieve hyperacidity and dyspepsia; also hyperphosphataemia. It is available as a liquid gel, and is not normally given to children under six years, except on medical advice.
✚▲ Side-effects/warnings: See ALUMINIUM HYDROXIDE.

Aludrox Tablets

(Warner Lambert Consumer Healthcare; Pfizer) is a proprietary, non-prescription compound preparation of the ANTACID agents aluminium hydroxide, magnesium carbonate, and magnesium hydroxide. It can be used to relieve hyperacidity and dyspepsia, and is available as tablets. It is not normally given to children under six years, except on medical advice.
✚▲ Side-effects/warnings: See ALUMINIUM HYDROXIDE; MAGNESIUM CARBONATE; MAGNESIUM HYDROXIDE.

aluminium acetate

is an ASTRINGENT which is used primarily to clean sites of infection and inflammation, particularly weeping or suppurating wounds or sores, for haemorrhoids, for eczema, and for infections of the outer ear. Administration is topical.
✪ Related entry: Xyloproct.

aluminium chloride

is a powerful ANTIPERSPIRANT with ASTRINGENT properties. It can be used to treat hyperhidrosis

(excessive sweating). Administration is topical.
✚ Side-effects: There may be skin irritation.
▲ Warnings: Keep away from the eyes; do not shave the armpits or use hair-removing creams for 12 hours after application.
✪ **Related entries: Anhydrol Forte; Driclor; Driclor Solution.**

aluminium hydroxide

is an ANTACID which, because it is relatively insoluble in water, has a long duration of action. It can be used for the symptomatic relief of dyspepsia, hyperacidity, gastritis, peptic ulcers, and oesophageal reflux. It can also be used to treat elevated levels of phosphates in the blood (hyperphosphataemia), for instance in renal failure. Administration is oral.
✚ Side-effects: Aluminium salts may cause constipation and sometimes nausea and vomiting.
▲ Warnings: It should not be administered to patients with hypophosphataemia (low blood phosphates); and use with caution in those with porphyria. It may decrease the absorption of a number of other drugs, including ANTIBIOTIC (particularly TETRACYCLINES), ANTIFUNGAL and ACE INHIBITOR drugs.
✪ **Related entries: Actonorm Gel; Actonorm Powder; Algicon; Alu-Cap; Aludrox Liquid; Aludrox Tablets; Asilone Antacid Liquid; Asilone Antacid Tablets; Asilone Heartburn Liquid; Asilone Heartburn Tablets; Asilone Suspension; Dijex Suspension; Dijex Tablets; Entrotabs; Gastrocote Liquid; Gastrocote Tablets; Gaviscon 250; Gaviscon 500 Lemon Flavour Tablets; Kolanticon Gel; Maalox Plus; Maalox TC Tablets and Suspension; Mucaine; Mucogel Suspension; Pyrogastrone; Topal.**

Alupent

(Boehringer Ingelheim) is a proprietary, prescription-only preparation of the BETA-RECEPTOR STIMULANT orciprenaline sulphate. It can be used as a BRONCHODILATOR in reversible obstructive airways disease, as an ANTI-ASTHMATIC treatment. It is available as tablets and a sugar-free syrup.
✚▲ Side-effects/warnings: See ORCIPRENALINE SULPHATE.

alverine citrate

is an ANTISPASMODIC which is used orally to treat spasm in the gastrointestinal tract and in dysmenorrhoea (period pain). It is given orally.
✚ Side-effects: These are relatively rare, but there have been reports of nausea, headache, pruritus, rash, and dizziness.
▲ Warnings: It should not be administered to patients who suffer from paralytic ileus or certain other intestinal disorders; and is administered with care to those who are pregnant or breast-feeding.
✪ **Related entries: Relaxyl Capsules; Spasmonal; Spasmonal Fibre.**

amantadine hydrochloride

is a prescription-only ANTIPARKINSONISM drug used to treat the disease, but is not used to treat the parkinsonian symptoms induced by some drugs. It also has some ANTIVIRAL activity and has been used to prevent infection with the influenza A_2 virus (but not other influenza viruses) and in the treatment of herpes zoster (shingles). Administration is oral.
✚ Side-effects: These include restlessness and inability to concentrate; there may also be dizziness and insomnia, gastrointestinal disturbances, oedema, blood disorders, skin discoloration, anorexia, hallucinations, and blurred vision.
▲ Warnings: It should not be administered to patients who suffer from gastric ulcers or from epilepsy, who are pregnant or breast-feeding, or who suffer from certain serious kidney disorders. Administer with caution to patients who suffer from certain heart, liver or kidney disorders, psychosis, who are in a state of confusion. Withdrawal of treatment in Parkinson's disease must be gradual. It may effect performance of skilled tasks, such as driving.
✪ **Related entry: Symmetrel.**

Amaryl

(Hoechst Marion Roussel; Aventis Pharma) is a proprietary, prescription-only preparation of the SULPHONYLUREA glimepiride. It can be used in DIABETIC TREATMENT of Type II diabetes (non-insulin-dependent diabetes mellitus; NIDDM; maturity-onset diabetes). It is available as tablets.
✚▲ Side-effects/warnings: See GLIMEPIRIDE.

AmBisome

(Gilead) is a proprietary, prescription-only preparation of the ANTIFUNGAL drug amphotericin, which is in an unusual lipid

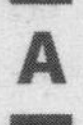

formulation (encapsulated in liposomes) that is intended to minimize toxicity, and can be used for severe systemic infections. It is available in a form for intravenous infusion.
✚▲ Side-effects/warnings: See AMPHOTERICIN.

Ambre Solaire
(Garnier) is the name of a range of proprietary, non-prescription SUNSCREEN lotions. Total screen, sun intolerant skin lotion (UVA and UVB protection; UVB-SPF60) contains avobenzone, octocrylene, drometrizole, trisiloxone, terephthalydene dicamphor sulphonic acid and TITANIUM DIOXIDE. A patient whose skin condition requires this sort of preparation may be prescribed it at the discretion of their doctor.
✚▲ Side-effects/warnings: TITANIUM DIOXIDE.

amethocaine
see TETRACAINE.

Ametop
(Smith & Nephew Healthcare) is a proprietary, non-prescription preparation of the LOCAL ANAESTHETIC tetracaine. It can be used by topical application to the site of venepuncture or venous cannulation, and is available as a gel.
✚▲ Side-effects/warnings: See TETRACAINE.

amfebutamone
see BUPROPION.

Amias
(AstraZenica, Takeda) is a proprietary, prescription-only preparation of the ANGIOTENSIN-RECEPTOR BLOCKER candesartan cilexetil. It can be used as an ANTIHYPERTENSIVE, and is available as tablets.
✚▲ Side-effects/warnings: See CANDESARTAN CILEXETIL.

amifostine
is a specialist ANTIDOTE used to reduce neutropenia-related risk of infection due to treatment of ovarian carcinoma with CYCLOPHOSPHAMIDE or CISPLATIN. Also, to reduce nephrotoxicity due to cisplatin, and to prevent xerostomia during radiotherapy for the head and neck in cancer. Administration is by intravenous infusion.
✚ Side-effects: Hypotension, nausea and vomiting, flushing, chills, dizziness, sleepiness, hiccups and sneezing; rarely convulsions.
✪ **Related entry: Ethyol.**

amikacin
is a broad-spectrum ANTIBACTERIAL and (AMINOGLYCOSIDE) ANTIBIOTIC (a derivative of kanamycin). It is used primarily against serious infections caused by Gram-negative bacteria that prove to be resistant to the more widely used aminoglycoside GENTAMICIN. Administration is by injection.
✚▲ Side-effects/warnings: See GENTAMICIN.
✪ **Related entry: Amikin.**

Amikin
(Bristol-Myers Squibb) is a proprietary, prescription-only preparation of the ANTIBACTERIAL and (AMINOGLYCOSIDE) ANTIBIOTIC amikacin (as sulphate). It is available in forms for injection and intravenous infusion.
✚▲ Side-effects/warnings: See AMIKACIN.

Amilamont
(Rosemont) is a proprietary, prescription-only preparation of the *(potassium-sparing)* DIURETIC amiloride hydrochloride. It can be used to treat oedema, ascites in cirrhosis of the liver, heart failure (in conjunction with other diuretics) and as an ANTIHYPERTENSIVE. It is available as an oral solution.
✚▲ Side-effects/warnings: See AMILORIDE HYDROCHLORIDE.

Amil-Co
(IVAX) is a proprietary, prescription-only compound preparation of the *(potassium-sparing)* DIURETIC amiloride hydrochloride and the THIAZIDE diuretic hydrochlorothiazide (a combination called co-amilozide 5/50). It can be used to treat oedema and as an ANTIHYPERTENSIVE. It is available as tablets.
✚▲ Side-effects/warnings: See AMILORIDE HYDROCHLORIDE; HYDROCHLOROTHIAZIDE.

Amilmaxco 5/50
(Ashbourne) is a proprietary, prescription-only compound preparation of the *(potassium-sparing)* DIURETIC amiloride hydrochloride and the THIAZIDE diuretic hydrochlorothiazide (a combination called co-amilozide 5/50). It can be used to treat oedema and as an ANTIHYPERTENSIVE. It is available as tablets.

✚▲ Side-effects/warnings: See AMILORIDE HYDROCHLORIDE; HYDROCHLOROTHIAZIDE.

amiloride hydrochloride

is a weak, *potassium-sparing* DIURETIC which retains potassium in the body and is therefore used as an alternative to, or commonly in combination with, other diuretics such as the THIAZIDE and *loop diuretics* (which normally cause a loss of potassium from the body). It can be used to treat heart failure, oedema, ascites in liver cirrhosis, and as an ANTIHYPERTENSIVE (combined with other drugs, eg a BETA-BLOCKER). Administration is oral.
✚ Side-effects: Gastrointestinal upsets, skin rashes, dry mouth, confusion (particularly in the elderly), postural hypotension (fall in blood pressure on standing); raised blood potassium and lowered blood sodium.
▲ Warnings: It should not be administered to patients who have high blood potassium levels, who are taking potassium supplements or who have kidney failure. Administer with care to patients who are pregnant or breast-feeding, have diabetes or are elderly.
✪ Related entries: Amilamont; Amil-Co; Amilmaxco 5/50; Aridil; Burinex A; co-amilofruse 10/80; co-amilofruse 2.5/20; co-amilofruse 5/40; co-amilozide 2.5/25; co-amilozide 5/50; Froop-Co; Fru-Co; Frumil; Frumil Forte; Frumil LS; Kalten; Lasoride; Moducren; Moduret 25; Moduretic; Navispare.

aminacrine hydrochloride

(aminoacridine hydrochloride) is an (ANTIBACTERIAL) ANTISEPTIC incorporated into preparations that are used to treat mouth ulcers.
✚▲ Side-effects/warnings: Reasonably safe in normal topical use at recommended concentrations.
✪ Related entries: Medijel Gel; Medijel Pastels.

aminoacridine hydrochloride

see AMINACRINE HYDROCHLORIDE.

aminobenzoic acid

is an unusual drug, sometimes classed as one of the B-complex vitamins. It is also used as a SUNSCREEN because it helps to protect the skin from ultraviolet radiation. For this reason, aminobenzoic acid is present in some suntan lotions and also in some barrier preparations to ward off the harmful effects of repeated radiotherapy. Administration is topical.
▲ Warnings: Protection is temporary, so creams and lotions must be reapplied every so often. Preparations containing aminobenzoates may cause photosensitivity reactions (and are less used than at one time).
✪ Related entry: Spectraban Lotion.

aminoglutethimide

is used to treat breast cancer. It is an ENZYME INHIBITOR and is thought to work as an *indirect* HORMONE ANTAGONIST, by inhibiting steroid hormone synthesis in the body, especially the conversion of the sex hormone ANDROGEN to the sex hormone OESTROGEN, so may be used as an ANTICANCER drug for breast cancer (and sometimes prostate cancer). Since it inhibits the formation of corticosteroid in the adrenal gland, it may also be used to treat Cushing's disease caused by cancer of the adrenal gland, which results in the excessive release of CORTICOSTEROID hormones in the body. Administration is oral.
✚ Side-effects: Drowsiness, lethargy, unsteadiness, rashes and allergic manifestations, fever, nausea and diarrhoea, thyroid gland disturbances and blood disorders, liver enzyme disturbances, headache, sleep problems, and others.
▲ Warnings: It should not be given to pregnant or breast-feeding women; administer with caution to patients with adrenal hypofunction. There will be blood pressure, blood count and thyroid monitoring during treatment.
✪ Related entry: Orimeten.

aminoglycoside ▣

drugs make up a chemical class of ANTIBIOTIC that have ANTIBACTERIAL activity and are all *bactericidal* (that is, they kill bacteria rather than merely inhibiting their growth). Although they can be used against some Gram-positive bacteria, they are used primarily to treat serious infections caused by Gram-negative bacteria.

Aminoglycosides are not absorbed from the gut (unless there is damage), so they must be administered by injection, or by topical application in the case of the toxic members (eg NEOMYCIN SULPHATE). However, they all share a number of common toxic properties (ie side-effects) and, because they are excreted via the

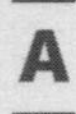

kidneys, a potentially dangerous accumulation can occur in patients with impaired kidney function. Toxic effects are related to the dose and one of the most serious is ototoxicity (impaired hearing and balance). See AMIKACIN; FRAMYCETIN SULPHATE; GENTAMICIN; NEOMYCIN SULPHATE; NETILMICIN; STREPTOMYCIN; TOBRAMYCIN.

aminophylline

is a BRONCHODILATOR which is used as an ANTI-ASTHMATIC for acute severe asthma and reversible airways obstruction (chronic obstructive airways disease). It is chemically classed as a *xanthine* and is a chemical combination of theophylline (with ethylenediamine to make it more water-soluble). Administration is either oral or by injection.

✚▲ Side-effects/warnings: See THEOPHYLLINE; but the ethylenediamine component can cause allergic reactions in the skin.

✪ **Related entries: Amnivent 225 SR; Min-I-Jet Aminophylline; Norphyllin SR; Phyllocontin Continus.**

aminosalicylate 🅱

agents are a chemical class of drugs that contain a 5-aminosalicylic acid component. They are used to maintain remission of the symptoms of ulcerative colitis, also to treat active Crohn's disease; also, they can be used to treat rheumatoid arthritis.

The drugs in this group include MESALAZINE, which is 5-aminosalicylic acid itself, OLSALAZINE SODIUM, which is two molecules of 5-aminosalicylic acid joined together, SULFASALAZINE, which combines within the one chemical both 5-aminosalicylic acid and the (SULPHONAMIDE) ANTIBACTERIAL sulfapyridine, and BALSALAZIDE DISODIUM which is a pro-drug of 5-aminosalicylic acid.

The aminosalicylate component causes characteristic side-effects such as diarrhoea, salicylate hypersensitivity and kidney effects (interstitial nephritis); whereas sulphasalazine also has sulphonamide-related side-effects, including rashes, blood disorders, oligospermia (lack of sperm) and lupoid syndrome. The sensitivity of individual patients to one or other chemical component partly determines the most suitable treatment. Patients taking aminosalicylates should tell their doctor if they have any unexplained bruising, bleeding, sore throat, fever or malaise, because of possible effects on the blood that may mean treatment should be stopped.

amiodarone hydrochloride

is a potentially toxic drug which is used as an ANTI-ARRHYTHMIC to treat certain severe irregularities of the heartbeat, especially in cases where, for one reason or another, alternative drugs cannot be used. Administration is either oral or by injection.

✚ Side-effects: These are many and include: photosensitivity, deposits on the cornea; neurological effects; muscle damage; nausea, vomiting; blood disturbances, rashes and impaired vision and others.

▲ Warnings: It should not be administered to patients with certain heart irregularities; thyroid disorders; certain liver and kidney disorders; or to those who are pregnant or breast-feeding. There should be regular testing of thyroid, liver and lung function. Its use is initiated under specialist supervision.

✪ **Related entry: Cordarone X.**

amisulpride

is an ANTIPSYCHOTIC drug (one of a group sometimes termed *atypical antipsychotics*) which can be used for the treatment of symptoms of schizophrenia, often in patients who do not respond to, or who can not tolerate, conventional antipsychotic drugs. It is taken orally.

✚ Side-effects: Of the 'atypical' antipsychotics these include weight gain, dizziness, postural hypotension and fainting, extrapyramidal symptoms (usually mild and transient, but occasionally tardive dyskinesia on long-term administration). Amisulpride may also cause insomnia, anxiety and agitation, drowsiness and gastrointestinal disorders; effects on the breast, menstrual cycle, sexual function, and heart.

▲ Warnings: Atypical antipsychotics are used with caution in patients with cardiovascular disease, history of epilepsy, the elderly and Parkinson's disease; they may affect performance of skilled tasks including driving. Also, caution in kidney impairment. Amisulpride should not be used in women who are pregnant or breast-feeding, or in phaeochromocytoma or prolactin-dependent tumours. There is significant interaction with a number of other drugs, and

effects of alcohol may be enhanced.
✪ **Related entry: Solian.**

amitriptyline hydrochloride

is an ANTIDEPRESSANT of the TRICYCLIC class. It has quite marked SEDATIVE properties, which may be of benefit to agitated or violent patients. Along with other members of this class, it has pronounced ANTICHOLINERGIC (ANTIMUSCARINIC) side-effects. It has also be used in post-herpatic neuralgia and some other types of neuropathic pain, including diabetic neuropathy, and has been used more generally in ANTIMIGRAINE treatment to prevent attacks. A further use is to prevent bed-wetting by children and in the management of unstable bladder conditions. Administration can be either oral or by injection.
✚ Side-effects: Common effects include loss of intricacy in movement or thought (affecting driving ability), sedation, dry mouth, blurred vision and constipation; there may also be difficulty in urinating, sweating, irregular heartbeat, behavioural disturbances, a rash, a state of confusion and changes in appetite and libido, effects on the breast and testicles, cardiovascular, liver and blood disorders, also convulsions.
▲ Warnings: It should not be administered to patients who suffer from certain heart disorders, severe liver disorders, psychosis or mania. It should be administered with caution to patients who suffer from diabetes, epilepsy, liver, heart or thyroid disease, phaeochromocytoma, closed-angle glaucoma or urinary retention; or who are pregnant or breast-feeding. Withdrawal of treatment must be gradual. The effects of alcohol are potentiated.
✪ **Related entries: Elavil; Lentizol; Triptafen.**

Amix

(Ashbourne)is a proprietary, prescription-only preparation of the broad-spectrum ANTIBACTERIAL and (PENICILLIN) ANTIBIOTIC amoxicillin. It can be used to treat systemic bacterial infections, and is available as capsules and an oral suspension.
✚▲ Side-effects/warnings: See AMOXICILLIN.

amlodipine besilate

(amlodipine besylate) is a CALCIUM-CHANNEL BLOCKER which can be used as an ANTIHYPERTENSIVE and as an ANTI-ANGINA drug in the prevention of attacks. Administration is oral.
✚ Side-effects: Flushing, nausea, dizziness, headache, oedema, and fatigue. There may be rashes, an excessive growth of the gums, blood and gastrointestinal upsets, aches and pains, and other side-effects.
▲ Warnings: Administer with caution to patients with liver impairment. Not used in pregnancy, breast-feeding or certain heart disorders.
✪ **Related entry: Istin.**

amlodipine besylate

see AMLODIPINE BESILATE.

Ammonaps

(Orphan Europe) is a proprietary, prescription-only preparation of sodium phenylbutyrate (a salt of the amino acid phenylbutyric acid) which is used as a METABOLIC DISORDER TREATMENT for urea cycle disturbances. It is available as tablets and granules.
✚▲ Side-effects/warnings: See SODIUM PHENYLBUTYRATE.

Ammonia and Ipecacuanha Mixture, BP

is a non-proprietary, non-prescription compound preparation of the EXPECTORANT ammonium bicarbonate and ipecacuanha tincture (together with liquorice liquid extract). It can be used to promote the expulsion of excess bronchial secretions, and is taken orally as a liquid preparation.
✚▲ Side-effects/warnings: See IPECACUANHA.

ammonium chloride

is used as an EXPECTORANT and is sometimes incorporated into cough treatments, though evidence of its efficacy is lacking. It is a mild DIURETIC and is used in some preparations to relieve premenstrual water retention. Also, it can cause metabolic acidosis and so can be used to correct metabolic alkalosis. It has some use in the therapeutic acidification of urine, which increases the rate of the excretion of some drugs and poisons and is therefore effectively an ANTIDOTE.
✚▲ Side-effects/warnings: It is regarded as safe when used for normal occasional use.
✪ **Related entries: Adult Meltus Night Time;Bronalin Expectorant Linctus; Histalix Syrup.**

A

ammonium salicylate
is a (NSAID) that has COUNTER-IRRITANT, or RUBEFACIENT, actions and can be applied to the skin for symptomatic relief of pain in underlying organs, for instance in rheumatic and other musculoskeletal disorders. Administration is topical. See also SALICYLATE; SALICYLIC ACID.
✚▲ Side-effects/warnings: See NSAID, though normally little is absorbed into the circulation and local side-effects are limited to mild irritation. It should not be used on broken skin or mucous membranes.
✪ **Related entry: Radian B Muscle Lotion.**

Amnivent 225 SR
(Ashbourne) is a proprietary, non-prescription preparation of the BRONCHODILATOR aminophylline. It can be used as an ANTI-ASTHMATIC, and is available as modified-release tablets.
✚▲ Side-effects/warnings: See AMINOPHYLLINE.

amobarbital
(amylobarbitone) is a BARBITURATE which is used as a HYPNOTIC, but only when absolutely necessary, to treat severe and intractable insomnia in patients who are already taking barbiturates. It can also be used as an ANTI-EPILEPTIC for severe episodes in specialist epilepsy centres. Administration can be either oral or by injection. Preparations containing amobarbital are on the Controlled Drugs list.
✚▲ Side-effects/warnings: See BARBITURATE.
✪ **Related entries: Amytal; Sodium Amytal; Tuinal.**

amoebicidal
agents are ANTIMICROBIAL drugs that are used to treat infection by the microscopic protozoan organisms known as amoebae, which cause such disorders as amoebic dysentery and hepatic amoebiasis. The best-known and most-used amoebicidal is the (AZOLE) METRONIDAZOLE. See also CLIOQUINOL, DILOXANIDE FUROATE, TINIDAZOLE and ANTIMALARIAL.

Amoram
(Eastern) is a proprietary, prescription-only preparation of the broad-spectrum ANTIBACTERIAL and (PENICILLIN) ANTIBIOTIC amoxicillin. It can be used to treat systemic bacterial infections, and is available as capsules and an oral suspension.
✚▲ Side-effects/warnings: See AMOXICILLIN.

amorolfine
is an ANTIFUNGAL drug that differs chemically from other antifungals (it is a morpholone derivative that interferes with fungal sterol synthesis). It can be used topically to treat fungal skin infections, such as foot mycosis. It is used by topical application.
✚ Side-effects: There may be an occasional short-lived burning sensation, reddening and itching of the skin.
▲ Warnings: It should be administered with caution in pregnancy or breast-feeding; avoid applying to mucous membranes, eyes and ears. Avoid using nail varnish or tasting nails when using the nail lacquer.
✪ **Related entry: Loceryl.**

amoxapine
is an ANTIDEPRESSANT of the TRICYCLIC group, and can be used to treat depressive illness. Administration is oral.
✚▲ Side-effects/warnings: See AMITRIPTYLINE HYDROCHLORIDE; but has less sedative actions. There may also be menstrual irregularities, breast enlargement in men, milk production (galactorrhoea) in women, and, rarely, tardive dyskinesia.
✪ **Related entry: Asendis.**

amoxicillin
(amoxycillin) is a broad-spectrum, penicillin-like ANTIBACTERIAL and ANTIBIOTIC drug, which is closely related to AMPICILLIN. It is readily absorbed orally (better than ampicillin) and is used to treat many infections (due to both Gram-positive and Gram-negative bacteria), especially infections of the urogenital tracts, the upper respiratory tract and the middle ear. It is also sometimes used to prevent infection following dental surgery, to prevent endocarditis, to treat Lyme disease in children and (in combination with other drugs) to treat long-standing *Helicobacter pylori* infection associated with peptic ulcers.

However, it is not *penicillinase-resistant*, as it is inactivated by penicillinase enzymes produced by Gram-positive bacteria such as *Stapylococcus aureus* and common Gram-negative bacteria such as *Escherichia coli*. For this reason, it is

sometimes combined with CLAVULANIC ACID, which is an inhibitor of penicillinase enzymes. Administration can be either oral, or by injection or intravenous infusion.
✚▲ Side-effects/warnings: See AMPICILLIN.
✪ Related entries: Almodan; Amix; Amoram; Amoxil; Augmentin; co-amoxiclav; Galenamox; HeliClear; Rimoxallin.

Amoxil
(Bencard; GSK) is a proprietary, prescription-only preparation of the broad-spectrum ANTIBACTERIAL and (PENICILLIN) ANTIBIOTIC amoxicillin. It can be used to treat systemic bacterial infections, and is available as capsules, a syrup for dilution, an oral suspension for children, a sugar-free powder in sachets and in a form for injection.
✚▲ Side-effects/warnings: See AMOXICILLIN.

amoxycillin
see AMOXICILLIN.

Amphocil
(Cambridge) is a proprietary, prescription-only preparation of the ANTIFUNGAL drug amphotericin, in a formulation as a lipid colloidal dispersion (with sodium cholesteryl sulphate) that is intended to minimize toxicity, and can be used for severe systemic fungal infections. It is available in a form for intravenous infusion.
✚▲ Side-effects/warnings: See AMPHOTERICIN.

amphotericin
(amphotericin B) is a broad-spectrum ANTIFUNGAL which is a (*polyene*) ANTIBIOTIC. It can be used particularly to treat infection by most fungi and yeasts and is an extremely important drug in the treatment of systemic fungal infections, when it is given by intravenous infusion. However, it is a toxic drug and side-effects are common. There have been recent attempts to minimize toxicity (particularly to the kidney) by making a lipid formulation (encapsulated in liposomes) and a colloidal dispersion (with sodium cholesteryl sulphate) so that it can be used by injection for severe systemic or deep-seated fungal infections. For *Candida* (thrush) infections of the mouth or intestine, it can be taken orally as a suspension or lozenges.
✚ Side-effects: Parenteral treatment may cause nausea, vomiting, diarrhoea, anorexia, abdominal pain, headache, muscle and joint pain, kidney, heart, hearing, liver and blood disorders, and rash.
▲ Warnings: During treatment, tests on kidney and blood function are essential. Administer with care to patients who are pregnant, breast-feeding or have kidney impairment.
✪ Related entries: Abelcet; AmBisome; Amphocil; Fungilin; Fungizone.

amphotericin B
see AMPHOTERICIN.

ampicillin
is a broad-spectrum, penicillin-type ANTIBACTERIAL and ANTIBIOTIC drug. It is taken orally (though absorption is reduced by the presence of food in the stomach or intestines) and is used to treat many infections (due to both Gram-positive and Gram-negative bacteria), especially infections of the urogenital tracts, the respiratory tract, the middle ear, and also gonorrhoea and invasive salmonellosis. It is sometimes given as a compound preparation with FLUCLOXACILLIN, which is a combination called *co-fluampicil*. Administration is either oral or by injection.
✚ Side-effects: see BENZYLPENICILLIN. Also, diarrhoea is common; nausea; rarely, sensitivity reactions such as rashes (particularly in patients suffering from chronic lymphatic leukaemia). Allergic patients may suffer anaphylactic shock.
▲ Warnings: It should not be administered to patients who are known to be allergic to penicillin-type antibiotics in case anaphylactic shock ensues. It should be administered with caution to those with impaired kidney function.
✪ Related entries: co-fluampicil; Flu-Amp; Magnapen; Penbritin; Rimacillin.

amprenavir
is a recently introduced (*protease inhibitor*) ANTIVIRAL drug which is often used together with other antiretrovirals. It can be used in the treatment of progressive or advanced HIV infection in patients previously treated with other protease inhibitors. Administration is oral.
✚ Side-effects: There may be a rash (often starting in week two of treatment) and rarely Stevens-Johnson syndrome (an inflammatory condition). There may be gastrointestinal disturbances, including nausea, vomiting,

diarrhoea, abdominal discomfort, flatulence, and dyspepsia, and also headache, tremors, sleep disturbances, paraesthesia in the mouth, fatigue and mood disorders, including depression. There have been blood changes and metabolic effects reported especially of lipids (and redistribution of body fat), so levels of these and blood sugar will be monitored.
▲ Warnings: Amprenavir should not be used by those who are breast-feeding. Caution is needed in people with impaired liver function, or who are pregnant, diabetic or haemophiliacs. Vitamin E supplements should be avoided because vitamin E is included in the formulation; and the oral solution is not prescribed to people with liver or sever kidney impairment or who are pregnant. Treatment with amprenavir may have to be stopped if there is severe rash with other symptoms, but if the rash is not severe, treatment may be continued and antihistamines may be prescribed. There can be important interactions and possible serious adverse reactions if amprenavir is taken with some other drugs and also the herbal antidepressant St John's wort. Any prescription, over-the-counter medicines, supplements, herbal remedies or other alternative therapies that you are using, have recently used or plan to use should be discussed with your doctor or pharmacist before you take amprenavir. Important interactions will be detailed in the Patient Information Leaflet.
✪ **Related entry: Agenerase.**

amsacrine

is a (CYTOTOXIC) ANTICANCER drug which is used specifically in the treatment of acute myeloid leukaemia. Administration is by intravenous infusion.
✚▲ Side-effects/warnings: See CYTOTOXIC; there may also be heartbeat irregularities.
✪ **Related entry: Amsidine.**

Amsidine

(Goldshield) is a proprietary, prescription-only preparation of the ANTICANCER drug amsacrine. It can be used to treat acute myeloid leukaemia, and is available in a form for intravenous infusion.
✚▲ Side-effects/warnings: See AMSACRINE.

amylmetacresol

is an ANTISEPTIC used in preparations to spray or dissolve in the mouth.
✚▲ Side-effects/warnings: Considered to be safe in normal topical use at recommended concentrations.
✪ **Related entries: Mentholatum Antiseptic Lozenges; Strepsils Honey and Lemon; Strepsils Menthol and Eucalyptus; Strepsils Original; Strepsils Pain Relief Plus; Strepsils Sugar Free Lozenges; Strepsils with Vitamin C 100 mg.**

amylobarbitone

see AMOBARBITAL.

Amytal

(Flynn) is a proprietary, prescription-only preparation of the BARBITURATE amobarbital and is on the Controlled Drugs list. It can be used as a HYPNOTIC to treat persistent and intractable insomnia, and is available as tablets.
✚▲ Side-effects/warnings: See AMOBARBITAL.

Anabact

(CHS) is a proprietary, prescription-only preparation of the ANTIMICROBIAL metronidazole, which has both ANTIPROTOZOAL and ANTIBACTERIAL properties. It can be used to deodorize and treat fungating, malodorous tumours. It is available as a gel for topical application.
✚▲ Side-effects/warnings: See METRONIDAZOLE.

anabolic steroid 🅴

drugs are chemically derived from the male ANDROGEN (STEROID) HORMONE, TESTOSTERONE. They generally promote body growth and masculinization, and tend to oppose the actions of OESTROGEN hormones in the body. They have protein-building properties, but have generally not proved to be useful for this in medicine. However, they are abused by some athletes and body-builders to increase muscle mass. Used this way, they are rather toxic having serious effects on the liver, increase the risk of arteriosclerosis and coronary artery disease, and cause virilization in women. Medically, anabolic steroids have been given for osteoporosis in women but are no longer commonly recommended for this purpose. They can also be used to treat the vascular manifestations of Behçet's disease, for hereditary angioedema, to treat aplastic anaemia and to reduce the itching of chronic biliary obstruction. They are given by mouth or injection. See NANDROLONE.

Anacal Rectal Ointment

(Sankyo Pharma) is a proprietary, non-prescription preparation of heparinoid (with lauromacrogol). It can be used for the symptomatic relief of haemorrhoids, perianal eczema, itching, and anal fissures. It is available as an ointment and is not normally used for children, except on medical advice.

✚▲ Side-effects/warnings: See HEPARINOIDS.

Anacal Suppositories

(Sankyo Pharma) is a proprietary, non-prescription preparation of heparinoid (with lauromacrogol). It can be used for the symptomatic relief of haemorrhoids, perianal eczema, itching, and anal fissures. It is available as suppositories and is not normally used for children, except on medical advice.

✚▲ Side-effects/warnings: See HEPARINOIDS.

Anadin Analgesic Capsules, Maximum Strength

(Whitehall Laboratories) is a proprietary, non-prescription compound preparation of the (NSAID) NON-NARCOTIC ANALGESIC and ANTIRHEUMATIC aspirin and the STIMULANT caffeine. It can be used for the treatment of mild to moderate pain and for symptomatic relief of colds and flu. It is available as capsules and is not normally given to children, except on medical advice.

✚▲ Side-effects/warnings: See ASPIRIN; CAFFEINE.

Anadin Cold Control Capsules

(Whitehall Laboratories) is a proprietary, non-prescription compound preparation of the NON-NARCOTIC ANALGESIC and ANTIPYRETIC paracetamol, the SYMPATHOMIMETIC and DECONGESTANT phenylephrine hydrochloride and the STIMULANT caffeine. It can be used to relieve cold and flu symptoms. It is available as capsules and is not normally given to children, except on medical advice.

✚▲ Side-effects/warnings: See CAFFEINE; PARACETAMOL; PHENYLEPHRINE HYDROCHLORIDE.

Anadin Cold Control Flu Strength Hot Lemon

(Whitehall Laboratories) is a proprietary, non-prescription compound preparation of the NON-NARCOTIC ANALGESIC and ANTIPYRETIC paracetamol and the SYMPATHOMIMETIC and DECONGESTANT phenylephrine hydrochloride. It can be used to relieve cold and flu symptoms, and is available as a powder. It is not normally given to children, except on medical advice.

✚▲ Side-effects/warnings: See PARACETAMOL; PHENYLEPHRINE HYDROCHLORIDE.

Anadin Extra

(Whitehall Laboratories) is a proprietary, non-prescription compound preparation of the (NSAID) NON-NARCOTIC ANALGESIC and ANTIRHEUMATIC aspirin, the non-narcotic analgesic paracetamol, and the STIMULANT caffeine. It can be used for the treatment of pain, especially headaches, period, dental and rheumatic pain, and also to relieve cold and flu symptoms. It is available as capsule-shaped tablets and is not normally given to children, except on medical advice.

✚▲ Side-effects/warnings: See ASPIRIN; CAFFEINE; PARACETAMOL.

Anadin Extra Soluble Tablets

(Whitehall Laboratories) is a proprietary, non-prescription compound preparation of the (NSAID) NON-NARCOTIC ANALGESIC and ANTIRHEUMATIC aspirin, the non-narcotic analgesic paracetamol, and the STIMULANT caffeine. It can be used to treat mild to moderate pain, relieve swelling, stiffness and cold and flu symptoms. It is available as soluble tablets and is not normally given to children, except on medical advice.

✚▲ Side-effects/warnings: See ASPIRIN; CAFFEINE; PARACETAMOL.

Anadin Ibuprofen

(Whitehall Laboratories) is a proprietary, non-prescription preparation of the (NSAID) NON-NARCOTIC ANALGESIC and ANTIRHEUMATIC ibuprofen. It can be used for mild to moderate pain, dental, period and muscle pain. It is available as tablets and is not normally given to children, except on medical advice.

✚▲ Side-effects/warnings: See IBUPROFEN.

Anadin Paracetamol Tablets

(Whitehall Laboratories) is a proprietary, non-prescription compound preparation of the NON-NARCOTIC ANALGESIC and ANTIPYRETIC

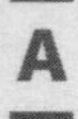

paracetamol. It can be used for mild to moderate pain such as period pain, headache and toothache, and the symptoms of colds and flu. It is available as tablets and is not normally given to children under six years, except on medical advice.
✚▲ Side-effects/warnings: See PARACETAMOL.

Anadin Tablets

(Whitehall Laboratories) is a proprietary, non-prescription compound preparation of the (NSAID) NON-NARCOTIC ANALGESIC, ANTIPYRETIC and ANTIRHEUMATIC aspirin and the STIMULANT caffeine. It can be used for mild to moderate pain, and the symptoms of feverish colds and flu. It is available as capsule-shaped tablets and is not normally given to children, except on medical advice.
✚▲ Side-effects/warnings: See ASPIRIN; CAFFEINE.

Anadin Ultra

(Whitehall Laboratories) is a proprietary, non-prescription compound preparation of the (NSAID) NON-NARCOTIC ANALGESIC and ANTIPYRETIC ibuprofen. It can be used for mild to moderate pain such as backache, headache, muscular pain, period pain and migraine, and the symptoms of feverish colds and flu. It is available as capsules, and is not normally given to children, except on medical advice.
✚▲ Side-effects/warnings: See IBUPROFEN.

anaemia treatment

involves the use of drugs to correct a deficiency of the oxygen-carrying capacity of red blood cells (anaemia). The type of treatment depends on the cause of the anaemia. For example, the drugs administered to treat iron-deficient anaemia are mainly salts of IRON and are used where there is deficiency of iron which is needed to synthesize haemoglobin in blood and a similar oxygen-carrier in muscles.

Dietary deficiency of iron in the diet, blood loss (eg due to disorders of menstruation or childbirth), and disease states that reduce the proper absorption of other nutrients (eg folic acid and vitamin B_{12} needed for red blood-cell production), can all lead to forms of anaemia. Iron supplements may be administered orally in one of several forms, as FERROUS FUMARATE, FERROUS GLUCONATE, FERROUS GLYCINE SULPHATE or FERROUS SULPHATE (and other salts), or *parenteral iron* by injection or intravenous infusion in the form of IRON SUCROSE and IRON SORBITAL preparations. Iron supplements are also used where there is deficiency of iron during pregnancy. The use of the B vitamin, FOLIC ACID and the B_{12} vitamin HYDROXOCOBALAMIN (also CYANOCOBALAMIN) are given for megaloblastic anaemias (including pernicious anaemia). The natural body factor EPOETIN (erythropoietin) is given when anaemia is due to the kidney's failure to stimulate red blood-cell production in the bone marrow (and after some forms of cancer chemotherapy).
▲ Warnings: Zinc, which is present in some mineral supplements, may reduce the absorption of iron.

anaesthetic

agents are used to reduce sensations, especially pain. LOCAL ANAESTHETIC drugs (eg LIDOCAINE HYDROCHLORIDE) affect a specific area and do not cause a loss of consciousness. GENERAL ANAESTHETIC drugs (eg halothane) do cause a loss of consciousness and the loss of sensation is a result of this. Local anaesthetics are a logical choice for minor and local surgical procedures, such as in dental surgery and vasectomy, because their duration of action can be short and there is less discomfort and medical risk.

However, local anaesthetics can also achieve a more extensive loss of sensation with nerve block (eg injected near to the nerve supplying a limb), or with spinal anaesthesia (eg epidural injection in childbirth) where loss of sensation in whole areas of the body allows major surgery. Local anaesthetics are particularly valuable in situations where general anaesthesia carries a high risk, or the conscious cooperation of the patient is required. General anaesthetics are normally used for more extensive surgical procedures. In modern anaesthetic practice, ANALGESIC, SEDATIVE or SKELETAL MUSCLE RELAXANT drugs are used in premedication or during the operation so that quite low doses of general anaesthetic are needed. See also NARCOTIC ANALGESIC.

analeptic

see RESPIRATORY STIMULANT.

analgesic

drugs relieve pain, and this can be achieved in

many ways. In this book the term analgesic is restricted to two main classes of drug. The first class are the NARCOTIC ANALGESIC drugs (eg MORPHINE SULPHATE), which have powerful actions on the central nervous system and alter the perception of pain. Because of the numerous possible side-effects, the most important of which is drug dependence (habituation or addiction), this class is usually used under strict medical supervision and preparations are normally available only on prescription. Other notable side-effects include depression of respiration, nausea and vomiting, sometimes hypotension, constipation, inhibition of coughing (ANTITUSSIVE action), and constriction of the pupils (miosis). Narcotic analgesics are used for different types and severities of pain. It is now recognized that the characteristic pharmacology of the narcotic analgesics follows from their action as mimics of the natural opioid neurotransmitters (enkephalins, endorphins, dynorphins) in nerves in the brain.

Other members of this class, also known as the OPIOID (or OPIATE) group, include CODEINE PHOSPHATE, DIAMORPHINE HYDROCHLORIDE (heroin), METHADONE HYDROCHLORIDE, PENTAZOCINE and PETHIDINE HYDROCHLORIDE.

The second class is the NON-NARCOTIC ANALGESIC, which are drugs that have no tendency to produce dependence, for example ASPIRIN, but are by no means free of side-effects. This class is referred to by many names, including *weak analgesics* (something of a misnomer in view of their powerful actions in treating inflammatory pain); and, in medical circles, a very large number are referred to as *non-steroidal, anti-inflammatory drugs*, abbreviated to NSAID (see NSAID). The latter term refers to the valuable anti-inflammatory action of some members of this class. These drugs are used for a variety of purposes, ranging from mild aches and pains (at lower dosages), to the treatment of rheumatoid arthritis (at higher dosages).

PARACETAMOL does not have strong anti-inflammatory actions, but is non-narcotic and, along with other drugs in this class, has ANTIPYRETIC action (the ability to lower raised body temperature when there is fever). The non-narcotic analgesics work by altering the synthesis of prostaglandins (natural local hormones (see LOCAL HORMONE) within the body) that tend to enhance pain.

Although this class of drugs has important actions and uses, all its members have side-effects of concern, which for aspirin-like drugs include gastrointestinal upsets ranging from dyspepsia to serious haemorrhage. Other examples of non-narcotic analgesics include IBUPROFEN and INDOMETHACIN. Drugs in this class are often used in combination with other analgesics (eg paracetamol with codeine) or with drugs of other classes (eg caffeine).

Apart from these two main classes, there are other drugs that are sometimes referred to as analgesic because of their ability to relieve pain. For example, LOCAL ANAESTHETIC drugs are referred to as *local analgesics* in the USA; and RUBEFACIENT, or COUNTER-IRRITANT, agents are sometimes called analgesics.

Anapen

(Lincoln) is a proprietary prescription-only preparation of adrenaline (epinephrine). It is used as a SYMPATHOMIMETIC and BRONCHODILATOR drug in emergency treatment of acute and severe bronchoconstriction and other symptoms of acute anaphylaxis (allergic reaction; eg an insect sting). It is available as an auto-injector for self-administration, which delivers a single intramuscular dose, in two versions, *Anapen 0.3 mg solution for injection* used for adults and *Anapen Junior 0.15 mg solution for injection* for children.

✚▲ Side-effects/warnings: See ADRENALINE ACID TARTRATE.

anastrozole

is an ANTICANCER drug which is used to treat advanced breast cancer in post-menopausal women. It is a non-steroidal compound that works as an *indirect* HORMONE ANTAGONIST by inhibiting the conversion of the male SEX HORMONES to the female sex hormones (ANDROGEN to OESTROGEN. Administration is oral.

✚ Side-effects: There may be drowsiness, sleepiness and lethargy (which at first may affect the ability to drive or operate machinery); weakness, rashes, vomiting and diarrhoea; hot flushes and headache; vaginal dryness, hair thinning, and loss of appetite has been reported.

▲ Warnings: It should not be used in those who are pregnant or breast-feeding, or with impaired kidney function or liver disease.

✪ Related entry: Arimidex.

A

Anbesol Adult Strength Gel

(SSL) is a proprietary, non-prescription compound preparation of the LOCAL ANAESTHETIC lidocaine hydrochloride and the ANTISEPTIC cetylpyridinium chloride (with chlorocresol). It can be used for the temporary relief of pain caused by mouth ulcers and denture irritation. It is available as a gel for topical application. It is not recommended for use in children.

✚▲ Side-effects/warnings: See CETYLPYRIDINIUM CHLORIDE; LIDOCAINE HYDROCHLORIDE.

Anbesol Liquid

(SSL) is a proprietary, non-prescription compound preparation of the LOCAL ANAESTHETIC lidocaine hydrochloride and the ANTISEPTIC cetylpyridinium chloride (with chlorocresol). It can be used for the temporary relief of pain caused by teething, mouth ulcers and denture irritation. It is available as a liquid for topical application.

✚▲ Side-effects/warnings: See CETYLPYRIDINIUM CHLORIDE; LIDOCAINE HYDROCHLORIDE.

Anbesol Teething Gel

(SSL) is a proprietary, non-prescription compound preparation of the LOCAL ANAESTHETIC lidocaine hydrochloride and the ANTISEPTIC cetylpyridinium chloride (with chlorocresol). It can be used for the temporary relief of pain caused by teething, mouth ulcers and denture irritation. It is available as a gel for topical application.

✚▲ Side-effects/warnings: See CETYLPYRIDINIUM CHLORIDE; LIDOCAINE HYDROCHLORIDE.

Ancotil

(ICN) is a proprietary, prescription-only preparation of the ANTIFUNGAL flucytosine. It can be used to treat systemic fungal infections (eg candidiasis), and is available in a form for intravenous infusion.

✚▲ Side-effects/warnings: See FLUCYTOSINE.

Andrews Antacid

(GSK Consumer Healthcare) is a proprietary, non-prescription compound preparation of the ANTACID agents calcium carbonate and magnesium carbonate. It can be used to relieve upset stomach, heartburn, indigestion, and trapped wind. It is available as chewable tablets and also in a flavoured version called *Andrews Antacid Fruit Flavour*. It is not normally given to children, except on medical advice.

✚▲ Side-effects/warnings: See CALCIUM CARBONATE; MAGNESIUM CARBONATE.

Androcur

(Schering Health) is a proprietary, prescription-only preparation of the ANTI-ANDROGEN cyproterone acetate, which is a sex HORMONE ANTAGONIST. It can be used to treat severe hypersexuality and sexual deviation in men. It is available as tablets.

✚▲ Side-effects/warnings: See CYPROTERONE ACETATE.

androgen 🅱

is one of a group of predominantly male (STEROID) SEX HORMONES, which stimulate the development of male sex organs and male secondary sexual characteristics. In men, they are produced primarily by the testes and the main form is called TESTOSTERONE. However, androgens are produced in both men and women by the adrenal glands and in women small quantities are also secreted by the ovaries. An excessive amount in women causes masculinization. Forms of the natural hormone and a number of synthetic androgens are used therapeutically (eg forms of testosterone and MESTEROLONE) to correct hormonal deficiency, for example, delayed puberty and replacement therapy in testicular failure, sometimes in menopausal women as part of HRT, and can also be used as ANTICANCER treatments for cancers linked to sex hormones (eg breast cancer in women). ANTI-ANDROGEN drugs inhibit the actions of androgens and are also used in medicine.

✚ Side-effects: Oedema, leading to weight gain, headache, depression, nausea, gastrointestinal problems, anxiety, weakness, changes in sexual behaviour, liver effects. Increased levels of calcium in the body may cause bone growth (and in younger patients may fuse bones before fully grown, resulting in short stature), there may be prostate gland disorders, reduced production of sperm, priapism in men (prolonged painful erection), and masculinization in women.

▲ Warnings: They should not be administered to male patients who suffer from nephrosis, cancer of the prostate gland or cancer of the breast; or to women who are pregnant or breast-feeding. Administer with caution to those with impaired function of the heart, liver or kidney, certain circulatory disorders and/or hypertension, epilepsy or diabetes, thyroid disorders or migraine. There may be anabolic effects (see ANABOLIC STEROID).

androgen antagonist

see ANTI-ANDROGEN.

Andropatch

(SmithKline Beecham; GSK) is a proprietary, prescription-only preparation of the ANDROGEN (male sex hormone) testosterone. It can be used to treat testosterone deficiency in men, and is available in the form of skin patches.
✚▲ Side-effects/warnings: See TESTOSTERONE.

Anectine

(GlaxoWellcome; GSK) is a proprietary, prescription-only preparation of the (*depolarizing*) SKELETAL MUSCLE RELAXANT suxamethonium chloride. It can be used to induce muscle paralysis during surgery, and is available in a form for injection.
✚▲ Side-effects/warnings: See SUXAMETHONIUM CHLORIDE.

Anexate

(Roche) is a proprietary, prescription-only preparation of the BENZODIAZEPINE antagonist flumazenil. It can be used to reverse the effects of benzodiazepines, and is available in a form for intravenous injection or intravenous infusion.
✚▲ Side-effects/warnings: See FLUMAZENIL.

Angettes 75

(Bristol-Myers Squibb) is a proprietary, non-prescription preparation of the ANTIPLATELET aggregation agent aspirin. It can be used to help prevent the formation of thrombi (blood clots) and is used particularly for problems relating to blocked blood vessels, such as following and to prevent heart attacks. It is available as tablets.
✚▲ Side-effects/warnings: See ASPIRIN.

Angeze

(Opus; Trinity) is a proprietary, non-prescription preparation of the VASODILATOR drug isosorbide mononitrate. It can be used as an ANTI-ANGINA drug, and is available as tablets.
✚▲ Side-effects/warnings: See ISOSORBIDE MONONITRATE.

Angeze SR

(Opus; Trinity) is a proprietary, prescription-only preparation of the VASODILATOR drug isosorbide mononitrate. It can be used as an ANTI-ANGINA drug, and is available as capsules.
✚▲ Side-effects/warnings: See ISOSORBIDE MONONITRATE.

Angilol

(DDSA) is a proprietary, prescription-only preparation of the BETA-BLOCKER propranolol hydrochloride. It can be used as an ANTIHYPERTENSIVE for raised blood pressure, as an ANTI-ANGINA treatment to relieve symptoms and to improve exercise tolerance and as an ANTI-ARRHYTHMIC to regularize heartbeat and to treat myocardial infarction. It may also be used as an ANTITHYROID drug for short-term treatment of thyrotoxicosis, as an ANTIMIGRAINE treatment to prevent attacks, as an ANXIOLYTIC, particularly for symptomatic relief of tremor and palpitations, and, with an ALPHA-ADRENOCEPTOR BLOCKER, in the acute treatment of phaeochromocytoma. It is available as tablets.
✚▲ Side-effects/warnings: See PROPRANOLOL HYDROCHLORIDE.

Angiopine

(Ashbourne) is a proprietary, prescription-only preparation of the CALCIUM-CHANNEL BLOCKER nifedipine. It can be used as an ANTI-ANGINA treatment in the prevention of attacks, and as an ANTIHYPERTENSIVE. It is available as capsules.
✚▲ Side-effects/warnings: See NIFEDIPINE.

Angiopine MR

(Ashbourne) is a proprietary, prescription-only preparation of the CALCIUM-CHANNEL BLOCKER nifedipine. It can be used as an ANTIHYPERTENSIVE, and is available as modified-release tablets.
✚▲ Side-effects/warnings: See NIFEDIPINE.

angiotensin-converting enzyme inhibitor

see ACE INHIBITOR.

A

angiotensin-receptor blocker 🄱 drugs work by blocking angiotensin receptors. Angiotensin II is a circulating HORMONE that is a powerful VASOCONSTRICTOR and so blocking its effects leads to a fall in blood pressure. Recently introduced drugs of this type include CANDESARTAN CILEXETIL, EPROSARTAN, IRBESARTAN, LOSARTAN POTASSIUM, TELMISARTAN and VALSARTAN, which can be used as ANTIHYPERTENSIVE agents. The general actions and uses are similar to those of an ACE INHIBITOR, but unlike some earlier ACE inhibitors they do not cause a persistent dry cough, so are used in patients who had to stop taking ACE inhibitors because of this cough.
▲ Warnings: Potassium supplements should be avoided when taking angiotensin-receptor blockers or there is a risk of hyperkalemia (high blood-potassium levels) developing.

Angiozem CR
(Ashbourne) is a proprietary, prescription-only preparation of the CALCIUM-CHANNEL BLOCKER diltiazem hydrochloride. It can be used as an ANTIHYPERTENSIVE and as an ANTI-ANGINA drug, and is available as modified-release tablets.
✚▲ Side-effects/warnings: See DILTIAZEM HYDROCHLORIDE.

Angitak
(Eastern) is a proprietary, non-prescription preparation of the VASODILATOR drug isosorbide dinitrate, which can be used as an ANTI-ANGINA drug. It is available as an aerosol spray.
✚▲ Side-effects/warnings: See ISOSORBIDE DINITRATE.

Angitil SR
(Trinity) is a proprietary, prescription-only preparation of the CALCIUM-CHANNEL BLOCKER diltiazem hydrochloride. It can be used as an ANTIHYPERTENSIVE and as an ANTI-ANGINA drug. It is available as modified-release capsules.
✚▲ Side-effects/warnings: See DILTIAZEM HYDROCHLORIDE.

Angitil XL
(Trinity) is a proprietary, prescription-only preparation of the CALCIUM-CHANNEL BLOCKER diltiazem hydrochloride. It can be used as an ANTIHYPERTENSIVE and as an ANTI-ANGINA drug. It is available as modified-release capsules.
✚▲ Side-effects/warnings: See DILTIAZEM HYDROCHLORIDE.

Anhydrol Forte
(Dermal Laboratories) is a proprietary, non-prescription preparation of aluminium chloride (as hexahydrate), which can be used as an ANTIPERSPIRANT to treat hyperhidrosis (excessive sweating). Available in a roll-on applicator.
✚▲ Side-effects/warnings: See ALUMINIUM CHLORIDE.

Anodesyn Ointment
(SSL) is a proprietary, non-prescription preparation of the LOCAL ANAESTHETIC lidocaine hydrochloride (with allantoin). It can be used for the symptomatic relief of the pain and itching of haemorrhoids, and is available as an ointment. It is not normally given to children, except on medical advice.
✚▲ Side-effects/warnings: See LIDOCAINE HYDROCHLORIDE.

Anodesyn Suppositories
(SSL) is a proprietary, non-prescription preparation of the LOCAL ANAESTHETIC lidocaine hydrochloride (with allantoin). It can be used for the symptomatic relief of the pain and itching of haemorrhoids, and is available as suppositories. It is not normally given to children, except on medical advice.
✚▲ Side-effects/warnings: See LIDOCAINE HYDROCHLORIDE.

Anquil
(Concord) is a proprietary, prescription-only preparation of the ANTIPSYCHOTIC benperidol. It can be used to treat and tranquillize psychotic patients, especially those with antisocial and deviant sexual behaviour, and is available as tablets.
✚▲ Side-effects/warnings: See BENPERIDOL.

Antabuse
(Alpharma) is a proprietary, prescription-only preparation of the ENZYME INHIBITOR disulfiram. It can be used to assist in the treatment of alcoholism, because, in combination with the consumption of even small quantities of alcohol, it causes unpleasant reactions: flushing, headache, palpitations, nausea and vomiting. It is available as tablets.
✚▲ Side-effects/warnings: See DISULFIRAM.

antacid

agents are used to neutralize the hydrochloric acid (gastric acid) that the stomach produces as part of the normal digestion of food. Overproduction of acid (hyperacidity) can cause the symptoms of dyspepsia (indigestion), which can be exacerbated by alcohol and NSAID drugs. Antacids give symptomatic relief of the dyspepsia and gastritis associated with peptic ulcers (gastric or duodenal ulcer), but do not allow actual healing of ulcers unless taken in sufficient quantities over long periods. A further painful condition is when there is regurgitation of acid and enzymes into the oesophagus ('oesophageal reflux'), which in the short term causes heartburn and in the long term can cause inflammation (reflux oesophagitis: common in hiatus hernia and pregnancy). Antacids taken alone effectively reduce acidity, but are commonly combined with other drugs (eg an ANTIFOAMING AGENT, DEMULCENT or ULCER-HEALING DRUG). Antacids themselves have side-effects; bicarbonates and carbonates tend to cause flatulence and belching; and some aluminium-containing antacids cause constipation, whereas magnesium-containing antacids can cause diarrhoea (so are often used in combination). Some preparations contain high concentrations of sodium, so should not be given to patients who are on a sodium-restricted diet.

▲ Warnings: Antacids should not be taken at the same time as some other drugs as they may impair absorption of the drug and therefore reduce the drug's efficacy. Affected drug classes include many ANTIBIOTIC and ANTIBACTERIAL agents (especially TETRACYCLINES), some ANTI-EPILEPTIC drugs (PHENYTOIN and GABAPENTIN), BISPHOSPHONATE drugs, CARDIAC GLYCOSIDE drugs, IRON preparations, ANGIOTENSIN-RECEPTOR BLOCKER and ACE INHIBITOR drugs.

See ALUMINIUM HYDROXIDE; CALCIUM CARBONATE; HYDROTALCITE; MAGNESIUM CARBONATE; MAGNESIUM HYDROXIDE; MAGNESIUM TRISILICATE; SODIUM BICARBONATE.

antagonist

– or more correctly receptor antagonist – is a term used to describe a group of drugs that have no pharmacological actions in their own right, but have profound actions because they actually block (physically occupy) RECEPTORS that normally allow natural mediators, or sometimes synthetic drugs, to have an effect. Many of the most widely used drugs in medicine are antagonists. Their most important property is that they can be used to prevent the actions of mediators within the body, including within the brain and can therefore be used to 'switch-off' systems that are not functioning correctly, for instance in a disease state caused by excessive amounts of neurotransmitters, local hormones (see LOCAL HORMONE) and hormones (see HORMONE). This very valuable property can be used in a range of applications from changing mood and psychological states of mind, through to preventing allergic responses. Some examples will illustrate this point.

BETA-BLOCKER (beta-adrenoceptor blocker) drugs are antagonists that prevent the action of ADRENALINE and NORADRENALINE by blocking the receptors called beta-adrenoceptors. They may be used as ANTIHYPERTENSIVE drugs, in ANTI-ARRHYTHMIC and ANTI-ANGINA treatment for the heart, as ANXIOLYTIC and ANTITHYROID agents, and in GLAUCOMA TREATMENT. The best-known and most-used beta-blockers include ACEBUTOLOL, OXPRENOLOL HYDROCHLORIDE, PROPRANOLOL HYDROCHLORIDE, and SOTALOL HYDROCHLORIDE, and as a class they are probably the single most-used drugs in medicine.

ANTIHISTAMINE (H_1-antagonist) drugs inhibit the effects in the body of the local hormone histamine by blocking receptors called H_1 receptors. Histamine is released as an allergic reaction to a substance, for example, pollen, insect bites and stings, contact with certain metal objects, or certain foods. Antihistamines can be given by mouth or applied topically to block many of the unpleasant or dangerous actions of histamine.

There is a second group of drugs that also inhibit histamine effects, but block a quite different class of receptor called the H_2 receptor, which is involved in (stomach) gastric acid secretion. This group is referred to as H_2-antagonists (see H_2-ANTAGONIST) and they are used in the treatment of ulcers (see ULCER-HEALING DRUG), for example, peptic ulcers. The H_2-antagonist drug RANITIDINE is probably the most prescribed individual drug in the world.

Other examples of antagonist drugs include ANTICHOLINERGIC, ANTI-ANDROGEN, ANTI-OESTROGEN and OPIOID ANTAGONIST agents.

antazoline

is an ANTIHISTAMINE which can be used for the

symptomatic relief of allergic symptoms such as allergic conjunctivitis in the eye. Administration is topical.
✚▲ Side-effects/warnings: See ANTIHISTAMINE.
✪ **Related entries: Otrivine-Antistin; Wasp-Eze Ointment.**

Antepsin
(Chugai) is a proprietary, prescription-only preparation of the CYTOPROTECTANT drug sucralfate. It can be used to treat gastric and duodenal ulcers, and is available as tablets and a suspension.
✚▲ Side-effects/warnings: See SUCRALFATE.

anthelminthic
see ANTHELMINTIC.

anthelmintic
(anthelminthic; antihelminthic) drugs are used to treat infestation by parasitic organisms of the helminth (worm) family. The threadworm, roundworm and tapeworm are the most common helminths responsible for infection in the UK. In warmer countries illnesses caused by helminths are a major problem, eg hookworm disease (caused by hookworms), bilharziasis (caused by schistosomes), and elephantiasis (caused by filaria). Most worms infest the intestines and diagnosis is often made by finding the worms in the faeces. Drugs can then be administered and the worms are killed or anaesthetized and then excreted. Complications arise if the worms migrate within the body, in which case the treatment becomes very unpleasant for the patient. In the case of threadworms, medication should be combined with hygienic measures (eg short fingernails) and the whole family should be treated.
Anthelmintics work by penetrating the cuticle of the worm or gaining access to its alimentary tract. Among the most useful and best-known anthelmintics are NICLOSAMIDE, PIPERAZINE, MEBENDAZOLE, and TIABENDAZOLE (thiabendazole).

Anthisan Bite and Sting Cream
(Aventis Pharma) is a proprietary, non-prescription preparation of the ANTIHISTAMINE mepyramine maleate. It can be used to relieve wasp and other insect stings and bites, and nettle rash, and is available as a cream.
✚▲ Side-effects/warnings: See MEPYRAMINE MALEATE.

Anthisan Plus Sting Relief Spray
(Aventis Pharma) is a proprietary, non-prescription compound preparation of the ANTIHISTAMINE mepyramine maleate and the LOCAL ANAESTHETIC benzocaine. It can be used to relieve wasp and other insect stings and bites, jellyfish stings and nettle stings. It is available as a spray.
✚▲ Side-effects/warnings: See BENZOCAINE; MEPYRAMINE MALEATE.

Anthrax Vaccine
(Public Health Laboratory Service) is a non-proprietary, prescription-only VACCINE preparation, which can be used to protect individuals exposed to anthrax-infected materials. It is available in a form for injection.
✚▲ Side-effects/warnings: See VACCINE.

anthrax vaccine
for IMMUNIZATION is required only by individuals who are exposed to anthrax-infected hides and carcasses, or who handle imported bone meal, fish meal and other feedstuffs. The VACCINE is a precipitate of antigen from *Bacillus anthracis*, which causes anthrax and can be administered by injection.
✚▲ Side-effects/warnings: See VACCINE.

anti-allergic
drugs relieve the symptoms of an allergic reaction that follows exposure to specific substances to which a patient is allergic. These substances may be endogenous (in the patient's body) or exogenous (present in the environment). Because allergic reactions generally cause the release of the natural LOCAL HORMONE histamine within the body, ANTIHISTAMINE drugs are often very effective for providing symptomatic relief.

For example, allergic skin reactions to foreign proteins, contact dermatitis and insect stings and bites, show characteristic symptoms – including pruritus (itching), urticaria (an itchy skin rash) and erythema (reddening of the skin) – and these often respond well to treatment with antihistamines (including local application in a cream). However, because allergic responses cause an inflammatory effect, many anti-allergic drugs also have ANTI-INFLAMMATORY properties.

For example, in the treatment of atopic (allergic) bronchial asthma, chronic (long-term) inhalation of a CORTICOSTEROID may prevent asthma attacks and the associated bronchoconstriction and congested airways. Similar anti-inflammatory protection from the symptoms of allergic asthma may be achieved by chronic inhalation of SODIUM CROMOGLICATE, which prevents the release of histamine and other substances (though exactly how it works is not clear). In the acute treatment of anaphylactic shock immediate treatment with three types of drugs is often required: an injection of a SYMPATHOMIMETIC, such as ADRENALINE, to dilate the bronchioles and stimulate the cardiovascular circulation; and administration of corticosteroids and antihistamines to counter other serious allergic reactions. In general, corticosteroids will suppress or mask inflammatory responses at most sites (including the skin), but these drugs have quite marked and serious side-effects and are only given systemically in serious conditions and are normally used topically only for short-term alleviation of symptoms.

anti-androgen

(androgen antagonist) agents are a class of drugs that are hormone antagonists (see HORMONE ANTAGONIST), which act directly to prevent the actions of the male sex hormone TESTOSTERONE at its target tissues. Examples of drugs acting directly include CYPROTERONE ACETATE, BICALUTAMIDE and FLUTAMIDE.

Also there is another group of drugs which have anti-androgen activity. They are hormone analogues which when given on a long-term basis, after an initial stimulation and sex hormone release phase, go on to give a therapeutically useful suppression of the formation, or inhibit the release, of various sex hormones including androgens. These are analogues of GONADORELIN, and here work as *indirect* hormone antagonists, which can be used as anti-androgens (BUSERELIN, GOSERELIN, LEUPRORELIN ACETATE, TRIPTORELIN). Anti-androgens are used therapeutically mainly as part of ANTICANCER treatment for conditions such as prostate and breast cancer, and also for endometriosis.

anti-angina

drugs are used to relieve the pain of angina pectoris, which is an intense pain originating from the heart and due to ischaemia (insufficient blood supply to the heart muscle) and is especially pronounced when the heart is working hard, as in *exercise angina*, or in unstable angina it can even occur when the person is resting. The disease state often results from atheroma, which is a disease state of the lining of the arteries of the heart where there is a build up of fatty deposits. The objective of drug treatment is to reduce the heart's workload and to prevent spasm or to dilate the arteries of the heart (the coronary arteries). Different drugs are used for the various different types of angina, and they are often given alongside specific treatment for the underlying atheromatous disease (eg with a LIPID-REGULATING DRUG such as the *statins*). Unloading can be achieved by stopping exercise, preventing the speeding of the heart and by dilating the coronary arteries.

BETA-BLOCKER drugs prevent the normal increase in heart rate seen in exercise by blocking the effect of ADRENALINE and NORADRENALINE on the heart, and are very effective in preventing anginal pain. Examples of beta-blockers include: ACEBUTOLOL, ATENOLOL, METOPROLOL TARTRATE, NADOLOL, OXPRENOLOL HYDROCHLORIDE, PINDOLOL, PROPRANOLOL HYDROCHLORIDE, SOTALOL HYDROCHLORIDE, TIMOLOL MALEATE.

VASODILATOR drugs (many of which are from the SMOOTH MUSCLE RELAXANT group) dilate blood vessels and thereby increase blood flow. For the acute treatment of anginal pain (and to a lesser extent in preventing angina attacks) the NITRATE drugs (eg GLYCERYL TRINITRATE, ISOSORBIDE DINITRATE, ISOSORBIDE MONONITRATE) are widely used.

CALCIUM-CHANNEL BLOCKER and POTASSIUM-CHANNEL ACTIVATOR drugs are a more recently introduced anti-angina treatment. In angina (especially unstable angina), there is a risk of myocardial infarction, so ASPIRIN, A HEPARIN, or one of the newer drugs (eg EPTIFIBATIDE OF TIROFIBAN) may be given to reduce this risk. The vasodilator drugs may act on the coronary arteries, peripheral small arteries and other blood vessels, which helps to reduce the workload on the heart. If drug treatment is not sufficient, then a coronary bypass operation may be needed. See also AMLODIPINE BESILATE; DILTIAZEM HYDROCHLORIDE; NICARDIPINE HYDROCHLORIDE; NIFEDIPINE; VERAPAMIL HYDROCHLORIDE.

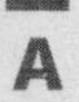

anti-anxiety
see ANXIOLYTIC.

anti-arrhythmic
(antidysrhythmic) drugs strengthen and regularize a heartbeat that has become unsteady and is not showing its usual pattern of activity. But because there are many ways in which the heartbeat can falter – atrial tachycardia, supraventricular arrhythmias, ventricular arrhythmias, ventricular tachycardia, atrial flutter or fibrillation, and the severe heartbeat irregularity that may follow a heart attack (myocardial infarction) – there is a variety of drugs available, each for a fairly specific use. The treatment of arrhythmias requires careful diagnosis as to the type of arrhythmia, including an electrocardiogram (ECG). The anti-arrhythmics that are used include CARDIAC GLYCOSIDE drugs (eg DIGOXIN and DIGITOXIN), CALCIUM-CHANNEL BLOCKER drugs (VERAPAMIL HYDROCHLORIDE), LOCAL ANAESTHETIC-related drugs (LIDOCAINE HYDROCHLORIDE, PROCAINAMIDE HYDROCHLORIDE); certain BETA-BLOCKER drugs (including ACEBUTOLOL, ATENOLOL, ESMOLOL HYDROCHLORIDE, METOPROLOL TARTRATE, NADOLOL, OXPRENOLOL HYDROCHLORIDE, SOTALOL HYDROCHLORIDE, TIMOLOL MALEATE); and a number of other drugs (including ADENOSINE, AMIODARONE HYDROCHLORIDE, BRETYLIUM TOSILATE, DISOPYRAMIDE, FLECAINIDE ACETATE, MEXILETINE HYDROCHLORIDE, MORACIZINE HYDROCHLORIDE, PHENYTOIN, PROPAFENONE HYDROCHLORIDE, QUINIDINE).

anti-asthmatic
drugs relieve the symptoms of bronchial asthma or prevent recurrent attacks. The symptoms of asthma include bronchoconstriction (a narrowing of the bronchioles of the airways, with consequent difficulty in exhaling), often with over-secretion of fluid by glands within the bronchioles, with coughing, wheezing and breathing difficulties (dyspnoea). Two main types of drugs are used: one group treat acute attacks; and the second prevent attacks (as prophylaxis). Bronchodilators (see BRONCHODILATOR), which are SMOOTH MUSCLE RELAXANT drugs, work by dilating and relaxing the bronchioles. The most commonly used are the BETA-RECEPTOR STIMULANT drugs (which are SYMPATHOMIMETIC), notably SALBUTAMOL and TERBUTALINE SULPHATE. The beta-receptor stimulants, normally inhaled, are mostly used for treating acute attacks (or immediately before exertion in exercise asthma) and are largely of a type that does not normally adversely stimulate the heart. Other bronchodilator drugs that work directly on the bronchioles include smooth muscle relaxants such as THEOPHYLLINE.

The second group of anti-asthmatic drugs do not directly cause bronchodilation, but because of their ANTI-INFLAMMATORY action they prevent the release of local inflammatory mediators, which contribute to attacks; so preventing asthma attacks and providing symptomatic relief. Examples of this group of anti-inflammatory drugs include the CORTICOSTEROID drugs, SODIUM CROMOGLICATE and LEUKOTRIENE-RECEPTOR ANTAGONIST drugs such as MONTELUKAST. These drugs are almost always taken over a period of time, both to prevent attacks and to reverse pathological changes, and preferably are inhaled so as to deliver the drug to where it is required and which helps limit side-effects. Indeed, a great deal of research has been done to design devices that are able to more efficiently deliver the inhaled droplets, or particles, of bronchodilator or anti-inflammatory drugs into the airways, particularly in an attempt to reach the narrower bronchioles.

There are some other drugs, such as KETOTIFEN and IPRATROPIUM BROMIDE, that are occasionally used to treat asthma (for instance, when the other types of drug are ineffective for some reason). ANTIHISTAMINE drugs, however, are now thought to be of no value, but are useful as ANTI-ALLERGIC treatments for hay fever or rashes. It is now generally agreed that anti-inflammatory drugs (eg corticosteroids) should be used early on in asthma treatment, rather than relying on the use of bronchodilators alone – which only treat the symptoms of the disease.

antibacterial
drugs are used to treat infections caused by bacteria, on which they have a selective toxic action. They can be used both topically (eg, on the skin or the eye) to treat infections of superficial tissues or systemically (carried by the blood after being swallowed or injected to the site of the infection). Many are ANTIBIOTIC drugs.

A distinction can be made between

bacteriostatic drugs, which act primarily by arresting bacterial growth (eg SULPHONAMIDE drugs, TETRACYCLINES, CHLORAMPHENICOL) and the *bactericidal* agents, which act primarily by killing bacteria (eg the AMINOGLYCOSIDE, CEPHALOSPORIN and PENICILLIN families and ISONIAZID and RIFAMPICIN). As bacteria are the largest and most diverse group of pathogenic (disease-causing) micro-organisms, antibacterials form the major constituent group of the ANTIMICROBIAL class.

antibiotic

agents are, strictly speaking, natural products secreted by micro-organisms into their environment where they inhibit the growth of competing micro-organisms of different types. But in common usage the term is often applied to any drug, natural or synthetic, that has a selectively toxic action on bacteria or similar non-nucleated, single-celled micro-organisms (including chlamydia, Rickettsia and mycoplasma) – but they are not effective against viruses.

However, the more accurate term for these drugs is ANTIMICROBIAL. Most modern antibiotics are, in fact, either completely or partly synthetic and not produced by natural organisms, but nevertheless they are generally modelled on natural substances.

When administered by an appropriate route, such as topically (eg to the skin or eyes) orally, by injection or by infusion, antibiotics kill micro-organisms such as bacteria – *bactericidal action* – or inhibit their growth – *bacteriostatic action*. The selectively toxic action on invading micro-organisms exploits differences between bacteria and their human host cells. Major target sites are the bacterial cell wall located outside the cell membrane (animal cells have only a cell membrane) or the bacterial ribosome (the protein-synthesizing organelle within its cell), which in micro-organisms is different from human cells. Antibiotic families such as the PENICILLIN and CEPHALOSPORIN classes (collectively known as the BETA-LACTAM group) attack the bacterial cell wall, whereas the AMINOGLYCOSIDE and tetracycline (see TETRACYCLINES) classes attack the ribosomes.

Viruses, which lack both cell walls and ribosomes, are therefore resistant to these and other types of antibiotic. Because there is such a diversity of pathogenic (disease-causing) micro-organisms, it is not surprising that specific infections are best treated using specific antibiotics developed to combat them.

Unfortunately, because of the widespread use of antibiotics, certain strains of common bacteria have developed resistance to antibiotics that were once effective against them and this has become a major problem. A mechanism by which bacteria become resistant is by the development of enzymes called *penicillinases*, which break down penicillins and so limit an antibiotic's action. It has proved possible both to use drugs that inhibit these enzymes and, more directly, to develop *penicillinase-resistant* antibiotics.

Another problem is the occurrence of *superinfections*, in which the use of a broad-spectrum antibiotic disturbs the normal, harmless bacterial population in the body, as well as the pathogenic ones. In mild cases this may allow, for example, an existing but latent oral or vaginal thrush infection to become worse, or mild diarrhoea to develop. In rare cases the superinfection that develops is more serious than the disorder for which the antibiotic was administered.

anticancer

drugs are used to treat cancer and most of them are CYTOTOXIC, that is, they work by interfering with cell replication or production, so preventing the growth of new cancerous tissue. Inevitably, this means that normal cell production is also affected, which causes serious side-effects. They are usually administered in combination in a group of treatments known collectively as *chemotherapy*, sometimes in combination with *radiotherapy* and/or surgery.

However, cytotoxic drugs are not always necessary in some types of cancer, for example where the growth of a tumour is dependent on sex hormone levels (as with some cases of breast cancer or cancer of the prostate gland), and here treatment with sex hormones opposite to the patient's own sex, or HORMONE ANTAGONIST drugs (eg TAMOXIFEN at oestrogen receptors), can be extremely beneficial (though the side-effects of some may be marked). Other drugs used directly or indirectly as adjuncts in cancer treatment include CORTICOSTEROID (eg PREDNISOLONE) and other IMMUNOSUPPRESSANT drugs, monoclonal antibodies (eg BASILIXIMAB), INTERFERON drugs (eg INTERFERON BETA), along with ANTI-EMETIC and ANALGESIC agents.

A

anticholinergic

drugs inhibit the action, release or production of the neurotransmitter ACETYLCHOLINE, which plays an important role in the nervous system. The term is commonly loosely used synonymously with the more precise term ANTIMUSCARINIC (drugs that block the actions of acetylcholine at *muscarinic* receptors). Anticholinergic drugs (of the antimuscarinic type) tend to relax smooth (involuntary) muscle, reduce the secretion of saliva, digestive juices and sweat, and dilate the pupil of the eye (mydriasis). They can therefore be used as ANTISPASMODIC drugs in the treatment of intestinal colic, for parkinsonian symptoms, for peptic ulcer, and to dilate the pupil for ophthalmic examinations. Other uses include reversal of the adverse effects of overdose with anticholinesterases (in medicine, agricultural accidental poisoning or warfare). However, the administration of such drugs is usually accompanied by side-effects, including dry mouth, dry skin, blurred vision, increased heart rate, constipation, and difficulty in urinating. A number of other types of drug, for instance ANTIHISTAMINE drugs, can also cause *anticholinergic side-effects.*

Examples of drugs used in medicine for their antimuscarinic anticholinergic actions include ATROPINE SULPHATE, BENZHEXOL HYDROCHLORIDE, BENZTROPINE MESILATE, BIPERIDEN, CO-PHENOTROPE, CYCLOPENTOLATE HYDROCHLORIDE, FLAVOXATE HYDROCHLORIDE, GLYCOPYRRONIUM BROMIDE, HYOSCINE BUTYLBROMIDE, HYOSCINE HYDROBROMIDE, IPRATROPIUM BROMIDE, MEBEVERINE HYDROCHLORIDE, ORPHENADRINE HYDROCHLORIDE, PROCYCLIDINE HYDROCHLORIDE, PROPANTHELINE BROMIDE and TROPICAMIDE.

The other main groups of anticholinergic drugs work at sites where acetylcholine interacts with *nicotinic* receptors (such as in the autonomic ganglia, skeletal neuromuscular junction, and central nervous system) and have quite different actions. See GANGLION-BLOCKER; SKELETAL MUSCLE RELAXANT.

anticholinesterase

drugs are ENZYME INHIBITOR agents. They inhibit certain enzymes (called cholinesterases) that are normally involved in the rapid break down of the natural neurotransmitter acetylcholine. Acetylcholine is released from cholinergic nerves and has many actions in the body. Consequently, since anticholinesterase drugs enhance the effects of acetylcholine on its release from these nerves, they may have a very wide range of actions and can be used for a variety of purposes.

In respect of their actions at the junction of nerves with skeletal (voluntary) muscles, anticholinesterases are used in the diagnosis and treatment of the muscle-weakness disease *myesthenia gravis.*

At the end of surgical operations in which certain SKELETAL MUSCLE RELAXANT drugs have been used, the anaesthetist is able to reverse the muscle paralysis by injecting an anticholinesterase.

In organs innervated by parasympathetic division of the autonomic nervous system, anticholinesterases cause an exaggeration of the nerves' actions – referred to as PARASYMPATHOMIMETIC actions – and they can be used for a number of purposes. These include stimulation of the bladder (in urinary retention). Recently, anticholinesterases have been introduced for the treatment of impaired mental cognition (see NOOTROPIC AGENT). However, anticholinesterases have a number of generally undesirable side-effects, such as slowing of the heart, constriction of the airways with excessive production of secretions, and actions in the brain.

In anticholinesterase poisoning, their diverse actions can be life-threatening. Chemicals with anticholinesterase properties are used as insecticides (and in chemical warfare), so an ANTIDOTE is required (eg PRALIDOXIME MESILATE and ATROPINE SULPHATE). See DISTIGMINE BROMIDE; DONEPEZIL; NEOSTIGMINE; PYRIDOSTIGMINE; RIVASTIGMINE.

anticoagulant

agents prevent the clotting of blood and help break up blood clots that have formed. The blood's own natural anticoagulant is HEPARIN, which is probably still the most effective anticoagulant known, but must be injected so is termed a *parenteral* anticoagulant. There are semisynthetic versions of heparin, called *low molecular weight heparins* (CERTOPARIN, DALTEPARIN SODIUM, ENOXAPARIN, TINZAPARIN SODIUM), that work for longer but still must be injected. Some other versions of heparin are called HEPARINOIDS, of which some are injected as anticoagulants (eg DANAPAROID SODIUM), whereas others are incorporated into topical ointments (and are thought to improve circulation in the skin, having here an anti-inflammatory or soothing action by an unclear mechanism).

Another natural parenteral anticoagulant is *hirudin* from the salivary glands of the medicinal leech, that works by inhibiting thrombin (which is necessary for the formation of blood clots). It is now replaced by a synthetic (recombinant) version and LEPIRUDIN.

Synthetic oral anticoagulants, such as WARFARIN SODIUM, ACENOCOUMAROL (nicoumalone) and PHENINDIONE, are available and some are widely used, but they take longer to act. They work by antagonizing the action of VITAMIN K.

Therapeutically, anticoagulants are used to prevent the formation of and to treat blood clots in conditions such as thrombosis and embolism, especially following surgery (eg to prevent deep-vein thrombosis). They are also used to prevent blood clots in patients fitted with a heart pacemaker or who have certain heart disorders.
▲ Warnings: Many drugs can influence the effect of anticoagulants and increase or reduce their therapeutic effects. Further, certain vitamins found in foodstuffs and in nutritional supplements can influence the effect of anticoagulants, so dietary advice will be given. Vitamin K can reduce the effect of anticoagulants (including ACENOCOUMAROL, PHENINDIONE and WARFARIN SODIUM) and in large doses VITAMIN E may potentiate the anticoagulant effects of, for example, warfarin sodium. Also, many other nutritional supplements and herbal remedies, including St John's wort, bromelain, chondroitin, garlic, ginkgo biloba, feverfew, fish oils, willow and ginseng, may interfere with the effectiveness of some anticoagulants.

anticonvulsant

is a term often used synonymously with ANTI-EPILEPTIC to describe drugs that are used to prevent the onset of epileptic seizures or to reduce their severity if they do occur, and to treat non-epileptic convulsive disorders. The best-known and most-used anticonvulsant is SODIUM VALPROATE, which is used to treat most forms of epilepsy, especially absence seizures. Other examples include CARBAMAZEPINE and PHENYTOIN, which are used to treat grand mal forms of epilepsy, and ETHOSUXIMIDE, which is used to treat absence seizures ('petit mal'). In every case, dosage must be adjusted to the requirements of each individual patient. Anticonvulsant drugs may also be used to treat other types of convulsions, for instance, in drug or chemical poisoning. However, some of these drugs, such as DIAZEPAM, are not effective or so suitable for treating epilepsy.
▲ Warnings: Folic acid, which is present in some nutritional supplements, and the herbal remedy St John's wort can reduce blood levels of some anticonvulsants, including PHENOBARBITAL, PHENYTOIN and others, so it should not be taken at the same time.

antidepressant

drugs are used to relieve the symptoms of depressive illness and are divided into three main groups. The first and oldest, group is the TRICYCLIC antidepressants (named after the chemical structure of the original members), such as AMITRIPTYLINE HYDROCHLORIDE, IMIPRAMINE HYDROCHLORIDE and DOXEPIN. They are effective in alleviating a number of depressive symptoms, but have ANTICHOLINERGIC side-effects. Most drugs of this class also have SEDATIVE properties, which in some is quite pronounced (especially amitriptyline hydrochloride, which may be beneficial in some anxious and agitated patients).

The second group consists of the MONOAMINE-OXIDASE INHIBITOR drugs (MAOIs), eg ISOCARBOXAZID, PHENELZINE and TRANYLCYPROMINE, which are now used less frequently because they have severe side-effects, particularly through interaction with constituents of foodstuffs.

The third type of antidepressant, and the most recently developed, is the SSRIS, for example FLUOXETINE, which are named after their mechanisms of action (*Selective Serotonin Re-uptake Inhibitors*). A number of newer antidepressants represent variations on this approach (see SSRI entry).

Also used is the amino acid TRYPTOPHAN, which may be used when other classes of antidepressant have not been effective, and LITHIUM, which is used to treat manic-depression and related illnesses and also for preventing certain types of recurrent depression. The ANTIPSYCHOTIC drug FLUPENTIXOL is

A

occasionally used (at a much lower dose) as a short-term antidepressant.

Treatment with antidepressants often takes some weeks to show maximal beneficial effects. (See individual class entries for more detail.)

▲ Warnings: Other types of antidepressants, including herbal or other remedies for depression, and in particular the herbal remedy St John's wort, and other non-prescription antidepressants medications should not be taken at the same time as any other medications for depression because serious adverse reactions can result.

antidiarrhoeal

drugs prevent the onset of diarrhoea, or assist in treating it if already present. The main medical treatment while diarrhoea lasts, however, is always the replacement of fluids and minerals (particularly sodium). However, because there is a perceived need on the part of the general public, antidiarrhoeal preparations are generally available without prescription. Many are adsorbent mixtures that bind faecal material into solid masses.

These mixtures include preparations containing KAOLIN or sometimes ACTIVATED CHARCOAL and METHYLCELLULOSE, which may also be useful in controlling faecal consistency for patients who have undergone colostomy or ileostomy. The main antidiarrhoeals are antimotility drugs, and work by reducing peristalsis (the movement of the intestine), which slows down the movement of faecal material. The OPIOID, such as CODEINE PHOSPHATE, MORPHINE SULPHATE, LOPERAMIDE HYDROCHLORIDE and DIPHENOXYLATE HYDROCHLORIDE, are very efficient at this. A first priority is to replace salts and water lost in diarrhoea and there are a number of preparations available containing sodium and potassium chloride to be taken orally (or sodium chloride and glucose, which works well because glucose enhances sodium absorption from the small intestine, and thus water as well).

Diarrhoea caused by inflammatory disorders, such as irritable bowel syndrome, ulcerative colitis and Crohn's disease may be relieved by treatment with CORTICOSTEROID or AMINOSALICYLATE drugs. When diarrhoea is caused by a bacterial infection (eg *Campylobacter*) and is severe, this is treated with an ANTIBIOTIC (eg ERYTHROMYCIN or CIPROFLOXACIN).

antidiuretic hormone

see VASOPRESSIN.

antidote

agents are used to counteract poisons or overdose with other drugs. They are used in a wide variety of circumstances and can work in many ways. First, the most straightforward and commonly used method is where the poison works by stimulating, or over-stimulating, a distinct pharmacological receptor, since here the appropriate receptor ANTAGONIST can be used to reduce or completely block the effects of the poison. For example, NALOXONE HYDROCHLORIDE is an OPIOID ANTAGONIST and can be used as an antidote to an overdose of an (OPIOID) NARCOTIC ANALGESIC (including DIAMORPHINE HYDROCHLORIDE; heroin) and being quick-acting it effectively reverses the respiratory depression, coma or convulsions that result from such an overdose. It can also be used at the end of operations to reverse respiratory depression caused by narcotic analgesics and in newborn babies where mothers have been given large amounts of opioid (such as PETHIDINE HYDROCHLORIDE) for pain-relief during labour.

Second, poisoning by some agents is best counteracted by using an antidote that binds to the poison, rendering it relatively inert and facilitating its excretion from the body. For example, a CHELATING AGENT is used as an antidote to metal poisoning because it chemically binds to certain metallic ions and other substances, making them less toxic and allowing their excretion from the body. Chelating agents are used to treat too high levels of metals of external origin (accidental or environmental), in METABOLIC DISORDER TREATMENT (eg high levels of copper in Wilson's disease) or other disease states (eg penicillamine in rheumatoid arthritis). Examples of chelating agents include DEFERIPRONE, DESFERRIOXAMINE MESILATE, DICOBALT EDETATE, DIMERCAPROL, PENICILLAMINE and SODIUM CALCIUM EDETATE.

An ANTIVENOM is an antidote to the poison in a snakebite, a scorpion's sting or a bite from any other poisonous creature (such as a spider). Normally, it is an ANTISERUM and is injected into the bloodstream for immediate relief (though it has its own adverse side-effects).

DIGIBIND is a proprietary drug that comprises antibody fragments that react with the glycosides and is used in the emergency treatment of an overdose of CARDIAC GLYCOSIDE drugs, eg DIGOXIN and DIGITOXIN.

ACETYLCYSTEINE and METHIONINE are used as antidotes to treat overdose poisoning by the ANALGESIC paracetamol. The initial symptoms of paracetamol poisoning usually settle within 24 hours, but give way to serious toxic effect on the liver which takes some days to develop. It is to prevent these latter effects that treatment is directed and is required immediately after overdose. The antidotes work by chemically reacting with toxic products made by the liver from paracetamol when it is taken in excessive amounts.

A different principle is used with ANTICHOLINESTERASE poisoning. These ENZYME INHIBITOR drugs are used in medicine, as insecticides and in chemical warfare. PRALIDOXIME MESILATE is an antidote that actually reactivates the cholinesterase enzyme after it has been poisoned and is highly effective (taken in conjunction with other drugs) in preventing the life-endangering chemical changes to certain anticholinesterases.

In all cases of poisoning, prompt action in using an antidote is necessary.

anti-D (Rh0) immunoglobulin

(anti-D immunoglobulin) for IMMUNIZATION is a SPECIFIC IMMUNOGLOBULIN which is used to prevent rhesus-negative mothers from making antibodies against fetal rhesus-positive cells that may pass into the mother's circulation during childbirth, miscarriage or abortion, or certain procedures such as amniocentesis (and sometimes for prophylaxis). The result of this is to protect a future child from haemolytic disease of the newborn. Anti-D (Rh0) immunoglobulin should be injected within a few days of birth, miscarriage or abortion.

✚▲ Side-effects/warnings: See IMMUNIZATION.

✪ Related entries: Anti-D (Rh0) Immunoglobulin[1]; Anti-D (Rh0) Immunoglobulin[2]; WinRho SDF.

Anti-D (Rh0) Immunoglobulin[1]

(Baxter Bioscience) is a proprietary, prescription-only preparation of anti-D Rh0 immunoglobulin. It can be used to prevent rhesus-negative mothers from making antibodies against fetal rhesus-positive cells that may pass into the mother's circulation during childbirth, so protecting a future child from haemolytic disease of the newborn. It can be injected both before and soon after birth. It is available in a form for injection.

✚▲ Side-effects/warnings: See ANTI-D (RHO) IMMUNOGLOBULIN.

Anti-D (Rh0) Immunoglobulin[2]

(RBTC; BPL; SNBTS) is a non-proprietary, prescription-only preparation of anti-D Rh0 immunoglobulin. It can be used to prevent rhesus-negative mothers from making antibodies against fetal rhesus-positive cells that may pass into the mother's circulation during childbirth, so protecting a future child from haemolytic disease of the newborn. It can be injected both before and soon after birth, miscarriage or abortion. It is available in a form for injection.

✚▲ Side-effects/warnings: See ANTI-D (RHO) IMMUNOGLOBULIN.

antidysrhythmic drug

see ANTI-ARRHYTHMIC.

anti-emetic 🅱

drugs prevent vomiting (emesis), whereas ANTINAUSEANT drugs are used to reduce or prevent the *sensation* of nausea that very often precedes the physical process of vomiting. In practice, there is considerable overlap between the two drug types, and the terms are often used interchangeably. Anti-emetics are used to help reduce the vomiting that accompanies radiotherapy and chemotherapy, and may help by actually preventing vomiting and aiding the passage of food out of the stomach; that is, they act as gastric MOTILITY STIMULANT drugs (eg METOCLOPRAMIDE HYDROCHLORIDE), and they also act at the 'chemoreceptor trigger-zone' in the brain. See ANTINAUSEANT.

anti-epileptic 🅱

drugs are used to prevent the occurrence of epileptic seizures. Some of these drugs work against other types of convulsion (non-epileptic convulsive disorders), so in the more general sense are termed ANTICONVULSANT. In order to prevent the occurrence of epileptic seizures on a chronic basis (often for many years), an effective concentration of the drug must be maintained in the blood plasma and so the dose varies according to each patient's requirements. Often, therapy starts with a low dose of drug, and this is gradually increased until seizures are controlled, and side-effects are acceptable. Generally, only one drug is required at any one time and the drug of choice depends on the type and severity of the epilepsy. CARBAMAZEPINE, PHENYTOIN and SODIUM VALPROATE are the drugs of choice for *tonic-clonic seizures* (grand mal) as part of a syndrome of primary generalized epilepsy; ETHOSUXIMIDE and sodium valproate are used for *absence seizures* (petit mal); and CLONAZEPAM, ethosuximide and sodium valproate for *myoclonic seizures.*

For other types of seizure, such as atypical absence, atonic and tonic seizures (often in childhood), phenytoin, sodium valproate, clonazepam, PHENOBARBITAL (phenobarbitone) or ethosuximide are often used. Other drugs sometimes used include ACETAZOLAMIDE, PIRACETAM, GABAPENTIN, TOPIRAMATE and TIAGABINE. These drugs as a whole have quite appreciable side-effects, and some are not recommended for use in women of childbearing age.

antifoaming agent 🅱

is a term used to describe a chemical that is incorporated into ANTACID preparations in order to lower surface tension so that small bubbles of froth coalesce into large bubbles, which allows the remedy to pass more easily through the intestine. They are commonly used to treat flatulence and a feeling of fullness and bloating. The most effective are silicone polymers such as DIMETICONE.

antifungal 🅱

agents are ANTIMICROBIAL drugs that are used to treat infections caused by fungal micro-organisms, and are often ANTIBIOTIC agents that are produced naturally or synthetically. Fungal infections are usually not a major problem in healthy, well-nourished individuals. However, superficial, localized infections such as thrush (caused by *Candida albicans*), athlete's foot and ringworm (caused by fungi of the dermatophyte group) are common. Severe infections occur most frequently in situations where the host's immunity is low, for example following immunosuppression for transplant surgery, or in AIDS.

Under such conditions fungi that are not normally pathogenic (disease-causing) can exploit their host's altered state and cause infection. Unfortunately, the most potent antifungal drugs also tend to be highly toxic and therefore severe systemic fungal infections remain an ever-present danger. NYSTATIN and AZOLE (imidazoles), such as CLOTRIMAZOLE, are often used for local treatment. AMPHOTERICIN and FLUCYTOSINE are reserved for systemic fungal infections. The commonest form of fungal infection in childhood is thrush, which usually occurs in the mouth and nappy area of infants and is usually treated with the topical application of MICONAZOLE.

antihelminthic

see ANTHELMINTIC.

antihistamine 🅱

drugs are of the H_1-antagonist type which inhibit the effects of histamine in the body. Histamine is released naturally as the result of a patient coming into contact with a substance to which he or she is allergic to, and causes various symptoms such as hay fever, urticaria, itching (pruritus) or even asthma-like bronchoconstriction.

Many agents can act as triggers for histamine release, including inhalation of pollen, insect bites and stings, contact with some metal objects, food constituents, food dye additives, a number of drug types (notably PENICILLIN-type ANTIBIOTIC drugs, LOCAL ANAESTHETIC drugs, MORPHINE SULPHATE and, potentially, all drugs of a protein or peptide nature) and many environmental factors. Consequently, antihistamines may be used for many purposes, but particularly for the symptomatic relief of allergy such as hay fever and urticaria, and in the acute treatment of anaphylactic shock.

Many antihistamines also have ANTI-EMETIC properties and are therefore used to prevent vomiting associated with travel sickness, vertigo or the effects of chemotherapy. All but some recently developed antihistamines produce drowsiness and this SEDATIVE action may be used to help induce sleep.

Conventionally, only the long established antihistamine drugs, which act on histamine H_1-receptors, are referred to by the general name *antihistamines* without qualification. However, somewhat confusingly, the newer and extensively prescribed drugs that can be used as ulcer-healing drugs (see ULCER-HEALING DRUG: eg CIMETIDINE and RANITIDINE) are also antihistamines, but they act on H_2-receptors that are involved in gastric secretion and so are referred to as H_2-ANTAGONIST drugs.

See ACRIVASTINE; ANTAZOLINE; AZATADINE MALEATE; AZELASTINE HYDROCHLORIDE; BROMPHENIRAMINE MALEATE; BUCLIZINE HYDROCHLORIDE; CETIRIZINE HYDROCHLORIDE; CHLORPHENAMINE MALEATE; CINNARIZINE; CLEMASTINE; CYCLIZINE; CYPROHEPTADINE HYDROCHLORIDE; DESLORATADINE; DIPHENHYDRAMINE HYDROCHLORIDE; DOXYLAMINE; FEXOFENADINE HYDROCHLORIDE; HYDROXYZINE HYDROCHLORIDE; KETOTIFEN; LEVOCABASTINE; LORATADINE; MECLOZINE HYDROCHLORIDE; MIZOLASTINE; PHENIRAMINE MALEATE; PIZOTIFEN; PROMETHAZINE HYDROCHLORIDE; PROMETHAZINE TEOCLATE; TRIMEPRAZINE TARTRATE; TRIPROLIDINE HYDROCHLORIDE.

✚ Side-effects: What is considered an unwanted effect depends on what the antihistamine is being used for (for example, when used as a sedative, sedation is the wanted effect). Following oral or systemic administration, there is commonly drowsiness, headache, impaired muscular coordination or dizziness, anticholinergic effects (dry mouth, blurred vision, urinary retention, gastrointestinal disturbances), occasional rashes and photosensitivity, palpitations and heart arrhythmias. Rarely, there may be paradoxical stimulation, especially in children (and convulsions in overdose), hypersensitivity reactions, blood disorders, liver disturbances, depression, sleep disturbances and hypotension.

▲ Warnings: Administer with caution to patients with epilepsy, hypertrophy of the prostate gland, urinary retention, glaucoma, liver disease or porphyria; or who are pregnant or breast-feeding. Those antihistamines with sedative actions may impair the performance of skilled tasks such as driving; and the sedative effect is enhanced by alcohol. See additional warnings under individual entries.

Some drugs, including ALCOHOL, ANTICHOLINERGIC, SEDATIVE and ANTIDEPRESSANT drugs, can increase the effects or side-effects, such as sedation, of antihistamines.

antihypertensive

drugs reduce hypertension (an elevation of arterial blood pressure above the normal range expected in a particular age group and sex) and so reduce a patient's risk of heart attacks, kidney failure or stroke. There are several large groups of drugs used as antihypertensives, each with a specific mode of action, but before any drugs are administered a check should be made on the patient's diet and lifestyle to see if therapy without drugs can be advised. DIURETIC drugs act as antihypertensives and often a mild diuretic may be all that is required.

If further treatment is necessary, any of the BETA-BLOCKER drugs may be used, with or without simultaneous administration of a diuretic. Other treatments include the use of a VASODILATOR, such as a CALCIUM-CHANNEL BLOCKER (eg NIFEDIPINE) or HYDRALAZINE HYDROCHLORIDE. Some antihypertensive drugs act on the brain centre responsible for controlling blood pressure (eg METHYLDOPA) and ADRENERGIC-NEURONE BLOCKER agents (eg DEBRISOQUINE) reduce the release of noradrenaline from sympathetic nerves, which are involved in controlling blood pressure. Other treatments include the ACE INHIBITOR, ANGIOTENSIN-RECEPTOR BLOCKER and POTASSIUM-CHANNEL ACTIVATOR drug groups. Individuals having antihypertensive treatment require regular medical checks and blood-pressure monitoring, and may have to take several antihypertensive drugs at one time to adequately control blood pressure. Also, a LIPID-REGULATING DRUG may be used to control deposition of lipids in the blood vessels (which makes a considerable adverse contribution to cardiovascular diseases).

▲ Warnings: Herbal remedies (including hawthorn and chaste tree) and some nutritional supplements can potentially interfere with antihypertensive medications.

anti-inflammatory

drugs are used to reduce inflammation – the body's response to injury. Although inflammation is essentially a normal defensive mechanism (eg a reaction to tissue injury, infection or inhalation of foreign proteins), the manifestations may be so serious and inappropriate, or involve such discomfort, that treatment with anti-inflammatory drugs is required. Inflammatory conditions can be acute (eg insect strings) or chronic (eg chronic asthma, dermatitis, and other skin conditions).

The NSAID (non-steroidal anti-inflammatory) drugs, such as ASPIRIN and IBUPROFEN, can give effective relief from inflammatory pain, tissue swelling, joint immobilization and can also lower raised body temperature, which means that they are often the first choice of treatment. They work by inhibiting the production and release in the body of pro-inflammatory LOCAL HORMONE mediators (the PROSTAGLANDIN family) and, used with care, can be relatively free of side-effects. For more serious conditions CORTICOSTEROID drugs may be required, but they can cause so many complications that they are normally only given by local application (eg as creams, or by inhalation into the lungs for asthma) with systemic injection reserved for emergencies, such as *anaphylactic shock*.

There are a number of other types of anti-inflammatory drugs, including SODIUM CROMOGLICATE, the ANTIRHEUMATIC drugs (which are used to relieve the pain and inflammation of rheumatoid arthritis and osteoarthritis), gold (in the form of SODIUM AUROTHIOMALATE), and PENICILLAMINE.

The IMMUNOSUPPRESSANT drugs (eg CYCLOPHOSPHAMIDE, CICLOSPORIN and METHOTREXATE) are reserved for the prevention of tissue rejection (eg in transplants) and are sometimes used to treat autoimmune diseases, such as rheumatoid arthritis and lupus, when they are unresponsive to less toxic drugs.

Other classes of drugs used to treat particular manifestations of inflammation include ANTIHISTAMINE drugs and drugs used to treat gout.

antimalarial

drugs are used to treat or prevent malaria. Malaria is caused by infection of the red blood cells by a small organism called a protozoan (of the genus *Plasmodium*), which is carried by several species of mosquito of the genus *Anopheles*. Infection occurs as a result of a mosquito's bite. The synthetic chemical class of drug most commonly used to treat or prevent infection is the *quinolines*; both *4-aminoquinolines*, of which CHLOROQUINE is the standard (see also MEFLOQUINE), and *8-aminoquinolines*, see PRIMAQUINE. However, in some parts of the world certain forms of the protozoan that causes malaria are resistant to chloroquine. In such cases, QUININE, the traditional remedy for malaria, is used (for treatment, but not for prophylaxis).

In general, drugs used for preventing malarial attacks include chloroquine, mefloquine, PROGUANIL HYDROCHLORIDE, PYRIMETHAMINE, DAPSONE and sometimes DOXYCYCLINE. Also ATOVAQUONE combined with PROGUANIL HYDROCHLORIDE can be used for prophylactic antimalarial treatment. For the treatment of acute attacks quinine, mefloquine, chloroquine and pyrimethamine are used (sometimes in combination with an ANTIBIOTIC.

Although the prevention of malaria by drugs cannot be guaranteed, administration of antimalarial drugs before, during and for a period after a trip to a tropical place is recommended for protection. See also PYRIMETHAMINE.

antimania

drugs are used to treat manic-depressive illness, which is characterized by periods of mood normality punctuated by episodes of *mania* and bouts of *depression*. Because of these mood swings around the norm, the disorder is sometimes called *bipolar disorder*. The manic phase may require acute treatment and here initially ANTIPSYCHOTIC (eg PHENOTHIAZINE) drugs are often administered. Thereafter LITHIUM, a very different psychoactive drug which acts as a mood stabilizer, may gradually be substituted in most patients and this can prevent or reduce the frequency and severity of both the manic and the depressive phases of the illness. Recently, valproic acid (as the semisodium salt) has been introduced for the treatment of manic episodes in manic-depressive illness.

antimicrobial

drugs are used to treat infections caused by microbes (micro-organisms), which includes the major classes of pathogenic (disease-causing) micro-organisms covered in this book – viruses, mycoplasma, mycobacteria, rickettsia, chlamydia, protozoa, bacteria and fungi (but not helminths; worms). The term therefore embraces ANTIBACTERIAL, ANTIBIOTIC, ANTIFUNGAL, ANTIMALARIAL, ANTIPROTOZOAL and ANTIVIRAL drugs.

antimigraine

drugs are used to treat migraine, which is a

specific, clinically recognized form of headache (which affects 10–15% of people) and not simply a particularly severe headache. Migraine attacks vary in form, but common characteristics include a throbbing pain confined to one side of the head (*unilateral headache*), nausea and vomiting, photophobia and a forewarning of an attack (an *aura*) up to 30 minutes before, consisting of visual disturbances and weakness or numbness of the limbs.

Drugs are used to help migraine sufferers (and also the related condition called 'cluster headache') in two quite distinct ways. One group of drugs is given chronically (ie long-term) in order to help prevent attacks (prophylactic use), for example, CALCIUM-CHANNEL BLOCKER drugs (eg NIFEDIPINE and VERAPAMIL HYDROCHLORIDE), BETA-BLOCKER drugs (eg METOPROLOL TARTRATE, NADOLOL, PROPRANOLOL HYDROCHLORIDE and TIMOLOL MALEATE), CYPROHEPTADINE HYDROCHLORIDE and METHYSERGIDE.

Attacks can last for several hours. All these drugs affect blood vessels in some way. The cause of migraine is not well understood, but during attacks blood vessels in the head and scalp are thought to narrow (constrict) before an attack and then widen (dilate) causing the pain during an attack. A second group of drugs may be used either at the *aura* stage or during the attack itself, and for maximum effect the speed of administration and subsequent absorption of the drug is an all-important factor. A number of ANALGESIC drugs can be used to offset the pain of an attack (eg ASPIRIN, CODEINE PHOSPHATE and PARACETAMOL) and are often incorporated into compound preparations together with a variety of drugs and drug types (eg CAFFEINE, BUCLIZINE HYDROCHLORIDE, DOXYLAMINE, ISOMETHEPTENE MUCATE, PIZOTIFEN).

Sometimes drugs with ANTINAUSEANT or ANTI-EMETIC properties are included (eg CYCLIZINE and METOCLOPRAMIDE HYDROCHLORIDE). Drugs that affect blood vessels can also be used during the attack stage, including the extensively used drug ERGOTAMINE TARTRATE and other ERGOT ALKALOID drugs, but these have been largely superseded by VASOCONSTRICTOR drugs of the 5-HT_1 receptor agonist type (sometimes called 'triptans'), including SUMATRIPTAN, ELETRIPAN, NARATRIPTAN, RIZATRIPTAN, ALMOTRIPTAN and ZOLMITRIPTAN which can achieve a rapid onset of action, some by self-injection. In all cases, the appropriate combination of drugs will vary from individual to individual and a certain amount of experimentation may be necessary to identify the factors that trigger a migraine attack (eg certain foods).

antimuscarinic 🅱

drugs are one of the main classes that make up the ANTICHOLINERGIC group of drugs. All the anticholinergic drugs act by inhibiting the action, release or production of the neurotransmitter ACETYLCHOLINE, which play an important part in the central and peripheral nervous systems. The term *anticholinergic* is commonly, and incorrectly, used synonymously with antimuscarinic, because so many antimuscarinics are used in medicine.

Drugs that block the actions of acetylcholine at *muscarinic* RECEPTORS (ie *anti*muscarinic drugs) tend to relax smooth muscle, reduce the secretion of saliva, digestive juices and sweat, and dilate the pupil of the eye. They may be used as ANTISPASMODIC, ANTIPARKINSONISM drugs (in the treatment of some symptoms of parkinsonian disease), ANTINAUSEANT or ANTI-EMETIC drugs in the treatment of motion sickness, to treat peptic ulcers, in ophthalmic examinations, and in antagonizing adverse effects of ANTICHOLINESTERASE agents (in medicine, agricultural accidental poisoning or warfare).

Examples of antimuscarinic anticholinergic drugs include: ATROPINE SULPHATE, BENZHEXOL HYDROCHLORIDE, BENZTROPINE MESILATE, BIPERIDEN, CO-PHENOTROPE, CYCLOPENTOLATE HYDROCHLORIDE, FLAVOXATE HYDROCHLORIDE, GLYCOPYRRONIUM BROMIDE, HYOSCINE BUTYLBROMIDE, HYOSCINE HYDROBROMIDE, IPRATROPIUM BROMIDE, ORPHENADRINE HYDROCHLORIDE, PROCYCLIDINE HYDROCHLORIDE, PROPANTHELINE BROMIDE and TROPICAMIDE.

The other main groups of anticholinergic drugs are the SKELETAL MUSCLE RELAXANT drugs (eg GALLAMINE TRIETHIODIDE) and GANGLION-BLOCKER agents. These drugs interact with *nicotinic* cholinergic receptors (at which NICOTINE is a powerful stimulant) rather than with *muscarinic* cholinergic receptors (which are powerfully stimulated by the plant ALKALOID muscarine; derived from the poisonous mushroom *Amanita muscaria*).

A

antinauseant

drugs are used to prevent or minimize the feeling of nausea and to reduce any subsequent vomiting. The type of drug used and the likelihood of its success, depends on the mechanism and origin of the nausea, which can be triggered in a number of ways. Motion sickness, or travel sickness, can often be prevented by taking before travelling antinauseants like the (ANTIMUSCARINIC) ANTICHOLINERGIC drug HYOSCINE HYDROBROMIDE, or the ANTIHISTAMINE drugs, eg MECLOZINE HYDROCHLORIDE.

Similar drugs may be used to treat nausea and other symptoms of labyrinthine disease (where the vestibular balance mechanisms of the inner ear are disturbed, eg Ménière's disease), though other drugs may also be necessary, such as CINNARIZINE and PHENOTHIAZINE drugs like PROCHLORPERAZINE.

A number of chemicals and drugs induce nausea and vomiting by an action involving the so-called *chemoreceptor trigger zone* within the brain; for instance, this is the most common side-effect when using the (OPIOID) NARCOTIC ANALGESIC morphine and so it may be combined with the antihistamine CYCLIZINE. The nausea and vomiting that is caused by chemotherapy and radiotherapy can be difficult to treat. However, some ANTI-EMETIC drugs, such as MOTILITY STIMULANT drugs (eg METOCLOPRAMIDE HYDROCHLORIDE), may be of some use by preventing vomiting and helping food out of the stomach.

Alternatively, there are some recently developed drugs that can also be effective, for instance, certain inhibitors of the actions of the mediator SEROTONIN (5-HT_3 antagonists) such as GRANISETRON, ONDANSETRON and TROPISETRON. The cannabis derivative NABILONE may be administered in difficult cases. Other drugs used sometimes include HALOPERIDOL and other butyrophenones, also CHLORPROMAZINE HYDROCHLORIDE in terminal illness.

anti-oestrogen

(oestrogen antagonist) is a term used to describe any of a class of HORMONE ANTAGONIST drugs that usually act directly to prevent the actions of female SEX HORMONES, the oestrogens (ESTRADIOL and ESTRIOL: see OESTROGEN), at RECEPTORS in their target tissues. Examples of drugs that act by the direct mechanism are TAMOXIFEN and TOREMIFENE. Also, some drugs can work indirectly as anti-oestrogens by inhibiting the formation or release of the hormone oestrogen. Examples of drugs which inhibit the conversion of androgens to oestrogens in the body (and therefore prevent the formation of oestrogens) are AMINOGLUTETHIMIDE, ANASTROZOLE and LETROZOLE.

antiparkinsonism

drugs are used to treat parkinsonism, which is the name used to describe the symptoms of several disorders of the central nervous system, including muscle tremor and rigidity (extrapyramidal symptoms), especially in the limbs. It is caused by an imbalance in the actions of the neurotransmitters ACETYLCHOLINE and DOPAMINE. In classic Parkinson's disease this is due to the degeneration of dopamine-containing nerves. However, what are known as parkinsonian extrapyramidal side-effects may be caused by treatment with several types of drugs, especially ANTIPSYCHOTIC drugs (eg HALOPERIDOL).

Treatment of parkinsonism may be with ANTICHOLINERGIC drugs (more accurately called ANTIMUSCARINIC; eg BENZHEXOL HYDROCHLORIDE, BENZTROPINE MESILATE, BIPERIDEN, PROCYCLIDINE HYDROCHLORIDE) or by drugs that increase the effects of dopamine (eg LEVODOPA, BROMOCRIPTINE, PERGOLIDE). The former class is more useful for controlling fine tremor, including that induced by drugs, and the latter class for overcoming difficulty in commencing movement and slowness brought about by degenerative disease. It is a difficult and often lengthy process to achieve the optimum dose in each patient and there are certain side-effects (such as confusion in the elderly) that occur with all the various treatments.

antiperspirant

agents help to prevent sweating. Medically, they are required only in cases of severe hyperhidrosis (excessive sweating), when some disorder of the sweat glands causes constant and streaming perspiration. In such cases, aluminium preparations such as ALUMINIUM CHLORIDE solution is an effective treatment and dusting powders may also be useful to dry the skin. Also various aluminium-containing ASTRINGENT salts are incorporated into preparations for minor fungal infections associated with sweating.

antiplatelet

drugs (also known as platelet-aggregation inhibitors or antithrombotic drugs) prevent the formation of blood clots (thrombi), that is, they reduce platelet aggregation. These drugs (eg ASPIRIN, taken at low doses) can be used as a preventive treatment (prophylactic use) in patients who are at risk, for instance, after a heart attack, stroke or bypass operation. However, this same action may also increase bleeding time and so patients receiving ANTICOAGULANT drugs should not normally have antiplatelet drugs as well. By decreasing platelet aggregation, antiplatelet drugs may beneficially inhibit thrombus formation on the arterial side of the circulation, where thrombi are formed by platelet aggregation and anticoagulant drugs have little effect. The antiplatelet DIPYRIDAMOLE seems to work by stopping platelets sticking to each other or to surgically inserted tubes or artificial heart valves. EPOPROSTENOL (prostacyclin) is a naturally occurring PROSTAGLANDIN present in the walls of blood vessels which has antiplatelet activity when administered therapeutically by intravenous infusion. Newly introduced drugs that work in novel ways to reduce clot formation include ABCIXIMAB, CLOPIDOGREL, EPTIFIBATIDE and TICLOPIDINE.

Antipressan

(Berk; APS) is a proprietary, prescription-only preparation of the BETA-BLOCKER atenolol. It can be used as an ANTIHYPERTENSIVE for raised blood pressure, as an ANTI-ANGINA treatment to relieve symptoms and improve exercise tolerance and as an ANTI-ARRHYTHMIC to regularize heartbeat and to treat myocardial infarction. Available as tablets.
✚▲ Side-effects/warnings: See ATENOLOL.

antiprotozoal

drugs are used to treat or prevent infections caused by micro-organisms called protozoa. The most important protozoa, in terms of illness and death, are those of the genus *Plasmodium*, which cause malaria (see ANTIMALARIAL). Other major protozoal diseases found in tropical countries include trypanosomiasis, leishmaniasis and amoebic dysentery. Protozoal infections more familiar in this country include toxoplasmosis, trichomoniasis and giardiasis. A common form of pneumonia is caused in immunosuppressed patients (including those suffering from AIDS) by the protozoan *Pneumocystis carinii* (which has some features of both protozoals and fungi). The drugs used to treat amoebic-protozoal infections are commonly referred to as AMOEBICIDAL drugs. See also ATOVAQUONE.

antipsychotic

(or neuroleptic) drugs calm and soothe patients without impairing consciousness. They are used mainly to treat psychologically disturbed patients, particularly those who manifest the complex behavioural patterns of schizophrenia, and also those with brain damage, toxic delirium and mania. In the short term, some can also be used as ANXIOLYTIC drugs to treat severe anxiety. Because they can affect mood, in the short term some may worsen depression, but in other cases there may be a useful ANTIDEPRESSANT effect with a beneficial elevation of mood. Antipsychotics with markedly depressant side-effects were at one time somewhat misleadingly known as major tranquillizers, since for example, in schizophrenics, the tranquillizing effect is of secondary importance, or for some even a debilitating side-effect.

Antipsychotics work by acting in the brain, principally as dopamine-receptor blockers, to change the balance of the effects there of the neurotransmitter DOPAMINE, which is intimately involved in mood. Because the balance of neurotransmitters in the brain is in a finely balanced state, there is a price to pay for interference with this, and drugs used to treat a neurological or psychological disorder illness inevitably have some undesirable side-effects. The antipsychotic drugs are particularly bad in this respect and can cause many important and unpleasant side-effects, of which some resemble Parkinson's disease (a condition whose pathology largely results from a depletion of dopamine in the brain). These antipsychotic drug side-effects, collectively called *extrapyramidal symptoms*, divide into two main groups: the *acute dystonias* that develop in the first few weeks and reverse on stopping the drug; or *tardive dyskinesia* which develops after months or years, and which does not reverse. Some of these acute dystonias resemble symptoms seen in Parkinson's disease, and are therefore termed 'parkinsonian symptoms'. These dystonias include tremor, slow movements and cog-wheel rigidity, akathisia ('restless-leg syndrome'), abnormal face movements (protruding tongue, head-turning and wryneck) and other manifestations. Most or all of these dystonias follow directly from the fact that antipsychotic drugs work by blocking dopamine receptors in the brain. Some of these side-effects can be controlled with other drugs or by careful control of dosage. Also, the so-called 'atypical' antipsychotics may have more restricted side-effects by virtue of a selectivity in which a set of dopamine receptors are blocked. Tardive dyskinesia (tardive means late) is a complex syndrome particularly characterized by sometimes disabling involuntary movements, and may resemble a worsening of the psychotic condition being treated. It develops only after prolonged usage of certain drugs but is not usually reversible and is a major problem in antipsychotic therapy. It may get worse if antipsychotic drug treatment is stopped. Its incidence depends greatly on dosage and the age of the treated individual (being greater in those over 50 years), and the drug used ('atypical' antipsychotics are better in this respect). Further side-effects of dopamine antagonists can be attributed to blockade of certain subsets of dopamine receptors in the brain, including breast swelling, pain and milk production in both sexes.

Other side-effects seen with certain antipsychotic drugs result from blockage of the actions of the neurotransmitter ACETYLCHOLINE. These ANTICHOLINERGIC (antimuscarinic) side-effects include a dry mouth, gastrointestinal and vision upsets, but are generally less marked with newer drugs.

There are nearly 30 antipsychotic drugs currently in use in the UK. These differ in their characteristics and side-effects. They are usually grouped and named according to their chemical structures. The biggest group is the PHENOTHIAZINE class which contains many different drugs (including drugs not used for their antipsychotic actions). For example, CHLORPROMAZINE HYDROCHLORIDE, PROMAZINE HYDROCHLORIDE, PERICYAZINE, PIPOTIAZINE PALMITATE, THIORIDAZINE, FLUPHENAZINE, PERPHENAZINE, PROCHLORPERAZINE, LEVOMEPROMAZINE (methotrimeprazine) and TRIFLUOPERAZINE. There are a number of further antipsychotic drugs that belong to yet other chemical groups, but in their spectrum of action these tend to resemble some of the phenothiazines and include the *butyrophenones* (BENPERIDOL, HALOPERIDOL); *diphenylbutylpiperidines* (PIMOZIDE); *thioxanthenes* (flupentixol); *zuclopenthixol*; *benzamides* (SULPIRIDE, OXYPERTINE, LOXAPINE). Some more recently introduced antipsychotics resist this chemical classification, and these 'atypical' antipsychotics may be better tolerated with less frequent extrapyramidal symptoms (and less raised levels of the pituitary hormone prolactin, hence the effects on the breasts) than with older antipsychotics (eg AMISULPRIDE, CLOZAPINE, OLANZAPINE, QUETIAPINE, RISPERIDONE, ZOTEPINE).

For more detailed side-effects see chlorpromazine hydrochloride, or individual antipsychotics.

Antipsychotic drugs may be given by mouth, by intravenous or intramuscular injection, or sometimes, in the form of special oily preparations, as a long-lasting deep-intramuscular 'depot' injection.

antipyretic

drugs are used to reduce raised body temperature, for example in fever, but they do not lower normal body temperature. The best-known and most-used antipyretics include certain NON-NARCOTIC ANALGESIC drugs such as ASPIRIN, PARACETAMOL and IBUPROFEN. See also NSAID.

antirabies immunoglobulin injection

see RABIES IMMUNOGLOBULIN.

antirheumatic

drugs are used to relieve the pain and inflammation of rheumatism and arthritis (particularly rheumatoid arthritis (antirheumatoid drugs) and osteoarthritis, and so they are also known as *anti-arthritic drugs*) and sometimes of other musculoskeletal disorders. The primary form of treatment is with NSAIDS (non-steroidal anti-inflammatory drugs), NON-NARCOTIC ANALGESIC drugs such as ASPIRIN, the aspirin-paracetamol ester BENORYLATE, also FENOPROFEN, IBUPROFEN, INDOMETHACIN and PHENYLBUTAZONE. CORTICOSTEROID drugs can also be used because they are anti-inflammatory (eg PREDNISOLONE). Finally, there are some drugs that seem to halt the progression of certain musculoskeletal disorders, for example AURANOFIN and SODIUM AUROTHIOMALATE (which both contain gold), PENICILLAMINE, SULFASALAZINE and also CHLOROQUINE and HYDROXYCHLOROQUINE SULPHATE. However, some of these drugs have unpleasant side-effects and others can take up to six months to have any effect. In cases where there is an autoimmune element to the disease, IMMUNOSUPPRESSANT drugs (eg AZATHIOPRINE, LEFLUMOMIDE, CYCLOPHOSPHAMIDE, CICLOSPORIN, DEXAMETHASONE, METHOTREXATE) can also be used.

antiseborrhoeic

drugs are used to treat seborrhoea, which is an excessive secretion of the oily substance sebum from the sebaceous glands of the skin, and the glands are often enlarged, especially beside the nose. Over-secretion is common in adolescence and often results in acne or seborrhoeic eczema. Dandruff often appears during the development of seborrhoeic eczema. Seborrhoeic dermatitis may respond to mild topical CORTICOSTEROID or topical ANTIFUNGAL drugs such as KETOCONAZOLE as a cream, or to a combination. Topical application of ZINC SULPHATE or LITHIUM SUCCINATE ointment can be effective. Also, COAL TAR, SALICYLIC ACID and SULPHUR preparations can be used for seborrhoeic dermatitis of the scalp by means of topical scalp preparations.

antiseptic

agents destroy micro-organisms or inhibit their activity to such an extent that they are less, or no longer, harmful to health. Antiseptics can be applied to the skin, burns or wounds to prevent infections and to limit the spread of pathogenic (disease-causing) micro-organisms. The term is often used synonymously with DISINFECTANT. However, the latter term can also apply to agents used on inanimate objects (such as surgical equipment, catheters etc.), as well as to agents used on the skin and other living tissue. Examples include: ETHANOL, AMINACRINE HYDROCHLORIDE, AMYLMETACRESOL, BENZALKONIUM CHLORIDE, CETRIMIDE, CETYLPYRIDINIUM CHLORIDE, CHLORHEXIDINE, CRYSTAL VIOLET, DEQUALINIUM CHLORIDE, DOMIPHEN BROMIDE, GLUTARALDEHYDE, HALQUINOL, HEXACHLOROPHANE, HEXETIDINE, HEXYLRESORCINOL, HYDROGEN PEROXIDE, IODINE, PHENOL, POTASSIUM PERMANGANATE, POVIDONE-IODINE, SILVER SULFADIAZINE, SODIUM HYPOCHLORITE, SODIUM PERBORATE, THYMOL, TRICLOSAN, TYROTHRICIN.

Antiseptic First Aid Cream

(Anglian Pharma) is a proprietary, non-prescription preparation of the ANTISEPTIC cetrimide. It can be used to cleanse skin and prevent infection of cuts, minor wounds, nappy rash and chapped hands. It is available as a cream.
✚▲ Side-effects/warnings: See CETRIMIDE.

antiserum

is a general term that is used to describe certain preparations of blood serum rich in particular antibodies. Antiserum preparations (*antisera*) are used to provide what is called *passive immunity* to diseases (as opposed to *active immunity* produced after vaccination), or some measure of beneficial treatment if the disease has already been contracted. The essence of passive immunity is the introduction of antibodies to the pathogenic organism, or to its toxin, into the patient's own blood.

The general term used to describe that part of a disease-causing entity which is recognized by the immune system is *antigen*. If an antigen is injected into an animal, the animal produces *antibodies* in response. An 'antiserum' is a preparation of animal blood serum containing these antibodies. Most antisera were prepared from the blood of antigen-treated horses, which were then purified and administered to humans to immunize them against disease. However, because they are *foreign* proteins, serious hypersensitivity reactions may result and, at the most extreme, cause anaphylactic shock. For this reason, such animal preparations are now only used when there is no real alternative, and have to a large extent been replaced by preparations of human antibodies separated from human blood serum, usually referred to simply as *immunoglobulins* (although this is not technically a correct term since all antibodies, including those produced by animals, are immunoglobulins): the term antisera is now generally applied to material prepared from animals. But the use of both immunoglobulins and antisera are ways of imparting passive immunity.

A

✪ Related entries: botulism antitoxin; diphtheria antitoxin.

antispasmodic

(or spasmolytic) drugs relieve spasm in smooth muscle (involuntary muscles, eg muscles in the respiratory tract and the intestinal walls) and form part of the group of drugs known collectively as SMOOTH MUSCLE RELAXANT drugs. Some are used as BRONCHODILATOR drugs (eg used in asthma), some relax the uterus so may be used to help relieve the discomfort of period pain, while others are used to relieve abdominal pain due to intestinal colic. They can also be used, along with other drugs, in the adjunct treatment of non-ulcer dyspepsia, diverticular disease, and irritable bowel syndrome. They include the (ANTIMUSCARINIC) ANTICHOLINERGIC drugs, such as ATROPINE SULPHATE, and agents such as MEBEVERINE HYDROCHLORIDE and ALVERINE CITRATE which act directly on smooth muscle to relax it.

antisympathetic

drugs act at some site or other within the sympathetic nervous system to reduce its overall effect. Since activity within this division of the (autonomic) nervous system controls blood pressure and heart rate, then drugs that act to reduce its activity cause a fall in blood pressure and so the main use of such drugs is in ANTIHYPERTENSIVE treatment.

There are several sites and mechanisms by which such drugs act. For example, METHYLDOPA acts mainly within the brain itself to reduce the activity of the sympathetic nervous system, while METIROSINE inhibits the enzymes that produce NORADRENALINE (norepinephrine; the sympathetic neurotransmitter) within nerves.

Another distinct class of drugs, the ADRENERGIC-NEURONE BLOCKER (DEBRISOQUINE and GUANETHIDINE MONOSULPHATE) work to interfere with the storage and release of noradrenaline, and CLONIDINE HYDROCHLORIDE decreases the amount that is released.

All these drugs have quite marked side-effects and some of them may be administered in conjunction with other classes of antihypertensives, for instance the DIURETIC drugs.

antitetanus immunoglobulin injection

see TETANUS IMMUNOGLOBULIN.

antithrombin III concentrate

is a human blood product with ANTICOAGULANT properties. It inhibits the action of several clotting enzymes that activate thrombin, which is necessary for the final stages of blood coagulation. In people with hereditary deficiency of this thrombin inhibitor (an uncommon condition), antithrombin III can be used in surgery or for other procedures to lower the risk of thromboembolism. Administration is by intravenous infusion.

✚▲ Side-effects/warnings: Flushing, headache; nausea; rarely, allergic reactions and fever.

✪ Related entry: Dried Antithrombin III.

antithrombotic

drugs prevent the formation of blood clots (thrombi). See ANTICOAGULANT; ANTIPLATELET.

antithyroid

drugs are used in the treatment of over-activity of the thyroid gland (hyperthyroidism; thyrotoxicosis). In thyrotoxicosis there is an excess secretion of THYROID HORMONES and this results in an exaggeration of the normal activity of the gland, which causes increased metabolic rate, raised body temperature, sweating, increased sensitivity to heat, nervousness, tremor, raised heart rate, tendency to fatigue, and sometimes loss of body weight with an increased appetite.

How the disease is treated depends on its origin. However, if it is severe the surgical removal of part of the gland may be necessary, though more commonly the gland is treated with radioactive iodine to reduce the number of cells.

In any event, drugs are used to either control the symptoms in the long term, or in the short term to prepare the gland for more radical intervention. A BETA-BLOCKER (eg NADOLOL and PROPRANOLOL HYDROCHLORIDE) may be used in the prevention of a number of the signs and symptoms of thyrotoxicosis. They work by blocking the effects of over-stimulation caused by the release of ADRENALINE and NORADRENALINE by thyroid hormones, but do not treat the cause of the problem in the thyroid gland itself.

Some other drugs (chemically thionamides, eg CARBIMAZOLE (most commonly used) and PROPYLTHIOURACIL act directly on the thyroid gland to reduce the production of the thyroid hormones, so treating the excess of thyroid

hormones in the blood. Iodine itself, which is chemically incorporated into the thyroid hormones THYROXINE and TRIIODOTHYRONINE, can be given (as AQUEOUS IODINE ORAL SOLUTION, or Lugol's solution) to suppress gland activity prior to thyroid surgery.
▲ Warnings: Some nutritional supplements and herbal remedies contain high levels of iodine (eg kelp), which can interfere with antithyroid treatment.

antitoxin

refers to antibody material raised to react with the *toxin* (including *exotoxin*) released by a bacterium (rather than to the bacterium itself, which is generally called ANTISERUM or IMMUNOGLOBULIN), and the same term (antitoxin) is used for antibodies raised to the toxins contained in snake or spider bites, and to *exotoxins* (a potent toxin that is released from a bacterial parasite to work at a distance). The antitoxin produced can be used to provide *passive immunity* to people who have been exposed, and works, in the short term only, as a sort of ANTIDOTE by neutralizing the toxin. However, since antitoxin material is generally produced in horses, hypersensitivity reactions are common (because the impure preparations contain 'foreign' horse protein). Snake and spider venom antitoxins are available from special centres, along with BOTULISM ANTITOXIN and DIPHTHERIA ANTITOXIN. See also ANTISERUM; IMMUNOGLOBULIN.

antitubercular

(or antituberculous) drugs are used in combination to treat tuberculosis. The initial phase of treatment usually involves three or more drugs (commonly ISONIAZID, RIFAMPICIN and PYRAZINAMIDE; sometimes ETHAMBUTOL HYDROCHLORIDE) in order to tackle the disease as efficiently as possible, while reducing the risk of encountering bacterial resistance.

If, after about two months, the first phase is successful, treatment usually continues with only two of the initial three drugs (often isoniazid and rifampicin). If treatment is not successful, for example, because the patient suffered intolerable side-effects or because the disease was resistant to the drugs, then other drugs are used. Treatment of tuberculosis with drugs is only necessary where the far more effective public health measure of vaccination has, for some reason, failed (see BCG VACCINE).

antituberculous

see ANTITUBERCULAR.

antitussive

drugs assist in the treatment of coughs. The term is usually used to describe only those drugs that suppress coughing, rather than drugs used to treat the cause of coughing. Cough suppressants include OPIOID drugs such as CODEINE PHOSPHATE, DEXTROMETHORPHAN HYDROBROMIDE and PHOLCODINE. They tend to cause constipation as a side-effect and so should not be used for prolonged periods.

Other types of drugs that are useful to use alongside cough-suppressants include the EXPECTORANT and DEMULCENT classes. Expectorants are used to decrease the viscosity of mucus or to increase the secretion of liquid mucus in dry, irritant, unproductive coughs. Expectorants include AMMONIUM CHLORIDE, GUAIFENESIN (guaiphenesin) and IPECACUANHA; and these are incorporated into many proprietary compound cough medicines. Sedative members of the ANTIHISTAMINE group are incorporated into many proprietary cough preparations, and they may work by drying up secretions or by virtue of being sedatives. Demulcents (eg glycerol, sugar or honey syrup) also help to reduce the viscosity of mucus and relieve dry, unproductive irritating coughs. All of these drugs are used to soothe coughs rather than to treat the underlying cause, such as an infection.

antivaricella-zoster immunoglobulin

see VARICELLA-ZOSTER IMMUNOGLOBULIN.

antivenom

(antivenin) is an antidote to the poison in a snakebite, a scorpion's sting or a bite from any other poisonous creature (such as a spider). Normally, it is an ANTITOXIN that is injected into the bloodstream for immediate relief. Identification of the poisonous creature is important so that the right antidote can be selected.

In the UK the only indigenous poisonous snake is the adder (*Vipera berus*), the poison of which can usually be treated by medical supportive therapy, but on occasion may require treatment with European Viper Venom Antiserum. Antivenoms have been prepared internationally for many foreign snakes, insects and spiders. Some of these are available in the UK for emergency use from regional centres in London, Liverpool and Oxford. They are given by injection or intravenous infusion.

✚▲ Side-effects/warnings: Treatment is under specialist conditions. Because antivenoms are themselves foreign proteins, hypersensitivity reactions (including anaphylactic shock) are not uncommon and may exacerbate the symptoms and distress caused by the bite itself, therefore antivenoms are only used where symptoms are severe.

antiviral

drugs are used to treat infections caused by viruses, which are micro-organisms much smaller than bacteria – so minute they cannot be seen under the normal (light) microscope. They can only replicate within the living cells of the host which they parasitize.

In terms of public health, prevention of viral infection is best achieved by vaccination (eg against poliomyelitis, rubella, measles and mumps, and some types of rabies), but continual mutation of other viruses makes vaccination more difficult (eg flu, the common cold, HIV). ANTIBIOTIC drugs are inactive against viruses, and treatment of infection is only possible with a few, relatively new, antiviral drugs. Mainly, the use of antivirals is restricted to preventive or disease-limitation treatment (eg ACICLOVIR (acyclovir) against *herpes viruses*). However, some antiviral drugs can be life-savers, especially in immunocompromised patients. A great deal of effort is currently being made to develop antivirals for use in the treatment of HIV infection, but AIDS treatment currently relies heavily on drugs active against bacterial, fungal or other microbial infections in these immunocompromised individuals.

Antivirals can be divided into groups on the basis of how they work. Most currently used antiviral drugs are only effective when the viruses are replicating. Some are *nucleoside analogues* (or related compounds) that resemble cellular molecules necessary to viral function or replication, often working as ENZYME INHIBITOR drugs against an essential viral enzyme because some viral enzymes are virus-specific, so antiviral drugs can target them without much affecting the human patient. For example, the group of antivirals modelled on the natural nucleosides involved in cell division and replication which work against the enzyme *reverse transcriptase* are termed *reverse transcriptase inhibitors* (eg DIDANOSINE, LAMIVUDINE, STAVUDINE, ZALCITABINE, ZIDOVUDINE (AZT)); and some even later drugs (the *non-nucleoside* group) which chemically are not actually nucleosides (eg EFAVIRENZ, NEVIRAPINE) but which also work as *reverse transcriptase inhibitors*. Other antivirals that prevent viral cell replication by inhibiting nucleic acid synthesis include FOSCARNET SODIUM, GANCICLOVIR and TRIBAVIRIN. The most recently introduced group of antivirals, the *protease inhibitors*, work as enzyme inhibitors acting against an enzyme (*HIV-1 protease*) that is essential for the replication of viruses. Examples of this group include AMPRENAVIR, INDINAVIR, lopinavir (see LOPINAVIR WITH RITONAVIR), NELFINAVIR, RITONAVIR and SAQUINAVIR. There are a number of other types of antivirals that work in a different way. The first extensively used antiviral drug – aciclovir – inhibits a viral enzyme called DNA polymerase. AMANTADINE HYDROCHLORIDE is active against influenza A virus (an action unrelated to its ANTIPARKINSONISM use), and interferons (see INTERFERON) act as IMMUNOMODULATOR agents that help the body's immunological response to viruses.

In clinical practice, antivirals are often grouped by the types of infection against which they are effective (rather than by mechanism of action). For instance, serious cytomegaloviral (CMV) infections may be contained by treatment with ganciclovir and foscarnet sodium. Infections due to the herpes viruses (eg cold sores, genital herpes, shingles and chickenpox) may be contained by early treatment with aciclovir, amantadine, FAMCICLOVIR, INOSINE PRANOBEX or VALACICLOVIR. HIV infections are increasingly being treated by several drug groups in combination, for instance *protease inhibitors* together with *reverse transcriptase inhibitors*. Many uses of antiviral drugs are for specialist treatment in hospital for serious infections and the profoundly ill. Full assessment of the patient's particular circumstances and suitability will be carried out, and explanation of the possible

(often marked) side-effects given.
▲ Warnings: The herbal remedy, St John's wort, which is used for depression, can reduce the blood concentration of some antiviral drugs such as NEVIRAPINE and EFAVIRENZ.

Anturan

(Novartis) is a proprietary, prescription-only preparation of sulfinpyrazone. It can be used to treat and prevent gout and hyperurea, and is available as tablets.
✚▲ Side-effects/warnings: See SULFINPYRAZONE.

Anugesic-HC

(Parke-Davis; Pfizer) is a proprietary, prescription-only compound preparation of the CORTICOSTEROID and ANTI-INFLAMMATORY hydrocortisone (as acetate) and the ASTRINGENT agents zinc oxide and bismuth oxide, benzyl benzoate (with Peru balsam) and the LOCAL ANAESTHETIC pramoxine hydrochloride. It can be used to treat haemorrhoids and inflammation in the anal region, and is available as a cream and suppositories.
✚▲ Side-effects/warnings: See BENZYL BENZOATE; BISMUTH OXIDE; HYDROCORTISONE; PRAMOXINE HYDROCHLORIDE; ZINC OXIDE.

Anusol Cream

(Warner Lambert Consumer Healthcare; Pfizer) is a proprietary, non-prescription compound preparation of the ASTRINGENT agents bismuth oxide and zinc oxide (with Peru balsam). It can be used to treat haemorrhoids and discomfort in the anal region, and is available as a cream. It is not recommended for use in children.
✚▲ Side-effects/warnings: See BISMUTH OXIDE; ZINC OXIDE.

Anusol-HC

(Kestrel; Pfizer) is a proprietary, prescription-only compound preparation of the CORTICOSTEROID and ANTI-INFLAMMATORY hydrocortisone (as acetate) and the ASTRINGENT or ANTISEPTIC agents bismuth oxide, benzyl benzoate and zinc oxide (with bismuth subgallate and Peru Balsam). It can be used to treat haemorrhoids and inflammation in the anal region, and is available as an ointment and as suppositories. It is not recommended for children. (A version is also available to the public without prescription.)
✚▲ Side-effects/warnings: See BENZYL BENZOATE; BISMUTH OXIDE; HYDROCORTISONE; ZINC OXIDE.

Anusol Ointment

(Warner Lambert Consumer Healthcare; Pfizer) is a proprietary, non-prescription compound preparation of the ASTRINGENT agents bismuth oxide, bismuth subgallate and zinc oxide (with Peru balsam). It can be used to treat haemorrhoids and discomfort in the anal region, and is available as an ointment. It is not recommended for use in children.
✚▲ Side-effects/warnings: See BISMUTH OXIDE; BISMUTH SUBGALLATE; ZINC OXIDE.

Anusol Plus HC Ointment

(Warner Lambert Consumer Healthcare; Pfizer) is a proprietary, non-prescription compound preparation of the CORTICOSTEROID and ANTI-INFLAMMATORY hydrocortisone (as acetate) and the ASTRINGENT or ANTISEPTIC agents bismuth oxide, benzyl benzoate and zinc oxide (with bismuth subgallate and Peru Balsam). It can be used to treat haemorrhoids and inflammation in the anal region, and is available as an ointment. It is not used for those under 18 years, except on medical advice.
✚▲ Side-effects/warnings: See BENZYL BENZOATE; BISMUTH OXIDE; HYDROCORTISONE; ZINC OXIDE.

Anusol Plus HC Suppositories

(Warner Lambert Consumer Healthcare; Pfizer) is a proprietary, non-prescription compound preparation of the CORTICOSTEROID and ANTI-INFLAMMATORY hydrocortisone (as acetate) and the ASTRINGENT and ANTISEPTIC agents bismuth oxide and zinc oxide, benzyl benzoate (with Peru Balsam). It can be used to treat haemorrhoids and inflammation in the anal region, and is available as suppositories. It is not used for those under 18 years, except on medical advice.
✚▲ Side-effects/warnings: See BENZYL BENZOATE; BISMUTH OXIDE; HYDROCORTISONE; ZINC OXIDE.

Anusol Suppositories

(Warner Lambert Consumer Healthcare; Pfizer) is a proprietary, non-prescription compound preparation of the ASTRINGENT agents bismuth subgallate, bismuth oxide and zinc oxide (with

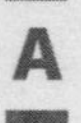

Peru balsam). It can be used to treat haemorrhoids and discomfort in the anal region, and is available as suppositories. It is not recommended for use in children.
✚▲ Side-effects/warnings: See BISMUTH OXIDE; ZINC OXIDE.

anxiolytic

drugs are used to relieve medically diagnosed anxiety states and are prescribed, usually short term, for patients whose anxiety is impeding its resolution by other therapies, such as psychotherapy. They are also used to relieve acute anxiety, for instance, before surgery. Treatment should be at the lowest dose effective and must not be prolonged, because psychological dependence and physical dependence (addiction) readily occurs and may make withdrawal difficult. The best-known and most-used anxiolytics are the BENZODIAZEPINE drugs (eg CHLORDIAZEPOXIDE, DIAZEPAM and LORAZEPAM) and other drugs such as MEPROBAMATE and some of the ANTIPSYCHOTIC drugs (at low doses). Additionally, BETA-BLOCKER drugs are sometimes used to treat anxiety by preventing the physical symptoms such as palpitations of the heart, sweating and tremor, which helps the patient to stop the chain reaction of worry to fear to panic. Some people in the performing arts use these drugs to control stage-fright symptoms. Some of these drugs take time to work and careful adjustment of the dose is required. Drugs of this class are sometimes, somewhat misleadingly, referred to as *minor tranquillizers.*

APD

see DISODIUM PAMIDRONATE.

APO-go

(Britannia) is a prescription-only preparation of the ANTIPARKINSONISM drug apomorphine hydrochloride. It is available in a form for injection.
✚▲ Side-effects/warnings: See APOMORPHINE HYDROCHLORIDE.

apomorphine hydrochloride

is an ANTIPARKINSONISM drug with similar actions to BROMOCRIPTINE and is used in a patient's *off* periods, which are not controlled by the drug levodopa. It is chemically related to MORPHINE SULPHATE, though it is not an ANALGESIC, and has been used as an emetic. Administration for Parkinson's disease is by injection. Recenty, it has been introduced in a form for use in IMPOTENCE TREATMENT for erectile dysfunction, when it is taken by the sublingual route (from where absorption is limited, and side-effects are less).
✚ Side-effects: These include dyskinesias (movement disorders) during *on* periods, nausea and vomiting, confusion, euphoria, light-headedness and hallucinations; yawning, drowsiness, rhinitis, pharyngitis, cough, flushing, taste disturbance, postural hypotension, blood disorders and cognitive impairment. Pain at site of injection. With sublingual use, the main side-effects are sweating and fainting, though these are not common.
▲ Warnings: It should not be administered to patients with central nervous system or respiratory depression, hypersensitivity to opioids, psychiatric disorders and dementia; or who are pregnant or breast-feeding. Administer with caution to those with respiratory, cardiovascular and hormone disorders, kidney impairment, and those who have a tendency to nausea and vomiting. For impotence treatment it should not be used where there is anatomical deformation of the penis (for instance, Peyronie's disease, cavernosal fibrosis, angulation), and it is not recommended for use in combination with other treatments for erectile dysfunction. It may impair the performance of skilled tasks (eg driving).
✪ Related entries: APO-go; Britaject; Uprima.

appetite suppressant

(anorectic) is a term used to describe agents (of two main types) that are mainly used as OBESITY TREATMENT drugs.

The first type works by acting on the brain, and a number of such drugs that have been used are related and have actions similar to the STIMULANT amfetamine (amphetamine). These include phentermine, fenfluramine, dexfenfluramine, dexamfetamine and metamfetamine. However, amphetamines can readily cause psychological dependence and preparations of such drugs are on the Controlled Drugs list. Recently, several such drugs have been shown to cause serious adverse side-effects (heart valve disorders and a serious risk of pulmonary hypertension) and consequently, in the UK all have been withdrawn from mainstream medical use (though are still available in a number of other countries). A new and different type of drug that works on the brain to modify appetite, represented by the recently introduced agent SIBUTRAMINE, acts by inhibiting reuptake of noradrenaline, serotonin and dopamine in the central nervous system (a similar activity to certain ANTIDEPRESSANT drugs).

The second type of appetite suppressants work by bulking out the food eaten so that the body feels it has actually taken more than it has. The main bulking agent used medically is METHYLCELLULOSE, while others also used are better known as (bulking-agent) LAXATIVE drugs, eg STERCULIA and ISPAGHULA HUSK. Both types of drug are intended to assist in the medical treatment of obesity, where the primary therapy is an appropriate diet.

apraclonidine

is an ALPHA-ADRENOCEPTOR STIMULANT that is selective for the $alpha_2$subtype of receptor. It is chemically a derivative of CLONIDINE HYDROCHLORIDE. It reduces the rate of production of aqueous humour in the eyeball and so can be used to control or prevent postoperative elevation of intraocular pressure (pressure in the eyeball) after laser surgery and in GLAUCOMA TREATMENT (particularly when other drugs have not been effective). Administration is topical as eye-drops.

✚ Side-effects: Dry mouth, taste disturbances, itching of the eye, discomfort (stop taking the drug if there is intolerance, such as oedema of lids and conjunctiva); headache, tiredness, dry nose; lid retraction, sometimes whitening of the conjunctiva and dilation of the pupil; systemic effects, since absorption may follow topical application, for instance on the cardiovascular system.

▲ Warnings: Avoid its use in patients with severe cardiovascular disease (including hypertension); administer with care to those with certain conditions including those of the cardiovascular, depression, or who are pregnant or breast-feeding.

✪ **Related entry: Iopidine.**

Apresoline

(Alliance) is a proprietary, prescription-only preparation of the VASODILATOR hydralazine hydrochloride. It can be used in long-term ANTIHYPERTENSIVE treatment and in hypertensive crisis. It is available as tablets and in a form for injection.

✚▲ Side-effects/warnings: See HYDRALAZINE HYDROCHLORIDE.

Aprinox

(Sovereign) is a proprietary, prescription-only preparation of the (THIAZIDE) DIURETIC bendroflumethiazide. It can be used, either on its own or in conjunction with other diuretics or drugs, in the treatment of oedema and as an ANTIHYPERTENSIVE. It is available as tablets.

✚▲ Side-effects/warnings: See BENDROFLUMETHIAZIDE.

aprotinin

is a natural ENZYME INHIBITOR that has antifibrinolytic activity by inhibiting the proteolytic enzymes that normally dissolve blood clots. Medically, it can be used to prevent life-threatening bleeding, for instance, in open-heart surgery, removal of tumours, in surgical procedures in patients with certain blood disorders (eg hyperplasminaemias) and after excess thrombolytic therapy. It is given by slow injection or intravenous infusion.

✚ Side-effects: Hypersensitivity reactions and occasionally inflammation of vein walls.

✪ **Related entry: Trasylol.**

Aprovel

(Bristol-Myers Squibb) is a proprietary, prescription-only preparation of the ANGIOTENSIN-RECEPTOR BLOCKER irbesartan. It can be used as an ANTIHYPERTENSIVE, and is available as tablets.

✚▲ Side-effects/warnings: See IRBESARTAN.

Apsin

(APS) is a proprietary, prescription-only preparation of the ANTIBACTERIAL and (PENICILLIN) ANTIBIOTIC phenoxymethylpenicillin. It can be used to treat a range of infections, and is available as tablets and an oral solution (as the potassium salt).

✚▲ Side-effects/warnings: See PHENOXYMETHYLPENICILLIN.

Apstil

(APS) is a proprietary, prescription-only preparation of the synthetic OESTROGEN

A

diethylstilbestrol. It can be used as an ANTICANCER drug to treat prostate cancer and breast cancer, and is available in the form of tablets.
✚▲ Side-effects/warnings: See DIETHYLSTILBESTROL.

Aquadrate

(Procter & Gamble) is a proprietary, non-prescription preparation of the HYDRATING AGENT urea. It can be used for dry, scaling or itching skin, and is available as a cream.
✚▲ Side-effects/warnings: See UREA.

Aquasept Skin Cleanser

(SSL) is a proprietary, non-prescription preparation of the ANTISEPTIC triclosan. It can be used to cleanse the skin and prevent infection, and is available as a topical solution.
✚▲ Side-effects/warnings: See TRICLOSAN.

Aqueous Iodine Oral Solution

(or Lugol's solution) is a non-proprietary, freshly made solution of iodine and potassium iodide in water. It is used by patients suffering from an excess of THYROID HORMONES in the bloodstream (thyrotoxicosis) prior to thyroid surgery. It is taken by mouth after dilution.
✚▲ Side-effects/warnings: See IODINE.

arachis oil

is peanut oil, used primarily as an EMOLLIENT in treating crusts on skin surfaces in conditions such as dandruff or cradle cap, and to soften ear wax; administration is topical as ear-drops to loosen wax. Also used as a LAXATIVE to soften impacted faeces in order to promote bowel movement; administration is oral. A number of proprietary preparations have recently substituted liquid paraffin in their formulation in place of arachis oil (since the former is less likely to cause allergic reactions).
✚▲ Side-effects/warnings: Traditionally considered safe (it is widely used as a cooking oil) but allergy to peanut products is now quite common, to the extent of anaphylaxis, and so there is a potential risk of allergic reaction. Some individuals (including some infants and children) need to avoid all products containing peanut oil products.
✪ Related entries: Cerumol Ear Drops; Earex Ear Drops; Fletchers' Arachis Oil Retention Enema; Hewletts Cream; Oilatum Cream; Siopel.

Aramine

(MSD) is a proprietary, prescription-only preparation of the SYMPATHOMIMETIC and VASOCONSTRICTOR metaraminol. It is most often used to raise blood pressure in people with hypotension. It is available in a form for injection or intravenous infusion.
✚▲ Side-effects/warnings: See METARAMINOL.

Aranesp

(Amgen) is a recently introduced proprietary, prescription-only preparation of DARBEPOETIN ALFA. It can be used in ANAEMIA TREATMENT for conditions such as those known to be associated with chronic renal failure. It is available in a number of forms for injection.
✚▲ Side-effects/warnings: See EPOETIN.

Arava

(Aventis Pharma) is a proprietary, prescription-only preparation of leflumomide, an IMMUNOSUPPRESSANT drug used as a disease-modifying ANTIRHEUMATIC. Its use is confined to specialist centres. It is available as tablets.
✚▲ Side-effects/warnings: See LEFLUMOMIDE.

Aredia Dry Powder

(Novartis) is a proprietary, prescription-only preparation of disodium pamidronate. It is used to treat bone disorders, and is available in a form for intravenous infusion.
✚▲ Side-effects/warnings: See DISODIUM PAMIDRONATE.

Aricept

(Eisai, Pfizer) is a prescription-only form of the ANTICHOLINESTERASE donepezil which can be used in DEMENTIA TREATMENT. Available as tablets.
✚▲ Side-effects/warnings: See DONEPEZIL.

Aridil

(CP) is a proprietary, prescription-only compound preparation of the (*potassium-sparing*) DIURETIC amiloride hydrochloride and the (*loop*) diuretic furosemide (frusemide) (a combination called co-amilofruse 10/80). It can be used to treat oedema. Available as tablets.
✚▲ Side-effects/warnings: See AMILORIDE HYDROCHLORIDE; FUROSEMIDE.

Arilvax

(Evans Medical) is a proprietary, prescription-only VACCINE preparation. It can be used to prevent infection by yellow fever, and is available

in a form for subcutaneous injection.
✚▲ Side-effects/warnings: See YELLOW FEVER VACCINE.

Arimidex
(AstraZeneca) is a proprietary, prescription-only preparation of the 'indirect' HORMONE ANTAGONIST anastrozole. It can be used as an ANTICANCER drug in the advanced stages of breast cancer in post-menopausal women, and is available as tablets.
✚▲ Side-effects/warnings: See ANASTROZOLE.

Arpicolin
(Rosemont) is a proprietary, prescription-only preparation of the ANTICHOLINERGIC (ANTIMUSCARINIC) procyclidine hydrochloride. It can be used in the treatment of parkinsonism, and is available as a syrup.
✚▲ Side-effects/warnings: See PROCYCLIDINE HYDROCHLORIDE.

Arret
(Johnson & Johnson • MSD) is a proprietary, non-prescription preparation of the (OPIOID) ANTIDIARRHOEAL loperamide hydrochloride. It can be used to relieve acute diarrhoea and its associated discomfort, and is available as capsules. It is not given to children, except on medical advice.
✚▲ Side-effects/warnings: See LOPERAMIDE HYDROCHLORIDE.

Artelac SDU
(Pharma-Global) is a proprietary, non-prescription preparation of HYPROMELLOSE. It can be used as artificial tears to treat dryness of the eyes due to disease, and is available as eye-drops.
✚▲ Side-effects/warnings: HYPROMELLOSE.

Arthrofen
(Ashbourne) is a proprietary, prescription-only preparation of the (NSAID) NON-NARCOTIC ANALGESIC and ANTIRHEUMATIC ibuprofen. It can be used to relieve pain, particularly that of rheumatic disease and other musculoskeletal disorders, period pain, and migraine. It is available as tablets.
✚▲ Side-effects/warnings: See IBUPROFEN.

Arthrosin
(Ashbourne) is a proprietary, prescription-only preparation of the (NSAID) NON-NARCOTIC ANALGESIC and ANTIRHEUMATIC naproxen. It can be used to relieve pain, particularly rheumatic and arthritic pain, to treat other musculoskeletal disorders, and period pain. It is available as tablets.
✚▲ Side-effects/warnings: See NAPROXEN.

Arthrotec
(Searle; Pharmacia) is a proprietary, prescription-only compound preparation of the powerful (NSAID) NON-NARCOTIC ANALGESIC and ANTIRHEUMATIC diclofenac sodium and an ULCER-HEALING DRUG the PROSTAGLANDIN misoprostol. It can be used to treat pain and inflammation in rheumatic disease. This preparation has a novel approach to minimizing the gastrointestinal side-effects of the NSAID by adding prostaglandin, which is the LOCAL HORMONE whose production has been reduced by the NSAID. Prostaglandins are necessary for correct blood circulation in the gastrointestinal tract and if their level is reduced gastrointestinal side-effects (such as ulceration) may occur. It is available as tablets (in two strengths).
✚▲ Side-effects/warnings: See DICLOFENAC SODIUM; MISOPROSTOL.

Arthroxen
(CP) is a proprietary, prescription-only preparation of the (NSAID) NON-NARCOTIC ANALGESIC and ANTIRHEUMATIC naproxen. It can be used to relieve pain and inflammation, particularly in rheumatism, arthritis and other musculoskeletal disorders, and period pain. It is available as tablets.
✚▲ Side-effects/warnings: See NAPROXEN.

artificial saliva
is used to make up a deficiency of saliva in conditions that cause a dry mouth. Common preparations include viscous constituents such as CARMELLOSE SODIUM, SORBITOL, gastric mucin, gum acacia, MALIC ACID and electrolytes, including potassium chloride, sodium chloride and potassium phosphates.

Arythmol
(Knoll) is a proprietary, prescription-only preparation of the ANTI-ARRHYTHMIC propafenone hydrochloride. It can be used to prevent and treat irregularities of the heartbeat,

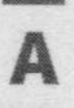

and is available as tablets.
✚▲ Side-effects/warnings: See PROPAFENONE HYDROCHLORIDE.

Asacol

(SmithKline Beecham; GSK) is a proprietary, prescription-only preparation of the AMINOSALICYLATE mesalazine. It can be used to treat patients who suffer from ulcerative colitis but who are unable to tolerate the more commonly used sulfasalazine. It is available as tablets, a foam enema and as suppositories.
✚▲ Side-effects/warnings: See MESALAZINE.

Asasantin Retard

(Boehringer Ingelheim) is a proprietary, prescription-only compound preparation of the ANTIPLATELET drugs dipyridamole and aspirin (low dose). It can be used to prevent thrombosis in the treatment of ischaemic stroke and ischaemic attacks. It is available in the form of capsules.
✚▲ Side-effects/warnings: See ASPIRIN; DIPYRIDAMOLE.

Ascabiol Emulsion

(Rhône-Poulenc Rorer; Aventis Pharma) is a proprietary, non-prescription preparation of benzyl benzoate, which is used as a SCABICIDAL for infestation by mites (scabies). It is available as an emulsion.
✚▲ Side-effects/warnings: See BENZYL BENZOATE.

ascorbic acid

(Vitamin C) is a VITAMIN that is essential for the development and maintenance of cells and tissues. It cannot be synthesized within the body and must be found in the diet (good food sources are vegetables and citrus fruits). Deficiency eventually leads to scurvy, but before that there is a lowered resistance to infection and other disorders may develop, particularly in the elderly. However, vitamin C supplements are rarely necessary with a normal, well-balanced diet. There have been claims that 'pharmacological' (high) doses help prevent colds and because of this it is incorporated into a number of cold remedies (though actually, not at particularly high doses). Administration is oral.
▲ Warnings: It is destroyed by over-cooking or through the action of ultraviolet light (ie sunlight). It may increase the absorption of some other drugs (eg iron preparations).
✪ Related entries: Beechams Cold and Flu Hot Blackcurrant; Beechams Cold and Flu Hot Lemon; Beechams Flu-Plus Hot Berry Fruits; Beechams Flu-Plus Hot Lemon; Ferfolic SV; Ferrograd C; Lemsip Cold + Flu Breathe Easy; Lemsip Pharmacy Flu Strength; Lemsip Sore Throat Anti-bacterial Citrus Fruits Lozenge; Lemsip Cold + Flu Max Strength Capsules; Lemsip Cold + Flu Original Lemon; Lemsip Pharmacy Flu Strength; Paracets Cold Relief Powders; Redoxon; Resolve; Strepsils with Vitamin C 100 mg.

Asendis

(Lederle; Wyeth) is a proprietary, prescription-only preparation of the (TRICYCLIC) ANTIDEPRESSANT amoxapine. It can be used to treat depressive illness, and is available as tablets.
✚▲ Side-effects/warnings: See AMOXAPINE.

Aserbine

(Goldshield) is a proprietary, non-prescription compound preparation of the ANTISEPTIC and KERATOLYTIC agents benzoic acid and salicylic acid with malic acid. It can be used as a desloughing agent in the treatment of superficial ulcers, burns and bedsores so that natural healing can take place. It is available as a cream and a solution.
✚▲ Side-effects/warnings: See BENZOIC ACID; MALIC ACID; SALICYLIC ACID: also, avoid contact with the eyes.

Asilone Antacid Liquid

(SSL) is a proprietary, non-prescription compound preparation of the ANTACID agents aluminium hydroxide and magnesium oxide, and the ANTIFOAMING AGENT dimeticone (as simeticone). It can be used to treat dyspepsia, flatulence and associated abdominal distension, heartburn (including heartburn that occurs with hiatus hernia, pregnancy and reflux oesophagitis), and to soothe the symptoms of peptic ulcers. It is available as a liquid, and is not normally given to children, except on medical advice.
✚▲ Side-effects/warnings: See ALUMINIUM HYDROXIDE; DIMETICONE.

Asilone Antacid Tablets

(SSL) is a proprietary, non-prescription

compound preparation of the ANTACID aluminium hydroxide and the ANTIFOAMING AGENT dimeticone (as simeticone). It can be used to treat dyspepsia, flatulence and associated abdominal distension, heartburn (including heartburn that occurs with hiatus hernia, pregnancy and reflux oesophagitis), and to soothe the symptoms of peptic ulcers. It is available as tablets and is not normally given to children under 12 years, except on medical advice.
✚▲ Side-effects/warnings: See ALUMINIUM HYDROXIDE; DIMETICONE.

Asilone Heartburn Liquid

(SSL) is a proprietary, non-prescription compound preparation of the ANTACID agents aluminium hydroxide, sodium bicarbonate, alginic acid (as sodium alginate) and magnesium trisilicate. It can be used to treat acid indigestion and heartburn (including heartburn that occurs with hiatus hernia, pregnancy and reflux oesophagitis). It is available as a liquid and is not normally given to children under six years, except on medical advice.
✚▲ Side-effects/warnings: See ALGINIC ACID; ALUMINIUM HYDROXIDE; MAGNESIUM TRISILICATE; SODIUM BICARBONATE.

Asilone Heartburn Tablets

(SSL) is a proprietary, non-prescription compound preparation of the ANTACID agents aluminium hydroxide, sodium bicarbonate and magnesium trisilicate, together with alginic acid. It can be used to give relief of acid indigestion and heartburn. It is available as tablets and is not normally given to children under six years, except on medical advice.
✚▲ Side-effects/warnings: See ALUMINIUM HYDROXIDE; MAGNESIUM TRISILICATE, SODIUM ALGINATE; SODIUM BICARBONATE.

Asilone Suspension

(SSL) is a proprietary, non-prescription compound preparation of the ANTACID agents aluminium hydroxide and magnesium oxide, and the ANTIFOAMING AGENT dimeticone (as simeticone). It can be used to treat dyspepsia, flatulence and associated abdominal distension, heartburn (including heartburn that occurs with hiatus hernia, pregnancy and reflux oesophagitis), and to soothe the symptoms of peptic ulcers. It is available as a suspension and is not normally given to children, except on medical advice.
✚▲ Side-effects/warnings: See ALUMINIUM HYDROXIDE; DIMETICONE.

Asilone Windcheaters

(SSL) is a proprietary, non-prescription preparation of the ANTIFOAMING AGENT dimeticone (as simeticone (simethicone)). It can be used for the symptomatic relief of bloating, flatulence and associated pain, and is available as capsules.
✚▲ Side-effects/warnings: See DIMETICONE.

Askit Powders

(Roche Consumer Health) is a proprietary, non-prescription compound preparation of the (NSAID) NON-NARCOTIC ANALGESIC, ANTIRHEUMATIC and ANTIPYRETIC drugs aspirin and aloxiprin (a buffered form of aspirin), and the STIMULANT caffeine. It can be used to treat mild to moderate pain (including rheumatic pain), to relieve swelling, flu symptoms and other feverish conditions. It is available as a powder and is not normally given to children, except on medical advice.
✚▲ Side-effects/warnings: See ALOXIPRIN; ASPIRIN; CAFFEINE.

Asmabec Clickhaler

(Celltech) is a proprietary, prescription-only preparation of the CORTICOSTEROID and ANTI-ASTHMATIC beclometasone dipropionate. It can be used to prevent asthmatic attacks, and is available in a dry powder for inhalation.
✚▲ Side-effects/warnings: See BECLOMETASONE DIPROPIONATE.

Asmasal Clickhaler

(Celltech) is a proprietary, prescription-only preparation of the BETA-RECEPTOR STIMULANT salbutamol. It can be used as a BRONCHODILATOR in reversible obstructive airways disease, as an ANTI-ASTHMATIC treatment, including exercise-induced asthma. It is available in the form of an inhalant powder (also *Asmasal Spacehaler* aerosol is available).
✚▲ Side-effects/warnings: See SALBUTAMOL.

Asmaven

(Berk; APS) is a proprietary, prescription-only preparation of the BETA-RECEPTOR STIMULANT salbutamol (as salbutamol sulphate). It can be

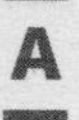

used as a BRONCHODILATOR in reversible obstructive airways disease, as an ANTI-ASTHMATIC treatment. It is available as tablets and an aerosol.
+▲ Side-effects/warnings: See SALBUTAMOL.

Aspav

(Alpham) is a proprietary, prescription-only preparation of the compound analgesic containing the mixed (OPIOID) NARCOTIC ANALGESIC alkaloids (including morphine and codeine) that make up the standard preparation called papaveretum, together with the (NSAID) NON-NARCOTIC ANALGESIC aspirin. It can be used to relieve pain, and is available as soluble tablets.
+▲ Side-effects/warnings: See ASPIRIN; PAPAVERETUM.

aspirin

or acetylsalicylic acid, is a well-known and widely used NSAID (non-steroidal anti-inflammatory drug), NON-NARCOTIC ANALGESIC and ANTIRHEUMATIC. As an analgesic it relieves mild to moderate pain, particularly headache, toothache and period pain.

It is a useful ANTIPYRETIC for reducing raised body temperature in the treatment of the common cold, fevers or flu. Aspirin reduces platelet aggregation, which allows its prophylactic (preventive) use, at a low dose, as an ANTIPLATELET treatment in those at risk (such as those who have already suffered a heart attack or following bypass surgery, as part of ANTI-ANGINA treatment). However, this same action may also increase bleeding time, so those taking ANTICOAGULANT drugs must avoid aspirin. In tablet form, aspirin irritates the stomach lining and may cause bleeding and ulceration; consequently forms of soluble aspirin are preferred.

Many proprietary forms combine aspirin with such drugs as codeine, paracetamol and ibuprofen. Administration is normally oral. Medicines containing aspirin are now no longer normally given to children (except for juvenile arthritis, Still's disease and on medical advice), because of a link with the rare, but serious, condition called Reye's syndrome (which causes inflammation of the brain and liver). Authorities recommend that aspirin is not taken by children or adolescents over 12 years who have a feverish or viral infection. Aspirin can produce the same allergic-like symptoms (including bronchospasm) that occur in many patients after taking NSAIDs, including bronchospasm in 'aspirin-sensitive' asthmatics. Administration can be either oral or topical.
+▲ Side-effects/warnings: See NSAID. Aspirin should not be used by women who are breast-feeding, or by anyone with gout or certain bleeding disorders (eg haemophilia). If taken in addition to other OTC or prescription NSAIDs (and some corticosteroids), side-effects are increased. ANTICOAGULANT agents may increase bleeding. The effects of ANTI-EPILEPTIC drugs (eg PHENYTOIN and SODIUM VALPROATE/valproic acid) may be increased.
✪ Related entries: Alka-Seltzer Original; Alka-Seltzer XS; Alka XS Go;Anadin Analgesic Capsules, Maximum Strength; Anadin Extra; Anadin Extra Soluble Tablets; Anadin Tablets; Angettes 75; Asasantin Retard; Askit Powders; Aspav; Aspro Clear; Beechams Powders; Caprin; co-codaprin; Codis 500; Disprin; Disprin Direct; Disprin Extra; Equagesic; Imazin XL; Maximum Strength Aspro Clear; MigraMax; Nu-Seals Aspirin; Nurse Sykes Powders; Phensic Original; Radian B Heat Spray; Veganin Tablets.

Aspro Clear

(Roche Consumer Health) is a proprietary, non-prescription preparation of the (NSAID) NON-NARCOTIC ANALGESIC, ANTIRHEUMATIC and ANTIPYRETIC aspirin. It can be used to treat various aches and pains and fevers, including the symptoms of colds and flu. It is available as effervescent, lemon-flavoured tablets and is not normally given to children, except on medical advice.
+▲ Side-effects/warnings: See ASPIRIN.

astringent 🅱

precipitate proteins and are used in lotions to harden and protect skin where there are minor abrasions. They can also be used in lozenges, mouthwashes, eye-drops, ear-drops and antiperspirants. Examples include ZINC OXIDE and salts of aluminium (ALUMINIUM ACETATE, ALUMINIUM CHLORIDE and ALUMINIUM HYDROXIDE.

AT 10

(Intrapharm) is a proprietary, prescription-only preparation of dihydrotachysterol, which is a

VITAMIN D analogue. It can be used in the treatment of hypocalcaemic tetany due to hypoparathyroidism, and is available as an oral solution.

✚▲ Side-effects/warnings: See DIHYDROTACHYSTEROL.

Atarax

(Pfizer) is a proprietary, prescription-only preparation of the ANTIHISTAMINE hydroxyzine hydrochloride, which has some additional ANXIOLYTIC properties. It can be used to relieve allergic symptoms, such as pruritus (itching and rashes), and also for the short-term treatment of anxiety. It is available as tablets.

✚▲ Side-effects/warnings: See HYDROXYZINE HYDROCHLORIDE.

Atenix

(Ashbourne) is a proprietary, prescription-only preparation of the BETA-BLOCKER atenolol. It can be used as an ANTIHYPERTENSIVE for raised blood pressure, as an ANTI-ANGINA treatment to relieve symptoms and improve exercise tolerance and as an ANTI-ARRHYTHMIC to regularize heartbeat and to treat myocardial infarction. It is available as tablets.

✚▲ Side-effects/warnings: See ATENOLOL.

AtenixCo

(Ashbourne) is a proprietary, prescription-only compound preparation of the BETA-BLOCKER atenolol and the DIURETIC chlortalidone (a combination called co-tenidone). It can be used as an ANTIHYPERTENSIVE for raised blood pressure, and is available as tablets.

✚▲ Side-effects/warnings: See ATENOLOL; CHLORTALIDONE.

atenolol

is a BETA-BLOCKER which can be used as an ANTIHYPERTENSIVE for raised blood pressure, as an ANTI-ANGINA treatment to relieve symptoms and to improve exercise tolerance and as an ANTI-ARRHYTHMIC to regularize heartbeat and after myocardial infarction. Administration can be either oral or by injection. It is also available as an antihypertensive treatment in the form of compound preparations with DIURETIC or CALCIUM-CHANNEL BLOCKER drugs.

✚▲ Side-effects/warnings: See PROPRANOLOL HYDROCHLORIDE.

✪ **Related entries: Antipressan; Atenix; AtenixCo; Beta-Adalat; co-tenidone; Kalten; Tenben; Tenchlor; Tenif; Tenoret 50; Tenoretic; Tenormin; Totaretic.**

Ativan

(Wyeth) is a proprietary, prescription-only preparation of the BENZODIAZEPINE lorazepam. It can be used as an ANXIOLYTIC in the short-term treatment of anxiety, as a HYPNOTIC in short-term treatment for insomnia, as an ANTI-EPILEPTIC in status epilepticus and as a SEDATIVE, including in postoperative premedication. It is available as tablets or in a form for injection.

✚▲ Side-effects/warnings: See LORAZEPAM.

atorvastatin

is a (*statin*) LIPID-REGULATING DRUG that can be used in hyperlipidaemia to reduce the levels, or change the proportions, of various lipids in the bloodstream. It is usually administered only to patients in whom a strict and regular dietary regime, alone, is not having the desired effect and in familial hypercholesterolaemia. Administration is oral.

✚▲ Side-effects/warnings: See SIMVASTATIN. Also reports of anorexia, insomnia, alopecia, impotence, chest pains, hypoglycaemia and hyperglycaemia, tingling in the extremities, effects on blood sugar; rarely angioedema and hepatitis. Patients should report any muscle pain, weakness or tenderness.

✪ **Related entry: Lipitor.**

atosiban

is one of a recently introduced type of drug, an OXYTOCIN-RECEPTOR ANTAGONIST, which can be used to prevent uncomplicated premature labour (between 24 and 33 weeks of gestation). It is given by intravenous infusion.

✚ Side-effects: Nausea and vomiting, tachycardia, hypotension, headache, hot flushes, dizziness, hyperglycaemia and reactions at the injection site. Less commonly, pruritus and rash, fever and insomnia.

▲ Warnings: Atosiban is a new specialist hospital drug and full patient assessment and monitoring will be carried out prior to, during and after its use.

✪ **Related entry: Tractocile.**

atovaquone

is an ANTIPROTOZOAL. It is used to treat

pneumonia caused by the protozoan (but fungal-like) micro-organism *Pneumocystis carinii* in patients whose immune system has been suppressed (either following transplant surgery or because of a disease such as AIDS). It is also available combined with proguanil hydrochloride for prophylactic antimalarial treatment. Administration is oral.
✚ Side-effects: Diarrhoea, nausea and vomiting, headache, insomnia, fever, rash, changes in liver function and effects on the blood.
▲ Warnings: Initial gastrointestinal upsets cause difficulties (eg in taking food). Administer with care to patients with impaired kidney or liver function, or who are pregnant. It should not be taken by patients who are breast-feeding.
✪ **Related entries: Malarone; Wellvone.**

atracurium besilate

(atracurium besylate) is a *non-depolarizing* SKELETAL MUSCLE RELAXANT. It can be used to induce muscle paralysis during surgery, and is administered by injection.
✚▲ Side-effects/warnings: It is a specialist drug used by anaesthetists in hospital.
✪ **Related entry: Tracrium.**

atracurium besylate

see ATRACURIUM BESILATE.

atropine sulphate

(hyoscyamine) is a powerful ANTICHOLINERGIC (acting at muscarinic receptors, an ANTIMUSCARINIC drug), sometimes referred to as a BELLADONNA ALKALOID because of its origin from the family of plants that include *Atropa belladonna* (deadly nightshade). It is able to depress certain functions of the autonomic nervous system which results in smooth muscle relaxation and is therefore a useful ANTISPASMODIC. It is commonly used during operations to dry up secretions and protect the heart.

It can also be used to cause a long-lasting dilation of the pupil of the eye for ophthalmic procedures. Atropine is able to decrease the secretion of gastric acid, but it has too many side-effects to make it suitable for routine treatment of peptic ulcers. It may also be used as an ANTIDOTE in organophosphate poisoning. Administration can be oral, topical or by injection.
✚ Side-effects: Depending on route of administration and dose, there may be dry mouth, difficulty in swallowing and thirst, dilation of the pupils and loss of ability to focus, increase in intraocular pressure (pressure in the eye-ball), dry skin with flushing, slowing then speeding of the heart, urgency then difficulty in urination, constipation, palpitations and heart arrhythmias. Rarely, there may be high temperature accompanied by delirium or hallucinations. When used as eye-drops, there may be other local side-effects such as stinging, irritation, conjunctivitis, contact dermatitis. Systemic side-effects on using eye-drops are more common in the elderly and children.
▲ Warnings: Depending on route and dose, it should not be administered to patients with closed-angle glaucoma, myasthenia gravis, prostate gland enlargement and certain gastrointestinal disorders; and used with caution in patients with urinary retention, ulcerative colitis, pyloric stenosis, or who are pregnant or breast-feeding, or have Down's syndrome. It may worsen gastro-oesophageal reflux and certain cardiovascular disorders.
✪ **Related entries: Actonorm Powder; co-phenotrope; Diarphen; Isopto Atropine; Lomotil; Minims Atropine Sulphate; Tropergen.**

Atrovent

(Boehringer Ingelheim) is a proprietary, prescription-only preparation of the ANTICHOLINERGIC and BRONCHODILATOR ipratropium bromide. It can be used to treat the symptoms of reversible airways obstructive disease, particularly chronic bronchitis, and is available as an aerosol and *Forte* aerosol, a breath-actuated aerosol inhaler (*Autohaler*), a powder for inhalation (*Aerocaps*) and as a nebulizer solution.
✚▲ Side-effects/warnings: See IPRATROPIUM BROMIDE.

Audax Ear Drops

(SSL) is a proprietary, non-prescription compound preparation of the LOCAL ANAESTHETIC choline salicylate (with glycerin). It can be used as a local pain-reliever in the outer or middle ear and as an aid to wax removal. It is available as ear-drops and is not normally given to children under one year, except on medical advice.
✚▲ Side-effects/warnings: See CHOLINE SALICYLATE.

Audicort

(Wyeth) is a proprietary, prescription-only compound preparation of the ANTI-INFLAMMATORY and CORTICOSTEROID triamcinolone (in the form of acetonide) and the ANTIBACTERIAL and (AMINOGLYCOSIDE) ANTIBIOTIC neomycin (as undecanoate). It can be used to treat infections of the outer ear, and is available as ear-drops.

✚▲ Side-effects/warnings: See NEOMYCIN SULPHATE; TRIAMCINOLONE.

Augmentin

(SmithKline Beecham; GSK) is a proprietary, prescription-only compound preparation of the broad-spectrum ANTIBACTERIAL and (PENICILLIN) ANTIBIOTIC amoxicillin (as trihydrate) and the PENICILLINASE INHIBITOR clavulanic acid (a combination known as co-amoxiclav). It can be used to treat a range of infections, and is available in a number of forms (one called *Augmentin-Duo*): as tablets, dispersible tablets, an oral suspension and in a form for injection or intravenous infusion.

✚▲ Side-effects/warnings: See AMOXICILLIN; CLAVULANIC ACID; CO-AMOXICLAV.

auranofin

is a form in which gold may be used as an ANTI-INFLAMMATORY and ANTIRHEUMATIC treatment. It is used to treat severe, progressive rheumatoid arthritis when NSAID treatment alone is not adequate. Administration is oral.

✚▲ Side-effects/warnings: See SODIUM AUROTHIOMALATE. There may also be diarrhoea; it should be administered with caution to patients with inflammatory bowel disease. In addition to the warning listed under sodium aurothiomalate, if there is conjunctivitis or hair loss, report this to your doctor. It will take several months for full therapeutic effects but if there is no improvement after nine months, treatment may be discontinued.

✪ Related entry: Ridaura.

Aureocort

(Lederle; Wyeth) is a proprietary, prescription-only compound preparation of the CORTICOSTEROID triamcinolone (in the form of acetonide) and the ANTIBACTERIAL and (TETRACYCLINES) ANTIBIOTIC chlortetracycline (as hydrochloride). It can be used to treat severe inflammatory skin disorders, including forms of eczema that are resistant to less powerful corticosteroids, and psoriasis. It is available as an ointment.

✚▲ Side-effects/warnings: See CHLORTETRACYCLINE; TRIAMCINOLONE.

Aureomycin

(Lederle; Wyeth) is a proprietary, prescription-only preparation of the ANTIBACTERIAL and (TETRACYCLINES) ANTIBIOTIC chlortetracycline (as hydrochloride). It can be used to treat eye and skin infections, and is available as an ophthalmic (eye) ointment and cream.

✚▲ Side-effects/warnings: See CHLORTETRACYCLINE.

Avandia

(SmithKline Beecham; GSK) is a recently introduced proprietary, prescription-only preparation of ROSIGLITAZONE (as maleate). It can be used in DIABETIC TREATMENT of Type II diabetes (non-insulin-dependent diabetes mellitus; NIDDM; maturity-onset diabetes), and is available as tablets.

✚▲ Side-effects/warnings: See ROSIGLITAZONE.

Avaxim

(Aventis Pasteur) is a proprietary, prescription-only VACCINE preparation of hepatitis A vaccine. It can be used to protect people at risk from infection with hepatitis A. It is available in a form for injection.

✚▲ Side-effects/warnings: see HEPATITIS A VACCINE.

Aveeno

(Bioglan) is a proprietary, non-prescription preparation of colloidal oatmeal and an EMOLLIENT base. It can be used for eczema, itching and other skin complaints, and is available as a cream, lotion and a bath oil.

Avloclor

(AstraZeneca) is a proprietary, prescription-only preparation of the ANTIMALARIAL drug chloroquine (as phosphate). It can be used to prevent or suppress certain forms of malaria and also as an ANTIRHEUMATIC to treat active rheumatoid arthritis (including juvenile arthritis), also discoid and systemic lupus erythematosus. It is available as tablets. (This

A

product also appears in a non-prescription preparation, as tablets or syrup, labelled for use in the prevention of malaria.)
+▲ Side-effects/warnings: See CHLOROQUINE.

AVOCA
(Bray) is a proprietary, non-prescription preparation of silver nitrate, a KERATOLYTIC agent (with potassium nitrate) which can be used to dissolve verrucas and common warts. It is available as a caustic pencil containing silver nitrate (along with an emery file, dressings and protector pads).
+▲ Side-effects/warnings: See SILVER NITRATE.

Avomine
(ManxPharma) is a proprietary, non-prescription preparation of the ANTIHISTAMINE promethazine teoclate (promethazine theoclate). It can be used as an ANTINAUSEANT for motion sickness, general nausea and labyrinthine disorders. It is available as tablets. It is not recommended for children under five years, except on medical advice.
+▲ Side-effects/warnings: See PROMETHAZINE TEOCLATE.

Avonex
(Biogen) is a proprietary, prescription-only preparation of the drug interferon (in the form of beta-1a). It can be used to treat relapsing-remitting multiple sclerosis. It is available in a form for intramuscular injection.
+▲ Side-effects/warnings: See INTERFERON.

Axid
(Lilly) is a proprietary, prescription-only preparation of the H_2-ANTAGONIST nizatidine. It can be used as an ULCER-HEALING DRUG for benign peptic ulcers (in the stomach or duodenum), gastro-oesophageal reflux, dyspepsia and associated conditions. It is available as capsules and in a form for injection.
+▲ Side-effects/warnings: See NIZATIDINE.

Axsain
(Elan) is a proprietary, non-prescription preparation of capsaicin, the main active principle of capsaicin oleoresin, which has a COUNTER-IRRITANT, or RUBEFACIENT, action. It can be applied to the skin for symptomatic relief of post-herpatic neuralgia and painful diabetic neuropathy (after lesions have healed), and is available as a cream.
+▲ Side-effects/warnings: See CAPSAICIN.

Azactam
(Squibb; Bristol-Myers Squibb) is a proprietary, prescription-only preparation of the ANTIBACTERIAL and (BETA-LACTAM) ANTIBIOTIC aztreonam. It can be used to treat severe infections, and is available in a form for injection.
+▲ Side-effects/warnings: See AZTREONAM.

Azamune
(Penn) is a proprietary, prescription-only preparation of the (CYTOTOXIC) IMMUNOSUPPRESSANT azathioprine. It can be used to treat tissue rejection in transplant patients and for a variety of autoimmune and inflammatory diseases, including as an ANTIRHEUMATIC. It is available as tablets.
+▲ Side-effects/warnings: See AZATHIOPRINE.

azapropazone
is a (NSAID) NON-NARCOTIC ANALGESIC and ANTIRHEUMATIC drug. It is used to treat only serious cases of rheumatoid arthritis, acute gout and certain rheumatic diseases of the spine (ankylosing spondylitis), because of its side-effects. Administration is oral.
+▲ Side-effects/warnings: See NSAID; but there is a high incidence of gastrointestinal disturbances, so it is restricted to use where other drugs have proved ineffective in serious inflammatory conditions. It is not to be used if there is inflammatory bowel disease or porphyria. There is also a seriously prolonged potentiation of the bleeding time when anticoagulants are being used. It should not be given to patients with gastric ulcers or kidney disease. It may cause rashes; also avoid strong sunlight (because of a risk of photosensitivity).
✪ Related entry: Rheumox.

azatadine maleate
is an ANTIHISTAMINE which can be used for the symptomatic relief of allergic symptoms such as hay fever and urticaria. Administration is oral.
+▲ Side-effects/warnings: See ANTIHISTAMINE. Because of its sedative side-effects, the performance of skilled tasks, such as driving, may be impaired.
✪ Related entry: Optimine.

A

azathioprine

is a powerful CYTOTOXIC and IMMUNOSUPPRESSANT. It is mainly used to reduce tissue rejection in transplant patients, but it can also be used to treat myasthenia gravis, rheumatoid arthritis, ulcerative colitis and several autoimmune diseases. Administration is either oral or by injection.

✚ Side-effects: These include hypersensitivity reactions, such as dizziness, malaise, nausea and vomiting, fever, muscular pains and shivering, joint pain, skin eruptions, hypotension with interstitial nephritis, changes in liver function, jaundice, heart arrhythmias, low blood pressure (requiring withdrawal of treatment), symptoms of bone marrow suppression, which should be reported (eg bleeding or bruising), or infection.

▲ Warnings: It is not to be given to patients with known sensitivity to azathioprine or mercaptopurine; or who are pregnant; monitoring is required throughout treatment with blood-count checks.

✪ **Related entries: Azamune; Immunoprin; Imuran; Oprisine.**

azelaic acid

is a drug which has mild ANTIBACTERIAL and KERATOLYTIC properties, and can be used to treat skin conditions such as acne. Administration is topical.

✚ Side-effects: Some patients experience skin irritation and sensitivity to light.

▲ Warnings: Avoid the eyes when applying. It should be administered with caution to patients who are pregnant or breast-feeding.

✪ **Related entry: Skinoren.**

azelastine hydrochloride

is an ANTIHISTAMINE which can be used for the symptomatic relief of allergic rhinitis (inflammation of the mucosal lining of the nose) and seasonal allergic conjunctivitis. Administration is topical in the form of a nasal spray and as eye-drops.

✚▲ Side-effects/warnings: See ANTIHISTAMINE; but any adverse effects are less severe when given locally. It may cause irritation and taste disturbances.

✪ **Related entries: Optilast; Rhinolast; Rhinolast Allergy.**

azidothymidine

see ZIDOVUDINE.

azithromycin

is an ANTIBACTERIAL and ANTIBIOTIC of the MACROLIDE group. It has more activity against Gram-negative organisms compared to erythromycin (though less against Gram-positive bacteria) and can be used as an alternative for people allergic to penicillin. It can be used to treat infections of the middle ear, the respiratory tract (including *H. influenzae*), the skin and soft tissues and genital chlamydia infections. It has a long duration of action and so usually it can be taken once a day. Administration is oral.

✚▲ Side-effects/warnings: See ERYTHROMYCIN, but it has less gastrointestinal effects. Administer with caution to patients who are pregnant or breast-feeding. It should not be used in patients with liver impairment. Also, dyspepsia, dizziness, anorexia, headache, photosensitivity, weakness, tingling, effects on liver and kidney, tinnitus.

✪ **Related entry: Zithromax.**

azole

is the name of an important group of synthetic drugs mainly used for their broad-spectrum ANTIFUNGAL activity, working against most fungi and yeasts. Others have some useful ANTIPROTOZOAL or weak ANTIBACTERIAL activity. They are thus all ANTIMICROBIAL drugs. They are thought to work by damaging the fungal cell membrane by inhibiting an enzyme called demethylase at concentrations harmless to the human. Conventionally, some of the azoles are further divided into chemical subclasses: *imidazoles*, *triazoles* and *benzimidazoles*.

The *imidazole* chemical group includes: CLOTRIMAZOLE, ECONAZOLE NITRATE, KETOCONAZOLE, METRONIDAZOLE, MICONAZOLE, TIABENDAZOLE, TINIDAZOLE, TIOCONAZOLE.

The *triazole* group includes: FLUCONAZOLE, ITRACONAZOLE, MEBENDAZOLE.

The *benzimidazole* group includes: TIABENDAZOLE.

Azopt

(Alcon) is a recently introduced proprietary, prescription-only preparation of the CARBONIC-ANHYDRASE INHIBITOR brinzolamide. It is used in GLAUCOMA TREATMENT and for ocular hypertension, and is available as eye-drops.

✚▲ Side-effects/warnings: See BRINZOLAMIDE.

AZT

see ZIDOVUDINE.

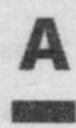

aztreonam

is an ANTIBACTERIAL and ANTIBIOTIC drug of the BETA-LACTAM group. It can be used to treat severe infections caused by Gram-negative bacteria, including *Pseudomonas aeruginosa*, *Haemophilus influenzae* (Hib), *Neisseria meningitidis*, lung infections in cystic fibrosis, gonorrhoea, cystitis, infections of the urinary tract, *Neisseria gonorrhoeae* Administration is by injection.

✚ Side-effects: Vomiting, nausea, diarrhoea and abdominal pain; altered taste and mouth ulcers; skin rashes; hepatitis, jaundice and blood disorders.

▲ Warnings: It should not be administered to patients who are pregnant or breast-feeding. It should be administered with caution in patients with certain liver or kidney disorders.

✪ **Related entry: Azactam.**

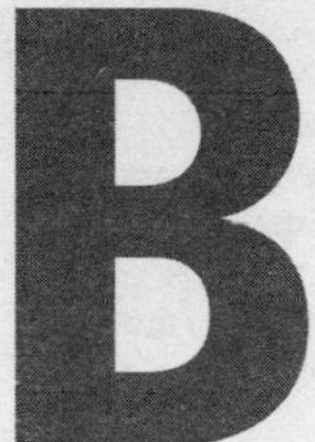

Bacillus Calmette-Guérin Vaccine, Percutaneous

(District Health Authorities; Farillon) (Tub/Vac/BCG (Perc)) is a non-proprietary, prescription-only preparation of BCG vaccine. It is administered percutaneously (multiple puncture through the skin).
✚▲ Side-effects/warnings: See BCG VACCINE.

Bacillus Calmette-Guérin Vaccine

(District Health Authorities; Farillon) (Dried Tub/Vac/BCG) is a non-proprietary, prescription-only preparation of BCG vaccine, and is available in a form for injection.
✚▲ Side-effects/warnings: See BCG VACCINE.

bacitracin zinc

is an ANTIBACTERIAL and ANTIBIOTIC drug (a polypeptide). It is commonly used for the treatment of infections of the skin and usually in combination with other antibiotics in the form of an ointment or spray for topical application.
✪ Related entries: Cicatrin; Polyfax.

baclofen

is a SKELETAL MUSCLE RELAXANT which is used for relaxing muscles that are in spasm, particularly when caused by an injury to or a disease of the central nervous system (eg multiple sclerosis). It works by an action on part of the central nervous system (spinal cord).

Administration is oral.

✚ Side-effects: Sedation, drowsiness, nausea; also, there may be light-headedness, fatigue, disturbances of gait, headache, hallucinations, euphoria, insomnia, depression, tremor, eye-flicker, tingling in the extremities, convulsions, muscle weakness and pain, depression of respiration and blood pressure, gastrointestinal and urinary disturbances; rarely, taste alterations, visual disorders, sweating, rash.
▲ Warnings: It is not used in people with peptic ulcer. Administer with caution to those with psychiatric disorders, impaired respiratory, liver or kidney function; epilepsy, porphyria, certain bladder dysfunction; or who are pregnant. Withdrawal of treatment should be gradual. It may affect the performance of skilled tasks, such as driving, because it causes drowsiness.
✪ Related entries: Baclospas; Balgifen; Lioresal.

Baclospas

(Ashbourne) is a proprietary, prescription-only preparation of the SKELETAL MUSCLE RELAXANT baclofen. It can be used to treat muscle spasm caused by an injury to or a disease of the central nervous system (eg multiple sclerosis), and is available as tablets.
✚▲ Side-effects/warnings: See BACLOFEN.

Bactroban

(Beecham; GSK) is a proprietary, prescription-only preparation of the ANTIBACTERIAL and ANTIBIOTIC mupirocin. It can be used to treat infections of the skin, and is available as an ointment and cream for topical application.
✚▲ Side-effects/warnings: See MUPIROCIN.

Bactroban Nasal

(Beecham; GSK) is a proprietary, prescription-only preparation of the ANTIBACTERIAL and ANTIBIOTIC mupirocin. It can be used to treat staphylococcal infections (including methoxycillin-resistant *Staphylococcus aureus*; MRSA) which is carried in and around the nostrils. It is available as an ointment for topical application.
✚▲ Side-effects/warnings: See MUPIROCIN.

BAL (British Anti-Lewisite)

see DIMERCAPROL.

Balgifen

(Berk; APS) is a proprietary, prescription-only preparation of the SKELETAL MUSCLE RELAXANT baclofen. It can be used to treat muscle spasm caused by an injury to or a disease of the central nervous system (eg multiple sclerosis), and is available as tablets.
✚▲ Side-effects/warnings: See BACLOFEN.

Balmosa Cream

(Pharmax) is a proprietary, non-prescription compound preparation of capsicum oleoresin, camphor, menthol and methyl salicylate, which

B

have COUNTER-IRRITANT, or RUBEFACIENT, actions. It can be applied to the skin for symptomatic relief of muscular rheumatism, fibrosis, lumbago and sciatica, and also for pain associated with unbroken chilblains. It is available as a cream.
✚▲ Side-effects/warnings: See CAMPHOR; CAPSICUM OLEORESIN; MENTHOL; METHYL SALICYLATE.

balsalazide disodium

is an AMINOSALICYLATE, a drug related to MESALAZINE and a pro-drug of 5-aminosalicylic acid, which can be used in the treatment of ulcerative colitis, particularly in patients sensitive to the sulphonamide content of SULPHASALAZINE. Administration is oral.
✚ Side-effects: Diarrhoea and abdominal pain, nausea and vomiting, headache; rarely, worsening of colitis, hepatitis, pancreatitis, blood disturbances, hypersensitivity reactions. Patients should tell their doctor if they have any unexplained bruising, bleeding, sore throat, fever or malaise, because of possible effects on the blood requiring treatment to be stopped.
▲ Warnings: It should not be administered to patients who are allergic to aspirin or other salicylates; it should be administered with caution to those who are pregnant or breast-feeding.
✪ **Related entry: Colazide.**

Bambec

(AstraZeneca) is a proprietary, prescription-only preparation of the BETA-RECEPTOR STIMULANT bambuterol hydrochloride. It can be used as a BRONCHODILATOR in reversible obstructive airways disease, such as an ANTI-ASTHMATIC treatment. It is available as tablets.
✚▲ Side-effects/warnings: See BAMBUTEROL HYDROCHLORIDE.

bambuterol hydrochloride

is a SYMPATHOMIMETIC and BETA-RECEPTOR STIMULANT which has good beta$_2$-receptor selectivity. It is mainly used as a BRONCHODILATOR in reversible obstructive airways disease, such as in ANTI-ASTHMATIC treatment. It is a pro-drug of TERBUTALINE SULPHATE (that is, it is converted to terbutaline within the body). Administration is oral.
✚▲ Side-effects/warnings: See SALBUTAMOL. It is not to be used by patients with certain kidney or liver disorders or who are pregnant.
✪ **Related entry: Bambec.**

Bansor Mouth Antiseptic

(Thornton & Ross) is a proprietary, non-prescription preparation of the ANTISEPTIC cetrimide. It can be used to treat sore gums, and is available as a solution to rub into the gums.
✚▲ Side-effects/warnings: See CETRIMIDE.

Baratol

(Shire) is a proprietary, prescription-only preparation of the ALPHA-ADRENOCEPTOR BLOCKER indoramin hydrochloride. It can be used as an ANTIHYPERTENSIVE, often in conjunction with other antihypertensives, and is available as tablets.
✚▲ Side-effects/warnings: See INDORAMIN.

barbiturate 🅱

is the name of a chemical class of drugs that are derived from barbituric acid and have a wide range of essentially depressant actions. They are much less used than they once were, but some are still used as HYPNOTIC, GENERAL ANAESTHETIC, ANTICONVULSANT and ANTI-EPILEPTIC drugs. They work by a direct action on the brain, depressing specific areas and may be slow- or fast-acting, but are all extremely effective. However, they can rapidly cause tolerance and then both psychological and physical dependence (addiction) may result, therefore they are used as infrequently as possible.

Moreover, prolonged use, even in small doses, can have serious toxic side-effects and in overdose they are lethal without specialist intervention. Barbiturates still in use include the hypnotic drugs AMOBARBITAL (amylobarbitone), butobarbital (butobarbitone) and secobarbital sodium (quinalbarbitone sodium); the anticonvulsant and anti-epileptic PHENO-BARBITAL (phenobarbitone) and methyl-phenobarbital (methylphenobarbitone); and the general anaesthetic thiopental sodium (thiopentone sodium). Their use as hypnotics is avoided wherever possible, and limited to severe intractable insomnia in patients are already taking barbiturates.
✚ Side-effects: Depending on the use, dose and type; there may be drowsiness, dizziness, unsteady gait, respiratory depression, headache, hypersensitivity reactions; there may be paradoxical excitement and confusion before sleep.

▲ Warnings: Dependence can readily occur (with withdrawal syndrome including rebound insomnia, anxiety, tremor and convulsions). Administer with caution to patients with certain lung, kidney or liver disorders. Withdrawal should be gradual. They are very dangerous in overdose. The effect of alcohol is enhanced, and they may cause drowsiness the next day, so driving ability may be impaired.

barrier cream

is a substance used to protect the skin against irritants, chapping, urine and faeces (nappy rash), bedsores and toxic substances. It is normally applied as an ointment or a cream (commonly in a WHITE SOFT PARAFFIN or LANOLIN oily base) and often incorporating a silicone (eg DIMETICONE).

basiliximab

is an IMMUNOSUPPRESSANT drug, a monoclonal antibody (a form of pure antibody produced by a type of molecular engineering) which prevents proliferation of the white blood cells, T-lymphocytes, which have an important role in immunity and cell rejection. It has recently been introduced for prophylaxis (prevention) of rejection in kidney transplantation. It is administered together with CICLOSPORIN and corticosteroids (see CORTICOSTEROID). Its use is confined to specialist centres. Administration is by intravenous infusion.

✚▲ Side-effects/warnings: This product is still under evaluation, and is used in specialist centres. It is not used in pregnancy or breast-feeding.

✪ Related entry: Simulect.

Baxan

(Bristol-Myers Squibb) is a proprietary, prescription-only preparation of the ANTIBACTERIAL and (CEPHALOSPORIN) ANTIBIOTIC cefadroxil. It can be used to treat many infections, and is available as capsules and an oral suspension.

✚▲ Side-effects/warnings: See CEFADROXIL.

Bazuka Extra Strength Gel

(DDD) is a proprietary, non-prescription preparation of the KERATOLYTIC agent salicylic acid. It can be used to remove warts, verrucas, corns and calluses, and is available as a gel.

✚▲ Side-effects/warnings: See SALICYLIC ACID.

Bazuka Gel

(DDD) is a proprietary, non-prescription preparation of the KERATOLYTIC agent salicylic acid (with lactic acid). It can be used to remove warts, verrucas, corns and calluses, and is available as a gel.

✚▲ Side-effects/warnings: See SALICYLIC ACID.

BCG vaccine

(bacillus Calmette-Guérin vaccine, BCG) for IMMUNIZATION is a VACCINE produced from *live* attenuated strain of the tuberculosis bacillus *Mycobacterium bovis*, which no longer causes the disease in humans, but stimulates formation in the body of the specific antibodies that react with the tuberculosis bacillus *Mycobacterium tuberculosis* and so can be used as an ANTITUBERCULAR vaccine. It is used for routine vaccination of children (aged 10-14) and in those at risk, such as those likely to come into contact with individuals with active respiratory tuberculosis, veterinary staff, and visitors to countries where there is a high incidence of TB. It is available as Tub/Vac/BCG, a dried preparation for intradermal injection or as Tub/Vac/BCG (Perc) for percutaneous administration, and as other preparations. In a different use, a *live* attenuated preparation prepared from the TICE strain of *Mycobacterium tuberculosis* has recently become available in a form for bladder instillation for use as an IMMUNOSTIMULANT or IMMUNOMODULATOR to help in the treatment of primary or recurrent bladder carcinoma *in situ* and for the prevention of recurrence following surgery.

✚▲ Side-effects/warnings: See VACCINE. When used in bladder cancer therapy, there may be urinary tract effects, such as cystitis, difficult, painful or increased frequency in urination; fever, flu-like symptoms, and occasionally hypersensitivity reactions. It is not used for people who have impaired immune responses, infections of the urinary tract, TB or who are pregnant or breast-feeding.

✪ Related entries: Bacillus Calmette-Guérin Vaccine; Bacillus Calmette-Guérin Vaccine, Percutaneous; OncoTICE; ImmuCyst.

becaplermin

is a form of human *platelet-derived growth factor* (PDGF), manufactured by recombinant technology. GROWTH FACTORS are proteins produced normally in tiny quantities by cells in

the body, acting as a sort of local hormone to modulate cell growth. Growth factors have complex effects on cells, but a topical preparation is under evaluation as an adjunct in the treatment of ulcers found in neuropathic diabetic disease. It is used as a topical preparation.
✚ Side-effects: Irritation, sometimes eruption, oedema.
▲ Warnings: Caution in malignant disease; osteomyelitis; avoid on infected sites, diseased arteries.
✪ Related entry: Regranex.

Beclazone
(IVAX) is a proprietary, prescription-only preparation of the CORTICOSTEROID and ANTI-ASTHMATIC beclometasone dipropionate. It can be used to prevent asthmatic attacks, and is available in an aerosol for inhalation.
✚▲ Side-effects/warnings: See BECLOMETASONE DIPROPIONATE.

Beclazone Easi-Breathe
(IVAX) is a proprietary, prescription-only preparation of the CORTICOSTEROID beclometasone dipropionate. It can be used to prevent asthma attacks and is available in forms for aerosol inhalation with breath-actuated units.
✚▲ Side-effects/warnings: See BECLOMETASONE DIPROPIONATE.

Becloforte
(A&H; GSK) is a proprietary, prescription-only preparation of the CORTICOSTEROID beclometasone dipropionate. It can be used to prevent asthma attacks, and is available in various forms with inhalers and a dry powder used with the *Diskhaler*.
✚▲ Side-effects/warnings: See BECLOMETASONE DIPROPIONATE.

beclometasone dipropionate
(beclomethasone dipropionate; BDP) is a CORTICOSTEROID which is used primarily as an ANTI-ASTHMATIC treatment to prevent attacks and also as an ANTI-INFLAMMATORY for severe skin inflammation (eg eczema and psoriasis) and for inflammatory conditions of the nasal mucosa (eg rhinitis). Administration as an anti-inflammatory preparation is by topical application as a cream or an ointment; as an anti-asthmatic it is administered by inhalation from an aerosol, as a powder for inhalation or as a suspension for nebulization, or an oral spray for nasal rhinitis.
✚▲ Side-effects/warnings: See CORTICOSTEROID; but serious systemic effects are unlikely with the low doses used. As a nasal spray it may cause sneezing and dryness and irritation of the nose and throat (with smell and taste disturbances), nose-bleeds. As a cream or ointment, there may be local skin effects. When inhaled, it may cause hoarseness and candidiasis of the throat and mouth. There may be hypersensitivity reactions such as bronchospasm, rash and angioedema.
✪ Related entries: AeroBec; Asmabec Clickhaler; Beclazone; Beclazone Easi-Breathe; Becloforte; Becodisks; Beconase; Beconase Allergy; Becotide; Care Hayfever Relief Nasal Spray; Filair; Nasobec Hayfever; Propaderm; Qvar; Ventide.

beclomethasone dipropionate
see BECLOMETASONE DIPROPIONATE.

Becodisks
(A&H; GSK) is a proprietary, prescription-only preparation of the CORTICOSTEROID and ANTI-ASTHMATIC beclometasone dipropionate. It can be used to prevent asthmatic attacks, and is available as a powder in discs for inhalation from a *Diskhaler* device.
✚▲ Side-effects/warnings: See BECLOMETASONE DIPROPIONATE.

Beconase
(A&H; GSK) is a proprietary, prescription-only preparation of the CORTICOSTEROID and ANTI-INFLAMMATORY beclometasone dipropionate. It can be used to relieve the symptoms of conditions such as hay fever and allergic and other types of rhinitis. Available as a nasal spray.
✚▲ Side-effects/warnings: See BECLOMETASONE DIPROPIONATE.

Beconase Allergy
(GlaxoWellcome; GSK) is a proprietary, non-prescription preparation of the CORTICOSTEROID and ANTI-INFLAMMATORY beclometasone dipropionate. It can be used to relieve the symptoms of conditions such as hay fever and rhinitis. It is available as a nasal spray. Not used for those under 18 years, except on medical advice.
✚▲ Side-effects/warnings: See BECLOMETASONE DIPROPIONATE.

B

Becotide

(A&H; GSK) is a proprietary, prescription-only preparation of the CORTICOSTEROID and ANTI-ASTHMATIC beclometasone dipropionate. It can be used to prevent asthmatic attacks, and is available in an aerosol for inhalation in three forms: *Becotide-50*, *Becotide-100* and *Becotide-200*.

✚▲ Side-effects/warnings: See BECLOMETASONE DIPROPIONATE.

Bedranol SR

(Lagap) is a proprietary, prescription-only preparation of the BETA-BLOCKER propranolol hydrochloride. It can be used as an ANTIHYPERTENSIVE for raised blood pressure, as an ANTI-ANGINA treatment to relieve symptoms and improve exercise tolerance and as an ANTI-ARRHYTHMIC to regularize heartbeat and to treat myocardial infarction. It can also be used as an ANTITHYROID drug for short-term treatment of thyrotoxicosis, as an ANTIMIGRAINE treatment to prevent attacks, as an ANXIOLYTIC, particularly for symptomatic relief of tremor and palpitations, and, with an ALPHA-ADRENOCEPTOR BLOCKER, in the acute treatment of phaeochromocytoma. It is available as modified-release capsules.

✚▲ Side-effects/warnings: See PROPRANOLOL HYDROCHLORIDE.

Beechams All-In-One

(GSK Consumer Healthcare) is a proprietary, non-prescription compound preparation of the ANTIPYRETIC and NON-NARCOTIC ANALGESIC paracetamol, the SYMPATHOMIMETIC and DECONGESTANT phenylephrine hydrochloride and the EXPECTORANT agent guaifenesin (guaiphenesin). It can be used for the symptomatic relief of colds, flu, aches and pains, and nasal congestion. It is available as a syrup and is not normally given to children, except on medical advice.

✚▲ Side-effects/warnings: See GUAIFENESIN; PARACETAMOL; PHENYLEPHRINE HYDROCHLORIDE.

Beechams Cold and Flu Hot Blackcurrant

(GSK Consumer Healthcare) is a proprietary, non-prescription compound preparation of the NON-NARCOTIC ANALGESIC and ANTIPYRETIC paracetamol, the SYMPATHOMIMETIC and DECONGESTANT phenylephrine hydrochloride and vitamin C (ascorbic acid). It can be used to relieve cold and flu symptoms, feverishness, nasal congestion, aches and pains. It is available as an oral powder and is not normally given to children, except on medical advice.

✚▲ Side-effects/warnings: See ASCORBIC ACID; PARACETAMOL; PHENYLEPHRINE HYDROCHLORIDE.

Beechams Cold and Flu Hot Lemon

(GSK Consumer Healthcare) is a proprietary, non-prescription compound preparation of the NON-NARCOTIC ANALGESIC and ANTIPYRETIC paracetamol, the SYMPATHOMIMETIC and DECONGESTANT phenylephrine hydrochloride and vitamin C (ascorbic acid). It can be used to relieve cold and flu symptoms, feverishness, nasal congestion, aches and pains. It is available as an oral powder and is not normally given to children, except on medical advice.

✚▲ Side-effects/warnings: See ASCORBIC ACID; PARACETAMOL; PHENYLEPHRINE HYDROCHLORIDE.

Beechams Cold and Flu Hot Lemon and Honey

(GSK Consumer Healthcare) is a proprietary, non-prescription compound preparation of the NON-NARCOTIC ANALGESIC and ANTIPYRETIC paracetamol, the SYMPATHOMIMETIC and DECONGESTANT phenylephrine hydrochloride and vitamin C (ascorbic acid). It can be used to relieve cold and flu symptoms, feverishness, nasal congestion, aches and pains. It is available as an oral powder and is not normally given to children, except on medical advice.

✚▲ Side-effects/warnings: See ASCORBIC ACID; PARACETAMOL; PHENYLEPHRINE HYDROCHLORIDE.

Beechams Flu-Plus Caplets

(GSK Consumer Healthcare) is a proprietary, non-prescription compound preparation of the ANTIPYRETIC and NON-NARCOTIC ANALGESIC paracetamol, the SYMPATHOMIMETIC and DECONGESTANT phenylephrine hydrochloride and the STIMULANT caffeine. It can be used for the symptomatic relief of mild to moderate pain, colds, flu, aches and pains and nasal congestion. It is available as caplets and is not normally given to children, except on medical advice.

B

+▲ Side-effects/warnings: See CAFFEINE; PARACETAMOL; PHENYLEPHRINE HYDROCHLORIDE.

Beechams Flu-Plus Hot Berry Fruits
(GSK Consumer Healthcare) is a proprietary, non-prescription compound preparation of the NON-NARCOTIC ANALGESIC paracetamol, the SYMPATHOMIMETIC and DECONGESTANT phenylephrine hydrochloride and vitamin C (ascorbic acid). It can be used for the symptomatic relief of mild to moderate pain, colds, flu, aches and pains, and nasal congestion. It is available as a powder and is not normally given to children, except on medical advice.
+▲ Side-effects/warnings: See ASCORBIC ACID; PARACETAMOL; PHENYLEPHRINE HYDROCHLORIDE.

Beechams Flu-Plus Hot Lemon
(GSK Consumer Healthcare) is a proprietary, non-prescription compound preparation of the NON-NARCOTIC ANALGESIC paracetamol, the SYMPATHOMIMETIC and DECONGESTANT phenylephrine hydrochloride and vitamin C (ascorbic acid). It can be used for the symptomatic relief of mild to moderate pain, colds, flu, aches and pains, and nasal congestion. It is available as a powder and is not normally given to children, except on medical advice.
+▲ Side-effects/warnings: See ASCORBIC ACID; PARACETAMOL; PHENYLEPHRINE HYDROCHLORIDE.

Beechams Powders
(GSK Consumer Healthcare) is a proprietary, non-prescription compound preparation of the (NSAID) NON-NARCOTIC ANALGESIC, ANTIPYRETIC and ANTIRHEUMATIC aspirin and the STIMULANT caffeine. It can be used for the symptomatic relief of mild to moderate pain, colds, flu, aches and pains (including the pain and inflammation of rheumatic disease) and period pain. It is available as tablets and is not normally given to children, except on medical advice.
+▲ Side-effects/warnings: See ASPIRIN; CAFFEINE.

Beechams Powders Capsules
(GSK Consumer Healthcare) is a proprietary, non-prescription compound preparation of the NON-NARCOTIC ANALGESIC paracetamol, the SYMPATHOMIMETIC and DECONGESTANT phenylephrine hydrochloride and the STIMULANT caffeine. It can be used for the symptomatic relief of mild to moderate pain, colds, flu, aches and pains, and nasal congestion. It is available as capsules and is not normally given to children under six years, except on medical advice.
+▲ Side-effects/warnings: See CAFFEINE; PARACETAMOL; PHENYLEPHRINE HYDROCHLORIDE.

Beechams Throat-Plus Blackcurrant Lozenges
(GSK Consumer Healthcare) is a proprietary, non-prescription compound preparation of the ANTISEPTIC agents hexylresorcinol and benzalkonium chloride. It can be used for the relief of painful sore throat and is available as lozenges. It is not normally given to children under seven years, except on medical advice.
+▲ Side-effects/warnings: See HEXYLRESORCINOL; BENZALKONIUM CHLORIDE.

Beechams Throat-Plus Lemon Lozenges
(GSK Consumer Healthcare) is a proprietary, non-prescription compound preparation of the ANTISEPTIC agents hexylresorcinol and benzalkonium chloride. It can be used for the relief of painful sore throat and is available as lozenges. It is not normally given to children under seven years, except on medical advice.
+▲ Side-effects/warnings: See HEXYLRESORCINOL; BENZALKONIUM CHLORIDE.

Beechams Veno's Expectorant
(GSK Consumer Healthcare) is a proprietary, non-prescription preparation of the EXPECTORANT agent guaifenesin (guaiphenesin) with glucose and treacle, and is used to treat symptoms of cough and chesty catarrh, especially after colds and flu, and to soothe a sore throat. It is not normally given to children under three years, except on medical advice.
+▲ Side-effects/warnings: See GLUCOSE; GUAIFENESIN.

Begrivac
(Wyeth) is a proprietary, prescription-only preparation of influenza VACCINE (split virion vaccine; Flu/Vac/Split). It can be used as immunization for the prevention of influenza,

and is available in a form for injection.
✚▲ Side-effects/warnings: See INFLUENZA VACCINE.

belladonna alkaloid

drugs are derived from solanaceous plants such as *Atropa belladonna* (deadly nightshade) and include the drugs ATROPINE SULPHATE (hyoscyamine) and HYOSCINE HYDROBROMIDE (scopolamine). These drugs have ANTICHOLINERGIC (more accurately ANTIMUSCARINIC) properties and are used for a variety of medical purposes. Poisoning due to eating the berries of *Atropa belladonna* is not uncommon, particularly in children. Indeed, it has been one of the more popular poisons throughout history, from the time of Imperial Rome to the Borgias in 15th-century Italy. The name *belladonna* literally means 'beautiful lady' and is thought to refer to the use of the plant as a cosmetic in ancient times, when it was used as eye-drops to dilate the pupils.
✚▲ Side-effects/warnings: See ATROPINE SULPHATE; HYOSCINE HYDROBROMIDE.
✪ **Related entries: Cuxson Gerrard Belladonna Plaster BP; Enterosan.**

Benadryl Allergy Relief

(Warner Lambert; Pfizer) is a proprietary, non-prescription preparation of the ANTIHISTAMINE acrivastine. It can be used to treat the symptoms of allergic disorders, such as hay fever and skin allergies, and is available as capsules. It is not to be used by children, or those over 65 years, except on medical advice.
✚▲ Side-effects/warnings: See ACRIVASTINE.

Benadryl Skin Allergy Relief Cream

(Warner Lambert; Pfizer) is a proprietary, non-prescription preparation of the ANTIHISTAMINE diphenhydramine hydrochloride, the COUNTER-IRRITANT, or rubefacient, camphor and the mild ASTRINGENT zinc oxide. It is available as a cream and can be used to treat the symptoms of irritation such as with sunburn, urticaria, prickly heat, nettle stings and insect bites and hives.
✚▲ Side-effects/warnings: See CAMPHOR; DIPHENHYDRAMINE HYDROCHLORIDE; ZINC OXIDE.

Benadryl Skin Allergy Relief Lotion

(Warner Lambert; Pfizer) is a proprietary, non-prescription preparation of the ANTIHISTAMINE diphenhydramine hydrochloride, the COUNTER-IRRITANT, or rubefacient, camphor and the mild ASTRINGENT zinc oxide. It is available as a lotion and can be used to treat the symptoms of irritation such as with sunburn, urticaria, prickly heat, nettle stings and insect bites and hives.
✚▲ Side-effects/warnings: See CAMPHOR; DIPHENHYDRAMINE HYDROCHLORIDE; ZINC OXIDE.

bendrofluazide

see BENDROFLUMETHIAZIDE.

bendroflumethiazide

(bendrofluazide) is a DIURETIC of the THIAZIDE class. It is used as an ANTIHYPERTENSIVE, either alone or in conjunction with other types of diuretic or other drugs (eg a BETA-BLOCKER). It can also be used in the treatment of oedema. Administration is oral.
✚ Side-effects: There may be mild gastrointestinal upsets, postural hypotension, reversible impotence; low blood potassium, sodium, magnesium and chloride; raised blood urea, glucose and lipids; gout, rarely photosensitivity, blood disorders, skin reactions and pancreatitis.
▲ Warnings: It should not be administered to patients with certain severe kidney or liver disorders. It should be administered with caution to the elderly, or who are pregnant or breast-feeding. It may aggravate diabetes or gout. Blood potassium levels should be monitored in patients taking thiazide diuretics, because they may deplete the body of potassium. It should not be used where there are abnormal levels of sodium and potassium or in Addison's disease. It may aggravate or exacerbate some other conditions (eg systemic lupus erythematosus).
✪ **Related entries: Aprinox; Berkozide; Centyl K; Corgaretic 40; Corgaretic 80; Inderetic; Inderex; Neo-NaClex; Neo-NaClex-K; Prestim; Tenben.**

BeneFIX

(Hyland Immuno) is a proprietary, prescription-only recombinant coagulation factor IX (nonocog alfa) which is prepared synthetically by molecular biology techniques. It can be used in treating patients with a deficiency in factor IX (haemophilia B). It is available in a form for intravenous infusion.
✚▲ Side-effects/warnings: See **factor IX fraction, dried.**

B

Benoral

(Sanofi-Synthelabo) is a proprietary, non-prescription preparation of the (NSAID) NON-NARCOTIC ANALGESIC and ANTIRHEUMATIC drug benorilate, which is derived from both ASPIRIN and PARACETAMOL. It can be used to treat mild to moderate pain, especially the pain of rheumatic disease and other musculoskeletal disorders, also to reduce fever. It is available as tablets, as granules in sachets for oral solution and as a sugar-free suspension.
✚▲ Side-effects/warnings: See BENORILATE.

benorilate

(benorylate) is a (NSAID) NON-NARCOTIC ANALGESIC and ANTIRHEUMATIC drug with ANTIPYRETIC actions. It is chemically derived from both ASPIRIN and PARACETAMOL, and these two pharmacologically active constituents are released into the bloodstream at different rates. It is used particularly to treat the pain of rheumatic disease and other musculoskeletal disorders and to lower a high temperature in fever. Administration is oral.
✚▲ Side-effects/warnings: See NSAID; but it is better tolerated and causes less gastrointestinal disturbances than the majority of this class.
✪ **Related entry: Benoral.**

benorylate

see BENORILATE.

benoxinate

see OXYBUPROCAINE HYDROCHLORIDE.

benperidol

is a powerful ANTIPSYCHOTIC and is chemically a butyrophenone. It is used to treat and tranquillize psychotic patients and is especially used for treating antisocial and deviant forms of sexual behaviour. Administration is oral.
✚▲ Side-effects/warnings: See HALOPERIDOL.
✪ **Related entry: Anquil.**

benserazide hydrochloride

is an ENZYME INHIBITOR which is administered therapeutically in combination with the drug LEVODOPA to treat parkinsonism, but not the parkinsonian symptoms induced by drugs (see ANTIPARKINSONISM). Benserazide prevents levodopa being too rapidly broken down in the body into dopamine and so allowing more levodopa to reach the brain to make up the deficiency of dopamine, which is the major cause of parkinsonian symptoms; therefore less levodopa is needed and there are less side-effects. It is only used in the combination of benserazide hydrochloride with levodopa known in medicine by the simplified name of CO-BENELDOPA. Administration of the combination is oral.
✚▲ Side-effects/warnings: See LEVODOPA.
✪ **Related entries: co-beneldopa; Madopar.**

Benuryl

(IDIS) is a non-proprietary, prescription-only preparation of probenecid available on a named-patient basis only. It can be used to prevent nephrotoxicity associated with the ANTIVIRAL drug CIDOFOVIR. It is available as tablets.
✚▲ Side-effects/warnings: See PROBENECID.

Benylin Chesty Coughs (Non-Drowsy)

(Warner Lambert; Pfizer) is a proprietary, non-prescription compound preparation of the EXPECTORANT guaifenesin (guaiphenesin) and menthol (as levomenthol). It can be used for the symptomatic relief of productive cough, and is available as a syrup. It is not normally given to children under six years, except on medical advice.
✚▲ Side-effects/warnings: See GUAIFENESIN; MENTHOL.

Benylin Chesty Coughs (Original)

(Warner Lambert; Pfizer) is a proprietary, non-prescription compound preparation of the ANTIHISTAMINE diphenhydramine hydrochloride and menthol (as levomenthol). It can be used for the symptomatic relief of cough and associated congestive symptoms, and is available as a syrup. It is not normally given to children under six years, except on medical advice.
✚▲ Side-effects/warnings: See DIPHENHYDRAMINE HYDROCHLORIDE; MENTHOL.

Benylin Children's Chesty Coughs

(Warner Lambert; Pfizer) is a proprietary, non-prescription compound preparation of the EXPECTORANT agent guaifenesin (guaiphenesin). It can be used for the symptomatic relief of productive coughs, and is available as an oral solution. It is not normally given to children

under one year, except on medical advice.
✚▲ Side-effects/warnings: See GUAIFENESIN.

Benylin Children's Coughs and Colds
(Warner Lambert; Pfizer) is a proprietary, non-prescription compound preparation of the ANTIHISTAMINE triprolidine hydrochloride, the ANTITUSSIVE dextromethorphan hydrobromide and menthol. It can be used for the symptomatic relief of persistent, dry, irritating coughs. Available as an oral syrup and not normally given to children under 12 months, except on medical advice.
✚▲ Side-effects/warnings: See DEXTROMETHORPHAN HYDROBROMIDE; MENTHOL; TRIPROLIDINE HYDROCHLORIDE.

Benylin Children's Dry Coughs
(Warner Lambert; Pfizer) is a proprietary, non-prescription preparation of the ANTITUSSIVE pholcodine. It can be used for the symptomatic relief of persistent, dry, irritating coughs. It is available as an oral solution, and is not normally given to children under one year, except on medical advice.
✚▲ Side-effects/warnings: See PHOLCODINE.

Benylin Children's Night Coughs
(Warner Lambert; Pfizer) is a proprietary, non-prescription compound preparation of the ANTIHISTAMINE diphenhydramine hydrochloride and menthol (as levomenthol). It can be used for the symptomatic relief of cough and its congestive symptoms, and for the treatment of hay fever and other allergic conditions of the upper respiratory tract. It is available as an oral solution and is not normally given to children under one year, except on medical advice.
✚▲ Side-effects/warnings: See DIPHENHYDRAMINE HYDROCHLORIDE; MENTHOL.

Benylin Cough and Congestion
(Warner Lambert; Pfizer) is a proprietary, non-prescription compound preparation of the ANTIHISTAMINE diphenhydramine hydrochloride, the ANTITUSSIVE dextromethorphan hydrobromide, the DECONGESTANT pseudoephedrine hydrochloride and menthol. It can be used for the symptomatic relief of cough and congestion with colds. It is available as a syrup and is not normally given to children under six years, except on medical advice.
✚▲ Side-effects/warnings: See DEXTROMETHORPHAN HYDROBROMIDE; DIPHENHYDRAMINE HYDROCHLORIDE; PSEUDOEPHEDRINE HYDROCHLORIDE; MENTHOL.

Benylin Day and Night
(Warner Lambert; Pfizer) is a proprietary, non-prescription preparation which can be used for the symptomatic relief of colds and flu. It is available in the form of two types of compound preparations in the same pack: a amber film-coated tablet (taken during the day) contains the NON-NARCOTIC ANALGESIC and ANTIPYRETIC paracetamol and the SYMPATHOMIMETIC phenylpropanolamine hydrochloride; a blue film-coated tablet (taken at night) contains paracetamol and the ANTIHISTAMINE diphenhydramine hydrochloride. It is not normally given to children, except on medical advice.
✚▲ Side-effects/warnings: See DIPHENHYDRAMINE HYDROCHLORIDE; PARACETAMOL; PHENYLPROPANOLAMINE HYDROCHLORIDE.

Benylin Dry Coughs (Non-Drowsy)
(Warner Lambert; Pfizer) is a proprietary, non-prescription preparation of the ANTITUSSIVE dextromethorphan hydrobromide. It can be used for the symptomatic relief of persistent, dry, irritating coughs. It is available as a syrup and is not normally given to children under six years, except on medical advice.
✚▲ Side-effects/warnings: See DEXTROMETHORPHAN HYDROBROMIDE.

Benylin Dry Coughs (Original)
(Warner Lambert; Pfizer) is a proprietary, non-prescription compound preparation of the ANTIHISTAMINE diphenhydramine hydrochloride, the ANTITUSSIVE dextromethorphan hydrobromide and menthol (as levomenthol). It can be used for the symptomatic relief of persistent, dry, irritating coughs. It is available as a syrup and is not normally given to children under six years, except on medical advice.
✚▲ Side-effects/warnings: See DEXTROMETHORPHAN HYDROBROMIDE; DIPHENHYDRAMINE HYDROCHLORIDE; MENTHOL.

Benylin Four Flu Liquid
(Warner Lambert; Pfizer) is a proprietary, non-

B

prescription compound preparation of the NON-NARCOTIC ANALGESIC and ANTIPYRETIC paracetamol, the SYMPATHOMIMETIC pseudoephedrine hydrochloride and the ANTIHISTAMINE diphenhydramine hydrochloride. It can be used for the symptomatic relief of colds and flu and coughs, and is available in the form of an oral liquid. It is not normally given to children under six years, except on medical advice.

✚▲ Side-effects/warnings: See DIPHENHYDRAMINE HYDROCHLORIDE; PARACETAMOL; PSEUDOEPHEDRINE HYDROCHLORIDE.

Benylin Four Flu Tablets

(Warner Lambert; Pfizer) is a proprietary, non-prescription compound preparation of the NON-NARCOTIC ANALGESIC and ANTIPYRETIC paracetamol, the SYMPATHOMIMETIC pseudoephedrine hydrochloride and the ANTIHISTAMINE diphenhydramine hydrochloride. It can be used for the symptomatic relief of colds and flu and coughs, and is available as tablets. It is not normally given to children under six years, except on medical advice.

✚▲ Side-effects/warnings: See DIPHENHYDRAMINE HYDROCHLORIDE; PARACETAMOL; PSEUDOEPHEDRINE HYDROCHLORIDE.

Benylin with Codeine

(Warner Lambert Consumer Healthcare; Pfizer) is a proprietary, non-prescription compound preparation of the ANTITUSSIVE codeine phosphate, the ANTIHISTAMINE diphenhydramine hydrochloride and menthol (as levomenthol). It can be used for the symptomatic relief of persistent, dry cough, and is available as a syrup. It is not normally given to children under six years, except on medical advice.

✚▲ Side-effects/warnings: See CODEINE PHOSPHATE; DIPHENHYDRAMINE HYDROCHLORIDE; MENTHOL.

benzalkonium chloride

is an ANTISEPTIC which has some KERATOLYTIC properties. It can be topically applied to remove hard, dead skin from around wounds or ulcers, or to dissolve warts. It can also be used on minor abrasions and burns and (in the form of lozenges) for mouth ulcers, gum disease and sore throats. For other than oral purposes, administration is topical in the form of a cream or (combined with bromine) as a paint.

✚▲ Side-effects/warnings: Avoid normal skin when using as a cream or paint.

✪ Related entries: Beechams Throat-Plus Blackcurrant Lozenges;Beechams Throat-Plus Lemon Lozenges; Bradosol Sugar-Free Cherry Menthol Lozenges; Bradosol Sugar-Free Original Citrus Lozenges; Conotrane; Dermol 500 Lotion; Dermol 200 Shower Emollient; Dettol Antiseptic Wash; Dettol Fresh; Drapolene Cream; Emulsiderm Emollient; Ionax Scrub; Ionil T; Mycil Ointment; Neo Baby Cream; Oilatum Junior Flare-Up; Timodine.

Benzamycin

(Bioglan) is a proprietary, prescription-only compound preparation of the ANTIBACTERIAL and (MACROLIDE) ANTIBIOTIC erythromycin and the KERATOLYTIC and ANTIMICROBIAL benzoyl peroxide. It can be used to treat acne, and is available as a gel for topical application.

✚▲ Side-effects/warnings: See BENZOYL PEROXIDE; ERYTHROMYCIN.

benzatropine mesylate

see BENZTROPINE MESILATE.

benzhexol hydrochloride

(trihexyphenidyl hydrochloride) is an ANTICHOLINERGIC (ANTIMUSCARINIC) drug which is used in the treatment of some types of parkinsonism (see ANTIPARKINSONISM). It increases mobility and decreases rigidity and tremor, and the tendency to produce an excess of saliva is also reduced, but it has only a limited effect on bradykinesia. Additionally, the drug has the capacity to treat these symptoms (extrapyramidal symptoms, but not tardive dyskinesia), in some cases, where they are produced by drugs. It is thought to work by correcting the over-effectiveness of the neurotransmitter ACETYLCHOLINE (cholinergic excess), which is caused by the deficiency of dopamine that occurs in parkinsonism. Administration, which may be in conjunction with other drugs used to relieve parkinsonism, is oral.

✚ Side-effects: Dry mouth, gastrointestinal disturbances, blurred vision, dizziness; frequently there is urinary retention, speeding of the heart,

sensitivity reactions or nervousness. Rarely, and only in susceptible patients, there may be confusion, excitement and psychological disturbance.
▲ Warnings: It should not be used in patients with urinary retention, closed-angle glaucoma, gastrointestinal obstruction. Administer with caution to those with impaired kidney or liver function, or cardiovascular disease. Withdrawal of treatment must be gradual. May effect skilled tasks (eg driving). There is an addictive liability because it can cause euphoria.
✪ Related entry: Broflex.

benzocaine

is a LOCAL ANAESTHETIC which is used by topical application to relieve pain in the skin surface or mucous membranes, particularly in or around the mouth (eg mouth ulcers) and throat, or (in combination with other drugs) in the ears. Administration is topical and in various forms.
▲ Warnings: Prolonged use should be avoided and some patients may experience sensitivity reactions.
✪ Related entries: AAA Mouth and Throat Spray; Anthisan Plus Sting Relief Spray; Burneze Spray; Dequacaine Lozenges; Intralgin; Lanacane Cream; Merocaine Lozenges; Rinstead Adult Gel; Solarcaine Cream; Solarcaine Lotion; Solarcaine Spray; Tyrozets; Ultra Chloraseptic; Wasp-Eze Spray.

benzodiazepine 🄱

drugs belong chemically to a large group of agents that have a marked effect upon the central nervous system. The effect varies according to the level of dose, the frequency of dosage and which member of the group is used. They have to varying degrees SEDATIVE, ANXIOLYTIC, HYPNOTIC, ANTICONVULSANT, ANTI-EPILEPTIC and SKELETAL MUSCLE RELAXANT actions. They can also cause amnesia which, in addition to their other properties, is a reason why they may be used as a postoperative medication in order to allow patients to forget unpleasant procedures. Benzodiazepines are used in the initial stages of LITHIUM treatment of mania, and for night terrors and sleep-walking in children. Benzodiazepines that are used as hypnotics have virtually replaced earlier drugs, such as the BARBITURATE class and CHLORAL HYDRATE, because they are just as effective but much safer in overdose.

There are now benzodiazepine ANTAGONIST drugs, such as FLUMAZENIL, that can be used to reverse some of the central nervous system effects of benzodiazepines, for instance, at the end of operations. It is now realized that dependence may result from prolonged use of benzodiazepines, and there may be a paradoxical increase in hostility and aggression in patients having long-term treatment.

The best-known and most-used benzodiazepines include DIAZEPAM (which can be used for many purposes, including to control anxiety, skeletal muscle relaxation during operations, to relieve withdrawal symptoms of addiction to other drugs (such as alcohol), the convulsions of epilepsy or for drug poisoning), NITRAZEPAM (a widely used hypnotic), CHLORDIAZEPOXIDE and LORAZEPAM (anxiolytic). See also ALPRAZOLAM; CLONAZEPAM; FLUNITRAZEPAM; FLURAZEPAM; LORMETAZEPAM; OXAZEPAM; TEMAZEPAM.
✚ Side-effects: Depending on use, dose and type; there may be drowsiness and light-headedness the day after treatment, confusion and impaired movement and coordination (particularly in the elderly), dependence, mental changes, memory loss, aggression; occasionally, vertigo, headache, hypotension, salivation changes, rashes, visual disturbances, changes in libido, urinary retention, liver and blood disorders, jaundice and gastrointestinal disorders.
▲ Warnings: Depending on use, dose and type; they should not be given to patients with respiratory depression or acute pulmonary insufficiency, psychosis or phobic or obsessional states. They are given with care to those with muscle weakness, history of alcohol or drug abuse, severe personality disorders, liver or kidney impairment; who are elderly or debilitated, or have porphyria, or who are pregnant or breast-feeding. Prolonged use carries a risk of dependence. In the presence of alcohol, benzodiazepines may cause serious respiratory depression. Drowsiness may affect driving skills.

Benzoic Acid Ointment, Compound, BP

is a non-proprietary, non-prescription compound preparation of the ANTIFUNGAL and KERATOLYTIC agents salicylic acid and benzoic acid. It is commonly used to treat patches of ringworm infection on the limbs, palms, soles of

B

feet and chest. It is available in the form of an ointment, which is also known as *Whitfield's Ointment*.
✚▲ Side-effects/warnings: See BENZOIC ACID; SALICYLIC ACID.

benzoic acid

has ANTIFUNGAL and KERATOLYTIC activity. It can be used to treat ringworm infections, and is incorporated into non-proprietary and proprietary ointments and creams.
✚▲ Side-effects/warnings: It is regarded as safe in normal topical use.
✪ **Related entries: Aserbine; Benzoic Acid Ointment, Compound, BP.**

benzoyl peroxide

is a KERATOLYTIC and ANTIMICROBIAL drug which is used in combination with other drugs to treat conditions like acne and skin infections such as athlete's foot. Administration is topical.
✚ Side-effects: Some patients experience skin irritation.
▲ Warnings: It should not be used to treat the skin disease of the facial blood vessels, rosacea. When applying, avoid the eyes, mouth and mucous membranes. It may bleach fabrics.
✪ **Related entries: Acnecide; Benzamycin; Brevoxyl; Oxy 10 Lotion; Oxy 5 Lotion; Oxy On-The-Spot; PanOxyl 10 Acnegel; PanOxyl 10 Lotion; PanOxyl 5 Acnegel; PanOxyl 5 Cream; PanOxyl 5 Lotion; PanOxyl Aquagel 10; PanOxyl Aquagel 2.5; PanOxyl Aquagel 5; PanOxyl Wash 10; Quinoderm Cream; Quinoderm Cream 5; Quinoderm Lotio-Gel 5%; Quinoped Cream.**

benzthiazide

is a DIURETIC of the THIAZIDE class. It is used in the treatment of oedema. Administration is oral.
✚▲ Side-effects/warnings: See BENDROFLUMETHIAZIDE.
✪ **Related entry: Dytide.**

benztropine mesilate

(benzatropine mesylate) is an ANTICHOLINERGIC (ANTIMUSCARINIC) drug which is used in the treatment of some types of parkinsonism (see ANTIPARKINSONISM). It increases mobility and decreases rigidity and tremor, and the tendency to produce an excess of saliva is also reduced, but it has only a limited effect on bradykinesia. Additionally, it has the capacity to treat these symptoms (extrapyramidal symptoms, but not tardive dyskinesia), in some cases, where they are produced by drugs. It is thought to work by correcting the over-effectiveness of the neurotransmitter ACETYLCHOLINE (cholinergic excess), which results from the deficiency of dopamine that occurs in parkinsonism. Administration, which may be with other drugs used to relieve parkinsonism, is either oral or by injection.
✚▲ Side-effects/warnings: See BENZHEXOL HYDROCHLORIDE; but it causes sedation rather than stimulation.
✪ **Related entry: Cogentin.**

benzydamine hydrochloride

has COUNTER-IRRITANT, OR RUBEFACIENT, action and can be used for the symptomatic relief of pain when applied to the skin, mouth ulcers and other sores or inflammation in the mouth and throat. Administration is by topical application.
✚ Side-effects: There may be stinging or numbness on initial oral application. Avoid broken skin and eyes. It should be discontinued if rash develops. If there is any appreciable systemic absorption, further side-effects may be seen.
✪ **Related entry: Difflam.**

benzyl benzoate

can be used either as a SCABICIDAL drug to treat infestation of the skin, chest and limbs by itch-mites (scabies) or as a PEDICULICIDAL to treat head lice infestation. It is also incorporated into suppositories and ointments for haemorrhoids (some with a CORTICOSTEROID). Administration is topical.
✚ Side-effects: There may be skin irritation, a burning sensation and occasionally a rash.
▲ Warnings: Administer with caution to patients who are pregnant or breast-feeding; avoid contact with the eyes, mucous membranes and broken skin. Because it is irritant, it is not normally recommended for children.
✪ **Related entries: Anugesic-HC; Anusol-HC; Anusol Plus HC Ointment; Anusol Plus HC Suppositories; Ascabiol Emulsion; Sudocrem Antiseptic Cream; Sudocream Antiseptic Healing Cream.**

benzylpenicillin

(penicillin G) is the chemical name for the ANTIBACTERIAL drug that was the first of the penicillins to be isolated and used as an

ANTIBIOTIC. Despite the many hundreds of antibiotics introduced since, it still remains the drug of choice in treating many severe infections, including those caused by sensitive strains of meningococcus (eg meningitis and septicaemia) and streptococcus (eg bacterial sore throat, scarlet fever and septicaemia), Lyme disease, in serious conditions when the micro-organism causing the disease has not be identified for certain (eg endocarditis) and to prevent bacterial infection following amputation.

It is usually injected because it is inactivated by digestive acids in the stomach. Its rapid excretion by the kidney also means frequent administration is necessary, unless long-acting preparations are used.
✚ Side-effects: Hypersensitivity reactions which can be serious (including urticaria, fever, joint pains, rashes, angioedema, anaphylaxis, serum sickness-like reactions, haemolytic anaemia, and kidney problems); blood changes; central nervous system toxicity reported, including convulsions (especially with high doses or in severe renal impairment); diarrhoea and colitis; tingling in the extremities with prolonged use.
▲ Warnings: It should not be administered to patients with known allergy to penicillins, and patients should take care to tell their doctors; use with care in patients with impaired kidney function.
✪ **Related entry: Crystapen.**

Berkozide
(Berk; APS) is a proprietary, prescription-only preparation of the (THIAZIDE) DIURETIC bendroflumethiazide. It can be used, either alone or in conjunction with other drugs, in the treatment of oedema and as an ANTIHYPERTENSIVE. It is available as tablets.
✚▲ Side-effects/warnings: See BENDROFLUMETHIAZIDE.

Beta-Adalat
(Bayer) is a proprietary, prescription-only compound preparation of the BETA-BLOCKER atenolol and the CALCIUM-CHANNEL BLOCKER nifedipine. It can be used as an ANTIHYPERTENSIVE for raised blood pressure and angina, and is available as capsules.
✚▲ Side-effects/warnings: See ATENOLOL; NIFEDIPINE.

beta-adrenoceptor-blocking drug 🅴
see BETA-BLOCKER.

beta-adrenoceptor stimulant 🅴
see BETA-RECEPTOR STIMULANT.

beta-agonist 🅴
see BETA-RECEPTOR STIMULANT.

beta-blocker 🅴
(beta-adrenoceptor-blocking) drugs inhibit some actions of the sympathetic nervous system by preventing the actions of ADRENALINE (epinephrine) and NORADRENALINE (norepinephrine) (HORMONE and neurotransmitter mediators, respectively) by blocking the RECEPTORS called beta-adrenoceptors on which they act. Correspondingly, ALPHA-ADRENOCEPTOR BLOCKER agents are drugs used to inhibit the remaining actions by occupying the other main class of adrenoceptor, alpha-adrenoceptors.

These two classes of adrenoceptor are responsible for the very widespread actions of adrenaline and noradrenaline in the body, both in normal physiology and in stress. For example, they speed the heart, constrict or dilate certain blood vessels (thereby increasing blood pressure) and suppress activity in the intestines. In general, they prepare the body for emergency action.

In disease, some of these actions may be inappropriate, exaggerated and detrimental to health, so beta-blockers may be used to restore a more healthy balance. Thus beta-blockers may be used as ANTIHYPERTENSIVE drugs to lower blood pressure when it is abnormally raised in cardiovascular disease; as ANTI-ARRHYTHMIC drugs to correct heartbeat irregularities; as ANTI-ANGINA drugs to prevent the pain of angina pectoris during exercise and to treat myocardial infarction (damage to heart muscle) associated with heart attacks; as ANTIMIGRAINE drugs (prophylaxis; to prevent migraine attacks); as ANXIOLYTIC drugs to reduce anxiety, particularly its manifestations such as tremor and a racing heart; as ANTITHYROID drugs, specifically, shortly before surgery to correct thyrotoxicosis and, in the form of eye-drops, as a GLAUCOMA TREATMENT to lower raised intraocular pressure.

However, there may be a price to pay, in as much as they will also block beta-receptors elsewhere in the body, thereby reducing the normal, beneficial actions of adrenaline and noradrenaline and these side-effects may well be undesirable. For instance, they may precipitate asthma attacks. Similarly, the blood flow in the extremities will often be reduced, so patients may complain of cold feet or hands.

The beta-blockers currently used include ACEBUTOLOL, ATENOLOL, BETAXOLOL HYDROCHLORIDE, BISOPROLOL FUMARATE, CARTEOLOL HYDROCHLORIDE, CARVEDILOL, CELIPROLOL HYDROCHLORIDE, ESMOLOL HYDROCHLORIDE, LABETALOL HYDROCHLORIDE, LEVOBUNOLOL HYDROCHLORIDE, METIPRANOLOL, METOPROLOL TARTRATE, NADOLOL, NEBIVOLOL, OXPRENOLOL HYDROCHLORIDE, PINDOLOL, PROPRANOLOL HYDROCHLORIDE, SOTALOL HYDROCHLORIDE and TIMOLOL MALEATE.

Different beta-blockers are used for different purposes, and there are a number of reasons for this. Some of them are relatively lipid soluble and some are relatively water soluble, and the latter are less likely to enter the fat of the brain cells so have less CNS effects such as sleep disturbances and nightmares (atenolol; celiprolol hydrochloride; nadolol; sotalol hydrochloride). Others have a small intrinsic ability to stimulate the heart, so cause less slowing of the heart or coldness in the extremities (acebutolol; celiprolol hydrochloride; pindolol; oxprenolol hydrochloride). Others again are more active on the heart than other sites such as the bronchioles (called *cardioselective*) so are more suitable for treating people who also have asthma, when there is no alternative (atenolol; betaxolol hydrochloride; bisoprolol fumarate; metoprolol tartrate; nebivolol). There are those that are regarded as safe when given topically to the eye in glaucoma treatment (since only a little drug is absorbed from eye-drops), but side-effects may still occur (betaxolol hydrochloride; carteolol hydrochloride; levobunolol hydrochloride; metipranolol). In general, recently introduced drugs are often only licensed for use in treating a single disorder (eg hypertension) where they have been most extensively tested. But if they prove to be well tolerated by patients, they may eventually be licensed for use in treating a range of disorders: the 'oldest' beta-blocker, propranolol hydrochloride, is used for about a dozen purposes. Beta-blockers are commonly given with other antihypertensives such as DIURETIC and CALCIUM-CHANNEL BLOCKER drugs.

✚▲ Side-effects/warnings: See PROPRANOLOL HYDROCHLORIDE. Some beta-blockers enter the brain less easily than others, and these will cause fewer sleep disturbances and nightmares (eg atenolol, celiprolol, nadolol and sotalol). These side-effects may occur when beta-blockers are used as eye-drops for glaucoma treatment, but less than when taken by mouth or injection. Some beta-blockers which work more specifically on the heart, have fewer general side-effects and are known as *cardioselective*.

Betacap

(Dermal) is a proprietary, prescription-only, preparation of the CORTICOSTEROID and ANTI-INFLAMMATORY betamethasone (as valerate). It can be used to treat severe, non-infective inflammation of the scalp, and is available in a 'Scalp application' water-miscible form.

✚▲ Side-effects/warnings: See BETAMETHASONE.

Beta-Cardone

(Celltech) is a proprietary, prescription-only preparation of the BETA-BLOCKER sotalol hydrochloride. It can be used as an ANTI-ARRHYTHMIC to regularize heartbeat in serious conditions, and is available as tablets.

✚▲ Side-effects/warnings: See SOTALOL HYDROCHLORIDE.

Betadine Antiseptic Paint

(SSL) is a proprietary, non-prescription preparation of the ANTISEPTIC povidone-iodine. It can be used to prevent and treat skin infections and is available as a topical paint.

✚▲ Side-effects/warnings: See POVIDONE-IODINE.

Betadine Dry Powder Spray

(SSL) is a proprietary, non-prescription preparation of the ANTISEPTIC povidone-iodine. It can be used to prevent and treat skin infections in wounds, cuts and burns. It is available as a topical spray and is not normally used on children under two years, except on medical advice.

✚▲ Side-effects/warnings: See POVIDONE-IODINE.

Betadine Gargle and Mouthwash

(SSL) is a proprietary, non-prescription preparation of the ANTISEPTIC povidone-iodine. It can be used to treat mouth and throat infections, and is available as a gargle. It is not normally given to children under six years, except on medical advice.

✚▲ Side-effects/warnings: See POVIDONE-IODINE.

Betadine Ointment

(SSL) is a proprietary, non-prescription

preparation of the ANTISEPTIC povidone-iodine. It can be used to prevent and treat skin infections in minor cuts and wounds and to treat infection in other skin conditions. It is available as an ointment and is not normally used on children under two years.

✚▲ Side-effects/warnings: See POVIDONE-IODINE.

Betadine Shampoo

(SSL) is a proprietary, non-prescription range of preparations of the ANTISEPTIC povidone-iodine and can be used to treat seborrhoeic conditions of the scalp associated with excess dandruff, impetigo and infected sores. It is available as a shampoo. It is not normally given to children under two years, except on medical advice.

✚▲ Side-effects/warnings: See POVIDONE-IODINE.

Betadine Skin Cleanser

(SSL) is a proprietary, non-prescription preparation of the ANTISEPTIC povidone-iodine. It is available as a skin cleanser solution for treating acne.

✚▲ Side-effects/warnings: See POVIDONE-IODINE.

Betadine Vaginal Gel

(SSL) is a proprietary, non-prescription preparation of the ANTISEPTIC povidone-iodine. It is available as a vaginal gel for the treatment of bacterial infections in the vagina and cervix. It is not used for children, except on medical advice.

✚▲ Side-effects/warnings: See POVIDONE-IODINE.

Betadine Vaginal Pessaries

(SSL) is a proprietary, non-prescription preparation of the ANTISEPTIC povidone-iodine. It is available as vaginal pessaries for the treatment of bacterial infections in the vagina and cervix. It is not used for children, except on medical advice.

✚▲ Side-effects/warnings: See POVIDONE-IODINE.

Betadine VC Kit

(SSL) is a proprietary, non-prescription preparation of the ANTISEPTIC povidone-iodine. It is available as a vaginal cleanser that may be used in combination with Betadine Vaginal Pessaries or Betadine Vaginal Gel for the treatment of bacterial infections in the vagina and cervix. It is not used for children, except on medical advice.

✚▲ Side-effects/warnings: See POVIDONE-IODINE.

Betaferon

(Schering Health) is a proprietary, prescription-only preparation of the IMMUNOMODULATOR interferon (in the form of beta-1b). It can be used to treat relapsing-remitting multiple sclerosis, and is available in a form for injection.

✚▲ Side-effects/warnings: See INTERFERON.

Betagan

(Allergan) is a proprietary, prescription-only preparation of the BETA-BLOCKER levobunolol hydrochloride. It can be used for GLAUCOMA TREATMENT, and is available as eye-drops.

✚▲ Side-effects/warnings: See LEVOBUNOLOL HYDROCHLORIDE.

betahistine hydrochloride

is an ANTINAUSEANT which is used to treat the vertigo, hearing loss and tinnitus (ringing in the ears) associated with Ménière's disease. Administration is oral.

✚ Side-effects: Gastrointestinal disturbances, headache, rash, itching.

▲ Warnings: It is not to be given to patients with phaeochromocytoma; it is administered with caution to those with peptic ulcer, asthma, or who are pregnant or breast-feeding.

✪ Related entry: Serc.

beta-lactam 🅴

is the chemical name of the group of ANTIBIOTIC drugs that have a certain chemical structure called a lactam ring. This extensive family includes the PENICILLIN class (whose generic names usually end *-cillin*; eg AMOXICILLIN, AMPICILLIN), the CEPHALOSPORIN class (whose names often include *cef* or *ceph*; eg CEFACLOR, CEFTAZIDIME), together with newer synthetic classes such as the *carbapenems* (eg IMIPENEM WITH CILASTATIN, MEROPENEM) and *monobactams* (eg AZTREONAM). A notable adverse reaction to this family of antibiotics is an allergic drug response, which can be dangerous. Allergy to one type of beta-lactam (eg penicillin) makes reaction to another likely, though not inevitable. Aside from allergy, the side-effects of some members of this class are relatively slight (eg diarrhoea is common, sometimes nausea) compared to some antibiotic classes.

Betaloc

(AstraZeneca) is a proprietary, prescription-only

preparation of the BETA-BLOCKER metoprolol tartrate. It can be used as an ANTIHYPERTENSIVE for raised blood pressure, as an ANTI-ANGINA treatment to relieve symptoms and improve exercise tolerance and as an ANTI-ARRHYTHMIC to regularize heartbeat and to treat myocardial infarction. It can also be used as an ANTITHYROID drug for short-term treatment of thyrotoxicosis and as an ANTIMIGRAINE to prevent attacks. It is available as tablets and in a form for injection.
✚▲ Side-effects/warnings: See METOPROLOL TARTRATE.

Betaloc-SA

(AstraZeneca) is a proprietary, prescription-only preparation of the BETA-BLOCKER metoprolol tartrate. It can be used as an ANTIHYPERTENSIVE for raised blood pressure and as an ANTIMIGRAINE treatment to prevent attacks. It is available as modified-release tablets (called *Durules*).
✚▲ Side-effects/warnings: See METOPROLOL TARTRATE.

betamethasone

is a CORTICOSTEROID with ANTI-INFLAMMATORY properties. It is used in the treatment of many kinds of inflammation, particularly inflammation associated with skin conditions, such as eczema and psoriasis, and of the eyes, ears or nose. It is also used to treat cerebral oedema (fluid retention in the brain) and congenital adrenal hyperplasia (abnormal growth of a part of the adrenal gland called the adrenal cortex). It is administered in several forms by different methods, depending on the form of the drug. Administration as *betamethasone* is either oral as tablets or by injection; as *betamethasone dipropionate*, by topical application as *betamethasone sodium phosphate* by topical application as eye-, ear- or nose-drops; and as *betamethasone valerate* also by topical application. Betamethasone is also available in several compound preparations with ANTIMICROBIAL and LOCAL ANAESTHETIC drugs.
✚▲ Side-effects/warnings: See CORTICOSTEROID. Serious systemic side-effects are unlikely with topical application, but there may be local skin reactions.
✪ Related entries: Betacap; Betnelan; Betnesol; Betnesol-N; Betnovate; Betnovate-C; Betnovate-N; Betnovate-RD; Bettamousse; Diprosalic; Diprosone; Fucibet; Lotriderm; Vista-Methasone; Vista-Methasone-N.

betamethasone dipropionate

see BETAMETHASONE.

betamethasone sodium phosphate

see BETAMETHASONE.

betamethasone valerate

see BETAMETHASONE.

Beta-Prograne

(Tillomed) is a proprietary, prescription-only preparation of the BETA-BLOCKER propranolol hydrochloride. It can be used as an ANTIHYPERTENSIVE for raised blood pressure, as an ANTI-ANGINA treatment to relieve symptoms and improve exercise tolerance and as an ANTI-ARRHYTHMIC to regularize heartbeat and to treat myocardial infarction. It can also be used as an ANTITHYROID drug for the short-term treatment of thyrotoxicosis, as an ANTIMIGRAINE treatment to prevent attacks, as an ANXIOLYTIC, particularly for symptomatic relief of tremor and palpitations, and, with an ALPHA-ADRENOCEPTOR BLOCKER, in the acute treatment of phaeochromocytoma. It is available as modified-release capsules.
✚▲ Side-effects/warnings: See PROPRANOLOL HYDROCHLORIDE.

beta-receptor stimulant 🄴

(beta-adrenoceptor stimulant; beta-adrenoceptor agonist; beta-agonist) drugs act at beta-receptors, which, along with alpha-adrenoceptors, are the sites that recognize and respond to the natural hormones and neurotransmitters (adrenaline and noradrenaline; also called epinephrine and norepinephrine) of the sympathetic nervous system. Drugs that activate this system, by whatever mechanism, are called sympathomimetics (see SYMPATHOMIMETIC). Notable actions of beta-receptor stimulants include bronchodilation, speeding and strengthening of the heartbeat and relaxation of contraction of the uterus and intestine. Importantly, differences in receptors at different sites allow selectivity of action.

For example, $beta_2$-receptor stimulant drugs are normally used as BRONCHODILATOR drugs in the treatment of asthma, chronic bronchitis and emphysema, since they can act within the respiratory tract without significant and

B

potentially dangerous parallel stimulation of the heart (which is a $beta_1$-receptor site). Examples of $beta_2$-stimulant drugs used to cause bronchodilation are SALBUTAMOL and TERBUTALINE SULPHATE. In contrast, $beta_1$-receptor stimulants may be used to stimulate the failing heart (though need to be used with care). Agents that are not selective between the two beta-receptor types are now less used (eg ISOPRENALINE, ORCIPRENALINE SULPHATE).

betaxolol hydrochloride

is a BETA-BLOCKER which can be used as an ANTI-HYPERTENSIVE for raised blood pressure taken orally. Also used in the form of eye-drops as a GLAUCOMA TREATMENT for chronic simple glaucoma.

✚▲ Side-effects/warnings: There may be some systemic absorption after using eye-drops, so some of the side-effects listed under PROPRANOLOL HYDROCHLORIDE may be seen. Dry eyes, stinging, redness, pain and some local allergic reactions, including conjunctivitis may also occur.

✪ **Related entries: Betoptic; Kerlone.**

bethanechol chloride

is a PARASYMPATHOMIMETIC which is used occasionally to stimulate motility in the intestines and to treat urinary retention (particularly following surgery). Administration is oral.

✚ Side-effects: Sweating, blurred vision, nausea and vomiting, intestinal colic and a slow heart rate.

▲ Warnings: It should not be administered to patients who suffer from urinary or intestinal obstruction, asthma, epilepsy, parkinsonism, thyroid or certain heart disorders, who have peptic ulceration or are pregnant.

✪ **Related entry: Myotonine.**

Betim

(ICN) is a proprietary, prescription-only preparation of the BETA-BLOCKER timolol maleate. It can be used as an ANTIHYPERTENSIVE for raised blood pressure, as an ANTI-ANGINA treatment to relieve symptoms and improve exercise tolerance and to treat myocardial infarction. It can also be used as an ANTIMIGRAINE treatment to prevent attacks. Available as tablets.

✚▲ Side-effects/warnings: See TIMOLOL MALEATE.

Betnelan

(Celltech) is a proprietary, prescription-only preparation of the CORTICOSTEROID and ANTI-INFLAMMATORY betamethasone. It can be used to treat inflammation, such as in rheumatic or allergic conditions, cerebral oedema and congenital adrenal hyperplasia. Available as tablets.

✚▲ Side-effects/warnings: See BETAMETHASONE.

Betnesol

(Celltech) is a proprietary, prescription-only preparation of the CORTICOSTEROID and ANTI-INFLAMMATORY betamethasone (as sodium phosphate). It can be used to treat local inflammation (eg of the ear, eye or nose) as well as more widespread rheumatic or allergic conditions. It is available as tablets, as ear-, eye- and nose-drops, an eye ointment and in a form for injection.

✚▲ Side-effects/warnings: See BETAMETHASONE.

Betnesol-N

(Celltech) is a proprietary, prescription-only compound preparation of the ANTI-INFLAMMATORY and CORTICOSTEROID betamethasone (as sodium phosphate) and the ANTIBACTERIAL and ANTIBIOTIC neomycin sulphate. It can be used to treat local inflammation, and is available as ear-, eye- and nose-drops and an eye ointment.

✚▲ Side-effects/warnings: See BETAMETHASONE; NEOMYCIN SULPHATE.

Betnovate

(GlaxoWellcome; GSK) is a proprietary, prescription-only preparation of the ANTI-INFLAMMATORY and CORTICOSTEROID betamethasone (as valerate). It can be used topically to treat severe non-infective inflammation of the skin, rectum and scalp. It is available as a cream, ointment, lotion and a scalp preparation. A rectal ointment is also available as a compound preparation of betamethasone (as valerate), the LOCAL ANAESTHETIC lidocaine hydrochloride and the SYMPATHOMIMETIC and VASOCONSTRICTOR phenylephrine hydrochloride.

✚▲ Side-effects/warnings: See BETAMETHASONE; LIDOCAINE HYDROCHLORIDE; PHENYLEPHRINE HYDROCHLORIDE.

Betnovate-C

(GlaxoWellcome; GSK) is a proprietary, prescription-only compound preparation of the

B

ANTI-INFLAMMATORY and CORTICOSTEROID betamethasone (as valerate) and the ANTIMICROBIAL clioquinol. It can be used topically to treat severe inflammation, including where there is infection such as skin eczema and psoriasis, and is available as a cream and ointment.
✚▲ Side-effects/warnings: See BETAMETHASONE; CLIOQUINOL.

Betnovate-N

(GlaxoWellcome; GSK) is a proprietary, prescription-only compound preparation of the ANTI-INFLAMMATORY and CORTICOSTEROID betamethasone (as valerate) and the ANTIBACTERIAL and ANTIBIOTIC neomycin sulphate. It can be used topically to treat severe inflammation, including where there is infection such as skin psoriasis and eczema, and is available as a cream and an ointment.
✚▲ Side-effects/warnings: See BETAMETHASONE; NEOMYCIN SULPHATE.

Betnovate-RD

(GlaxoWellcome; GSK) is a proprietary, prescription-only, preparation of the CORTICOSTEROID and ANTI-INFLAMMATORY betamethasone (as valerate). It can be used to treat severe, non-infective inflammation of the skin and scalp, and is available as a cream and an ointment.
✚▲ Side-effects/warnings: See BETAMETHASONE.

Betoptic

(Alcon) is a proprietary, prescription-only preparation of the BETA-BLOCKER betaxolol hydrochloride, and can be used, in forms of eye-drops, for GLAUCOMA TREATMENT.
✚▲ Side-effects/warnings: See BETAXOLOL HYDROCHLORIDE.

Bettamousse

(Celltech) is a proprietary, prescription-only, preparation of the CORTICOSTEROID and ANTI-INFLAMMATORY betamethasone (as valerate). It can be used to treat severe, non-infective inflammation of the scalp, and is available in a form for scalp application.
✚▲ Side-effects/warnings: See BETAMETHASONE.

bezafibrate

is a (*fibrate*) LIPID-REGULATING DRUG used in hyperlipidaemia to reduce the levels, or change the proportions, of various lipids in the bloodstream. Generally, it is administered only to patients in whom a strict and regular dietary regime, alone, is not having the desired effect. Administration is oral.
✚ Side-effects: There may be gastrointestinal effects (including nausea, abdominal pain, loss of appetite); skin complaints, including rashes and itching; and impotence. Occasionally, dizziness and vertigo, fatigue and headache, hair loss, and blood disorders.
▲ Warnings: Avoid administering to patients who have severely impaired kidney or liver function (eg alcoholics), disease of the gall bladder, or who are pregnant or breast-feeding. Patients should report any muscle weakness, pain or tenderness to their doctor.
✪ **Related entries: Bezalip; Bezalip-Mono.**

Bezalip

(Roche) is a proprietary, prescription-only preparation of the LIPID-REGULATING DRUG bezafibrate. It can be used in hyperlipidaemia to modify the proportions of various lipids in the bloodstream. It is available as tablets.
✚▲ Side-effects/warnings: See BEZAFIBRATE.

Bezalip-Mono

(Roche) is a proprietary, prescription-only preparation of the LIPID-REGULATING DRUG bezafibrate. It can be used in hyperlipidaemia to modify the proportions of various lipids in the bloodstream. It is available as tablets.
✚▲ Side-effects/warnings: See BEZAFIBRATE.

bicalutamide

is a HORMONE ANTAGONIST (an ANTI-ANDROGEN) which is used as an ANTICANCER drug used, sometimes with other drugs for the treatment of prostate cancer. Administration is oral.
✚ Side-effects: There may be hot flushes, growth and tenderness of breasts, weakness, pruritus, sleepiness, effects on the liver and cardiovascular system; other effects (more common in elderly) include dizziness, insomnia, decreased libido, impotence, anorexia, shortness of breath, gastrointestinal problems (such as flatulence, constipation and dyspepsia), hair loss, rashes, sweating, oedema, dry mouth, chest and abdominal pain.
▲ Warnings: Administer with caution to patients suffering certain liver disorders (liver function may be monitored).

✪ Related entry: Casodex.

BiCNU

(Bristol-Myers Squibb) is a proprietary, prescription-only preparation of the ANTICANCER drug carmustine. It can be used in the treatment of a range of cancers, and is available in a form for injection.

✚▲ Side-effects/warnings: See CARMUSTINE.

biguanide

drugs are a chemical class of orally administered HYPOGLYCAEMIC drugs (of which only METFORMIN HYDROCHLORIDE is available in the UK) which are used in DIABETIC TREATMENT for Type II diabetes (non-insulin-dependent diabetes mellitus; NIDDM; maturity-onset diabetes). How they work is complex, but it is thought to involve an effect on glucose uptake by skeletal muscle, glucose absorption and production.

BiNovum

(Janssen-Cilag) is a proprietary, prescription-only compound preparation which can be used as a (*biphasic*) ORAL CONTRACEPTIVE of the *COC* (standard strength) type that combines an OESTROGEN and a PROGESTOGEN, in this case ethinylestradiol and norethisterone. It is available as tablets in a calendar pack.

✚▲ Side-effects/warnings: See ETHINYLESTRADIOL; NORETHISTERONE.

Bioplex

(Provalis) is a proprietary, prescription-only preparation of the CYTOPROTECTANT drug carbenoxolone sodium. It can be used to treat mouth ulcers, and is available as granules to make up into a mouthwash.

✚▲ Side-effects/warnings: See CARBENOXOLONE SODIUM.

Bioral Gel

(Merck Consumer Health; Seven Seas) is a proprietary, non-prescription preparation of the ANTI-INFLAMMATORY carbenoxolone sodium. It can be used to treat mouth ulcers. Available as a gel.

✚▲ Side-effects/warnings: See CARBENOXOLONE SODIUM.

Biorphen

(Alliance) is a proprietary, prescription-only preparation of the ANTICHOLINERGIC orphenadrine hydrochloride. It can be used to relieve some of the symptoms of parkinsonism, especially muscle rigidity and the tendency to produce an excess of saliva (see ANTIPARKINSONISM). The drug also has the capacity to treat these symptoms, in some cases, where they are produced by drugs. It is available as an elixir.

✚▲ Side-effects/warnings: See ORPHENADRINE HYDROCHLORIDE.

biosynthetic human growth hormone

see SOMATROPIN.

biperiden

is an ANTICHOLINERGIC (ANTIMUSCARINIC) drug which is used in the treatment of some types of parkinsonism (see ANTIPARKINSONISM). It increases mobility and decreases rigidity and the tendency to produce an excess of saliva is also reduced, but it has only a limited effect on bradykinesia. Additionally, it has the capacity to treat these symptoms (extrapyramidal symptoms, but not tardive dyskinesia), in some cases, where they are produced by drugs. It is thought to work by correcting the over-effectiveness of the neurotransmitter ACETYLCHOLINE (cholinergic excess), which results from the deficiency of dopamine that occurs in parkinsonism. Because it also has some sedative properties, it is sometimes used in preference to the similar drug BENZHEXOL HYDROCHLORIDE. Administration, which may be in conjunction with other drugs used to relieve parkinsonism, is either oral or by injection.

✚▲ Side-effects/warnings: See BENZHEXOL HYDROCHLORIDE; but it may cause drowsiness; when administered by injection, it may cause hypotension.

✪ Related entry: Akineton.

biphasic insulin lispro

is a recombinant (biosynthetic) human insulin analogue, which is used in DIABETIC TREATMENT to maintain diabetic patients. It is available in biphasic form (containing mixed insulin lispro and insulin lispro protamine; having different rates of onset and offset of action) that is intermediate-acting. Administration is by injection.

B

✚▲ Side-effects/warnings: See INSULIN. There may be allergic reactions.
✪ **Related entry: Humalog Mix25; Humalog Mix50.**

biphasic isophane insulin

is a form of purified insulin which is prepared as a sterile buffered suspension of porcine insulin complexed with protamine in a solution of porcine insulin, or human insulin complex in a solution of human insulin. It is used in DIABETIC TREATMENT to maintain diabetic patients. It is available in vials for injection and has an intermediate duration of action.
✚▲ Side-effects/warnings: See INSULIN. There may be allergic reactions.
✪ **Related entries: Human Mixtard 10; Human Mixtard 20; Human Mixtard 30; Human Mixtard 30 ge; Human Mixtard 40; Human Mixtard 50; Humulin M2; Humulin M3; Humulin M5; Hypurin Porcine Biphasic Isophane 30/70 Mix; Pork Mixtard 30.**

bisacodyl

is a (*stimulant*) LAXATIVE which is used to promote defecation and relieve constipation. It seems to work by stimulating motility in the intestine (especially the rectal mucosa), but some medical authorities do not approve of the frequent use of *stimulant laxatives* (as compared to the relatively benign *bulking-agent laxatives*, which help establish good bowel habit). Medically, bisacodyl can be used to evacuate the colon prior to rectal examination or surgery. Administration is either oral as tablets (full effects are achieved after several hours) or topical as suppositories (with effects achieved within an hour).
✚ Side-effects: There may be abdominal cramps, griping, nausea or vomiting. Suppositories can sometimes cause local irritation.
▲ Warnings: It should not be administered to patients with intestinal obstruction.
✪ **Related entries: Dulco-lax Suppositories; Dulco-lax Tablets.**

bismuth chelate

see TRIPOTASSIUM DICITRATOBISMUTHATE.

bismuth oxide

is a mild ASTRINGENT agent which is used in the treatment of haemorrhoids, and is available as suppositories.
✚▲ Side-effects/warnings: It is regarded as safe in normal topical use.
✪ **Related entries: Anugesic-HC; Anusol Cream; Anusol Ointment; Anusol Plus HC Ointment; Anusol Plus HC Suppositories; Anusol Plus HC Suppositories; Anusol Suppositories.**

bismuth salicylate

(bismuth subsalicylate) can be used as an ANTACID and ANTIDIARRHOEAL agent in the treatment of stomach upsets. Administration is oral.
✚▲ Side-effects/warnings: It can liberate salicylate which can be absorbed, so side-effects of SALICYLATE may be experienced; see NSAID. Bismuth sulphide may be released in the gastrointestinal tract and this may darken faeces.
✪ **Related entry: Pepto-Bismol.**

bismuth subgallate

is a mild ASTRINGENT agent which is used in the treatment of haemorrhoids. Administration is topical as suppositories.
✚▲ Side-effects/warnings: It is regarded as safe in normal topical use.
✪ **Related entries: Anusol Ointment; Anusol Plus HC Suppositories.**

bismuth subsalicylate

see BISMUTH SALICYLATE.

Bisodol Extra Strong Mint

(Whitehall Laboratories) is a proprietary, non-prescription compound preparation of the ANTACID agents sodium bicarbonate, calcium carbonate and magnesium carbonate. It can be used to relieve indigestion, heartburn, dyspepsia, acidity and flatulence, and is available as chewable tablets.
✚▲ Side-effects/warnings: See CALCIUM CARBONATE; MAGNESIUM CARBONATE; SODIUM BICARBONATE.

Bisodol Heartburn Relief

(Whitehall Laboratories) is a proprietary, non-prescription compound preparation of the ANTACID sodium bicarbonate and magaldrate, and the DEMULCENT alginic acid. It can be used to relieve indigestion and heartburn. It is available as tablets and is not normally given to children under six years, except on medical advice.
✚▲ Side-effects/warnings: See ALGINIC ACID; SODIUM BICARBONATE.

Bisodol Indigestion Relief Powder

(Whitehall Laboratories) is a proprietary, non-prescription compound preparation of the ANTACID agents sodium bicarbonate and magnesium carbonate. It can be used to relieve indigestion, heartburn, dyspepsia, acidity and flatulence. It is available as a powder and is not normally given to children, except on medical advice.
✚▲ Side-effects/warnings: See MAGNESIUM CARBONATE; SODIUM BICARBONATE.

Bisodol Indigestion Relief Tablets

(Whitehall Laboratories) is a proprietary, non-prescription compound preparation of the ANTACID agents sodium bicarbonate, calcium carbonate and mixed magnesium carbonates. It can be used to relieve indigestion, heartburn, dyspepsia, acidity and flatulence. It is available as chewable tablets and is not normally given to children, except on medical advice.
✚▲ Side-effects/warnings: See CALCIUM CARBONATE; MAGNESIUM CARBONATE; SODIUM BICARBONATE.

Bisodol Wind Relief

(Whitehall) is a proprietary, non-prescription compound preparation of the ANTACID agents sodium bicarbonate, calcium carbonate and magnesium carbonate, and the ANTIFOAMING AGENT dimeticone (as simeticone (simethicone)). Used to relieve indigestion, heartburn, dyspepsia, acidity and flatulence, and is available as tablets.
✚▲ Side-effects/warnings: See CALCIUM CARBONATE; DIMETICONE; MAGNESIUM CARBONATE; SODIUM BICARBONATE.

bisoprolol fumarate

is a BETA-BLOCKER which can be used as an ANTIHYPERTENSIVE for raised blood pressure and as an ANTI-ANGINA treatment to relieve symptoms and increase exercise tolerance, and recently for heart failure treatment. Administration is oral.
✚▲ Side-effects/warnings: See PROPRANOLOL HYDROCHLORIDE.
✪ **Related entries: Cardicor; Emcor; Monocor; Monozide 10.**

bisphosphonate 🅱

(biphosphonate; diphosphonate) is the name of a chemical class of drug used as CALCIUM METABOLISM MODIFIER drugs to treat a number of conditions of disturbed calcium metabolism, including Paget's disease of the bone, malignant hypercalcaemia and osteoporosis, corticosteroid-induced osteoporosis and are being evaluated for use in treating bone pain associated with cancer metastases of the bone. These drugs are enzyme-resistant analogues of pyrophosphate, which is a natural physiological inhibitor of bone mineralization, and those used are DISODIUM ETIDRONATE, ALENDRONIC ACID, DISODIUM PAMIDRONATE, SODIUM CLODRONATE, TILUDRONIC ACID and ZOLEDRONIC ACID.
✚▲ Side-effects/warnings: Instructions on how to take bisphosphonate drugs need to be followed carefully. Calcium salts (eg CALCIUM CARBONATE) and IRON, which can be used for medical purposes or are contained in some multivitamin preparations, can reduce the absorption of some bisphosphonates so reducing their effectiveness.

Blemix

(Ashbourne) is a proprietary, prescription-only preparation of the ANTIBACTERIAL and (TETRACYCLINES) ANTIBIOTIC minocycline. It can be used to treat a wide range of infections, and is available as tablets.
✚▲ Side-effects/warnings: See MINOCYCLINE.

Bleo-Kyowa

(Kyowa Hakko) is a proprietary, prescription-only preparation of the (CYTOTOXIC) ANTICANCER drug bleomycin, used for various conditions, including squamous cell carcinoma. It is available in a form for injection.
✚▲ Side-effects/warnings: See BLEOMYCIN.

bleomycin

is a CYTOTOXIC drug (an ANTIBIOTIC in origin) which has wide use as an ANTICANCER treatment for leukaemias, lymphomas, solid tumours and squamous cell carcinoma. Administration is by injection.
✚▲ Side-effects/warnings: See CYTOTOXIC; but causes little bone marrow depression. Hypersensitivity reactions (chills and fevers) and effects on the lung and skin.
✪ **Related entry: Bleo-Kyowa.**

Blisteze

(DDD Ltd) is a proprietary, non-prescription

B

preparation of ammonia solution with phenol. It can be applied to cold sores, chapped and cracked lips, and is available as a cream for topical application.
▲ Warnings: See PHENOL.

Bocasan

(Oral-B Lab) is a proprietary, non-prescription preparation of the ANTISEPTIC sodium perborate. It can be used to cleanse and disinfect the mouth, and is available in a form for making up into a mouthwash. It is not normally given to children under five years, except on medical advice.
✚▲ Side-effects/warnings: See SODIUM PERBORATE.

Bonefos

(Boehringer Ingelheim) is a, proprietary, prescription-only preparation of sodium clodronate. It is used to treat high calcium levels associated with malignant tumours and bone lesions. It is available in a number of forms (one called *Bonefos Concentrate*), as tablets, capsules and in a form for intravenous infusion.
✚▲ Side-effects/warnings: See SODIUM CLODRONATE.

Bonjela Oral Pain-Relieving Gel

(Reckitt Benckiser Healthcare) is a proprietary, non-prescription compound preparation of the ANTISEPTIC cetylpyridinium chloride and choline salicylate. It can be applied to the mouth for symptomatic relief of pain from mouth ulcers, cold sores, denture irritation, inflammation of the tongue and teething in infants. It is available as a gel to be massaged in gently. It should not be given to babies under four months, except on medical advice.
✚▲ Side-effects/warnings: See CETYLPYRIDINIUM CHLORIDE; CHOLINE SALICYLATE. Excess use can cause ulcers under dentures.

Boots Dental Pain Relief

(Boots) is a proprietary, non-prescription compound analgesic preparation of the NON-NARCOTIC ANALGESIC paracetamol and the (OPIOID) NARCOTIC ANALGESIC dihydrocodeine tartrate. It can be used to relieve toothache and dental pain. It is available as tablets, and is not normally given to children.
✚▲ Side-effects/warnings: See DIHYDROCODEINE TARTRATE; PARACETAMOL.

Boots Diareze

(Boots) is a proprietary, non-prescription preparation of the (OPIOID) ANTIDIARRHOEAL loperamide hydrochloride. It can be used for the symptomatic relief of acute diarrhoea and its associated discomfort, and is available as capsules. It is not given to children, except on medical advice.
✚▲ Side-effects/warnings: See LOPERAMIDE HYDROCHLORIDE.

Boots Ibuprofen Gel

(Boots) is a proprietary, non-prescription preparation of the (NSAID) NON-NARCOTIC ANALGESIC and ANTIRHEUMATIC ibuprofen. It can be used to relieve backache, lumbago, strains and sprains and other musculoskeletal disorders, and is available as a gel for topical application. It is not normally given to children under 14 years, except on medical advice.
✚▲ Side-effects/warnings: See IBUPROFEN; but adverse effects on topical application are limited.

Boots Medicated Pain Relief Plaster

(Boots) is a proprietary, non-prescription preparation of methyl salicylate and camphor (which have COUNTER-IRRITANT, or RUBEFACIENT, actions) and menthol (as levomenthol) . It can be applied to the skin for symptomatic relief of underlying muscle or joint pain. It is available as a plaster for application to the skin, and is not normally used for children under 14 years, except on medical advice.
✚▲ Side-effects/warnings: See CAMPHOR; MENTHOL; METHYL SALICYLATE.

Boots Tension Headache Relief

(Boots) is a proprietary, non-prescription compound preparation of the NON-NARCOTIC ANALGESIC paracetamol, the (OPIOID) NARCOTIC ANALGESIC codeine phosphate, the ANTIHISTAMINE doxylamine (as succinate) and the STIMULANT caffeine. It can be used to treat tension headache. It is available as tablets and is not given to children, except on medical advice.
✚▲ Side-effects/warnings: See CAFFEINE; CODEINE PHOSPHATE; DOXYLAMINE; PARACETAMOL.

Botox

(Allergan) is a proprietary, prescription-only preparation of botulinum A toxin-haemagglutin complex, used to treating blepharospasm. It is available in a form for injection.

✚▲ Side-effects/warnings: See BOTULINUM TOXIN.

botulinum A toxin-haemagglutin complex

see BOTULINUM TOXIN.

botulinum toxin

is a type of exotoxin produced by culturing the bacterium *Clostridium botulinum*. Seven toxins can be isolated, falling into serotypes A–G. In nature, when involved in food poisoning, these neurotoxins can cause paralysis and death by preventing transmission of messages between nerves and muscles. Medically, toxins of the A (as botulinum A toxin-haemagglutin complex) and B (botulinum B toxin) groups are used. Botulinum A toxin-haemagglutin complex is mainly used for treating blepharospasm (involuntary tight contractions of the eyelids) and hemifacial (one-sided) facial spasm, deformities due to spasticity in cerebral palsy patients, and spasmodic torticollis (cervical dystonia; which is a condition where the head is inclined to one side because of abnormal muscle contraction in the neck). It can also can be used in cosmetic procedures to temporarily remove wrinkles. Botulinum B toxin can be used to treat spasmodic torticollis. Administration of the toxins is by local injection.

✚▲ Side-effects/warnings: This is a specialist type of drug with special warning and side-effects specific to each individual use.

✪ Related entries: Botox; Dysport; NeuroBloc.

botulism antitoxin

is a preparation that neutralizes the toxins produced by botulism bacteria (*Clostridium bolulinum* types A, B and E). It can therefore be used in a similar way to IMMUNIZATION to provide *passive immunity* to people who have been exposed to botulism in order to prevent them from developing the disease (though because it works by directly reacting with the toxin, its use is akin to the use of an ANTIDOTE). It is also given to the infected patient as a means of treatment. Hypersensitivity reactions are common and it is not effective against some strains of botulism. People will be tested for sensitivity first. Administration is by injection. It is available from local designated centres.

✚▲ Side-effects/warnings: See IMMUNIZATION. Sensitivity to the toxin will be checked before administration.

Bradosol Plus (Sugar Free)

(Novartis Consumer Health) is a proprietary, non-prescription compound preparation of the ANTISEPTIC agent DOMIPHEN BROMIDE and the LOCAL ANAESTHETIC lidocaine hydrochloride. It can be used for the symptomatic relief of a painful sore throat, and is available as lozenges. It is not normally given to children under 12 years, except on medical advice.

✚▲ Side-effects/warnings: See DOMIPHEN BROMIDE; LIDOCAINE HYDROCHLORIDE.

Bradosol Sugar-Free Cherry Menthol Lozenges

(Novartis Consumer Health) is a proprietary, non-prescription preparation of the ANTISEPTIC benzalkonium chloride, and can be used for the symptomatic relief of a painful sore throat. It is not normally given to children under five years, except on medical advice.

✚▲ Side-effects/warnings: See BENZALKONIUM CHLORIDE.

Bradosol Sugar-Free Original Citrus Lozenges

(Novartis Consumer Health) is a proprietary, non-prescription preparation of the ANTISEPTIC benzalkonium chloride, and can be used for the symptomatic relief of a painful sore throat. It is not normally given to children under five years, except on medical advice.

✚▲ Side-effects/warnings: See BENZALKONIUM CHLORIDE.

bran

is a natural *bulking-agent* LAXATIVE, which is commonly used to keep people 'regular' and to treat constipation. It works by increasing the overall mass of faeces (by retaining a lot of water) and so stimulating bowel movement (the full effect may not be achieved for many hours). As an excellent source of dietary fibre, bran is thought to reduce the risk of diverticular disease while actively assisting digestion. It is useful in managing patients with colostomy, ileostomy, haemorrhoids, chronic diverticular disease, irritable bowel syndrome and ulcerative colitis.

✚ Side-effects: Some patients cannot tolerate

B

bran, particularly those sensitive to gluten.
▲ Warnings: It should not be consumed if there is intestinal blockage or coeliac disease. Adequate fluid intake must be maintained to avoid faecal impaction.
✪ **Related entry: Trifyba.**

bretylium tosilate

(bretylium tosylate) can be used in ANTI-ARRHYTHMIC treatment of abnormal heart rhythms in resuscitation, where other therapies have not been successful. It also has ADRENERGIC-NEURONE BLOCKER actions, and as an ANTISYMPATHETIC prevents release of noradrenaline from sympathetic nerves. Administration is by injection.
✚ Side-effects: Hypotension; nausea and vomiting; tissue damage at the site of injection.
▲ Warnings: It should not be used in patients with phaeochromocytoma.
✪ **Related entry: Min-I-Jet Bretylate Tosylate.**

bretylium tosylate

see BRETYLIUM TOSILATE.

Brevibloc

(Baxter) is a proprietary, prescription-only preparation of the BETA-BLOCKER esmolol hydrochloride. It can be used as an ANTIHYPERTENSIVE during operations and as an ANTI-ARRHYTHMIC, in the short term, to regularize heartbeat. It is available in a form for injection.
✚▲ Side-effects/warnings: See ESMOLOL HYDROCHLORIDE.

Brevinor

(Searle; Pharmacia) is a proprietary, prescription-only compound preparation which can be used as a (*monophasic*) ORAL CONTRACEPTIVE of the *COC* (standard strength) type that combines an OESTROGEN and a PROGESTOGEN, in this case ethinylestradiol and norethisterone. It is available as tablets in a calendar pack.
✚▲ Side-effects/warnings: See ETHINYLESTRADIOL; NORETHISTERONE.

Brevoxyl

(Stiefel) is a proprietary, non-prescription preparation of the KERATOLYTIC and ANTIMICROBIAL benzoyl peroxide (4%). It can be used to treat acne, and is available as a cream for topical application.
✚▲ Side-effects/warnings: See BENZOYL PEROXIDE.

Brexidol

(Trinity) is a proprietary, prescription-only preparation of the (NSAID) NON-NARCOTIC ANALGESIC and ANTIRHEUMATIC piroxicam. It can be used to relieve pain, particularly rheumatic and also arthritic pain and inflammation, and to treat other acute musculoskeletal disorders. It is available as tablets.
✚▲ Side-effects/warnings: See PIROXICAM.

Bricanyl

(AstraZeneca) is a proprietary, prescription-only preparation of the BETA-RECEPTOR STIMULANT terbutaline sulphate. It can be used as a BRONCHODILATOR in reversible obstructive airways disease, as an ANTI-ASTHMATIC treatment. It is available as a syrup, tablets, modified-release tablets (*Bricanyl SA*), in a form for injection or intravenous infusion, as a metered aerosol used with a spacer device or a *Nebuhaler*, as a breath-actuated dry powder with an inhaler called a *Turbohaler*, in single-dose nebulization solution, and as a respirator solution (for use with a nebulizer or a ventilator). It can also be used as a means of slowing premature labour by injection.
✚▲ Side-effects/warnings: See TERBUTALINE SULPHATE.

brimonidine tartrate

is an ALPHA-ADRENOCEPTOR STIMULANT that is selective for the $alpha_2$subtype of receptor. It has recently been introduced into GLAUCOMA TREATMENT (for open-angle glaucoma and ocular hypertension, particularly when other drugs have not been effective or are not appropriate) when it is applied as eye-drops.
✚ Side-effects: Eye reactions include dilation of the blood vessels of the eye, burning, stinging, blurring, itching, allergy, eyelid inflammation, conjunctivitis, photophobia and a number of other local reactions. If absorbed there may be dry mouth, headache, taste alteration, dizziness, fatigue, occasionally drowsiness, rarely depression, dryness of the nose, palpitations, and hypersensitivity reactions.
▲ Warnings: Care should be taken where there is severe cardiovascular disease; coronary or cerebral insufficiency, Raynaud's syndrome,

postural hypotension, depression, liver or kidney impairment; and in pregnancy and breast-feeding. Drowsiness may affect performance of skilled tasks (eg driving).
✪ **Related entry: Alphagan.**

brinzolamide

is a CARBONIC-ANHYDRASE INHIBITOR which is used in GLAUCOMA TREATMENT because it reduces the formation of aqueous humour in the eye. It is also used for ocular hypertension and open-angle glaucoma, alone, or in combination with beta-blockers. Administration is topical.
✚ Side-effects: It may irritate the eye and cause disturbances of taste; less often it has been reported to cause nausea, dyspepsia, dry mouth, nose bleeds, coughing up of blood, rhinitis, pharyngitis, bronchitis, breathing difficulties and/or chest pain, paraesthesia, depression, dizziness, headache, hair loss and skin reactions such as dermatitis and erosion of the cornea.
▲ Warnings: Brinzolamide is not suitable for people who have impaired kidney function or some types of acidosis of the blood when it is associated with high chloride levels, and is not used in women who are breast-feeding. It should be used with caution in people who have impaired liver functioning or who are pregnant.
✪ **Related entry: Azopt.**

Britaject

(Britannia) is a prescription-only preparation of the ANTIPARKINSONISM drug apomorphine hydrochloride. It is available in a form for injection.
✚▲ Side-effects/warnings: See APOMORPHINE HYDROCHLORIDE.

BritLofex

(Britannia) is a proprietary, prescription-only preparation of the drug lofexidine hydrochloride. It can be used to alleviate the symptoms of OPIOID withdrawal, and is available as tablets.
✚▲ Side-effects/warnings: See LOFEXIDINE HYDROCHLORIDE.

Broflex

(Alliance) is a proprietary, prescription-only preparation of the ANTICHOLINERGIC benzhexol hydrochloride. It can be used in the treatment of parkinsonism, and is available as a syrup.
✚▲ Side-effects/warnings: See BENZHEXOL HYDROCHLORIDE.

Brolene Eye Drops

(Aventis Pharma) is a proprietary, non-prescription preparation of the ANTIBACTERIAL propamidine isethionate. It can be used to treat infections of the eyelids or conjunctiva, and is available as eye-drops.
✚▲ Side-effects/warnings: See PROPAMIDINE ISETHIONATE.

Brolene Eye Ointment

(Aventis Pharma) is a proprietary, non-prescription preparation of the ANTIBACTERIAL dibrompropamidine isethionate. It can be used to treat infections of the eyelids or conjunctiva, and is available as an eye ointment.
✚▲ Side-effects/warnings: See DIBROMPROPAMIDINE ISETHIONATE.

bromocriptine

is an ERGOT ALKALOID and is used to treat parkinsonism (but not the parkinsonian symptoms caused by certain drug therapies: see ANTIPARKINSONISM). It works by stimulating the DOPAMINE receptors in the brain (it is a DOPAMINE-RECEPTOR STIMULANT) and so is different to the more commonly used treatment with levodopa, which is converted to dopamine in the body. It is therefore particularly useful in the treatment of patients who, for one reason or another, cannot tolerate levodopa. Occasionally, the two drugs are combined. Bromocriptine has alternative uses (some related to its ability to inhibit prolactin secretion by the pituitary gland): to treat delayed puberty caused by hormonal insufficiency; to relieve certain menstrual disorders, infertility, or to reduce or halt milk production (in galactorrhoea), prolactinoma (tumour of the pituitary gland, leading to excess prolactin secretion) and to treat cyclical benign breast disease; and sometimes for treating acromegaly (over-secretion of the anterior pituitary gland due to a tumour). Administration is oral.
✚ Side-effects: There may be nausea, vomiting, constipation, headache, dizziness (especially on rising from sitting or lying down – postural hypotension), spasm in the blood vessels of the extremities and drowsiness. High dosage may cause hallucinations, a state of confusion, leg cramps and a variety of other rare reactions.
▲ Warnings: There are certain circumstances when it can not be used, especially in or after

B

pregnancy. Care is needed in cardiovascular or menstrual disorders, porphyria and Raynaud's syndrome. Full, regular monitoring of various body systems is essential during treatment. If used to prevent milk production but fails to work, women should not then breast-feed.
✪ **Related entry: Parlodel.**

brompheniramine maleate
is an ANTIHISTAMINE which is used to treat the symptoms of allergic conditions such as hay fever and urticaria, and is also used, in combination with other drugs, in the treatment of coughs. Administration is oral.
✚▲ Side-effects/warnings: See ANTIHISTAMINE. Because of its sedative side-effects, the performance of skilled tasks, such as driving, may be impaired.
✪ **Related entries: Dimotane Co; Dimotane Co Paediatric; Dimotane Expectorant.**

Bronalin Decongestant Elixir
(SSL) is a proprietary, non-prescription preparation of the DECONGESTANT pseudoephedrine hydrochloride. It can be used for the symptomatic relief of flu and cold symptoms, catarrh, blocked sinuses, rhinitis and hay fever, and is available as an oral liquid. It is not normally given to children under two years, except on medical advice.
✚▲ Side-effects/warnings: See PSEUDOEPHEDRINE HYDROCHLORIDE.

Bronalin Expectorant Linctus
(SSL) is a proprietary, non-prescription preparation of the ANTIHISTAMINE diphenhydramine hydrochloride and the EXPECTORANT ammonium chloride (with sodium citrate). It can be used for the symptomatic relief of deep chesty coughs and colds, and is available as an oral solution. It is not normally given to children under six years, except on medical advice.
✚▲ Side-effects/warnings: See AMMONIUM CHLORIDE; DIPHENHYDRAMINE HYDROCHLORIDE; SODIUM CITRATE.

Bronalin Junior Linctus
(SSL) is a proprietary, non-prescription preparation of the ANTIHISTAMINE diphenhydramine hydrochloride (and sodium citrate). It can be used for the symptomatic relief of coughs and colds. Available as an oral solution, it is not normally given to children under one year, except on medical advice.
✚▲ Side-effects/warnings: See DIPHENHYDRAMINE HYDROCHLORIDE; SODIUM CITRATE.

bronchodilator 🅱
drugs relax the smooth muscle of the bronchioles (air passages in the lungs), so allowing air to flow more easily in or out (the latter being the major problem in obstructive airways disease). There are a number of conditions that cause bronchospasm (spasm in the bronchial muscles) and increased secretion of mucus and hence blockage, but the most common are asthma and chronic bronchitis. The type of drug mainly used to treat bronchospasm is a BETA-RECEPTOR STIMULANT (SYMPATHOMIMETIC) agent. These drugs (eg SALBUTAMOL and TERBUTALINE SULPHATE) work by stimulating beta-adrenoceptors on the smooth muscle of the airways, which normally respond to adrenal hormones and sympathetic nerve neurotransmitters (adrenaline and noradrenaline; also called epinephrine and norepinephrine). Other types of bronchodilator, such as the xanthine compounds AMINOPHYLLINE and THEOPHYLLINE, act directly on the smooth muscle of the bronchioles. Also used are inhaled (ANTIMUSCARINIC) ANTICHOLINERGIC drugs (eg IPRATROPIUM BROMIDE and OXITROPIUM BROMIDE) which may be of value in certain respiratory states including chronic bronchitis. All classes of drugs are best administered directly to the airways (except in an emergency) in the form of aerosols, ventilator sprays or nebulizing mists, because this minimizes side-effects (since less of the drug is absorbed into the bloodstream).

Brufen
(Knoll) is a proprietary, prescription-only preparation of the (NSAID) NON-NARCOTIC ANALGESIC and ANTIRHEUMATIC ibuprofen. It can be used to relieve pain, particularly the pain of rheumatic disease and other musculoskeletal disorders. It is available as tablets, a syrup for dilution and effervescent granules.
✚▲ Side-effects/warnings: See IBUPROFEN.

Brufen Retard
(Knoll) is a proprietary, prescription-only

preparation of the (NSAID) NON-NARCOTIC ANALGESIC and ANTIRHEUMATIC ibuprofen. It can be used to relieve pain and inflammation, particularly the pain of rheumatic disease and other musculoskeletal disorders, and is available as modified-release tablets.
✚▲ Side-effects/warnings: See IBUPROFEN.

Brulidine

(Manx) is a proprietary, non-prescription preparation of the (ANTIBACTERIAL) ANTISEPTIC dibrompropamidine isethionate. It can be used to treat minor burns and abrasions and nappy rash, and is available as a cream for topical application.
✚▲ Side-effects/warnings: See DIBROMPROPAMIDINE ISETHIONATE.

Buccastem

(Reckitt & Colman; Reckitt Benckiser) is a proprietary, prescription-only preparation of prochlorperazine (as maleate). It can be used as an ANTINAUSEANT and ANTI-EMETIC to relieve nausea and vomiting. It can also be used as an ANTIPSYCHOTIC to treat schizophrenia and other psychoses and for the short-term treatment of acute anxiety. It is available as buccal tablets (placed between the upper lip and gum and left to dissolve).
✚▲ Side-effects/warnings: See PROCHLORPERAZINE.

buclizine hydrochloride

is an ANTIHISTAMINE which is included in a proprietary ANTIMIGRAINE treatment as an ANTI-EMETIC. Administration is oral.
✚▲ Side-effects/warnings: See ANTIHISTAMINE.
✪ **Related entry: Migraleve; Migraleve Pink.**

Budenofalk

(Provalis) is a proprietary, prescription-only preparation of the CORTICOSTEROID budesonide. It can be used for the induction of remission in mild to moderate Crohn's disease affecting the ileum or ascending colon. It is available as capsules.
✚▲ Side-effects/warnings: See BUDESONIDE.

budesonide

is a CORTICOSTEROID with ANTI-INFLAMMATORY and ANTI-ALLERGIC properties, which is used to treat and prevent attacks of asthma, allergic and vasomotor rhinitis and nasal polyps. Administration is by inhalation or a nasal spray, or topically as a cream or ointment. It is now also used for the induction of remission in mild to moderate Crohn's disease affecting the ileum or ascending colon, when it is administered orally, and as an enema for acute attacks of ulcerative colitis.
✚▲ Side-effects/warnings: See BECLOMETHASONE DIPROPIONATE.
✪ **Related entries: Budenofalk; Entocort; Pulmicort; Rhinocort Aqua.**

bumetanide

is a powerful DIURETIC, one of the class of *loop diuretics.* It can be used to treat oedema, and low urine production due to kidney failure (oliguria). Administration is either oral or by injection.
✚▲ Side-effects/warnings: See FRUSEMIDE; there may also be muscle pain.
✪ **Related entries: Burinex; Burinex A; Burinex K.**

bupivacaine hydrochloride

is a LOCAL ANAESTHETIC with a long duration of action. It is an amide derivative of another local anaesthetic lidocaine hydrochloride, and is particularly long-lasting. It is commonly used for spinal anaesthesia, including epidural injection (especially during labour) and also for nerve block and by local infiltration. Administration is by injection.
✚▲ Side-effects/warnings: See LIDOCAINE HYDROCHLORIDE.
✪ **Related entries: Bupivicaine; Marcain; Marcain with Adrenaline.**

Bupivicaine

(Antigen) is a non-proprietary, prescription-only preparation of the LOCAL ANAESTHETIC bupivacaine hydrochloride. It can be used particularly when a prolonged course of treatment is required, particularly for spinal anaesthesia, including epidural injection (especially during labour). Administration is by injection or infusion.
✚▲ Side-effects/warnings: See: BUPIVACAINE HYDROCHLORIDE.

buprenorphine

is a NARCOTIC ANALGESIC, an OPIOID, which is long-acting (its effects last longer than morphine) and used to treat moderate to severe pain, including during surgical operations. Preparations of buprenorphine are on the

B

Controlled Drugs list, because it can cause dependence (addiction). It has some OPIOID ANTAGONIST properties and so may be dangerous to use in combination with other narcotic analgesics, and can precipitate withdrawal symptoms in those habituated to, for instance, high doses of morphine or diamorphine. But it can be used as part of substitute therapy for those dependent on moderate doses of opioids. Administration is oral in the form of tablets placed sublingually (under the tongue) or by injection.
✚▲ Side-effects/warnings: See OPIOID. It may cause vomiting.
✪ **Related entries: Subutex; Temgesic.**

bupropion

(amfebutamone) is a newly introduced drug which can be is used to help in giving up smoking (in combination with motivational support). It works by inhibiting nerve uptake of monoamine neurotransmitter chemicals in the brain (especially) DOPAMINE and to a lesser extent SEROTONIN and NORADRENALINE) – a similar action to some antidepressants (though bupropion is chemically different to other drugs with this action). In fact, bupropion is used as an ANTIDEPRESSANT in some other countries. It is taken orally.
✚ Side-effects: Bupropion can cause gastrointestinal disturbances, dry mouth, insomnia, tremor, reduced ability to concentrate, headache, dizziness, depression, agitation and anxiety and sweating. It may cause hypersensitivity reactions such as a rash and pruritus, and also fever, taste disturbances and less commonly chest pain, weakness, increased heart rate and hypertension, flushing, anorexia and disturbances of vision and hearing (such as tinnitus). Rarely, it can cause postural hypotension, seizures and Stevens-Johnson syndrome (an inflammatory condition).
▲ Warnings: Bupropion is not prescribed to people who have a history of epilepsy, eating disorders, manic-depressive (bipolar) disorder; CNS tumours, who are pregnant or breast-feeding. It is used with care in the elderly, people who have liver or kidney impairment or with a predisposition to seizures, which includes people taking certain other drugs, diabetics, people with anorexia or who have experienced head trauma or have a history of abusing alcohol. Bupropion may impair the ability to perform skilled tasks such as driving.
✪ **Related entry: Zyban.**

Burinex

(Leo) is a proprietary, prescription-only preparation of the (*loop*) DIURETIC bumetanide. It can be used to treat oedema, and is available as tablets.
✚▲ Side-effects/warnings: See BUMETANIDE.

Burinex A

(Leo) is a proprietary, prescription-only compound preparation of the (*loop*) DIURETIC bumetanide and the *potassium-sparing* diuretic amiloride hydrochloride. It can be used to treat oedema. It is available as tablets.
✚▲ Side-effects/warnings: See AMILORIDE HYDROCHLORIDE; BUMETANIDE.

Burinex K

(Leo) is a proprietary, prescription-only compound preparation of the (*loop*) DIURETIC bumetanide and the potassium supplement POTASSIUM CHLORIDE. It can be used to treat oedema. It is available as tablets.
✚▲ Side-effects/warnings: See BUMETANIDE; POTASSIUM CHLORIDE.

Burneze Spray

(SSL) is a proprietary, non-prescription preparation of the LOCAL ANAESTHETIC benzocaine. It can be used to treat local pain and skin irritation, burns and scalds (on unbroken skin), and is available as a spray.
✚▲ Side-effects/warnings: See BENZOCAINE.

Buscopan

(Boehringer Ingelheim) is a proprietary, prescription-only preparation of the ANTICHOLINERGIC hyoscine butylbromide, which can be used as an ANTISPASMODIC to treat gastrointestinal and genitourinary tract disorders. It is available as tablets and in a form for injection. (Tablets are also available and can be obtained without a prescription under certain conditions.)
✚▲ Side-effects/warnings: See HYOSCINE BUTYLBROMIDE.

Buscopan Tablets

(Boehringer Ingelheim) is a proprietary, non-

prescription preparation of the ANTISPASMODIC hyoscine (as hyoscine-N-butylbromide). It can be used to relieve the symptoms of irritable bowel syndrome and period pain, and other conditions where there is spasm of the genitourinary or gastrointestinal tract. It is available as tablets and is not given to children under six years, except on medical advice.
✚▲ Side-effects/warnings: See HYOSCINE BUTYLBROMIDE.

buserelin
is an analogue of the hypothalamic hormone GONADORELIN (gonadothrophin-releasing hormone; GnRH). Injected in a pulsitile manner, in the short term it mimics the physiological response to GnRH and so stimulates release of gonadothrophins from the pituitary gland. Thus, it may be used in the treatment of infertility (prior to IVF). Paradoxically, when given long-term, following this initial stimulatory phase, there is a prolonged reduction of secretion of gonadotrophins, and this in turn results in reduced secretion of sex hormones by the ovaries or testes; so it is sometimes termed an *indirect* ANTI-ANDROGEN or ANTI-OESTROGEN. Because of this latter action, buserelin can also be used to treat endometriosis, and as an ANTICANCER drug to treat cancer of the prostate gland. It can be given as a nasal spray (because it is absorbed into the systemic circulation from the nasal mucosa) or by injection.
✚ Side-effects: Depending on sex and use, there may be menstruation-like and breakthrough bleeding and symptoms similar to the menopause (sweating, hot flushes, headache, palpitations, vaginal dryness). There may be mood changes; back, muscle and abdominal pain; changes to breast size and tenderness; nervousness, tiredness and sleep disturbances; ovarian cysts; skin disturbances (eg acne, rashes); constipation; blurred vision; vaginal discharge; tingling and sensitivity in fingers and toes; and changes in body hair. In men: there may be effects on bones, hair loss, fatigue, hearing disorders. In men and women: there may be changes in libido; dizziness; vomiting; headache. There may be irritation on using the nasal spray.
▲ Warnings: It is not to be used in pregnancy or when breast-feeding, or where there is vaginal bleeding of unknown origin. Some men initially experience increased tumour growth, to the extent of compressing the spinal cord and additional drugs may be necessary to counteract this. Care is necessary in certain bone diseases, depression, diabetes and hypotension.
✪ **Related entries: Suprecur; Suprefact.**

Buspar
(Bristol-Myers Squibb) is a proprietary, prescription-only preparation of the ANXIOLYTIC buspirone hydrochloride. It can be used for the short-term treatment of anxiety, and is available as tablets.
✚▲ Side-effects/warnings: See BUSPIRONE HYDROCHLORIDE.

buspirone hydrochloride
is an ANXIOLYTIC which works as serotonin receptor stimulant in the brain. It can be used for the short-term treatment of anxiety. Administration is oral.
✚ Side-effects: Nausea, dizziness, headache, nervousness, excitement, light-headedness; rarely, effects on the heart, chest pain, drowsiness, dry mouth, confusion, fatigue or sweating.
▲ Warnings: It should not be given to patients with epilepsy, severe liver or kidney impairment; or who are pregnant or breast-feeding. It may impair the performance of skilled tasks, such as driving; avoid alcohol because its effects may be enhanced.
✪ **Related entry: Buspar.**

busulfan
(busulphan) is an (*alkylating agent*) CYTOTOXIC drug which is used as an ANTICANCER treatment, particularly for chronic myeloid leukaemia. It works by direct interference with the DNA. Administration is oral.
✚▲ Side-effects/warnings: See CYTOTOXIC. Hyperpigmentation of the skin is common.
✪ **Related entry: Myleran.**

busulphan
see BUSULFAN.

Butacote
(Novartis) is a proprietary, prescription-only preparation of the (NSAID) NON-NARCOTIC ANALGESIC and ANTIRHEUMATIC phenylbutazone. Because of its sometimes severe side-effects, it is used solely in the treatment of ankylosing spondylitis under medical supervision in hospitals.

Administration is oral.
✚▲ Side-effects/warnings: See PHENYLBUTAZONE.

butobarbital

(butobarbitone) is a BARBITURATE which is used only when absolutely necessary as a HYPNOTIC to treat severe and intractable insomnia in patients who are already taking barbiturates. Administration is oral. Preparations containing butobarbitone are on the Controlled Drugs list.
✚▲ Side-effects/warnings: See BARBITURATE.
✪ Related entry: Soneryl.

butobarbitone

see BUTOBARBITAL.

Buttercup Infant Cough Syrup

(Warner Lambert Consumer Healthcare; Pfizer) is a proprietary, non-prescription preparation of the EXPECTORANT ipecacuaha and menthol. It can be used for the symptomatic relief of chesty, dry, tickly or bronchial coughs, and is available as a syrup. It is not normally given to children under one year, except on medical advice.
✚▲ Side-effects/warnings: See IPECACUANHA; MENTHOL.

Buttercup Syrup (Original Flavour)

(Warner Lambert Consumer Healthcare; Pfizer) is a proprietary, non-prescription preparation of capsicum tincture and squill liquid extract, which can be used to give relief for coughs, sore throats and hoarseness. It is available as a syrup and is not normally given to children under two years, except on medical advice.
✚▲ Side-effects/warnings: See CAPSAICIN.

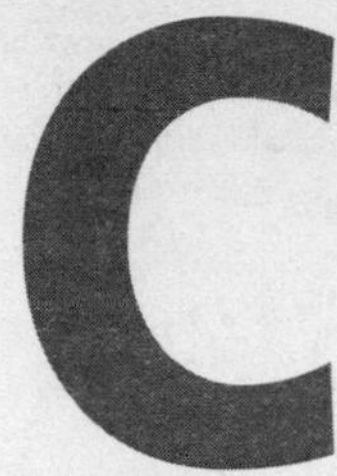

Cabaser

(Pharmacia) is a proprietary, prescription-only preparation of the drug cabergoline. It is used primarily to treat parkinsonism, but not the parkinsonian symptoms caused by certain drug therapies (see ANTIPARKINSONISM). Available as tablets.

✚▲ Side-effects/warnings: See CABERGOLINE.

Cabdriver's Adult Cough Linctus

(Merck Consumer Health; Seven Seas) is a proprietary, non-prescription compound preparation of the (OPIOID) ANTITUSSIVE dextromethorphan hydrobromide, with aromatic oils and menthol. It can be used for the symptomatic relief of chesty coughs, such as those associated with colds and bronchitis. It is available as a linctus and is not given to children.

✚▲ Side-effects/warnings: See DEXTROMETHORPHAN HYDROBROMIDE; MENTHOL.

cabergoline

works by stimulating the DOPAMINE receptors in the brain (a DOPAMINE-RECEPTOR STIMULANT), with properties similar to BROMOCRIPTINE. It is used for ANTIPARKINSONISM (usually with LEVODOPA), and in hormonal disorders such as preventing milk production and other disorders due to excess secretion of the hormone PROLACTIN. Administration is oral.

✚▲ Side-effects/warnings: See BROMOCRIPTINE. The side-effects are somewhat different and there may be gastrointestinal and epigastric pain and other side-effects. Do not use in pregnancy.

✪ Related entries: Cabaser; Dostinex.

Caelyx

(Schering-Plough) is a proprietary, prescription-only preparation of the ANTICANCER drug doxorubicin hydrochloride. It can be used to treat AIDS-related Kaposi's sarcoma. It is available in a form encapsulated in liposomes for intravenous infusion.

✚▲ Side-effects/warnings: See DOXORUBICIN HYDROCHLORIDE.

Cafergot

(Alliance) is a proprietary, prescription-only compound preparation of the VASOCONSTRICTOR ergotamine tartrate and the STIMULANT caffeine. It can be used as an ANTIMIGRAINE treatment for acute attacks. Available as tablets and suppositories.

✚▲ Side-effects/warnings: See CAFFEINE; ERGOTAMINE TARTRATE.

caffeine

is a weak central nervous system STIMULANT, which is present in tea, coffee and some soft drinks. It is also included in many analgesic preparations, partly in the belief that it speeds absorption. Administration is oral.

✚ Side-effects: Excessive doses may cause headache, either during treatment or on withdrawal, and also anxiety.

✪ Related entries: Alka-Seltzer XS; Alka XS Go;Anadin Analgesic Capsules, Maximum Strength; Anadin Cold Control Capsules; Anadin Extra; Anadin Extra Soluble Tablets; Anadin Tablets; Askit Powders; Beechams Flu-Plus Caplets; Beechams Powders; Beechams Powders Capsules; Boots Tension Headache Relief; Cafergot; Do-Do Chesteze; Feminax; Hedex Extra Tablets; Lemsip Cold + Flu Max Strength Capsules; Migril; Nurse Sykes Powders; Panadol Extra Soluble Tablets; Panadol Extra Tablets; Paracets Plus Capsules; Phensic Original; Propain Caplets; Pro-plus Tablets; Solpadeine Capsules; Solpadeine Soluble Tablets; Solpadeine Tablets; Syndol; Yeast-vite.

Calabren

(Berk; APS) is a proprietary, prescription-only preparation of the SULPHONYLUREA glibenclamide. It can be used in DIABETIC TREATMENT of Type II diabetes (non-insulin-dependent diabetes mellitus; NIDDM; maturity-onset diabetes) and works by augmenting what remains of INSULIN production in the pancreas. It is available as tablets.

✚▲ Side-effects/warnings: See GLIBENCLAMIDE.

Calamine and Coal Tar Ointment, BP

is a non-proprietary, non-prescription

C

compound preparation of calamine, zinc oxide and coal tar. It can be used by topical application to treat chronic eczema and psoriasis, and to relieve itching. It is available as an ointment.
✚▲ Side-effects/warnings: See CALAMINE; COAL TAR.

calamine

is a suspension containing mainly (basic) zinc carbonate (with added ferric oxide) and has a mild ASTRINGENT action. It is incorporated into several preparations that are used to cool and soothe itching skin in conditions such as pruritus, eczema and psoriasis, and is also used in some EMOLLIENT preparations. Administration is by topical application.
✚▲ Side-effects/warnings: It is regarded as safe in normal topical use.
✪ Related entries: Calamine and Coal Tar Ointment, BP; Care Calamine Lotion; Vasogen Cream.

Calanif

(Berk; APS) is a proprietary, prescription-only preparation of the CALCIUM-CHANNEL BLOCKER nifedipine. It can be used as an ANTI-ANGINA treatment in the prevention of attacks, and peripheral vascular disease (Raynaud's phenomenon). It is available as capsules.
✚▲ Side-effects/warnings: See NIFEDIPINE.

Calceos

(Thames) is a proprietary, non-prescription compound preparation of the VITAMIN colecalciferol (cholecalciferol; vitamin D_3) and calcium (in the form of calcium carbonate). It is used to treat VITAMIN D deficiency, and is available in the forms of tablets.
✚▲ Side-effects/warnings: See CALCIUM CARBONATE; COLECALCIFEROL.

Calcicard CR

(Norton) is a proprietary, prescription-only preparation of the CALCIUM-CHANNEL BLOCKER diltiazem hydrochloride. It can be used as an ANTIHYPERTENSIVE and as an ANTI-ANGINA drug, and is available as modified-release tablets.
✚▲ Side-effects/warnings: See DILTIAZEM HYDROCHLORIDE.

Calcichew

(Shire) is a proprietary, non-prescription preparation of calcium carbonate. It can be used as a MINERAL SUPPLEMENT for calcium in cases of deficiency, and is available as chewable tablets (in two strengths, the stronger called *Calichew Forte*).
✚▲ Side-effects/warnings: See CALCIUM CARBONATE.

Calcichew D3

(Shire) is a proprietary, non-prescription compound preparation of the VITAMIN colecalciferol (cholecalciferol; vitamin D_3) and calcium (in the form of calcium carbonate). It can be used as a MINERAL SUPPLEMENT for supplementation in malnutrition, prevention and treatment of calcium and vitamin D deficiency. It is available in the forms of chewable tablets (in two strengths, the stronger called *Calichew D3 Forte*).
✚▲ Side-effects/warnings: See CALCIUM CARBONATE; COLECALCIFEROL.

Calcidrink

(Shire) is a proprietary, non-prescription preparation of calcium carbonate. It can be used as a MINERAL SUPPLEMENT for calcium in cases of deficiency, and is available as effervescent granules.
✚▲ Side-effects/warnings: See CALCIUM CARBONATE.

calciferol

see ERGOCALCIFEROL.

Calcijex

(Abbott) is a proprietary, prescription-only preparation of calcitriol, and can be used in vitamin D deficiency. It is available in a form for injection.
✚▲ Side-effects/warnings: See CALCITRIOL.

Calciparine

(Sanofi-Synthelabo) is a proprietary, prescription-only preparation of the ANTICOAGULANT heparin calcium. It can be used to treat various forms of thrombosis, and is available in a form for injection.
✚▲ Side-effects/warnings: See HEPARIN.

calcipotriol

is a vitamin-D derivative widely used to treat plaque psoriasis. It is available in forms for topical application.
✚ Side-effects: Local irritation, various skin irritations (itching, dermatitis, reddening,

photosensitivity); raised blood calcium.

▲ Warnings: It is not suitable for people with disorders of calcium metabolism. Administer with caution during pregnancy; avoid contact with the face. Wash hands thoroughly after use.

✪ **Related entry: Dovonex.**

calcitonin

is a thyroid hormone (see THYROID HORMONES) produced and secreted by the thyroid gland at the base of the neck. Its function is to lower the levels of calcium and phosphate in the blood and together with the correspondingly opposite action of PARATHYROID HORMONE (parathormone) which plays a complex role, along with VITAMIN D, in regulating these levels. Therapeutically, calcitonin itself is used to lower blood levels of calcium when they are abnormally high (hypercalcaemia), to treat Paget's disease of the bone and when there is cancer. However, the porcine form has been withdrawn (it tends to cause antibody formation) and the salmon form alone is used in the UK at the time of writing, and this is referred to as SALCATONIN or 'calcitonin (salmon)'.

calcitriol

(1,25-dihydroxycolecalciferol; 1,25-dihydroxycholecalciferol) is a synthesized form of vitamin D which is used to make up vitamin D deficiency in the body, such as in the treatment of certain forms of osteoporosis in postmenopausal women. and hypocalcaemia (low blood calcium) in dialysis patients with chronic renal failure. Administration is oral or by injection.

✚▲ Side-effects/warnings: See VITAMIN D.

✪ **Related entries: Calcijex; Rocaltrol.**

Calcium-500

(Martindale) is a proprietary, non-prescription preparation of calcium carbonate. It can be used as a MINERAL SUPPLEMENT for calcium in cases of deficiency, and is available as tablets.

✚▲ Side-effects/warnings: See CALCIUM CARBONATE.

Calcium and Ergocalciferol Tablets

is a non-proprietary, non-prescription compound preparation of the VITAMIN ergocalciferol (vitamin D_2) and calcium (in the form of calcium lactate and calcium phosphate). It can be used as a vitamin and MINERAL SUPPLEMENT in the treatment of nutritional or absorptive deficiencies. Administration is oral.

✚▲ Side-effects/warnings: See ERGOCALCIFEROL.

calcium antagonist 🅱

see CALCIUM-CHANNEL BLOCKER.

calcium carbonate

or chalk, is used therapeutically as an ANTACID. It is incorporated into many proprietary preparations that are used to relieve hyperacidity, dyspepsia and for the symptomatic relief of heartburn and symptoms of peptic ulcer. It is also used by mouth in the treatment of hyperphosphataemia (abnormally raised levels of phosphates in the blood). Administration is oral.

✚ Side-effects: Treatment with calcium carbonate as an antacid may cause belching (due to carbon dioxide).

▲ Warnings: Its prolonged use as an antacid can induce tolerance and eventually cause renewed acid secretion. There may also be abnormally high levels of calcium in the blood. Antacids may impair the absorption of other drugs.

✪ **Related entries: Actonorm Powder; Adcal-D3; Andrews Antacid; Bisodol Extra Strong Mint; Bisodol Indigestion Relief Tablets; Bisodol Wind Relief; Calceos; Calcichew; Calcichew D3; Calcidrink; Calcium-500; Didronel PMO; Digestif Rennie Peppermint Flavour; J Collis Browne's Tablets; Liquid Gaviscon; Ossopan; Peptac Liquid; Remegel Original; Rennie Deflatine; Rennie Duo; Rennie Rap-Eze; Sandocal; Setlers Antacid Peppermint Tablets; Setlers Heartburn and Indigestion Liquid; Titralac; Tums Assorted Fruit Flavours.**

calcium-channel blocker 🅱

(calcium antagonist; calcium-entry blocker) drugs are being increasingly used in therapeutics. They work by blocking entry of calcium through channels (specialized 'pores' in a cell's membrane) that admit calcium ions from the fluid surrounding cells to the interior of the cell. Since calcium has very profound activities within cells (such as increasing muscle contraction and electrical excitability), these drugs have powerful effects on cell function. Their main uses include: a direct SMOOTH MUSCLE RELAXANT action causing dilation of blood vessels and effects on heart muscle, which has led to their widespread use as ANTIHYPERTENSIVE drugs (eg AMLODIPINE BESILATE, ISRADIPINE, LACIDIPINE,

LERCANIDIPINE HYDROCHLORIDE, NICARDIPINE HYDROCHLORIDE, NIFEDIPINE, NISOLDIPINE and VERAPAMIL HYDROCHLORIDE); in ANTI-ANGINA treatment (eg amlodipine besylate, DILTIAZEM HYDROCHLORIDE, nicardipine hydrochloride, nifedipine and verapamil hydrochloride); as ANTI-ARRHYTHMIC agents (eg verapamil hydrochloride); in the prevention of damage to the brain due to ischaemia (lack of blood supply) following subarachnoid haemorrhage (a form of stroke, by reducing the risk of cerebral vasospasm which could lead to neurological damage) (eg NIMODIPINE); for Raynaud's phenomenon (nicardipine hydrochloride); and after myocardial infarction when beta-blockers are not appropriate (verapamil hydrochloride).
✚▲ Side-effects/warnings: See individual entries, but note that grapefruit juice should be avoided with certain members of this group because it effects metabolism of the drug.

calcium-entry blocker

see CALCIUM-CHANNEL BLOCKER.

calcium folinate

(calcium leucovorin) is the usual form in which FOLINIC ACID (a derivative of folic acid, which is a vitamin of the VITAMIN B complex) is administered as a supplement to patients who are susceptible to some of the toxic effects caused by the folate-antagonist activity of certain anticancer drugs, especially METHOTREXATE. It is also used, along with the ANTICANCER drug fluorouracil, to treat colorectal cancer. Administration is either oral or by injection or intravenous infusion.
✚ Side-effects: Rarely, fever after injections.
✪ **Related entries: Lederfolin; Refolinon; Sodiofolin.**

calcium leucovorin

see CALCIUM FOLINATE.

calcium levofolinate

(calcium levoleucovorin) is an alternate form of CALCIUM FOLINATE which is a vitamin of the vitamin-B complex (see VITAMIN B). It is, in fact, a salt of one isomer of FOLINIC ACID. (An alternative form, disodium folinate, is used as an alternative.) Forms of folinic acid are administered as a supplement to patients who are susceptible to some of the toxic effects caused by the folate-antagonist activity of certain anticancer drugs, especially METHOTREXATE. They are also used, along with the ANTICANCER drug FLUOROURACIL, to treat colorectal cancer. Administration is by injection or intravenous infusion.
✚▲ Side-effects/warnings: See CALCIUM FOLINATE.
✪ **Related entry: Isovorin.**

calcium levoleucovorin

see CALCIUM LEVOFOLINATE.

calcium metabolism modifier

drugs alter the metabolism and therefore the levels of calcium in the body. Calcium has an important role in most body processes and there are many ways in which it can be disrupted in disease. PARATHYROID HORMONE (parathormone; parathyrin; PTH) is a HORMONE secreted by the parathyroid gland, and increases the concentration of calcium (and decreases phosphate) in the blood (but is not currently used therapeutically). CALCITONIN is a hormone from the thyroid gland (and is quite unrelated to THYROXINE, and is secreted by different cells). Calcitonin lowers calcium levels in the blood, and its action is balanced in the body by corresponding opposite action of parathyroid hormone from the adjacent parathyroid gland. Calcitonin is used in therapeutics to lower blood levels of calcium when they are abnormally high (hypercalcaemia), to treat Paget's disease of the bone and for some sorts of cancer. It works by reducing calcium uptake of bone and has effects on the kidney. Preparations for clinical use include synthetic SALCATONIN (salmon calcitonin) though natural porcine (pig) calcitonin has been available. It is also expected to become available more widely in the synthetic human form.

Vitamin D (used as synthetic CALCITRIOL) acts with parathyroid hormone to mobilize bone calcium and by increasing calcium absorption from the intestine. Vitamin D occurs in a number of natural forms, including COLECALCIFEROL (cholecalciferol; D_3) and ERGOCALCIFEROL (D_2). It increases the absorption of calcium (and, to a lesser extent, phosphorus) from the intestine, to deposit it in the bones. A deficiency of vitamin D therefore results in bone deficiency disorders, eg rickets in children. Therapeutic replacement of vitamin D in cases of severe deficiency requires quantities of the vitamin best provided by one of the synthetic vitamin-D analogues such as ALFACALCIDOL and DIHYDROTACHYSTEROL.

Calcium forms used therapeutically to counter too low levels, include the mineral supplements CALCIUM CARBONATE, calcium gluconate, calcium lactate and calcium bicarbonate.

A drug series that chemically are *bisphosphonates* (diphosphonates) are used to treat a number of conditions of disturbed calcium metabolism, including Paget's disease of the bone, malignant hypercalcaemia and osteoporosis, and are being evaluated for use in treating bone pain associated cancer metastases of the bone. These drugs include DISODIUM ETIDRONATE, DISODIUM PAMIDRONATE and SODIUM CLODRONATE. Also, oestrogens (see OESTROGEN) are used in prevention of post-menopausal osteoporosis.

Calcium Resonium

(Sanofi-Synthelabo) is a proprietary, non-prescription preparation of calcium polystyrene sulphonate, which is a resin that can be used to treat high blood potassium levels. It is available in the form of a powdered resin for use as a rectal enema or by mouth.
✚▲ Side-effects/warnings: See POLYSTYRENE SULPHONATE RESINS.

calcium salts

are soluble forms of this metallic element which is essential for the normal growth and development of the body, especially (in the form of calcium phosphate) of the bones and teeth. Its level in blood is regulated by the opposing actions of the thyroid hormone CALCITONIN and the parathyroid HORMONE parathormone. Its uptake from food is enhanced by vitamin D (calciferol). Good food sources include most dairy products. Salts of calcium used therapeutically for deficiency when dietary intake is not sufficient (eg in old age due to poor absorption which can contribute to osteoporosis) include the ANTACID salt CALCIUM CARBONATE and a MINERAL SUPPLEMENT such as calcium gluconate and calcium lactate. It is also used in cardiac resuscitation.
▲ Warnings: Deficiency of vitamin D leads to calcium deficiency and corresponding bone, blood and nerve and muscle disorders. Conversely, excess calcium in the body may cause the formation of stones (calculi, generally composed of calcium oxalate), particularly in the kidney or gall bladder. It may cause gastrointestinal disturbances and effects on the heart.

Calcium-Sandoz

(Alliance) is a proprietary, non-prescription preparation of calcium glubionate and calcium lactobionate. It can be used as a MINERAL SUPPLEMENT in cases of calcium deficiency or when extra calcium is required. It is available as a syrup.
✚▲ Side-effects/warnings: See CALCIUM CARBONATE.

Calcort

(Shire) is a proprietary, prescription-only preparation of the CORTICOSTEROID deflazacort. It can be used as an ANTI-INFLAMMATORY agent for the suppression of inflammatory and allergic conditions, and is available as tablets.
✚▲ Side-effects/warnings: See DEFLAZACORT.

Calgel Teething Gel

(Warner Lambert Consumer Healthcare; Pfizer) is a proprietary, non-prescription compound preparation of the LOCAL ANAESTHETIC lidocaine hydrochloride and the ANTISEPTIC cetylpyridinium chloride. It can be used for the temporary relief of pain caused by teething in babies from three months, and is available as a gel for topical application.
✚▲ Side-effects/warnings: See CETYLPYRIDINIUM CHLORIDE; LIDOCAINE HYDROCHLORIDE.

Califig California Syrup of Figs

(Merck Consumer Health; Seven Seas) is a proprietary, non-prescription preparation of the (*stimulant*) LAXATIVE senna. It can be used to relieve constipation. Available as a viscous liquid, it is not normally given to children under one year, except on medical advice.
✚▲ Side-effects/warnings: See SENNA.

Califig Herbal Laxative Tablets with Senna

(Merck Consumer Healthcare; Seven Seas) is a proprietary, non-prescription preparation of the (*stimulant*) LAXATIVE senna with dandelion root and peppermint oil. It can be used to relieve constipation. Available as tablets, it is not normally given to children under seven years, except on medical advice.
✚▲ Side-effects/warnings: See PEPPERMINT OIL; SENNA.

Calimal Antihistamine Tablets

(Sussex) is a proprietary, non-prescription

preparation of the ANTIHISTAMINE chlorphenamine maleate (chlorpheniramine maleate). It can be used to treat allergic conditions such as hay fever, food allergies and urticaria, and is available as tablets. It is not normally given to children under six years, except on medical advice.
✚▲ Side-effects/warnings: See CHLORPHENAMINE MALEATE.

Calmurid

(Galderma) is a proprietary, non-prescription compound preparation of lactic acid and the HYDRATING AGENT urea. It can be used for dry, scaly or hard skin, and is available as a cream.
✚▲ Side-effects/warnings: See UREA.

Calmurid HC

(Galderma) is a proprietary, prescription-only compound preparation of the CORTICOSTEROID and ANTI-INFLAMMATORY hydrocortisone and the HYDRATING AGENT urea (with lactic acid). It can be used as a treatment for mild inflammation of the skin, and dry, scaling and itchy skin caused by conditions such as eczema, and is available as a cream for topical application.
✚▲ Side-effects/warnings: See HYDROCORTISONE; UREA.

Calpol Infant Suspension

(Warner Lambert Consumer Healthcare; Pfizer) is a proprietary, non-prescription preparation of the NON-NARCOTIC ANALGESIC paracetamol. It can be used to treat mild to moderate pain (including teething pain) and as an ANTIPYRETIC (for instance, to reduce fever after vaccination, when it can be used in two-month-old babies). It is available as a liquid suspension and is not normally given to infants under three months, except on medical advice.
✚▲ Side-effects/warnings: See PARACETAMOL.

Calpol Infant Suspension Sachets

(Warner Lambert Consumer Healthcare; Pfizer) is a proprietary, non-prescription preparation of the NON-NARCOTIC ANALGESIC paracetamol. It can be used to treat mild to moderate pain (including teething pain) and as an ANTIPYRETIC (for instance, to reduce fever after vaccination, when it can be used in two-month-old babies). It is available as a suspension in sachets and is not normally given to infants under three months, except on medical advice.
✚▲ Side-effects/warnings: See PARACETAMOL.

Calpol Six Plus Sugar Free/Colour Free Suspension

(Warner Lambert Consumer Healthcare; Pfizer) is a proprietary, non-prescription preparation of the NON-NARCOTIC ANALGESIC and ANTIPYRETIC paracetamol. It can be used to treat mild to moderate pain and to reduce fever in children. However, it is not normally given to children under six years, except on medical advice. It is available in the form of a liquid suspension.
✚▲ Side-effects/warnings: See PARACETAMOL.

Calpol Six Plus Suspension

(Warner Lambert Consumer Healthcare; Pfizer) is a proprietary, non-prescription preparation of the NON-NARCOTIC ANALGESIC and ANTIPYRETIC paracetamol. It can be used to treat mild to moderate pain and to reduce fever in children. However, it is not normally given to children under six years, except on medical advice. It is available in the form of an orange-flavoured liquid suspension.
✚▲ Side-effects/warnings: See PARACETAMOL.

Calpol Sugar-Free Infant Suspension

(Warner Lambert Consumer Healthcare; Pfizer) is a proprietary, non-prescription preparation of the NON-NARCOTIC ANALGESIC paracetamol. It can be used to treat mild to moderate pain (including teething pain) and as an ANTIPYRETIC (for instance, to reduce fever after vaccination, when it can be used in two-month-old babies). It is available as a liquid suspension and is not normally given to infants under three months, except on medical advice.
✚▲ Side-effects/warnings: See PARACETAMOL.

Calpol Sugar-Free Infant Suspension Sachets

(Warner Lambert Consumer Healthcare; Pfizer) is a proprietary, non-prescription preparation of the NON-NARCOTIC ANALGESIC paracetamol. It can be used to treat mild to moderate pain (including teething pain) and as an ANTIPYRETIC (for instance, to reduce fever after vaccination, when it can be used in two-month-old babies). It is available as a liquid suspension in sachets and is not normally given to infants under three months, except on medical advice.

✚▲ Side-effects/warnings: See PARACETAMOL.

Calsynar

(Rhône-Poulenc Rorer; Aventis Pharma) is a proprietary, prescription-only preparation of the thyroid hormone (see THYROID HORMONES) calcitonin, in the form of salcatonin (*calcitonin* (*salmon*)). It can be used to lower blood levels of calcium when they are abnormally high (hypercalcaemia). It is available in a form for injection.

✚▲ Side-effects/warnings: See SALCATONIN.

Camcolit

(Norgine) is a proprietary, prescription-only preparation of the ANTIMANIA drug lithium (as lithium carbonate). It can be used to prevent and treat mania, manic-depressive bouts and recurrent depression, and is available as tablets (in two strengths; *Camcolit 250* and *Camcolit 400*).

✚▲ Side-effects/warnings: See LITHIUM.

camphor

is an aromatic substance with mild COUNTER-IRRITANT, or RUBEFACIENT, properties. It is incorporated into a number of topical preparations that are used to help relieve itchiness and for the symptomatic relief of muscular pains and rheumatism, fibrosis, lumbago, sciatica and skin irritation. It is also available in a capsule whose contents are sprinkled on bed linen for inhaling.

✚▲ Side-effects/warnings: It is regarded as safe in normal topical or inhalant use, but avoid cuts or abraded skin.

✪ Related entries: Balmosa Cream; Benadryl Skin Allergy Relief Cream; Benadryl Skin Allergy Relief Lotion; Boots Medicated Pain Relief Plaster; Earex Ear Drops; Mentholatum Vapour Rub; PR Heat Spray; Radian B Heat Spray; Radian B Muscle Lotion; Radian B Muscle Rub; Scholl Corn and Callous Removal Liquid; Scholl Seal and Heal Verruca Removal Gel; TCP Antiseptic Ointment; Tiger Balm Red (Extra Strength); Tiger Balm White (Regular Strength); Tixycolds Cold and Hayfever Inhalant Capsules; Vicks Inhaler; Vicks Vaporub; Woodward's Baby Chest Rub.

Campral EC

(Lipha) is a proprietary, prescription-only preparation of acamprosate calcium, a drug used to treat alcoholic patients. It is available as tablets.

✚▲ Side-effects/warnings: See ACAMPROSATE CALCIUM.

Campto

(Rhône-Poulenc Rorer; Aventis Pharma) is a proprietary, prescription-only preparation of the ANTICANCER drug irinotecan hydrochloride. It can be used to treat colorectal cancer, and is available in a form for intravenous infusion.

✚▲ Side-effects/warnings: See IRINOTECAN HYDROCHLORIDE.

candesartan cilexetil

is an ANGIOTENSIN-RECEPTOR BLOCKER and acts as a VASODILATOR. Candesartan cilexetil is, in fact, a pro-drug of candesartan, to which it is converted in the body. It can be used as an ANTIHYPERTENSIVE. Administration is oral.

✚▲ Side-effects/warnings: See LOSARTAN POTASSIUM. Also, respiratory tract and flu-like symptoms including rhinitis; altered liver function, back muscle and joint pain, headache, nausea and rash. Not to be used in breast-feeding or severe liver impairment. Caution in liver or kidney impairment, or some heart valve disorders.

✪ Related entry: Amias.

Candiden Cream

(Akita) is a proprietary, non-prescription preparation of the ANTIFUNGAL drug clotrimazole. It can be used particularly to treat fungal infections such as athlete's foot, ringworm, vaginal thrush, candidial balanitis and nappy rash. It is available as a cream.

✚▲ Side-effects/warnings: See CLOTRIMAZOLE.

Candiden Vaginal Tablet

(Akita) is a proprietary, non-prescription preparation of the ANTIFUNGAL drug clotrimazole. It can be used particularly to treat vaginal thrush. It is available as a vaginal tablet, and is not given to children, except on medical advice.

✚▲ Side-effects/warnings: See CLOTRIMAZOLE.

Canesten

(Bayer Consumer Care) is the name of several proprietary preparations of the ANTIFUNGAL drug clotrimazole. They can be used to treat fungal infections, particularly vaginal candidiasis (thrush) and skin infections such as nappy rash and balanitis (infection of the glans penis). The

preparations are available in several forms and strengths, including a skin cream, an ear solution, a dusting powder, a vaginal cream, vaginal tablets (pessaries) and thrush cream. Most of these products are now available on a non-prescription basis for stated conditions, though their use will generally follow medical diagnosis, but *Caneston-HC* (which contains hydrocortisone) is available only on prescription. The various preparations are detailed under separate headings.
✚▲ Side-effects/warnings: See CLOTRIMAZOLE.

Canesten AF Cream
(Bayer) is a proprietary, non-prescription preparation of the ANTIFUNGAL drug clotrimazole. It can be used to treat fungal and *Candida* skin infections, particularly athlete's foot infections. It is available as a cream for topical application.
✚▲ Side-effects/warnings: See CLOTRIMAZOLE.

Canesten AF Powder
(Bayer) is a proprietary, non-prescription preparation of the ANTIFUNGAL drug clotrimazole. It can be used to treat fungal and *Candida* skin infections, particularly athlete's foot infections. It is available as a powder for topical application.
✚▲ Side-effects/warnings: See CLOTRIMAZOLE.

Canesten AF Spray
(Bayer) is a proprietary, non-prescription preparation of the ANTIFUNGAL drug clotrimazole. It can be used to treat athlete's foot, and is available as a spray for topical application.
✚▲ Side-effects/warnings: See CLOTRIMAZOLE.

Canesten Combi
(Bayer) is a proprietary, non-prescription preparation of the ANTIFUNGAL drug clotrimazole. It can be used to treat fungal and *Candida* skin infections, particularly vaginal thrush. It is available as a pack containing cream and a pessary with applicator for intra-vaginal application. It is not normally for children under 16 or those over 60, except on medical advice.
✚▲ Side-effects/warnings: See CLOTRIMAZOLE.

Canesten Cream
(Bayer) is a proprietary, non-prescription preparation of the ANTIFUNGAL drug clotrimazole. It can be used to treat fungal and *Candida* skin infections, particularly ringworm, nappy rash (caused by candida), balanitis and vulvitis. Available as a cream for topical application.
✚▲ Side-effects/warnings: See CLOTRIMAZOLE.

Canesten Dermatological Powder
(Bayer) is a proprietary, non-prescription preparation of the ANTIFUNGAL drug clotrimazole. It can be used to treat fungal and *Candida* skin infections, such as sweat rash, jock itch, ringworm, nappy rash and body infections. It is available as a powder for application to items of clothing and footware.
✚▲ Side-effects/warnings: See CLOTRIMAZOLE.

Canesten Dermatological Spray
(Bayer) is a proprietary, non-prescription preparation of the ANTIFUNGAL drug clotrimazole. It can be used to treat fungal skin infections, including nappy rash, sweat rash, jock itch and ringworm. It is available as a spray for topical application.
✚▲ Side-effects/warnings: See CLOTRIMAZOLE.

Canesten-HC
(Bayer Consumer Care) is a proprietary, prescription-only compound preparation of the CORTICOSTEROID hydrocortisone and the ANTIFUNGAL drug clotrimazole. It can be used to treat fungal infections, particularly those associated with inflammation, and is available as a cream for topical application.
✚▲ Side-effects/warnings: See CLOTRIMAZOLE; HYDROCORTISONE.

Canesten Hydrocortisone
(Bayer Consumer Care) is a proprietary, non-prescription-only compound preparation of the CORTICOSTEROID hydrocortisone and the ANTIFUNGAL drug clotrimazole. It can be used to treat fungal infections, particularly those associated with inflammation, such as candidal intertrigo and athlete's foot. It is available as a cream for topical application, and is not given to children under ten years, except on medical advice.
✚▲ Side-effects/warnings: See CLOTRIMAZOLE; HYDROCORTISONE.

Canesten Oasis
(Bayer) is a proprietary, non-prescription, preparation of sodium bicarbonate, sodium carbonate, sodium citrate and citric acid. It can be

used to make the urine more alkaline in treating cystitis in adult women. It is available as an oral powder. It is not normally used by males or children, except on medical advice.
✚▲ Side-effects/warnings: See SODIUM BICARBONATE; SODIUM CARBONATE; SODIUM CITRATE.

Canesten Once
(Bayer) is a proprietary, non-prescription preparation of the ANTIFUNGAL drug clotrimazole. It can be used to treat the *Candida* infection vaginal thrush. It is available as a vaginal cream with applicator. It is not normally given to children under 16 years or women over 60 years, except on medical advice.
✚▲ Side-effects/warnings: See CLOTRIMAZOLE.

Canesten Pessary
(Bayer) is a proprietary, non-prescription preparation of the ANTIFUNGAL drug clotrimazole. It can be used to treat the *Candida* infection vaginal thrush. It is not given to children under 16 years or women over 60 years, except on medical advice. It is available as a vaginal tablet.
✚▲ Side-effects/warnings: See CLOTRIMAZOLE.

Canesten Thrush Cream
(Bayer) is a proprietary, non-prescription preparation of the ANTIFUNGAL drug clotrimazole. It can be used to treat the *Candida* infection candidal vulvitis and as an additional treatment of candidal vaginitis. It is available as a cream for topical application. It is not recommended for children under 16 years or women over 60 years, except on medical advice.
✚▲ Side-effects/warnings: See CLOTRIMAZOLE.

Capasal Therapeutic Shampoo
(Demal) is a proprietary, non-prescription compound preparation of salicylic acid and coal tar (in coconut oil). It is used to treat dry scalp conditions such as seborrhoeic eczema, seborrhoeic dermatitis, dandruff psoriasis and cradle cap in infants, and is available as a shampoo.
✚▲ Side-effects/warnings: See COAL TAR; SALICYLIC ACID.

Capastat
(Dista; Lilly) is a proprietary, prescription-only preparation of the ANTIBIOTIC and ANTITUBERCULAR drug capreomycin (as sulphate). It can be used to treat tuberculosis, and is available in a form for injection.
✚▲ Side-effects/warnings: See CAPREOMYCIN.

capecitabine
is an (*antimetabolite*) CYTOTOXIC drug which is used as an ANTICANCER treatment primarily of solid tumours (eg of the colon and breast) and malignant skin lesions. It is a pro-drug (that is, it is converted in the body to) of FLUOROURACIL, which prevents the cancer cells from replicating and so prevents the growth of the cancer. It is particularly useful for metastatic colorectal cancer. It is taken orally.
✚▲ Side-effects/warnings: See CYTOTOXIC; but serious toxicity is unusual.
✪ **Related entry: Xeloda.**

Caplenal
(Berk; APS) is a proprietary, prescription-only preparation of the ENZYME INHIBITOR allopurinol, which is a XANTHINE-OXIDASE INHIBITOR. It can be used to treat excess uric acid in the blood and to prevent renal stones and attacks of gout. It is available as tablets.
✚▲ Side-effects/warnings: See ALLOPURINOL.

Capoten
(Squibb; Bristol-Myers Squibb) is a proprietary, prescription-only preparation of the ACE INHIBITOR captopril. It can be used as an ANTIHYPERTENSIVE and in HEART FAILURE TREATMENT, usually in conjunction with other classes of drug. It is available as tablets.
✚▲ Side-effects/warnings: See CAPTOPRIL.

Capozide
(Squibb; Bristol-Myers Squibb) is a proprietary, prescription-only compound preparation of the ACE INHIBITOR captopril and the DIURETIC hydrochlorothiazide, a combination called CO-ZIDOCAPT. It can be used as an ANTIHYPERTENSIVE, and is available as tablets (in two strengths, one called *LS tablets*).
✚▲ Side-effects/warnings: See CAPTOPRIL; HYDROCHLOROTHIAZIDE.

capreomycin
is an ANTIBACTERIAL and (polypeptide) ANTIBIOTIC drug. It is used specifically in the treatment of tuberculosis that proves to be

C

resistant to the first-line drugs (see ANTITUBERCULAR), or in cases where those drugs are not tolerated. Administration is by injection (alongside other drugs).
✚ Side-effects: There may be kidney toxicity and impaired hearing with tinnitus or vertigo; sometimes there are sensitivity reactions, such as rashes or urticaria, blood changes, pain at injection site.
▲ Warnings: It should not be administered to patients who are pregnant; administer with caution to those who have impaired liver or kidney function or sense of hearing (functions that should be monitored during treatment), or who are breast-feeding.
✪ **Related entry: Capastat.**

Caprin

(Sinclair) is a proprietary, prescription-only preparation of aspirin, available in two strengths. The low-dose version (75mg) is used as an ANTIPLATELET aggregation drug to help prevent certain cardiovascular diseases, including heart attack. The high-dose version (300mg) is used as an (NSAID) NON-NARCOTIC ANALGESIC and ANTIRHEUMATIC drug, and can be used to treat mild to moderate pain and to relieve flu and cold symptoms, rheumatism and lumbago (and is also available in limited quantities for sale without prescription). Both preparations are available in the form of tablets.
✚▲ Side-effects/warnings: See ASPIRIN.

capsaicin

is the active principle of capsicum, which is often used medically in the form of the resin called CAPSICUM OLEORESIN and is a pungent extract from capsicum peppers. Both capsicum resin and capsaicin are incorporated into medicines with RUBEFACIENT, or COUNTER-IRRITANT, actions, and when rubbed in topically to the skin cause a feeling of warmth that offsets the pain from underlying muscles, joints or internal organs. They can also be used to treat some types of neuropathic pain and post-herpatic pain.
✚ Side-effects: There may be local irritation.
▲ Warnings: It should not be used on inflamed or broken skin, or on mucous membranes. Keep away from the eyes. It causes burning in the initial stages of treatment, avoid taking a hot bath or shower just before or after applying.
✪ **Related entries: Axsain; Buttercup Syrup (Original Flavour).**

capsicum oleoresin

or capsicum resin, is a pungent extract from capsicum peppers. The active principle of these 'hot' peppers, which are also used for culinary purposes as chilli and cayenne pepper, is CAPSAICIN. Both capsicum resin and capsaicin are incorporated into medicines with RUBEFACIENT, or COUNTER-IRRITANT, action, and when rubbed in topically to the skin, cause a feeling of warmth that offsets the pain from underlying muscles, joints or internal organs.
✚ Side-effects: There may be local irritation, and it can cause an intense burning sensation when first used.
▲ Warnings: It should not be used on inflamed or broken skin, or on mucous membranes. Keep away from the eyes.
✪ **Related entries: Algipan Rub; Balmosa Cream; Jackson's Indian Brandee; Radian B Muscle Rub; Ralgex Cream; Ralgex Stick; Zacin.**

Capsuvac

(Galen) is a proprietary, prescription-only preparation of co-danthramer 50/60, which is a (*stimulant*) LAXATIVE based on dantron and docusate sodium. It can be used to relieve constipation and to prepare patients for abdominal procedures. It is available as capsules.
✚▲ Side-effects/warnings: See DANTRON; DOCUSATE SODIUM.

Capto-co

(Alpharm; IVAX) is a proprietary, prescription-only compound preparation of the ACE INHIBITOR captopril and the DIURETIC hydrochlorothiazide, a combination called CO-ZIDOCAPT. It can be used as an ANTIHYPERTENSIVE, and is available as tablets.
✚▲ Side-effects/warnings: See CAPTOPRIL; HYDROCHLOROTHIAZIDE.

captopril

is an ACE INHIBITOR. It is a powerful VASODILATOR which can be used as an ANTIHYPERTENSIVE and in congestive HEART FAILURE TREATMENT. It is often used in conjunction with other classes of drug, particularly (THIAZIDE) DIURETIC. Additionally, it can be used following myocardial infarction (damage to heart muscle, usually after a heart attack) and in diabetic nephropathy (kidney disease) in insulin-dependent diabetes.

Administration is oral.
✚ Side-effects: See ACE INHIBITOR. Also tachycardia, weight loss, rash, photosensitivity, flushing and acidosis. A number of other, rarer, side-effects have been reported.
▲ Warnings: See ACE INHIBITOR. Also, it should not be given to patients who are breast-feeding, or have porphyria.
✪ **Related entries: Acepril; Acezide; Capoten; Capozide; Capto-co; co-zidocapt; Ecopase; Kaplon; Tensopril.**

Carace

(DuPont; Bristol-Myers Squibb) is a proprietary, prescription-only preparation of the ACE INHIBITOR lisinopril. It can be used as an ANTIHYPERTENSIVE and in HEART FAILURE TREATMENT. It is available as tablets.
✚▲ Side-effects/warnings: See LISINOPRIL.

Carace Plus

(DuPont; Bristol-Myers Squibb) is a proprietary, prescription-only compound preparation of the ACE INHIBITOR lisinopril and the DIURETIC hydrochlorothiazide. It can be used as an ANTIHYPERTENSIVE, and is available as tablets (*Carace 10 Plus* and *Carace 20 Plus*).
✚▲ Side-effects/warnings: See HYDROCHLOROTHIAZIDE; LISINOPRIL.

carbachol

is a PARASYMPATHOMIMETIC drug which is used in GLAUCOMA TREATMENT to lower pressure in the eyeball (while constricting the pupil) and to treat urinary retention (particularly following surgery; though this use has largely been superseded by catherization). Administration can be oral, topical (to the eye) or by injection.
✚▲ Side-effects/warnings: See BETHANECHOL CHLORIDE. Systemic effects do not apply, or are rare, when application is to the eye. When used for glaucoma treatment, there may be browache and headache, which may get worse in the weeks following treatment. There may also be blurred vision, itching, burning and smarting, and other effects on the eye. Blurring may affect ability to perform skilled tasks such as driving.
✪ **Related entry: Isopto Carbachol.**

Carbalax

(Pharmax) is a proprietary, non-prescription preparation of the (*osmotic*) LAXATIVE sodium acid phosphate. It can be used to relieve constipation and to evacuate the rectum prior to abdominal procedures, and is available as an effervescent suppository. It is not normally given to children, except on medical advice.
✚▲ Side-effects/warnings: See SODIUM ACID PHOSPHATE.

carbamazepine

is an ANTICONVULSANT and ANTI-EPILEPTIC drug which is used in the preventive treatment of most forms of epilepsy (except absence seizures), to relieve the pain of trigeminal neuralgia (a searing pain from the trigeminal nerve in the face), in the management of manic-depressive illness resistant to lithium, in the treatment of diabetes insipidus, and sometimes for painful diabetic neuropathy. Administration is either oral or by suppositories.
✚ Side-effects: These are many and diverse, and include water retention, skin disorders, sedation, nausea and vomiting, dizziness, drowsiness, headache, unsteady gait, confusion and agitation (particularly in the elderly), visual disturbances and double or blurred vision, hair loss, cardiovascular and gastrointestinal disturbances, mental disturbances, blood and liver disorders, growth of breasts in men, impotence, aggression and depression.
▲ Warnings: It should not be administered to patients who suffer from certain heart defects, porphyria or bone marrow depression. Use with caution in those with certain impaired liver, kidney or heart function, a history of blood reactions to other drugs, glaucoma or who are pregnant or breast-feeding. Seek medical advice if fever, bruising, bleeding, sore throat, rash or mouth ulcers occur. Withdrawal should be gradual.
✪ **Related entries: Epimaz; Tegretol; Teril CR; Timonil Retard.**

carbaril

see CARBARYL.

carbaryl

(carbaril) is a PEDICULICIDAL drug which is used in the treatment of head lice. Administration is topical.
✚ Side-effects: Skin irritation.
▲ Warnings: Avoid contact with the eyes and broken or infected skin. Certain formulations should not be used by asthmatics or those with eczema. Its use should be limited.
✪ **Related entry: Carylderm.**

C

carbenoxolone sodium
is derived from LIQUORICE and is a synthetic derivative of glycyrrhizinic acid. It has been used as an ULCER-HEALING DRUG because it has a cytoprotectant action, though it has been replaced by more effective types of drug. However, because of its cytoprotective action it is still used to treat oesophageal ulceration and inflammation, and also mouth lesions and ulcers. Oral administration can be in the form of chewable tablets or as a liquid and in both cases with incorporated antacids. It may also be used locally as a gel or mouthwash to soothe mouth ulcers.
✚ Side-effects: There may be oedema, raised blood potassium levels (leading to muscle damage and other problems).
▲ Warnings: It should not be administered to patients with cardiac failure, certain liver or kidney disorders, with hyperkalaemia (raised blood potassium) or who are pregnant. Use with caution in patients with hypertension or heart, liver or kidney disease.
✪ Related entries: Bioplex; Bioral Gel; Pyrogastrone.

carbidopa
is a drug that is administered in combination with levodopa to treat parkinsonism, but not the parkinsonian symptoms induced by other drugs (see ANTIPARKINSONISM). It is levodopa that actually has the major effect, but carbidopa is an ENZYME INHIBITOR that blocks the break down of levodopa to dopamine in the body before it reaches the brain where it carries out its function. The presence of carbidopa allows the dose of levodopa to be at a minimum and so minimizes potentially severe side-effects and speeds the therapeutic response. Administration of carbidopa and levodopa is oral as single-compound tablets called CO-CARELDOPA.
✚▲ Side-effects/warnings: See LEVODOPA.
✪ Related entries: co-careldopa; Half Sinemet CR; Sinemet; Sinemet CR.

carbimazole
is a drug that acts as an indirect HORMONE ANTAGONIST, by reducing the production and output of the THYROID HORMONES from the thyroid gland, therefore treating an excess in the blood of thyroid hormones and the symptoms that it causes (thyrotoxicosis). Treatment may be on a maintenance basis over a long period (with dosage adjusted to optimum effect) or prior to surgical removal of the thyroid gland. Administration is oral.
✚ Side-effects: There may be rash, nausea and headache, gastrointestinal disturbances, occasionally, jaundice, hair loss, blood disorders, joint pain.
▲ Warnings: It should be administered with caution to patients who are pregnant, breast-feeding or who have certain liver disorders. Patients should tell their doctor if a sore throat develops, because this may be a sign of a rare, but serious, adverse effect of carbimazole on the bone marrow.
✪ Related entry: Neo-Mercazole.

carbocisteine
is a MUCOLYTIC drug which is used to reduce the viscosity of sputum and thus acts as an EXPECTORANT in patients with disorders of the upper respiratory tract, such as chronic asthma and bronchitis. Administration is oral.
✚ Side-effects: Sometimes gastrointestinal upsets and rashes.
▲ Warnings: It should not be used by people with peptic ulcers.
✪ Related entry: Mucodyne.

Carbo-Dome
(Lagap) is a proprietary, prescription-only preparation of coal tar. It can be used by topical application to treat psoriasis, and is available as a cream.
✚▲ Side-effects/warnings: See COAL TAR.

carbomer
(polyacrylic acid) is a synthetic agent which can be used in artificial tears where there is dryness of the eye due to a disease, such as keratoconjunctivitis. It is available as a liquid or gel for application to the eye.
✪ Related entries: GelTears; Pilogel; Viscotears.

Carbomix
(Penn) is a proprietary, non-prescription preparation of activated charcoal. It can be used to treat patients suffering from poisoning or a drug overdose, and is available as a powder.
✚▲ Side-effects/warnings: See ACTIVATED CHARCOAL.

carbonic-anhydrase inhibitor 🅱
drugs have enzyme-inhibitor actions (see

ENZYME INHIBITOR) against the enzyme *carbonic anhydrase*, which is present throughout the body and has an important role in the control of acid-base balance (pH). Medical applications of carbonic anhydrase inhibitors include as a weak DIURETIC to treat systemic oedema (accumulation of fluid in the tissues), as a GLAUCOMA TREATMENT in reducing fluid (aqueous humour) and intraocular pressure in the eye (the pressure in the eyeball), as an ANTI-EPILEPTIC in some types of epilepsy, and in prevention of mountain sickness (an unlicensed use). See ACETAZOLAMIDE and DORZOLAMIDE.

carboplatin

is a (*platinum compound*) CYTOTOXIC drug (derived from cisplatin) which is used as an ANTICANCER treatment specifically for cancer of the ovary. Administration is by injection.
✚▲ Side-effects/warnings: See CYTOTOXIC.
✪ Related entry: Paraplatin.

carboprost

is used to treat haemorrhage following childbirth, which is caused by the muscles of the uterus losing their tone. It is an analogue of PROSTAGLANDIN (a synthetic form related to $PGF_2\alpha$), which is a LOCAL HORMONE naturally involved in controlling the muscles of the uterus. It is generally used in patients who are unresponsive to ERGOMETRINE MALEATE and OXYTOCIN. Administration is by injection.
✚ Side-effects: There may be nausea, headache and dizziness, vomiting and diarrhoea, flushing, chills and hyperthermia. There may be raised blood pressure, oedema of the lungs, shortness of breath and sweating. There may be pain at the site of injection.
▲ Warnings: Use with caution in patients with a history of glaucoma, anaemia, jaundice, epilepsy, asthma, abnormal blood pressure (high or low) and uterine scars or any other predisposition to uterine rupture. It should not be used in patients with acute pelvic inflammatory disease; heart, kidney, lung or liver disorders.
✪ Related entry: Hemabate.

Cardene

(Yamanouchi) is a proprietary, prescription-only preparation of the CALCIUM-CHANNEL BLOCKER nicardipine hydrochloride. It can be used as an ANTIHYPERTENSIVE and as an ANTI-ANGINA drug in the prevention of attacks. Available as capsules.
✚▲ Side-effects/warnings: See NICARDIPINE HYDROCHLORIDE.

Cardene SR

(Yamanouchi) is a proprietary, prescription-only preparation of the CALCIUM-CHANNEL BLOCKER nicardipine hydrochloride. It can be used as an ANTIHYPERTENSIVE and is available as modified-release capsules.
✚▲ Side-effects/warnings: See NICARDIPINE HYDROCHLORIDE.

cardiac glycoside

is the name of a class of drugs derived from the leaf of the *Digitalis* foxgloves. These drugs have a pronounced effect on the failing heart by increasing the force of contraction and so have been commonly used for their CARDIAC STIMULANT actions to increase the force in HEART FAILURE TREATMENT. They can also correct certain abnormal heart rhythms (eg atrial fibrillation and atrial flutter) and are therefore used as an ANTI-ARRHYTHMIC treatment. However, today, these drugs are used far less often, because doses that are useful therapeutically are close to those that are toxic, so dose must be carefully adjusted in the individual. A digitalis antidote for use in overdose, DIGOXIN-SPECIFIC ANTIBODY FRAGMENT, is available. Examples of cardiac glycosides include DIGOXIN and DIGITOXIN.
▲ Warnings: Many herbal remedies and nutritional supplements (eg VITAMIN D, hawthorn, magnesium salts, St John's wort) can potentially interfere with the action of cardiac glycosides.

cardiac stimulant

drugs are used in medicine to stimulate the rate or the force of the heartbeat, but only when it is weak as a result of some disease state or in medical emergencies. CARDIAC GLYCOSIDE drugs have a pronounced effect on the failing heart, increasing the force of contraction and so have been widely prescribed in HEART FAILURE TREATMENT. A number of SYMPATHOMIMETIC drugs can be used directly to stimulate the heart through their BETA-RECEPTOR STIMULANT properties (eg ADRENALINE, ISOPRENALINE, DOPAMINE and DOBUTAMINE HYDROCHLORIDE), or DOPAMINE-RECEPTOR STIMULANT properties (eg DOPEXAMINE HYDROCHLORIDE), or a mixture of these. There is likely to be increased use of PHOSPHODIESTERASE INHIBITOR drugs specific for the form of this enzyme in the heart (type III), since drugs of this type (eg ENOXIMONE and MILRINONE) have a stimulatory action on heart muscle (myocardium) and can be used in severe congestive heart failure. Most of these drugs tend to be reserved for acute emergencies, such as cardiogenic shock, septic shock, during heart surgery and in cardiac infarction and cardiac arrest.

Cardicor

(Merck) is a proprietary, prescription-only preparation of the BETA-BLOCKER bisoprolol fumarate. It has been introduced as a HEART FAILURE TREATMENT, usually in conjunction with other drugs. It is available as tablets.
+▲ Side-effects/warnings: See BISOPROLOL FUMARATE.

Cardilate MR

(IVAX) is a proprietary, prescription-only preparation of the CALCIUM-CHANNEL BLOCKER nifedipine. It can be used as an ANTI-ANGINA treatment in the prevention of attacks and as an ANTIHYPERTENSIVE. It is available as tablets.
+▲ Side-effects/warnings: See NIFEDIPINE.

Cardinol

(CP) is a proprietary, prescription-only preparation of the BETA-BLOCKER propranolol hydrochloride. It can be used as an ANTIHYPERTENSIVE for raised blood pressure, as an ANTI-ANGINA treatment to relieve symptoms and improve exercise tolerance and as an ANTI-ARRHYTHMIC to regularize heartbeat and to treat myocardial infarction. It can also be used as an ANTITHYROID drug for short-term treatment of thyrotoxicosis, as an ANTIMIGRAINE treatment to prevent attacks, as an ANXIOLYTIC, particularly for symptomatic relief of tremor and palpitations, and, with an ALPHA-ADRENOCEPTOR BLOCKER, in the acute treatment of phaeochromocytoma. Available as tablets.
+▲ Side-effects/warnings: See PROPRANOLOL HYDROCHLORIDE.

Cardura

(Pfizer) is a proprietary, prescription-only preparation of the ALPHA-ADRENOCEPTOR BLOCKER doxazosin. It can be used as an ANTIHYPERTENSIVE, often in conjunction with other antihypertensives, and for benign prostatic hyperplasia (BPH). It is available as tablets.
+▲ Side-effects/warnings: See DOXAZOSIN.

Cardura XL

(Pfizer) is a proprietary, prescription-only preparation of the ALPHA-ADRENOCEPTOR BLOCKER doxazosin. It can be used as an ANTIHYPERTENSIVE (often in conjunction with other antihypertensives) and for benign prostatic hyperplasia (BPH). It is available as tablets.
+▲ Side-effects/warnings: See DOXAZOSIN.

Care Aqueous Cream

(Thornton & Ross) is a proprietary, non-prescription compound preparation of liquid paraffin, petroleum jelly and phenoxyethanol. It can be used as an emollient for dry skin conditions and to relieve symptoms of dry or chapped hands. It is available as a cream.
+▲ Side-effects/warnings: See LIQUID PARAFFIN.

Care Calamine Lotion

(Thornton & Ross) is a proprietary, non-prescription preparation of the mild ASTRINGENT agents calamine and zinc oxide. It is available as a lotion and can be used to treat the symptoms of sunburn and minor skin conditions.
+▲ Side-effects/warnings: See CALAMINE; ZINC OXIDE.

Care Clotrimazole Cream 1%

(Thornton & Ross) is a proprietary, non-prescription preparation of the ANTIFUNGAL drug clotrimazole. It can be used particularly to treat fungal infections such as athlete's foot, ringworm, nappy rash and nail infections. It is available as a cream and is not normally used for children, except on medical advice.
+▲ Side-effects/warnings: See CLOTRIMAZOLE.

Care Cystitis Relief

(Thornton & Ross) is a proprietary, non-prescription, preparation of sodium citrate (as dihydrate). It can be used to make the urine more alkaline in the treatment of cystitis. It is available as an oral powder, and is not normally used for men or children, except on medical advice.
+▲ Side-effects/warnings: See SODIUM CITRATE.

Care Extra Strength Ibuprofen Tablets 400mg

(Thornton & Ross) is a proprietary, non-

prescription compound preparation of the (NSAID) NON-NARCOTIC ANALGESIC and ANTIPYRETIC ibuprofen. It can be used for relief of backache, headache, muscular pain, period pain and migraine, and the symptoms of feverishness and colds and flu. It is available as tablets and is not normally given to children under 12 years, except on medical advice.
✚▲ Side-effects/warnings: See IBUPROFEN.

Care Extra Strength Long Lasting Pain Relief

(Thornton & Ross) is a proprietary, non-prescription compound preparation of the (NSAID) NON-NARCOTIC ANALGESIC and ANTIPYRETIC ibuprofen. It can be used for relief of pain of non-serious arthritic conditions, backache, headache, muscular pain, period pain and migraine, and the symptoms of feverishness and colds and flu. It is available as capsules and is not normally given to children under 12 years, except on medical advice.
✚▲ Side-effects/warnings: See IBUPROFEN.

Care Glycerin Suppositories for Adults

(Thornton & Ross) is a proprietary, non-prescription preparation of the LAXATIVE glycerol. It can be used for the relief of constipation. Available as a suppository. Not normally given to children, except on medical advice.
✚▲ Side-effects/warnings: See GLYCEROL.

Care Glycerin Suppositories for Children

(Thornton & Ross) is a proprietary, non-prescription preparation of the LAXATIVE glycerol. It can be used to relieve constipation. Available as a suppository, it is not normally given to infants, except on medical advice.
✚▲ Side-effects/warnings: See GLYCEROL.

Care Glycerin Suppositories for Infants

(Thornton & Ross) is a proprietary, non-prescription preparation of the LAXATIVE glycerol. It can be used to relieve constipation, and is available as a suppository for infants.
✚▲ Side-effects/warnings: See GLYCEROL.

Care Hayfever Relief Nasal Spray

(Thornton & Ross) is a proprietary, non-prescription compound preparation of the ANTI-INFLAMMATORY corticosteroid beclometasone dipropionate. It can be used for hay fever, and is available as a nasal spray. It is not normally given to children or adolescents under 18 years, except on medical advice.
✚▲ Side-effects/warnings: BECLOMETASONE DIPROPIONATE.

Care Ibuprofen Gel

(Thornton & Ross) is a proprietary, non-prescription preparation of the (NSAID) NON-NARCOTIC ANALGESIC and ANTIRHEUMATIC ibuprofen. It can be used to treat pain and inflammation, especially pain from arthritis and rheumatism, backache, sprains and strains, and other musculoskeletal disorders, and is available as a gel for topical application. It is not given to children under 14, except on medical advice.
✚▲ Side-effects/warnings: See IBUPROFEN; but adverse effects on topical application are limited.

Care Ibuprofen Tablets 200mg

(Thornton & Ross) is a proprietary, non-prescription compound preparation of the (NSAID) NON-NARCOTIC ANALGESIC and ANTIPYRETIC ibuprofen. It can be used for relief of backache, headache, muscular pain, period pain and migraine, and the symptoms of feverishness and colds and flu. It is available as tablets and is not normally given to children under 12 years, except on medical advice.
✚▲ Side-effects/warnings: See IBUPROFEN.

Care Loperamide Hydrochloride Capsules 2 mg

(Thornton & Ross) is a proprietary, non-prescription preparation of the (OPIOID) ANTIDIARRHOEAL loperamide hydrochloride. It can be used to relieve the symptoms of acute diarrhoea and its associated discomfort, and is available as capsules. It is not given to children under 12 years, except on medical advice.
✚▲ Side-effects/warnings: See LOPERAMIDE HYDROCHLORIDE.

Care Pholcodine Linctus

(Thornton & Ross) is a proprietary, non-prescription preparation of the ANTITUSSIVE pholcodine. It can be used for the relief of dry or irritating coughs, and is available as a linctus. It is not normally given to children under five years,

except on medical advice.
✚▲ Side-effects/warnings: See PHOLCODINE.

Care Potassium Citrate Mixture
(Thornton & Ross) is a proprietary, non-prescription, preparation of potassium citrate. It can be used to make the urine more alkaline in the treatment of cystitis and minor urinary tract infections. It is available as an oral powder, and is not given to children under one year, except on medical advice.
✚▲ Side-effects/warnings: See POTASSIUM CITRATE.

Care Senna Laxative Tablets
(Thornton & Ross) is a proprietary, non-prescription preparation of the (*stimulant*) LAXATIVE senna. It can be used to relieve constipation. Available as tablets, it is not normally given to children under five years, except on medical advice.
✚▲ Side-effects/warnings: See SENNA.

Carisoma
(Forest) is a proprietary, prescription-only preparation of the SKELETAL MUSCLE RELAXANT carisoprodol. It can be used to treat muscle spasm, and is available as tablets.
✚▲ Side-effects/warnings: See CARISOPRODOL.

carisoprodol
is a SKELETAL MUSCLE RELAXANT which can be used for relaxing muscles that are in spasm. It works by an action on the central nervous system. Administration is oral.
✚▲ Side-effects/warnings: See MEPROBAMATE; but with carisoprodol drowsiness is less common. It is not used in patients with porphyria.
✪ **Related entry: Carisoma.**

carmellose sodium
(sodium carboxymethyl cellulose) is a substance that is used as the basis for a paste or a powder which is spread or sprinkled over lesions in or around the mouth in order to provide a protective barrier and relieve some of the discomfort while lesions heal. Also, it is incorporated into mouth spray preparations for dry mouth (eg due to Sicca syndrome, certain drug treatments, after radiotherapy etc.). It can also be used as eye-drops for dry eye conditions. It is applied topically.
✚▲ Side-effects/warnings: It is regarded as safe in normal topical use.
✪ **Related entries: Celluvisc; Glandosane; Luborant; Orabase; Orahesive; Salivace.**

carmustine
is an (*alkylating agent*) CYTOTOXIC drug which works by direct interference with DNA and so prevents normal cell replication. It is used as an ANTICANCER drug to treat some myelomas, lymphomas and brain tumours. Administration is by injection.
✚▲ Side-effects/warnings: See CYTOTOXIC.
✪ **Related entry: BiCNU.**

Carnation Callous Caps
(Cuxson Gerrard) is a proprietary, non-prescription preparation of the KERATOLYTIC agent salicylic acid. It can be used to treat calluses, and is available as medicated dressing. It is not normally given to children under 16 years, except on medical advice.
✚▲ Side-effects/warnings: See SALICYLIC ACID.

Carnation Corn Caps
(Cuxson Gerrard) is a proprietary, non-prescription preparation of the KERATOLYTIC agent salicylic acid. It can be used to treat hard corns, and is available as adhesive dressing. It is not normally given to children under 15 years, except on medical advice.
✚▲ Side-effects/warnings: See SALICYLIC ACID.

Carnation Verruca Treatment
(Cuxson Gerrard) is a proprietary, non-prescription preparation of the KERATOLYTIC agent salicylic acid. It can be used to treat verrucas, and is available as adhesive dressing. It is not normally given to children under six years or adults over 50 years, except on medical advice.
✚▲ Side-effects/warnings: See SALICYLIC ACID.

carnitine
(L-carnitine) is an amino acid used to treat carnitine deficiency, either as a METABOLIC DISORDER TREATMENT where there is a primary deficiency due to an inborn error of metabolism, or where there is a secondary deficiency in haemodialysis patients. It is given orally or by injection.
✚ Side-effects: Nausea, vomiting, abdominal pain, diarrhoea, body odour.

▲ Warnings: Use with care where there is kidney impairment, pregnancy and breast-feeding. Levels of carnitine in blood and urine may be monitored.
✪ **Related entry: Carnitor.**

Carnitor

(Shire) is a proprietary, prescription-only preparation of the amino acid carnitine which is used to treat deficiency, either as a METABOLIC DISORDER TREATMENT or in haemodialysis patients. It is available as an oral liquid (one form for children) and in a form for injection.
✚▲ Side-effects/warnings: See CARNITINE.

carteolol hydrochloride

is a BETA-BLOCKER which can be used as a GLAUCOMA TREATMENT for chronic simple glaucoma. It is thought to work by slowing the rate of production of the aqueous humour in the eye. Administration is topical.
✚ Side-effects: There may be some systemic absorption after using eye-drops, so some of the side-effects listed under PROPRANOLOL HYDROCHLORIDE may be seen. Dry eyes, stinging, redness, pain and some local allergic reactions, including conjunctivitis, may also occur.
▲ Warnings: In view of possible systemic absorption, dangerous side-effects should be borne in mind; in particular, the danger of bronchospasm in asthmatics and interactions with some CALCIUM-CHANNEL BLOCKER.
✪ **Related entry: Teoptic.**

carvedilol

is a BETA-BLOCKER that is a VASODILATOR and can be used as an ANTIHYPERTENSIVE and as an ANTI-ANGINA treatment to relieve symptoms. It is sometimes used under specialist advice (in combination with other types of drug) in chronic HEART FAILURE TREATMENT. Administration is oral.
✚▲ Side-effects/warnings: See PROPRANOLOL HYDROCHLORIDE. Also, postural hypotension, dizziness, headache, fatigue, gastrointestinal disturbances, slowing of the heart, oedema, painful and tingling extremities, dry mouth and eyes, eye irritation or disturbed vision, sleep disturbances, impotence, disturbances of urination, stuffy nose and wheezing, flu-like symptoms, heart and blood changes.
✪ **Related entry: Eucardic.**

Carylderm

(SSL) is a proprietary, prescription-only preparation of the PEDICULICIDAL carbaryl. It can be used to treat infestations of lice, and is available as a liquid (water base) and a lotion (alcohol base).
✚▲ Side-effects/warnings: See CARBARYL.

Casodex

(AstraZeneca) is a proprietary, prescription-only preparation of the anti-androgen, HORMONE ANTAGONIST bicalutamide. It can be used as an ANTICANCER drug to treat cancer of the prostate, and is available as tablets.
✚▲ Side-effects/warnings: See BICALUTAMIDE.

castor oil

has EMOLLIENT properties and is found in some skin preparations and BARRIER CREAM products. It was once used as a (*stimulant*) LAXATIVE but is now obsolete. It is used in a polyethoxylated form in some drug formulations for injection.
✚▲ Side-effects/warnings: It is normally safe and relatively free of side-effects on topical application, but the polyethoxylated form has been associated with anaphylaxis on injection. As a laxative, its irritant properties are powerful, and it can induce labour.

Catapres

(Boehringer Ingelheim) is a proprietary, prescription-only preparation of the ANTISYMPATHETIC clonidine hydrochloride. It can be used as an ANTIHYPERTENSIVE and ANTIMIGRAINE treatment, and is available as tablets and in a form for injection.
✚▲ Side-effects/warnings: See CLONIDINE HYDROCHLORIDE.

Caverject

(Pharmacia) is a PROSTAGLANDIN, alprostadil (PGE_1). It is a prescription-only IMPOTENCE TREATMENT for men to manage penile erectile dysfunction. It available in a form for injection and is administered by intracavernosal injection into the penis.
✚▲ Side-effects/warnings: See ALPROSTADIL.

Ceanel Concentrate

(Quinoderm) is a proprietary, non-prescription compound preparation of the ANTISEPTIC cetrimide and the ANTIFUNGAL undecenoic acid

(with phenylethyl alcohol). It can be used as an adjunct in the treatment of psoriasis (including of the trunk and limbs) and other non-infective scalp conditions, and also for dandruff. It is available as a shampoo.
✚▲ Side-effects/warnings: See CETRIMIDE; UNDECENOIC ACID.

Cedocard-Retard

(Pharmacia) is a proprietary, non-prescription preparation of the VASODILATOR drug isosorbide dinitrate, which can be used as an ANTI-ANGINA drug. It is available as modified-release tablets in two strengths (*Retard-20 tablets; Retard-40 tablets*).
✚▲ Side-effects/warnings: See ISOSORBIDE DINITRATE.

cefaclor

is a broad-spectrum ANTIBACTERIAL and ANTIBIOTIC drug. It is one of the 'second-generation' CEPHALOSPORIN class, and is now primarily used to treat Gram-positive and Gram-negative bacterial infections of the respiratory and urinary tracts. It is used particularly for urinary tract infections that do not respond to other drugs. Administration is oral.
✚ Side-effects: Nausea, vomiting, diarrhoea, headache, colitis, sensitivity reactions that may be serious (from rashes to anaphylaxis), blood and liver disturbances, behavioural and nervous disturbances.
▲ Warnings: It should not be administered to patients who are sensitive to penicillins and cephalosporins. Do not use in patients with porphyria and use with caution in those who are pregnant or breast-feeding.
✪ **Related entries: Distaclor; Distaclor MR; Keftid.**

cefadroxil

is a broad-spectrum ANTIBACTERIAL and ANTIBIOTIC drug. It is one of the 'first-generation' CEPHALOSPORIN class, and is now primarily used to treat bacterial infections, especially of the urinary tract, that do not respond to other drugs. Administration is oral.
✚▲ Side-effects/warnings: See CEFACLOR.
✪ **Related entry: Baxan.**

cefalexin

(cephalexin) is a broad-spectrum ANTIBACTERIAL and ANTIBIOTIC drug. It is one of the 'first-generation' orally active CEPHALOSPORIN class, and can be used to treat a wide range of bacterial infections, particularly of the urinary tract. Administration is oral.
✚▲ Side-effects/warnings: See CEFACLOR.
✪ **Related entries: Ceporex; Keflex; Kiflone; Tenkorex.**

cefamandole

(cephamandole) is a broad-spectrum ANTIBACTERIAL and ANTIBIOTIC drug. It is one of the 'second-generation' CEPHALOSPORIN class, and is less susceptible to inactivation by bacterial penicillinases than others in its class and is therefore effective against a greater range of Gram-negative bacteria, for example, penicillin-resistant *Neisseria gonorrhoeae* and *Haemophilus influenzae*. It can be used to treat a wide range of bacterial infections, particularly of the skin and soft tissues, the genitourinary and upper respiratory tracts and middle ear. It is also used to prevent infection during surgery. Administration is by injection.
✚▲ Side-effects/warnings: See CEFACLOR.
✪ **Related entry: Kefadol.**

cefazolin

(cephazolin) is a broad-spectrum ANTIBACTERIAL and ANTIBIOTIC drug. It is one of the 'first-generation' CEPHALOSPORIN class, and can be used to treat a wide range of bacterial infections. Administration is by injection.
✚▲ Side-effects/warnings: See CEFACLOR.
✪ **Related entry: Kefzol.**

cefixime

is a broad-spectrum ANTIBACTERIAL and (CEPHALOSPORIN) ANTIBIOTIC drug. It is used to treat acute bacterial infections. It has a longer duration of action than many other cephalosporin taken by mouth. Administration is oral.
✚▲ Side-effects/warnings: See CEFACLOR.
✪ **Related entry: Suprax.**

cefotaxime

is a broad-spectrum ANTIBACTERIAL and ANTIBIOTIC drug. It is one of the 'third-generation' CEPHALOSPORIN class, and can be used to treat a wide range of bacterial infections, including the urinary tract, for meningitis and gonorrhoea. It can also be used to prevent infection during surgery. Administration is by injection.
✚▲ Side-effects/warnings: See CEFACLOR.

✪ **Related entry: Claforan.**

cefoxitin

is a broad-spectrum ANTIBACTERIAL and ANTIBIOTIC drug. It is one of the 'second-generation' CEPHALOSPORIN class, and can be used to treat a wide range of bacterial infections, particularly abdominal sepsis such as peritonitis, urinary tract gonorrhoea and before operations. Administration is by injection.

✚▲ Side-effects/warnings: See CEFACLOR.

✪ **Related entry: Mefoxin.**

cefpirome

is a broad-spectrum ANTIBACTERIAL and ANTIBIOTIC drug, a member of the CEPHALOSPORIN class. It is used to treat urinary-tract, skin and respiratory tract infections and particularly for severe infections including bacteraemia and infections in neutropenic patients. Administration is by injection.

✚▲ Side-effects/warnings: See CEFACLOR; also, there may be taste disturbances.

✪ **Related entry: Cefrom.**

cefpodoxime

is a broad-spectrum ANTIBACTERIAL and (CEPHALOSPORIN) ANTIBIOTIC. It can be used to treat bacterial infections of the respiratory tract, including bronchitis and pneumonia, skin and soft tissue infections, tonsillitis, urinary tract infections, gonorrhoea, particularly those that are recurrent, chronic or resistant to other drugs. Administration is oral.

✚▲ Side-effects/warnings: See CEFACLOR.

✪ **Related entry: Orelox.**

cefprozil

is a broad-spectrum ANTIBACTERIAL and ANTIBIOTIC drug. It is one of the second-generation CEPHALOSPORIN class, and can be used to treat a range of bacterial infections, particularly upper respiratory-tract infections, acute exacerbation of chronic bronchitis, middle ear infections (otitis media), and skin and soft tissue infections. Administration is oral.

✚▲ Side-effects/warnings: See CEFACLOR.

✪ **Related entry: Cefzil.**

cefradine

(cephradine) is a broad-spectrum ANTIBACTERIAL and ANTIBIOTIC drug. It is one of the 'first-generation' CEPHALOSPORIN class, and can be used to treat a wide range of bacterial infections, and is also used to prevent infection during surgery. Administration is either oral or by injection.

✚▲ Side-effects/warnings: See CEFACLOR.

✪ **Related entries: Nicef; Velosef.**

Cefrom

(Hoechst Marion Roussel; Aventis Pharma) is a proprietary, prescription-only preparation of the ANTIBACTERIAL and (CEPHALOSPORIN) ANTIBIOTIC cefpirome. It can be used to treat serious infections, and is available in a form for intravenous injection.

✚▲ Side-effects/warnings: See CEFPIROME.

ceftazidime

is a broad-spectrum ANTIBACTERIAL and ANTIBIOTIC drug. It is one of the 'third-generation' CEPHALOSPORIN class, and is among the most effective of the cephalosporins against bacterial infections. It can be used particularly to treat infections of the skin and soft tissues, the urinary and respiratory tracts, the ear, nose and throat (eg *Pseudomonal* lung infections in cystic fibrosis) and to prevent infection following surgery. It can also be used to treat infection in patients whose immune systems are defective. Administration is by injection.

✚▲ Side-effects/warnings: See CEFACLOR.

✪ **Related entries: Fortum; Kefadim.**

ceftriaxone

is a broad-spectrum ANTIBACTERIAL and ANTIBIOTIC drug. It is a 'third-generation' CEPHALOSPORIN, and can be used to treat a wide range of Gram-negative bacterial infections, including gonorrhoea. It can also be used to prevent infections during surgery. It has a much longer duration of action than others of this class. Administration is by injection.

✚▲ Side-effects/warnings: See CEFACLOR. Administer with caution to patients with certain liver disorders.

✪ **Related entry: Rocephin.**

cefuroxime

is a broad-spectrum ANTIBACTERIAL and ANTIBIOTIC drug. It is one of the 'second-generation' CEPHALOSPORIN class, and can be used to treat a wide range of bacterial infections,

C

particularly Gram-negative infections of the urinary, respiratory and genital tracts, meningitis, Lyme disease and *Haemophilus influenzae* and *Neisseria gonorrhoeae*. It can also be used to prevent infection following surgery. Administration is either oral or by injection.
✚▲ Side-effects/warnings: See CEFACLOR.
✪ **Related entries: Zinacef; Zinnat.**

Cefzil
(Bristol-Myers Squibb) is a proprietary, prescription-only preparation of the ANTIBACTERIAL and (CEPHALOSPORIN) ANTIBIOTIC cefprozil. It can be used to treat a range of bacterial infections, and is available as tablets and an oral suspension.
✚▲ Side-effects/warnings: See CEFACLOR.

Celance
(Lilly) is a proprietary, prescription-only preparation of pergolide, which can be used as an ANTIPARKINSONISM drug. It is available as tablets.
✚▲ Side-effects/warnings: See PERGOLIDE.

Celebrex
(Searle; Pharmacia) is a recently introduced proprietary, prescription-only preparation of the (NSAID) NON-NARCOTIC ANALGESIC and ANTIRHEUMATIC celecoxib. It can be used to treat the pain and inflammation of osteoarthritis and rheumatoid arthritis, and is available as capsules.
✚▲ Side-effects/warnings: See CELECOXIB.

celecoxib
is a recently introduced (NSAID) NON-NARCOTIC ANALGESIC and ANTIRHEUMATIC drug, one of a new type (cyclo-oxygenase 2 selective inhibitors), which is used to treat the pain and inflammation of osteoarthritis and rheumatoid arthritis. Administration is oral.
✚ Side-effects: Flatulence, insomnia, inflammation of the pharynx and/or sinusitis. Celecoxib may also cause inflammation of the mouth, constipation, heart palpitations, psychological effects such as anxiety and/or depression, fatigue, paraesthesia and muscle cramps. Occasionally, it may cause hair loss and alteration in the sense of taste.
▲ Warnings: See NSAID. It is not used in people with sulphonamide sensitivity, kidney impairment, inflammatory bowel disease or congestive heart failure. Authorities recommend that it is not to be used routinely for all patients with rheumatoid arthritis or osteoarthritis, but should be used in preference to more commonly used NSAIDs only for certain people. For instance, those who have a history of gastroduodenal ulcer and other digestive system disorders or people who are taking other medicines (including standard NSAIDs) which increase the risk of gastrointestinal effects.
✪ **Related entry: Celebrex.**

Celectol
(Pantheon) is a proprietary, prescription-only preparation of the BETA-BLOCKER celiprolol hydrochloride. It can be used as an ANTIHYPERTENSIVE for raised blood pressure, and is available as tablets.
✚▲ Side-effects/warnings: See CELIPROLOL HYDROCHLORIDE.

Celevac
(Shire) is a proprietary, non-prescription preparation of the (*bulking-agent*) LAXATIVE methylcellulose. It can be used to treat a number of gastrointestinal disorders and also as an APPETITE SUPPRESSANT in the treatment of obesity. It is available as tablets.
✚▲ Side-effects/warnings: See METHYLCELLULOSE.

celiprolol hydrochloride
is a BETA-BLOCKER that is a VASODILATOR and can be used as an ANTIHYPERTENSIVE for raised blood pressure. Administration is oral.
✚▲ Side-effects/warnings: See LABETALOL HYDROCHLORIDE. There may also be headache, sleepiness, fatigue, nausea, bronchospasm and slowing of the heart.
✪ **Related entry: Celectol.**

CellCept
(Roche) is a proprietary, prescription-only preparation of the (CYTOTOXIC) IMMUNOSUPPRESSANT mycophenolate mofetil. It can be used to treat tissue rejection in transplant patients, and is available as capsules and a form for intravenous infusion.
✚▲ Side-effects/warnings: See MYCOPHENOLATE MOFETIL.

Celluvisc
(Allergan) is a proprietary, non-prescription

preparation of carmellose sodium. It can be used as artificial tears where there is dryness of the eye due to disease. It is available as eye-drops.
✚▲ Side-effects/warnings: See: CARMELLOSE SODIUM.

Centyl K

(Leo) s a proprietary, prescription-only compound preparation of the (THIAZIDE) DIURETIC bendroflumethiazide (bendrofluazide) and the potassium supplement potassium chloride. It can be used in as an ANTIHYPERTENSIVE and to treat oedema. It is available as tablets.
✚▲ Side-effects/warnings: See BENDROFLUMETHIAZIDE; POTASSIUM CHLORIDE.

cephalexin

see CEFALEXIN.

cephalosporin

is the name of a group of ANTIBIOTIC drugs that are chemically part of the BETA-LACTAM class. They are broad-spectrum ANTIBACTERIAL drugs that act against both Gram-positive and Gram-negative bacteria. Their chemical structure bears a strong resemblance to that of the penicillins as they both contain a beta-lactam ring, hence their classification as *beta-lactam antibiotics*. The similarity in structure extends to their mechanism of action: both classes inhibit the synthesis of the bacterial cell wall, so killing growing bacteria – they are *bactericidal*.

As a group, the cephalosporins are generally active against streptococci, staphylococci and a number of Gram-negative bacteria, including many coliforms. Examples of the original, 'first-generation' cephalosporins are CEFRADINE and CEFADROXIL. Some 'second-generation' cephalosporins (eg CEFUROXIME and CEFAMANDOLE) are resistant to inactivation by bacterial penicillinase (beta-lactamase) enzymes, which widens their range of action to include treating sensitive Gram-negative organisms, including *Haemophilus influenzae*.

Some of the latest, 'third-generation', cephalosporins (eg CEFOTAXIME, CEFTAZIDIME) act as antibacterials against certain Gram-negative bacteria (eg *Haemophilus influenzae*) and pseudomonal infections (eg *Pseudomonas aeruginosa*). Many cephalosporins are actively excreted by the kidney and therefore reach considerably higher concentrations in the urine than in the blood. For this reason, they may be used to treat infections of the urinary tract where they work as they are being excreted. In general, cephalosporins are rarely the drug of first choice, but provide a useful alternative, or reserve option, in particular situations. The cephalosporins currently used are relatively non-toxic and well-tolerated, and only occasional blood-clotting problems, superinfections and hypersensitivity reactions occur (only 10% of patients allergic to penicillin show sensitivity to cephalosporins).

cephamandole

see CEFAMANDOLE.

cephazolin

see CEFAZOLIN.

cephradine

see CEFRADINE.

Ceporex

(GlaxoWellcome; GSK) is a proprietary, prescription-only preparation of the ANTIBACTERIAL and (CEPHALOSPORIN) ANTIBIOTIC cefalexin. It can be used to treat many infections, including of the urogenital tract, and is available as capsules, tablets and a syrup.
✚▲ Side-effects/warnings: See CEFALEXIN.

Ceprotin

(Baxter) is a proprietary prescription-only preparation of a natural ANTICOAGULANT, protein C concentrate, and is used in patients with congenital protein C deficiency.
✚▲ Side-effects/warnings: See PROTEIN C CONCENTRATE.

Cerebrovase

(Ashbourne) is a proprietary, prescription-only preparation of the ANTIPLATELET drug dipyridamole. It can be used to prevent thrombosis, and is available as tablets.
✚▲ Side-effects/warnings: See DIPYRIDAMOLE.

Cerezyme

(Genzyme) is a proprietary, prescription-only preparation of the enzyme imiglucerase, which is produced by recombinant DNA technology and used as a specialist replacement in the METABOLIC DISORDER TREATMENT of the enzyme deficiency

disease, Gaucher's disease. It is available in a form for intravenous infusion.
✚▲ Side-effects/warnings: See IMIGLUCERASE.

certoparin

is a *low molecular weight* heparin and is used as an ANTICOAGULANT. It has some advantages over heparin (longer duration of action), for instance, when used for prophylaxis of deep-vein thrombosis. Administration is by injection.
✚▲ Side-effects/warnings: See HEPARIN.
✪ **Related entry: Alphaparin.**

Cerumol Ear Drops

(LAB) is a proprietary, non-prescription compound preparation of the ANTISEPTIC agent chlorbutol (chlorobutanol) and arachis oil (with paradichlorobenzene). It can be used to remove earwax, and is available as ear-drops.
✚▲ Side-effects/warnings: See ARACHIS OIL; CHLORBUTOL.

cetirizine hydrochloride

is a recently developed ANTIHISTAMINE with less side-effects (such as sedation) than some of the older members of this class. It can be used for the symptomatic relief of allergic symptoms such as hay fever and urticaria. Administration is oral.
✚▲ Side-effects/warnings: See ANTIHISTAMINE. Administer with caution to patients with kidney impairment. The incidence of sedation and anticholinergic side-effects is low. It should not be used in pregnancy or breast-feeding.
✪ **Related entry: Zirtek Allergy.**

Cetraben Emollient Cream

(Sankyo) is a proprietary, non-prescription compound preparation of liquid paraffin, white soft paraffin and several other constituents. It can be used as an EMOLLIENT for inflammed, damaged, dry or chapped skin, including eczema, and is available as a cream.
✚▲ Side-effects/warnings: See LIQUID PARAFFIN; WHITE SOFT PARAFFIN.

cetrimide

is an ANTISEPTIC and DISINFECTANT which is used therapeutically (often in combination with CHLORHEXIDINE) for cleansing the skin and scalp, burns and wounds and, as a cream, as a soap substitute for conditions such as acne and seborrhoea. It is also used for minor cuts and abrasions, and for cold sores. It is applied topically.
✚ Side-effects: There may be skin irritation.
▲ Warnings: Avoid contact with eyes and body cavities.
✪ **Related entries: Antiseptic First Aid Cream; Bansor Mouth Antiseptic; Ceanel Concentrate; Dermidex Cream; Drapolene Cream; Hibicet Hospital Concentrate; Lypsyl Cold Sore Gel; Neo Baby Cream; Savlon Antiseptic Cream; Savlon Antiseptic Liquid; Siopel; Steripod Chlorhexidine/Cetrimide; Tisept; Travasept 100.**

cetrorelix

is a HORMONE ANTAGONIST which indirectly inhibits release of gonadotrophins (LH & FSH). It is used in the treatment of infertility by assisted reproductive techniques (IVF). Administration is by injection.
✚ Side-effects: Nausea, headache, reaction at the injection site.
▲ Warnings: Should not be used in pregnancy or breast-feeding, kidney or liver impairment.
✪ **Related entry: Cetrotide.**

Cetrotide

(Serono) is a proprietary, prescription-only preparation of cetrorelix, a drug that affects the release of gonadotrophins and is used in the treatment of infertility by assisted reproductive techniques (IVF). It is available in a form for injection.
✚▲ Side-effects/warnings: See CETRORELIX.

cetylpyridinium chloride

is an ANTISEPTIC which is used as a mouthwash or gargle for oral hygiene and minor throat infections. It is available in various topical forms as a gel, lozenges and an oral solution.
✚▲ Side-effects/warnings: Reasonably safe in normal topical use at recommended concentrations.
✪ **Related entries: Adult Meltus Expectorant for Chesty Coughs and Catarrh; Adult Meltus Expectorant with Decongestant; Anbesol Adult Strength Gel; Anbesol Liquid; Anbesol Teething Gel; Bonjela Oral Pain-Relieving Gel; Calgel Teething Gel; Dentinox Teething Gel; Junior Meltus Expectorant for Chesty Coughs and Catarrh; Junior Meltus Sugar and Colour Free Expectorant; Merocaine Lozenges; Merocet Gargle/Mouthwash; Merocets Lozenges; Merocets Plus Lozenges; Rinstead Adult Gel;**

Rinstead Sugar Free Pastilles; Rinstead Teething Gel; Woodward's Teething Gel.

chalk
see CALCIUM CARBONATE.

Charcodote
(Dominion) is a proprietary, non-prescription preparation of activated charcoal. It can be used to treat patients suffering from poisoning or a drug overdose. It is available as an oral suspension.
✚▲ Side-effects/warnings: See ACTIVATED CHARCOAL.

chelating agent 🅱
is the term used to describe a drug that can be used as an ANTIDOTE mainly in metal poisoning. Chelating agents work by chemically binding to certain metallic ions and other substances, making them less toxic and allowing the body to excrete (remove) them. They are used to reduce unacceptably high levels of metals of external origin (accidental or environmental) and in METABOLIC DISORDER TREATMENT (eg of copper in Wilson's disease) and to treat disease states (eg deferiprone or desferrioxamine for iron overload in thalassaemia). See DEFERIPRONE; DESFERRIOXAMINE MESILATE; DICOBALT EDETATE; DIMERCAPROL; SODIUM CALCIUM EDETATE.

Chemotrim
(Rosemont) is a proprietary, prescription-only compound preparation of the (SULPHONAMIDE) ANTIBACTERIAL sulfamethoxazole and the sulphonamide-like antibacterial trimethoprim, which is a combination known as co-trimoxazole. It can be used to treat bacterial infections, and is available as a paediatric oral suspension.
✚▲ Side-effects/warnings: See CO-TRIMOXAZOLE.

Chemydur 60XL
(Sovereign) is a proprietary, prescription-only preparation of the VASODILATOR drug isosorbide mononitrate. It can be used as an ANTI-ANGINA drug, and is available as modified-release tablets.
✚▲ Side-effects/warnings: See ISOSORBIDE MONONITRATE.

Chimax
(Chiron) is a proprietary, prescription-only preparation of the anti-androgen, HORMONE ANTAGONIST flutamide. It can be used as an ANTICANCER drug to treat cancer of the prostate, and is available as tablets.
✚▲ Side-effects/warnings: See FLUTAMIDE.

Chirocaine
(Abbott) is a proprietary, prescription-only preparation of the LOCAL ANAESTHETIC levobupivacaine hydrochloride. It can be used particularly when a prolonged course of treatment is required. It is available in several forms for injection.
✚▲ Side-effects/warnings: See LEVOBUPIVACAINE HYDROCHLORIDE.

Chloractil
(DDSA) is a proprietary, prescription-only preparation of the (PHENOTHIAZINE) ANTIPSYCHOTIC chlorpromazine hydrochloride. It can be used in patients undergoing behavioural disturbances, who are psychotic (especially schizophrenics) or showing severe anxiety where a degree of sedation is useful. It can also be used as an ANTINAUSEANT and ANTI-EMETIC to relieve nausea and vomiting, and for intractable hiccup. It is available as tablets.
✚▲ Side-effects/warnings: See CHLORPROMAZINE HYDROCHLORIDE.

Chloral Elixir, Paediatric, BP
is a non-proprietary, prescription-only preparation of the HYPNOTIC drug chloral hydrate, which is used to treat insomnia, and is available as an elixir for children.
✚▲ Side-effects/warnings: See CHLORAL HYDRATE.

Chloral Mixture, BP
is a non-proprietary, prescription-only preparation of the HYPNOTIC drug chloral hydrate, which is used to treat insomnia. It is available as an oral solution.
✚▲ Side-effects/warnings: See CHLORAL HYDRATE.

chloral betaine
see CLORAL BETAINE.

chloral hydrate
is a short-term SEDATIVE and HYPNOTIC drug. It used to be considered to be particularly useful in

inducing sleep in children or elderly patients. Administration is usually oral.

✚ Side-effects: Stomach irritation, abdominal distension and flatulence; occasionally, rashes, vertigo and light-headedness, headache, blood and movement changes and excitement (eg night terror, delirium). Dependence can occur with prolonged use.

▲ Warnings: It should not be used by patients with severe heart disease, inflammation of the stomach, or severely impaired function of the liver or kidneys, who are pregnant or breast-feeding. It should be administered with caution to those with respiratory disorders, or who have a history of personality disorders, drug abuse or porphyria. Avoid contact with the skin or mucous membranes.

✪ **Related entries: cloral betaine; Chloral Elixir, Paediatric, BP; Chloral Mixture, BP; Welldorm.**

chlorambucil

is an (*alkylating agent*) CYTOTOXIC drug which is used as an ANTICANCER treatment, particularly for chronic lymphocytic leukaemia, lymphomas and ovarian cancer and Hodgkin's disease. It works by interfering with the DNA and so preventing normal cell replication. It is also used as an IMMUNOSUPPRESSANT in the treatment of rheumatoid arthritis. Administration is oral.

✚▲ Side-effects/warnings: See CYTOTOXIC.

✪ **Related entry: Leukeran.**

chloramphenicol

is a broad-spectrum ANTIBACTERIAL and ANTIBIOTIC drug, which can be used to treat many forms of infection. However, the serious side-effects caused by its systemic use mean that it is normally restricted to certain severe infections, such as typhoid fever and, in particular, infections caused by *Haemophilus influenzae*. It is useful in treating conditions such as bacterial conjunctivitis, otitis externa or many types of skin infection, because it is applied topically to the eyes, ears or skin and therefore its toxicity is not encountered. Topical administration is by eye-drops, ear-drops or a cream. Systemic administration is either oral or by injection.

✚ Side-effects: These depend on the route of administration. When used systemically there may be nausea, vomiting, diarrhoea; certain types of neuritis. Systemic treatment may cause serious damage to the bone marrow, which results in blood disorders, and other serious side-effects. When used topically, there may be stinging of the eyes (eye-drops) and sensitivity reactions to vehicle (eye-drops).

▲ Warnings: It should not be administered to patients who are pregnant, breast-feeding or have porphyria. Administer with caution to those with impaired liver or kidney function. Prolonged or repeated use should be avoided. Regular blood counts are essential when it is used systemically.

✪ **Related entries: Actinac; Chloromycetin; Kemicetine; Minims Chloramphenicol; Sno Phenicol.**

Chlorasol

(SSL) is a proprietary, non-prescription preparation of the ANTISEPTIC sodium hypochlorite. It can be used as a cleanser to treat skin infections and particularly for cleansing wounds and ulcers. It is available as a solution.

✚▲ Side-effects/warnings: See SODIUM HYPOCHLORITE.

chlorbutol

(chlorobutanol) is used in some inhalation preparations, and (as a preservative) in some drug preparations for removing earwax.

✚▲ Side-effects/warnings: It is regarded as safe in normal topical use.

✪ **Related entries: Cerumol Ear Drops; Dermidex Cream; Karvol Decongestant Capsules; Karvol Decongestant Drops; Monphytol.**

chlordiazepoxide

is a BENZODIAZEPINE which can be used as an ANXIOLYTIC in the short-term treatment of anxiety and, in conjunction with other drugs, in the treatment of acute alcohol withdrawal symptoms. Administration is oral.

✚▲ Side-effects/warnings: See BENZODIAZEPINE.

✪ **Related entries: Librium; Tropium.**

chlorhexidine

is an ANTISEPTIC and DISINFECTANT agent which is a constituent in many preparations. It can be used prior to surgery and in obstetrics, but is used mainly (as chlorhexidine gluconate, chlorhexidine acetate, or chlorhexidine hydrochloride) either as a mouthwash for oral hygiene or as a dressing for minor skin wounds and infections. It can also be used for instillation in the bladder to relieve minor infections.

✚ Side-effects: Some patients experience sensitivity reactions. It may cause irritation, burning and blood in the urine when used to irrigate the bladder.

▲ Warnings: Avoid contact with the eyes and delicate body tissues.

✪ **Related entries: Acriflex Cream; Chlorohex; Corsodyl Dental Gel; Corsodyl Original Mouthwash; Corsodyl Spray; CX Antiseptic Dusting Powder; Dermol 200 Shower Emollient; Dermol 500 Lotion; Eludril; Hibicet Hospital Concentrate; Hibisol; Hibitane; Hydrex; Instillagel; Mycil Powder; Naseptin; Nystaform; Nystaform-HC; pHiso-Med; Savlon Antiseptic Cream; Savlon Antiseptic Liquid; Savlon Antiseptic Wound Wash; Steripod Chlorhexidine; Steripod Chlorhexidine/Cetrimide; Tisept; Travasept 100; Unisept.**

chlormethiazole

see CLOMETHIAZOLE.

chlormethine hydrochloride

(mustine hydrochloride) is an (*alkylating agent*) CYTOTOXIC drug which is used as an ANTICANCER drug in the treatment of the Hodgkin's disease. Administration is by intravenous infusion.

✚▲ Side-effects/warnings: See CYTOTOXIC. There may be severe vomiting.

chlorobutanol

see CHLORBUTOL.

Chlorohex

(Colgate-Palmolive) is a proprietary, non-prescription preparation of the ANTISEPTIC chlorhexidine (as gluconate). It can be used by topical application for oral hygiene and plaque prevention, and is available as a mouthwash (in two strengths *1200* and *2000*).

✚▲ Side-effects/warnings: See CHLORHEXIDINE.

Chloromycetin

(Goldshield) is a proprietary, prescription-only preparation of the broad-spectrum ANTIBACTERIAL and ANTIBIOTIC chloramphenicol, used for bacterial infections in the eye. It is available as an eye ointment and eye-drops.

✚▲ Side-effects/warnings: See CHLORAMPHENICOL.

chloroquine

is a (*4-aminoquinoline*) ANTIMALARIAL drug which is used as an AMOEBICIDAL to treat and to prevent contraction of malaria. In certain areas of the world strains of *Plasmodium falciparum* and others have recently exhibited resistance to chloroquine, so an alternative therapy is now advised. Chloroquine is also used as an ANTIRHEUMATIC to slow the progress of rheumatic disease (eg rheumatoid arthritis and lupus erythematosus). Administration is either oral or by injection.

✚ Side-effects: There may be nausea and vomiting, headache; gastrointestinal disturbance; some patients itch and break out in a rash. Susceptible patients may suffer psychotic episodes, blood disorders, damage to the eyes and effects to the hair.

▲ Warnings: An assessment will be made, and depending on use; administer with caution to those with porphyria, G6PD deficiency, psoriasis or who are pregnant, have certain kidney, liver or gastrointestinal disorders, or neurological disorders. Ophthalmic checks should be made for long-term patients. It is very toxic in overdose.

✪ **Related entries: Avloclor; Nivaquine; Paludrine/Avloclor.**

chloroxylenol

is an ANTISEPTIC agent. It can be used for many purposes, including to prevent minor staphylococcal infections of the skin, and is incorporated into preparations to soften ear wax. Administration is topical as a dilute solution.

✚ Side-effects: Rarely, there may be sensitivity reactions.

▲ Warnings: It should not be used on areas of raw or badly burned skin.

✪ **Related entries: Dettol Antiseptic Cream; Dettol Liquid; Rinstead Adult Gel; TCP First Aid Antiseptic Cream; Wax Wane Ear Drops.**

chlorphenamine maleate

(chlorpheniramine maleate) is an ANTIHISTAMINE used to treat the symptoms of allergic conditions, such as hay fever and urticaria, and also occasionally in emergencies to treat anaphylactic shock. Administration is either oral or by injection.

✚▲ Side-effects/warnings: See ANTIHISTAMINE. Because of its sedative side-effects, the performance of skilled tasks, such as driving, may be impaired. Injections may be irritant and cause short-lasting hypotension and stimulation of the

central nervous system. There may be tinnitus and skin reactions.
✪ Related entries: Calimal Antihistamine Tablets; Contac 400; Haymine; Piriton; Piriton Allergy Tablets; Piriton Syrup; Tixylix Cough and Cold.

chlorpheniramine maleate

see CHLORPHENAMINE MALEATE.

chlorpromazine hydrochloride

is chemically an important member of the PHENOTHIAZINE group and has a number of actions and uses. It is used as an ANTIPSYCHOTIC and has marked sedative effects that make it a useful treatment for schizophrenia and other psychoses, particularly during violent behavioural disturbances. It can also be used as an ANXIOLYTIC in the short-term treatment of severe anxiety, and to remedy an intractable hiccup. Additionally, it has an important use as an ANTINAUSEANT and ANTI-EMETIC to relieve nausea and vomiting, particularly in terminal illness. Administration can be either oral, by suppositories or by injection.
✚ Side-effects: They may be many and include drowsiness, apathy, pallor, insomnia, nightmares, depression (or, rarely, agitation), hypothermia (but occasionally raised body temperature), extrapyramidal symptoms (and, on prolonged administration, occasionally tardive dyskinesia); *muscarinic* ANTICHOLINERGIC side-effects including dry mouth, nasal constriction, difficulty in urination, constipation, blurred vision; cardiovascular effects; respiratory depression; changes in hormone function (irregular menstruation, growth of breasts, abnormal milk production, impotence, weight gain), sensitivity reactions, blood changes, photosensitization, contact sensitization, rashes, jaundice and alterations in liver function, and skin; rarely, neuroleptic malignant syndrome, lupus erythematosus-like syndrome; eye changes. Intramuscular injection may be painful.
▲ Warnings: It should not be given to patients with bone marrow depression, or phaeochromocytoma. Administer with care to those with certain vascular and respiratory disease sates, parkinsonism and epilepsy, liver and kidney problems, a history of jaundice, blood disorders, myasthenia gravis, hypothyroidism, hypertrophy of the prostate gland, closed-angle glaucoma; or who are pregnant or breast-feeding. Withdrawal of treatment should be gradual. Because of its sedative effects, the performance of skilled tasks may be impaired. The effects of alcohol may be enhanced.
✪ Related entries: Chloractil; Largactil.

chlorpropamide

is a SULPHONYLUREA which is used in DIABETIC TREATMENT of Type II diabetes mellitus (non-insulin-dependent diabetes mellitus; NIDDM; maturity-onset diabetes). It works by augmenting what remains of INSULIN production in the pancreas and its effect lasts longer than that of most similar drugs. Unusually for a sulphonylurea, chlorpropamide can also be used as a DIABETES INSIPIDUS TREATMENT, though only mild forms caused by pituitary or thalamic malfunction, because it also reduces frequency of urination. Administration is oral.
✚▲ Side-effects/warnings: See GLIBENCLAMIDE; but has appreciably more side-effects. The consumption of alcohol may cause flushing and nausea.

chlorquinaldol

is an ANTIMICROBIAL which is included in some preparations that incorporate a CORTICOSTEROID and are used for treatment of inflammatory skin conditions.
✚▲ Side-effects/warnings: It is regarded as safe in normal topical use.
✪ Related entry: Locoid C.

chlortalidone

(chlorthalidone) is a DIURETIC related to the THIAZIDE. It is used to treat oedema, hypertension, ascites due to cirrhosis, in chronic HEART FAILURE treatment; and, unlike most thiazide diuretics, in diabetes insipidus treatment. Administration is oral.
✚▲ Side-effects/warnings: See BENDROFLUMETHIAZIDE.
✪ Related entries: AtenixCo; co-tenidone; Hygroton; Kalspare; Tenchlor; Tenoret 50; Tenoretic; Totaretic.

chlortetracycline

is a broad-spectrum ANTIBACTERIAL and (TETRACYCLINES) ANTIBIOTIC. It can be used to treat many forms of infection including chlamidial infections (eg trachoma), especially of the eye and skin. Administration (as

chlortetracycline hydrochloride) is topical or oral.
✚▲ Side-effects/warnings: See TETRACYCLINE. Although topical application would not usually cause most of these side-effects, but local sensitivity reactions may occur.
✪ **Related entries: Aureocort; Aureomycin; Deteclo.**

chlorthalidone
see CHLORTALIDONE.

cholecalciferol
see COLECALCIFEROL.

cholestyramine
see COLESTYRAMINE.

choline salicylate
is a NSAID (non-steroidal anti-inflammatory drug) that has COUNTER-IRRITANT, OT RUBEFACIENT, actions and can be applied to the skin for symptomatic relief of pain in underlying structures. It can be used by topical application in the mouth or ears to relieve, for example, the pain of teething or ulcers. Administration is topical. See also SALICYLATE; SALICYLIC ACID.
✚▲ Side-effects/warnings: See NSAID; though normally little is absorbed into the circulation and local side-effects are limited to mild irritation. Excessive use in babies for teething upsets has resulted in poisoning.
✪ **Related entries: Audax Ear Drops; Bonjela Oral Pain-Relieving Gel; Dinnefords Teejel Gel; Earex Plus Ear Drops.**

Choragon
(Ferring) is a proprietary, prescription-only preparation of the HORMONE human chorionic gonadotrophin (human chorionic gonadotropin; HCG). It can be used to treat delayed puberty in boys, and also women who are suffering from specific hormonal deficiency for infertility. It is available in a form for injection.
✚▲ Side-effects/warnings: See CHORIONIC GONADOTROPHIN.

choriogonadotropin alpha
(a form of human chorionic gonadotrophin; HCG) is secreted by the chorionic tissue of the placenta, and so is obtained from the urine of pregnant women. Its main actions are the same as those of LUTEINISING HORMONE (LH). It can be used as an infertility treatment in women with proven hypopituitarism, and also to correct deficiencies in prepubertal males, including aiding decent of testicles and to treat delayed puberty (though use of testosterone for this purpose is more usual). Administration is by injection.
✚ Side-effects: Nausea and vomiting, pain in the abdomen, sleepiness, headache, overstimulation of the ovary; rarely, irritability, depression, breast pain and there is a possibility of ectopic pregnancy. There may be reactions at the site of injection.
▲ Warnings: It is not used in women with ovarian enlargement or cysts (except when due to polycyctic ovary disease), tumours of pituitary and hypothalamus, recent previous ectopic pregnancy, thromboembolytic disorders, tumours of the breast, pituitary and hypothalamus. Before it is prescribed, the doctor will exclude certain causes of infertility to assess its suitability.
✪ **Related entry: Ovitrelle.**

chorionic gonadotrophin
(human chorionic gonadotrophin; human chorionic gonadotropin; HCG) is secreted by the chorionic tissue of the placenta, and so is obtained from the urine of pregnant women. Its main actions are the same as those of LUTEINISING HORMONE (LH). It can be used as an infertility treatment in women with proven hypopituitarism, and to treat delayed puberty (though use of testosterone for this purpose may be preferred). Administration is by injection.
✚ Side-effects: Depending on use and sex, there may be oedema, tiredness and mood changes, headache; breast enlargement in males; multiple pregnancy, reactions at site of injection.
▲ Warnings: It should be given with caution to patients with certain heart or kidney disorders, asthma, epilepsy or migraine.
✪ **Related entries: Choragon; Pregnyl; Profasi.**

chorionic gonadotropin
see CHORIONIC GONADOTROPHIN.

Chymol Emollient Balm
(Anglian Pharma) is a proprietary, non-prescription preparation of methyl salicylate which has COUNTER-IRRITANT, OT RUBEFACIENT, actions (together with eucalyptus oil, terpineol

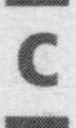

and phenol). It can be applied to bruises, chapped and sore skin, chilblains and sprains for symptomatic relief. It is available as an ointment.
✚▲ Side-effects/warnings: See METHYL SALICYLATE.

Cicatrin

(GlaxoWellcome; GSK) is a proprietary, prescription-only preparation of the (AMINOGLYCOSIDE) neomycin sulphate and the ANTIBIOTIC bacitracin zinc. It can be used to treat skin infections, and is available as a cream and a dusting-powder.
✚▲ Side-effects/warnings: See BACITRACIN ZINC; NEOMYCIN SULPHATE.

ciclosporin

(cyclosporin) is an IMMUNOSUPPRESSANT drug which is used particularly to limit tissue rejection during and following organ transplant surgery. It can also be used to treat severe, active rheumatoid arthritis and some skin conditions such as severe, resistant atopic dermatitis and (under special supervision) psoriasis. It has very little effect on the blood-cell producing capacity of the bone marrow, but does have kidney toxicity.
Administration is either oral or by injection or intravenous infusion.
✚ Side-effects: These depend on the use and route of administration, and include, most dangerously, kidney effects (nephrotoxicity), also changes in blood enzymes, disturbances in liver and cardiovascular function, excessive hair growth, gastrointestinal disturbances, lethargy, tremor, gum growth, oedema, fatigue and tingling sensations in the hands and feet and a number of others.
▲ Warnings: Treatment with ciclosporin inevitably leaves the body vulnerable to infection. It should be administered with caution to patients who are pregnant or breast-feeding, or with porphyria. Body functions (liver, kidney and cardiovascular system) should be monitored. When used by mouth, grapefruit or grapefruit juice should be avoided for one hour before (and during) taking ciclosporin by mouth. It should not be given to patients with abnormal kidney function, uncontrolled hypertension, infections or malignancy.

Ciclosporin interacts with a large number of other conventional drugs, alternative remedies or supplements where either the therapeutic effect of the drugs taken can be changed or there may be adverse reactions, some of which can be serious. For example, potassium supplements should be avoided when taking ciclosporin or there is a risk of hyperkalemia (high blood potassium levels) developing and St John's wort can reduce the blood concentration and hence the effectiveness of ciclosporin. Any prescription, over-the-counter medicines, supplements, herbal remedies or other alternative therapies that you are using, have recently used or plan to use should be discussed with your doctor or pharmacist before you take ciclosporin. Important interactions will be detailed in the Patient Information Leaflet.
✪ Related entries: Neoral; Sandimmun; SangCya.

cidofovir

is an ANTIVIRAL drug used in the treatment of life-threatening or sight-threatening cytomegalovirus (CMV) retinitis infections in AIDS patients. It can be given with the drug PROBENECID to prolong its action.
Administration is by intravenous infusion.
✚ Side-effects: Kidney toxicity; vomiting, fever, hair-loss, nausea, effects on blood and eyes.
▲ Warnings: It is a specialist drug, and there will be full assessment and patient monitoring throughout treatment.
✪ Related entry: Vistide.

Cidomycin

(Hoechst Marion Roussel; Aventis Pharma) is a proprietary, prescription-only preparation of the ANTIBACTERIAL and (AMINOGLYCOSIDE) ANTIBIOTIC gentamicin (as sulphate). It can be used to treat many forms of infection, particularly serious infections by Gram-negative bacteria. It is available in various forms for injection.
✚▲ Side-effects/warnings: See GENTAMICIN.

cilastatin

is an ENZYME INHIBITOR that inhibits an enzyme in the kidney which breaks down the ANTIBACTERIAL and (BETA-LACTAM) ANTIBIOTIC imipenem, and so prolongs and enhances the antibiotic's effects. Cilastatin and imipenem are administered together in a preparation called impenem with cilastatin. Administration is by injection.
✚▲ Side-effects/warnings: See IMIPENEM WITH CILASTATIN.
✪ Related entry: Primaxin.

cilazapril

is an ACE INHIBITOR. It is a powerful VASODILATOR that can be used as an ANTIHYPERTENSIVE, and in congestive HEART FAILURE TREATMENT, often in conjunction with other classes of drug, particularly DIURETIC drugs. Administration is oral.

✚ Side-effects: See ACE INHIBITOR. Also shortness of breath and bronchitis.

▲ Warnings: See ACE INHIBITOR. Also not used in ascites.

✪ **Related entry: Vascace.**

Cilest

(Janssen-Cilag) is a proprietary, prescription-only compound preparation which can be used as a (*monophasic*) ORAL CONTRACEPTIVE of the *COC* (standard strength) type that combines an OESTROGEN and PROGESTOGEN, in this case ethinylestradiol and norgestimate. It is available as tablets in a calendar pack.

✚▲ Side-effects/warnings: See ETHINYLESTRADIOL; NORGESTIMATE.

Ciloxan

(Alcon) is a proprietary, prescription-only preparation of the (QUINOLONE) ANTIBIOTIC-like ANTIBACTERIAL ciprofloxacin. It can be used to treat a variety of infections, and also corneal ulcers. It is available as eye-drops.

✚▲ Side-effects/warnings: See CIPROFLOXACIN.

cimetidine

is an effective and much-prescribed H_2-ANTAGONIST and ULCER-HEALING DRUG. It is used to assist in the treatment of benign peptic (gastric and duodenal) ulcers, to relieve heartburn in cases of reflux oesophagitis, Zollinger-Ellison syndrome and a variety of conditions where reduction of acidity is beneficial. It works by reducing the secretion of gastric acid (by acting as a histamine receptor H_2-receptor antagonist), so reducing erosion and bleeding from peptic ulcers and allowing them a chance to heal. However, treatment with cimetidine should not be given before full diagnosis of gastric bleeding or serious pain has been carried out, because its action in restricting gastric secretions may possibly mask the presence of other serious disorders such as stomach cancer. Cimetidine can also be used to treat ulceration induced by NSAID treatment. Administration can be oral, or by injection or infusion. (Although it is a prescription-only drug when used for the treatment of ulcers and related conditions, it can be sold over-the-counter in limited quantities and dosage for occasional indigestion and heartburn for people over sixteen years.)

✚▲ Side-effects/warnings: See H_2-ANTAGONIST. Also, occasionally, hair loss, speeding of the heart and kidney changes. Cimetidine (but not the other available H_2-antagonists) inhibits some enzymes (such as the microsomal oxidative system of the liver), and because of this, it can potentiate the effects of a number of other drugs: this is of special importance in patients stabilized on the drugs warfarin, theophylline, tricyclic antidepressants, nifedipine and phenytoin. Cimetedine can cause confusion in the elderly. Sometimes it causes gynaecomastia in men (growth of breasts), and, rarely, decrease in sexual function.

✪ **Related entries: Acitak; Dyspamet; Galenamet; Peptimax; Phimetin; Tagamet; Tagamet 100; Ultec; Zita.**

Cinazière

(Ashbourne) is a proprietary, non-prescription preparation of the ANTIHISTAMINE cinnarizine. It can be used as an ANTINAUSEANT to treat nausea and vomiting caused by the vertigo and loss of balance that is experienced in vestibular disease and also for motion sickness in travelling. It is available as tablets.

✚▲ Side-effects/warnings: See CINNARIZINE.

cinchocaine

(dibucaine hydrochloride) is a LOCAL ANAESTHETIC which is used to relieve pain, particularly in dental surgery but also in the skin or mucous membranes (eg rectally for haemorrhoids). Administration is by topical application.

✚▲ Side-effects/warnings: See LIDOCAINE HYDROCHLORIDE.

✪ **Related entries: Proctosedyl; Scheriproct; Ultraproct; Uniroid-HC.**

cinchona alkaloid 🅴

drugs are chemically complex substances extracted from the bark of the cinchona tree (it is also known as Peruvian, Jesuit's bark or Cardinal's bark). The best-known cinchona alkaloid is QUININE, which has been used for many centuries to treat fevers and is still used in the treatment of malaria. It has a bitter taste and is incorporated into non-medicinal drinks to mask its flavour. People who are sensitive to it or who consume large quantities of 'tonic water' may experience one of its more marked side-effects, which is tinnitus (a ringing in the ears). The other main cinchona alkaloid is QUINIDINE (which is chemically similar to quinine, but is its other isomer) which is used as an ANTI-ARRHYTHMIC to treat heartbeat irregularities (supraventricular arrhythmias).

cineole

is a constituent of several natural aromatic oils (extracted from eucalyptus and other sources) and is chemically a TERPENE. It is commonly used in inhalations intended to clear the nasal or catarrhal congestion associated with colds, rhinitis (inflammation of the nasal mucous membrane) or sinusitis. It is also included in some COUNTER-IRRITANT, or RUBEFACIENT, preparations that are rubbed into the skin to relieve muscle or joint pain, and in a preparation used for dissolution of gallstones or kidney stones.
✚▲ Side-effects/warnings: It is regarded as safe in normal topical use, but avoid using it on cuts or abraded skin.
✪ Related entries: Dubam Cream; Rowatinex.

cinnarizine

has ANTIHISTAMINE properties and is used for a number of purposes. It is mainly used as an ANTINAUSEANT (and thus an ANTI-EMETIC), for example, in the treatment of vestibular balance disorders (especially vertigo, tinnitus, nausea and vomiting in Ménière's disease) and motion sickness. Quite separately, it has VASODILATOR properties that affect the blood vessels of the hands and feet and so is sometimes used to try and improve the circulation in peripheral vascular disease (Raynaud's phenomenon). Administration is oral.
✚▲ Side-effects/warnings: See CYCLIZINE. May also cause fatigue and skin reactions. Rarely, extra-pyramidal symptoms (movement disorders) in the elderly. Do not administer to those with porphyria.
✪ Related entries: Cinazière; Stugeron 15 Tablets; Stugeron Forte.

Cipramil

(Lundbeck) is a proprietary, prescription-only preparation of the (SSRI) ANTIDEPRESSANT citalopram, which has fewer sedative effects than some other antidepressants. It is available as tablets and oral drops.
✚▲ Side-effects/warnings: See CITALOPRAM.

ciprofibrate

is a (*fibrate*) LIPID-REGULATING DRUG used in hyperlipidaemia to modify the proportions of various lipids in the bloodstream. Generally, it is administered only to patients in whom a strict and regular dietary regime, alone, is not having the desired effect. Administration is oral.
✚▲ Side-effects/warnings: See BEZAFIBRATE. Patients should report any muscle weakness, pain or tenderness to their doctor.
✪ Related entry: Modalim.

ciprofloxacin

is a (QUINOLONE) ANTIBIOTIC-like ANTIBACTERIAL. It can be used to treat infections in patients who are allergic to PENICILLIN or whose strain of bacterium is resistant to standard antibiotics. It is active against Gram-negative bacteria, including salmonella, *Shigella*, *Campylobacter*, *Neisseria* and *Pseudomonas*; and to a lesser extent against Gram-positive bacteria of the streptococcal family (eg *S. pneumoniae*, *Enterococcus faecalis*. It is used to treat infections of the urinary, gastrointestinal and respiratory tracts, gonorrhoea and septicaemia. But usually only when these cases are resistant to more conventional agents. It can also be used to prevent infection during surgical procedures, and is used topically for eye infections. Administration can be oral, topical or by injection.
✚▲ Side-effects/warnings: See QUINOLONE. Other side-effects include difficulty in swallowing, flatulence, liver and kidney impairment, effects on the heart and tinnitus. An adequate fluid intake should be maintained.
✪ Related entries: Ciloxan; Ciproxin.

Ciproxin

(Bayer) is a proprietary, prescription-only preparation of the (QUINOLONE) ANTIBIOTIC-like ANTIBACTERIAL ciprofloxacin. It can be used to treat a variety of infections, for example, of the urinary tract and gonorrhoea. It is available as tablets, a suspension and for intravenous infusion.
✚▲ Side-effects/warnings: See CIPROFLOXACIN.

C

cisatracurium
is a *non-depolarizing* SKELETAL MUSCLE RELAXANT (and is a form of ATRACURIUM BESILATE) which can be used to induce muscle paralysis (of medium duration) during surgery. Administered by injection.
✚▲ Side-effects/warnings: It is a specialist drug used by anaesthetists in hospital.
✪ **Related entry: Nimbex.**

cisplatin
is a (*platinum compound*) CYTOTOXIC drug (an organic complex of platinum) that works by damaging the DNA of replicating cells and so can be used as an ANTICANCER drug in the treatment of certain solid tumours, including ovarian cancer and testicular teratoma. Administration is by injection.
✚▲ Side-effects/warnings: See CYTOTOXIC; but also severe nausea and vomiting, kidney damage, toxicity to the ear (tinnitus, hearing-loss), myelosuppression and peripheral nerve effects.

citalopram
is a (SSRI) ANTIDEPRESSANT which is used to treat depressive illness and has the advantage over some earlier antidepressants because it has relatively fewer SEDATIVE and ANTICHOLINERGIC (ANTIMUSCARINIC) side-effects. It can also be used to treat panic disorders. It may take some weeks to reach full effect and offset on discontinuation is also slow. Administration is oral.
✚▲ Side-effects/warnings: See SSRI. Also, there may be palpitations, speeding of the heart, postural hypotension, yawning, coughing; confusion, difficulty in concentrating and memory loss; migraine, hypersensitivity reactions (eg rash, pruritus, muscle pain), tingling in the extremities, visual and taste disturbance, increased salivation, rhinitis, ringing in the ears; urination disorders have also been reported. Increased appetite and weight gain have been reported with citalopram (unlike other SSRIs).
✪ **Related entry: Cipramil.**

Citanest
(AstraZeneca) is a proprietary, prescription-only preparation of the LOCAL ANAESTHETIC prilocaine hydrochloride. It can be used for various types of anaesthesia, and is available in forms for injection.
✚▲ Side-effects/warnings: See PRILOCAINE HYDROCHLORIDE.

Citanest with Octapressin
(AstraZeneca) is a proprietary, prescription-only compound preparation of the LOCAL ANAESTHETIC prilocaine hydrochloride and the VASOCONSTRICTOR felypressin. It can be used in dental surgery, and is available in a form for injection.
✚▲ Side-effects/warnings: See FELYPRESSIN; PRILOCAINE HYDROCHLORIDE.

Citramag
(Bioglan) is a proprietary, non-prescription preparation of the (*osmotic*) LAXATIVE magnesium carbonate. It can be used as a bowel cleansing solution to clear the bowel before radiological examination, colonoscopy or colonic surgery, and is available as an effervescent powder.
✚▲ Side-effects/warnings: See MAGNESIUM CARBONATE.

cladribine
is an (*antimetabolite*) CYTOTOXIC which is used as an ANTICANCER treatment for hairy cell leukaemia, also chronic lymphocytic leukaemia in certain patients. Administration is by injection.
✚▲ Side-effects/warnings: See CYTOTOXIC.
✪ **Related entry: Leustat.**

Claforan
(Hoechst Marion Roussel; Aventis Pharma) is a proprietary, prescription-only preparation of the ANTIBACTERIAL and (CEPHALOSPORIN) ANTIBIOTIC cefotaxime. It can be used to treat a range of infections, and is available in a form for injection.
✚▲ Side-effects/warnings: See CEFOTAXIME.

clarithromycin
is an ANTIBACTERIAL and (MACROLIDE) ANTIBIOTIC which is a derivative of erythromycin, and is usually given to patients who are allergic to PENICILLIN. It can be used to treat skin, soft tissue and respiratory tract infections, otis media infections and for *Helicobacter pylori* infection (see ULCER-HEALING DRUG). Administration can be oral or by injection.
✚▲ Side-effects/warnings: See ERYTHROMYCIN, but fewer gastrointestinal effects. Administer with caution to patients who are pregnant or breast-feeding. There may be headache, effects on

taste and smell, inflammation of the tongue and mouth, also dizziness, muscle and joint aches, vertigo, tinnitus, anxiety, confusion, nightmares, psychosis and others.
✪ **Related entries: HeliClear; HeliMet; Klaricid.**

Clarityn
(Schering-Plough) is a proprietary, prescription-only preparation of the ANTIHISTAMINE loratadine. It can be used to treat the symptoms of allergic disorders, such as hay fever and urticaria, and is available as a syrup.
✚▲ Side-effects/warnings: See LORATADINE.

Clarityn Allergy Eyedrops
(Schering-Plough Consumer Health) is a proprietary, non-prescription preparation of the ANTI-ALLERGIC sodium cromoglicate. It can be used to treat the symptoms of allergic disorders, such as seasonal allergic conjunctivitis, for example, in hay fever, and is available as eye-drops.
✚▲ Side-effects/warnings: See SODIUM CROMOGLICATE.

Clarityn Allergy Syrup
(Schering-Plough Consumer Health) is a proprietary, non-prescription preparation of the ANTIHISTAMINE loratadine. It can be used to treat the symptoms of allergic disorders, such as hay fever, rhinitis, sneezing, itching eyes and urticaria, and is available as a syrup. It is not usually given to children under two years, except on medical advice.
✚▲ Side-effects/warnings: See LORATADINE.

Clarityn Allergy Tablets
(Schering-Plough Consumer Health) is a proprietary, non-prescription preparation of the ANTIHISTAMINE loratadine. It can be used to treat the symptoms of allergic disorders, such as hay fever, rhinitis and urticaria, and is available as tablets. It is not normally given to children.
✚▲ Side-effects/warnings: See LORATADINE.

clavulanic acid
is chemically an ANTIBIOTIC but is only weakly ANTIBACTERIAL and is used instead as a PENICILLINASE INHIBITOR to combat bacterial resistance. It works as an ENZYME INHIBITOR by inhibiting the penicillinase enzymes ('beta-lactamases') that are produced by some bacteria. These enzymes can inactivate many antibiotics of the penicillin family, such as amoxicillin and ticarcillin, and so prevent the antibiotics from working. Clavulanic acid is therefore used in combination with AMOXICILLIN or TICARCILLIN.
✚▲ Side-effects/warnings: Cholestatic jaundice (particularly in the elderly); caution in liver impairment (liver function may be monitored), or pregnancy.
✪ **Related entries: Augmentin; co-amoxiclav; Timentin.**

Clearasil Treatment Cream Regular (Colourless)
(Procter & Gamble) is a proprietary, non-prescription preparation of the ANTISEPTIC triclosan and sulphur. It can be used to treat acne, spots and pimples, and is available as a cream for topical application. (Also available as *Cover Up*.)
✚▲ Side-effects/warnings: See TRICLOSAN; SULPHUR.

clemastine
is an ANTIHISTAMINE which can be used for the symptomatic relief of allergic symptoms, such as hay fever and urticaria. Administration is oral.
✚▲ Side-effects/warnings: See ANTIHISTAMINE. Because of its sedative side-effects, the performance of skilled tasks, such as driving, may be impaired. It is used with care in pregnancy and breast-feeding.
✪ **Related entries: Tavegil.**

Clexane
(Rhône-Poulenc Rorer; Aventis Pharma) is a proprietary, prescription-only preparation of the ANTICOAGULANT enoxaparin, which is a low molecular weight version of heparin. It can be used for long-duration prevention of venous thrombo-embolism, particularly in orthopaedic use. It is available in a form for injection.
✚▲ Side-effects/warnings: See ENOXAPARIN.

Climagest
(Novartis) is a proprietary, prescription-only compound preparation of estradiol (as valerate; an OESTROGEN) and norethisterone (a PROGESTOGEN). It can be used to treat menopausal problems, including in HRT (hormone replacement therapy), and is available as tablets in two strengths (*1-mg* and *2-mg*).
✚▲ Side-effects/warnings: See NORETHISTERONE; ESTRADIOL.

Climaval

(Novartis) is a proprietary, prescription-only preparation of the OESTROGEN estradiol (as valerate). It can be used in HRT, and is available as tablets.
✚▲ Side-effects/warnings: See ESTRADIOL.

Climesse

(Novartis) is a proprietary, prescription-only compound preparation of estradiol (an OESTROGEN) and norethisterone (as acetate; a PROGESTOGEN). It can be used in HRT. Available as tablets.
✚▲ Side-effects/warnings: See NORETHISTERONE; ESTRADIOL.

clindamycin

is an ANTIBACTERIAL and ANTIBIOTIC drug which is used to treat infections of bones and joints, peritonitis (inflammation of the peritoneal lining of the abdominal cavity). It is active against many anaerobic bacteria (including *Bacteroides fragilis* and Gram-positive cocci (including penicillin-resistant *Staphylocci*). It can also be used topically to treat acne and also vaginal infections. However, it is not widely used because of its serious side-effects (though these depend on the route of administration). Administration can be oral, by topical application or by injection.
✚ Side-effects: These depend on the route of administration. If diarrhoea or colitis appear during treatment, administration must be halted (see below). There may be nausea and vomiting; abdominal discomfort; jaundice, liver dysfunction; blood disorders.
▲ Warnings: Depending on the route of administration, it should not be administered to patients suffering from diarrhoea; and if diarrhoea or other symptoms of colitis appear during treatment, administration must be stopped. This is because clindamycin greatly alters the normal balance of bacteria in the gut and in a few cases this allows a superinfection by the anaerobe *Clostridium difficile*, which causes a form of colitis that can be serious. It should be administered with caution to those with certain liver or kidney disorders, or who are pregnant or breast-feeding.
✪ Related entries: Dalacin; Dalacin C; Dalacin T; Zindaclin.

Clinitar

(CHS) is a proprietary, prescription-only preparation of coal tar. It can be used by topical application to treat scalp psoriasis, dandruff and seborrhoeic dermatitis, and is available as a shampoo.
✚▲ Side-effects/warnings: See COAL TAR.

Clinoril

(MSD) is a proprietary, prescription-only preparation of the (NSAID) NON-NARCOTIC ANALGESIC and ANTIRHEUMATIC sulindac. It can be used to treat rheumatic conditions and other musculoskeletal disorders and acute gout. It is available as tablets.
✚▲ Side-effects/warnings: See SULINDAC.

clioquinol

is an ANTIMICROBIAL drug which is chemically an iodine-containing member of the 8-hydroxyquinoline group. It can be used as an ANTIFUNGAL agent, and its primary use is to treat *Candida* fungal infections of the skin and outer ear. Administration is topical as drops, creams, ointments and anal suppositories.
✚ Side-effects: Some patients experience sensitivity reactions.
✪ Related entries: Betnovate-C; Locorten-Vioform; Synalar C; Vioform-Hydrocortisone.

Clivarine

(ICN) is a recently introduced proprietary, prescription-only preparation of the ANTICOAGULANT reviparin sodium, which is a low molecular weight version of heparin. It can be used for long-duration prevention of deep-vein thrombosis. It is available in a form for subcutaneous injection.
✚▲ Side-effects/warnings: See REVIPARIN SODIUM.

clobazam

is a BENZODIAZEPINE which is used as an ANXIOLYTIC in the short-term treatment of anxiety. It can also be used, in conjunction with other drugs, as an ANTI-EPILEPTIC treatment. Administration is oral.
✚▲ Side-effects/warnings: See BENZODIAZEPINE.
✪ Related entry: Frisium.

clobetasol propionate

is an extremely powerful CORTICOSTEROID with ANTI-INFLAMMATORY properties. It is used to treat severe, non-infective inflammation of the skin caused by conditions such as eczema and psoriasis, especially in cases where less powerful steroid treatments have failed. Administration is by topical application.

✚▲ Side-effects/warnings: See CORTICOSTEROID; though systemic side-effects are unlikely with topical application when applied correctly, but there may be local skin reactions. The amount applied to the skin each week should be below a certain maximum amount. The instructions for application should be followed carefully.

✪ **Related entries: Dermovate; Dermovate-NN.**

clobetasone butyrate

is a moderately potent CORTICOSTEROID with ANTI-INFLAMMATORY properties. It is used in the treatment of severe inflammation of the skin caused by conditions such as eczema and certain types of dermatitis, especially as a maintenance treatment between courses of more potent corticosteroids. Administration is by topical application.

✚▲ Side-effects/warnings: See CORTICOSTEROID; though serious systemic effects are unlikely with topical application, but there may be local skin reactions or effects on the eye. As eye-drops, it can be used under expert supervision to treat inflammation (eg following surgery).

✪ **Related entries: Cloburate; Eumovate; Trimovate.**

Cloburate

(Dominion) is a proprietary, prescription-only preparation of the CORTICOSTEROID and ANTI-INFLAMMATORY clobetasone butyrate. It can be used to treat non-infective and severe inflammation of the eye (eg after surgery), and is available as eye-drops.

✚▲ Side-effects/warnings: See CLOBETASONE BUTYRATE.

clofazimine

is an ANTIBACTERIAL which is used, in combination with dapsone and rifampicin, in the treatment of the major form of leprosy. The fact that the treatment requires no fewer than three drugs is due to the increasing resistance shown by the leprosy bacterium. Administration is oral.

✚ Side-effects: There may be nausea and vomiting, diarrhoea and abdominal pain, tiredness, headache. The skin and urine may have a reddish tinge, skin lesions, hair, body fluids and faeces may be discoloured. There may be rash, skin itching, dry eyes and a number of other side-effects.

▲ Warnings: It should be administered with caution to patients with impaired kidney or liver function. Regular tests on both functions will be made.

✪ **Related entry: Lamprene.**

clofibrate

is a (*fibrate*) LIPID-REGULATING DRUG used in hyperlipidaemia to reduce the levels, or change the proportions, of various lipids in the bloodstream. Generally, it is administered only to patients in whom a strict and regular dietary regime, alone, is not having the desired effect. Administration is oral.

✚▲ Side-effects/warnings: See BEZAFIBRATE. Also, may form stones in the gall bladder, so its use is usually restricted to patients who have had a cholecystectomy. Patients should report any muscle weakness, pain or tenderness to their doctor.

clomethiazole

(chlormethiazole) has a number of uses: as a HYPNOTIC for treating severe insomnia (especially in elderly patients because it is relatively free of a 'hangover' effect); as an ANTICONVULSANT and ANTI-EPILEPTIC to treat status epilepticus and eclampsia; and to reduce the symptoms of withdrawal from alcohol (under strict medical supervision). Administration is either oral or by injection.

✚ Side-effects: Nasal congestion, sneezing, irritation of the conjunctiva of the eyes and nose, headache, excitement, confusion, gastrointestinal upsets, rashes and urticaria, anaphylaxis, blood and liver changes, or dependence.

▲ Warnings: It should not be given to patients with acute pulmonary insufficiency, or who are alcoholics who continue to drink. Use with care in patients with heart or respiratory disease, or impaired liver or kidney function, or who have a history of drug abuse. Withdrawal of treatment should be gradual. It may cause drowsiness the next day, which can impair the performance of skilled tasks, such as driving. The effects of alcohol may be enhanced.

✪ **Related entry: Heminevrin.**

Clomid

(Aventis Pharma) is a proprietary, prescription-only preparation of the HORMONE ANTAGONIST

clomifene citrate, which is an ANTI-OESTROGEN. It can be used to treat infertility due to ovulatory failure, and is available as tablets.
✚▲ Side-effects/warnings: See CLOMIFENE CITRATE.

clomifene citrate
(clomiphene citrate) is a sex HORMONE ANTAGONIST (an ANTI-OESTROGEN) which is used as a fertility treatment in women whose condition is linked to the persistent presence of oestrogens and a consequent failure to ovulate (characterized by sparse or infrequent periods). Clomiphene prevents the action of oestrogens and this increases secretion of GONADOTROPHIN hormones, which cause ovulation. Administration is oral.
✚ Side-effects: Multiple births may result. Hot flushes, nausea, vomiting, visual disturbances, dizziness and insomnia, breast tenderness, weight gain, rashes, and hair loss may occur.
▲ Warnings: It should not be administered to patients with ovarian cysts; certain liver disorders; abnormal uterine bleeding; or who are pregnant. It is not normally used for more than six menstrual cycles. It is used with care in women with certain gynaecological conditions.
✪ **Related entry: Clomid.**

clomiphene citrate
see CLOMIFENE CITRATE.

clonazepam
is a BENZODIAZEPINE which is used as an ANTICONVULSANT and ANTI-EPILEPTIC for all forms of epilepsy, myoclonus and status epilepticus. Administration can be either oral or by injection.
✚▲ Side-effects/warnings: See BENZODIAZEPINE; but is not to be used in patients with certain lung disorders.
✪ **Related entry: Rivotril.**

clonidine hydrochloride
is an ANTISYMPATHETIC drug which decreases the release of NORADRENALINE (norepinephrine) from sympathetic nerves. It can be used as an ANTIHYPERTENSIVE, an ANTIMIGRAINE treatment (for reducing the incidence of attacks) and for vascular headaches and menopausal flushing (however, authorities are not convinced of its efficacy for these purposes). Also, there is some use for it in treating the symptoms (tics) of Gilles de la Tourette syndrome. Administration is either oral or by injection.
✚ Side-effects: Sedation, dizziness, headache, depression or euphoria; dry mouth; fluid retention; rashes; nausea and constipation; blood disorders; slow heart rate, poor circulation in the extremities; rarely, there may be impotence. Clonidine used for migraine may cause insomnia and aggravate depression.
▲ Warnings: It is given with caution to those with depression, porphyria or peripheral vascular disease. The drug may cause drowsiness and impair the ability to drive or operate machinery. Effects of alcohol may be enhanced. Withdrawal of treatment should be gradual.
✪ **Related entries: Catapres; Dixarit.**

clopamide
is a (THIAZIDE) DIURETIC which can be used as an ANTIHYPERTENSIVE in conjunction with BETA-BLOCKER. Administration is oral.
✚▲ Side-effects/warnings: See BENDROFLUMETHIAZIDE.
✪ **Related entry: Viskaldix.**

clopidogrel
is an ANTIPLATELET (antithrombotic) drug which is used to prevent thrombosis (blood-clot formation), but does not have an ANTICOAGULANT action. It works by stopping platelets sticking to one another or to the walls of blood vessels. It is used to reduce complications in patients with history of atherosclerotic disease (ischaemic stroke, myocardial infarction or peripheral arterial disease). Administration is oral.
✚ Side-effects: There may be haemorrhage (including in the gastrointestinal tract and within the skull); also abdominal discomfort, nausea, vomiting, constipation or diarrhoea, stomach and duodenal ulcers; headache, dizziness, vertigo, tingling in the extremities; skin rash and itching; liver and biliary disorders, and changes in blood.
▲ Warnings: It should not be used when there is actual bleeding, or in breast-feeding. Avoid for first few days after heart attacks or ischaemic stroke. It is not recommended in unstable angina or after certain heart operations or procedures, or in other cases where patients at risk of increased bleeding from trauma or surgery. Use with caution in pregnancy, liver or kidney liver impairment.

C

✪ **Related entry: Plavix.**

Clopixol
(Lundbeck) is a proprietary, prescription-only preparation of the ANTIPSYCHOTIC zuclopenthixol dihydrochloride, and can be used for the long-term maintenance of schizophrenia and other psychoses. It is available as tablets (as zuclopenthixol dihydrochloride) and a depot deep intramuscular injection called (as zuclopenthixol decanoate). There is also a range of *Clopixol* preparations which differ in their duration of action and may be used according to the length of treatment intended.
✚▲ Side-effects/warnings: See ZUCLOPENTHIXOL.

Clopixol Acuphase
(Lundbeck) is a proprietary, prescription-only preparation of the ANTIPSYCHOTIC zuclopenthixol acetate. It can be used for short-term management of acute psychosis and mania or exacerbation of a chronic psychotic disorder. It is available in a form for depot deep intramuscular injection.
✚▲ Side-effects/warnings: See ZUCLOPENTHIXOL.

Clopixol Conc.
(Lundbeck) is a proprietary, prescription-only preparation of the ANTIPSYCHOTIC zuclopenthixol decanoate, and can be used for long-term maintenance of schizophrenia and other psychoses. It is available in a form for depot deep intramuscular injection.
✚▲ Side-effects/warnings: See ZUCLOPENTHIXOL.

cloral betaine
(chloral betaine) is an alternative form of the SEDATIVE and HYPNOTIC chloral hydrate, with similar properties. Administration is oral.
✚▲ Side-effects/warnings: See CHLORAL HYDRATE.
✪ **Related entry: Welldorm.**

cloral hydrate
see CHLORAL HYDRATE.

clorazepate dipotassium
(dipotassium clorazepate) is a BENZODIAZEPINE which is used as an ANXIOLYTIC in the short-term treatment of anxiety. Administration is oral.
✚▲ Side-effects/warnings: See BENZODIAZEPINE.
✪ **Related entry: Tranxene.**

Clostet
(Evans Vaccines) (Tet/Vac/Ads) is a non-proprietary, prescription-only VACCINE preparation of adsorbed tetanus vaccine. It can be used for active IMMUNIZATION against tetanus, and is available in a form for injection.
✚▲ Side-effects/warnings: See ADSORBED TETANUS VACCINE.

Clotam
(Provalis) is a proprietary, prescription-only preparation of the (NSAID) NON-NARCOTIC ANALGESIC tolfenamic acid. It can be used to relieve acute attacks of migraine pain. It is available as tablets.
✚▲ Side-effects/warnings: See TOLFENAMIC ACID.

clotrimazole
is an (AZOLE) ANTIMICROBIAL and ANTIFUNGAL drug (that works by interfering with amino acid transport in the invading organisms). It can be used in topical application to treat fungal infections (including *Candida* organisms) of the skin and mucous membranes (especially the vagina, outer ear and toes). Administration is by topical application.
✚ Side-effects: Rarely, there may be a burning sensation or irritation; a very few patients experience sensitivity reactions.
✪ **Related entries: Candiden Cream; Candiden Vaginal Tablet; Canesten; Canesten AF Cream; Canesten AF Powder; Canesten Combi; Canesten Cream; Canesten Dermatological Spray; Canesten Hydrocortisone; Canesten Once; Canesten Pessary; Canesten Dermatological Powder; Canesten AF Spray; Canesten Thrush Cream; Canesten-HC; Care Clotrimazole Cream 1%; Lotriderm.**

clozapine
is an ANTIPSYCHOTIC drug (one of a group sometimes termed 'atypical' antipsychotics) which can be used for the treatment of schizophrenia in patients who do not respond to, or who can not tolerate, conventional antipsychotic drugs. Because clozapine can cause serious blood disorders, its use is restricted to patients registered with the Clozaril Patient Monitoring Service. Administration is oral.

✚ Side-effects: Of the atypical antipsychotics these include weight gain, dizziness, postural hypotension and fainting, extrapyramidal symptoms (usually mild and transient, but occasionally tardive dyskinesia on long-term administration). Also, for clozapine initiation of treatment is in hospital, blood counts are monitored. Patients should report any symptoms of infection immediately. Withdrawal is gradual. There are significant interactions with other drugs.
▲ Warnings: Atypical antipsychotics are used with caution in patients with cardiovascular disease, history of epilepsy, and Parkinson's disease; they may affect performance of skilled tasks (including driving). They should not be given to some patients, including people who are pregnant or breast-feeding, or who have certain kidney, liver or heart disease. It can be used with caution in angle-closure glaucoma, kidney impairment and prostatic hypertrophy.
✪ **Related entry: Clozaril.**

Clozaril

(Novartis) is a proprietary, prescription-only preparation of the ANTIPSYCHOTIC clozapine. It can be used to treat schizophrenics who are unresponsive to other drugs, and is subject to special monitoring because of its potentially severe effects on the blood. It is available as tablets.
✚▲ Side-effects/warnings: See CLOZAPINE.

Coal Tar and Salicylic Acid Ointment, BP

is a non-proprietary, non-prescription preparation of coal tar, salicylic acid and soft white and liquid paraffin. It can be used by topical application to treat chronic eczema and psoriasis, and is available as an ointment.
✚▲ Side-effects/warnings: See COAL TAR; LIQUID PARAFFIN; SALICYLIC ACID.

Coal Tar Paste, BP

is a non-proprietary, non-prescription preparation of coal tar (in zinc paste). It can be used by topical application to treat chronic eczema and psoriasis and to relieve itching. It is available as an ointment.
✚▲ Side-effects/warnings: See COAL TAR.

coal tar

is a black, viscous liquid obtained by the distillation of coal. It is used on the skin to reduce inflammation and itching and also has some KERATOLYTIC properties. Therapeutically, it is used to treat psoriasis and chronic atopic eczema, and as an ANTISEBORRHOEIC for seborrhoeic dermatitis, where it is used in solution at a concentration determined by a patient's condition and response. It is a constituent in many non-proprietary and proprietary preparations, especially pastes.
✚ Side-effects: Skin irritation, an acne-like rash and sensitivity to light.
▲ Warnings: Avoid contact with broken or inflamed skin and the eyes. Coal tar stains skin, hair and fabric.
✪ **Related entries: Alphosyl 2 in 1 Shampoo; Alphosyl HC; Calamine and Coal Tar Ointment, BP; Coal Tar and Salicylic Acid Ointment, BP; Coal Tar Paste, BP; Capasal Therapeutic Shampoo; Carbo-Dome; Clinitar; Cocois; Exorex Lotion; Ionil T; Pentrax; Polytar AF; Polytar Emmollient; Polytar Liquid; Polytar Plus; Pragmatar; Psoriderm; Psorin; Zinc and Coal Tar Paste, BP.**

co-amilofruse 2.5/20

is a simplified name for the compound preparation of the (*potassium-sparing*) DIURETIC amiloride hydrochloride and the (*loop*) diuretic furosemide (frusemide), in the ratio of 2.5:20 (mg), for treating oedema. It is given orally.
✚▲ Side-effects/warnings: See AMILORIDE HYDROCHLORIDE; FUROSEMIDE.
✪ **Related entry: Frumil LS.**

co-amilofruse 5/40

is a simplified name for the compound preparation of the (*potassium-sparing*) DIURETIC amiloride hydrochloride and the (*loop*) diuretic furosemide (frusemide), in the ratio of 5:40, for treating oedema. It is given orally.
✚▲ Side-effects/warnings: See AMILORIDE HYDROCHLORIDE; FUROSEMIDE.
✪ **Related entries: Froop-Co; Fru-Co; Frumil; Lasoride.**

co-amilofruse 10/80

is a simplified name for the compound preparation of the (*potassium-sparing*) DIURETIC amiloride hydrochloride and the (*loop*) diuretic furosemide (frusemide), in the ratio of 10:80 (mg), for treating oedema. It is given orally.
✚▲ Side-effects/warnings: See AMILORIDE HYDROCHLORIDE; FUROSEMIDE.

✪ **Related entries: Aridil; Frumil Forte.**

co-amilozide 2.5/25

is a simplified name for the compound preparation of the (*potassium-sparing*) DIURETIC amiloride hydrochloride and the THIAZIDE diuretic hydrochlorothiazide, in the ratio 2.5:25 (mg), for treating oedema. It is given orally.
✚▲ Side-effects/warnings: See AMILORIDE HYDROCHLORIDE; HYDROCHLOROTHIAZIDE.
✪ **Related entry: Moduret 25.**

co-amilozide 5/50

is a simplified name for the compound preparation of the (*potassium-sparing*) DIURETIC amiloride hydrochloride and the THIAZIDE diuretic hydrochlorothiazide, in the ratio 5:50 (mg), for treating oedema. It is given orally.
✚▲ Side-effects/warnings: See AMILORIDE HYDROCHLORIDE; HYDROCHLOROTHIAZIDE.
✪ **Related entries: Amil-Co; Amilmaxco 5/50; Moduretic.**

co-amoxiclav

is a simplified name for the compound preparation of the broad-spectrum ANTIBACTERIAL and (PENICILLIN) ANTIBIOTIC amoxicillin and the ENZYME INHIBITOR clavulanic acid (in the form of its potassium salt). Clavulanic acid interferes with the action of beta-lactamase and so makes amoxicillin *penicillinase resistant* when it is used against *Staphylococcus aureus*, *Haemophilus influenzae* and certain other bacteria that would otherwise inactivate the antibiotic. Co-amoxiclav can be used to treat many infections, including those of the upper respiratory tract, of the ear, nose and throat and of the urogenital tracts. Administration is either oral or by injection.
✚▲ Side-effects/warnings: See AMOXICILLIN; CLAVULANIC ACID. There is evidence of cholestatic jaundice (particularly in the elderly). Administer with caution to patients with liver impairment, jaundice, certain blood disorders; or who are pregnant or breast-feeding. There may be skin reactions, stained teeth, dizziness, headache and other side-effects.
✪ **Related entry: Augmentin.**

CoAprovel

(Bristol-Myers Squibb) is a proprietary, prescription-only compound preparation of the ANGIOTENSIN-RECEPTOR BLOCKER irbesartan and the (THIAZIDE) DIURETIC hydrochlorothiazide. It can be used as an ANTIHYPERTENSIVE, and is available as tablets.
✚▲ Side-effects/warnings: See HYDROCHLOROTHIAZIDE; IRBESARTAN.

Cobalin-H

(Link) is a proprietary, prescription-only preparation of the VITAMIN hydroxocobalamin. It can be used as an ANAEMIA TREATMENT to correct deficiency of vitamin B_{12}, including pernicious anaemia, and is available in a form for injection.
✚▲ Side-effects/warnings: See HYDROXOCOBALAMIN.

co-beneldopa

is a simplified name for the compound preparation of the ANTIPARKINSONISM drug levodopa and the ENZYME INHIBITOR benserazide hydrochloride (in a ratio of benzeride/levodopa 1:4). It is used to treat parkinsonism, but not the parkinsonian symptoms induced by drugs. Benserazide prevents levodopa from being broken down too rapidly in the body (into dopamine) and so allowing more of it to reach the brain to make up the deficiency of dopamine, which is the cause of parkinsonian symptoms. Administration is oral.
✚▲ Side-effects/warnings: See LEVODOPA.
✪ **Related entry: Madopar.**

Co-Betaloc

(Searle; Pharmacia) is a proprietary, prescription-only compound preparation of the BETA-BLOCKER metoprolol tartrate and the (THIAZIDE) DIURETIC hydrochlorothiazide. It can be used as an ANTIHYPERTENSIVE for raised blood pressure, and is available as tablets.
✚▲ Side-effects/warnings: See HYDROCHLOROTHIAZIDE; METOPROLOL TARTRATE.

Co-Betaloc SA

(Searle; Pharmacia) is a proprietary, prescription-only compound preparation of the BETA-BLOCKER metoprolol tartrate and the (THIAZIDE) DIURETIC hydrochlorothiazide. It can be used as an ANTIHYPERTENSIVE for raised blood pressure, and is available as modified-release tablets.

✚▲ Side-effects/warnings: See HYDROCHLOROTHIAZIDE; METOPROLOL TARTRATE.

cocaine

is a central nervous system STIMULANT which rapidly causes dependence (addiction). Therapeutically, it can be used as a LOCAL ANAESTHETIC for otolaryngology (ears, nose, throat) procedures when it is applied topically, sometimes with adrenaline, for example, to the nasal mucosa.

✚▲ Side-effects/warnings: It is a specialist drug usually used under hospital conditions. There is stimulation of the central nervous system, sympathomimetic effects and heart arrhythmias. It is not used in patients with porphyria.

co-careldopa

is a simplified name for the compound preparation of the ANTIPARKINSONISM drug levodopa and the ENZYME INHIBITOR carbidopa (the proportion of carbidopa to levodopa varies). It is used to treat parkinsonism, but not the parkinsonian symptoms induced by drugs. Carbidopa prevents levodopa from being broken down too rapidly in the body (into dopamine) and so allowing more of it to reach the brain to make up the deficiency of dopamine, which is the cause of parkinsonian symptoms. Administration is oral.

✚▲ Side-effects/warnings: See LEVODOPA.

✪ **Related entries: Half Sinemet CR; Sinemet; Sinemet CR.**

co-codamol

is a compound analgesic preparation of the (OPIOID) NARCOTIC ANALGESIC codeine phosphate and the NON-NARCOTIC ANALGESIC paracetamol; in either a ratio of 8:500 (mg) – *co-codamol 8/500*, or the stronger 30:500 (mg) – *co-codamol 30/500*. The 8/500 preparation is available on a non-prescription basis (as it has a lower codeine content) either as one of an extensive range of generic preparations or in proprietary forms that cannot be prescribed under the National Health Service. The 30/500 and 60/1000 preparations are available only on prescription and should be used with caution, especially in the elderly.

✚▲ Side-effects/warnings: See CODEINE PHOSPHATE; PARACETAMOL.

✪ **Related entries: Kapake; Panadeine Tablets; Paracodol Capsules; Paracodol Tablets; Parake; Solpadeine Capsules; Solpadeine Max; Solpadeine Soluble Tablets; Solpadeine Tablets; Solpadol; Tylex.**

co-codaprin

(co-codaprin 8/400) is a compound analgesic preparation of the weak (OPIOID) NARCOTIC ANALGESIC codeine phosphate and the (NSAID) NON-NARCOTIC ANALGESIC and ANTIRHEUMATIC aspirin; in a ratio of 8:400 (mg). Administration is oral.

✚▲ Side-effects/warnings: See ASPIRIN; CODEINE PHOSPHATE.

Cocois

(Celltech) is a proprietary, non-prescription compound preparation of salicylic acid, coal tar and sulphur (in coconut oil). It is used to treat scaly scalp disorders such as eczema and psoriasis, and is available as a scalp ointment. It is not normally given to children under six years, except on medical advice.

✚▲ Side-effects/warnings: See COAL TAR; SALICYLIC ACID; SULPHUR.

Codafen Continus

(Napp) is a proprietary, prescription-only compound analgesic preparation of the (NSAID) NON-NARCOTIC ANALGESIC and ANTIRHEUMATIC ibuprofen and the (OPIOID) NARCOTIC ANALGESIC codeine phosphate (in higher amounts than in proprietary, non-prescription compound analgesics). It can be used in particular for treating the pain of musculoskeletal disorders. Available as modified-release tablets.

✚▲ Side-effects/warnings: See CODEINE PHOSPHATE; IBUPROFEN.

Codalax

(Napp) is a proprietary, prescription-only preparation of CO-DANTHRAMER 25/200, which is a (*stimulant*) LAXATIVE based on dantron and poloxamer '188'. It can be used to treat constipation and to prepare patients for abdominal procedures, and is available as an oral suspension.

✚▲ Side-effects/warnings: See DANTRON; POLOXAMER '188'.

Codalax Forte

(Napp) is a proprietary, prescription-only

C

preparation of CO-DANTHRAMER 75/1000, which is a (*stimulant*) LAXATIVE based on dantron and poloxamer '188'. It can be used to treat constipation and to prepare patients for abdominal procedures, and is available as an oral suspension.
✚▲ Side-effects/warnings: See DANTRON; POLOXAMER '188'.

co-danthramer 25/200

is the general name for a non-proprietary, prescription-only compound preparation of the (*stimulant*) LAXATIVE danthron and poloxamer '188'. Administration is oral.
✚▲ Side-effects/warnings: See DANTRON; POLOXAMER '188'. Some preparations of co-danthramer turn the urine red.
✪ **Related entries: Ailax; Codalax; Danlax.**

co-danthramer 75/1000

is the general name for non-proprietary, prescription-only compound preparations of the (*stimulant*) LAXATIVE dantron and poloxamer '188'. Administration is oral.
✚▲ Side-effects/warnings: See DANTRON; POLOXAMER '188'. Some preparations of co-danthramer turn the urine red.
✪ **Related entry: Codalax Forte.**

co-danthrusate 50/60

is the general name for non-proprietary, prescription-only compound preparations of the (*stimulant*) LAXATIVE dantron and docusate sodium. Administration is oral.
✚▲ Side-effects/warnings: See DANTRON; DOCUSATE SODIUM.
✪ **Related entries: Capsuvac; Normax.**

codeine phosphate

is an (OPIOID) NARCOTIC ANALGESIC that is an analgesic. Codeine is a common but often minor constituent of non-proprietary and proprietary preparations used to relieve mild to moderate pain. It is also an ANTITUSSIVE and is incorporated with other drugs into a number of cough-and-cold preparations. The drug also has the capacity to reduce intestinal motility and so can be used as an ANTIDIARRHOEAL and antimotility treatment. Administration is normally oral. Codeine phosphate tablets (that is, codeine alone without addition of a major proportion of other constituents) are available only on prescription, and travellers going abroad may require a doctor's letter explaining why they are required. (Preparations of codeine for injection are on the Controlled Drugs list.)
✚▲ Side-effects/warnings: See OPIOID. Tolerance occurs readily, though dependence (addiction) is relatively unusual. Serious adverse effects with the doses of codeine contained in over-the-counter preparations, are relatively rare. Codeine and alcohol ingestion should not be combined because of potentiation of effects, including sleepiness and respiratory depression.
✪ **Related entries: Benylin with Codeine; Boots Tension Headache Relief; co-codamol; co-codaprin; Codafen Continus; Codis 500; Dimotane Co; Dimotane Co Paediatric; Famel Original Cough Syrup; Feminax; Galcodine; Galcodine Paediatric; Kaodene; Kapake; Migraleve; Migraleve Pink; Migraleve Yellow; Nurofen Plus; Panadeine Tablets; Panadol Ultra; Paracodol Capsules; Paracodol Tablets; Parake; Propain Caplets; Pulmo Bailly; Robitussin Night-Time; Solpadeine Capsules; Solpadeine Max; Solpadeine Soluble Tablets; Solpadeine Tablets; Solpadol; Solpaflex Tablets; Syndol; Tylex; Veganin Tablets.**

co-dergocrine mesilate

(co-dergocrine mesylate) is a VASODILATOR drug mixture which affects the blood vessels of the brain. It consists of a mixture of dihydroergocornine mesilate, dihydroergocristine mesilate and alpha- and beta-dihydroergocryptine mesilates, which have alpha-adrenoceptor blocking actions (see ALPHA-ADRENOCEPTOR BLOCKER). It has been claimed to be a NOOTROPIC AGENT, improving brain function; but clinical results of psychological tests during and following treatment have neither proved nor disproved such a claim. It is for the treatment of senile dementia that the drug is most frequently used. Administration is oral.
✚ Side-effects: There may be gastrointestinal disturbances, dizziness, flushing, a blocked nose, headache, rash, postural hypotension (in patients with hypertension).
▲ Warnings: It should be administered with caution to patients who have a very slow heart rate.
✪ **Related entry: Hydergine.**

co-dergocrine mesylate

see CO-DERGOCRINE MESILATE.

Codis 500

(Reckitt Benckiser Healthcare) is a proprietary, non-prescription compound analgesic preparation of the (NSAID) NON-NARCOTIC ANALGESIC and ANTIRHEUMATIC aspirin and the (OPIOID) NARCOTIC ANALGESIC codeine phosphate. It can be used to relieve mild to moderate pain and high body temperature. It is available as soluble tablets and is not normally given to children, except on medical advice.

+▲ Side-effects/warnings: See ASPIRIN; CODEINE PHOSPHATE.

cod-liver oil

has EMOLLIENT properties and is one of the constituents of a proprietary compound preparation that is administered by topical application to the skin in the form of a cream. At one time cod-liver oil was commonly used as a source of VITAMIN A and VITAMIN D, but now HALIBUT-LIVER OIL is preferred.

+▲ Side-effects/warnings: It is regarded as safe in normal topical use.

✪ **Related entry: Morhulin Ointment.**

co-dydramol

is a prescription-only compound analgesic preparation of the (OPIOID) NARCOTIC ANALGESIC dihydrocodeine tartrate and the NON-NARCOTIC ANALGESIC paracetamol; in a ratio of 10:500 (mg) – though some similar non-prescription and prescription-only preparations have somewhat different amounts of the two analgesics. This compound analgesic has the advantages and disadvantages of both drugs. It can be particularly dangerous in overdose because of the (opioid) dihydrocodeine tartrate component. It is available as tablets.

+▲ Side-effects/warnings: See DIHYDROCODEINE TARTRATE; PARACETAMOL.

✪ **Related entries: Galake; Paramol Tablets.**

co-fluampicil

is a simplified name for the compound preparation of the broad-spectrum, penicillin-like ANTIBACTERIAL and ANTIBIOTIC ampicillin and the *penicillinase-resistant*, penicillin-like antibacterial and antibiotic flucloxacillin. It can be used to treat severe mixed infections where penicillin-resistant bacterial infection is probable. Administration is either oral or by injection.

+▲ Side-effects/warnings: See AMPICILLIN; FLUCLOXACILLIN.

✪ **Related entries: Flu-Amp; Magnapen.**

co-flumactone 25/25

is a simplified name for the compound preparation of the (*aldosterone-antagonist* and *potassium-sparing*) DIURETIC spironolactone and the (*potassium-depleting* THIAZIDE) diuretic hydroflumethiazide, in the ratio 25:25 (mg), for treating oedema. It is given orally.

+▲ Side-effects/warnings: See HYDROFLUMETHIAZIDE; SPIRONOLACTONE.

✪ **Related entry: Aldactide 25.**

co-flumactone 50/50

is a simplified name for the compound preparation of the (*aldosterone-antagonist* and *potassium-sparing*) DIURETIC spironolactone and the (*potassium-depleting* THIAZIDE) diuretic hydroflumethiazide, in the ratio of 50:50 (mg), for treating oedema. It is given orally.

+▲ Side-effects/warnings: See HYDROFLUMETHIAZIDE; SPIRONOLACTONE.

✪ **Related entry: Aldactide 50.**

Cogentin

(MSD) is a proprietary, prescription-only preparation of the ANTICHOLINERGIC benztropine mesilate. It can be used in the treatment of parkinsonism, and is available as tablets and in a form for injection.

+▲ Side-effects/warnings: See BENZTROPINE MESILATE.

Colazide

(Shire) is a proprietary, prescription-only preparation of the AMINOSALICYLATE balsalazide disodium. It can be used to treat patients who suffer from ulcerative colitis but who are unable to tolerate the more commonly used sulphasalazine. It is available as capsules.

+▲ Side-effects/warnings: See BALSALAZIDE DISODIUM.

colchicine

is a drug derived from the autumn crocus *Colchicum autumnale*. It is used in the treatment of gout, particularly as a short-term, introductory measure to prevent acute attacks during initial treatment with other drugs (eg ALLOPURINOL) that reduce uric acid levels in the blood.

Administration is oral.
✚ Side-effects: Nausea, vomiting and abdominal pain. High or excessive dosage may lead to gastrointestinal bleeding and diarrhoea, rashes and liver or kidney damage. Rarely, peripheral nerve disorders, loss of hair or blood disorders.
▲ Warnings: Do not use in those who are pregnant or breast-feeding. Administer with caution to patients with gastrointestinal disease, impaired liver or kidney function.

colecalciferol

(cholecalciferol; vitamin D_3) is one of the natural forms of calciferol (vitamin D) which is found particularly in fish oil (eg tuna). It is vitamin D_3 but in medicine it is usually referred to as colecalciferol, and is used to make up deficiencies. Administration can be oral or by injection.
✚▲ Side-effects/warnings: See VITAMIN D.
✪ **Related entries: Adcal-D3; Calceos; Calcichew D3; Crampex Tablets.**

Colestid

(Pharmacia) is a proprietary, prescription-only preparation of the LIPID-REGULATING DRUG colestipol hydrochloride. It can be used in hyperlipidaemia to reduce the levels, or change the proportions, of lipids in the bloodstream. It is available as granules (in two forms) to be taken with liquids.
✚▲ Side-effects/warnings: See COLESTIPOL HYDROCHLORIDE.

colestipol hydrochloride

is a resin that binds bile acids and lowers LDL-cholesterol. It is used as a LIPID-REGULATING DRUG in hyperlipidaemia to reduce the levels, or change the proportions, of various lipids in the bloodstream. It is usually administered only to patients in whom a strict and regular dietary regime, alone, is not having the desired effect. Administration is oral.
✚▲ Side-effects/warnings: See CHOLESTYRAMINE. Other drugs should be taken 4-6 hours after, or 1 hour before, colestipol hydrochloride (it can affect absorption of other drugs).
✪ **Related entry: Colestid.**

colestyramine

(cholestyramine) is a resin that binds bile acids in the gut which reduces absorption of bile salts from the gut which results in changed cholesterol metabolism in the liver. It can be used as a LIPID-REGULATING DRUG in hyperlipidaemia to reduce the levels, or change the proportions, of various lipids in the bloodstream. It has various other uses, including as an ANTIDIARRHOEAL and in certain biliary disturbances (including pruritus in biliary obstruction, or biliary cirrhosis). Generally, it is administered only to patients in whom a strict and regular dietary regime, alone, is not having the desired effect. Administration is oral.
✚ Side-effects: These are not common because the drug is not absorbed into the body from the intestine, but there may be gastrointestinal upsets including nausea and vomiting; flatulence with abdominal discomfort, constipation (or sometimes diarrhoea). (Prolonged use may lead to vitamin K deficiency with increased bleeding.)
▲ Warnings: It should not be administered to patients who suffer from complete blockage of the bile ducts. Prolonged treatment may require simultaneous administration of fat-soluble vitamins and folic acid. Care is required in pregnancy and breast-feeding.
✪ **Related entries: Questran; Questran Light.**

Colifoam

(Stafford-Miller; GSK) is a proprietary, prescription-only preparation of the CORTICOSTEROID hydrocortisone (as acetate). It can be used to treat inflammation with colitis and proctitis, and is available as a foam and applied with an aerosol.
✚▲ Side-effects/warnings: See HYDROCORTISONE.

colistin

(polymyxin E) is an ANTIBACTERIAL and ANTIBIOTIC drug which is a comparatively toxic member of the POLYMYXIN family. It is active against Gram-negative bacteria, including *Pseudomonas aeruginosa*, and can be used in topical application (as colistin sulphate) to treat infections of the skin. However, in certain conditions and under strict supervision, the drug may be administered orally (primarily to sterilize the bowel and is not absorbed) or by injection (in the form colistimethate sodium (colistin sulphomethate sodium)), eye-drops. intravenous infusion or inhalation (as an adjunct to standard

antibiotic treatment).
✚ Side-effects: These depend on route of administration. When given systemically, there may be breathlessness, vertigo, numbness round the mouth and muscular weakness and a tingling sensation. Rarely, slurred speech, confusion and visual disturbances, kidney effects; bronchospasm when inhaled.
▲ Warnings: It should not be administered to patients who suffer from the neuromuscular disease myasthenia gravis, or who are pregnant or breast-feeding. It should be administered with caution to those who suffer from impaired kidney function or porphyria. Large areas of skin should not be treated in topical use.
✪ Related entry: Colomycin.

Colofac

(Solvay) is a proprietary, prescription-only preparation of the ANTISPASMODIC mebeverine hydrochloride. It can be used to treat gastrointestinal disorders where there is spasm such as irritable bowel syndrome, and is available as tablets and an oral suspension.
✚▲ Side-effects/warnings: See MEBEVERINE HYDROCHLORIDE.

Colofac 100

(Solvay Healthcare) is a proprietary, non-prescription preparation of the ANTISPASMODIC mebeverine hydrochloride. It can be used for symptomatic relief of gastrointestinal colicky pain, and is available as tablets. It is not recommended for children under ten years.
✚▲ Side-effects/warnings: See MEBEVERINE HYDROCHLORIDE.

Colofac IBS

(Solvay Healthcare) is a proprietary, non-prescription preparation of the ANTISPASMODIC mebeverine hydrochloride. It can be used for symptomatic relief of irritable bowel syndrome, and is available as tablets. It is not recommended for children under ten years.
✚▲ Side-effects/warnings: See MEBEVERINE HYDROCHLORIDE.

Colofac MR

(Solvay) is a proprietary, prescription-only preparation of the ANTISPASMODIC mebeverine hydrochloride. It can be used to treat gastrointestinal spasm such as irritable bowel syndrome, and is available as modified-release capsules.
✚▲ Side-effects/warnings: See MEBEVERINE HYDROCHLORIDE.

Colomycin

(Forest) is a proprietary, prescription-only preparation of the ANTIBACTERIAL and (POLYMYXIN) ANTIBIOTIC colistin. It can be used by topical application to treat bacterial skin infections, and also by mouth and by injection for other purposes.
✚▲ Side-effects/warnings: See COLISTIN.

Colpermin

(Pharmacia) is a proprietary, non-prescription preparation of the ANTISPASMODIC peppermint oil. It can be used to relieve the discomfort of abdominal colic and distension, particularly in irritable bowel syndrome, and is available as capsules. It is not given to children under 15 years, except on medical advice.
✚▲ Side-effects/warnings: See PEPPERMINT OIL.

Combivent

(Boehringer Ingelheim) is a proprietary, prescription-only compound preparation of the SYMPATHOMIMETIC and BETA-RECEPTOR STIMULANT salbutamol (as sulphate) and the ANTICHOLINERGIC ipratropium bromide, which both have BRONCHODILATOR properties. It can be used in obstructive airways disease, and is available in a metered-dose *Autoinhaler*, as an aerosol and a nebulizer solution.
✚▲ Side-effects/warnings: See SALBUTAMOL; IPRATROPIUM BROMIDE.

Combivir

(GlaxoWellcome; GSK) is a proprietary, prescription-only compound preparation of the ANTIVIRAL agents lamivudine and zidovudine. It can be used in the treatment of HIV infection, and is available as tablets.
✚▲ Side-effects/warnings: See LAMIVUDINE; ZIDOVUDINE.

co-methiamol

is a combination of the NON-NARCOTIC ANALGESIC and ANTIPYRETIC paracetamol and the amino acid METHIONINE (an antidote to paracetamol overdose). It can be used to provide relief from painful and feverish conditions, such

as period pain, toothache, cold and flu symptoms, and to reduce high body temperature (especially for patients likely to overdose). Administration is oral.
✚▲ Side-effects/warnings: See PARACETAMOL.
✪ **Related entry: Paradote.**

Compound Thymol Glycerin, BP

is a non-proprietary, non-prescription preparation of GLYCEROL and THYMOL (with colour and flavouring). It can be used as a mouthwash for oral hygiene.

Compound W

(SSL) is a proprietary, non-prescription preparation of the KERATOLYTIC agent salicylic acid. It can be used to remove warts and verrucas, and is available as a liquid. It is not normally given to children under six years, except on medical advice.
✚▲ Side-effects/warnings: See SALICYLIC ACID.

Comtess

(Orion) is a proprietary, prescription-only preparation of the ANTIPARKINSONISM drug entacapone. It can be used to assist in the treatment of the symptoms of parkinsonism, and is available as tablets.
✚▲ Side-effects/warnings: See ENTACAPONE.

Condyline

(Ardern) is a proprietary, prescription-only preparation of the KERATOLYTIC agent podophyllum. It can be used in men to treat and remove penile warts, and in women warts on the external genitalia. It is available as a solution for topical application.
✚▲ Side-effects/warnings: See PODOPHYLLUM.

conjugated oestrogens

are OESTROGEN obtained from the urine of pregnant mares, which are used in HRT (hormone replacement therapy). Administration is oral.
✚▲ Side-effects/warnings: See OESTROGEN.
✪ **Related entries: Premarin; Premique; Prempak-C.**

Conotrane

(Yamanouchi) is a proprietary, non-prescription preparation of the ANTISEPTIC benzalkonium chloride (with dimeticone '350'). It can be used to relieve nappy and urinary rash and skin (pressure) sores, and is available as a cream.
✚▲ Side-effects/warnings: See BENZALKONIUM CHLORIDE; DIMETICONE.

Contac 400

(GSK Consumer Healthcare) is a proprietary, non-prescription compound preparation of the SYMPATHOMIMETIC and DECONGESTANT phenylpropanolamine hydrochloride and the ANTIHISTAMINE chlorphenamine maleate (chlorpheniramine maleate). It can be used for symptomatic relief of a blocked and runny nose due to hay fever, colds and sinusitis. It is available as capsules, and is not normally given to children, except on medical advice.
✚▲ Side-effects/warnings: See CHLORPHENAMINE MALEATE; PHENYLPROPANOLAMINE HYDROCHLORIDE.

Contimin

(Berk; APS) is a proprietary, prescription-only preparation of the ANTICHOLINERGIC oxybutynin hydrochloride. It can be used as an ANTISPASMODIC in the treatment of urinary disorders such as incontinence. It is available as tablets.
✚▲ Side-effects/warnings: See OXYBUTYNIN HYDROCHLORIDE.

contraceptive 🄱

is a term used to describe drugs, methods or devices that prevent conception. Contraceptive drugs include types of ORAL CONTRACEPTIVE preparations (most notably the Pill), which contain either a hormonal combination of PROGESTOGENS plus an OESTROGEN (combined oral contraceptive pill; *COC*), just a progestogen (progesterone-only contraceptive pill; *POP*) or parenteral contraceptives (progesterone-only preparations given by injection or implantation and renewable every three months). SPERMICIDAL CONTRACEPTIVE preparations contain drugs that kill sperm and/or prevent sperm motility within the vagina or cervix, and should only be used in combination with barrier methods of contraception (such as a condom or diaphragm). Post-coital emergency contraception consists of a high dose of a combined preparation of oestrogen and progestogen, or progestogen alone (known as the 'morning-after pill'). Traditional intra-uterine contraceptive devices are not normally regarded as drugs (and are not within the scope of this book), but have a copper wire or ring incorporated which is thought to be pharmacologically active in changing production of local mediators (especially the PROSTAGLANDIN family), which effect implantation. However, a hormonal contraceptive (*intra-uterine progestogen-only contraceptive*) is available, where the progestogen (LEVONORGESTREL) is released directly into the uterine cavity from a plastic storage device which is inserted (by the doctor) into the uterine cavity. All contraceptives that involve the use of drugs produce side-effects and expert advice is required to identify the form ideally suited to an individual's circumstances.

Convulex

(Pharmacia) is a proprietary, prescription-only preparation of the ANTICONVULSANT and ANTI-EPILEPTIC sodium valproate (actually in the form of valproic acid). It is a valuable drug in the treatment of epilepsy, and is available as capsules.
✚▲ Side-effects/warnings: See SODIUM VALPROATE.

Copaxone

(Teva) is a proprietary, prescription-only preparation of the recently introduced IMMUNOMODULATOR glatiramer acetate. It can be used to reduce the frequency of relapses in people with relapsing-remitting multiple sclerosis, and is available in a form for subcutaneous injection.
✚▲ Side-effects/warnings: See GLATIRAMER ACETATE.

co-phenotrope

is a compound preparation of the ANTIDIARRHOEAL and OPIOID diphenoxylate hydrochloride and the ANTICHOLINERGIC (ANTIMUSCARINIC) atropine sulphate (in the proportion 2.5:0.025 (mg)). It can be used to treat acute diarrhoea, and chronic diarrhoea such as in mild chronic ulcerative colitis, but dependency may occur with prolonged use. It is available as tablets and a sugar-free liquid.
✚▲ Side-effects/warnings: See ATROPINE SULPHATE; DIPHENOXYLATE HYDROCHLORIDE. Children are particularly susceptible to overdose.
✪ **Related entries: Diarphen; Lomotil; Tropergen.**

co-prenozide

is the name given to a compound preparation of the BETA-BLOCKER oxprenolol hydrochloride and the (THIAZIDE) DIURETIC cyclopenthiazide (more fully called *co-prenozide 160/0.25*). It can be used as an ANTIHYPERTENSIVE for raised blood pressure.
✚▲ Side-effects/warnings: See CYCLOPENTHIAZIDE; OXPRENOLOL HYDROCHLORIDE.

co-proxamol

is a compound analgesic preparation of the (OPIOID) NARCOTIC ANALGESIC dextropropoxyphene hydrochloride and the NON-NARCOTIC ANALGESIC paracetamol; in a ratio of 32.5:325 (mg). It is available in generic and proprietary preparations, and has the advantages and disadvantages of both drugs. It is particularly dangerous to overdose because of the (opioid) dextropropoxyphene component. Administration is oral.
✚▲ Side-effects/warnings: See DEXTROPROPOXYPHENE HYDROCHLORIDE; PARACETAMOL.
✪ **Related entries: Cosalgesic; Distalgesic.**

Coracten SR

(Celltech) is a proprietary, prescription-only preparation of the CALCIUM-CHANNEL BLOCKER nifedipine. It can be used as an ANTI-ANGINA treatment in the prevention of attacks and as an ANTIHYPERTENSIVE. It is available as capsules.
✚▲ Side-effects/warnings: See NIFEDIPINE.

Coracten XL

(Celltech) is a proprietary, prescription-only preparation of the CALCIUM-CHANNEL BLOCKER nifedipine. It can be used as an ANTI-ANGINA treatment in the prevention of attacks and as an ANTIHYPERTENSIVE. It is available as modified-release capsules.
✚▲ Side-effects/warnings: See NIFEDIPINE.

Cordarone X

(Sanofi-Synthelabo) is a proprietary, prescription-only preparation of the ANTI-ARRHYTHMIC amiodarone hydrochloride. It can be used to treat heartbeat irregularities, and is available as tablets and in a form for injection.
✚▲ Side-effects/warnings: See AMIODARONE HYDROCHLORIDE.

Cordilox

(IVAX) is a proprietary, prescription-only

preparation of the CALCIUM-CHANNEL BLOCKER verapamil hydrochloride. It can be used as an ANTIHYPERTENSIVE, as an ANTI-ANGINA treatment in the prevention of attacks and as an ANTI-ARRHYTHMIC to correct heart irregularities. It is available as tablets and in a form for injection.
✚▲ Side-effects/warnings: See VERAPAMIL HYDROCHLORIDE.

Cordilox MR

(IVAX) is a proprietary, prescription-only preparation of the CALCIUM-CHANNEL BLOCKER verapamil hydrochloride. It can be used as an ANTIHYPERTENSIVE and as an ANTI-ANGINA treatment in the prevention of attacks. It is available as modified-release tablets.
✚▲ Side-effects/warnings: See VERAPAMIL HYDROCHLORIDE.

Corgard

(Sanofi-Synthelabo) is a proprietary, prescription-only preparation of the BETA-BLOCKER nadolol. It can be used as an ANTIHYPERTENSIVE for raised blood pressure, as an ANTI-ANGINA treatment to relieve symptoms and improve exercise tolerance, and as an ANTI-ARRHYTHMIC to regularize heartbeat and to treat myocardial infarction. It can also be used as an ANTIMIGRAINE treatment to prevent attacks and as an ANTITHYROID for short-term treatment of thyrotoxicosis. It is available as tablets.
✚▲ Side-effects/warnings: See NADOLOL.

Corgaretic 40

(Sanofi-Synthelabo) is a proprietary, prescription-only compound preparation of the BETA-BLOCKER nadolol and the DIURETIC bendroflumethiazide. It can be used as an ANTIHYPERTENSIVE for raised blood pressure, and is available as tablets.
✚▲ Side-effects/warnings: See BENDROFLUMETHIAZIDE; NADOLOL.

Corgaretic 80

(Sanofi-Synthelabo) is a proprietary, prescription-only compound preparation of the BETA-BLOCKER nadolol and the DIURETIC bendroflumethiazide. It can be used as an ANTIHYPERTENSIVE for raised blood pressure, and is available as tablets.
✚▲ Side-effects/warnings: See BENDROFLUMETHIAZIDE; NADOLOL.

Corlan

(Celltech) is a proprietary, non-prescription preparation of the CORTICOSTEROID and ANTI-INFLAMMATORY hydrocortisone (as sodium succinate). It can be used to treat ulcers and sores in the mouth, and is available as lozenges.
✚▲ Side-effects/warnings: See HYDROCORTISONE.

Coroday MR

(Generics) is a proprietary, prescription-only preparation of the CALCIUM-CHANNEL BLOCKER nifedipine. It can be used as an ANTI-ANGINA treatment in the prevention of attacks and as an ANTIHYPERTENSIVE. It is available as tablets.
✚▲ Side-effects/warnings: See NIFEDIPINE.

Coro-Nitro Pump Spray

(Roche) is a proprietary, non-prescription preparation of the VASODILATOR and ANTI-ANGINA drug glyceryl trinitrate. It can be used to treat and prevent angina pectoris, and is available in the form of a sublingual (beneath the tongue) aerosol spray in metered doses.
✚▲ Side-effects/warnings: See GLYCERYL TRINITRATE.

Corsodyl Dental Gel

(GSK Consumer Healthcare) is a proprietary, non-prescription preparation of the ANTISEPTIC chlorhexidine (as gluconate). It can be used by topical application to treat inflammation and infections of the mouth, such as candida and ulcers, and for oral hygiene. Available as a dental gel.
✚▲ Side-effects/warnings: See CHLORHEXIDINE.

Corsodyl Original Mouthwash

(GSK Consumer Healthcare) is a proprietary, non-prescription preparation of the ANTISEPTIC chlorhexidine (as gluconate). It can be used by topical application to treat inflammation and infections of the mouth, such as candida and ulcers, and for oral hygiene. It is available as a mouthwash (one version in mint flavour).
✚▲ Side-effects/warnings: See CHLORHEXIDINE.

Corsodyl Spray

(GSK Consumer Healthcare) is a proprietary, non-prescription preparation of the ANTISEPTIC chlorhexidine (as gluconate). It can be used by topical application to treat inflammation and infections of the mouth, such as candida and ulcers. It is available as a oral spray.

✚▲ Side-effects/warnings: See CHLORHEXIDINE.

corticosteroid

hormones are steroid hormones secreted by the cortex (outer part) of the adrenal glands, or are synthetic substances that closely resemble the natural forms. There are two main types, *glucocorticoids* and *mineralocorticoids*. The latter assist in maintaining the salt-and-water balance of the body. Corticosteroids such as the glucocorticoids HYDROCORTISONE and the mineralocorticoid FLUDROCORTISONE ACETATE can be given to patients for replacement therapy where there is a deficiency, in Addison's disease or following adrenalectomy or hypopituitarism. The glucocorticoids are potent ANTI-INFLAMMATORY and ANTI-ALLERGIC drugs and are frequently used to treat inflammatory and/or allergic reactions of the skin and airways; also in neoplastic disease in combination with cytotoxic drugs, and uses elsewhere, such as anti-inflammatory/immunosuppressive therapy in chronic illnesses such as rheumatic arthritis and other connective tissue disorders (eg lupus and inflammatory bowel disease). Compound preparations are available that contain both an ANTIBACTERIAL or ANTIFUNGAL with an anti-inflammatory corticosteroid, and can be used in conditions where an infection is also present. However, these preparations must be used with caution because the corticosteroid component diminishes the patient's natural immune response to the infective agent. Absorption of a high dose of corticosteroid over a period of time may also cause undesirable, systemic side-effects. See ALCLOMETASONE DIPROPIONATE; BECLOMETASONE DIPROPIONATE; BETAMETHASONE; BUDESONIDE; CLOBETASOL PROPIONATE; CLOBETASONE BUTYRATE; CORTISONE ACETATE; DEFLAZACORT; DESOXIMETASONE; DEXAMETHASONE; DIFLUCORTOLONE VALERATE; FLUMETHASONE PIVALATE; FLUNISOLIDE; FLUOCINOLONE ACETONIDE; FLUOCINONIDE; FLUOCORTOLONE; FLUOROMETHOLONE; FLUDROXYCORTIDE; FLUTICASONE PROPIONATE; HALCINONIDE; METHYLPREDNISOLONE; MOMETASONE FUROATE; PREDNISOLONE; RIMEXOLONE and TRIAMCINOLONE.

✚ Side-effects: Unwanted effects are likely with high doses or prolonged use, but most should not occur with replacement therapy. *Mineralocorticoid* adverse effects include hypertension, sodium and water retention and potassium loss. *Glucocorticoid* adverse effects include high blood sugar and possibly diabetes, osteoporosis, avascular necrosis, mental disturbances, euphoria but sometimes depression, muscle wasting, weakness, menstrual disorders, blood disorders, possibly peptic ulceration. Corticosteroids may also cause Cushing's syndrome, suppressed growth in children and adrenal atrophy. If administered during pregnancy, they may affect adrenal gland development in the child. When given by inhalation, there may be oral thrush. When taken nasally, there may be dryness, irritation of the nose, ulceration, rarely glaucoma, changes in smell and taste, and hypersensitivity reactions. Used as eye-drops, there may be effects on the eye such as cataracts (after prolonged use), or glaucoma (in susceptible patients) with some corticosteroids. When used on skin, there may be local side-effects such as worsening of untreated infection, skin reactions (eg dermatitis, acne).

▲ Warnings: Because the symptoms of infection may be masked, signs should be looked for, and infections treated (eg with combined preparations). For long-term treatment, or at high doses, there will be a full assessment and counselling will be done. Withdrawal of treatment must be gradual. Patients on corticosteroid therapy will be fully medically counselled on the effects of drug treatment and precautions, and will be given a *steroid card* with general advice.

corticotrophin

see CORTICOTROPIN.

corticotropin

(corticotrophin) or adrenocorticotrophic hormone (ACTH) is a HORMONE produced and secreted by the pituitary gland in order to control the production and secretion of other hormones – CORTICOSTEROID – from the adrenal glands, generally as a response to stress. Therapeutically, synthetic corticotrophin analogues (eg TETRACOSACTIDE (tetracosactide) have been used to cause the production of extra corticosteroids in the treatment of inflammatory conditions, such as rheumatoid arthritis and Crohn's disease, but

C

now are usually used only to test the function of the adrenal glands.

cortisol
is another name for HYDROCORTISONE.

cortisone acetate
is a CORTICOSTEROID hormone with ANTI-INFLAMMATORY properties and has both *glucocorticoid* and *mineralocorticoid* activity. It can therefore be used to make up for hormonal deficiency (especially relating to the salt-and-water balance in the body), for instance, following surgical removal of the adrenal glands. Administration is oral.
✚▲ Side-effects/warnings: See CORTICOSTEROID.
✪ **Related entry: Cortisyl.**

Cortisyl
(Hoechst Marion Roussel; Aventis Pharma) is a proprietary, prescription-only preparation of the CORTICOSTEROID and ANTI-INFLAMMATORY cortisone acetate. It can be used in replacement therapy to make up hormonal deficiency, for instance, following surgical removal of one or both of the adrenal glands. It is available as tablets.
✚▲ Side-effects/warnings: See CORTISONE ACETATE.

Cosalgesic
(Alpharma) is a proprietary, prescription-only compound analgesic preparation of the (OPIOID) NARCOTIC ANALGESIC dextropropoxyphene hydrochloride and the NON-NARCOTIC ANALGESIC paracetamol (a combination called co-proxamol). It can be used to treat many types of pain, and is available as tablets.
✚▲ Side-effects/warnings: See DEXTROPROPOXYPHENE HYDROCHLORIDE; PARACETAMOL.

Cosmegen Lyovac
(MSD) is a proprietary, prescription-only preparation of the ANTICANCER drug dactinomycin. It is used particularly to treat cancer in children, and is available in a form for injection.
✚▲ Side-effects/warnings: See DACTINOMYCIN.

Cosopt
(MSD) is a proprietary, prescription-only compound preparation of the CARBONIC-ANHYDRASE INHIBITOR dorzolamide combined with the BETA-BLOCKER timolol (as maleate). It is used in GLAUCOMA TREATMENT to treat raised intraocular pressure in open-angle glaucoma, or types of glaucoma when beta-blockers alone are not adequate. It is available as eye-drops.
✚▲ Side-effects/warnings: See DORZOLAMIDE; TIMOLOL MALEATE.

Cosuric
(DDSA) is a proprietary, prescription-only preparation of the ENZYME INHIBITOR allopurinol, which is a XANTHINE-OXIDASE INHIBITOR. It can be used to treat excess uric acid in the blood and to prevent renal stones and attacks of gout. It is available as tablets.
✚▲ Side-effects/warnings: See ALLOPURINOL.

co-tenidone
is a compound preparation of the BETA-BLOCKER atenolol and the DIURETIC chlortalidone (in two different proportions called *co-tenidone 50/12.5* and *co-tenidone 100/25*). It can be used as an ANTIHYPERTENSIVE for raised blood pressure, and is available as tablets.
✚▲ Side-effects/warnings: See ATENOLOL; CHLORTALIDONE.
✪ **Related entries: AtenixCo; Tenchlor; Tenoret 50; Tenoretic; Totaretic.**

co-triamterzide 50/25
is a simplified name for the compound preparation of the (*potassium-sparing*) DIURETIC triamterene and the (THIAZIDE) diuretic hydrochlorothiazide; in the ratio 50:25 (mg).
✚▲ Side-effects/warnings: See HYDROCHLOROTHIAZIDE; TRIAMTERENE.
✪ **Related entries: Dyazide; TriamaxCo; Triam-Co.**

co-trimoxazole
is a simplified name for the compound preparation of the (SULPHONAMIDE) ANTIBACTERIAL sulfamethoxazole and the similar, but not related, antibacterial trimethoprim (a folic acid inhibitor); in the ratio of 5:1. It is thought that each drug enhances the action of the other, giving a combined effect greater than the sum of the two. Although there is little substantial evidence to support this, the combination remains a very useful antibacterial preparation. It is used to treat and prevent the

spread of infections of the urinary tract, chronic bronchitis, toxoplasmosis, nocardiosis and acute otis media in children. It is also used as an antiprotozoal agent to treat or prevent *Pneumocystis carinii* pneumonia, an opportunistic infection seen in immunocompromised patients such as those suffering from HIV infection. Administration is either oral or by injection.
✚ Side-effects: These are largely due to the sulphonamide and may include nausea and vomiting; diarrhoea and rashes. Blood and skin disorders, allergic reactions, aches and pains, and others.
▲ Warnings: It should not be administered to patients who are pregnant or who have certain liver or kidney disorders. It should be administered with caution to patients who are elderly, pregnant or breast-feeding. Adequate fluid intake must be maintained. Prolonged treatment requires regular blood counts.
✪ Related entries: Chemotrim; Fectrim; Septrin.

counter-irritant

preparations, also called RUBEFACIENT, cause a feeling of warmth and offset the pain from underlying muscle and joints or viscera when rubbed in topically to the skin. Some are rubbed onto the gums (eg in teething babies) where they have a LOCAL ANAESTHETIC or *local analgesic* actions. A number of them are aromatic or volatile oils. How these agents act is uncertain, but the reddening of the skin (denoted by the name *rube*facient) indicates a dilatation of the blood vessels which gives a soothing feeling of warmth. The term counter-irritant refers to the idea that irritation of the sensory nerve endings alters or offsets pain in the underlying muscle or joints that are served by the same nerves. See CAPSAICIN; CAPSICUM OLEORESIN; CHOLINE SALICYLATE; ETHYL SALICYLATE; GLYCOL SALICYLATE; METHYL SALICYLATE; MENTHOL; SALICYLIC ACID; TURPENTINE OIL.

Coversyl

(Servier) is a proprietary, prescription-only preparation of the ACE INHIBITOR perindopril. It can be used as an ANTIHYPERTENSIVE and in HEART FAILURE TREATMENT. Available as tablets.
✚▲ Side-effects/warnings: See PERINDOPRIL.

Covonia Bronchial Balsam

(Thornton & Ross) is a proprietary, non-prescription compound preparation of the (OPIOID) ANTITUSSIVE dextromethorphan hydrobromide, and menthol. It can be used for the symptomatic relief of non-productive coughs, such as those associated with colds and bronchitis. It is available as a linctus and is not normally given to children under six years, except on medical advice.
✚▲ Side-effects/warnings: See DEXTROMETHORPHAN HYDROBROMIDE; MENTHOL.

Covonia Night Time Formula

(Thornton & Ross) is a proprietary, non-prescription compound preparation of the (OPIOID) ANTITUSSIVE dextromethorphan hydrobromide and the ANTIHISTAMINE diphenhydramine hydrochloride. It can be used for the night-time relief of non-productive coughs and congestion, such as those associated with colds. It is available as a sugar-free oral solution and is not normally given to children, except on medical advice.
✚▲ Side-effects/warnings: See DEXTROMETHORPHAN HYDROBROMIDE; DIPHENHYDRAMINE HYDROCHLORIDE.

Cozaar

(MSD) is a proprietary, prescription-only preparation of the ANGIOTENSIN-RECEPTOR BLOCKER losartan potassium. It can be used as an ANTIHYPERTENSIVE treatment, and is available as tablets.
✚▲ Side-effects/warnings: See LOSARTAN POTASSIUM.

Cozaar-Comp

(MSD) is a proprietary, prescription-only preparation of the ANGIOTENSIN-RECEPTOR BLOCKER losartan potassium, and the (THIAZIDE) DIURETIC hydrochlorothiazide. It can be used as an ANTIHYPERTENSIVE treatment, and is available as tablets.
✚▲ Side-effects/warnings: See HYDROCHLOROTHIAZIDE; LOSARTAN POTASSIUM.

co-zidocapt

is the name given to a compound preparation of the ACE INHIBITOR captopril and the DIURETIC hydrochlorothiazide (in the proportion 12.5/25). It can be used as an ANTIHYPERTENSIVE, taken orally.

C

+▲ Side-effects/warnings: See CAPTOPRIL; HYDROCHLOROTHIAZIDE.

Crampex Tablets

(SSL) is a proprietary, non-prescription preparation of the VASODILATOR niacin (nicotinic acid) with the VITAMIN colecalciferol (vitamin D_3) and the MINERAL SUPPLEMENT calcium gluconate. It can be taken for night muscle cramps, and is available as tablets. It is not given to children, except on medical advice.
+▲ Side-effects/warnings: See COLECALCIFEROL; NICOTINIC ACID.

Creon

(Solvay) is a proprietary, non-prescription preparation of the digestive enzyme pancreatin. It can be used to compensate for deficiencies of digestive juices that are normally supplied by the pancreas, and is available as enteric-coated granules.
+▲ Side-effects/warnings: See PANCREATIN.

Creon 10 000

(Solvay) is a proprietary, non-prescription preparation of the digestive enzyme pancreatin. It can be used to compensate for deficiencies of digestive juices that are normally supplied by the pancreas, and is available as capsules (in a higher strength than *Creon*).
+▲ Side-effects/warnings: See PANCREATIN.

Creon 25 000

(Solvay) is a proprietary, prescription-only preparation of the digestive enzyme pancreatin. It can be used to compensate for deficiencies of digestive juices that are normally supplied by the pancreas, and is available as capsules containing enteric-coated granules (in a higher strength than *Creon*).
+▲ Side-effects/warnings: See PANCREATIN.

Crinone

(Serono) is a proprietary, prescription-only preparation of the PROGESTOGEN progesterone. It can be used to treat many hormonal deficiency disorders in women associated with progesterone deficiency, for menopausal symptoms and for treating infertility, including *in vitro* fertilization. It is available in a form of vaginal gel in various strengths.
+▲ Side-effects/warnings: See PROGESTERONE.

cristantaspase

is an enzyme called asparaginase which is used as a ANTICANCER treatment almost exclusively for acute lymphoblastic leukaemia. Administration is by injection.
+▲ Side-effects/warnings: See CYTOTOXIC. Also there may be nausea, vomiting, central nervous system depression and changes in liver function and blood lipids (requiring monitoring, including of the urine for glucose) and anaphylaxis.
✪ **Related entry: Erwinase.**

Crixivan

(MSD) is a proprietary, prescription-only preparation of the ANTIVIRAL indinavir. It can be used in the treatment of HIV infection, and is available as capsules.
+▲ Side-effects/warnings: See INDINAVIR.

Cromogen Easi-Breathe

(IVAX) is a proprietary, prescription-only preparation of sodium cromoglicate (sodium cromoglycate). It can be used in ANTI-ASTHMATIC treatment. It is available in forms for aerosol inhalation including a liquid (*Steri-Neb*).
+▲ Side-effects/warnings: See SODIUM CROMOGLICATE.

crotamiton

has antipruritic activity and so is used to relieve pruritus (itching) of the skin (though its efficacy has been questioned). It also has SCABICIDAL (acaricide) activity and is used sometimes to eliminate the scabies infestation (though there are more effective agents) and to treat the itching after elimination. Administration is topical.
+▲ Side-effects/warnings: There can be hypersensitivity reactions. It should not be used on broken skin, in acute exudative dermatoses, or near the eyes. Breast-feeding mothers should avoid using it around the nipple area. Some formulations not recommended for pregnant women.
✪ **Related entries: Eurax Cream; Eurax HC Cream; Eurax Lotion; Eurax-Hydrocortisone.**

crystal violet

(gentian violet; methyl violet; methylrosanilium chloride) is a dye with astringent and oxidizing properties which is used as an ANTISEPTIC. It is occasionally administered to treat certain bacterial and fungal skin infections or abrasions

and minor wounds. Administration is usually by topical application. As a non-proprietary, antiseptic paint preparation, it is used specifically to prepare skin for surgery.
✚ Side-effects: It may cause mucosal ulcerations.
▲ Warnings: It should not be applied to mucous membranes or broken skin. It stains clothes as well as skin.

Crystapen

(Britannia) is a proprietary, prescription-only preparation of the ANTIBACTERIAL and (PENICILLIN) ANTIBIOTIC benzylpenicillin (as sodium). It can be used to treat a wide range of infections. It is available in a form for injection or intravenous infusion.
✚▲ Side-effects/warnings: See BENZYLPENICILLIN.

Cuplex

(Smith & Nephew Healthcare) is a proprietary, non-prescription preparation of the KERATOLYTIC agent salicylic acid (together with lactic acid and copper acetate). It can be used to remove warts and corns and calluses, and is available as a gel.
✚▲ Side-effects/warnings: See SALICYLIC ACID.

Cuprofen Ibuprofen Tablets

(SSL) is a proprietary, non-prescription preparation of the (NSAID) NON-NARCOTIC ANALGESIC and ANTIRHEUMATIC ibuprofen. It can be used to relieve headache, period pain, muscular pain, dental pain, feverishness and cold and flu symptoms. It is available as tablets and is not normally given to children, except on medical advice.
✚▲ Side-effects/warnings: See IBUPROFEN.

Cuprofen Tablets Maximum Strength

(SSL) is a proprietary, non-prescription preparation of the (NSAID) NON-NARCOTIC ANALGESIC and ANTIRHEUMATIC drug ibuprofen. It can be used to relieve headache, period pain, muscular pain, dental pain, feverishness and cold and flu symptoms. It is available as tablets and is not normally given to children.
✚▲ Side-effects/warnings: See IBUPROFEN.

Curatoderm

(Crookes) is a proprietary, prescription-only preparation of derivative tacalcitol, a VITAMIN D analogue which can be used as a skin treatment for plaque psoriasis. It is available as an ointment.
✚▲ Side-effects/warnings: See TACALCITOL.

Cutivate

(GlaxoWellcome; GSK) is a proprietary, prescription-only preparation of the CORTICOSTEROID fluticasone propionate. It can be used to treat skin disorders, including dermatitis and eczemas that are unresponsive to less potent corticosteroids, and is available as a cream and ointment.
✚▲ Side-effects/warnings: See FLUTICASONE PROPIONATE.

Cuxson Gerrard Belladonna Plaster BP

(Cuxson Gerrard) is a proprietary, non-prescription preparation of the ANTICHOLINERGIC belladonna (see BELLADONNA ALKALOID) in the form of a self-adhesive skin plaster. It can be used to relieve aches and pains such as sciatica and rheumatism. It is not normally given to children under ten years, people with glaucoma, or in pregnancy or breast-feeding (or those allergic to plasters).
✚▲ Side-effects/warnings: See BELLADONNA ALKALOID.

CX Antiseptic Dusting Powder

(Adams) is a proprietary, non-prescription preparation of the ANTISEPTIC chlorhexidine (as acetate). It can be used as a dusting powder by topical application for disinfecting skin.
✚▲ Side-effects/warnings: See CHLORHEXIDINE.

cyanocobalamin

is a form of vitamin B_{12} which is readily found in most normal, well-balanced diets (for example, in fish, eggs, liver and red meat). Vegans, who eat no animal products at all, may eventually suffer from deficiency of this vitamin. A deficiency of vitamin B_{12} eventually causes megaloblastic anaemia where large deformed red blood-cells are produced, and this leads to degeneration of nerves in the central and peripheral nervous systems and abnormalities of epithelia (particularly the lining of the mouth and gut). Apart from poor diet, deficiency can also be caused by the lack of an *intrinsic factor* necessary for absorption in the stomach (pernicious anaemia) and by various malabsorption syndromes in the gut (sometimes due to drugs). Deficiencies are normally rectified by giving the HYDROXOCOBALAMIN form of vitamin B_{12}), since it has a longer duration of action in the body so necessitating less frequent administration (important when given by injection). Cyanocobalamin itself is rarely given by injection, but is still available as a single vitamin to be taken orally. There is no real beneficial effect for inclusion of vitamin B_{12} (as cyanocobalamin) in the many proprietary multivitamin 'tonic' preparations.

✚▲ Side-effects/warnings: There may be skin itching in overdose; also fever, chills, hot flushes, dizziness, allergic reactions.

✪ **Related entries: Cytacon; Cytamen.**

Cyclimorph

(GlaxoWellcome; GSK) is a proprietary, prescription-only preparation of the (OPIOID) NARCOTIC ANALGESIC morphine tartrate and the ANTI-EMETIC cyclizine tartrate. It can be used to treat moderate to severe pain. It is available, in two strengths (*Cyclimorph-10* and *Cyclimorph-15*) for injection and is on the Controlled Drugs list.

✚▲ Side-effects/warnings: See MORPHINE SULPHATE; CYCLIZINE.

cyclizine

is an ANTIHISTAMINE and ANTINAUSEANT which can be used to treat nausea, vomiting, vertigo, motion sickness and disorders of the balance function of the inner-ear (labyrinthine disorders). It can be combined with ANTIMIGRAINE treatments and analgesics to reduce nausea. Administration is either oral or by injection.

✚ Side-effects: See ANTIHISTAMINE; there may also be drowsiness, occasional dry mouth and blurred vision.

▲ Warnings: It is not used in severe heart failure. Drowsiness may impair the performance of skilled tasks, such as driving; avoid alcohol because its effects may be enhanced.

✪ **Related entries: Cyclimorph; Diconal; Migril; Valoid.**

Cyclodox

(Berk; APS) is a proprietary, prescription-only preparation of the ANTIBACTERIAL and (TETRACYCLINES) ANTIBIOTIC doxycycline. It can be used to treat a wide variety of infections, and is available as capsules.

✚▲ Side-effects/warnings: See DOXYCYCLINE.

Cyclogest

(Shire) is a proprietary, prescription-only preparation of the PROGESTOGEN progesterone. It can be used to treat many conditions of hormonal deficiency in women, including postnatal depression and premenstrual syndrome, and is available as (vaginal or anal) pessaries.

✚▲ Side-effects/warnings: See PROGESTERONE.

cyclopenthiazide

is a (THIAZIDE) DIURETIC which can be used as an ANTIHYPERTENSIVE (either alone or in conjunction with different types of diuretic or other drugs) and in the treatment of oedema, including as part of HEART FAILURE treatment. Administration is oral.

✚▲ Side-effects/warnings: See BENDROFLUMETHIAZIDE.

✪ **Related entries: Navidrex; Navispare; Trasidrex.**

cyclopentolate hydrochloride

is an ANTICHOLINERGIC (ANTIMUSCARINIC) drug which can be used to dilate the pupil and paralyse the focusing of the eye for ophthalmic examination. Administration is topical as eye-drops.

✚▲ Side-effects/warnings: See ATROPINE SULPHATE. When applied locally it has few side-effects, but it should not be used in patients with raised intraocular pressure (it may precipitate glaucoma).

✪ **Related entries: Minims Cyclopentolate; Mydrilate.**

cyclophosphamide

is an (*alkylating agent*) CYTOTOXIC drug which is used as an ANTICANCER treatment of chronic lymphocytic leukaemia, lymphomas and some solid tumours. It works by interfering with DNA and so preventing normal cell replication. It can also be used as an IMMUNOSUPPRESSANT in the treatment of complicated rheumatoid arthritis and other connective tissue diseases such as vasculitis. Administration is either oral or by injection.

✚▲ Side-effects/warnings: See CYTOTOXIC. Avoid its use in patients with porphyria; rarely, it may cause haemorrhagic cystitis.

✪ **Related entry: Endoxana.**

Cyclo-Progynova

(ASTA Medica) is a proprietary, prescription-only compound preparation estradiol (as valerate; an OESTROGEN) and norgestrel (a PROGESTOGEN). It can be used in HRT and osteoporosis prophylaxis, and is available as tablets in two strengths (*1-mg* and *2-mg*).
✚▲ Side-effects/warnings: See NORGESTREL; ESTRADIOL.

Cycloserine

(Lilly) is a proprietary, prescription-only preparation of the ANTIBACTERIAL cycloserine. It can be used as an ANTITUBERCULAR treatment for drug-resistant tuberculosis. It is available as capsules.
✚▲ Side-effects/warnings: See CYCLOSERINE.

cycloserine

is an ANTIBACTERIAL drug which is used specifically as an ANTITUBERCULAR treatment for tuberculosis that is resistant to the powerful drugs ordinarily used first, or in cases where those drugs are not tolerated. Administration is oral.
✚ Side-effects: There may be headache, dizziness and vertigo, drowsiness, depression, convulsions, tremor, allergic dermatitis and effects on blood components and the liver.
▲ Warnings: It should not be administered to patients with epilepsy, alcoholism, depressive illness, anxiety or psychosis, porphyria or severe kidney impairment; it should be administered with caution to those with impaired kidney function, or who are pregnant or breast-feeding. Blood, kidney and liver function should be monitored.
✪ Related entry: Cycloserine.

cyclosporin

see CICLOSPORIN.

Cyklokapron

(Pharmacia) is a proprietary, prescription-only preparation of the antifibrinolytic tranexamic acid. It can be used to stop bleeding in circumstances such as dental extraction in a haemophiliac patient or menorrhagia (excessive menstrual bleeding). It may also be used in treating hereditary angioedema and for thrombolytic (eg streptokinase) overdose. It is available as tablets in a form for injection.
✚▲ Side-effects/warnings: See TRANEXAMIC ACID.

Cymalon

(SSL) is a proprietary, non-prescription, preparation of sodium bicarbonate, sodium carbonate, sodium citrate and citric acid. It can be used to make the urine more alkaline in treating cystitis in adult women. It is available as an oral powder.
✚▲ Side-effects/warnings: See SODIUM BICARBONATE; SODIUM CARBONATE; SODIUM CITRATE.

Cymevene

(Roche) is a proprietary, prescription-only preparation of the ANTIVIRAL ganciclovir. It can be used to treat serious viral infections in immunocompromised patients. It is available as capsules and in a form for intravenous infusion.
✚▲ Side-effects/warnings: See GANCICLOVIR.

cyproheptadine hydrochloride

is an ANTIHISTAMINE which can be used for the symptomatic relief of allergic symptoms such as hay fever and urticaria. It differs from other antihistamines in having additional actions as an antagonist of SEROTONIN and as a CALCIUM-CHANNEL BLOCKER, and is useful in a wider range of conditions, including as an ANTIMIGRAINE agent for the prevention of attacks. Administration is oral.
✚▲ Side-effects/warnings: See ANTIHISTAMINE. It may cause weight gain. Because of its sedative side-effects, the performance of skilled tasks, such as driving, may be impaired. It should not be used by breast-feeding women, and should be used with care in pregnancy.
✪ Related entry: Periactin.

Cyprostat

(Schering Health) is a proprietary, prescription-only preparation of the ANTI-ANDROGEN cyproterone acetate, which is a sex HORMONE ANTAGONIST. It can be used as an adjunct in ANTICANCER treatment (eg prostate cancer). It is available as tablets.
✚▲ Side-effects/warnings: See CYPROTERONE ACETATE.

cyproterone acetate

is a sex HORMONE ANTAGONIST, an ANTI-ANDROGEN, which reduces the effects of male sex hormones (androgens) in the body. It is used as an ANTICANCER treatment for cancer of the

prostate gland. It can also be used for the treatment of hypersexuality or sexual deviation in men, in whom the drug causes a condition of reversible sterility through a reduction in the production of sperm. Additionally, it can be used (in a compound preparation also containing oestrogen) to treat acne and excess body hair (hirsutism) in women. Administration is oral.
✚ Side-effects: Concentration and speed of thought and movement may be affected; breathlessness; weight changes; fatigue and lethargy. Hormonal effects include changes in hair-growth patterns and enlargement of the breasts and inhibition of sperm production in men. There may be osteoporosis and liver problems (function will be monitored).
▲ Warnings: Depending on use, it should not be administered, or should be administered with care, to patients who have sickle-cell anaemia, severe diabetes, liver disease or severe depression; who have a history of thrombosis; who are pregnant; or who are adolescent boys (in whom bone growth and testicular development may be arrested). It should be administered with caution to those with diabetes or insufficient secretion of adrenal hormones, or who are breast-feeding. There will be careful assessment before treatment of patient suitability, and regular checks on liver function, adrenal gland function, blood counts and determination of glucose levels. Because it may cause tiredness and lethargy, the performance of skilled tasks such as driving may be impaired.
✪ Related entries: Androcur; Cyprostat; Dianette.

Cystagon
(Orphan Europe) is proprietary, prescription-only preparation of the amino acid mercapatamine which is used as a METABOLIC DISORDER TREATMENT for nephropathic cystinosis. It is available in capsules which can be opened and sprinkled on food.
✚▲ Side-effects/warnings: See MERCAPATAMINE.

cysteamine
see MERCAPATAMINE.

Cysticide
(Merck) is a proprietary, prescription-only preparation of the ANTHELMINTIC drug praziquantel, and can be used in treating schistosome and tapeworm infestation. Taken orally.
✚▲ Side-effects/warnings: See PRAZIQUANTEL.

Cystopurin
(Roche Consumer Health) is a proprietary, non-prescription, preparation of potassium citrate. It can be used to relieve the symptoms of cystitis. It is available as an oral powder. It is not normally given to children under six years, except on medical advice.
✚▲ Side-effects/warnings: See SODIUM BICARBONATE; SODIUM CARBONATE; SODIUM CITRATE.

Cystrin
(Sanofi-Synthelabo) is a proprietary, prescription-only preparation of the ANTICHOLINERGIC oxybutynin hydrochloride. It can be used as an ANTISPASMODIC in the treatment of urinary disorders such as incontinence. It is available as tablets.
✚▲ Side-effects/warnings: See OXYBUTYNIN HYDROCHLORIDE.

Cytacon
(Goldshield) is a proprietary, prescription-only preparation of the VITAMIN cyanocobalamin. It can be used to prevent or correct diagnosed clinical deficiency of vitamin B_{12} (eg in vegans), and is available in the form of tablets and an oral liquid.
✚▲ Side-effects/warnings: See CYANOCOBALAMIN.

Cytamen
(Celltech) is a proprietary, prescription-only preparation of cyanocobalamin, vitamin B_{12}, and is available in a form for injection.
✚▲ Side-effects/warnings: See CYANOCOBALAMIN.

cytarabine
is an (*antimetabolite*) CYTOTOXIC drug which is used as an ANTICANCER treatment primarily of acute myeloblastic leukaemia. It works by interfering with pyrimidine synthesis (a chemical needed for cell replication/DNA) and so prevents cell replication. Administration is by injection.
✚▲ Side-effects/warnings: See CYTOTOXIC.
✪ Related entry: Cytosar.

cytoprotectant
drugs have the capacity to protect the gastric

mucosa (the lining of the stomach) from the normal stomach contents of acid and enzymes, which can cause erosion and pain in peptic ulcers (gastric and duodenal ulcers). They may be used as long-term ulcer-healing drugs (see ULCER-HEALING DRUG), as well as affording short-term relief from discomfort and helping relieve stress-ulceration. They may also be used to treat oesophageal ulceration and inflammation. Examples of cytoprotectants include: CARBENOXOLONE SODIUM; *bismuth salts*; and TRIPOTASSIUM DICITRATOBISMUTHATE (bismuth chelate) and SUCRALFATE.

Cytosar

(Pharmacia) is a proprietary, prescription-only preparation of the ANTICANCER drug cytarabine. It can be used to treat leukaemia, and is available in a form for injection.
✚▲ Side-effects/warnings: See CYTARABINE.

Cytotec

(Pharmacia) is a proprietary, prescription-only preparation of the synthetic PROSTAGLANDIN analogue misoprostol. It can be used to treat gastric and duodenal ulcers, and is available as tablets.
✚▲ Side-effects/warnings: See MISOPROSTOL.

cytotoxic 🅴

agents are used mainly in the treatment of cancer and are the biggest group of ANTICANCER drugs. They have the essential property of preventing cell replication and so inhibiting the growth of cancerous tumours or of excess production of cells (eg blood cells) in body fluids. There are several mechanisms by which they do this, but in every case they inevitably also affect the growth of normal (non-cancerous) healthy cells and cause toxic side-effects.

The most-used cytotoxics are the *alkylating agents*, which work by interfering with the action of DNA in cell replication (eg BUSULFAN, CARMUSTINE, CHLORAMBUCIL, CYCLOPHOSPHAMIDE, ESTRAMUSTINE PHOSPHATE, IFOSFAMIDE, LOMUSTINE, MELPHALAN, CHLORMETHINE HYDROCHLORIDE, THIOTEPA, TREOSULFAN). The VINCA ALKALOIDS are also effective cytotoxic drugs and work by arresting division (metaphase of miosis) in new-forming cells (eg vinblastine sulphate, vincristine sulphate, vindesine sulphate, vinorelbine). However, they have severe side-effects (such as damage to peripheral nerves) which limits their use.

A number of cytotoxics are ANTIBIOTIC in origin, but ANTIMICROBIAL actions do not contribute an important part of their action, they work by a direct action on DNA (eg ACLARUBICIN, BLEOMYCIN, DACTINOMYCIN, DAUNORUBICIN, DOXORUBICIN HYDROCHLORIDE, EPIRUBICIN HYDROCHLORIDE, IDARUBICIN HYDROCHLORIDE, MITOMYCIN, MITOXANTRONE (mitozantrone), PENTOSTATIN).

A number of cytotoxics are referred to as *antimetabolites* because they combine with cellular components and interfere with the metabolic pathways involved in DNA synthesis and so preventing cellular division (CLADRIBINE, CYTARABINE, FLUDARABINE PHOSPHATE, FLUDARABINE PHOSPHATE, GEMCITABINE, MERCAPTOPURINE, METHOTREXATE, RALTITREXED, TIOGUANINE).

A new advance has been the development of the *taxane* drugs based on a chemical found in the yew tree, and these show promise in the treatment of ovarian and breast cancer (eg PACLITAXEL, DOCETAXEL).

A further new group is the *topoisomerase I inhibitors* which act on an enzyme involved in DNA replication, eg IRINOTECAN HYDROCHLORIDE and TOPOTECAN.

There are some cytotoxics that are not only administered in anticancer treatment, but also are used as IMMUNOSUPPRESSANT drugs to limit tissue rejection during and following transplant surgery and in the treatment of autoimmune diseases, such as rheumatoid arthritis and lupus erythematosus. Of these, some are, in practice, used for both purposes (eg chlorambucil, cyclophosphamide), and others for immunosuppression alone (eg AZATHIOPRINE, CICLOSPORIN, METHOTREXATE).

As mentioned, cytotoxic anticancer drugs cause profound changes in cellular metabolism in the body. They inevitably also affect the growth of normal healthy cells and cause many toxic side-effects. Normally, *myelosuppression* (a reduction in blood-cell production of the bone marrow, including leukocytes and hence decreased resistance to infection) is one of the most serious side-effects; but conversely, this is the very cytotoxic effect harnessed in cytotoxic drug treatment of leukaemias. Some of the serious discomfort experienced by individuals undergoing cancer treatment, for instance

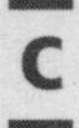

nausea, vomiting and hair loss, can be minimized by careful adjustment of chemotherapy and radiotherapy regimens. Also, side-effects in common include impaired wound healing, depression of growth in children, and damage to the lining (epithelium) of the gastrointestinal tract, sterility, kidney damage, and some may be carcinogenic themselves. Recently, there have been significant advances in drug adjunct therapy used to reduce side-effects. In particular, use of ANTI-EMETIC / ANTINAUSEANT drugs such as ONDANSETRON have revolutionized anticancer treatment with the platinum-containing group of drugs (CARBOPLATIN, CISPLATIN) which are particularly prone to cause nausea and vomiting.

✚▲ Side-effects/warnings: The treatment of cancer is very complex and is carried out by specialists (oncologists). A full assessment of patient suitability will be carried out, along with counselling and explanations of what side-effects are to be expected, and what to look out for.

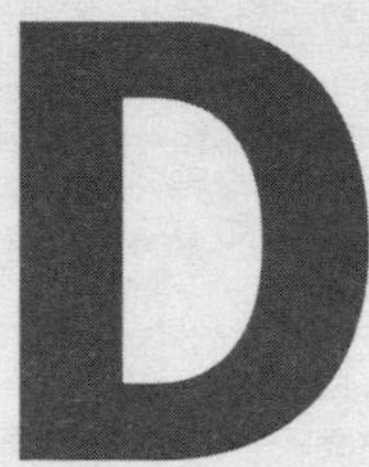

dacarbazine

is a CYTOTOXIC which is used comparatively rarely because of its high toxicity. It may be administered to treat the skin (mole) cancer melanoma and, in combination with other ANTICANCER drugs, in some soft-tissue sarcomas and the lymphatic cancer Hodgkin's disease. Administration is by injection.
✚▲ Side-effects/warnings: See CYTOTOXIC. There is intense nausea and vomiting; myelosuppression.
✪ **Related entry: DTIC-Dome.**

daclizumab

is an IMMUNOSUPPRESSANT drug, a monoclonal antibody (a form of pure antibody produced by a type of molecular engineering) which is a specific CYTOTOXIC that prevents proliferation of white blood cells, T-lymphocytes, which have an important role in immunity and cell rejection. It has recently been introduced for prophylaxis of rejection in kidney transplantation. It is administered together with CICLOSPORIN and CORTICOSTEROID drugs. Its use is confined to specialist centres. Administration is by intravenous infusion.
✚▲ Side-effects/warnings: This product is still under evaluation. Not used in pregnancy or breast-feeding.
✪ **Related entry: Zenapax.**

dactinomycin

(actinomycin D) is a CYTOTOXIC (an ANTIBIOTIC in origin) which is used as an ANTICANCER drug, particularly to treat cancer in children. Administration is by injection.
✚▲ Side-effects/warnings: See CYTOTOXIC; similar side-effects to DOXORUBICIN HYDROCHLORIDE, but with less heart toxicity.
✪ **Related entry: Cosmegen Lyovac.**

Daktacort

(Janssen-Cilag) is a proprietary, prescription-only compound preparation of the CORTICOSTEROID hydrocortisone and the (AZOLE) ANTIFUNGAL miconazole (as nitrate). It can be used to treat skin infections with inflammation, and is available as a cream and an ointment for topical application.
✚▲ Side-effects/warnings: See HYDROCORTISONE; MICONAZOLE.

Daktarin

(Janssen-Cilag) is a proprietary, prescription-only preparation of the (AZOLE) ANTIFUNGAL miconazole. It can be used to treat both systemic and skin-surface fungal infections, and is available in the form of a number of types of preparation including an oral gel. (There are other forms for topical application that are available without prescription.)
✚▲ Side-effects/warnings: See MICONAZOLE.

Daktarin Cream

(Janssen-Cilag) is a proprietary, non-prescription preparation of the (AZOLE) ANTIFUNGAL miconazole (as nitrate). It can be used for the prevention and treatment of fungal (and associated bacterial) infections of the skin, such as infected nappy rash. It is available as a cream for topical application.
✚▲ Side-effects/warnings: See MICONAZOLE.

Daktarin Dual Action Cream

(Janssen-Cilag) is a proprietary, non-prescription preparation of the (AZOLE) ANTIFUNGAL miconazole (as nitrate). It can be used for the prevention and treatment of athlete's foot, and is available as a cream.
✚▲ Side-effects/warnings: See MICONAZOLE.

Daktarin Dual Action Powder

(Janssen-Cilag) is a proprietary, non-prescription preparation of the (AZOLE) ANTIFUNGAL miconazole (as nitrate). It can be used for the prevention and treatment of the fungal infection athlete's foot. It is available as a powder for application to articles in contact with the affected region.
✚▲ Side-effects/warnings: See MICONAZOLE.

Daktarin Dual Action Spray Powder

(Janssen-Cilag) is a proprietary, non-prescription preparation of the (AZOLE) ANTIFUNGAL miconazole (as nitrate). It can be used for the prevention and treatment of the fungal infection

D

athlete's foot, and is available as a powder spray for application to the skin, clothes and shoes. It is not used for children, except on medical advice.
✚▲ Side-effects/warnings: See MICONAZOLE.

Daktarin Gold Cream

(Janssen-Cilag) is a proprietary, non-prescription preparation of the (AZOLE) ANTIFUNGAL ketoconazole. It can be used for the prevention and treatment of fungal infections of the skin, such as athlete's foot, jock itch and intertrigo. It is available as a cream for topical application.
✚▲ Side-effects/warnings: See KETOCONAZOLE.

Daktarin Oral Gel

(Janssen-Cilag) is a proprietary, non-prescription preparation of the (AZOLE) ANTIFUNGAL miconazole (as base). It can be used for the prevention and treatment of fungal infections of the oropharynx (mouth and throat), and is available as an oral gel for use by adults and children.
✚▲ Side-effects/warnings: See MICONAZOLE.

Daktarin Powder

(Janssen-Cilag) is a proprietary, non-prescription preparation of the (AZOLE) ANTIFUNGAL miconazole (as nitrate). It can be used for the prevention and treatment of fungal (and associated bacterial) infections of the skin, including nappy rash. It is available as a powder for application to the skin and clothes.
✚▲ Side-effects/warnings: See MICONAZOLE.

Dalacin

(Pharmacia) is a proprietary, prescription-only preparation of the ANTIBACTERIAL and ANTIBIOTIC clindamycin. It can be used to treat vaginal infections, and is available as a cream.
✚▲ Side-effects/warnings: See CLINDAMYCIN; the vaginal cream may damage latex condoms and diaphragms.

Dalacin C

(Pharmacia) is a proprietary, prescription-only, preparation of the ANTIBACTERIAL and ANTIBIOTIC clindamycin. It can be used to treat systemic infections. It is available as capsules and in a form for injection.
✚▲ Side-effects/warnings: See CLINDAMYCIN.

Dalacin T

(Pharmacia) is a proprietary, prescription-only preparation of the ANTIBACTERIAL and ANTIBIOTIC clindamycin. It can be used to treat acne, and is available as a lotion and a solution for topical application.
✚▲ Side-effects/warnings: See CLINDAMYCIN.

Dalmane

(ICN) is a proprietary, prescription-only preparation of the (BENZODIAZEPINE) HYPNOTIC flurazepam, which can be used to treat insomnia in cases where some degree of sedation during the daytime is acceptable. Administration is oral.
✚▲ Side-effects/warnings: See FLURAZEPAM.

dalteparin sodium

is a *low molecular weight* heparin which is used as an ANTICOAGULANT. It has some advantages over heparin when used in the long-term prevention of venous thrombo-embolism, particularly in orthopaedic use. Administration is by injection.
✚▲ Side-effects/warnings: See HEPARIN.
✪ **Related entry: Fragmin.**

danaparoid sodium

is a version of heparin, called a heparinoid (see HEPARINOIDS), that is used as an ANTICOAGULANT. It has some advantages over heparin when used for prevention of deep-vein thrombosis, particularly in orthopaedic surgery. It may be used in some patients who are hypersensitive to heparin itself. Administration is by injection.
✚▲ Side-effects/warnings: See HEPARIN. There may also be thrombocytopenia, liver changes, hypersensitivity, osteoporosis and pain or tissue damage at injection site. Administer with care to patients who are pregnant, breast-feeding, or have certain liver or kidney disorders and asthma. (Sulphite in ampoules may lead to hypersensitivity reactions, eg bronchospasm.)
✪ **Related entry: Orgaran.**

danazol

is a drug that inhibits output of GONADOTROPHIN homones. It has weak androgen activity, plus HORMONE ANTAGONIST actions as an ANTI-OESTROGEN and antiprogestogen. It can be used to treat endometriosis (the presence of areas of uterus-lining, endometrium, outside the uterus); gynaecomastia (the development of breasts on a male); menorrhagia (excessive menstrual flow) and other menstrual disorders; benign breast cysts and breast pain, and other conditions where reduction in sex hormone production would be beneficial. Administration is oral.

✚ Side-effects: These are many and include, backache, dizziness, flushing, weight gain, gastrointestinal disturbances, headache, menstrual disorders, nervousness, rash, flushing, reduction in breast size, muscle spasm, hair loss, masculinization in women (oily skin, acne, hair growth, voice changes, enlarged clitoris), blood disorders, visual disturbances, jaundice and insulin resistance, fluid retention and others.

▲ Warnings: It is not be administered to those who are pregnant or breast-feeding; have severe kidney, heart or liver impairment, thromboembolytic disease or porphyria. It is used with caution in patients with certain heart, liver or kidney disorders, diabetes, epilepsy, migraine, hypertension, thrombosis, blood disorders and others.

✪ Related entry: Danol.

Danlax

(Sovereign) is a proprietary, prescription-only preparation of CO-DANTHRAMER 25/200, which is a (*stimulant*) LAXATIVE based on dantron and poloxamer '188'. It can be used to treat constipation and to prepare patients for abdominal procedures, and is available as an oral suspension.

✚▲ Side-effects/warnings: See DANTRON; POLOXAMER '188'.

Danol

(Sanofi-Synthelabo) is a proprietary, prescription-only preparation of danazol, which is used to treat conditions such as inflammation of the endometrial lining of the uterus, gynaecomastia and menstrual disorders. It is available as capsules.

✚▲ Side-effects/warnings: See DANAZOL.

danthron

see DANTRON.

Dantrium

(Procter & Gamble Pharm.) is a proprietary, prescription-only preparation of the SKELETAL MUSCLE RELAXANT dantrolene sodium. It can be used for relieving severe spasticity of muscles in spasm, and is available as capsules and in a form for injection (*Dantrium Intravenous*).

✚▲ Side-effects/warnings: See DANTROLENE SODIUM.

dantrolene sodium

is a SKELETAL MUSCLE RELAXANT which acts directly on skeletal muscle and can be used for relieving severe spasticity of muscles in spasm and is also used in the treatment of malignant hyperthermia (a rare, but serious, complication of anaesthesia). Administration is either oral or by injection.

✚▲ Side-effects/warnings: It is a specialist drug normally used in hospital.

✪ Related entry: Dantrium.

dantron

(danthron) is a (*stimulant*) LAXATIVE. It is used to promote defecation and so relieve constipation, and seems to work by stimulating motility in the intestine. Therapeutically, it is used for constipation in geriatric practice (particularly analgesic-induced constipation in the terminally ill) and in cardiac failure and coronary thrombosis (to avoid the patients having to strain). It is also available in compound preparations with DOCUSATE SODIUM (CO-DANTHRUSATE 50/60) or poloxamer '188'. Administration is oral.

✚ Side-effects: There may be abdominal pain, griping, nausea or vomiting. The urine may be coloured red. Prolonged contact with the skin may cause irritation (eg in incontinent patients).

▲ Warnings: It should not be taken when pregnant or breast-feeding. It is mainly restricted to use in the elderly and in terminally ill patients.

✪ Related entries: Ailax; Codalax; co-danthramer 25/200; co-danthramer 75/1000; Codalax; Codalax Forte; Danlax; Normax.

Daonil

(Hoechst Marion Roussel; Aventis Pharma) is a proprietary, prescription-only preparation of the SULPHONYLUREA glibenclamide. It can be used in DIABETIC TREATMENT of Type II diabetes (non-insulin-dependent diabetes mellitus; NIDDM; maturity-onset diabetes), and is available as tablets (at twice the strength of SEMI-DAONIL tablets).

✚▲ Side-effects/warnings: See GLIBENCLAMIDE.

dapsone

is a (SULPHONE) ANTIBACTERIAL drug which is

D

used in leprosy treatment, also sometimes used to treat dermatitis herpetiformis or, in combination with the ENZYME INHIBITOR pyrimethamine (under the name *Maloprim*), to prevent travellers in tropical regions from contracting malaria. Administration is either oral or by injection.
✚ Side-effects: These are rare at low doses (when used for leprosy), but with higher dosage there may be nausea, vomiting and headache, insomnia, anorexia, hepatitis, nerve disorders and blood changes.
▲ Warnings: It should be administered with caution to patients with anaemia, porphyria, G6PH deficiency, certain heart or lung diseases; or who are pregnant or breast-feeding. Patients should be aware of the signs of blood disorders and report to their doctor if they have symptoms such as rash, mouth ulcers, sore throat, bruising or bleeding.
✪ Related entry: Maloprim.

Daraprim

(GlaxoWellcome; GSK) is a proprietary, prescription-only preparation of the ANTIMALARIAL drug pyrimethamine. It can be used to prevent or treat malaria in combination with other drugs, but is not administered as the sole agent of prevention. It is taken as tablets.
✚▲ Side-effects/warnings: See PYRIMETHAMINE.

darbepoetin alfa

is a recently introduced derivative of epoetin, synthesized by recombinant techniques, which lasts longer and may be administered less frequently than epoetin, but has similar actions. It is used in ANAEMIA TREATMENT for types of anaemia such as those known to be associated with erythropoietin deficiency in chronic renal failure. It is administered by intravenous or subcutaneous injection.
✚▲ Side-effects/warnings: See EPOETIN.
✪ Related entry: Aranesp.

daunorubicin

is a CYTOTOXIC drug (of ANTIBIOTIC origin) with properties similar to doxorubicin. It is used as an ANTICANCER treatment particularly for advanced HIV-related Kaposi's sarcoma and for acute leukaemias. Administration is by injection or as a liposomal formulation for intravenous infusion (for Kaposi's sarcoma).
✚▲ Side-effects/warnings: See CYTOTOXIC.
✪ Related entry: DaunoXome.

DaunoXome

(Gilead) is a proprietary, prescription-only preparation of the ANTICANCER drug daunorubicin. It can be used to treat Kaposi's sarcoma, and is available in a liposomal form for intravenous infusion.
✚▲ Side-effects/warnings: See DAUNORUBICIN.

Day Nurse Capsules

(GSK Consumer Healthcare) is a proprietary, non-prescription compound preparation of the NON-NARCOTIC ANALGESIC and ANTIPYRETIC paracetamol, the SYMPATHOMIMETIC and DECONGESTANT phenylpropanolamine hydrochloride and the ANTITUSSIVE dextromethorphan hydrobromide. It can be used to relieve cold and flu symptoms, and is available as capsules. It is not normally given to children, except on medical advice.
✚▲ Side-effects/warnings: See DEXTROMETHORPHAN HYDROBROMIDE; PARACETAMOL; PHENYLPROPANOLAMINE HYDROCHLORIDE.

Day Nurse Liquid

(GSK Consumer Healthcare) is a proprietary, non-prescription compound preparation of the NON-NARCOTIC ANALGESIC and ANTIPYRETIC paracetamol, the SYMPATHOMIMETIC and DECONGESTANT phenylpropanolamine hydrochloride and the ANTITUSSIVE dextromethorphan hydrobromide. It can be used to relieve cold and flu symptoms, and is available as a liquid. It is not normally given to children under six years, except on medical advice.
✚▲ Side-effects/warnings: See DEXTROMETHORPHAN HYDROBROMIDE; PARACETAMOL; PHENYLPROPANOLAMINE HYDROCHLORIDE.

DDAVP

(Ferring) is a proprietary, prescription-only preparation of desmopressin, which is an analogue of the pituitary HORMONE vasopressin (ADH). It is administered primarily to diagnose or to treat pituitary-originated diabetes insipidus. It can be used for some other diagnostic tests, to boost the blood concentration of blood-clotting factors in haemophiliac patients and to treat bed-wetting. It is available (as the acetate) in the form

of tablets, as nose-drops (it is absorbed into the systemic circulation from the nasal mucosa) and in a form for injection.
✚▲ Side-effects/warnings: See DESMOPRESSIN.

DDC
see ZALCITABINE.

DDI
see DIDANOSINE.

Debrisoquine
(Cambridge) is a proprietary, prescription-only preparation of the ADRENERGIC-NEURONE BLOCKER debrisoquine. It can be used as an ANTIHYPERTENSIVE for moderate to severe high blood pressure, and is available as tablets.
✚▲ Side-effects/warnings: See DEBRISOQUINE.

debrisoquine
is an ADRENERGIC-NEURONE BLOCKER, which is an ANTISYMPATHETIC class of drug that prevents the release of noradrenaline (norepinephrine) from sympathetic nerves. It can be used, sometimes in combination with other antihypertensive drugs, as an ANTIHYPERTENSIVE for moderate to severe high blood pressure, especially when other forms of treatment have failed. Administration is oral.
✚▲ Side-effects/warnings: See GUANETHIDINE MONOSULPHATE; except it does not cause diarrhoea.
✪ Related entry: Debrisoquine.

Decadron
(MSD) is a proprietary, prescription-only preparation of the CORTICOSTEROID and ANTI-INFLAMMATORY dexamethasone. It can be used in the suppression of allergic and inflammatory conditions in shock, diagnosis of Cushing's disease, congenital adrenal hyperplasia and cerebral oedema. It is available as tablets.
✚▲ Side-effects/warnings: See DEXAMETHASONE.

Deca-Durabolin
(Organon) is a proprietary, prescription-only preparation of the ANABOLIC STEROID nandrolone (as decanoate). It can be used to treat aplastic anaemia and sometimes osteoporosis in postmenopausal women. It is available in a form for injection.
✚▲ Side-effects/warnings: See NANDROLONE.

De-capeptyl sr
(Ipsen) is a proprietary, prescription-only preparation of the HORMONE triptorelin and can be used as an ANTICANCER treatment for cancer of the prostate gland and for endometriosis, and is available in a form for injection.
✚▲ Side-effects/warnings: See TRIPTORELIN.

decongestant ⊟
drugs are administered to relieve or reduce the symptoms of congestion of the airways and/or nose. NASAL DECONGESTANT drugs are generally applied in the form of nose-drops or as a nasal spray. This method of administration avoids the tendency of such drugs to have side-effects, such as raising the blood pressure, though some are administered orally.

Most decongestants are (ALPHA-ADRENOCEPTOR STIMULANT) SYMPATHOMIMETIC drugs which work by constricting blood vessels in the mucous membranes of the airways and nasal cavity, so reducing the thickness of this nasal lining, improving drainage and possibly decreasing mucus and fluid secretions. However, rhinitis, especially when caused by an allergy (eg hay fever), is usually dealt with by using ANTIHISTAMINE drugs, which inhibit the detrimental and congestive effects of histamine released by an allergic response, or by drugs, and so inhibit the allergic response itself and therefore effectively reduce inflammation (eg a CORTICOSTEROID or SODIUM CROMOGLICATE).

Decongestants are often included in compound preparations that are used to treat colds and which may contain a number of other constituents. However, most people are unaware of this, but it is important to realize that the vasoconstriction, speeding of the heart and hypertension often caused by sympathomimetic drugs are detrimental and potentially dangerous in a number of cardiovascular disorders. Further, sympathomimetics can have serious interactions with a number of other drug classes, especially MAOI antidepressant drugs. Decongestants can be inhaled to minimize systemic side-effects (important for those with cardiovascular problems), but it is believed that is 'rebound' congestion phase follows the beneficial decongestant phase.

Decubal Clinic
(Alpharma) is a proprietary, non-prescription

D

EMOLLIENT compound preparation of glycerol, wool fat, the water-repellent silicone dimeticone and isopropyl myristate. It can be used for dry skin conditions, including ichthyosis, psoriasis, dermatitis and hyperkeratosis, and is available as a cream.
✚▲ Side-effects/warnings: See DIMETICONE; GLYCEROL; WOOL FAT.

Deep Freeze Cold Gel

(Mentholatum) is a proprietary, non-prescription preparation of menthol which has COUNTER-IRRITANT, or RUBEFACIENT, actions. It can be applied to the skin for symptomatic relief of underlying muscle or joint pain and stiffness. It is available as a gel for topical application and is not normally used for children under five years, except on medical advice.
✚▲ Side-effects/warnings: See MENTHOL.

Deep Freeze Spray

(Mentholatum) is a proprietary, non-prescription preparation of menthol which has COUNTER-IRRITANT, or RUBEFACIENT, actions. It can be applied to the skin for symptomatic relief of underlying muscle or joint pain, stiffness, bruises and sprains. It is available as an aerosol spray for topical application and is not normally used for children under six years, except on medical advice.
✚▲ Side-effects/warnings: See MENTHOL.

Deep Heat Massage Liniment

(Mentholatum) is a proprietary, non-prescription compound preparation of menthol and methyl salicylate, which both have COUNTER-IRRITANT, or RUBEFACIENT, actions. It can be applied to the skin for symptomatic relief of underlying muscle or joint pain and stiffness. It is available as a liquid emulsion for topical application and is not normally used for children under five years, except on medical advice.
✚▲ Side-effects/warnings: See MENTHOL; METHYL SALICYLATE.

Deep Heat Maximum Strength

(Mentholatum) is a proprietary, non-prescription compound preparation of menthol and methyl salicylate, which both have COUNTER-IRRITANT, or RUBEFACIENT, actions. It can be applied to the skin for symptomatic relief of underlying muscle or joint pain and stiffness. It is available as an emulsion cream for topical application and is not normally used for children under five years.
✚▲ Side-effects/warnings: See MENTHOL; METHYL SALICYLATE.

Deep Heat Rub

(Mentholatum) is a proprietary, non-prescription compound preparation of menthol, methyl salicylate, eucalyptus oil and turpentine oil, which have COUNTER-IRRITANT, or RUBEFACIENT, actions. It can be applied to the skin for symptomatic relief of underlying muscle or joint pain and stiffness. It is available as a liquid emulsion for topical application and is not normally used for children under five years, except on medical advice.
✚▲ Side-effects/warnings: See MENTHOL; METHYL SALICYLATE; TURPENTINE OIL.

Deep Heat Spray

(Mentholatum) is a proprietary, non-prescription compound preparation of methyl salicylate, ethyl salicylate and 2-hydroxyethyl salicylate, which have COUNTER-IRRITANT, or RUBEFACIENT, actions, and the VASODILATOR methyl nicotinate. It can be applied to the skin for symptomatic relief of underlying muscle pain, bursitis and tendonitis. It is available as a spray for topical application and is not normally used for children under five years.
✚▲ Side-effects/warnings: See ETHYL SALICYLATE; METHYL SALICYLATE; METHYL NICOTINATE.

Deep Relief

(Mentholatum) is a proprietary, non-prescription compound preparation of the NSAID ibuprofen and menthol (as levomenthol) which has COUNTER-IRRITANT, or RUBEFACIENT, actions. It can be applied to the skin for symptomatic relief of underlying muscle or joint pain, such as rheumatic pain, strains and sprains. It is available as a gel for topical application and is not normally used for children, except on medical advice.
✚▲ Side-effects/warnings: See MENTHOL; IBUPROFEN.

deferiprone

is a CHELATING AGENT which is used as an ANTIDOTE for the treatment of iron overload in patients with thalassaemia major, in whom

DESFERRIOXAMINE MESILATE is contraindicated or is not tolerated. Administration is oral.

✚ Side-effects: Gastrointestinal disturbances; red-brown urine discoloration; joint conditions; also blood dyscrasias (particularly agranulocytosis) have been reported.

▲ Warnings: Deferiprone is not to be used during pregnancy or if breast-feeding. It is used with caution in those with kidney and liver impairment; and in neutropenia (with monitoring of neutrophil count; treatment is discontinued if neutropenia develops). Patients and their carers should be told how to recognize signs of neutropenia. Immediate medical attention should be sought if symptoms such as fever or sore throat develop.

✪ Related entry: Ferriprox.

deferoxamine mesylate

see DESFERRIOXAMINE MESILATE.

deflazacort

is a CORTICOSTEROID which has predominantly *glucocorticoid* activity. It can be used as an ANTI-INFLAMMATORY for a variety of inflammatory and allergic disorders. Administration is oral.

✚▲ Side-effects/warnings: See CORTICOSTEROID.

✪ Related entry: Calcort.

Delfen

(Janssen-Cilag) is a proprietary, non-prescription SPERMICIDAL CONTRACEPTIVE for use in combination with barrier methods of contraception (such as a condom). It is available as a foam containing nonoxinol.

✚▲ Side-effects/warnings: See NONOXINOL.

Delph

(Fenton) is the name of a range of proprietary, non-prescription SUNSCREEN preparations with (UVA and UVB protection; UVB-SPF 15–30) containing titanium dioxide, also hydroxybenzoates (parabens), ethylhexyl p-methoxycinnamate, oxybenzone, avobenzone and imidurea. The preparations are available as lotions. A patient whose skin condition requires this sort of preparation may be prescribed it at the discretion of his or her doctor.

✚▲ Side-effects/warnings: See TITANIUM DIOXIDE.

Deltacortril Enteric

(Pfizer) is a proprietary, prescription-only preparation of the CORTICOSTEROID and ANTI-INFLAMMATORY prednisolone. It can be used to treat inflammatory conditions, particularly those affecting the joints and soft tissues. It is available as tablets.

✚▲ Side-effects/warnings: See PREDNISOLONE.

Deltastab

(Sovereign) is a proprietary, prescription-only preparation of the CORTICOSTEROID and ANTI-INFLAMMATORY prednisolone. It can be used to treat inflammatory conditions, particularly those affecting the joints and soft tissues. It is available in a form for injection.

✚▲ Side-effects/warnings: See PREDNISOLONE.

demeclocycline hydrochloride

is a broad-spectrum ANTIBACTERIAL and ANTIBIOTIC drug, which is one of the TETRACYCLINES. It can be used to treat many kinds of infection, but particularly those of the respiratory tract, the gastrointestinal and genitourinary tracts, acne, syphilis, urethritis, chronic bronchitis, and a wide variety of soft-tissue infections. Administration is oral. It is also used, quite separately to its use as an antibiotic, as a HORMONE ANTAGONIST to treat over-secretion of antidiuretic hormone (ADH) through an action on the kidney.

✚▲ Side-effects/warnings: See TETRACYCLINE; but the incidence of photosensitivity is greater.

✪ Related entries: Deteclo; Ledermycin.

dementia treatment 🅱

seeks to restore some of the cognitive brain function agents lost in the group of neurological diseases referred to as *dementia*, characterized by a general decline in all areas of mental ability. Causes include brain tumours, stroke, syphilis, head injury, pernicious anaemia and alcoholism. Some dementias are due to *cerebrovascular disease* where the blood supply to the brain is impaired. For this reason claimed nootropic agents (cognition enhancers, memory enhancers or 'smart drugs': see NOOTROPIC AGENT) include cerebral vasodilators such as PAPAVERINE, BETA-ADRENOCEPTOR STIMULANT drugs (eg isoxsuprine), CALCIUM-CHANNEL BLOCKER drugs (eg NIMODIPINE) and certain ERGOT ALKALOID drugs with alpha-adrenoceptor blocking actions (eg CO-DERGOCRINE MESILATE). Another class of drugs claimed to have nootropic actions include agents

D

chemically resembling PIRACETAM (Nootropil), which were reported to improve mental function in tests, possibly by potentiating the effects of the neurotransmitter glutamate.

Alzheimer's disease and similar neurodegenerative diseases have long been proposed to involve defective function of neurones (cholinergic neurones) in the central nervous system (with impaired release or action of the neurotransmitter, ACETYLCHOLINE). For this reason ANTICHOLINESTERASE drugs (eg the 'atypical' agent tacrine) have been used in trials aimed at enhancing cholinergic nerve function (though at the price of extensive side-effects). The drugs DONEPEZIL and RIVASTIGMINE are anticholinesterases intended for the symptomatic treatment of mild to moderate dementia of Alzheimer's disease only, where they may slow the rate of cognitive and non-cognitive deterioration in about half of patients treated (though it has no effect in patients with other causes of confusion or dementia).

Demix

(Ashbourne) is a proprietary, prescription-only preparation of the ANTIBACTERIAL and (TETRACYCLINES) ANTIBIOTIC doxycycline. It can be used to treat infections of many kinds, and is available as capsules.

✚▲ Side-effects/warnings: See DOXYCYCLINE.

Demser

(MSD) is a proprietary, prescription-only preparation of the ANTISYMPATHETIC metirosine. It can be used in the preoperative treatment of phaeochromocytoma, and is available (on a named-patient basis only) as capsules.

✚▲ Side-effects/warnings: See METIROSINE.

demulcent

are agents or preparations that soothe or protect mucous membranes and help relieve pain and irritation. They work by forming a protective film and are incorporated into ANTACID preparations for protecting the gastric mucosa (stomach lining) and into mouthwashes, gargles etc., to soothe the membranes of the mouth. The most commonly used demulcent agent is ALGINIC ACID or one of its alginate salts. Syrup, honey and GLYCEROL also soothe mucous membranes.

De-Noltab

(Yamanouchi) is a proprietary, non-prescription preparation of the CYTOPROTECTANT tripotassium dicitratobismuthate. It can be used as an ULCER-HEALING DRUG for benign peptic ulcers in the stomach and duodenum, and is available as tablets.

✚▲ Side-effects/warnings: See TRIPOTASSIUM DICITRATOBISMUTHATE.

Dentinox Cradle Cap Treatment Shampoo

(DDD) is a proprietary, non-prescription compound preparation containing the SURFACTANT or detergent agents sodium lauryl ether sulphate and sodium lauryl ether sulphosuccinate. It can be used for treating cradle cap in infants, and is available as a shampoo.

✚▲ Side-effects/warnings: See SODIUM LAURYL SULPHATE.

Dentinox Infant Colic Drops

(DDD) is a proprietary, non-prescription preparation of the ANTIFOAMING AGENT dimeticone (as simeticone). It can be used to relieve wind and griping pain in infants (from birth onwards), and is available as an oral suspension.

✚▲ Side-effects/warnings: See DIMETICONE.

Dentinox Teething Gel

(DDD) is a proprietary, non-prescription compound preparation of the LOCAL ANAESTHETIC lidocaine hydrochloride and the ANTISEPTIC cetylpyridinium chloride. It can be used for the temporary relief of pain caused by teething in babies, and is available as a gel for topical application.

✚▲ Side-effects/warnings: See CETYLPYRIDINIUM CHLORIDE; LIDOCAINE HYDROCHLORIDE.

Dentomycin

(Blackwell) is a proprietary, prescription-only preparation of the ANTIMICROBIAL minocycline, which has ANTIBACTERIAL actions. It can be used for the treatment of local infections in dental surgery, and is available as a gel.

✚▲ Side-effects/warnings: See MINOCYCLINE.

Depakote

(Sanofi-Synthelabo) is a recently introduced proprietary, prescription-only preparation of valproic acid (in the form of semisodium

valproate). It is used in this form for the treatment of mania associated with manic-depressive illness (bipolar disorder), and is available as tablets.
✚▲ Side-effects/warnings: See SODIUM VALPROATE.

Depixol

(Lundbeck) is a proprietary, prescription-only preparation of the ANTIPSYCHOTIC flupentixol. It can be used to treat patients suffering from psychotic disorders (including schizophrenia), especially those with a type of psychosis that renders them apathetic and withdrawn. It can also be used for short-term treatment of depressive illness. It is available as tablets (as dihydrochloride) and in forms for depot deep intramuscular injection (as decanoate).
✚▲ Side-effects/warnings: See FLUPENTIXOL.

Depixol Conc.

(Lundbeck) is a proprietary, prescription-only preparation of the ANTIPSYCHOTIC flupentixol (as decanoate). It can be used in the maintenance of patients suffering from schizophrenia and other psychotic disorders. It is available in a form for depot deep intramuscular injection.
✚▲ Side-effects/warnings: See FLUPENTIXOL.

Depixol Low Volume

(Lundbeck) is a proprietary, prescription-only preparation of the ANTIPSYCHOTIC flupentixol (as decanoate). It can be used in the maintenance of patients suffering from schizophrenia and other psychotic disorders. It is available in a form for depot deep intramuscular injection.
✚▲ Side-effects/warnings: See FLUPENTIXOL.

Depo-Medrone

(Pharmacia) is a proprietary, prescription-only preparation of the CORTICOSTEROID and ANTI-INFLAMMATORY methylprednisolone (as acetate). It can be used to relieve allergic and inflammatory disorders, particularly of the joints and soft tissues, and also to treat cerebral oedema. It is available in a form for injection.
✚▲ Side-effects/warnings: See METHYLPREDNISOLONE.

Depo-Medrone with Lidocaine

(Pharmacia) is a proprietary, prescription-only compound preparation of the CORTICOSTEROID and ANTI-INFLAMMATORY methylprednisolone (as acetate) and the LOCAL ANAESTHETIC lidocaine hydrochloride. It can be used to treat inflammation in the joints (for example, in rheumatic disease) or soft tissue, and is available in a form for injection.
✚▲ Side-effects/warnings: See LIDOCAINE HYDROCHLORIDE; METHYLPREDNISOLONE.

Deponit

(Schwarz) is a proprietary, non-prescription preparation of the VASODILATOR and ANTI-ANGINA drug glyceryl trinitrate. It can be used to treat and prevent angina pectoris. It is available as a self-adhesive dressing (patch; in two strengths *4* and *10*) and so when placed on the chest the drug is absorbed through the skin and helps to give lasting relief.
✚▲ Side-effects/warnings: See GLYCERYL TRINITRATE.

Depo-Provera

(Pharmacia) is a proprietary, prescription-only preparation of the PROGESTOGEN medroxyprogesterone acetate. It can be used as a long-lasting *progesterone-only* (*POP*) CONTRACEPTIVE preparation (administered by intramuscular injection every three months). It is available in a form for injection.
✚▲ Side-effects/warnings: See MEDROXYPROGESTERONE ACETATE.

Dequacaine Lozenges

(Crookes Healthcare) is a proprietary, non-prescription compound preparation of the ANTISEPTIC dequalinium chloride and the LOCAL ANAESTHETIC benzocaine in the form of lozenges. It can be used to relieve the discomfort of a severe sore throat. It is not normally given to children, except on medical advice.
✚▲ Side-effects/warnings: See BENZOCAINE; DEQUALINIUM CHLORIDE.

Dequadin Lozenges

(Crookes Healthcare) is a proprietary, non-prescription preparation of the ANTISEPTIC dequalinium chloride. It can be used to treat common infections of the mouth and throat. It is not normally given to children under ten years, except on medical advice.
✚▲ Side-effects/warnings: See DEQUALINIUM CHLORIDE.

dequalinium chloride

is a mild ANTISEPTIC agent with ANTIBACTERIAL and weak ANTIFUNGAL properties. It can be used to treat infections of the mouth and throat, and administration is oral. It is also available in some compound preparations combined with LOCAL ANAESTHETIC drugs.
✚▲ Side-effects/warnings: Considered safe in normal topical use at recommended concentrations.
✪ **Related entries: Dequacaine Lozenges; Dequadin Lozenges; Labosept Pastilles.**

Derbac-M Liquid

(SSL) is a proprietary, non-prescription preparation of the SCABICIDAL and PEDICULICIDAL drug malathion. It can be used to treat infestations of the scalp and pubic hair by lice (pediculosis) or of the skin by the itch-mite (scabies). It is available as a liquid and is not normally used for infants under six months, except on medical advice.
✚▲ Side-effects/warnings: See MALATHION.

Dermacort Cream

(Sankyo Pharma) is a proprietary, non-prescription preparation of the CORTICOSTEROID and ANTI-INFLAMMATORY hydrocortisone. It can be used to treat mild, inflammatory skin conditions, such as irritant contact dematitis, moderate eczema and insect bites. It is available as a cream for topical application. Not normally given to children under ten, except on medical advice.
✚▲ Side-effects/warnings: See HYDROCORTISONE.

Dermalo

(Dermal) is a proprietary, non-prescription preparation of liquid paraffin, along with acetylated wool alcohol. It has EMOLLIENT action and can be used for contact dermatitis and dry skin conditions. It is available as a bath oil.
✚▲ Side-effects/warnings: See LIQUID PARAFFIN.

Dermestril

(Straken) is a proprietary, prescription-only preparation of the OESTROGEN estradiol. It can be used in HRT and is available as self-adhesive skin patches (in varying strengths).
✚▲ Side-effects/warnings: See ESTRADIOL.

Dermestril-Septem

(Strakan) is a proprietary, prescription-only preparation of the OESTROGEN estradiol. It can be used for menopausal symptoms as part of HRT, and is available in the form of skin patches.
✚▲ Side-effects/warnings: See ESTRADIOL.

Dermidex Cream

(SSL) is a proprietary, non-prescription compound preparation of the LOCAL ANAESTHETIC lidocaine (as base) and the ANTISEPTIC cetrimide and chlorbutanol (with aluminium chlorhydroxyallantoinate). It can be used for the temporary relief of pain caused by minor scratches and soreness, bites and stings, and is available as a cream. Not normally given to children under four, except on medical advice.
✚▲ Side-effects/warnings: See CETRIMIDE; LIDOCAINE HYDROCHLORIDE.

Dermol 200 Shower Emollient

(Dermal) is a proprietary, non-prescription preparation of the ANTISEPTIC benzalkonium chloride and chlorhexidine hydrochloride (with liquid paraffin and isopropyl myristate). It can be used for dry and pruritic skin conditions including eczema and dermatitis, and is available as a shower emollient.
✚▲ Side-effects/warnings: See BENZALKONIUM CHLORIDE; CHLORHEXIDINE; LIQUID PARAFFIN.

Dermol 500 Lotion

(Dermal) is a proprietary, non-prescription preparation of the ANTISEPTIC benzalkonium chloride and chlorhexidine hydrochloride (with liquid paraffin and isopropyl myristate). It can be used for dry and pruritic skin conditions including eczema and dermatitis, and is available as a skin lotion.
✚▲ Side-effects/warnings: See BENZALKONIUM CHLORIDE; CHLORHEXIDINE; LIQUID PARAFFIN.

Dermovate

(GlaxoWellcome; GSK) is a proprietary, prescription-only preparation of the CORTICOSTEROID and ANTI-INFLAMMATORY clobetasol propionate. It can be used for the short-term treatment of severe, inflammatory skin disorders, such as eczema and psoriasis, that are resistant to weaker corticosteroids. It is used topically and available as a cream, an ointment and a scalp application for topical application.
✚▲ Side-effects/warnings: See CLOBETASOL PROPIONATE.

D

Dermovate-NN

(GlaxoWellcome; GSK) is a proprietary, prescription-only compound preparation of the CORTICOSTEROID clobetasol propionate, the ANTIBACTERIAL and (AMINOGLYCOSIDE) ANTIBIOTIC neomycin sulphate and the ANTIFUNGAL and antibiotic nystatin. It can be used, in the short term, to treat severe inflammation of the skin in which infection is also present. It is available as an ointment and a cream for topical application.
✚▲ Side-effects/warnings: See CLOBETASOL PROPIONATE; NEOMYCIN SULPHATE; NYSTATIN.

desensitizing vaccine 🅱

preparations contain particular allergens (substances to which a patient has an allergic reaction to) which are administered, in progressive doses, to reduce the degree of allergic reaction the patient suffers when exposed to the allergen following treatment – a procedure called *hyposensitization*. For example, preparations of grass pollens are administered for the treatment of hay fever, or bee venom or wasp venom to protect against the effects of subsequent stings. The mechanism by which they work is not clear. They are given by injection (usually subcutaneous).
✚ Side-effects: Allergic reactions, especially in small children.
▲ Warnings: They are not to be used in patients who are pregnant, young children, or those who have acute asthma or feverish conditions. A heavy meal must not be eaten before treatment. Injections should be administered under close medical supervision and in locations where emergency facilities for full cardiorespiratory resuscitation are immediately available (in case of anaphylactic reaction), and patients need to be monitored for at least an hour after administration.
✪ **Related entries: Pharmalgen; Pollinex.**

Deseril

(Alliance) is a proprietary, prescription-only preparation of methysergide. It can be used under specialist supervision in hospital, as an ANTIMIGRAINE treatment to prevent severe, recurrent migraine and similar headaches in patients for whom other forms of treatment have failed. It is available as tablets.
✚▲ Side-effects/warnings: See METHYSERGIDE.

Desferal

(Novartis) is a proprietary, prescription-only preparation of the CHELATING AGENT desferrioxamine mesilate. It can be used as an ANTIDOTE to treat iron poisoning and iron overload. It is available in a form for injection.
✚▲ Side-effects/warnings: See DESFERRIOXAMINE MESILATE.

desferrioxamine mesilate

(deferoxamine mesilate) is a CHELATING AGENT which is used as an ANTIDOTE to treat IRON poisoning or an overload of iron in the tissues (eg in aplastic anaemia due to repeated blood transfusions), and also can be used to treat aluminium overload (eg in kidney dialysis patients). Administration is by injection.
✚ Side-effects: There may be pain at the site of injection, gastrointestinal disturbances, hypotension, heart rate changes, anaphylaxis, convulsions, dizziness, disturbances in vision and hearing and skin, heart and liver disorders.
▲ Warnings: Depending on use, it should be avoided in patients with kidney impairment; or who are pregnant or breast-feeding.
✪ **Related entry: Desferal.**

desloratadine

is a recently developed ANTIHISTAMINE which has less sedative side-effects than some older members of its class. It is a metabolite of LORATADINE. It can be used for the symptomatic relief of allergic symptoms, such as hay fever and urticaria. Administration is oral.
✚▲ Side-effects/warnings: See ANTIHISTAMINE. But the incidence of sedative and anticholinergic effects is low; nevertheless, it may impair the performance of skilled tasks, such as driving. It should not be given to patients who are pregnant or breast-feeding.
✪ **Related entry: Neoclarityn.**

desmopressin

is one of two major analogues of the antidiuretic HORMONE vasopressin (ADH), which naturally reduces urine production. It is used to diagnose or to treat certain (pituitary-originated, or 'cranial') types of diabetes insipidus, to test renal function, in DIABETES INSIPIDUS TREATMENT, or to prevent bed-wetting. For these purposes it is preferred to VASOPRESSIN because it is not a VASOCONSTRICTOR and has a longer duration of

D

action. It is also used to boost blood concentrations of some blood-clotting factors (VIII) in haemophiliac patients. Administration can be oral, or topical as nose-drops or a nasal spray (it is absorbed into the systemic circulation from the nasal mucosa) or by injection.
✚▲ Side-effects/warnings: See VASOPRESSIN, but depend on what it is being used for, and it has a longer duration of action. There is less rise in blood pressure, but nevertheless care is needed in patients with certain cardiovascular or kidney disorders, or hypertension. Fluid retention and raised sodium levels may occur unless fluid intake is restricted. There may be vomiting, stomach pain, headache and nosebleeds; also, congestion and rhinitis with the nasal spray.
✪ **Related entries: DDAVP; Desmospray; Desmotabs; Nocutil.**

Desmospray
(Ferring) is a proprietary, prescription-only preparation of desmopressin, which is an analogue of the pituitary HORMONE vasopressin (ADH). It is administered in pituitary-originated DIABETES INSIPIDUS TREATMENT. It can be used for some other diagnostic tests, to test kidney function, and to prevent bed-wetting. It is available as a nasal spray (it is absorbed into the systemic circulation from the nasal mucosa).
✚▲ Side-effects/warnings: See DESMOPRESSIN.

Desmotabs
(Ferring) is a proprietary, prescription-only preparation of desmopressin, which is an analogue of the pituitary HORMONE vasopressin (ADH). It is used in (pituitary-originated) DIABETES INSIPIDUS TREATMENT. It can also be used to prevent bed-wetting. It is available (as desmopressin acetate) as tablets.
✚▲ Side-effects/warnings: See DESMOPRESSIN.

desogestrel
is a PROGESTOGEN that is used as a constituent of the *combined* ORAL CONTRACEPTIVE preparations that contain an OESTROGEN and a progestogen. Administration is oral.
✚▲ Side-effects/warnings: See PROGESTOGEN.
✪ **Related entries: Marvelon; Mercilon.**

desoximetasone
(desoxymethasone) is a CORTICOSTEROID with ANTI-INFLAMMATORY properties. It is used in the treatment of severe, acute inflammation of the skin and chronic skin disorders, such as psoriasis. Administration is by topical application.
✚▲ Side-effects/warnings: See CORTICOSTEROID; though serious systemic effects are unlikely with topical application, but there may be local skin reactions.
✪ **Related entry: Stiedex.**

desoxymetasone
see DESOXIMETASONE.

desquamating agent
see KERATOLYTIC.

Destolit
(Norgine) is a proprietary, prescription-only preparation of ursodeoxycholic acid. It is used to dissolve gallstones, and is available as tablets.
✚▲ Side-effects/warnings: See URSODEOXYCHOLIC ACID.

Deteclo
(Lederle; Wyeth) is a proprietary, prescription-only compound preparation of the ANTIBACTERIAL and (TETRACYCLINES) ANTIBIOTIC chlortetracycline (as hydrochloride), tetracycline (as hydrochloride) and demeclocycline hydrochloride. It can be used to treat many kinds of infection, and is available as tablets.
✚▲ Side-effects/warnings: See CHLORTETRACYCLINE; DEMECLOCYCLINE HYDROCHLORIDE; TETRACYCLINE.

Detrunorm
(Schering-Plough) is a proprietary, prescription-only preparation of the ANTICHOLINERGIC propiverine hydrochloride. It can be used as an ANTISPASMODIC in the treatment of urinary disorders such as incontinence. Available as tablets.
✚▲ Side-effects/warnings: See PROPIVERINE HYDROCHLORIDE.

Detrusitol
(Pharmacia) is a proprietary, prescription-only preparation of the ANTICHOLINERGIC tolterodine tartrate. It can be used as an ANTISPASMODIC in the treatment of urinary disorders such as incontinence. It is available as tablets.
✚▲ Side-effects/warnings: See TOLTERODINE TARTRATE.

Detrusitol XL

(Pharmacia) is a proprietary, prescription-only preparation of the anticholinergic tolterodine tartrate. It can be used as an ANTISPASMODIC in the treatment of urinary disorders such as incontinence. It is available as modified-release capsules.

✚▲ Side-effects/warnings: See TOLTERODINE TARTRATE.

Dettol Antiseptic Cream

(Reckitt Benckiser Healthcare) is a proprietary, non-prescription preparation of the ANTISEPTIC triclosan and chloroxylenol (with edetic acid). It can be used to cleanse wounds and skin to prevent infection, and is available as a cream.

✚▲ Side-effects/warnings: See CHLOROXYLENOL; TRICLOSAN.

Dettol Antiseptic Wash

(Reckitt Benckiser Healthcare) is a proprietary, non-prescription preparation of the ANTISEPTIC benzalkonium chloride. It can be used to cleanse skin wounds, insect bites, grazes and blisters to prevent infection, and is available as a spray.

✚▲ Side-effects/warnings: See BENZALKONIUM CHLORIDE.

Dettol Fresh

(Reckitt Benckiser Healthcare) is a proprietary, non-prescription preparation of the ANTISEPTIC benzalkonium chloride. It can be used to cleanse wounds and skin to prevent infection, and is available as a liquid.

✚▲ Side-effects/warnings: See BENZALKONIUM CHLORIDE.

Dettol Liquid

(Reckitt Benckiser Healthcare) is a proprietary, non-prescription preparation of the ANTISEPTIC and DISINFECTANT chloroxylenol. It can be used as a cleanser to treat skin infections and particularly for cleansing wounds and ulcers. It is available as a solution.

✚▲ Side-effects/warnings: See CHLOROXYLENOL.

dexamethasone

is a CORTICOSTEROID with ANTI-INFLAMMATORY properties. It is used for a variety of purposes, including the suppression of inflammatory and allergic disorders, in the treatment of shock, in the diagnosis of Cushing's disease, to treat congenital adrenal hyperplasia, cerebral oedema and in rheumatic disease to relieve pain and to increase mobility and decrease deformity of joints. It is used in several forms: dexamethasone, dexamethasone sodium phosphate and dexamethasone isonicotinate. Administration can be oral, topical or by injection, in eye-drops to treat local inflammation, ear drops for otitis externa eczema; also with other drugs to prevent nausea and vomiting prior to treatment with chemotherapy.

✚▲ Side-effects/warnings: See CORTICOSTEROID; although serious systemic effects are unlikely with topical application; there may be local reactions.

✪ **Related entries: Decadron; Dexa-Rhinaspray Duo; Dexsol; Maxidex; Maxitrol; Minims Dexamethasone; Otomize; Sofradex; Tobradex.**

dexamfetamine sulphate

(dexamphetamine sulphate) is a drug that, in adults, works directly on the brain as a STIMULANT and can be used to treat narcolepsy (a condition involving irresistible attacks of sleep during the daytime). Paradoxically, in children it has more of a sedative action and can be used (under specialist supervision) in the treatment of hyperactivity. It is on the Controlled Drugs list because of its addictive potential. Administration is oral.

✚ Side-effects: Insomnia, irritability, restlessness, night terrors, euphoria, tremor, dizziness, headache, dependence, tolerance, psychosis, gastrointestinal symptoms, anorexia, growth retardation in children, dry mouth, sweating and effects on the cardiovascular system, and others.

▲ Warnings: It should not be administered to patients with heart disease, hypertension, hyperexcitability states, hyperthyroidism, history of drug abuse, glaucoma, extrapyramidal disorders, or who are pregnant or breast-feeding. Avoid alcohol because of the potential of unpredictable reactions. Growth will be monitored. It may impair the performance of skilled tasks, such as driving. Withdrawal of treatment should be gradual.

✪ **Related entry: Dexedrine.**

Dexa-Rhinaspray Duo

(Boehringer Ingelheim) is a proprietary, prescription-only compound preparation of the ANTI-INFLAMMATORY and CORTICOSTEROID dexamethasone (as isonicotinate) and the

SYMPATHOMIMETIC and VASOCONSTRICTOR tramazoline hydrochloride. It can be used to treat allergic rhinitis, and is available as a spray for nasal inhalation.
✚▲ Side-effects/warnings: See DEXAMETHASONE; TRAMAZOLINE HYDROCHLORIDE.

Dexedrine
(Celltech) is a proprietary, prescription-only preparation of the powerful STIMULANT dexamfetamine sulphate, and is on the Controlled Drugs list. It can be used to treat narcolepsy in adults and medically diagnosed hyperactivity in children. It is available as tablets.
✚▲ Side-effects/warnings: See DEXAMFETAMINE SULPHATE.

dexketoprofen
is a (NSAID) NON-NARCOTIC ANALGESIC and ANTIRHEUMATIC drug which can be used to treat short-term treatment of mild to moderate pain including dysmenorrhoea. Administration is oral.
✚▲ Side-effects/warnings: See NSAID.
✪ **Related entry: Keral.**

Dexsol
(Rosemont) is a non-proprietary, prescription-only preparation of the CORTICOSTEROID and ANTI-INFLAMMATORY dexamethasone. It can be used in the suppression of allergic and inflammatory conditions, in the treatment of shock, congenital adrenal hyperplasia, cerebral oedema and in the diagnosis of Cushing's disease. It is available as an oral solution.
✚▲ Side-effects/warnings: See DEXAMETHASONE.

dextromethorphan hydrobromide
is an (OPIOID) ANTITUSSIVE which is used alone or in combination with other drugs in linctuses, syrups and lozenges to relieve dry or painful coughs.
✚▲ Side-effects/warnings: See OPIOID; but at correct dosage side-effects are rare.
✪ **Related entries: Actifed Compound Linctus; Adult Meltus for Dry Tickly Coughs and Catarrh; Benylin Children's Coughs and Colds; Benylin Cough and Congestion; Benylin Dry Coughs (Non-Drowsy); Benylin Dry Coughs (Original); Cabdriver's Adult Cough Linctus; Covonia Bronchial Balsam; Covonia Night Time Formula; Day Nurse Capsules; Day Nurse Liquid; Junior Meltus for Dry Tickly Coughs and Catarrh; Night Nurse Capsules; Night Nurse Liquid; Robitussin Dry Cough; Strepsils Cough Lozenges; Sudafed Linctus; Vicks Medinite; Vicks Vaposyrup for Dry Coughs.**

dextromoramide
is an (OPIOID) NARCOTIC ANALGESIC drug that is a synthetic derivative of morphine. It can be used to treat severe and intractable pain, and is less sedating and shorter acting than morphine. Its proprietary forms are on the Controlled Drugs list because, as with morphine, it is potentially addictive. Administration can be either oral or topical as suppositories.
✚▲ Side-effects/warnings: See OPIOID.
✪ **Related entry: Palfium.**

dextropropoxyphene hydrochloride
is an (OPIOID) NARCOTIC ANALGESIC which is used to treat pain anywhere in the body. It is usually combined with other analgesics (especially paracetamol or aspirin) as a compound analgesic. Administration of the drug on its own is oral.
✚▲ Side-effects/warnings: See OPIOID. It is not to be used in patients with porphyria or suicidal tendencies or with a history of addiction. It is particularly dangerous in overdose.
✪ **Related entries: co-proxamol; Cosalgesic; Distalgesic; Doloxene**

dextrose
or dextrose monohydrate is another term for glucose.

DF118 Forte
(Martindale) is a proprietary, prescription-only preparation of the (OPIOID) NARCOTIC ANALGESIC dihydrocodeine tartrate. It can be used to treat moderate to severe pain, and is available as tablets.
✚▲ Side-effects/warnings: See DIHYDROCODEINE TARTRATE.

DHC Continus
(Napp) is a proprietary, prescription-only preparation of the (OPIOID) NARCOTIC ANALGESIC dihydrocodeine tartrate. It can be used to treat moderate to severe pain, and is available as modified-release tablets.
✚▲ Side-effects/warnings: See DIHYDROCODEINE TARTRATE.

Diabetamide

(Ashbourne) is a proprietary, prescription-only preparation of the SULPHONYLUREA glibenclamide. It is used in DIABETIC TREATMENT of Type II diabetes (non-insulin-dependent diabetes mellitus; NIDDM; maturity-onset diabetes), and is available as tablets.

✚▲ Side-effects/warnings: See GLIBENCLAMIDE.

diabetes insipidus treatment 🅱

involves the administration of drugs to counteract the under-production of, or decreased kidney response to, ANTIDIURETIC HORMONE (ADH; also called VASOPRESSIN) secreted by the pituitary gland, which is a characteristic of diabetes insipidus. Vasopressin itself may be used, but must be given by injection (it is a peptide that is broken down in the gastrointestinal tract). The analogue DESMOPRESSIN (a synthetic peptide) can be administered in the form of a nasal spray (it is absorbed into the systemic circulation from the nasal mucosa) and also can be given by mouth. Diabetes insipidus is a rare disease and has no connection at all with diabetes mellitus, which is also a HORMONE disorder, but due to the under-production of INSULIN (not ADH) by the pancreas gland. However, in both conditions symptoms include thirst and a production of large quantities of dilute urine.

diabetes mellitus treatment

see DIABETIC TREATMENT.

diabetic treatment 🅱

(*diabetes mellitus* treatment) uses two types of drug. The first treatment involves the use of ORAL HYPOGLYCAEMIC drugs. These are synthetic agents taken by mouth to reduce the levels of glucose (sugar) in the bloodstream and are used primarily in the treatment of Type II diabetes (non-insulin-dependent diabetes mellitus; NIDDM; maturity-onset diabetes) when there is still some residual capacity in the pancreas for the production of the HORMONE insulin. The main oral hypoglycaemics used, sometimes in combination, are the SULPHONYLUREA (eg CHLORPROPAMIDE, GLIBENCLAMIDE, GLICLAZIDE, GLIMEPIRIDE, GLIPIZIDE, GLIQUIDONE, TOLBUTAMIDE) and BIGUANIDE drugs (METFORMIN HYDROCHLORIDE). Repaglinide is a newly introduced oral drug that works by stimulating insulin release from the pancreas. Also, ACARBOSE and GUAR GUM may be used by mouth to help control Type II diabetes.

The second treatment involves the administration of INSULIN, which is mainly used in Type I diabetes (insulin-dependent diabetes mellitus; IDDM; juvenile-onset diabetes) and must be injected. There are many insulin preparations available and the difference between them is mainly their duration of action. For the unrelated disorder, diabetes insipidus, see DIABETES INSIPIDUS TREATMENT.

▲ Warnings: A number of other drugs taken at the same time can potentially interact with diabetic treatments, altering their effectiveness and causing adverse reactions (some serious). For example, the gout treatment drug SULFINPYRAZONE, certain NSAIDS, ANTIFUNGAL agents (eg FLUCONAZOLE and MICONAZOLE) and ANTIBACTERIAL agents (eg CHLORAMPHENICOL) may enhance the effects of sulphonylurea hypoglycaemic drugs. Many other drugs potentially can interact with sulphonylureas and other types of diabetic treatments, including with insulin. Also, some nutritional supplements and herbal remedies, such as Aloe vera, alpha-lipoic acid, guar gum and chromium, can potentially interfere with the efficacy of diabetic treatments.

DIAGLYK

(Generics) is a proprietary, prescription-only preparation of the SULPHONYLUREA gliclazide. It is used in DIABETIC TREATMENT of Type II diabetes (non-insulin-dependent diabetes mellitus; NIDDM; maturity-onset diabetes), and is available as tablets.

✚▲ Side-effects/warnings: See GLICLAZIDE.

Diah-Limit

(Wallis) is a proprietary, non-prescription preparation of the (OPIOID) ANTIDIARRHOEAL loperamide hydrochloride. It can be used for the symptomatic relief of acute diarrhoea and its associated discomfort, and is available as capsules. It is not given to children except on medical advice.

✚▲ Side-effects/warnings: See LOPERAMIDE HYDROCHLORIDE.

Dialar

(Lagap) is a proprietary, prescription-only preparation of the BENZODIAZEPINE diazepam. It

can be used as an ANXIOLYTIC in the short-term treatment of anxiety, as a HYPNOTIC to relieve insomnia, as an ANTICONVULSANT and ANTI-EPILEPTIC for status epilepticus and for febrile convulsions in children, as a SEDATIVE in preoperative medication, as a SKELETAL MUSCLE RELAXANT and to assist in the treatment of alcohol withdrawal symptoms. It is available as an oral solution (in two strengths).
✚▲ Side-effects/warnings: See DIAZEPAM.

Diamicron
(Servier) is a proprietary, prescription-only preparation of the SULPHONYLUREA gliclazide. It is used in DIABETIC TREATMENT of Type II diabetes (non-insulin-dependent diabetes mellitus; NIDDM; maturity-onset diabetes), and is available as tablets.
✚▲ Side-effects/warnings: See GLICLAZIDE.

Diamicron MR
(Servier) is a proprietary, prescription-only preparation of the SULPHONYLUREA gliclazide. It is used in DIABETIC TREATMENT of Type II diabetes (non-insulin-dependent diabetes mellitus; NIDDM; maturity-onset diabetes), and is available as tablets.
✚▲ Side-effects/warnings: See GLICLAZIDE.

diamorphine hydrochloride
is the chemical name of heroin hydrochloride (a chemical derivative of morphine) and is a powerful (OPIOID) NARCOTIC ANALGESIC. It can be used in the treatment of moderate to severe pain (though it has a shorter duration of action than morphine), including management of the pain and anxiety of myocardial infarction (by intravenous injection). It is also occasionally used as an ANTITUSSIVE to treat severe and painful cough and for acute airways oedema (especially in the treatment of terminal lung cancer). Its use quickly tends to tolerance and then dependence (addiction). Administration is oral (tablets or linctus) or by injection. All preparations are on the Controlled Drugs list.
✚▲ Side-effects/warnings: See OPIOID, but it may cause less nausea and hypotension.

Diamox
(Wyeth) is a proprietary, prescription-only preparation of the CARBONIC-ANHYDRASE INHIBITOR acetazolamide. It is mainly used in GLAUCOMA TREATMENT. It is available as tablets, as a modified-release capsules (*Diamox SR*) and in a form for injection.
✚▲ Side-effects/warnings: See ACETAZOLAMIDE.

Dianette
(Schering Health) is a proprietary, prescription-only compound preparation of the OESTROGEN hormone ethinylestradiol and the ANTI-ANDROGEN cyproterone acetate. It can be used in women, in certain circumstances, to treat severe acne, and is available as tablets.
✚▲ Side-effects/warnings: See CYPROTERONE ACETATE; ETHINYLESTRADIOL.

Diarphen
(Mepra-pharm; Co-Pharma) is a proprietary, prescription-only compound preparation of the (OPIOID) ANTIDIARRHOEAL diphenoxylate hydrochloride and the ANTICHOLINERGIC atropine sulphate (a combination called co-phenotrope). It can be used to treat chronic diarrhoea, for example, in mild chronic ulcerative colitis. Dependence may occur with prolonged use. Available as tablets.
✚▲ Side-effects/warnings: See ATROPINE SULPHATE; DIPHENOXYLATE HYDROCHLORIDE.

Diasorb
(Norton Healthcare) is a proprietary, non-prescription preparation of the (OPIOID) ANTIDIARRHOEAL loperamide hydrochloride. It can be used for the symptomatic relief of acute diarrhoea and its associated discomfort, and is available as capsules. Not given to children except on medical advice.
✚▲ Side-effects/warnings: See LOPERAMIDE HYDROCHLORIDE.

Diazemuls
(Alpharma) is a proprietary, prescription-only preparation of the BENZODIAZEPINE diazepam. It can be used as an ANXIOLYTIC in the short-term treatment of acute severe anxiety, as an ANTICONVULSANT and ANTI-EPILEPTIC for status epilepticus, as a SEDATIVE in preoperative medication, as a SKELETAL MUSCLE RELAXANT and to assist in the treatment of alcohol withdrawal symptoms. It is available in a form for injection.
✚▲ Side-effects/warnings: See DIAZEPAM.

diazepam
is chemically a BENZODIAZEPINE. It can be used as

an ANXIOLYTIC in the short-term treatment of anxiety, as a HYPNOTIC in the short term to relieve insomnia, as an ANTICONVULSANT and ANTI-EPILEPTIC for convulsions due to poisoning and status epilepticus, for treating febrile convulsions in children, for the control of panic attacks, for night terror and sleepwalking in children, as a SEDATIVE in preoperative medication, as a SKELETAL MUSCLE RELAXANT and to assist in the treatment of alcohol withdrawal symptoms. Administration can be oral, rectal or by injection.
✚▲ Side-effects/warnings: See BENZODIAZEPINE. When injected, there may be pain, inflammation and swelling at the injection site.
✪ **Related entries: Dialar; Diazemuls; Diazepam Rectubes; Rimapam; Stesolid; Tensium; Valclair; Valium.**

Diazepam Rectubes

(CP) is a proprietary, prescription-only preparation of the BENZODIAZEPINE diazepam. It can be used as an ANXIOLYTIC in the short-term treatment of anxiety, as a HYPNOTIC to relieve insomnia, as an ANTICONVULSANT for febrile convulsions in children when the oral route is not appropriate. Available as a rectal solution (rectal tubes).
✚▲ Side-effects/warnings: See DIAZEPAM.

diazoxide

has two separate actions and uses. First, it is a VASODILATOR that can lower blood pressure rapidly on injection and can therefore be used as an ANTIHYPERTENSIVE in treating acute hypertensive crisis. Second, it is a hyperglycaemic drug and can be used by mouth to treat chronic hypoglycaemia (abnormally low levels of glucose in the bloodstream), for example, where a pancreatic tumour causes excessive secretion of INSULIN. Administration is either oral or by injection.
✚ Side-effects: There may be nausea and vomiting, hypotension, loss of appetite, oedema, heart rhythm irregularities and increased heart rate and hyperglycaemia; movement disorders, excessive growth of hair with chronic treatment.
▲ Warnings: Administer with caution to patients with reduced blood supply to the heart, certain kidney disorders, who are pregnant or in labour. During prolonged treatment, regular monitoring of blood constituents and blood pressure is required.
✪ **Related entries: Eudemine (injection); Eudemine (tablets).**

Dibenyline

(Goldshield) is a proprietary, prescription-only preparation of the ALPHA-ADRENOCEPTOR BLOCKER phenoxybenzamine hydrochloride. It can be used, in conjunction with a BETA-BLOCKER, as an ANTIHYPERTENSIVE in hypertensive crises in phaeochromocytoma and severe shock. It is available as capsules.
✚▲ Side-effects/warnings: See PHENOXYBENZAMINE HYDROCHLORIDE.

dibromopropamidine isethionate

see DIBROMPROPAMIDINE ISETHIONATE.

dibrompropamidine isethionate

(dibromopropamidine isethionate) is an ANTIBACTERIAL (and ANTIFUNGAL) agent which is used specifically to treat infections of the eyelids or conjunctiva, including the amoebic infection acanthamoeba keratitis (sometimes with additional drugs). Administration is topical.
✪ **Related entries: Brolene Eye Ointment; Brulidine; Golden Eye Ointment.**

dibucaine hydrochloride

see CINCHOCAINE.

dichlorophen

is an ANTIBACTERIAL and ANTIFUNGAL agent (with some ANTHELMINTIC activity) which is incorporated into a treatment for athlete's foot. Administration is topical.
✪ **Related entry: Mycota Spray.**

diclofenac sodium

is a (NSAID) NON-NARCOTIC ANALGESIC and ANTIRHEUMATIC drug. It is used to treat pain and inflammation in rheumatic disease and other musculoskeletal disorders (such as juvenile arthritis and gout). It is also used in some ophthalmic procedures. It is being increasingly used to treat pain immediately after certain surgical procedures, and for ureteric colic, usually by injection (or suppositories). Administration can be oral, topical as suppositories, or by injection.
✚▲ Side-effects/warnings: See NSAID. Avoid its use in patients with porphyria. There may be local irritation if using suppositories, or pain at the site of injection.
✪ **Related entries: Acoflam; Arthrotec; Dicloflex; Diclomax Retard; Diclomax SR; Diclovol; Diclozip;**

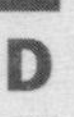

Enzed; Flamrase; Lofensaid; Motifene 75 mg; Pennsaid; Rhumalgan CR; Solaraze; Volraman; Voltarol; Voltarol Emulgel; Voltarol Ophtha.

Dicloflex
(Dexcel Pharma) is a proprietary, prescription-only preparation of the (NSAID) NON-NARCOTIC ANALGESIC and ANTIRHEUMATIC diclofenac sodium. It can be used to treat arthritic and rheumatic pain, other musculoskeletal disorders and acute gout. It is available as tablets.
✚▲ Side-effects/warnings: See DICLOFENAC SODIUM.

Diclomax Retard
(Parke-Davis; Pfizer) is a proprietary, prescription-only preparation of the (NSAID) NON-NARCOTIC ANALGESIC and ANTIRHEUMATIC diclofenac sodium. It can be used to treat arthritic and rheumatic pain and inflammation and other musculoskeletal disorders. It is available as modified-release capsules.
✚▲ Side-effects/warnings: See DICLOFENAC SODIUM.

Diclomax SR
(Parke-Davis; Pfizer) is a proprietary, prescription-only preparation of the (NSAID) NON-NARCOTIC ANALGESIC and ANTIRHEUMATIC diclofenac sodium. It can be used to treat arthritic and rheumatic pain and inflammation and other musculoskeletal disorders. It is available as modified-release capsules.
✚▲ Side-effects/warnings: See DICLOFENAC SODIUM.

Diclovol
(Arun) is a prescription-only, proprietary version of the (NSAID) NON-NARCOTIC ANALGESIC and ANTIRHEUMATIC diclofenac sodium. It can be used to treat arthritic and rheumatic pain and inflammation and other musculoskeletal disorders. It is available as tablets.
✚▲ Side-effects/warnings: See DICLOFENAC SODIUM.

Diclozip
(Ashbourne) is a prescription-only, proprietary version of the (NSAID) NON-NARCOTIC ANALGESIC and ANTIRHEUMATIC diclofenac sodium. It can be used to treat arthritic and rheumatic pain and inflammation and other musculoskeletal disorders. It is available as tablets.
✚▲ Side-effects/warnings: See DICLOFENAC SODIUM.

dicobalt edetate
is used as an ANTIDOTE to acute cyanide poisoning. It acts as a CHELATING AGENT by binding to cyanide to form a compound that can be excreted from the body. Administration by injection.
✚ Side-effects: Vomiting, effects on the heart and blood pressure.
▲ Warnings: Because of its toxicity, it is normally used only when the patient is losing, or has lost, consciousness.

Diconal
(CeNeS) is a proprietary, prescription-only compound preparation of the (OPIOID) NARCOTIC ANALGESIC dipipanone hydrochloride and the ANTIHISTAMINE and ANTINAUSEANT cyclizine hydrochloride. It can be used to treat moderate to severe pain, and is available as tablets. It is on the Controlled Drugs list.
✚▲ Side-effects/warnings: See CYCLIZINE; DIPIPANONE.

dicyclomine hydrochloride
see DICYLOVERINE HYDROCHLORIDE.

dicyloverine hydrochloride
(dicyclomine hydrochloride) is an ANTICHOLINERGIC (ANTIMUSCARINIC) drug which can be used as an ANTISPASMODIC for the symptomatic relief of muscle spasm in the gastrointestinal tract. Administration is oral.
✚▲ Side-effects/warnings: See ATROPINE SULPHATE.
✪ Related entries: Kolanticon Gel; Merbentyl; Merbentyl 20.

Dicynene
(Delandale) is a proprietary, prescription-only preparation of etamsylate, which is a HAEMOSTATIC drug that can be used in certain situations where antifibrinolytic drugs might be administered. It can be used for a variety of purposes, including bleeding in premature infants and in menorrhagia. It is taken as tablets and in a form for injection.
✚▲ Side-effects/warnings: See ETAMSYLATE.

didanosine
(ddI; DDI) is a (*reverse transcriptase*) ANTIVIRAL

which can be used in the treatment of HIV infection. It is mainly administered in combination with other antivirals to patients who are intolerant to, or have not benefited from, other antivirals. Administration is oral.

✚ Side-effects: Pancreatitis, peripheral neuropathy (eg loss of feeling in the feet), raised uric acid levels in the blood (monitoring is necessary). Other possible side-effects include nausea, headache, vomiting, confusion, insomnia, fever and headache, dry mouth, effects on the eye, skin rashes.

▲ Warnings: It is a specialist drug, and there will be full assessment and patient monitoring throughout treatment. It should not be given to those who are breast-feeding. It should be administered with caution where there is a history of pancreatitis, in peripheral neuropathy, where there is raised blood uric acid and in those who have impaired liver or kidney function; and to patients who are pregnant.

✪ **Related entry: Videx; Videx EC.**

Didronel

(Procter & Gamble Pharm.) is a proprietary, prescription-only preparation of disodium etidronate. It can be used to reduce the rate of bone turnover in treating the condition known as Paget's disease of the bone. It is available as tablets.

✚▲ Side-effects/warnings: See DISODIUM ETIDRONATE.

Didronel PMO

(Procter & Gamble Pharm.) is a proprietary, prescription-only compound preparation of the CALCIUM METABOLISM MODIFIER disodium etidronate and calcium carbonate. It can be used in the prevention and treatment of osteoporosis, in postmenopausal women (especially where HRT is inappropriate), and prevention and treatment of corticosteroid-induced osteoporosis. It is available as tablets (in two forms given in cycles).

✚▲ Side-effects/warnings: See CALCIUM CARBONATE; DISODIUM ETIDRONATE.

diethylamine salicylate

is a NSAID that has COUNTER-IRRITANT, or RUBEFACIENT, actions and can be applied to the skin for symptomatic relief of pain in underlying organs, for instance in rheumatic and other musculoskeletal disorders. Administration is topical.

✚▲ Side-effects/warnings: See NSAID, though normally little is absorbed into the circulation and local side-effects are limited to mild irritation. It should not be used on broken skin or mucous membranes. See also SALICYLATE; SALICYLIC ACID.

✪ **Related entries: Algesal; Lloyd's Cream; Transvasin Heat Spray.**

diethylcarbamazine

is an ANTHELMINTIC drug, effective against microfilariae and adults of tropical diseases *Loa loa, Wuchereria bancrofti* and *Brugia malayi*. usually gives a radical cure for these infections. Administration is oral.

✚ Side-effects: In heavy infections there may be a febrile reaction, and in heavy *Loa loa* infection there is a small risk of encephalopathy.

▲ Warnings: In cases of febrile complications, treatment must be given under careful supervision and stopped at the first sign of cerebral involvement (specialist advice necessary).

✪ **Related entry: Hetrazan.**

diethylstilbestrol

(diethylstilboestrol; stilbestrol; stilboestrol) is a synthetic OESTROGEN. It is useful in HRT (hormone replacement therapy) in women during the menopause. It is sometimes used in low dosage as an ANTICANCER treatment for cancer of the prostate gland in men and in women for breast cancer. Administration can be either oral or as pessaries.

✚ Side-effects: Nausea, thrombosis, fluid retention. In men, breast growth and impotence; in women, bleeding on withdrawal. There may be high blood calcium levels and bone pain when used for breast cancer.

▲ Warnings: It should not be administered to patients with certain cardiovascular or liver disorders.

✪ **Related entries: Apstil; Tampovagan.**

Differin

(Galderma) is a proprietary, prescription-only preparation of adapalene (a RETINOID). It can be used for the treatment of mild to moderate acne and is available as a cream and gel that is applied to the skin.

✚▲ Side-effects/warnings: See ADAPALENE.

D

Difflam
(3M) is a proprietary, non-prescription preparation of benzydamine hydrochloride, which has a COUNTER-IRRITANT, or RUBEFACIENT, action. It can be used for symptomatic relief of pain on the skin, mouth ulcers and other sores or inflammation in the mouth and throat. It is available as a cream for topical application and as a liquid mouthwash or spray.
+▲ Side-effects/warnings: See BENZYDAMINE HYDROCHLORIDE.

Diflucan
(Pfizer) is a proprietary, prescription-only preparation of the ANTIFUNGAL fluconazole. It can be used to treat candidiasis (thrush) of the vagina, mouth and other tissue areas. It is available as capsules, an oral suspension and in a form for intravenous infusion. (It can also be sold to the public without prescription, subject to limits of a single capsule for women of 16-60 years.)
+▲ Side-effects/warnings: See FLUCONAZOLE.

Diflucan One
(Warner Lambert Consumer Healthcare; Pfizer) is a proprietary, non-prescription preparation of the ANTIFUNGAL fluconazole. It can be used to treat vaginal thrush, and is available as capsules. It is not normally given to children, except on medical advice.
+▲ Side-effects/warnings: See FLUCONAZOLE.

diflucortolone valerate
is a CORTICOSTEROID with ANTI-INFLAMMATORY properties. It is used in the treatment of severe, inflammatory skin disorders, such as eczema and psoriasis, that are unresponsive to weaker corticosteroids. Administration is by topical application.
+▲ Side-effects/warnings: See CORTICOSTEROID; though serious systemic effects are unlikely with topical application, but there may be local skin reactions.
✪ **Related entry: Nerisone.**

diflunisal
is a (NSAID) NON-NARCOTIC ANALGESIC and ANTIRHEUMATIC drug derived from aspirin, but is quite powerful and with a longer duration of action. It can be used in the treatment of pain and inflammation (especially in rheumatic disease and other musculoskeletal disorders) and for period pain. Administration is oral.
+▲ Side-effects/warnings: See NSAID. Administer with care to patients who are breast-feeding.
✪ **Related entry: Dolobid.**

Diftavax
(Aventis Pasteur) is a proprietary, prescription-only VACCINE preparation of adsorbed diphtheria and tetanus vaccine for adults (DT/Vac/Ads for Adults and Adolescents), which combines (toxoid) vaccines for diphtheria and tetanus vaccine adsorbed onto a mineral carrier. It is available in a form for injection.
+▲ Side-effects/warnings: See DIPHTHERIA VACCINE; TETANUS VACCINE.

Digestif Rennie Peppermint Flavour
(Roche Consumer Health) is a proprietary, non-prescription compound preparation of the ANTACID agents calcium carbonate and magnesium carbonate. It can be used to relieve acid indigestion, heartburn, upset stomach, dyspepsia, biliousness and overindulgence. It is available as tablets and is not normally given to children under six, except on medical advice.
+▲ Side-effects/warnings: See CALCIUM CARBONATE; MAGNESIUM CARBONATE.

Digibind
(GlaxoWellcome; GSK) is a proprietary, prescription-only preparation of digoxin-specific antibody fragment which can be used as an ANTIDOTE to overdosage by the CARDIAC GLYCOSIDE drugs digoxin and digitoxin. It is administered for emergency use by injection.
+▲ Side-effects/warnings: See DIGOXIN-SPECIFIC ANTIBODY FRAGMENT.

digitoxin
is a CARDIAC GLYCOSIDE derived from the leaves of *Digitalis* foxgloves. It can be used as a CARDIAC STIMULANT, because it increases the force of contraction in HEART FAILURE TREATMENT and as an ANTI-ARRHYTHMIC to treat certain heartbeat irregularities. Administration is oral.
+▲ Side-effects/warnings: See DIGOXIN.

digoxin
is derived from the leaves of *Digitalis* foxgloves

and is the most-used of the CARDIAC GLYCOSIDE class. It can be used as a CARDIAC STIMULANT, because it increases the force of contraction in HEART FAILURE TREATMENT, and as an ANTI-ARRHYTHMIC to treat certain heartbeat irregularities. Administration is either oral or by injection.
✚ Side-effects: There are serious and common side-effects (the minimization of which depends on finding a suitable dosage schedule in each patient and regular monitoring): loss of appetite, nausea and vomiting, with a consequent weight loss; diarrhoea and abdominal pain; visual disturbances; fatigue, confusion, delirium and hallucinations. Overdosage may lead to arrhythmias or heart block.
▲ Warnings: It should be administered with caution to patients who have had a recent heart attack, certain arrhythmias and heart conditions, hypothyroidism, who are elderly, or have impaired kidney function. Regular monitoring of the blood potassium level is usual.
✪ **Related entries: Lanoxin; Lanoxin-PG.**

digoxin-specific antibody fragment
comprises antibody fragments that react with the glycosides, and can be used as an ANTIDOTE to overdosage by the CARDIAC GLYCOSIDE drugs digoxin and digitoxin. It is administered for emergency use by injection.
✚▲ Side-effects/warnings: It is used under specialist conditions only.
✪ **Related entry: Digibind.**

dihydrocodeine tartrate
is an (OPIOID) NARCOTIC ANALGESIC which is similar to CODEINE PHOSPHATE but more powerful. It is also available in some compound analgesic preparations (eg in co-dydramol, where it is combined with paracetamol).
Administration is either oral or sometimes by injection, preparations for which are on the Controlled Drugs list.
✚▲ Side-effects/warnings: See OPIOID.
✪ **Related entries: co-dydramol; Boots Dental Pain Relief; DF118 Forte; DHC Continus; Galake; Paramol Tablets; Remedeine.**

dihydrotachysterol
is a synthetic form of vitamin D (related to D_2 and D_3) which is used to make up body deficiencies of this vitamin. Administration is oral.
✚▲ Side-effects/warnings: See VITAMIN D.
✪ **Related entry: AT 10.**

Dijex Suspension
(SSL) is a proprietary, non-prescription compound preparation of the ANTACID agents aluminium hydroxide and magnesium hydroxide. It can be used to relieve acid indigestion and dyspepsia, and is available as a liquid suspension. It is not normally given to children under six years, except on medical advice.
✚▲ Side-effects/warnings: See ALUMINIUM HYDROXIDE; MAGNESIUM HYDROXIDE.

Dijex Tablets
(SSL) is a proprietary, non-prescription compound preparation of the ANTACID agents aluminium hydroxide and magnesium carbonate. It can be used to relieve acid indigestion and dyspepsia, and is available as tablets. It is not normally given to children under five years, except on medical advice.
✚▲ Side-effects/warnings: See ALUMINIUM HYDROXIDE; MAGNESIUM CARBONATE.

Dilcardia SR
(Generics) is a proprietary, prescription-only preparation of the CALCIUM-CHANNEL BLOCKER diltiazem hydrochloride. It can be used as an ANTIHYPERTENSIVE and as an ANTI-ANGINA drug. It is available as modified-release capsules.
✚▲ Side-effects/warnings: See DILTIAZEM HYDROCHLORIDE.

diloxanide furoate
is an ANTIPROTOZOAL and AMOEBICIDAL drug. It can be used to treat chronic infection of the intestine by amoebae (*Entamoeba histolytic*) that cause amoebic dysentery. Administration is oral.
✚ Side-effects: Flatulence; vomiting, pruritus (skin itching) and/or urticaria. It is not used in pregnant or breast-feeding women.

diltiazem hydrochloride
is a CALCIUM-CHANNEL BLOCKER drug which can be used in ANTIHYPERTENSIVE treatment and also as an ANTI-ANGINA drug in the prevention and treatment of attacks. Administration is oral.
✚ Side-effects: These include effects on the heart, hypotension, flushing, dizziness and malaise, headache, depression, swelling of the ankles,

gastrointestinal disturbances, rashes and altered liver function.
▲ Warnings: It is administered with caution to patients with certain liver, kidney or heart and blood disorders; and with abnormal blood states. It should not be given to patients who are pregnant or breast-feeding.
✪ Related entries: Adizem-SR; Adizem-XL; Angiozem CR; Angitil SR; Angitil XL; Calcicard CR; Dilcardia SR; Dilzem SR; Dilzem XL; Optil; Optil SR; Optil XL; Slozem; Tildiem; Tildiem LA; Tildiem Retard; Viazem XL.

Dilzem SR

(Elan) is a proprietary, prescription-only preparation of the CALCIUM-CHANNEL BLOCKER diltiazem hydrochloride. It can be used as an ANTIHYPERTENSIVE and as an ANTI-ANGINA treatment, and is available as modified-release capsules.
✚▲ Side-effects/warnings: See DILTIAZEM HYDROCHLORIDE.

Dilzem XL

(Elan) is a proprietary, prescription-only preparation of the CALCIUM-CHANNEL BLOCKER diltiazem hydrochloride. It can be used as an ANTI-HYPERTENSIVE and as an ANTI-ANGINA treatment, and is available as modified-release capsules.
✚▲ Side-effects/warnings: See DILTIAZEM HYDROCHLORIDE.

dimercaprol

(BAL) is a CHELATING AGENT which is used as an ANTIDOTE to poisoning with antimony, arsenic, bismuth, gold, mercury, thallium and (with sodium calcium edetate) lead. Administration is by injection.
✚ Side-effects: Hypertension, increase in heart rate, sweating, malaise, nausea and vomiting, excessive tears, constriction of the throat and chest, burning sensation (eyes and mouth), headache, muscle spasms, pain in the abdomen, tingling in extremities, pain and abscess at injection site.
▲ Warnings: It is not to be given to patients with severe liver impairment; administer with care to those with hypertension, kidney damage, or who are pregnant or breast-feeding.

dimeticone

(dimethicone) is a water-repellent silicone which is used as an ANTIFOAMING AGENT and, when taken orally, is thought to reduce flatulence while protecting mucous membranes. It is also a constituent in many BARRIER CREAM products that can be used to protect against irritation or chapping (eg nappy rash). *Dimeticone activated* is also known as *simeticone*.
▲ Warnings: Do not use topically on acutely inflamed or weeping skin.
✪ Related entries: Actonorm Gel; Altacite Plus; Asilone Antacid Liquid; Asilone Antacid Tablets; Asilone Suspension; Asilone Windcheaters; Bisodol Wind Relief; Conotrane; Decubal Clinic; Dentinox Infant Colic Drops; E45 Emollient Bath Oil; Imodium Plus; Infacol; Kolanticon Gel; Maalox Plus; Setlers Wind-eze; Siopel; Sprilon; Timodine; Vaseline Dermacare; Vasogen Cream; Woodward's Colic Drops.

Dimetriose

(Florizel) is a proprietary, prescription-only preparation of gestrinone, which is used to treat conditions such as endometriosis. It is available as capsules.
✚▲ Side-effects/warnings: See GESTRINONE.

Dimotane Co

(Whitehall Laboratories) is a proprietary, non-prescription compound preparation of the ANTITUSSIVE codeine phosphate, the ANTIHISTAMINE brompheniramine maleate and the SYMPATHOMIMETIC and VASOCONSTRICTOR pseudoephedrine hydrochloride. It can be used for the symptomatic relief of dry coughs associated with colds. It is available as a liquid and is not given to children under two years.
✚▲ Side-effects/warnings: See BROMPHENIRAMINE MALEATE; CODEINE PHOSPHATE; PSEUDOEPHEDRINE HYDROCHLORIDE.

Dimotane Co Paediatric

(Whitehall Laboratories) is a proprietary, non-prescription compound preparation of the ANTITUSSIVE codeine phosphate, the ANTIHISTAMINE brompheniramine maleate and the SYMPATHOMIMETIC and VASOCONSTRICTOR pseudoephedrine hydrochloride. It can be used for the symptomatic relief of dry coughs associated with colds and other respiratory disorders in children. It is available as a liquid and is not given to children under two years of age,

except on medical advice.
✚▲ Side-effects/warnings: See BROMPHENIRAMINE MALEATE; CODEINE PHOSPHATE; PSEUDOEPHEDRINE HYDROCHLORIDE.

Dimotane Expectorant

(Whitehall Laboratories) is a proprietary, non-prescription compound preparation of the EXPECTORANT agent guaifenesin (guaiphenesin), the ANTIHISTAMINE brompheniramine maleate and the SYMPATHOMIMETIC and DECONGESTANT pseudoephedrine hydrochloride. It can be used for the symptomatic relief of upper respiratory tract disorders, and is available as a liquid. It is not normally given to children under two years, except on medical advice.
✚▲ Side-effects/warnings: See BROMPHENIRAMINE MALEATE; GUAIFENESIN; PSEUDOEPHEDRINE HYDROCHLORIDE.

Dindevan

(Goldshield) is a proprietary, prescription-only preparation of the ANTICOAGULANT phenindione. It can be used to treat and prevent thrombosis, and is available as tablets.
✚▲ Side-effects/warnings: See PHENINDIONE.

Dinnefords Teejel Gel

(SSL) is a proprietary, non-prescription compound preparation of the ANTISEPTIC cetalkonium chloride and the COUNTER-IRRITANT, or RUBEFACIENT, choline salicylate. It can be applied to the mouth for the symptomatic relief of pain from mouth ulcers, cold sores, denture irritation, inflammation of the tongue and teething in infants. Not normally given to children under four months, except on medical advice.
✚▲ Side-effects/warnings: See CHOLINE SALICYLATE.

dinoprostone

is the PROSTAGLANDIN E_2, which has the effect of causing contractions in the muscular walls of the uterus. It is used to induce labour and occasionally as an ABORTIFACIENT. Administration can be oral, topical or by injection.
✚ Side-effects: There may be vomiting, flushing and shivering, headache and dizziness. Also, a raised temperature may occur after intravenous injection. Otherwise, nausea, diarrhoea, severe contractions of the uterus and increased white blood cell count. There will be uterine pain.
▲ Warnings: It is a specialist hospital drug given under close supervision, and an assessment will be made of the patient's suitability, especially with regard to asthma, glaucoma, liver and kidney impairment.
✪ Related entries: Propess; Prostin E2.

Diocalm

(SSL) is a proprietary, non-prescription preparation of the (OPIOID) ANTIDIARRHOEAL morphine (as hydrochloride), along with attapulgite (magnesium aluminium silicate) and activated attapulgite. It can be used to relieve occasional diarrhoea and its associated pain and discomfort, and is available as tablets. It is not normally given to children under six years, except on medical advice.
✚▲ Side-effects/warnings: See MORPHINE SULPHATE.

Diocalm Ultra

(SSL) is a proprietary, non-prescription preparation of the (OPIOID) ANTIDIARRHOEAL loperamide hydrochloride. It can be used for the symptomatic relief of acute diarrhoea and its associated discomfort. It is available as capsules. It is not given to children, except on medical advice.
✚▲ Side-effects/warnings: See LOPERAMIDE HYDROCHLORIDE.

Diocaps

(Berk; APS) is a proprietary, prescription-only preparation of the (OPIOID) ANTIDIARRHOEAL loperamide hydrochloride. It can be used for the symptomatic relief of acute diarrhoea and its associated discomfort, and is available as capsules. It is not given to children, except on medical advice.
✚▲ Side-effects/warnings: See LOPERAMIDE HYDROCHLORIDE.

Dioctyl

(Schwarz) is a proprietary, non-prescription preparation of the (*stimulant*) LAXATIVE docusate sodium. It can be used to relieve constipation and also to evacuate the rectum prior to abdominal procedures. It is available as capsules.
✚▲ Side-effects/warnings: See DOCUSATE SODIUM.

D

dioctyl sodium sulphosuccinate
see DOCUSATE SODIUM.

Dioderm
(Dermal) is a proprietary, prescription-only preparation of the CORTICOSTEROID and ANTI-INFLAMMATORY hydrocortisone. It can be used to treat mild, inflammatory skin conditions, such as eczema, and is available as a cream for topical application.
✚▲ Side-effects/warnings: See HYDROCORTISONE.

Dioralyte Natural
(Aventis Pharma) is a proprietary, non-prescription, preparation of sodium chloride, potassium chloride, sodium citrate (disodium hydrogen citrate) and glucose. It can be used as an electrolyte and water replacement in dehydration, for example in ANTIDIARRHOEAL treatment, and is available as an oral powder.
✚▲ Side-effects/warnings: See GLUCOSE; POTASSIUM CHLORIDE; SODIUM CHLORIDE; SODIUM CITRATE.

Dioralyte Relief
(Aventis Pharma) is a proprietary, non-prescription, preparation of sodium chloride, potassium chloride, sodium citrate and pre-cooked rice powder. It can be used as an electrolyte and water replacement in dehydration, for example in ANTIDIARRHOEAL treatment, and is available as an oral powder. It is only given to infants between three months and one year with medical advice.
✚▲ Side-effects/warnings: See POTASSIUM CHLORIDE; SODIUM CHLORIDE; SODIUM CITRATE.

Dioralyte Tablets Raspberry Flavour
(Aventis Pharma) is a proprietary, non-prescription, preparation of sodium chloride, potassium chloride, sodium bicarbonate, citric acid and glucose. It can be used as an electrolyte and water replacement in dehydration, for example in ANTIDIARRHOEAL treatment, and is available as an oral powder.
✚▲ Side-effects/warnings: See GLUCOSE; POTASSIUM CHLORIDE; SODIUM BICARBONATE; SODIUM CHLORIDE.

Diovan
(Novartis) is a proprietary, prescription-only preparation of the ANGIOTENSIN-RECEPTOR BLOCKER valsartan. It can be used as an ANTIHYPERTENSIVE, and is available as capsules.
✚▲ Side-effects/warnings: See VALSARTAN.

Dipentum
(Pharmacia) is a proprietary, prescription-only preparation of the AMINOSALICYLATE olsalazine sodium. It can be used to treat patients who suffer from ulcerative colitis, and is available as tablets and capsules.
✚▲ Side-effects/warnings: See OLSALAZINE SODIUM.

diphenhydramine hydrochloride
is an ANTIHISTAMINE which can be used for the symptomatic relief of allergic symptoms, such as hay fever and urticaria, and is incorporated into a number of proprietary cough and cold preparations. It has marked SEDATIVE properties and can be used to relieve occasional insomnia in adults. It is used orally or topically.
✚▲ Side-effects/warnings: See ANTIHISTAMINE. Because of its sedative side-effects, the performance of skilled tasks, such as driving, may be impaired. The effects of alcohol may be enhanced.
✪ **Related entries: Adult Meltus Night Time; Benadryl Skin Allergy Relief Cream; Benadryl Skin Allergy Relief Lotion;Benylin Chesty Coughs (Original); Benylin Children's Night Coughs; Benylin Cough and Congestion; Benylin Day and Night; Benylin Dry Coughs (Original); Benylin Four Flu Liquid; Benylin Four Flu Tablets; Benylin with Codeine; Bronalin Expectorant Linctus; Bronalin Junior Linctus; Covonia Night Time Formula; Histalix Syrup; Histergan Cream; Histergan Syrup; Junior Meltus Night Time; Medised Infant; Nytol; Nytol One-a-Night; Panadol Night; Paxidorm Syrup; Paxidorm Tablets; Propain Caplets; Tixycolds Syrup.**

diphenoxylate hydrochloride
is an (OPIOID) ANTIDIARRHOEAL drug which is used to treat diarrhoea. It is commonly used in combination with atropine sulphate to form a preparation known as CO-PHENOTROPE.
✚ Side-effects: See OPIOID; overdosage causes sedation. Prolonged use may lead to impaired gastrointestinal function and eventual dependence.
✪ **Related entries: co-phenotrope; Diarphen; Lomotil; Tropergen.**

diphosphonate

see BISPHOSPHONATE.

Diphtheria Antitoxin

(Communicable Disease Surveillance Centre) (Dip/Ser) is a proprietary, prescription-only preparation of diphtheria antitoxin. It can be used to treat suspected cases of diphtheria, and is available in a form for injection.

✚▲ Side-effects/warnings: See IMMUNIZATION.

diphtheria antitoxin

(Dip/Ser) is a preparation that neutralizes the toxins produced by diphtheria bacteria (*Corynebacterium diphtheriae*). It is not used for prevention (most people will have been immunized to diphtheria; see IMMUNIZATION), but only to provide *passive immunity* to people who have been exposed to suspected outbreaks or contact with patients infected with diphtheria. Since the antitoxin is produced in horses, hypersensitivity reactions are common. Administration is by injection. (See also DIPHTHERIA VACCINE.)

✚▲ Side-effects/warnings: See IMMUNIZATION.

✪ **Related entry: Diphtheria Antitoxin.**

diphtheria vaccine

for IMMUNIZATION is a VACCINE preparation of inactivated, but still antigenic, toxins (toxoid) of the diphtheria bacteria *Corynebacterium diphtheriae* that provides active immunity to diphtheria. This particular vaccine works mainly by promoting development of antitoxins (see ANTITOXIN) in the individual (ie that bind to and inactivate the *toxin* produced by the bacterium – rather than the bacterium itself). In most instances, it is not administered alone, but as a constituent in the *triple vaccine* ADSORBED DIPHTHERIA, TETANUS AND PERTUSSIS VACCINE (DTPer/Vac/Ads), or as a *double vaccine* ADSORBED DIPHTHERIA AND TETANUS VACCINE (DT/Vac/Ads). They are used for the primary immunization of children. Administration is by injection.

✚▲ Side-effects/warnings: See VACCINE.

✪ **Related entries: ACT-HIB DTP dc; Adsorbed Diphtheria and Tetanus Vaccine; Adsorbed Diphtheria and Tetanus Vaccine for Adolescents and Adults; Adsorbed Diphtheria, Tetanus and Pertussis Vaccine; Adsorbed Diphtheria, Tetanus and [whole-cell] Pertussis Vaccine; Adsorbed Diphtheria Vaccine; Adsorbed Diphtheria Vaccine for Adults and Adolescents; Adsorbed Diphtheria Vaccine for Adults and Adolescents; Diftavax; Infanrix-HIB.**

dipipanone

is a rapidly acting and powerful (OPIOID) NARCOTIC ANALGESIC. It is used in combination with an ANTI-EMETIC (the antihistamine cyclizine) to relieve short-term, moderate and severe pain. Its proprietary form is on the Controlled Drugs list. Administration (in the form of dipipanone hydrochloride) is oral.

✚▲ Side-effects/warnings: See OPIOID. It is less sedating than morphine.

✪ **Related entry: Diconal.**

dipivefrine hydrochloride

is a derivative of the SYMPATHOMIMETIC adrenaline and is a pro-drug that is converted in the body into adrenaline. It is used in GLAUCOMA TREATMENT to reduce intraocular pressure (pressure in the eyeball) and is administered instead of adrenaline because it is thought to pass more rapidly through the cornea. Administration is topical.

✚▲ Side-effects/warnings: See ADRENALINE.

✪ **Related entry: Propine.**

dipotassium clorazepate

see CLORAZEPATE DIPOTASSIUM.

Diprobath

(Schering-Plough) is a proprietary, non-prescription preparation of liquid paraffin (and isopropyl myristate). It can be used as an EMOLLIENT for dry skin conditions, including dermatitis and eczema. It is available as a bath oil.

✚▲ Side-effects/warnings: See LIQUID PARAFFIN.

Diprosalic

(Schering-Plough) is a proprietary, prescription-only compound preparation of the CORTICOSTEROID and ANTI-INFLAMMATORY betamethasone (as dipropionate) and the KERATOLYTIC salicylic acid. It can be used to treat severe inflammatory skin disorders, such as eczema and psoriasis. It is available as an ointment and a scalp lotion for topical application.

✚▲ Side-effects/warnings: See BETAMETHASONE; SALICYLIC ACID.

D

Diprosone
(Schering-Plough) is a proprietary, prescription-only preparation of the CORTICOSTEROID and ANTI-INFLAMMATORY betamethasone (as dipropionate). It can be used to treat severe inflammatory skin disorders, such as eczema and psoriasis. It is available as a cream, an ointment and a lotion for topical application.
✚▲ Side-effects/warnings: See BETAMETHASONE.

Dip/Ser
is an abbreviation for DIPHTHERIA ANTITOXIN.

dipyridamole
is an ANTIPLATELET (antithrombotic) drug which is used to prevent thrombosis (blood-clot formation), but does not have an ANTICOAGULANT action. It seems to work by stopping platelets sticking to one another or to surgically inserted tubes and valves (particularly artificial heart valves). Administration is either oral or by injection.
✚ Side-effects: There may be gastrointestinal disturbances, headache and low blood pressure, increased heart rate, muscle ache, hot flushes, rash and itching.
▲ Warnings: It may cause hypotension or worsen migraine. There may be dangerous interactions with adenosine (which is used in heart conditions as an anti-arrhythmic). Administer with caution to patients with certain heart disorders.
✪ Related entries: Asasantin Retard; Cerebrovase; Persantin.

Dirythmin SA
(AstraZeneca) is a proprietary, prescription-only preparation of the ANTI-ARRHYTHMIC disopyramide (as disopyramide phosphate), and is available as modified-release tablets (*Durules*).
✚▲ Side-effects/warnings: See DISOPYRAMIDE.

disinfectant 🅱
agents are used to destroy micro-organisms, or inhibit their activity to such extent that they are less or no longer harmful to health. The term can be applied to agents used on inanimate objects (including surgical equipment, catheters etc.) as well as to preparations that are used to treat the skin and living tissue (although in the latter case the name ANTISEPTIC is often used instead). Examples include CETRIMIDE, CHLORHEXIDINE, HEXACHLOROPHANE, GLUTARALDEHYDE, PHENOL, POTASSIUM PERMANGANATE, POVIDONE-IODINE, SODIUM HYPOCHLORITE and TRICLOSAN.

Disipal
(Yamanouchi) is a proprietary, prescription-only preparation of the ANTICHOLINERGIC orphenadrine hydrochloride. It can be used to relieve some of the symptoms of parkinsonism, especially muscle rigidity and the tendency to produce an excess of saliva (see ANTIPARKINSONISM). It also has the capacity to treat these conditions, in some cases, where they are produced by drugs. It is available as tablets.
✚▲ Side-effects/warnings: See ORPHENADRINE HYDROCHLORIDE.

disodium etidronate
is a CALCIUM METABOLISM MODIFIER, a BISPHOSPHONATE used to treat disorders of bone metabolism due to HORMONE disorders, to prevent and treat osteoporosis in post-menopausal women, to prevent and treat osteoporosis caused by corticosteroid treatment, and to treat Paget's disease of the bone. It is also available in a compound preparation with calcium carbonate to prevent or treat osteoporosis in postmenopausal women (where HRT is not suitable) and corticosteroid-induced osteoporosis. Administration is either oral or by injection.
✚ Side-effects: These include nausea and diarrhoea, skin reactions, abdominal pain and constipation, headache. With high dosage, there may be increased bone pain and the risk of fractures.
▲ Warnings: Administer with caution to patients with certain kidney disorders. It is not for use in pregnancy or breast-feeding. Food should be avoided two hours before and after taking disodium etidronate.
✪ Related entries: Didronel; Didronel PMO.

disodium pamidronate
(formerly called aminohydroxypropylidenediphosphonate disodium (APD)) is a CALCIUM METABOLISM MODIFIER, a BISPHOSPHONATE used to treat disorders of bone metabolism due to HORMONE disorders and malignant tumour-induced high blood calcium levels (hypercalcaemia) including Paget's disease of the bone and pain due to bone

metastases secondary to cancers including breast cancer. Administration is by injection.

✚ Side-effects: There may be nausea and diarrhoea, low blood calcium, gastrointestinal and blood upsets and transient fever. Also flu-like symptoms, bone and muscle pain, headache, dizziness, tiredness, rash and others.

▲ Warnings: Administer with caution to patients with certain kidney or heart disorders, or who have had thyroid surgery. It is not for use in pregnancy or breast-feeding. Because it may cause dizziness or sleepiness, patients should not drive or operate machinery immediately after treatment.

✪ **Related entry: Aredia Dry Powder.**

disopyramide

is an ANTI-ARRHYTHMIC drug which is used to regularize the heartbeat, especially ventricular arrhythmias following a heart attack (myocardial infarction). Administration, as disopyramide or disopyramide phosphate, can be either oral or by slow intravenous injection or infusion.

✚ Side-effects: There may be hypotension, gastrointestinal disturbances, dry mouth, blurred vision, urinary retention and effects on the heart.

▲ Warnings: It should be administered with caution to patients with certain kidney or liver disorders, glaucoma or who are pregnant or breast-feeding. It should not be given to patients with certain heart disorders.

✪ **Related entries: Dirythmin SA; Rythmodan; Rythmodan Retard.**

Disprin

(Reckitt Benckiser Healthcare) is a proprietary, non-prescription preparation of the (NSAID) NON-NARCOTIC ANALGESIC and ANTIRHEUMATIC aspirin. It can be used to treat mild to moderate pain and to relieve flu and cold symptoms, rheumatism and lumbago. It is available as soluble tablets and is not normally given to children, except on medical advice.

✚▲ Side-effects/warnings: See ASPIRIN.

Disprin Direct

(Reckitt Benckiser Healthcare) is a proprietary, non-prescription preparation of the (NSAID) NON-NARCOTIC ANALGESIC and ANTIRHEUMATIC aspirin. It can be used to treat mild to moderate pain, to relieve flu and cold symptoms and feverishness, and pain from headaches, migraine and period pain. It is available as tablets to be dispersed under the tongue and is not normally given to children, except on medical advice.

✚▲ Side-effects/warnings: See ASPIRIN.

Disprin Extra

(Reckitt Benckiser Healthcare) is a proprietary, non-prescription compound analgesic preparation of the (NSAID) NON-NARCOTIC ANALGESIC and ANTIRHEUMATIC aspirin and the non-narcotic analgesic paracetamol. It can be used to treat mild to moderate pain, relieve rheumatic aches and pains and flu and cold symptoms. It is available as tablets and is not normally given to children, except on medical advice.

✚▲ Side-effects/warnings: See ASPIRIN; PARACETAMOL.

Disprol Paracetamol Suspension

(Reckitt Benckiser Healthcare) is a proprietary, non-prescription preparation of the NON-NARCOTIC ANALGESIC and ANTIPYRETIC paracetamol. It can be used to treat mild to moderate pain (including teething), relieve flu and cold symptoms and feverishness, and to reduce high body temperature, for example after vaccination. It is available as a suspension (and in sachets) and is not normally given to children under three months, except for babies who develop fever after vaccination.

✚▲ Side-effects/warnings: See PARACETAMOL.

Disprol Soluble Paracetamol Tablets

(Reckitt Benckiser Healthcare) is a proprietary, non-prescription preparation of the NON-NARCOTIC ANALGESIC and ANTIPYRETIC paracetamol (for children). It can be used to treat mild to moderate pain (including teething), relieve flu and cold symptoms, feverishness and to reduce high body temperature. It is available as effervescent tablets and is not normally given to children under one year, except on medical advice.

✚▲ Side-effects/warnings: See PARACETAMOL.

Distaclor

(Dista; Lilly) is a proprietary, prescription-only preparation of the ANTIBACTERIAL and (CEPHALOSPORIN) ANTIBIOTIC cefaclor (as monohydrate). It can be used to treat a wide range of bacterial infections, eg pneumonia and

urinary tract infections. It is available as capsules and an oral suspension.
✚▲ Side-effects/warnings: See CEFACLOR.

Distaclor MR

(Dista; Lilly) is a proprietary, prescription-only preparation of the ANTIBACTERIAL and (CEPHALOSPORIN) ANTIBIOTIC cefaclor (as monohydrate). It can be used to treat a wide range of bacterial infections (eg pneumonia, urinary tract), and is available as modified-release tablets.
✚▲ Side-effects/warnings: See CEFACLOR.

Distalgesic

(Dista; Lilly) is a proprietary, prescription-only compound analgesic preparation of the (OPIOID) NARCOTIC ANALGESIC dextropropoxyphene hydrochloride and the NON-NARCOTIC ANALGESIC paracetamol (a combination known as CO-PROXAMOL). It can be used to relieve pain, and is available as tablets.
✚▲ Side-effects/warnings: See DEXTROPROPOXYPHENE HYDROCHLORIDE; PARACETAMOL.

Distamine

(Dista; Lilly) is a proprietary, prescription-only preparation of the CHELATING AGENT penicillamine. It can be used as an ANTIDOTE to copper or lead poisoning, as a METABOLIC DISORDER TREATMENT to reduce copper levels in Wilson's disease, also in severe rheumatoid arthritis. It is available as tablets.
✚▲ Side-effects/warnings: See PENICILLAMINE.

distigmine bromide

is an ANTICHOLINESTERASE drug which enhances the effects of the neurotransmitter acetylcholine (and certain cholinergic drugs). Because of this, it has PARASYMPATHOMIMETIC actions and can be used to stimulate the bladder to treat certain types of urinary retention. It can also be used to treat the neuromuscular transmission disorder *myasthenia gravis*. Administration is oral.
✚▲ Side-effects/warnings: See NEOSTIGMINE. It should be administered with caution to patients with hyperthyroidism.
✪ **Related entry: Ubretid.**

disulfiram

is an ENZYME INHIBITOR, which blocks a stage in the breakdown of ETHYL ALCOHOL (ethanol) in the body with a resultant accumulation in a metabolite (acetaldehyde). If even only a very small amount of alcohol is taken, disulfiram causes very unpleasant reactions – such as flushing, headache, palpitations, nausea and vomiting. Therefore, if an alcoholic takes disulfiram on a regular basis there is a powerful disincentive to drink alcoholic beverages. Administration is oral.
✚ Side-effects: Initially there may be drowsiness and fatigue; nausea and vomiting; bad breath, reduced libido; rarely, there may be psychiatric problems, skin reactions, peripheral nerve and liver damage.
▲ Warnings: It is a specialist drug and a full assessment and counselling will be carried out before prescription. The effects that disulphiram causes, if even a small amount of alcohol is taken, are potentially very dangerous, so simultaneous use of medications or toiletries containing forms of alcohol should also be avoided.
✪ **Related entry: Antabuse.**

Dithranol Ointment, BP

is a non-proprietary, prescription-only preparation of dithranol. It can be used for subacute and chronic psoriasis, and is available as an ointment. (Weaker than 1% dithranol ointment can be sold to the public without prescription.)
✚▲ Side-effects/warnings: See DITHRANOL.

Dithranol Paste, BP

is a non-proprietary, non-prescription preparation of dithranol. It can be used for subacute and chronic psoriasis, and is available as a paste.
✚▲ Side-effects/warnings: See DITHRANOL.

dithranol

is the most powerful drug presently used to treat chronic or milder forms of psoriasis in topical application and is incorporated into a number of preparations. Lesions are covered for a period with a dressing on which there is a preparation of dithranol in weak solution; the concentration is adjusted to suit individual response and tolerance of the associated skin irritation. It is thought to work by inhibiting cell division (antimitotic) and may be used in combination with a KERATOLYTIC or with agents that have a moisturizing effect (such as UREA). It may also be used in some preparations as dithranol triacetate. Application is topical (including as a scalp gel).

✚ Side-effects: Irritation and a local sensation of burning. Note that fair skin is more sensitive than dark.

▲ Warnings: It is not suitable for the treatment of acute forms of psoriasis. It stains skin, hair and fabrics. Avoid contact with healthy and sensitive areas of skin and the eyes.

✪ Related entries: Dithranol Ointment, BP; Dithranol Paste, BP; Dithrocream; Micanol; Psorin.

dithranol triacetate

see DITHRANOL.

Dithrocream

(Dermal) is a proprietary, non-prescription preparation of dithranol. It can be used to treat subacute and chronic psoriasis, and is available as an ointment in four strengths: 0.1% , 0.25%, 0.5% and 1%. A stronger version, 2%, is available only on prescription.

✚▲ Side-effects/warnings: See DITHRANOL.

Ditropan

(Sanofi-Synthelabo) is a proprietary, prescription-only preparation of the ANTICHOLINERGIC oxybutynin hydrochloride. It can be used as an ANTISPASMODIC in the treatment of urinary disorders such as incontinence, and is available as tablets and an elixir.

✚▲ Side-effects/warnings: See OXYBUTYNIN HYDROCHLORIDE.

Ditropan XL

(Sanofi-Synthelabo) s a proprietary, prescription-only preparation of the ANTICHOLINERGIC oxybutynin hydrochloride. It can be used as an ANTISPASMODIC in the treatment of urinary disorders, such as incontinence, and is available as modified-release tablets.

✚▲ Side-effects/warnings: See OXYBUTYNIN HYDROCHLORIDE.

Diumide-K Continus

(ASTA Medica) is a proprietary, prescription-only compound preparation of the (*loop*) DIURETIC furosemide (frusemide) and the potassium supplement POTASSIUM CHLORIDE. It can be used to treat oedema, and is available as tablets, which should be swallowed whole with plenty of fluid at mealtimes or when in an upright posture.

✚▲ Side-effects/warnings: See FUROSEMIDE; POTASSIUM CHLORIDE.

diuretic 🅳

drugs are used to reduce excess fluid in the body by increasing the excretion of water and mineral salts (sodium) by an action on the kidney, so increasing urine production (hence 'water tablets'). They have a wide range of uses, because oedema due to excess fluid in sites such as the lungs, ankles and eyeballs is a symptom of a number of disorders. Reducing oedema is, in itself, of benefit in some of these disorders; and diuretic drugs may be used in acute pulmonary (lung) oedema, congestive heart failure, some liver and kidney disorders, glaucoma and in certain electrolyte disturbances such as hypercalcaemia (raised calcium levels) and hyperkalaemia (raised potassium levels). Their most common use is as ANTIHYPERTENSIVE drugs, where their action of reducing oedema is of value in relieving the load on the heart, which then (over some days or weeks) gives way to a beneficial reduction in blood pressure (some of which appears to be associated with a VASODILATOR action).

In relation to their specific actions and uses, the diuretics are divided into a number of distinct classes. *Osmotic diuretics* (eg MANNITOL) are inert compounds secreted into the kidney proximal tubules and are not resorbed and therefore carry water and salts with them into the urine. *Loop diuretics* (eg FRUSEMIDE and BUMETANIDE) have a very vigorous action on the loop of Henlé (inhibiting resorption of sodium, chloride and water and also some potassium) and are used especially in heart failure. *Thiazide* and *thiazide-like* diuretics (eg HYDROCHLOROTHIAZIDE and XIPAMIDE) are the most commonly used and have a moderate action in inhibiting sodium reabsorption at the distal tubule of the kidney, allowing their prolonged use as antihypertensives. But they may cause potassium loss from the blood to the urine, which needs correction (sometimes through using preparations that combine the diuretic and a potassium salt in tablets). *Potassium-sparing*

D

diuretics (eg AMILORIDE HYDROCHLORIDE, TRIAMTERENE and SPIRONOLACTONE) have a weak action on the distal tubule of the kidney and – as the name suggests – cause retention of potassium, making them suitable for combination with some of the other diuretic classes and for some specific conditions. *Aldosterone antagonists* (eg potassium canrenoate and spironolactone) work by blocking the action of the normal mineralocorticoid hormone aldosterone, and this makes them suitable for treating oedema associated with aldosteronism, liver failure and certain heart conditions. *Carbonic anhydrase inhibitors* (eg ACETAZOLAMIDE) are weak diuretics and are now rarely used to treat systemic oedema, though they are useful in reducing fluid in the anterior chamber of the eye which causes glaucoma. In the treatment of hypertension, diuretics are commonly used in combination with other classes of drugs, particularly the BETA-BLOCKER class.
▲ Warnings: Calcium salts (eg CALCIUM CARBONATE) or VITAMIN D should not be taken at the same time as thiazide diuretics because this can result in hypercalcaemia (high blood calcium levels). Potassium supplements (including potassium chloride used as a table salt substitute) should be avoided when taking potassium-sparing diuretics because there is a risk of hyperkalemia (high blood potassium levels).

Diurexan

(ASTA Medica) is a proprietary, prescription-only preparation of the (THIAZIDE-like) DIURETIC xipamide. It can be used, either alone or in conjunction with other drugs, in the treatment of oedema and as an ANTIHYPERTENSIVE. Available as tablets.
✚▲ Side-effects/warnings: See XIPAMIDE.

Dixarit

(Boehringer Ingelheim) is a proprietary, prescription-only preparation of the ANTISYMPATHETIC clonidine hydrochloride. It can be used in ANTIMIGRAINE treatment for reducing the frequency of attacks, and is available as tablets.
✚▲ Side-effects/warnings: See CLONIDINE HYDROCHLORIDE.

dobutamine hydrochloride

is a CARDIAC STIMULANT with BETA-RECEPTOR STIMULANT (SYMPATHOMIMETIC) and DOPAMINE-RECEPTOR STIMULANT properties. It is used to treat serious heart disorders, including cardiogenic shock, septic shock, during open-heart surgery and in cardiac infarction. It works by increasing the heart's force of contraction. Administration is by intravenous infusion.
✚▲ Side-effects/warnings: It is a specialist drug used under hospital conditions.
✪ **Related entries: Dobutrex; Posiject.**

Dobutrex

(Lilly) is a proprietary, prescription-only preparation of the CARDIAC STIMULANT dobutamine hydrochloride, which has SYMPATHOMIMETIC and BETA-RECEPTOR STIMULANT properties. It can be used to treat serious heart disorders, including cardiogenic shock, septic shock, during heart surgery and in cardiac infarction. It works by increasing the heart's force of contraction. It is available in a form for intravenous infusion.
✚▲ Side-effects/warnings: See DOBUTAMINE HYDROCHLORIDE.

docetaxel

is a CYTOTOXIC drug, the first of a new group of drugs termed the *taxanes*, which is used as an ANTICANCER treatment of (anthracycline-resistant) breast cancer and non-small cell lung cancer. Administration is by intravenous infusion.
✚▲ Side-effects/warnings: See CYTOTOXIC. Also fluid retention (eg leg oedema) may be marked.
✪ **Related entry: Taxotere.**

docusate sodium

(dioctyl sodium sulphosuccinate) is a weak (SURFACTANT) LAXATIVE, with both *stimulant* and *faecal softener* properties. It is particularly effective when combined in preparations with DANTHRON. It is used to relieve constipation and also to evacuate the rectum prior to abdominal radiological procedures. It is a constituent of many proprietary compound laxatives because it seems to have few adverse side-effects. It works like a surfactant, by applying a very thin film of low surface tension (similar to a detergent) over the surface of the intestinal wall. It can also be used to dissolve and remove earwax and is a constituent of proprietary ear-drop preparations. Administration is either oral or topical (eg by enema).

✚ Side-effects: It may cause abdominal cramps.

▲ Warnings: Rectal preparations should not be used in patients with haemorrhoids or an anal fissures.

✪ **Related entries: co-danthrusate 50/60; Capsuvac; Dioctyl; Docusol; Fletchers' Enemette; Molcer Ear Drops; Norgalax Micro-enema; Normax; Waxsol Ear Drops.**

Docusol

(Typharm) is a proprietary, non-prescription preparation of the (*stimulant*) LAXATIVE docusate sodium. It can be used to relieve constipation and also to evacuate the rectum prior to abdominal procedures. It is available as a syrup (in two strengths, the weaker one is for children).

✚▲ Side-effects/warnings: See DOCUSATE SODIUM.

Do-Do Chesteze

(Novartis Consumer Health) is a proprietary, non-prescription compound preparation of the SYMPATHOMIMETIC and DECONGESTANT ephedrine hydrochloride, the BRONCHODILATOR theophylline (anhydrous) and the STIMULANT caffeine. It can be used to relieve bronchial cough, wheezing and breathlessness, and to help clear the chest after infections. It is available as tablets and is not normally given to children under 12 years, except on medical advice.

✚▲ Side-effects/warnings: See CAFFEINE; EPHEDRINE HYDROCHLORIDE; THEOPHYLLINE.

Dolmatil

(Sanofi-Synthelabo) is a proprietary, prescription-only preparation of the ANTIPSYCHOTIC sulpiride. It can be used to treat schizophrenia and also other conditions that may cause tremor, tics, involuntary movements or utterances (such as in Gilles de la Tourette syndrome). It is available as tablets.

✚▲ Side-effects/warnings: See SULPIRIDE.

Dolobid

(MSD) is a proprietary, prescription-only preparation of the (NSAID) NON-NARCOTIC ANALGESIC and ANTIRHEUMATIC diflunisal. It can be used to treat moderate to mild pain, the pain of rheumatic disease and other musculoskeletal disorders and period pain. It is available as tablets. (Antacid tablets containing aluminium hydroxide should be avoided since they interfere with absorption of preparations of Dolobid.)

✚▲ Side-effects/warnings: See DIFLUNISAL.

Doloxene

(Lilly) is a proprietary, prescription-only preparation of the (OPIOID) NARCOTIC ANALGESIC dextropropoxyphene hydrochloride. It can be used to treat mild to moderate pain, and is available as capsules.

✚▲ Side-effects/warnings: See DEXTROPROPOXYPHENE HYDROCHLORIDE.

domiphen bromide

is an ANTISEPTIC which is used as a mouthwash or gargle for oral hygiene, and is available as lozenges.

✚▲ Side-effects/warnings: Considered safe in normal topical use at recommended concentrations.

✪ **Related entry: Bradosol Plus (Sugar Free).**

Domperamol

(Servier) is a proprietary, prescription-only compound preparation of the ANTI-EMETIC and ANTINAUSEANT domperidone (as maleate) and the NON-NARCOTIC ANALGESIC paracetamol. It can be used as an ANTIMIGRAINE treatment for acute mild to moderate migraine attacks, and is available as tablets.

✚▲ Side-effects/warnings: See DOMPERIDONE; PARACETAMOL.

domperidone

is an ANTI-EMETIC and ANTINAUSEANT which is thought to work, in part, as a DOPAMINE-RECEPTOR ANTAGONIST, and is used particularly to relieve nausea and vomiting in patients undergoing treatment with CYTOTOXIC drugs. It is also used to prevent vomiting in patients treated for parkinsonism with the drugs levodopa or bromocriptine and to relieve nausea associated with migraine attacks. It hastens emptying of the stomach (so is a motility stimulant), so helps to protect against stomach acid escaping upwards into the gullet and can be used to treat heartburn and dyspepsia. Administration is either oral or topical (as suppositories).

✚ Side-effects: Occasionally, spontaneous milk production in women or the development of feminine breasts in men may occur; rashes and changes in libido.

▲ Warnings: It should be administered with

caution to those who suffer from impaired kidney function, or who are pregnant or breast-feeding. May cause acute dystonic reactions (especially in young females and children).
✪ **Related entries: Domperamol; Motilium; Motilium 10.**

donepezil

is an ANTICHOLINESTERASE used for the symptomatic treatment of mild to moderate dementia of Alzheimer's disease. It is thought only to slow the rate of cognitive deterioration in about half of patients treated. Authorities have identified those patients that may benefit by assessing what is known as a mini mental-state examination (MMSE) score. Diagnosis and treatment is initiated by specialists with assessment throughout treatment. It is available in a form for oral administration.
✚ Side-effects: Diarrhoea, muscle cramps, less frequently nausea, vomiting, fatigue, insomnia, dizziness; effects on the heart and gastrointestinal systems, and psychiatric disturbances.
▲ Warnings: It should be used with care in certain heart conduction abnormalities; in patients at risk of developing peptic ulcers; in obstructive airways disease (including asthma); and avoided in pregnancy or breast-feeding.
✪ **Related entry: Aricept**

Dopacard

(Elan) is a proprietary, prescription-only preparation of the CARDIAC STIMULANT dopexamine hydrochloride. It can be used for the treatment of heart conditions where moderate stimulation of the force of heartbeat with vasodilatation is required in heart failure associated with heart surgery. It is available in a form for intravenous infusion.
✚▲ Side-effects/warnings: See DOPEXAMINE HYDROCHLORIDE.

dopamine

is a neurotransmitter and is chemically a catecholamine (like ADRENALINE and NORADRENALINE). It is both an intermediate product in the biosynthetic pathway in the brain and sympathetic nervous system that manufactures and stores noradrenaline and adrenaline, and a neurotransmitter in its own right in relaying nerve messages. It is particularly concentrated in the brain and in the adrenal glands. It is possible that some psychoses may in part be caused by abnormalities in the metabolism of dopamine, because drugs that prevent some of its actions (DOPAMINE-RECEPTOR ANTAGONIST drugs; eg CHLORPROMAZINE HYDROCHLORIDE, HALOPERIDOL, PIMOZIDE) can be used as ANTIPSYCHOTIC drugs to relieve some schizophrenic symptoms. Conversely, drugs that lead to increased dopamine production or concentrations in the brain (eg LEVODOPA) play an important part in the therapy of parkinsonism and drugs that mimic some aspects of the action of dopamine in the brain (eg BROMOCRIPTINE) can be used both for ANTIPARKINSONISM treatment and to relieve a number of hormone disorders. In the periphery (that is, in the body rather than the brain), DOPAMINE HYDROCHLORIDE may be administered therapeutically as a CARDIAC STIMULANT in the treatment of the cardiogenic shock associated with a myocardial infarction or heart surgery, when its beneficial actions are thought to result partly through actions as a BETA-RECEPTOR STIMULANT in the heart and partly at dopamine receptors in blood vessels.

dopamine hydrochloride

is the chemical form of the naturally occurring DOPAMINE that is used in medicine as a CARDIAC STIMULANT in the treatment of cardiogenic shock associated with cardiac infarction or heart surgery. Administration is by intravenous infusion.
✚▲ Side-effects/warnings: It is a specialist drug used under hospital conditions.
✪ **Related entry: Select-A-Jet Dopamine.**

dopamine-receptor antagonist

agents act to block or prevent the actions of DOPAMINE in the body. In practice they are only used to act against natural (endogenous) dopamine acting as a neurotransmitter, mainly in the brain. It is likely that some psychoses involve abnormalities in the production, metabolism or actions of dopamine, and because of this, drugs such as the dopamine-receptor antagonists that reduce the influence of dopamine in certain nerve pathways in the brain can be used as ANTIPSYCHOTIC drugs to relieve some schizophrenic symptoms (eg CHLORPROMAZINE HYDROCHLORIDE, HALOPERIDOL, PIMOZIDE).

Because the balance of neurotransmitters in the brain is in a finely tuned state, there is a price to pay for interference with this, and drugs used to treat a neurological or psychological disorder illness, inevitably have some undesirable side-effects. Dopamine is closely involved in mediating other body functions apart from mood, especially in controlling motor (muscle) co-ordination, and because of this, dopamine antagonist antipsychotic drugs cause many important and unpleasant side-effects, of which some resemble Parkinson's disease (a condition whose pathology largely results from a depletion of dopamine in the brain). There are other uses for dopamine receptor antagonists, for instance DOMPERIDONE is an ANTI-EMETIC and ANTI-NAUSEANT which is thought to work, in part, as a dopamine receptor antagonist, and is used particularly to relieve nausea and vomiting in patients undergoing treatment with CYTOTOXIC drugs.

dopamine-receptor stimulant 🅴

drugs act to mimic the actions of DOPAMINE in the body, where it is a neurotransmitter, mainly in the brain. Some such drugs act directly at dopamine RECEPTORS and others act indirectly leading to increased dopamine production or concentrations in the brain. The most important example of the latter is LEVODOPA which is converted into dopamine in the body, and which is very extensively used in ANTIPARKINSONISM treatment (it works because in Parkinson's disease there is shortage of dopamine in the brain). There are also therapeutic drugs that act directly on dopamine receptors, notably BROMOCRIPTINE (also CABERGOLINE, LISURIDE MALEATE, PERGOLIDE, PRAMIPEXOLE, QUINAGOLIDE, ROPINIROLE) which may also be used in antiparkinsonism treatment, as well as in the treatment and relief of a number of hormone disorders. In the periphery (that is, in the body rather than the brain), DOPAMINE HYDRO-CHLORIDE may be administered therapeutically as a CARDIAC STIMULANT in the treatment of the cardiogenic shock associated with a myocardial infarction or heart surgery, when its beneficial actions are thought to result partly through actions as a BETA-RECEPTOR STIMULANT in the heart and partly at dopamine receptors in blood vessels. The dopamine analogues DOPEXAMINE HYDROCHLORIDE and DOBUTAMINE HYDRO-CHLORIDE have similar cardiac stimulant actions.

dopexamine hydrochloride

is a CARDIAC STIMULANT that is used for the treatment of heart conditions where moderate stimulation of the force of heartbeat with vasodilatation is required, such as in heart failure associated with heart surgery. Its beneficial actions are thought to result partly through actions as a BETA-RECEPTOR STIMULANT in the heart and partly as a DOPAMINE-RECEPTOR STIMULANT in peripheral blood vessels which beneficially increases kidney perfusion. It is available in a form for intravenous infusion.
✚▲ Side-effects/warnings: It is a specialist drug used under hospital conditions.
✪ **Related entry: Dopacard.**

Dopram

(Anpharm) is a proprietary, prescription-only preparation of the RESPIRATORY STIMULANT doxapram hydrochloride. It can be used to relieve severe respiratory difficulties in patients with chronic obstructive airways disease or who undergo respiratory depression following major surgery, under specialist conditions. It is available in a form for intravenous infusion or injection.
✚▲ Side-effects/warnings: See DOXAPRAM HYDROCHLORIDE.

Doralese

(SmithKline Beecham; GSK) is a proprietary, prescription-only preparation of the ALPHA-ADRENOCEPTOR BLOCKER indoramin. It can be used to treat urinary retention, for example, in benign prostatic hyperplasia. Available as tablets.
✚▲ Side-effects/warnings: See INDORAMIN.

dornase alfa

is a version, manufactured by genetic engineering, of a naturally occurring human enzyme which breaks down deoxyribonucleic acid (DNA) and is used in cystic fibrosis to improve lung function. It is given by inhalation.
✚ Side-effects: There may be inflammation of the pharynx with voice changes, chest pain; occasionally laryngitis, rashes and conjunctivitis.
▲ Warnings: Use with caution in pregnancy.
✪ **Related entry: Pulmozyme.**

dorzolamide

is a CARBONIC-ANHYDRASE INHIBITOR which is used in GLAUCOMA TREATMENT because it reduces the formation of aqueous humour in the eye, and ocular hypertension, alone, or in combination with BETA-BLOCKER drugs. Administration is topical.

✚ Side-effects: Blurred vision, stinging, burning and itching of the eye, tear formation; eyelid inflammation and conjunctivitis; headache and nausea; rarely rash and certain other side-effects reported; bitter taste from drug travelling down the lacrimal duct to the back of the mouth.

▲ Warnings: It should not be administered to patients who are pregnant or breast-feeding. There may be systemic absorption after using as eye-drops. It should not be used in liver or severe kidney impairment, or in certain disorders where there are raised levels of chloride in the blood.

✪ **Related entries: Cosopt; Trusopt.**

Dostinex

(Pharmacia & Upjohn; Pharmacia) is a proprietary, prescription-only preparation of cabergoline. It is used in ANTIPARKINSONISM treatment, also it may be used to treat a number of other hormonal disorders. It is available as tablets.

✚▲ Side-effects/warnings: See CABERGOLINE.

dosulepin hydrochloride

(dothiepin hydrochloride) is an ANTIDEPRESSANT of the TRICYCLIC group. It can be used to treat depressive illness, especially in cases where some degree of sedation is required. Administration is oral.

✚▲ Side-effects/warnings: See AMITRIPTYLINE HYDROCHLORIDE.

✪ **Related entries: Dothapax; Prepadine; Prothiaden.**

Dothapax

(Ashbourne) is a proprietary, prescription-only preparation of the (TRICYCLIC) ANTIDEPRESSANT dosulepin hydrochloride. It can be used to treat depressive illness, especially in cases where some degree of sedation is required. It is available as tablets and capsules.

✚▲ Side-effects/warnings: See DOSULEPIN HYDROCHLORIDE.

dothiepin hydrochloride

see DOSULEPIN HYDROCHLORIDE.

Doublebase

(Dermal) is a proprietary, non-prescription preparation of liquid paraffin (and isopropyl myristate). It can be used as an EMOLLIENT for dry chapped or itchy skin conditions, and is available as a gel.

✚▲ Side-effects/warnings: See LIQUID PARAFFIN.

Dovonex

(Leo) is a proprietary, prescription-only preparation of calcipotriol. It can be used for plaque psoriasis, and is available as an ointment, a cream and a scalp solution.

✚▲ Side-effects/warnings: See CALCIPOTRIOL.

doxapram hydrochloride

is a RESPIRATORY STIMULANT (analeptic) which is used to relieve severe respiratory difficulties in patients who suffer from chronic obstructive airways disease, or who undergo respiratory depression following major surgery in hospital. Administration is by injection or intravenous infusion.

✚▲ Side-effects/warnings: Increase in blood pressure and heart rate, dizziness, sweating and others. It is used under specialist conditions.

✪ **Related entry: Dopram.**

doxazosin

is a selective ALPHA-ADRENOCEPTOR BLOCKER which is used as an ANTIHYPERTENSIVE, often in conjunction with other antihypertensives (eg BETA-BLOCKER or (THIAZIDE) DIURETIC drugs). It can also be used to treat urinary retention in benign prostatic hyperplasia (BPH). Administration is oral.

✚ Side-effects: Postural hypotension; dizziness and vertigo, headache, fatigue, muscle weakness, oedema, sleepiness, nausea, rhinitis. Less frequently there may be abdominal discomfort, diarrhoea and vomiting, agitation, muscle tremor, rash and pruritus. Rarely, there may be blurred vision, nose-bleed, blood changes, liver problems and jaundice, urinary incontinence; prolonged erection and impotence reported.

▲ Warnings: Because of postural hypotension, care is needed with initial dosing; caution in liver impairment; pregnancy or breast-feeding.

✪ **Related entry: Cardura; Cardura XL.**

doxepin

is an ANTIDEPRESSANT of the TRICYCLIC group. It can be used, as doxepin hydrochloride, to treat depressive illness, especially in cases where some degree of sedation is required, when administration is oral. Also, since it also acts as an ANTIHISTAMINE, it may be used in the form of a cream for the treatment of pruritus (itching) associated with eczema.

✚▲ Side-effects/warnings: See AMITRIPTYLINE HYDROCHLORIDE. It should not be used if breast-feeding. When used as a cream, side-effects should be relatively minor though there may be skin sensitization, also sufficient may be absorbed to cause drowsiness, so performance of skilled tasks, eg driving, may be affected. Avoid application to large skin areas.

✪ **Related entries: Sinequan; Xepin.**

doxorubicin hydrochloride

is a CYTOTOXIC drug (an ANTIBIOTIC in origin) which is used as an ANTICANCER treatment particularly for acute leukaemia, lymphomas and some solid tumours and Kaposi's sarcoma in AIDS patients. Administration is by injection, intravenous infusion or bladder instillation.

✚▲ Side-effects/warnings: See CYTOTOXIC. Administer with care to patients with cardiovascular disease because it has effects on the heart.

✪ **Related entries: Caelyx; Doxorubicin Rapid Dissolution; Doxorubicin Solution for Injection.**

Doxorubicin Rapid Dissolution

(Pharmacia) is a proprietary, prescription-only preparation of the ANTICANCER drug doxorubicin hydrochloride. It is used to treat a range of cancers, and is available in a form for intravenous injection.

✚▲ Side-effects/warnings: See DOXORUBICIN HYDROCHLORIDE.

Doxorubicin Solution for Injection

(Pharmacia) is a proprietary, prescription-only preparation of the (CYTOTOXIC) ANTICANCER drug doxorubicin hydrochloride. It is used to treat a range of cancers, and is available in a form for intravenous injection.

✚▲ Side-effects/warnings: See DOXORUBICIN HYDROCHLORIDE.

doxycycline

is a broad-spectrum ANTIBACTERIAL and ANTIBIOTIC drug which is one of the TETRACYCLINES. It can be used to treat many kinds of infection, for example, of the respiratory and genital tracts, acne, chronic sinusitis, prostatitis and Lyme disease. It can also be used, in combination with other drugs, to treat brucellosis and pelvic inflammatory disease, and skin rosacea. It is also used as an ANTIMALARIAL in the prophylaxis of malaria. Administration is oral.

✚▲ Side-effects/warnings: See TETRACYCLINE; it can be used in patients with kidney impairment, but not with porphyria.

✪ **Related entries: Cyclodox; Demix; Doxylar; Vibramycin; Vibramycin D.**

doxylamine

is an ANTIHISTAMINE which is incorporated into a proprietary ANALGESIC and 'cold-cure' preparations. Administration is oral.

✚▲ Side-effects/warnings: See ANTIHISTAMINE.

✪ **Related entries: Syndol; Vicks Medinite.**

Doxylar

(Lagap) is a proprietary, prescription-only preparation of the ANTIBACTERIAL and (TETRACYCLINES) ANTIBIOTIC doxycycline. It can be used to treat infections of many kinds, and is available as capsules.

✚▲ Side-effects/warnings: See DOXYCYCLINE.

Dozic

(Rosemont) is a proprietary, prescription-only preparation of the ANTIPSYCHOTIC haloperidol. It can be used to treat psychoses, such as schizophrenia. It can also be used in the short-term treatment of severe anxiety and to treat some involuntary motor disturbances (and also intractable hiccup). It is available as an oral liquid.

✚▲ Side-effects/warnings: See HALOPERIDOL.

Drapolene Cream

(Warner Lambert Consumer Healthcare; Pfizer) is a proprietary, non-prescription compound preparation of the ANTISEPTIC benzalkonium chloride and cetrimide. It can be used to relieve nappy rash, the effects of the weather and to dress minor burns and wounds. It is available as a cream.

✚▲ Side-effects/warnings: See BENZALKONIUM CHLORIDE; CETRIMIDE.

Driclor

(Stiefel) is a proprietary, non-prescription

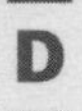

preparation of the ANTIPERSPIRANT aluminium chloride (as hexahydrate). It can be used as an antiperspirant to treat hyperhidrosis (excessive sweating), and is available in a roll-on applicator.
✚▲ Side-effects/warnings: See ALUMINIUM CHLORIDE.

Driclor Solution
(Stiefel) is a proprietary, non-prescription preparation of the ANTIPERSPIRANT aluminium chloride (as hexahydrate). It can be used as an antiperspirant to treat hyperhidrosis (excessive sweating), and is available as a solution.
✚▲ Side-effects/warnings: See ALUMINIUM CHLORIDE.

Dried Antithrombin III
(BPL) is a non-proprietary, prescription-only preparation of the natural ANTICOAGULANT antithrombin III concentrate. It can be used to treat a hereditary deficiency of this thrombin inhibitor and prevent thromboembolism, and is available in a form for intravenous infusion.
✚▲ Side-effects/warnings: See ANTITHROMBIN III CONCENTRATE.

Dried Tub/Vac/BCG
see BACILLUS CALMETTE-GUÉRIN VACCINE.

Dristan Nasal Spray
(Whitehall Laboratories) is a proprietary, non-prescription preparation of the SYMPATHOMIMETIC oxymetazoline hydrochloride. It can be used as a NASAL DECONGESTANT to relieve rhinitis in a head cold, and is available as a nasal spray. It is not normally given to children under six years, except on medical advice.
✚▲ Side-effects/warnings: See OXYMETAZOLINE HYDROCHLORIDE.

Drogenil
(Schering-Plough) is a proprietary, prescription-only preparation of the anti-androgen, HORMONE ANTAGONIST flutamide. It can be used as an ANTICANCER drug to treat cancer of the prostate. It is available as tablets.
✚▲ Side-effects/warnings: See FLUTAMIDE.

Dromadol SR
(IVAX) is a proprietary, prescription-only preparation of the (OPIOID) NARCOTIC ANALGESIC tramadol hydrochloride. It can be used to relieve pain, and is available as modified-release tablets.
✚▲ Side-effects/warnings: See TRAMADOL HYDROCHLORIDE.

Dromadol XL
(IVAX) is a proprietary, prescription-only preparation of the (OPIOID) NARCOTIC ANALGESIC tramadol hydrochloride. It can be used to relieve pain, and is available as modified-release tablets.
✚▲ Side-effects/warnings: See TRAMADOL HYDROCHLORIDE.

DTIC-Dome
(Bayer) is a proprietary, prescription-only preparation of the ANTICANCER drug dacarbazine. It can be used in the treatment of several types of cancer, and is available in a form for injection.
✚▲ Side-effects/warnings: See DACARBAZINE.

DTPer/Vac/Ads
see ADSORBED DIPHTHERIA, TETANUS AND PERTUSSIS VACCINE.

DT/Vac/Ads
see ADSORBED DIPHTHERIA AND TETANUS VACCINE.

Dubam Cream
(Wallace) is a proprietary, non-prescription compound preparation of methyl salicylate, cineole and menthol, which have COUNTER-IRRITANT, or RUBEFACIENT, actions. It can be used for the symptomatic relief of underlying muscle or joint pain, and is available as a cream for topical application to the skin. It is not normally given to children under six years, except on medical advice.
✚▲ Side-effects/warnings: See CINEOLE; METHYL SALICYLATE; MENTHOL.

Dulco-lax Perles
(Boehringer Ingelheim) is a proprietary, non-prescription preparation of the (*stimulant*) LAXATIVE sodium picosulfate. It can be used for the relief of constipation, and is available as perles (capsules). (Note: The brand name Dulco-lax is also used for picosulfate capsules.)
✚▲ Side-effects/warnings: See SODIUM PICOSULFATE.

Dulco-lax Suppositories
(Boehringer Ingelheim) is a proprietary, non-prescription preparation of the (*stimulant*) LAXATIVE bisacodyl. It can be used for constipation and is available as suppositories for adults and children over ten years. Another version for children under ten years is available under medical supervision. (Note: The brand name Dulco-lax is also used for picosulfate capsules.)
+▲ Side-effects/warnings: See BISACODYL.

Dulco-lax Tablets
(Boehringer Ingelheim) is a proprietary, non-prescription preparation of the (*stimulant*) LAXATIVE bisacodyl. It can be used for constipation and is available as tablets. It is not normally given to children under ten years, except on medical advice. (Note: The brand name Dulco-lax is also used for capsules and suppositories.)
+▲ Side-effects/warnings: See BISACODYL.

Duofilm
(Stiefel) is a proprietary, non-prescription preparation of the KERATOLYTIC salicylic acid (with lactic acid). It can be used to remove warts, and is available as a liquid paint. It is not normally given to children under two years, except on medical advice.
+▲ Side-effects/warnings: See SALICYLIC ACID.

Duovent
(Boehringer Ingelheim) is a proprietary, prescription-only compound preparation of the SYMPATHOMIMETIC and BETA-RECEPTOR STIMULANT fenoterol hydrobromide and the ANTICHOLINERGIC ipratropium bromide, which both have BRONCHODILATOR properties. It can be used as an ANTI-ASTHMATIC and chronic bronchitis treatment, and is available in a metered-dose *Autoinhaler*, as an aerosol and a nebulizer solution (use of which version depends on diagnosis).
+▲ Side-effects/warnings: See FENOTEROL HYDROBROMIDE; IPRATROPIUM BROMIDE.

Duphalac Solution
(Solvay Healthcare) is a proprietary, non-prescription preparation of the (*osmotic*) LAXATIVE lactulose. It can be used to relieve constipation, and is available as an oral solution.
+▲ Side-effects/warnings: See LACTULOSE.

Duphaston
(Solvay) is a proprietary, prescription-only preparation of the PROGESTOGEN dydrogesterone. It can be used to treat many conditions of hormonal deficiency in women, including menstrual problems, premenstrual syndrome, endometriosis, recurrent miscarriage and infertility, and as part of HRT. It is available (also in a packaging called *Duphaston HRT*) as tablets.
+▲ Side-effects/warnings: See DYDROGESTERONE.

Duragel
(SSL) is a proprietary, non-prescription preparation of the SPERMICIDAL CONTRACEPTIVE drug nonoxinol. It is available as a vaginal gel and it should be used in conjunction with barrier methods of contraception. Its use is not applicable to children or the elderly.
+▲ Side-effects/warnings: See NONOXINOL.

Duraphat
(Colgate-Palmolive) is a proprietary, non-prescription preparation of sodium fluoride that can be used in children over six years for protection against dental caries in areas where water is not fluoridated. It is available as a weekly dental rinse or mouthwash.
+▲ Side-effects/warnings: see FLUORIDE.

Durogesic
(Janssen-Cilag) is a proprietary, prescription-only preparation of the (OPIOID) NARCOTIC ANALGESIC fentanyl and is on the Controlled Drugs list. It can be used to treat moderate to severe pain, and is available as skin patches.
+▲ Side-effects/warnings: See FENTANYL. It is applied to dry, non-hairy skin on the torso or upper-arm. Replace after 72 hours.

Dutonin
(Bristol-Myers Squibb) is a proprietary, prescription-only preparation of the 'atypical' ANTIDEPRESSANT nefazodone hydrochloride, which is used to treat depressive illness. It is available as tablets.
+▲ Side-effects/warnings: See NEFAZODONE.

Dyazide
(Goldshield) is a proprietary, prescription-only compound preparation of the (THIAZIDE)

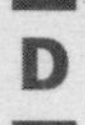

DIURETIC hydrochlorothiazide and the (*potassium-sparing*) diuretic triamterene (a combination called co-triamterzide 50/25). It can be used in the treatment of oedema and as an ANTIHYPERTENSIVE. It is available as tablets.
✚▲ Side-effects/warnings: See HYDROCHLOROTHIAZIDE; TRIAMTERENE; also, urine may be coloured blue.

dydrogesterone

is a PROGESTOGEN, an analogue of the sex hormone PROGESTERONE, which is used to treat many conditions of hormonal deficiency in women, including menstrual problems, premenstrual syndrome, displacement of uterus-lining tissue (endometriosis), recurrent miscarriage and infertility and as part of HRT. Administration is oral.
✚▲ Side-effects/warnings: See PROGESTOGEN. May cause breakthrough bleeding.
✪ **Related entries: Duphaston; Femapak; Femoston.**

Dynamin

(Berk; APS) is a proprietary, non-prescription preparation of the VASODILATOR drug isosorbide mononitrate. It can be used as an ANTI-ANGINA drug, and is available as tablets.
✚▲ Side-effects/warnings: See ISOSORBIDE MONONITRATE.

Dysman 250

(Ashbourne) is a proprietary, prescription-only preparation of the (NSAID) NON-NARCOTIC ANALGESIC and ANTIRHEUMATIC mefenamic acid. It can be used to treat pain and inflammation in rheumatoid arthritis, osteoarthritis and other musculoskeletal disorders and period pain. It is available as capsules (also a stronger one called 'Dysman 500').
✚▲ Side-effects/warnings: See MEFENAMIC ACID.

Dyspamet

(Goldshield) is a proprietary, prescription-only preparation of the H_2-ANTAGONIST cimetidine. It can be used as an ULCER-HEALING DRUG for benign peptic ulcers (in the stomach or duodenum), gastro-oesophageal reflux, dyspepsia and associated conditions. It is available as chewable tablets and as an oral suspension.
✚▲ Side-effects/warnings: See CIMETIDINE.

Dysport

(Ipsen) is a proprietary, prescription-only preparation of botulinum A toxin-haemagglutin complex, used to treat blepharospasm. It is available in a form for injection.
✚▲ Side-effects/warnings: See BOTULINUM TOXIN.

Dytac

(Goldshield) is a proprietary, prescription-only preparation of the (*potassium-sparing*) DIURETIC triamterene. It can be used to treat oedema, and is available as capsules.
✚▲ Side-effects/warnings: See TRIAMTERENE.

Dytide

(Goldshield) is a proprietary, prescription-only compound preparation of the (THIAZIDE) DIURETIC benzthiazide and the (*potassium-sparing*) diuretic triamterene. It can be used to treat oedema, and is available as capsules.
✚▲ Side-effects/warnings: See BENZTHIAZIDE; TRIAMTERENE.

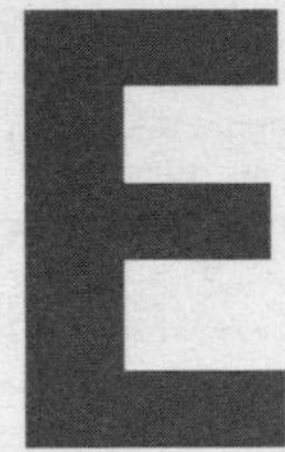

E45
(Crookes) is a proprietary, non-prescription compound preparation of liquid paraffin, white soft paraffin and hypoallergenic anhydrous lanolin. It can be used as an EMOLLIENT for dry skin conditions and is available in various forms including *Cream* and *Lotion*. There are also sun protection products.
✚▲ Side-effects/warnings: See LANOLIN; LIQUID PARAFFIN; WHITE SOFT PARAFFIN.

E45 Emollient Bath Oil
(Crookes) is a proprietary, non-prescription cream preparation of mineral oils and (cetyl) dimeticone. It can be used for symptomatic relief of eczema and pruritus associated with dry skin, and is available as a bath oil.
✚▲ Side-effects/warnings: See DIMETICONE.

E45 Emollient Wash Cream
(Crookes) is a proprietary, non-prescription cream preparation of EMOLLIENT mineral oils and zinc oxide. It can be used for symptomatic relief of eczema and pruritus associated with dry skin, and is available as a bath oil.
✚▲ Side-effects/warnings: See ZINC OXIDE.

E45 Itch Relief Cream
(Crookes) is a proprietary, non-prescription cream preparation of urea and lauromacrogol. It can be used as a HYDRATING AGENT for dry skin, scaling and itching skin.
✚▲ Side-effects/warnings: See UREA.

E45 Sun Lotion
(Crookes) is the name of a range of proprietary, non-prescription SUNSCREEN lotions. They contain titanium dioxide and zinc oxide, which provide protection from ultraviolet radiation (factors 15-50; but with both UVA and UVB protection).
✚▲ Side-effects/warnings: TITANIUM DIOXIDE; ZINC OXIDE.

Earex Ear Drops
(SSL) is a proprietary, non-prescription compound preparation of arachis oil with almond oil and camphor oil. It can be used as a local pain-reliever in the outer or middle ear and as an aid to wax removal.
✚▲ Side-effects/warnings: See ARACHIS OIL; CAMPHOR.

Earex Plus Ear Drops
(SSL) is a proprietary, non-prescription preparation of the COUNTER-IRRITANT, or RUBEFACIENT, choline salicylate and glycerol. It can be used as a local pain-reliever for outer or middle ear conditions and as an aid to wax removal. It is not normally given to children under one year, except on medical advice.
✚▲ Side-effects/warnings: See CHOLINE SALICYLATE; GLYCEROL.

Ebufac
(DDSA) is a proprietary, prescription-only preparation of the (NSAID) NON-NARCOTIC ANALGESIC and ANTIRHEUMATIC ibuprofen. It can be used to relieve pain, particularly the pain of rheumatic disease and other musculoskeletal disorders, and is available as tablets.
✚▲ Side-effects/warnings: See IBUPROFEN.

Econacort
(Squibb; Bristol-Myers Squibb) is a proprietary, prescription-only compound preparation of the CORTICOSTEROID hydrocortisone and the ANTIFUNGAL econazole nitrate. It can be used to treat inflammation in which there is fungal infection, and is available as a cream for topical application.
✚▲ Side-effects/warnings: See ECONAZOLE NITRATE; HYDROCORTISONE.

econazole nitrate
is a broad-spectrum (AZOLE imidazoles) ANTIFUNGAL which can be used to treat fungal infections of the skin, nails (eg tinea pedis) or mucous membranes, such as vaginal candidiasis. Administration is by creams, ointments, vaginal inserts (pessaries), or lotions.
✚▲ Side-effects/warnings: See CLOTRIMAZOLE.
✪ **Related entries: Econacort; Ecostatin; Gyno-Pevaryl; Pevaryl.**

E

Economycin
(DDSA) is a proprietary, prescription-only preparation of the ANTIBACTERIAL and (TETRACYCLINES) ANTIBIOTIC tetracycline (as hydrochloride). It can be used to treat a wide range of infections, and is available as capsules.
✚▲ Side-effects/warnings: See TETRACYCLINE.

Ecopase
(Goldshield) is a proprietary, prescription-only preparation of the ACE INHIBITOR captopril. It can be used as an ANTIHYPERTENSIVE and in HEART FAILURE TREATMENT, usually in conjunction with other classes of drug. It is available as tablets.
✚▲ Side-effects/warnings: See CAPTOPRIL.

Ecostatin
(Squibb; Bristol-Myers Squibb) is a proprietary, prescription-only preparation of the ANTIFUNGAL econazole nitrate. It can be used primarily to treat fungal infections of the skin and mucous membranes, especially of the vagina and vulva. It is available as a cream, vaginal pessaries (the stronger form is called *Ecostatin 1*) and a *Twinpack* with pessaries and cream (the cream – and some of the other preparations subject to certain restrictions – are available without prescription).
✚▲ Side-effects/warnings: See ECONAZOLE NITRATE.

Ednyt
(Dominion) a proprietary, prescription-only preparation of the ACE INHIBITOR enalapril maleate. It can be used as an ANTIHYPERTENSIVE and in HEART FAILURE TREATMENT, and is available as tablets.
✚▲ Side-effects/warnings: See ENALAPRIL MALEATE.

Edronax
(Pharmacia) is a proprietary, prescription-only preparation of the (*selective noradrenaline re-uptake blocker*) ANTIDEPRESSANT reboxetine (as maleate) used to treat depressive illness. It is available as tablets.
✚▲ Side-effects/warnings: See REBOXETINE.

edrophonium chloride
is an ANTICHOLINESTERASE drug which enhances the effects of the neurotransmitter acetylcholine (and of certain cholinergic drugs). It has a short duration of action and can be used in the diagnosis of myasthenia gravis and at the termination of operations to reverse the actions of neuromuscular blocking agents (when it is often administered with ATROPINE SULPHATE). Administration is by injection.
✚▲ Side-effects/warnings: See NEOSTIGMINE.

Efalith
(Scotia) is a proprietary, prescription-only compound preparation of the ANTISEBORRHOEIC lithium succinate and the ASTRINGENT zinc sulphate. It can be used for seborrhoeic dermatitis, and is available as an ointment.
✚▲ Side-effects/warnings: See LITHIUM SUCCINATE; ZINC SULPHATE.

Efamast
(Pharmacia) is a proprietary, prescription-only preparation of gamolenic acid (in evening primrose oil). It can be used to relieve breast pain (mastalgia), and is available as capsules (in two strengths).
✚▲ Side-effects/warnings: See GAMOLENIC ACID.

efavirenz
is a (*non-nucleoside* group of *reverse transcriptase inhibitor*) ANTIVIRAL drug which can be used in the treatment of HIV infection, normally in combination with other antiviral drugs. Administration is oral.
✚ Side-effects: Rash; dizziness, headache, insomnia, sleepiness, disturbing dreams, fatigue, impaired concentration, depression, psychotic state; nausea; raised blood lipids, liver enzyme changes; diarrhoea and pancreatitis reported.
▲ Warnings: It is not used in breast-feeding women. Care is necessary in those with impaired liver or kidney function.
✪ **Related entry: Sustiva.**

Efcortelan
(GlaxoWellcome; GSK) is a proprietary, prescription-only preparation of the CORTICOSTEROID and ANTI-INFLAMMATORY drug hydrocortisone. It can be used to treat mild inflammatory skin conditions, such as eczema, and is available as a cream and an ointment.
✚▲ Side-effects/warnings: See HYDROCORTISONE.

Efcortesol
(Sovereign) is a proprietary, prescription-only

preparation of the CORTICOSTEROID and ANTI-INFLAMMATORY hydrocortisone (as sodium phosphate). It can be used to treat inflammation, especially inflammation caused by allergy (eg anaphylactic shock) and to treat shock. It is available in a form for injection.
✚▲ Side-effects/warnings: See HYDROCORTISONE.

Efexor

(Wyeth) is a proprietary, prescription-only preparation of the 'atypical' ANTIDEPRESSANT venlafaxine. It can be used to treat depressive illness, and is available as tablets and modified-release capsules (Efexor XL).
✚▲ Side-effects/warnings: See VENLAFAXINE.

Effercitrate

(Typharm) is a proprietary, non-prescription preparation of potassium citrate. It is a proprietary equivalent of Potassium Citrate Mixture BP. It can be used as an alkalizing agent to relieve discomfort of mild urinary tract infection and to make the urine alkaline. It is available as effervescent tablets for an oral solution.
✚▲ Side-effects/warnings: See POTASSIUM CITRATE.

eformoterol fumarate

see FORMOTEROL FUMARATE.

Efudix

(ICN) is a proprietary, prescription-only preparation of the ANTICANCER drug fluorouracil. It can be used to treat skin lesions, and is available as a cream for topical application.
✚▲ Side-effects/warnings: See CYTOTOXIC.

8Y

(BPL) is a proprietary, prescription-only preparation of dried human factor VIII fraction. It acts as a HAEMOSTATIC to reduce or stop bleeding in the treatment of disorders in which bleeding is prolonged and potentially dangerous (mainly haemophilia A). It is available in a form for intravenous injection or infusion.
✚▲ Side-effects/warnings: See FACTOR VIII FRACTION (DRIED).

Elantan

(Schwarz)is a proprietary, prescription-only preparation of the VASODILATOR drug isosorbide mononitrate. It can be used as an ANTI-ANGINA drug, and is available as tablets in a non-prescription preparation, *Elantan 10* and two prescription-only preparations, *Elantan 20* and *Elantan 40*.
✚▲ Side-effects/warnings: See ISOSORBIDE MONONITRATE.

Elantan LA

(Schwarz) is a proprietary, non-prescription preparation of the VASODILATOR drug isosorbide mononitrate. It can be used as an ANTI-ANGINA drug, and is available as modified-release capsules in two forms, *Elantan LA 25* and *Elantan LA 50*.
✚▲ Side-effects/warnings: See ISOSORBIDE MONONITRATE.

Elavil

(DDSA) is a proprietary, prescription-only preparation of the (TRICYCLIC) ANTIDEPRESSANT amitriptyline hydrochloride. It can be used to treat depressive illness, especially in cases where some degree of sedation is required, and has also been used to treat bed-wetting by children at night. It is available as tablets.
✚▲ Side-effects/warnings: See AMITRIPTYLINE HYDROCHLORIDE.

Eldepryl

(Orion) is a proprietary, prescription-only preparation of the ANTIPARKINSONISM drug selegiline. It can be used in the treatment of the symptoms of parkinsonism, and is available as tablets and an oral liquid.
✚▲ Side-effects/warnings: See SELEGILINE.

Eldisine

(Lilly) is a proprietary, prescription-only preparation of the ANTICANCER drug vindesine sulphate. It can be used to treat a range of cancers, and is available in a form for injection.
✚▲ Side-effects/warnings: See VINDESINE SULPHATE.

eletripan

is a recently introduced (TRIPTAN) ANTIMIGRAINE drug, which is used to treat acute migraine attacks (but not to prevent them). It works as a vasoconstrictor through acting as a serotonin-receptor stimulant (selective for serotonin 5-HT_1 receptors), producing a rapid constriction of blood vessels surrounding the

E

brain. Administration is oral.
✚ Side-effects: See SUMATRIPTAN for general side-effects of drugs of this class. It is a new drug and not all side-effects are yet clear.
▲ Warnings: See SUMATRIPTAN for general warnings for drugs of this class. It is not used for people with severe liver or kidney impairment, or the elderly. It should not be used together with certain enzyme-inhibiting drugs including ketoconazole, itraconazole, erythromycin, clarithromycin, also protease-inhibitors (ritonavir, indinavir and nelfinavir).
✪ Related entry: Relpax.

Elleste-Duet

(Searle; Pharmacia) is a proprietary, prescription-only compound preparation of the OESTROGEN estradiol and the PROGESTOGEN norethisterone. It can be used in HRT, and is available as tablets in two strengths (*1-mg* and *2-mg*). Also available in a form called *Elleste-Duet Conti*.
✚▲ Side-effects/warnings: See NORETHISTERONE; ESTRADIOL.

Elleste Solo

(Searle; Pharmacia) is a proprietary, prescription-only preparation of the OESTROGEN estradiol. It can be used in HRT, and is available as tablets (in varying strengths).
✚▲ Side-effects/warnings: See ESTRADIOL.

Elleste-Solo

(Searle; Pharmacia) is a proprietary, prescription-only preparation of the OESTROGEN estradiol. It can be used in HRT, and is available as tablets in two strengths.
✚▲ Side-effects/warnings: See ESTRADIOL.

Elleste Solo MX

(Searle; Pharmacia) is a proprietary, prescription-only preparation of the OESTROGEN estradiol. It can be used in HRT, and is available as self-adhesive skin patches (in varying strengths).
✚▲ Side-effects/warnings: See ESTRADIOL.

Ellimans Universal Embrocation

(SSL) is a proprietary, non-prescription preparation of turpentine oil (with acetic acid). It has a COUNTER-IRRITANT, or RUBEFACIENT, action and can be applied to the skin for symptomatic relief of underlying muscle or joint pain. It is available as an embrocation for topical application and is not normally used for children under 12 years, except on medical advice.
✚▲ Side-effects/warnings: See TURPENTINE OIL.

Elocon

(Schering-Plough) is a proprietary, prescription-only preparation of the CORTICOSTEROID drug mometasone furoate. It can be used to treat severe inflammatory skin disorders such as eczemas and psoriasis. It is available as a cream, ointment and scalp lotion.
✚▲ Side-effects/warnings: See MOMETASONE FUROATE.

Eloxatin

(Sanofi-Synthelabo) is a proprietary, prescription-only preparation of the ANTICANCER drug oxaliplatin. It can be used in the treatment of colorectal cancer, and is available in a form for injection.
✚▲ Side-effects/warnings: See OXALIPLATIN.

Eltroxin

(Goldshield) is a proprietary, prescription-only preparation of levothyroxine sodium, which is a form of thyroid hormone. It can be used to make up a hormonal deficiency and to treat associated symptoms, and is available as tablets.
✚▲ Side-effects/warnings: See LEVOTHYROXINE SODIUM.

Eludril

(Ceuta) is a proprietary, non-prescription preparation of the antiseptic chlorhexidine (as gluconate) and chlorbutanol. It can be used by topical application to treat minor throat infections, to prevent plaque formation, for oral hygiene and to disinfect dentures. It is available as a mouthwash or gargle.
✚▲ Side-effects/warnings: See CHLORHEXIDINE.

Elyzol

(Alpharma) is a proprietary, prescription-only preparation of the ANTIMICROBIAL metronidazole, which has ANTIBACTERIAL and ANTIPROTOZOAL actions. It can be used for the treatment of local infections in the mouth, and is available as a gel.
✚▲ Side-effects/warnings: See METRONIDAZOLE.

Emadine

(Alcon) is a proprietary, prescription-only

preparation of the ANTI-INFLAMMATORY drug emedastine which can be used for seasonal allergic conjunctivitis. It is available as eye-drops.
✚▲ Side-effects/warnings: See EMEDASTINE.

Emblon
(Berk; APS) is a proprietary, prescription-only preparation of the sex HORMONE ANTAGONIST tamoxifen, which, because it inhibits the effect of OESTROGEN, is used primarily as an ANTICANCER treatment for cancers that depend on the presence of oestrogen in women, particularly breast cancer. It can also be used to treat certain conditions of infertility, and is available as tablets.
✚▲ Side-effects/warnings: See TAMOXIFEN.

Emcor
(Merck) is a proprietary, prescription-only preparation of the BETA-BLOCKER bisoprolol fumarate. It can be used as an ANTIHYPERTENSIVE for raised blood pressure and as an ANTI-ANGINA treatment to relieve symptoms and improve exercise tolerance. It is available as tablets.
✚▲ Side-effects/warnings: See BISOPROLOL FUMARATE.

emedastine
is an ANTI-INFLAMMATORY drug introduced recently for seasonal allergic conjunctivitis. Administration is as eye-drops.
✚ Side-effects: Short-lived burning or stinging; local oedema, blurred vision, inflammation of the cornea, irritation, dry eye, tears, photophobia; headache, and rhinitis occasionally reported.
✪ Related entry: Emadine.

Emeside
(LAB) is a proprietary, prescription-only preparation of the ANTICONVULSANT and ANTI-EPILEPTIC ethosuximide. It can be used to treat absence (petit mal), myoclonic and some other types of seizure, and is available as capsules and a syrup.
✚▲ Side-effects/warnings: See ETHOSUXIMIDE.

emetic 🅴
emetic drugs, or other agents, cause vomiting (emesis). Emetics are used primarily to treat poisoning by non-corrosive substances when the patient is conscious, especially drugs taken in overdose. Some affect the vomiting centre in the brain and/or irritate the gastrointestinal tract. Among the best-known and most-used emetics is IPECACUANHA, but several drugs used as EXPECTORANT can, in higher concentrations, also cause emesis.

Emfib
(Berk; APS) is a proprietary, prescription-only preparation of the LIPID-REGULATING DRUG gemfibrozil. It can be used in hyperlipidaemia to modify the proportions, of various lipids in the bloodstream. It is available as capsules.
✚▲ Side-effects/warnings: see GEMFIBROZIL.

Emflex
(Berk; APS) is a proprietary, prescription-only preparation of the (NSAID) NON-NARCOTIC ANALGESIC and ANTIRHEUMATIC acemetacin. It can be used to treat the pain of rheumatic and other musculoskeletal disorders and for postoperative pain. It is available as capsules.
✚▲ Side-effects/warnings: See ACEMETACIN.

Emla
(AstraZeneca) is a proprietary, prescription-only compound preparation of the LOCAL ANAESTHETIC lidocaine hydrochloride and prilocaine hydrochloride. It can be used for surface anaesthesia, including preparation for injections, and is available as a cream.
✚▲ Side-effects/warnings: See LIDOCAINE HYDROCHLORIDE; PRILOCAINE HYDROCHLORIDE.

emollient 🅴
agents soothe, soften and moisturize the skin, particularly when it is dry and scaling. They are usually emulsions of water, fats, waxes and oils; these may be animal or plant products (eg LANOLIN, wool oil, ARACHIS OIL or mineral oil preparations, LIQUID PARAFFIN, WHITE SOFT PARAFFIN, YELLOW SOFT PARAFFIN). They can be used alone to help hydrate the skin, or combined with a HYDRATING AGENT such as UREA. A notable example of a skin condition that may be treated with emollients is atopic eczema, when the skin is very dry. Emollients can be applied as creams, ointments, lotions or added to bath water. Such preparations contain preservatives (eg parabens) which in some patients may worsen the condition by causing contact allergic dermatitis, and similarly some patients are allergic to some of the major constituents (particularly lanolin or WOOL FAT). There are a

E

number of additives that may help itchiness (eg MENTHOL, CAMPHOR and PHENOL) and some preparations have a beneficial ASTRINGENT action (eg ZINC OXIDE or CALAMINE). In conditions that also involve a skin infection, emollients may have an ANTIMICROBIAL or ANTIFUNGAL drug added to them, or, in cases of severe inflammation, ANTI-INFLAMMATORY and CORTICOSTEROID drugs may be incorporated.

Emulsiderm Emollient

(Dermal) is a proprietary, non-prescription preparation of the ANTISEPTIC benzalkonium chloride and the skin EMOLLIENT liquid paraffin (with isopropyl myristate), and is used for treating dry skin conditions, eczema and psoriasis. It is available as a liquid emulsion that can be added to a bath or applied directly.
+▲ Side-effects/warnings: See BENZALKONIUM CHLORIDE; LIQUID PARAFFIN.

Emulsifying Ointment, BP

is a non-proprietary, non-prescription compound preparation formulation comprising a combination of wax, white soft paraffin and liquid paraffin. It can be used as a base for medications that require topical application.
+▲ Side-effects/warnings: See LIQUID PARAFFIN; WHITE SOFT PARAFFIN.

enalapril maleate

is an ACE INHIBITOR and acts as a VASODILATOR. It can be used as an ANTIHYPERTENSIVE, in congestive HEART FAILURE TREATMENT and to prevent ischaemia (lack of blood supply) in patients with left ventricular failure. It is often used in conjunction with other classes of drug, particularly (THIAZIDE) DIURETIC drugs. Administration is oral.
+▲ Side-effects/warnings: See ACE INHIBITOR. Also palpitations, irregular heart beats, angina and chest pains, fainting, myocardial infarction; cerebrovascular accident, anorexia; skin effects, confusion, depression, nervousness, muscle weakness, drowsiness, insomnia, blurred vision, ringing in the ears, sweating and flushing, impotence, hair loss, breathing difficulties and muscle cramps. It is not used in porphyria.
✪ **Related entries: Ednyt; Innovace; Innozide.**

Endekay

(Manx) is a proprietary, non-prescription preparation of sodium fluoride that can be used in children for protection against teeth decay and dental caries in areas where water is not fluoridated. It is available as tablets (*Fluotabs* in different strengths and flavours for two- to four-year olds), as paediatric drops for taking by mouth (*Fluodrops* for two-week to two-year olds), a daily topical mouthrinse, and a daily fluoride mouthrinse for children over 6 years and adults.
+▲ Side-effects/warnings: See FLUORIDE.

Endekay Fluodrops

(Manx) is a proprietary, non-prescription preparation of sodium fluoride which can be used in areas where the amount of fluoride in the water supply is less than 0.3 ppm (parts per million). It is available as drops and can be used to strengthen tooth enamel in order to resist tooth decay.
+▲ Side-effects/warnings: See FLUORIDE.

Endoxana

(ASTA Medica) is a proprietary, prescription-only preparation of the (CYTOTOXIC) ANTICANCER drug cyclophosphamide. It can be used to treat chronic lymphocytic leukaemia, lymphomas and some solid tumours. It is available as tablets and a form for injection.
+▲ Side-effects/warnings: See CYCLOPHOSPHAMIDE.

Engerix B

(SmithKline Beecham; GSK) is a proprietary, prescription-only VACCINE preparation of hepatitis B vaccine (rby), prepared from yeast cells by recombinant DNA techniques. It can be used to protect people at risk from infection with hepatitis B, and is available in a form for injection.
+▲ Side-effects/warnings: See HEPATITIS B VACCINE.

Eno

(SmithKline Beecham; GSK Consumer Healthcare) is a proprietary, non-prescription compound preparation of the ANTACID agents sodium carbonate and sodium bicarbonate together with citric acid. It can be used for the symptomatic relief of indigestion, flatulence and nausea. It is available as a powder for making up as a sparkling drink (also available in a form called *Lemon Eno*). It is not normally given to

children, except on medical advice.
✚▲ Side-effects/warnings: See SODIUM CARBONATE; SODIUM BICARBONATE.

enoxaparin

is a *low molecular weight* heparin. It has some advantages as an ANTICOAGULANT when used for long-duration prevention of venous thrombo-embolism, particularly in orthopaedic use. Administration is by injection.
✚▲ Side-effects/warnings: See HEPARIN.
✪ Related entry: Clexane.

enoximone

is a PHOSPHODIESTERASE INHIBITOR and is used in congestive HEART FAILURE TREATMENT, especially where other drugs have been unsuccessful. Administration is by intravenous injection or intravenous infusion.
✚ Side-effects: There may be irregular heart beats, hypotension, headache, nausea and vomiting, insomnia, chills and fever, diarrhoea, retention of urine and pain in the limbs.
▲ Warnings: It should be given with caution to patients with certain forms of heart failure and vascular disease. The blood pressure and electrocardiogram should be monitored. It is given with care to those with kidney impairment, or who are pregnant or breast-feeding.
✪ Related entry: Perfan.

entacapone

is an ENZYME INHIBITOR which is used in ANTIPARKINSONISM treatment because it inhibits one of the enzymes that break down the neurotransmitter DOPAMINE in the brain. It is thought that dopamine deficiency in the brain causes Parkinson's disease. It can be used to treat the symptoms of parkinsonism, in combination with LEVODOPA (which is converted to dopamine in the brain) together with a further enzyme inhibitor (CARBIDOPA or BENSERAZIDE HYDROCHLORIDE) to reduce fluctuations in motor muscle function at the end of dose periods. Administration is oral.
✚ Side-effects: Nausea and vomiting, abdominal pain, constipation or diarrhoea, red-brown coloured urine, dry mouth, involuntary body movements; dizziness; anaemia reported; rarely changed liver enzymes.
▲ Warnings: Entacapone should not be given to pregnant or breast-feeding women, or to anyone with liver impairment, phaeochromocytoma or certain concurrent diseases. Iron can reduce the absorption of entacapone and so its effectiveness may be reduced.
✪ Related entry: Comtess.

Enterosan

(Monmouth) is a proprietary, non-prescription preparation of the (OPIOID) ANTIDIARRHOEAL morphine (as hydrochloride), kaolin and the ANTICHOLINERGIC Belladonna extract (see BELLADONNA ALKALOID). It can be used for the symptomatic relief of occasional diarrhoea and its associated pain and discomfort, colic and acute gastroenteritis. It is available as tablets, and is not normally given to children, except on medical advice.
✚▲ Side-effects/warnings: See BELLADONNA ALKALOID; KAOLIN; MORPHINE SULPHATE.

Entocort

(AstraZeneca) is a proprietary, prescription-only preparation of the CORTICOSTEROID budesonide. It can be used for the induction of remission in mild to moderate Crohn's disease affecting the ileum and ascending colon, in the form of capsules (*CR capsules*), or for ulcerative colitis in the form of an enema.
✚▲ Side-effects/warnings: See BUDESONIDE.

Entrotabs

(Monmouth) is a proprietary, non-prescription preparation of the ANTACID aluminium hydroxide (with attapulgite and pectin). It can be used for the symptomatic relief of stomach upsets and diarrhoea, and is available as chewable tablets. It is not normally given to children under six years, except on medical advice.
✚▲ Side-effects/warnings: See ALUMINIUM HYDROXIDE.

Enzed

(Kent) is a prescription-only, proprietary version of the (NSAID) NON-NARCOTIC ANALGESIC and ANTIRHEUMATIC diclofenac sodium. It can be used to treat arthritic and rheumatic pain and inflammation and other musculoskeletal disorders. It is available as tablets.
✚▲ Side-effects/warnings: See DICLOFENAC SODIUM.

enzyme inhibitor

drugs work by inhibiting enzymes, which are

proteins that play an essential part in the metabolism by acting as catalysts in specific, necessary biochemical reactions. Certain drugs have been developed that act only on certain enzymes and so can be used to manipulate the biochemistry of the body. For example, ANTICHOLINESTERASE drugs (eg NEOSTIGMINE and PYRIDOSTIGMINE) inhibit enzymes called cholinesterases, which are normally involved in the rapid breakdown of ACETYLCHOLINE (an important neurotransmitter). Acetylcholine is released from cholinergic nerves and has many actions throughout the body. Consequently, since anticholinesterase drugs enhance the effects of acetylcholine on its release from these nerves, they can have a wide range of actions. Their actions at the junction of nerves with skeletal (voluntary) muscles are used in the diagnosis and treatment of the muscle weakness disease myasthenia gravis; also, at the end of surgical operations in which SKELETAL MUSCLE RELAXANT drugs have been used, the anaesthetist is able to reverse the muscle paralysis by injecting an anticholinesterase. In organs innervated by parasympathetic division of the autonomic nervous system, anticholinesterases cause an exaggeration of the nerves' actions, known as PARASYMPATHOMIMETIC actions and can be used for a number of purposes, such as stimulation of the bladder (in cases of urinary retention). However, anticholinesterases have a number of undesirable side-effects, including slowing of the heart, constriction of the airways with excessive production of secretions and actions in the brain. In anticholinesterase poisoning, their diverse actions can be life-threatening. Chemicals with anticholinesterase properties are used as insecticides and in chemical warfare. ANTIDOTE agents are available to treat cases of poisoning, for example, due to a farming accident.

MONOAMINE-OXIDASE INHIBITOR drugs, or MAOIs, (eg ISOCARBOXAZID, PHENELZINE and TRANYLCYPROMINE) are one of the three major classes of ANTIDEPRESSANT. They work by inhibiting an enzyme in the brain that metabolizes monoamines (including NORADRENALINE and SEROTONIN), which results in a change of mood. However, this same enzyme detoxifies other amines, so if certain foods are eaten or medicines taken that contain amines (eg sympathomimetic amines in cough and cold treatments), then dangerous side-effects could occur. MOCLOBEMIDE is a newly introduced MAOI which is an inhibitor of only one type of monoamine oxidase (type A) and is claimed to show less potentiation of the amine in foodstuffs.

ACE INHIBITOR (angiotensin-converting enzyme inhibitor) drugs, such as CAPTOPRIL, ENALAPRIL MALEATE or RAMIPRIL, are used in ANTIHYPERTENSIVE treatment and HEART FAILURE TREATMENT. They work by inhibiting the conversion of the natural circulating HORMONE angiotensin I to angiotensin II and because the latter form is a potent VASOCONSTRICTOR, the overall effect is vasodilation with a HYPOTENSIVE action.

Further examples of enzyme inhibitors include the CARBONIC-ANHYDRASE INHIBITOR drugs (which are used for their DIURETIC actions and in GLAUCOMA TREATMENT), the PHOSPHODIESTERASE INHIBITOR drugs (for congestive heart failure treatment), CARBIDOPA (in ANTIPARKINSONISM treatment), CLAVULANIC ACID (to prolong and enhance the effects of certain ANTIBIOTIC drugs) and DISULFIRAM (which is used in the treatment of alcoholism).

enzymes

are proteins that play an essential part in the body's processes by acting as catalysts in specific, necessary biochemical reactions. Their physiological functions range from digestion of food within the digestive tract, formation of hormones and neurotransmitters, through to synthesis of proteins and other structural elements of the body.

Impaired function of enzymes underlies many (particularly familial) diseases, and may cause some food intolerances that require special diets (eg phenylketonuria and favism). Specialized enzymes are involved in the metabolism and detoxification of chemicals, including drugs, that are foreign to the body. Impaired capacity of these enzymes (which again is often familial) may make persons hypersensitive to these chemicals, and is a prominent cause of adverse drug reactions (eg G6PD deficiency, porphyria) and metabolism by liver enzymes is often slower in the young, the elderly and in liver disease (including cirrhosis).

Many drugs (see ENZYME INHIBITOR) have been developed that in exerting their beneficial effects, achieve selectivity of action through affecting only certain enzymes and so can be used to manipulate the biochemistry of the body (eg MONOAMINE-OXIDASE INHIBITOR, ANTICHOLINESTERASE and PHOSPHODIESTERASE INHIBITOR drugs). In a few instances enzymes, themselves, are used as drugs, but their chemical nature makes it difficult to deliver them to their proposed sites of action. Also, because they are proteins, in most cases derived from animals, there are commonly serious allergic side-effects.

Some FIBRINOLYTIC drugs are enzymes and are administered by injection or infusion to dissolve blood clots in the treatment of life-threatening conditions, such as acute myocardial infarction, venous thrombi, pulmonary embolism and clots in the eye (eg ALTEPLASE).

A number of enzymes have been given by mouth with food to supplement deficiencies in production of the body's own proteolytic (protein-digesting) enzymes. This approach, however, is not generally very successful and such agents tend to erode the upper gastrointestinal tract (eg PANCREATIN, which is isolated from the pancreas of a cow or pig). Other proteolytic enzymes have diverse uses, for example, dissolving wound debris, by inhalation into the lungs to liquefy viscous sputum. Other enzymes that dissolve connective tissue are used in the treatment of skin extravastion injuries such as burns and inflammatory injuries (to promote reabsorption of excess fluids and blood), to increase the permeability of soft tissues to injected drugs and in ophthalmological practice (eg HYALURONIDASE).

IMIGLUCERASE is an enzyme that is used as a replacement in the specialist treatment of Gaucher's disease, which is a genetically determined enzyme-deficiency disease that affects the spleen, liver, bone marrow and lymph nodes. Enzymes also can be used in ANTICANCER therapy (eg asparaginase; an enzyme isolated from the *E. coli* bacterium).

Epaderm

(SSL) is a proprietary, non-prescription preparation of the EMOLLIENT yellow soft paraffin and emulsifying wax. It can be used to moisturize dry skin, and is available as an ointment.

✚▲ Side-effects/warnings: See YELLOW SOFT PARAFFIN; LIQUID PARAFFIN.

Epanutin

(Parke-Davis; Pfizer) is a proprietary, prescription-only preparation of the ANTICONVULSANT and ANTI-EPILEPTIC phenytoin. It can be used to treat and prevent most forms of seizure and also the pain of trigeminal (facial) neuralgia. It is available as capsules, chewable tablets (*Epanutin Infatabs*) and as a liquid suspension.

✚▲ Side-effects/warnings: See PHENYTOIN.

Epanutin Ready Mixed Parenteral

(Parke-Davis; Pfizer) is a proprietary, prescription-only preparation of the ANTICONVULSANT and ANTI-EPILEPTIC phenytoin. It can be used in the emergency treatment of status epilepticus and convulsive seizures during neurosurgical operations. It is available in a form for injection.

✚▲ Side-effects/warnings: See PHENYTOIN.

Epaxal

(MASTA) is a proprietary, prescription-only VACCINE preparation of hepatitis A vaccine. It can be used to protect people at risk from infection with hepatitis A, and is available in a form for injection.

✚▲ Side-effects/warnings: See HEPATITIS A VACCINE.

ephedrine hydrochloride

is an ALKALOID that is a SYMPATHOMIMETIC drug (also called an *indirect sympathomimetic*, because it works indirectly through the release of NORADRENALINE (also called norepinephrine) from sympathetic nerve endings). It is occasionally used as a BRONCHODILATOR, for instance in asthma. It is a VASOCONSTRICTOR and is used as a NASAL DECONGESTANT. Sometimes it is used to raise the blood pressure in emergencies where other methods have not worked. It is incorporated into proprietary hay fever and decongestant preparations. Administration can be either oral or topical.

✚ Side-effects: There may be changes in heart rate and blood pressure, anxiety, restlessness, tremor, insomnia, dry mouth, cold fingertips and toes and changes in the prostate gland. When used as a nasal decongestant, it may cause irritation in the nose.

▲ Warnings: Administer with caution to patients with certain heart, kidney and thyroid disorders, diabetes and hypertension; care should be taken to avoid interaction with other drugs (especially MAOI ANTIDEPRESSANT drugs in case of

hypertensive crisis).
✪ Related entries: Do-Do Chesteze; Haymine.

Ephynal

(Roche Consumer Health) is a proprietary, non-prescription preparation of alpha tocopheryl acetate. It can be used to treat vitamin E deficiency, and is available in the form of tablets.
✚▲ Side-effects/warnings: See ALPHA TOCOPHERYL ACETATE.

Epilim

(Sanofi-Synthelabo) is a proprietary, prescription-only preparation of the ANTICONVULSANT and ANTI-EPILEPTIC sodium valproate. It can be used to treat all forms of epilepsy, and is available as tablets, a liquid and a syrup.
✚▲ Side-effects/warnings: See SODIUM VALPROATE.

Epilim Chrono

(Sanofi-Synthelabo) is a proprietary, prescription-only preparation of the ANTICONVULSANT and ANTI-EPILEPTIC sodium valproate. It can be used to treat epilepsy, and is available as modified-release tablets.
✚▲ Side-effects/warnings: See SODIUM VALPROATE.

Epilim Intravenous

(Sanofi-Synthelabo) is a proprietary, prescription-only preparation of the ANTICONVULSANT and ANTI-EPILEPTIC sodium valproate. It can be used to treat epilepsy, and is available in a form for injection.
✚▲ Side-effects/warnings: See SODIUM VALPROATE.

Epimaz

(IVAX) is a proprietary, prescription-only preparation of the ANTICONVULSANT and ANTI-EPILEPTIC carbamazepine. It can be used to treat most forms of epilepsy (except absence seizures), trigeminal neuralgia and in the management of manic-depressive illness. It is available as tablets.
✚▲ Side-effects/warnings: See CARBAMAZEPINE.

epinephrine

see ADRENALINE ACID TARTRATE.

EpiPen

(ALK-Abello) is a proprietary, prescription-only preparation of adrenaline acid tartrate (epinephrine). It is used as a SYMPATHOMIMETIC and BRONCHODILATOR drug in emergency treatment of acute and severe bronchoconstriction and other symptoms of acute anaphylaxis (allergic reaction; eg an insect sting). It is available as an auto-injector, which delivers a single intramuscular dose, and also as a version for children, *Epipen Jr Auto-injector*.
✚▲ Side-effects/warnings: See ADRENALINE ACID TARTRATE.

epirubicin hydrochloride

is a CYTOTOXIC drug (an ANTIBIOTIC in origin) which is used as an ANTICANCER treatment of breast and certain bladder tumours. Administration is by injection or bladder instillation.
✚▲ Side-effects/warnings: See CYTOTOXIC; but it also has cardiac toxicity.
✪ Related entries: Pharmorubicin Rapid Dissolution; Pharmorubicin Solution for Injection.

Epivir

(GlaxoWellcome; GSK) is a proprietary, prescription-only preparation of the ANTIVIRAL lamivudine. It can be used in the treatment of HIV infection, and is available as tablets and as an oral solution.
✚▲ Side-effects/warnings: See LAMIVUDINE.

epoetin

is a form of human erythropoietin synthesized by recombinant techniques. It is used as an ANAEMIA TREATMENT for the type of anaemia such as those known to be associated with erythropoietin deficiency in chronic renal failure, and in people undergoing some forms of cancer chemotherapy. It is available as epoetin alpha and beta and is administered by injection.
✚ Side-effects: Cardiovascular symptoms including high blood pressure (hypertension) and cardiac complications; allergy reactions, flu-like symptoms, skin reactions and effects on the blood. A migraine-like headache must be reported immediately to a doctor.
▲ Warnings: It should not be administered to patients with uncontrolled hypertension. Administer with care to patients with poorly controlled blood pressure, a history of convulsions, vascular disease, liver failure or a malignant disease; or who are pregnant or breast-feeding.

✪ **Related entries: Aranesp; Eprex; NeoRecormon.**

Epogam

(Pharmacia) is a proprietary, prescription-only preparation of gamolenic acid (in evening primrose oil). It can be used for the symptomatic relief of atopic eczema, and is available as capsules (in two strengths called *Epogam 40* and *Epogam 80*); also as *Epogam paediatric capsules*.
✚▲ Side-effects/warnings: See GAMOLENIC ACID.

epoprostenol

(prostacyclin) is a PROSTAGLANDIN present naturally in the walls of blood vessels. When administered therapeutically by intravenous infusion it has ANTIPLATELET or antithrombotic activity and so inhibits blood coagulation by preventing the aggregation of platelets. It is also a potent VASODILATOR. Its main use is to act as an ANTITHROMBOTIC during procedures such as kidney dialysis (though it has a very short lifetime in the body). It is administered by infusion.
✚ Side-effects: Flushing, hypotension and headache. Also, pallor, sweating, slowing of the heart at high doses.
▲ Warnings: It must be administered in continuous intravenous infusion because it is rapidly removed from the blood. Blood monitoring is essential, especially when there is simultaneous administration of heparin.
✪ **Related entry: Flolan.**

Eppy

(Chauvin) is a proprietary, prescription-only preparation of the SYMPATHOMIMETIC adrenaline acid tartrate (epinephrine). It is used to treat glaucoma, and is available as eye-drops.
✚▲ Side-effects/warnings: See ADRENALINE ACID TARTRATE.

Eprex

(Janssen-Cilag) is a proprietary, prescription-only preparation of epoetin alpha (synthesized human erythropoietin alpha). It can be used as an ANAEMIA TREATMENT in conditions such as those associated with chronic renal failure. It is available in a form for injection.
✚▲ Side-effects/warnings: See EPOETIN.

eprosartan

is an ANGIOTENSIN-RECEPTOR BLOCKER, which is a class of drugs that work by blocking angiotensin receptors. Angiotensin II is a circulating HORMONE that is a powerful VASOCONSTRICTOR and so blocking its effects leads to a fall in blood pressure. Therefore eprosartan can be used as an ANTIHYPERTENSIVE. Administration is oral.
✚▲ Side-effects/warnings: See LOSARTAN POTASSIUM.
✪ **Related entry: Teveten.**

Epsom salt(s)

see MAGNESIUM SULPHATE.

eptifibatide

is an ANTIPLATELET (antithrombotic) drug which is used to prevent thrombosis (blood-clot formation). It works by stopping platelets sticking to one another or to the walls of blood vessels. It can be used (together with heparin and aspirin) to prevent thrombosis in myocardial infarction, and as part of ANTI-ANGINA treatment. Administration is by intravenous injection or infusion.
✚▲ Side-effects/warnings: Used only under hospital specialist supervision.
✪ **Related entry: Integrilin.**

Equagesic

(Wyeth) is a proprietary compound preparation of the ANXIOLYTIC and SEDATIVE drug meprobamate, the NSAID ANALGESIC aspirin and the OPIOID analgesic ethoheptazine citrate, and is on the Controlled Drugs list. It can be used primarily for the short-term treatment of pain, and is available as tablets.
✚▲ Side-effects/warnings: See ASPIRIN; ETHOHEPTAZINE CITRATE; MEPROBAMATE.

Equilon

(Chefaro) is a proprietary, non-prescription preparation of the ANTISPASMODIC mebeverine hydrochloride. It can be used for the relief from gastrointestinal spasm such as irritable bowel syndrome, and is available as tablets. It is not normally given to children under ten years, except on medical advice.
✚▲ Side-effects/warnings: See MEBEVERINE HYDROCHLORIDE.

Equilon Herbal

(Chefaro) is a proprietary, non-prescription preparation of the ANTISPASMODIC peppermint

E

oil. It can be used to give relief from irritable bowel syndrome, and is available as capsules. It is not recommended for children.

✚▲ Side-effects/warnings: See PEPPERMINT OIL.

ergocalciferol

(calciferol, vitamin D_2) is one of the natural forms of calciferol (vitamin D) which are formed in plants by the action of sunlight. It is vitamin D_2 but in medicine it is usually referred to as ergocalciferol or simply calciferol, and is used to make up deficiencies (often with calcium). Administration can be either oral or by injection.

✚▲ Side-effects/warnings: See VITAMIN D.

✪ **Related entry: Calcium and Ergocalciferol Tablets.**

ergometrine maleate

is an alkaloid VASOCONSTRICTOR and uterine stimulant which is used routinely in obstetric practice. It is administered to women in childbirth to speed up the third stage of labour (the delivery of the placenta), as a measure to prevent excessive postnatal bleeding and also bleeding due to incomplete abortion (when it may be combined with OXYTOCIN).

Administration is either oral or by injection.

✚ Side-effects: There may be nausea and vomiting; palpitations, breathlessness, slowing of the heart beat, headache, dizziness; abdominal and chest pain; rarely, cardiovascular complications.

▲ Warnings: It is not be administered to those with vascular disease, certain kidney, liver, heart or lung disorders, sepsis, severe hypertension or eclampsia. It should be administered with caution to those with heart disease, hypertension, blood disorders, multiple pregnancy or porphyria.

✪ **Related entry: Syntometrine.**

ergot alkaloid 🅱

is the term used to describe any of a group of alkaloids (see ALKALOID) derived, directly isolated or semisynthetically modified, from a mould or fungus called *Claviceps purpurea*, which grows on infected damp rye. These alkaloids are powerful VASOCONSTRICTOR substances that narrow the blood vessels in the fingers and toes, in particular, and cause a tingling sensation that progressively develops into pain then gangrene. Ergot poisoning was known as St Anthony's Fire and was caused by eating bread made from rye contaminated with ergot. In medicine, the dose of individual alkaloids is adjusted carefully to avoid the development of the more serious side-effects. ERGOTAMINE TARTRATE is the principal vasoconstrictor used in medicine and is mainly given as an ANTIMIGRAINE treatment. ERGOMETRINE MALEATE is used to contract the uterus in the last stages of labour and to minimize post-partum haemorrhage (it is the drug of choice because its effects on blood vessels are less pronounced). Some notable examples of semisynthetic ergot derivatives, which are used for a variety of purposes, include BROMOCRIPTINE, CO-DERGOCRINE MESILATE, ERGOTAMINE TARTRATE, PERGOLIDE, METHYSERGIDE and LISURIDE MALEATE (lisuride maleate). All the ergot alkaloids are chemically derivatives of lysergide acid, and lysergide (lysergic acid diethylamide) is the medical name for LSD.

ergotamine tartrate

is a vegetable ALKALOID which is given to patients who suffer from migraine that is not relieved by the ordinary forms of painkilling drug. It is most effective if administered during the aura – the initial symptoms – of an attack and probably works as a VASOCONSTRICTOR on the cranial arteries. However, although the pain may be relieved, other symptoms, such as the visual disturbances and nausea, may not (but other drugs may be used to treat these symptoms separately). Repeated treatment may, in some patients, cause ergot poisoning, which can cause gangrene of the fingers and toes and confusion. So the frequency with which ergotamine is taken must be carefully limited.

Administration is orally or topically as suppositories.

✚ Side-effects: Vomiting, nausea, vertigo, abdominal pain and diarrhoea, cramps, effects on the heart including pain. Repeated high dosage may cause confusion, gangrene and peritoneal fibrosis.

▲ Warnings: It is not to be used in prophylaxis of migraine attacks. If there is numbness or tingling in the extremities, stop treatment and seek medical advice. It is not to be used in patients who are pregnant or breast-feeding, who have vascular disease (eg Raynaud's disease), certain kidney or liver disorders, severe hypertension, porphyria, sepsis or hyperthyroidism. There can

be serious interactions with other drugs (eg the antimigraine drug SUMATRIPTAN).
✪ **Related entries: Cafergot; Migril.**

Ervevax

(SmithKline Beecham; GSK) is a proprietary, prescription-only VACCINE preparation for the prevention of rubella (German measles). It is available in a form for injection.
✚▲ Side-effects/warnings: See RUBELLA VACCINE.

Erwinase

(Ipsen) is a proprietary, prescription-only preparation of the ANTICANCER drug cristantaspase. It can be used in the treatment of leukaemia, and is available in a form for injection.
✚▲ Side-effects/warnings: See CRISTANTASPASE.

Eryacne

(Galderma) is a proprietary, prescription-only preparation of the ANTIBACTERIAL and (MACROLIDE) ANTIBIOTIC erythromycin. It can be used to treat acne, and is available as a gel for topical application.
✚▲ Side-effects/warnings: See ERYTHROMYCIN.

Erymax

(Elan) is a proprietary, prescription-only preparation of the ANTIBACTERIAL and (MACROLIDE) ANTIBIOTIC erythromycin. It can be used to treat and prevent many forms of infection, and is available as capsules.
✚▲ Side-effects/warnings: See ERYTHROMYCIN.

Erythrocin

(Abbott) is a proprietary, prescription-only preparation of the ANTIBACTERIAL and (MACROLIDE) ANTIBIOTIC erythromycin. It can be used to treat and prevent many forms of infection, and is available as tablets.
✚▲ Side-effects/warnings: See ERYTHROMYCIN.

erythromycin

is an ANTIBACTERIAL and ANTIBIOTIC drug which is an original member of the MACROLIDE group. It has a similar spectrum of action to PENICILLIN, but acts in a different way (macrolides work by inhibiting microbial protein synthesis). It is effective against many Gram-positive bacteria including streptococci (infections of the soft tissue and respiratory tract), mycoplasma (pneumonia), *Legionella* (legionnaires' disease) and chlamydia (urethritis). It can also be used in the treatment of acne, rosacea and chronic prostatitis and to prevent diphtheria and whooping cough. Its principal use is as an alternative to penicillin in individuals who are allergic to that drug. However, bacterial resistance to erythromycin is quite common. Administration is either by injection or oral (tablets are coated to prevent the drug being inactivated in the stomach).
✚ Side-effects: Depending on the route of administration, there may be nausea and vomiting, abdominal discomfort and diarrhoea after large doses; allergic sensitivity reactions including rashes (urticaria); reversible hearing loss after large doses; jaundice on prolonged use.
▲ Warnings: Use with caution in patients with certain heart, liver or kidney disorders; or who are pregnant or breast-feeding, or have porphyria.
✪ **Related entries: Aknemycin Plus; Benzamycin; Eryacne; Erymax; Erythrocin; Erythroped; Erythroped A; Isotrexin; Rommix; Stiemycin; Tiloryth; Zineryt.**

Erythroped

(Abbott) is a proprietary, prescription-only preparation of the ANTIBACTERIAL and (MACROLIDE) ANTIBIOTIC erythromycin. It can be used to treat and prevent many forms of infection, and is available as a suspension in several forms, *Erythroped SF Forte* or *PI SF.*
✚▲ Side-effects/warnings: See ERYTHROMYCIN.

Erythroped A

(Abbott) is a proprietary, prescription-only preparation of the ANTIBACTERIAL and (MACROLIDE) ANTIBIOTIC erythromycin. It can be used to treat and prevent many forms of infection, and is available as tablets.
✚▲ Side-effects/warnings: See ERYTHROMYCIN.

Eskamel

(Goldshield) is a proprietary, non-prescription compound preparation of the KERATOLYTIC agent resorcinol and sulphur. It can be used to treat acne, and is available as a cream.
✚▲ Side-effects/warnings: See RESORCINOL; SULPHUR.

Esmeron

(Organon) is a proprietary, prescription-only

E

preparation of the (*non-depolarizing*) SKELETAL MUSCLE RELAXANT rocuronium bromide. It can be used to induce muscle paralysis during surgery, and is available in a form for injection.
✚▲ Side-effects/warnings: See ROCURONIUM BROMIDE.

esmolol hydrochloride

is a BETA-BLOCKER which can be used as an ANTIHYPERTENSIVE for raised blood pressure and heart rate during operations and as an ANTI-ARRHYTHMIC, in the short term, to regularize heartbeat. Administration is by injection.
✚▲ Side-effects/warnings: See PROPRANOLOL HYDROCHLORIDE.
✪ **Related entry: Brevibloc.**

esomeprazole

is an ULCER-HEALING DRUG. It works as an inhibitor of gastric acid secretion in the parietal (acid-producing) cells of the stomach lining by acting as a PROTON-PUMP INHIBITOR. It is used for the treatment of benign gastric and duodenal ulcers, gastro-oesophageal reflux disease and duodenal ulcer associated with *Helicobacter pylori*. Administration is oral.
✚▲ Side-effects/warnings: See PROTON-PUMP INHIBITOR. Also reported, dermatitis. It should be used with caution in those with kidney impairment.
✪ **Related entry: Nexium.**

Estracombi

(Novartis) is a proprietary, prescription-only compound preparation of estradiol (an OESTROGEN) and norethisterone (as acetate; a PROGESTOGEN). It can be used to treat menopausal problems, including in HRT, and is available as skin patches of two types.
✚▲ Side-effects/warnings: See NORETHISTERONE; ESTRADIOL.

Estracyt

(Pharmacia) is a proprietary, prescription-only preparation of the ANTICANCER drug estramustine phosphate. It can be used to treat cancer of the prostate gland. Available as capsules.
✚▲ Side-effects/warnings: See ESTRAMUSTINE PHOSPHATE.

Estraderm MX

(Novartis) is a proprietary, prescription-only preparation of the OESTROGEN estradiol. It can be used in HRT, and is available in the form of skin patches.
✚▲ Side-effects/warnings: See ESTRADIOL.

Estraderm TTS

(Novartis) is a proprietary, prescription-only preparation of the OESTROGEN estradiol. It can be used in HRT, and is available as skin patches.
✚▲ Side-effects/warnings: See ESTRADIOL.

estradiol

(oestradiol) is the main female sex hormone (see SEX HORMONES) produced and secreted by the ovaries. It is an OESTROGEN and is used therapeutically to make up hormonal deficiencies, for instance, in HRT (hormone replacement therapy). Administration can be oral, by injection, implants, skin patches and nasal spray (which can also be used by directing the spray between the cheek and gum above the upper cheek in women who have a severely blocked nose).
✚▲ Side-effects/warnings: See OESTROGEN.
✪ **Related entries: Adgyn Combi; Adgyn Estro; Aerodiol; Climagest; Climaval; Climesse; Cyclo-Progynova; Dermestril; Dermestril-Septem; Elleste Solo; Elleste Solo MX; Elleste-Duet; Elleste-Solo; Estracombi; Estraderm MX; Estraderm TTS; Estrapak 50; Estring; Evorel; Femapak; Fematrix; Femoston; FemSeven; Hormonin; Indivina; Kliofem; Kliovance; Menorest; Menoring-50; Nuvelle; Nuvelle Continuous; Nuvelle TS; Oestrogel; Progynova; Progynova TS; Sandrena; Tridestra; Trisequens; Vagifem; Zumenon.**

Estradiol Implants

(Organon) is a proprietary, prescription-only preparation of the OESTROGEN estradiol. It can be used in HRT, and is available in the form of an implant.
✚▲ Side-effects/warnings: See ESTRADIOL.

estramustine phosphate

is an (*alkylating agent*) CYTOTOXIC drug and an OESTROGEN. It can be used as an ANTICANCER drug to treat cancer of the prostate gland, and is administered orally.
✚▲ Side-effects/warnings: See CYTOTOXIC. It causes some feminization in men (eg growth of breasts), altered liver function and cardiovascular disorders.

E

✪ Related entry: Estracyt.

Estrapak 50

(Novartis) is a proprietary, prescription-only compound preparation of estradiol (an OESTROGEN) and norethisterone (a PROGESTOGEN). It can be used in HRT, and is available as a calendar pack of skin patches and tablets.

✚▲ Side-effects/warnings: See NORETHISTERONE; ESTRADIOL.

Estring

(Pharmacia) is a proprietary, prescription-only preparation of the OESTROGEN estradiol. It can be used in HRT to treat urogenital complaints in postmenopausal women, and is available as a vaginal ring.

✚▲ Side-effects/warnings: See ESTRADIOL.

estriol

(oestriol) is a female sex hormone, a natural OESTROGEN, produced and secreted mainly by the ovaries. It is used therapeutically to make up hormonal deficiencies (sometimes in combination with a PROGESTOGEN) and to treat menstrual, menopausal or other gynaecological problems (such as infertility). Administration is either oral or by topical application.

✚▲ Side-effects/warnings: See OESTROGEN.

✪ Related entries: Hormonin; Ortho-Gynest; Ovestin.

estropipate

(piperazine oestrone sulphate) is an OESTROGEN, which is used in HRT (hormone replacement therapy) and osteoporosis prophylaxis. Administration is oral.

✚▲ Side-effects/warnings: See OESTROGEN.

✪ Related entry: Harmogen.

etamsylate

(ethamsylate) is a HAEMOSTATIC drug which can be used in some situations where antifibrinolytic drugs might be used, though it appears not to work in the way such drugs normally do (ie preventing clot formation). It seems to improve platelet adhesion (stickiness) and reduce capillary bleeding, and can be used for bleeding in premature infants and menorrhagia (excessive menstrual bleeding). Administration is either oral or by injection.

✚ Side-effects: Headache, nausea and rashes.

▲ Warnings: It should not be administered to patients with porphyria.

✪ Related entry: Dicynene.

ethambutol hydrochloride

is an ANTIBACTERIAL which is used as an ANTITUBERCULAR treatment for tuberculosis that is resistant to other types of drug. It is used mainly in combination (to cover resistance and for maximum effect) with other antitubercular drugs, such as ISONIAZID or RIFAMPICIN. Administration is oral.

✚ Side-effects: These are rare and mostly in the form of visual disturbances (such as loss of acuity or colour-blindness), effects on nerves, rash and itching, blood changes.

▲ Warnings: It should not be administered to children under six years or to patients who suffer from nerve disorders of the eyes. Administer with caution to patients with poor kidney function, the elderly or who are pregnant. Eye tests are advised during treatment.

ethamsylate

see ETAMSYLATE.

ethanol

is the name of a class of compounds that are derived from hydrocarbons. The best-known alcohol is ETHYL ALCOHOL, or ethanol. Although not commonly used in medicine, the actions of ethanol are similar to a number of drugs that depress the central nervous system and is therefore similar to SEDATIVE or HYPNOTIC drugs. The apparent stimulation experienced by many users is usually due to the loss of social inhibitions (ie an inhibiting rather than a stimulating action). Although it *can* be used as a hypnotic drug, it can also cause rebound wakefulness during the night.

Ethanol has quite a strong DIURETIC action, which can also lead to a disrupted night's sleep. There is also a marked dilation of blood vessels (particularly of the face) which can lead to a profound and potentially dangerous loss of body heat in cold weather. An equally dangerous and sometimes lethal side-effect is that vomiting is stimulated at higher doses and a protective reflex is inhibited which can lead to the inhalation of vomit. For medical purposes, a strong solution of ethanol can be used as an ANTISEPTIC (particularly to prepare skin before injection) or as a preservative. Ethanol can also be administered by intravenous infusion to delay labour.

ethanolamine oleate

(monoethanolamine oleate) is used in sclerotherapy, which is a technique to treat varicose veins by the injection of an irritant solution. Administration is by slow injection.

✚ Side-effects: Some patients experience allergic sensitivity reactions.

▲ Warnings: Leakage of the drug into the tissues at the site of injection may cause tissue damage. It should not be injected into patients whose varicose veins are already inflamed or so painful as to prevent walking, who are obese or are taking oral contraceptives.

✪ Related entry: Ethanolamine Oleate Injection.

Ethanolamine Oleate Injection

(Celltech) is a non-proprietary, prescription-only preparation of ethanolamine oleate. It can be used in sclerotherapy, which is a technique to treat varicose veins by the injection of an irritant solution. It is available in a form for slow injection.

✚▲ Side-effects/warnings: See ETHANOLAMINE OLEATE.

Ethimil MR

(Genus) is a proprietary, prescription-only preparation of the CALCIUM-CHANNEL BLOCKER verapamil hydrochloride. It can be used as an ANTIHYPERTENSIVE, as an ANTI-ANGINA treatment in the prevention of attacks. It is available as modified-release tablets.

✚▲ Side-effects/warnings: See VERAPAMIL HYDROCHLORIDE.

ethinylestradiol

(ethinyloestradiol) is a synthetic OESTROGEN which has been used to make up hormonal deficiencies – sometimes in combination with a PROGESTOGEN – to treat menstrual, menopausal or other gynaecological problems, and is also a constituent of many ORAL CONTRACEPTIVE preparations. It can also be used as an ANTICANCER drug in men with cancer of the prostate; and rarely (under specialist care) for hereditary haemorrhagic telangiectasia (hereditary condition of distended blood capillaries and bleeding). One form is available as a compound preparation with CYPROTERONE ACETATE for the treatment of acne. It can also be used in anticancer treatment for breast cancer. Administration is oral.

✚▲ Side-effects/warnings: These depend on use; also, see OESTROGEN. There may be nausea and vomiting. A common effect is weight gain, generally through fluid or sodium retention in the tissues. The breasts may become tender and enlarged. There may also be headache and/or depression; sometimes a rash; thrombosis; in men, feminizing effects including breast enlargement and impotence.

✪ Related entries: BiNovum; Brevinor; Cilest; Dianette; Eugynon 30; Femodene; Femodene ED; Femodette; Loestrin 20; Loestrin 30; Logynon; Logynon ED; Marvelon; Mercilon; Microgynon 30; Minulet; Norimin; Ovran; Ovran 30; Ovranette; Ovysmen; Synphase; Triadene; Tri-Minulet; Trinordiol; TriNovum.

Ethmozine

(Shire) is a proprietary, prescription-only preparation of the ANTI-ARRHYTHMIC moracizine hydrochloride. It can be used to treat irregularities of the heartbeat, and is available (on a named-patient basis only) as tablets.

✚▲ Side-effects/warnings: See MORACIZINE HYDROCHLORIDE.

ethoheptazine citrate

is an (OPIOID) NARCOTIC ANALGESIC related to PETHIDINE HYDROCHLORIDE which is used only in a compound preparation with other drugs. Administration is oral.

✚▲ Side-effects/warnings: See OPIOID.

✪ Related entry: Equagesic.

ethosuximide

is an ANTICONVULSANT and ANTI-EPILEPTIC which can be used mainly to treat absence (petit mal), myoclonic and some other types of seizure. Administration is oral.

✚ Side-effects: These include gastrointestinal disturbances, drowsiness, dizziness, movement disturbances, headache, hiccup, depression or mild euphoria, rashes, liver and kidney changes, effects on blood and psychotic states; also a number of other side-effects.

▲ Warnings: It should be administered with caution to patients with porphyria, kidney or

liver impairment, or who are pregnant or breast-feeding. The withdrawal of treatment should be gradual. If symptoms such as sore throat, fever, bruising or mouth ulcers occur, medical help should be sought.
✪ **Related entries: Emeside; Zarontin.**

ethyl alcohol

or ethanol, is the form of alcohol that is produced by the fermentation of sugar by yeast and which is found in alcoholic drinks. Therapeutically, it is used as a solvent in some medicines and as an ANTISEPTIC.
✚▲ Side-effects/warnings: See ETHANOL.

ethyl nicotinate

is a VASODILATOR which can be used to help improve blood circulation. It can be used with other constituents in compound preparations for topical use in the mouth or ears to relieve the pain of teething, ulcers or minor scratches. Administration is by topical application.
✚▲ Side-effects/warnings: It is regarded as safe in normal topical use at correct dosage.
✪ **Related entries: PR Heat Spray; Transvasin Heat Rub.**

ethyl salicylate

is a NSAID (non-steroidal anti-inflammatory drug) with COUNTER-IRRITANT, or RUBEFACIENT, actions and can be applied to the skin for symptomatic relief of pain in underlying organs, for instance in rheumatic and other musculoskeletal disorders. Administration is topical.
✚▲ Side-effects/warnings: See NSAID, though normally little is absorbed into the circulation and local side-effects are limited to mild irritation. It should not be used on broken skin or mucous membranes. See also SALICYLATE; SALICYLIC ACID.
✪ **Related entries: Deep Heat Spray; PR Heat Spray; Ralgex Stick.**

ethynodiol diacetate

see ETYNODIOL DIACETATE.

Ethyol

(Schering-Plough) is a proprietary, prescription-only preparation of amifostine, a specialist drug used as an ANTIDOTE to reduce complications in treatment of cancers with CYCLOPHOSPHAMIDE or CISPLATIN. It is available in a form for intravenous infusion.
✚▲ Side-effects/warnings: See AMIFOSTINE.

etidronate

see DISODIUM ETIDRONATE.

etodolac

is a (NSAID) NON-NARCOTIC ANALGESIC and ANTIRHEUMATIC drug. It is used primarily to treat the pain and inflammation of rheumatoid arthritis and osteoarthritis. Administration is oral.
✚▲ Side-effects/warnings: See NSAID.
✪ **Related entry: Lodine SR.**

etonogestrel

is a PROGESTOGEN which is used as an ORAL CONTRACEPTIVE in the form of an implant.
✚▲ Side-effects/warnings: See PROGESTOGEN.
✪ **Related entry: Implanton.**

Etopophos

(Bristol-Myers Squibb) is a proprietary, prescription-only preparation of the (CYTOTOXIC) ANTICANCER drug etoposide. It can be used in the treatment of cancers, particularly lymphoma or small cell carcinoma of the bronchus, also cancer of the testicle. It is available in a form for injection.
✚▲ Side-effects/warnings: See ETOPOSIDE.

etoposide

is an ANTICANCER drug which is used primarily to treat small cell lung cancer, lymphomas and cancer of the testes. It works in much the same way as the VINCA ALKALOIDS by disrupting the replication of cancer cells and so preventing further growth. Administration is either oral or by injection.
✚▲ Side-effects/warnings: See CYTOTOXIC.
✪ **Related entries: Etopophos; Vepesid.**

etynodiol diacetate

(ethynodiol diacetate) is a PROGESTOGEN which is used as a constituent of the PROGESTOGEN-only (*POP*) type ORAL CONTRACEPTIVE pills. Administration is oral.
✚▲ Side-effects/warnings: See PROGESTOGEN.
✪ **Related entry: Femulen.**

Eucardic

(Roche) is a proprietary, prescription-only

E

preparation of the BETA-BLOCKER carvedilol. It can be used as an ANTIHYPERTENSIVE, in the treatment of angina pectoris (see ANTI-ANGINA) and in HEART FAILURE TREATMENT. It is available as tablets.
✚▲ Side-effects/warnings: See CARVEDILOL.

Eucerin

(Beiersdorf) is a proprietary, non-prescription preparation of the HYDRATING AGENT urea. It can be used for dry skin conditions such as eczema, and is available as a cream and lotion.
✚▲ Side-effects/warnings: See UREA.

Eudemine (injection)

(Goldshield) is a proprietary, prescription-only preparation of diazoxide. It can be used, when administered by injection, as a VASODILATOR and ANTIHYPERTENSIVE to treat hypertensive crisis. It is available in a form for rapid intravenous injection.
✚▲ Side-effects/warnings: See DIAZOXIDE.

Eudemine (tablets)

(Celltech) is a proprietary, prescription-only preparation of diazoxide. It can be used, when taken orally, as a hyperglycaemic to treat chronic hypoglycaemia. It is available as tablets.
✚▲ Side-effects/warnings: See DIAZOXIDE.

Euglucon

(Hoechst Marion Roussel; Aventis Pharma) is a proprietary, prescription-only preparation of the SULPHONYLUREA glibenclamide. It is used in DIABETIC TREATMENT of Type II diabetes (non-insulin-dependent diabetes mellitus; NIDDM; maturity-onset diabetes). It is available as tablets.
✚▲ Side-effects/warnings: See GLIBENCLAMIDE.

Eugynon 30

(Schering Health) is a proprietary, prescription-only compound preparation which can be used as a (*monophasic*) ORAL CONTRACEPTIVE of the *COC* (standard strength) type that combines an OESTROGEN and a PROGESTOGEN, in this case ethinylestradiol and levonorgestrel. It is available as tablets in a calendar pack.
✚▲ Side-effects/warnings: See ETHINYLESTRADIOL; LEVONORGESTREL.

Eumovate

(GlaxoWellcome; GSK) is a proprietary, prescription-only preparation of the CORTICOSTEROID and ANTI-INFLAMMATORY clobetasone butyrate. It can be used to treat non-infective and severe inflammation of the skin caused by conditions such as eczema and various forms of dermatitis. It is used particularly as a maintenance treatment between courses of more potent corticosteroids. It is available as a cream and an ointment.
✚▲ Side-effects/warnings: See CLOBETASONE BUTYRATE.

Eurax Cream

(Novartis Consumer Health) is a proprietary, non-prescription preparation of crotamiton. It has antipruritic activity and so can be used to treat itching (pruritus) dry skin conditions such as dermatitis, eczema, heat rash and in the treatment for scabies. It is available as a cream. It is not normally given to children under three years, except on medical advice.
✚▲ Side-effects/warnings: See CROTAMITON.

Eurax HC Cream

(Novartis Consumer Health) is a proprietary, non-prescription compound preparation of the CORTICOSTEROID and ANTI-INFLAMMATORY hydrocortisone and antipruritic crotamiton. It is used to treat itching (eg in scabies) and inflammation of the skin, and is available as a cream for topical application. It is not normally given to children under ten years, except on medical advice.
✚▲ Side-effects/warnings: See CROTAMITON; HYDROCORTISONE.

Eurax-Hydrocortisone

(Novartis Consumer Health) is a proprietary, prescription-only compound preparation of the CORTICOSTEROID and ANTI-INFLAMMATORY hydrocortisone and antipruritic crotamiton. It is used to treat itching (eg in eczema) and inflammation of the skin, and is available as a cream for topical application.
✚▲ Side-effects/warnings: See CROTAMITON; HYDROCORTISONE.

Eurax Lotion

(Novartis Consumer Health) is a proprietary, non-prescription preparation of crotamiton. It has antipruritic activity so can be used to treat itching due to sunburn, dermatitis, eczema, heat rash and as treatment for scabies. It is available as a lotion. It is not normally used by pregnant women or children under three years, except on medical advice.

✚▲ Side-effects/warnings: See CROTAMITON.

Evista

(Lilly) is a proprietary, prescription-only preparation of raloxifene hydrochloride which has some OESTROGEN activity at some sites in the body, and is used as a form of HRT (hormone replacement therapy) for the prevention of vertebral fractures in postmenopausal women with increased risk of osteoporosis. It is available as tablets.

✚▲ Side-effects/warnings: See RALOXIFENE HYDROCHLORIDE.

Evorel

(Janssen-Cilag) is a proprietary, prescription-only compound preparation of estradiol (an OESTROGEN) and norethisterone (a PROGESTOGEN). It can be used in HRT, and is available in the form of skin patches in various forms (called *Evorel Conti, Evorel Pak, Evorel Sequi.*

✚▲ Side-effects/warnings: See ESTRADIOL; NORETHISTERONE.

Exelderm

(Bioglan) is a proprietary, prescription-only preparation of the ANTIFUNGAL sulconazole nitrate. It can be used to treat fungal skin infections, particularly tinea, and is available as a cream for topical application.

✚▲ Side-effects/warnings: See SULCONAZOLE NITRATE.

Exelon

(Novartis) is a prescription-only form of the ANTICHOLINESTERASE rivastigmine which can be used in DEMENTIA TREATMENT. It is available as capsules and as an oral solution.

✚▲ Side-effects/warnings: See RIVASTIGMINE.

Ex-Lax Senna

(Novartis Consumer Health) is a proprietary, non-prescription preparation of the (stimulant) LAXATIVE senna. It can be used to relieve constipation, and is available as a chocolate bar. It is not normally given to children under six years, except on medical advice.

✚▲ Side-effects/warnings: See SENNA.

Exocin

(Allergan) is a proprietary, prescription-only preparation of the (QUINOLONE) antibiotic-like ANTIBACTERIAL ofloxacin. It can be used to treat bacterial infections of the eye, and is available as eye-drops.

✚▲ Side-effects/warnings: See OFLOXACIN.

Exorex Lotion

(Pharmax) is a proprietary, non-prescription preparation of coal tar in an emulsion. It can be used to treat psoriasis of the skin and scalp, and is available as a lotion.

✚▲ Side-effects/warnings: See COAL TAR.

expectorant 🅴

is the term used to describe medicated liquids intended to change the viscosity of sputum (phlegm), so making it more watery and easier to cough up (an action of mucolytics). In high dosage, most expectorants can be used as emetics (to provoke vomiting), which leads to the traditional suggestion that they act as expectorants by stimulating nerves in the stomach to cause reflex secretion of fluid by the bronchioles in the lungs. However, it is not known for sure how they act and, further, there is considerable doubt about their clinical efficacy. Examples include IPECACUANHA, GUAIFENESIN (guaiphenesin) and AMMONIUM CHLORIDE.

Exterol Ear Drops

(Dermal) is a proprietary, non-prescription preparation of the ANTISEPTIC agent HYDROGEN PEROXIDE in a complex with UREA in glycerol. It can be used to dissolve and wash out earwax, and is available as ear-drops.

✚▲ Side-effects/warnings: See GLYCEROL; HYDROGEN PEROXIDE; UREA.

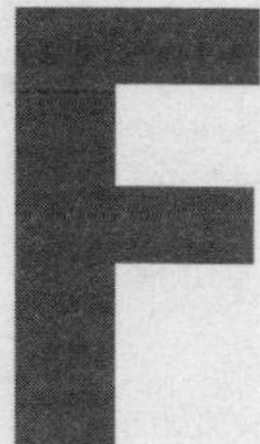

factor IX fraction, dried

is prepared from human blood plasma. It may also contain clotting factor II, VII and X. It is a HAEMOSTATIC used in treating patients with a deficiency in factor IX (Christmas Factor), haemophilia B. It is available in a form for intravenous infusion.

✚ Side-effects: There may be allergic reactions with fever or chills.

▲ Warnings: Risk of thrombosis (blood clots); it should not be used in conditions of uncontrolled generalized clotting (disseminated intravascular coagulation).

✪ **Related entries: AlphaNine; BeneFIX; HT Defix; Mononine; Replenine-VF.**

factor VIIa (recombinant)

is a preparation of recombinant human antihaemophilic factor VII. It acts as a HAEMOSTATIC drug to reduce or stop bleeding and is used to treat disorders in which bleeding is prolonged and potentially dangerous, usually patients with inhibitors to factors VIII and IX. Administration is by injection.

✪ **Related entry: NovoSeven.**

factor VIII fraction (dried)

(human antihaemophilic fraction, dried) is a dried principle prepared from blood plasma obtained from healthy human donors. It acts as a HAEMOSTATIC drug to reduce or stop bleeding, and is administered by intravenous infusion or injection to treat disorders in which bleeding is prolonged and potentially dangerous (mainly haemophilia A).

✚ Side-effects: There may be allergic reactions with fever or chills; rarely raised fibrin levels in the blood are seen.

▲ Warnings: Clotting within blood vessels is possible after large or frequent doses (in blood groups A, B and AB).

✪ **Related entries: Alphanate; Kogenate; Liberate; Monoclate-P; Replenate; 8Y.**

factor VIII fraction (octocog alfa)

is a preparation of recombinant human antihaemophilic factor VIII. It acts as a HAEMOSTATIC drug to reduce or stop bleeding, and is administered by intravenous infusion or injection to treat disorders in which bleeding is prolonged and potentially dangerous (mainly haemophilia A).

✚▲ Side-effects/warnings: See FACTOR VIII FRACTION (DRIED).

✪ **Related entries: Kogenate; Recombinate; ReFacto.**

factor VIII inhibitor bypassing fraction

is prepared from blood plasma obtained from healthy human donors and used as a HAEMO-STATIC in patients with factor VIII inhibitors. There is also a porcine preparation of antihaemophilic factor for patients with inhibitors to human factor VIII available. It is available, only on prescription, in a form for intravenous infusion.

✪ **Related entry: Hyate C.**

famciclovir

is an ANTIVIRAL drug similar to ACICLOVIR (acyclovir), but which can be given less often. It is a pro-drug of PENCICLOVIR. It is used to treat infection caused by herpes zoster and for recurrent genital herpes. Administration is oral.

✚ Side-effects: Headache, nausea and vomiting, sometimes dizziness, hallucinations and confusion, rash.

▲ Warnings: It should be administered with caution to patients who are pregnant or breast-feeding, or who have impaired kidney function.

✪ **Related entry: Famvir.**

Famel Original Cough Syrup

(SSL) is a proprietary, non-prescription preparation of the (OPIOID) ANTITUSSIVE codeine phosphate. It can be used to relieve a dry, troublesome cough, and is available as a linctus. It is not normally given to children, except on medical advice.

✚▲ Side-effects/warnings: See CODEINE PHOSPHATE.

famotidine

is an H_2-ANTAGONIST and ULCER-HEALING DRUG.

It can be used to assist in the treatment of benign peptic (gastric and duodenal) ulcers, to relieve heartburn in cases of reflux oesophagitis, Zollinger-Ellison syndrome and a variety of conditions where reduction of acidity is beneficial. It works by reducing the secretion of gastric acid (by acting as a histamine receptor H_2-receptor antagonist), so reducing erosion and bleeding from peptic ulcers and allowing them a chance to heal. However, treatment with famotidine should not begin before a full diagnosis of gastric bleeding or serious pain has been completed, because its action in restricting gastric secretions may possibly mask the presence of stomach cancer. Administration is oral. (Although it is a prescription-only drug when used for the treatment of ulcers and related conditions, it can be sold over-the-counter in limited quantities and dosage for occasional indigestion and heartburn for people over sixteen years.)

✚▲ Side-effects/warnings: See H_2-ANTAGONIST. Also, rarely, there may be anxiety, rash and skin toxicity, loss of appetite, dry mouth. It is not used for children.

✪ **Related entries: Pepcid; Pepcid AC.**

Famvir

(Novartis) is a proprietary, prescription-only preparation of the ANTIVIRAL famciclovir. It can be used to treat infections caused by herpes zoster simplex, and is available as tablets.

✚▲ Side-effects/warnings: See FAMCICLOVIR.

Fansidar

(Roche) is a proprietary, prescription-only compound preparation of the ANTIMALARIAL drug pyrimethamine and the SULPHONAMIDE sulfadoxine. It can be used to treat patients who are seriously ill with malaria, and is available as tablets.

✚▲ Side-effects/warnings: See PYRIMETHAMINE; SULFADOXINE.

Fareston

(Orion) is a proprietary, prescription-only preparation of the sex HORMONE ANTAGONIST toremifene (as citrate). It inhibits the effect of OESTROGEN and because of this is used as an ANTICANCER treatment of hormone-dependent metastatic breast cancer in postmenopausal women. It is available as tablets.

✚▲ Side-effects/warnings: See TOREMIFENE.

Farlutal

(Pharmacia) is a proprietary, prescription-only preparation of the synthetic PROGESTOGEN medroxyprogesterone acetate. It can be used as an ANTICANCER treatment for cancer of the endometrium of the uterus, breast, kidney and sometimes prostate in men. It is available as tablets (in two forms) and in a form for injection.

✚▲ Side-effects/warnings: See MEDROXYPROGESTERONE ACETATE.

Fasigyn

(Pfizer) is a proprietary, prescription-only preparation of the ANTIBACTERIAL and ANTIPROTOZOAL tinidazole. It can be used to treat anaerobic bacterial and protozoal infections. It is available as tablets.

✚▲ Side-effects/warnings: See TINIDAZOLE.

Fasturtec

(Sanofi-Synthelabo) is a proprietary, prescription-only preparation of the enzyme (see ENZYMES) rasburicase. It can be used to prevent or treat acute rise in blood urea which is caused by chemotherapy for blood cancers. It is available in a form for intravenous infusion.

✚▲ Side-effects/warnings: See RASBURICASE.

Faverin

(Solvay) is a proprietary, prescription-only preparation of the (SSRI) ANTIDEPRESSANT fluvoxamine maleate, also used for obsessive-compulsive disorders. It is available as tablets.

✚▲ Side-effects/warnings: See FLUVOXAMINE MALEATE.

Fectrim

(DDSA) is a proprietary, prescription-only compound preparation of the (SULPHONAMIDE) ANTIBACTERIAL sulfamethoxazole and the antibacterial trimethoprim, which is a combination called co-trimoxazole. It can be used to treat bacterial infections, and is available as soluble tablets; a stronger preparation, *Fectrim Forte*, is also available.

✚▲ Side-effects/warnings: See CO-TRIMOXAZOLE.

Fefol

(Celltech) is a proprietary, non-prescription

F

compound preparation of ferrous sulphate and folic acid. It can be used as an IRON and folic acid supplement during pregnancy, and is available as modified-release capsules (called *Spansules*).
✚▲ Side-effects/warnings: See FERROUS SULPHATE; FOLIC ACID.

felbinac

is a (NSAID) NON-NARCOTIC ANALGESIC and ANTIRHEUMATIC drug. (It is the active drug to which FENBUFEN is converted in the body.) It is used by topical application.
✚▲ Side-effects/warnings: See NSAID.
✪ **Related entries: Traxam; Traxam Pain Relief Gel.**

Feldene

(Pfizer) is a proprietary, prescription-only preparation of the (NSAID) NON-NARCOTIC ANALGESIC and ANTIRHEUMATIC piroxicam. It can be used to treat acute gout, arthritic and rheumatic pain and other musculoskeletal disorders. It is available as capsules, soluble tablets, as suppositories and in a form for injection. It is also available as a preparation called *Feldene Melt*, which can be taken by placing on the tongue or swallowing.
✚▲ Side-effects/warnings: See PIROXICAM.

Feldene P Gel

(Warner Lambert Consumer Healthcare; Pfizer) is a proprietary, non-prescription preparation of the (NSAID) NON-NARCOTIC ANALGESIC and ANTIRHEUMATIC piroxicam, which also has COUNTER-IRRITANT, or RUBEFACIENT, actions. It can be applied topically to the skin for symptomatic relief of underlying muscle or joint pain, and is available as a gel. It is not normally given to children, except on medical advice.
✚▲ Side-effects/warnings: See PIROXICAM; but adverse effects on topical application are limited.

felodipine

is a CALCIUM-CHANNEL BLOCKER which is used as an ANTIHYPERTENSIVE and as an ANTI-ANGINA drug to prevent attacks. Administration is oral.
✚ Side-effects: These include flushing, headache and fatigue; dizziness, palpitations; rashes; oedema. There may be an excessive growth of the gums.
▲ Warnings: It should be administered with care to patients with certain liver or heart disorders or who are breast-feeding. Treatment may have to be stopped if there are certain side-effects such as ischaemic pain (pain due to lack of blood supply). Do not use in pregnancy. Grapefruit juice should be avoided since it affects metabolism of the drug.
✪ **Related entries: Plendil; Triapin.**

felypressin

is an analogue of vasopressin and is a VASOCONSTRICTOR and can be incorporated into LOCAL ANAESTHETIC preparations to prolong their duration of action. It is given by injection.
✚▲ Side-effects/warnings: See VASOPRESSIN.
✪ **Related entry: Citanest with Octapressin.**

Femapak

(Solvay) is a proprietary, prescription-only preparation that is a combination pack in two strengths containing patches of *Fematrix*, which release the OESTROGEN estradiol, and tablets of *Duphaston*, which release the PROGESTOGEN (dydrogesterone). It can be used to treat many conditions of hormonal deficiency in women, including menopausal symptoms as part of HRT.
✚▲ Side-effects/warnings: See DYDROGESTERONE, ESTRADIOL.

Femara

(Novartis) is a proprietary, prescription-only preparation of the sex HORMONE ANTAGONIST letrozole. It inhibits the effect of OESTROGEN and because of this is used as an ANTICANCER treatment of hormone-dependent breast cancer in postmenopausal women. It is available as tablets.
✚▲ Side-effects/warnings: See LETROZOLE.

Fematrix

(Solvay) is a proprietary, prescription-only preparation that releases the OESTROGEN estradiol. It can be used to treat menopausal symptoms as part of HRT and for prophylaxis against osteoporosis. It is available as patches in two strengths.
✚▲ Side-effects/warnings: See ESTRADIOL.

Feminax

(Roche Consumer Health) is a proprietary, non-prescription compound analgesic preparation of the NON-NARCOTIC ANALGESIC paracetamol, the NARCOTIC ANALGESIC codeine phosphate, the STIMULANT caffeine and the ANTICHOLINERGIC

and ANTISPASMODIC hyoscine hydrobromide. It can be used specifically to relieve period pain, and is available as capsules.
✚▲ Side-effects/warnings: See CAFFEINE; CODEINE PHOSPHATE; HYOSCINE HYDROBROMIDE; PARACETAMOL.

Femodene

(Schering Health) is a proprietary, prescription-only compound preparation which can be used as a (*monophasic*) ORAL CONTRACEPTIVE of the *COC* (standard strength) type that combines an OESTROGEN and a PROGESTOGEN, in this case ethinylestradiol and gestodene. It is available as tablets in a calendar pack.
✚▲ Side-effects/warnings: See ETHINYLESTRADIOL; GESTODENE.

Femodene ED

(Schering Health) is a proprietary, prescription-only compound preparation which can be used as a (*monophasic*) ORAL CONTRACEPTIVE of the *COC* (standard strength) type that combines an OESTROGEN and a PROGESTOGEN, in this case ethinylestradiol and gestodene. It is available as tablets in a calendar pack.
✚▲ Side-effects/warnings: See ETHINYLESTRADIOL; GESTODENE.

Femodette

(Schering Health) is a proprietary, prescription-only compound preparation that can be used as a (*monophasic*) ORAL CONTRACEPTIVE (and also for certain menstrual problems) of the *COC* (low strength) type that combines an OESTROGEN and a PROGESTOGEN, in this case ethinylestradiol and gestodene. It is available as tablets.
✚▲ Side-effects/warnings: See GESTODENE; ETHINYLESTRADIOL.

Femoston

(Solvay) is a proprietary, prescription-only preparation that is a combination pack containing tablets of both the OESTROGEN estradiol and the PROGESTOGEN dydrogesterone. They are available in various dosage and release combinations (*1/10, 2/10; 2/20*; -conti). They can be used to treat many conditions of hormonal deficiency in women, including menopausal symptoms as part of HRT.
✚▲ Side-effects/warnings: See DYDROGESTERONE; ESTRADIOL.

FemSeven

(Merck) is a proprietary, prescription-only preparation that releases the OESTROGEN estradiol. It can be used to treat menopausal symptoms as part of HRT (including osteoporosis prevention). It is available as patches in various strengths.
✚▲ Side-effects/warnings: See ESTRADIOL.

Femulen

(Pharmacia) is a proprietary, prescription-only preparation which can be used as an ORAL CONTRACEPTIVE of the PROGESTOGEN-only pill (*POP*) type and contains etynodiol diacetate. It is available as tablets in a calendar pack.
✚▲ Side-effects/warnings: See ETYNODIOL DIACETATE.

Fenbid

(Goldshield) is a proprietary, prescription-only preparation of the (NSAID) NON-NARCOTIC ANALGESIC and ANTIRHEUMATIC ibuprofen. It can be used to treat pain and inflammation, especially pain from arthritis and rheumatism and other musculoskeletal disorders, and is available as modified-release capsules (*Spansules*).
✚▲ Side-effects/warnings: See IBUPROFEN.

Fenbid Forte Gel

(Goldshield) is a proprietary, prescription-only preparation of the (NSAID) NON-NARCOTIC ANALGESIC and ANTIRHEUMATIC ibuprofen. It can be used to treat all kinds of pain and inflammation, especially pain from arthritis and rheumatism and other musculoskeletal disorders, and is available as a gel for topical application.
✚▲ Side-effects/warnings: See IBUPROFEN; but with topical application there are few side-effects. Avoid contact with broken skin. Discontinue if a rash appears.

fenbufen

is a (NSAID) NON-NARCOTIC ANALGESIC and ANTIRHEUMATIC drug. It has effects similar to those of aspirin and is used particularly in the treatment of the pain of rheumatoid arthritis and osteoarthritis. (It is a pro-drug of FELBINAC which is also used.) Administration is oral.
✚▲ Side-effects/warnings: See NSAID. It is thought to cause less gastrointestinal bleeding than other NSAIDs. However, it has a greater risk of causing rashes and allergic lung disorders.
✪ **Related entry: Lederfen.**

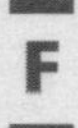

Fennings Children's Cooling Powders

(Anglian Pharma) is a proprietary, non-prescription preparation of the NON-NARCOTIC ANALGESIC paracetamol. It can be used for reducing temperature and relieving the symptoms of painful or feverish conditions, such as toothache, headache, colds and flu. It is available as a powder and is not normally given to children under three months, except on medical advice.

✚▲ Side-effects/warnings: See PARACETAMOL.

Fennings Little Healers

(Anglian Pharma) is a proprietary, non-prescription preparation of the EXPECTORANT ipecacuaha which can be used for coughs associated with colds and catarrh. It is available as tablets and is not normally given to children under five years, except on medical advice.

✚▲ Side-effects/warnings: See IPECACUANHA.

fenofibrate

is a (*fibrate*) LIPID-REGULATING DRUG used in hyperlipidaemia to reduce the levels, or change the proportions, of various lipids in the bloodstream. Generally, it is administered only to patients in whom a strict and regular dietary regime, alone, is not having the desired effect. Administration is oral.

✚▲ Side-effects/warnings: See BEZAFIBRATE. It is not to be used in patients with gall bladder disease, severe kidney or liver disorders; or who are pregnant or breast-feeding. Also, rash, photosensitivity, liver effects (so liver function tests are carried out). Patients should report any muscle weakness, pain or tenderness to their doctor.

✪ **Related entry: Lipantil; Supralip 160.**

Fenoket

(Hawgreen) is a proprietary, prescription-only preparation of the (NSAID) NON-NARCOTIC ANALGESIC and ANTIRHEUMATIC ketoprofen. It can be used to relieve the pain of arthritis and rheumatism and other musculoskeletal disorders, and is available as modified-release capsules.

✚▲ Side-effects/warnings: See KETOPROFEN.

fenoprofen

is a (NSAID) NON-NARCOTIC ANALGESIC and ANTIRHEUMATIC drug. It can be used to treat and relieve pain and inflammation, particularly the pain of arthritis and rheumatism and other musculoskeletal disorders. Administration is oral.

✚▲ Side-effects/warnings: See NSAID. Gastrointestinal side-effects are relatively common. Also, there may be nasopharyngitis, upper respiratory tract infections and cystitis.

✪ **Related entry: Fenopron.**

Fenopron

(Typharm) is a proprietary, prescription-only preparation of the (NSAID) NON-NARCOTIC ANALGESIC and ANTIRHEUMATIC fenoprofen. It can be used to treat and relieve pain and inflammation, particularly the pain of arthritis and rheumatism and other musculoskeletal disorders. It is available as tablets in two strengths, *Fenopron 300* and *Fenopron 600*.

✚▲ Side-effects/warnings: See FENOPROFEN.

fenoterol hydrobromide

is a SYMPATHOMIMETIC and BETA-RECEPTOR STIMULANT. It is mainly used as a BRONCHODILATOR in reversible obstructive airways disease and as an ANTI-ASTHMATIC treatment. Administration is by aerosol.

✚▲ Side-effects/warnings: See SALBUTAMOL. (Users will be cautioned not to exceed the stated dose and if a previously effective dose fails to relieve symptoms, they should consult their doctor.)

✪ **Related entry: Duovent.**

Fenox Nasal Drops

(SSL) is a proprietary, non-prescription preparation of the SYMPATHOMIMETIC and DECONGESTANT phenylephrine hydrochloride. It can be used for the symptomatic relief of nasal congestion associated with colds, catarrh, sinusitis and hay fever. It is available as viscous nose-drops and is not normally given to children under five years, except on medical advice.

✚▲ Side-effects/warnings: See PHENYLEPHRINE HYDROCHLORIDE.

Fenox Nasal Spray

(SSL) is a proprietary, non-prescription preparation of the SYMPATHOMIMETIC and DECONGESTANT phenylephrine hydrochloride. It can be used for the symptomatic relief of nasal congestion associated with colds, catarrh,

sinusitis and hay fever. It is available as a nasal spray and is not normally given to children under five years, except on medical advice.
+▲ Side-effects/warnings: See PHENYLEPHRINE HYDROCHLORIDE.

fentanyl

is an (OPIOID) NARCOTIC ANALGESIC which can be used to treat moderate to severe pain (mainly in operative procedures, but also cancer), to enhance the effect of general anaesthetics and to depress spontaneous respiration in patients having their breathing assisted. Administration is either by intravenous injection or infusion, or transdermally as skin patches. Its proprietary preparations are on the Controlled Drugs list.
+▲ Side-effects/warnings: See OPIOID.
✪ **Related entries: Actiq; Durogesic; Sublimaze.**

Fentazin

(Goldshield) is a proprietary, prescription-only preparation of the ANTIPSYCHOTIC perphenazine. It can be used to treat severe schizophrenia and other psychoses, and also as an ANTINAUSEANT and ANTI-EMETIC to relieve nausea and vomiting. It is available as tablets.
+▲ Side-effects/warnings: See PERPHENAZINE.

fenticonazole nitrate

is an (AZOLE) ANTIFUNGAL drug. It can be used to treat fungal infections including vaginal candidiasis. Administration is by topical application.
+▲ Side-effects/warnings: See CLOTRIMAZOLE. Occasionally, local irritation.
✪ **Related entry: Lomexin.**

Feospan

(Celltech) is a proprietary, non-prescription preparation of ferrous sulphate. It can be used as an IRON supplement in iron-deficiency ANAEMIA TREATMENT, and is available as modified-release capsules (spansules).
+▲ Side-effects/warnings: See FERROUS SULPHATE.

Ferfolic SV

(Sinclair) is a proprietary, prescription-only preparation of ascorbic acid; ferrous gluconate; folic acid. It can be used as an IRON supplement in ANAEMIA TREATMENT and as a folic acid supplement during pregnancy. Available as tablets.
+▲ Side-effects/warnings: See ASCORBIC ACID; FERROUS GLUCONATE; FOLIC ACID.

ferric ammonium citrate

is a drug rich in IRON which is used in iron-deficiency ANAEMIA TREATMENT to restore iron to the body, for example, to prevent deficiency in pregnancy.
+▲ Side-effects/warnings: See FERROUS SULPHATE.
✪ **Related entries: Lexpec with Iron; Lexpec with Iron-M.**

Ferriprox

(Swedish Orphan Int AB) is a newly introduced proprietary, prescription-only preparation of the CHELATING AGENT deferiprone. It can be used as an ANTIDOTE for the treatment of iron overload in patients with thalassaemia. It is available as tablets.
+▲ Side-effects/warnings: See DEFERIPRONE.

Ferrograd

(Abbott) is a non-prescription proprietary preparation of ferrous sulphate. It can be used as an IRON supplement in iron-deficiency ANAEMIA TREATMENT, and is available as modified-release tablets (called *Filmtabs*).
+▲ Side-effects/warnings: See FERROUS SULPHATE.

Ferrograd C

(Abbott) is a proprietary, non-prescription compound preparation of ferrous sulphate and ascorbic acid. It can be used as an IRON supplement for anaemia, and is available as modified-release capsules (called *Filmtabs*).
+▲ Side-effects/warnings: See ASCORBIC ACID; FERROUS SULPHATE.

Ferrograd Folic

(Abbott) is a proprietary, non-prescription compound preparation of ferrous sulphate and folic acid. It can be used as an IRON and folic acid supplement during pregnancy, and is available as tablets (*Filmtabs*).
+▲ Side-effects/warnings: See FERROUS SULPHATE; FOLIC ACID.

Ferrous Sulphate Oral Solution, Paediatric, BP

(paediatric ferrous sulphate mixture) is a non-

F

proprietary, non-prescription preparation of ferrous sulphate. It can be used as an IRON supplement in iron-deficiency ANAEMIA TREATMENT, and is available as a flavoured solution.

✚▲ Side-effects/warnings: See FERROUS SULPHATE.

Ferrous Sulphate Tablets, Compound

is a non-proprietary, non-prescription preparation of ferrous sulphate (with copper sulphate and manganese sulphate). It can be used as an IRON supplement in iron-deficiency anaemias, and is available as tablets.

✚▲ Side-effects/warnings: See FERROUS SULPHATE.

ferrous fumarate

is a drug rich in IRON which is used in iron-deficiency ANAEMIA TREATMENT to restore iron to the body or to prevent deficiency. Administration is oral.

✚▲ Side-effects/warnings: See FERROUS SULPHATE.

✪ **Related entries: Fersaday; Fersamal; Galfer; Galfer FA; Givitol; Pregaday.**

ferrous gluconate

is a drug rich in IRON which is used in iron-deficiency ANAEMIA TREATMENT to restore iron to the body or to prevent deficiency. Administration is oral.

✚▲ Side-effects/warnings: See FERROUS SULPHATE.

✪ **Related entry: Ferfolic SV.**

ferrous glycine sulphate

is a drug rich in IRON which is used in iron-deficiency ANAEMIA TREATMENT to restore iron to the body or to prevent deficiency. Administration is oral.

✚▲ Side-effects/warnings: See FERROUS SULPHATE.

✪ **Related entry: Plesmet.**

ferrous sulphate

is a drug rich in IRON which is used in iron-deficiency ANAEMIA TREATMENT to restore iron to the body or to prevent deficiency. Administration is oral.

✚ Side-effects: May cause gastrointestinal upset, nausea and abdominal cramps; altered bowel habits, diarrhoea or constipation especially in the elderly; there may be vomiting.

▲ Warnings: Iron preparations are best absorbed on an empty stomach, but may cause fewer gastrointestinal upsets if taken with food. Iron salts reduce the absorption of several drugs, including TETRACYCLINES. Stools may be discoloured. Severe toxic effects can occur if large amounts are ingested.

✪ **Related entries: Fefol; Feospan; Ferrograd; Ferrograd C; Ferrograd Folic; Ferrous Sulphate Oral Solution, Paediatric, BP; Ferrous Sulphate Tablets, Compound; Slow-Fe; Slow-Fe Folic.**

Fersaday

(Goldshield) is a proprietary, non-prescription preparation of ferrous fumarate. It can be used as an IRON supplement in iron-deficiency ANAEMIA TREATMENT, and is available as tablets.

✚▲ Side-effects/warnings: See FERROUS FUMARATE.

Fersamal

(Goldshield) is a proprietary, non-prescription preparation of ferrous fumarate. It can be used as an IRON supplement in iron-deficiency ANAEMIA TREATMENT, and is available as tablets and a syrup.

✚▲ Side-effects/warnings: See FERROUS FUMARATE.

fexofenadine hydrochloride

is a recently developed ANTIHISTAMINE drug with less sedative side-effects than some older members of its class. It is the active metabolite of terfenadine (which was formerly used), and can be used for the symptomatic relief of allergic symptoms such as chronic idiopathic urticaria and hay fever. Administration is oral.

✚▲ Side-effects/warnings: See ANTIHISTAMINE. Although the incidence of sedative and anticholinergic effects is low, there may still be drowsiness and dizziness which may impair the performance of skilled tasks such as driving. It should not be used by breast-feeding women, and should be used with care in pregnancy. It is not yet clear whether it shares some of the adverse side-effects of terfenadine.

✪ **Related entries: Telfast 120; Telfast 180.**

fibrinolytic

(or thrombolytic) drugs break up or disperse thrombi (blood clots). They work by activating the breaking down of the protein fibrin, which is the main constituent of many blood clots, and thus break up the thrombus. They can be used rapidly in serious conditions, such as life-threatening venous thrombi, pulmonary embolism and clots in the eye, particularly to re-open the occluded coronary arteries that are occluded in myocardial infarction. See ALTEPLASE; RETEPLASE; STREPTOKINASE; TENECTEPLASE. They are injected or intravenously infused.

✚ Side-effects: Nausea, vomiting and bleeding. There may be allergic reaction, such as a rash and a high temperature (with streptokinase and antistreplase; the others are not antigenic).

▲ Warnings: It should not be administered to patients with disorders of coagulation, or after recent surgery; who are liable to bleed (vaginal bleeding, peptic ulceration, recent trauma or surgery); with acute pancreatitis, or oesophageal varices. Administer with caution to patients who are pregnant.

Fibro-Vein

(STD Pharmaceutical) is a proprietary, prescription-only preparation of sodium tetradecyl sulphate. It is used in scleropathy, which is a technique to treat varicose veins by the injection of an irritant solution, and is available in a form for injection.

✚▲ Side-effects/warnings: See SODIUM TETRADECYL SULPHATE.

Filair

(3M) is a proprietary, prescription-only preparation of the CORTICOSTEROID and ANTI-ASTHMATIC beclometasone dipropionate. It can be used to prevent asthmatic attacks, and is available in an aerosol for inhalation (also in a stronger version called *Filair Forte*).

✚▲ Side-effects/warnings: See BECLOMETASONE DIPROPIONATE.

filgrastim

(recombinant human granulocyte-colony stimulating factor; G-CSF) is a specialist drug used to reduce neutropenia (a shortage of neutrophil white blood-cells in the circulation) by stimulating their production when this has been reduced during chemotherapy in ANTICANCER treatment, and this may reduce the incidence of associated sepsis. Administration is by injection or intravenous infusion.

✚▲ Side-effects/warnings: These are many. This is a specialist drug used only after full evaluation under hospital conditions.

✪ Related entry: Neupogen.

finasteride

is an ENZYME INHIBITOR which acts as an (*indirect*) ANTI-ANDROGEN, an indirect sex hormone antagonist (see SEX HORMONES; ANTAGONIST), which can be used to treat benign prostatic hyperplasia (BPH) in men. It has recently become available in a lower-dose form for use in treating male-pattern baldness. Administration is oral.

✚ Side-effects: Impotence, decreased libido and ejaculation disorders; breast tenderness and enlargement; symptoms of hypersensitivity reactions (eg rash and lip swelling).

▲ Warnings: Use with caution in patients with urinary obstruction, or cancer of the prostate. It is recommended that a condom is used during sexual intercourse because the drug may enter the woman in semen and have adverse effects; also women should handle the tablets with care.

✪ Related entry: Propecia; Proscar.

Flagyl

(Hawgreen) is a proprietary, prescription-only preparation of the ANTIMICROBIAL metronidazole, which has ANTIBACTERIAL and ANTIPROTOZOAL actions. It can be used to treat a wide range of infections, and is available as tablets, suppositories and in a form for injection.

✚▲ Side-effects/warnings: See METRONIDAZOLE.

Flagyl Compak

(Hawgreen) is a proprietary, prescription-only compound preparation of the ANTIMICROBIAL metronidazole, which has ANTIBACTERIAL properties and the ANTIFUNGAL and ANTIBIOTIC nystatin. It can be used to treat mixed infections of the vagina, including trichomoniasis and candidiasis, and is available as vaginal pessaries.

✚▲ Side-effects/warnings: See METRONIDAZOLE; NYSTATIN.

Flagyl S

(Hawgreen) is a proprietary, prescription-only preparation of the ANTIMICROBIAL metronidazole, which has ANTIBACTERIAL and ANTIPROTOZOAL properties. It can be used to treat a wide range of infections, and is available as a suspension.

✚▲ Side-effects/warnings: See METRONIDAZOLE.

Flamatrol

(Berk; APS) is a proprietary, prescription-only

preparation of the (NSAID) NON-NARCOTIC ANALGESIC and ANTIRHEUMATIC piroxicam. It can be used to relieve pain and inflammation, particularly rheumatic and arthritic pain and to treat other musculoskeletal disorders (including juvenile arthritis) and acute gout. It is available as capsules.
✚▲ Side-effects/warnings: See PIROXICAM.

Flamazine
(S&N Health) is a proprietary, prescription-only preparation of the ANTIBACTERIAL silver sulfadiazine. It can be used to treat wounds, burns and ulcers, bedsores and skin-graft donor sites. It is available as a cream.
✚▲ Side-effects/warnings: See SILVER SULFADIAZINE.

Flamrase
(Berk; APS) is a proprietary, prescription-only preparation of the (NSAID) NON-NARCOTIC ANALGESIC and ANTIRHEUMATIC diclofenac sodium. It can be used to treat pain and inflammation, particularly arthritic and rheumatic pain and other musculoskeletal disorders. It is available as tablets and modified-release capsules (*Flamrase SR*).
✚▲ Side-effects/warnings: See DICLOFENAC SODIUM.

flavoxate hydrochloride
is an ANTICHOLINERGIC (ANTIMUSCARINIC) drug which can be used as an ANTISPASMODIC to treat urinary frequency and incontinence. Administration is oral.
✚▲ Side-effects/warnings: See OXYBUTYNIN HYDROCHLORIDE; but it usually has fewer side-effects.
✪ Related entry: Urispas 200.

Flaxedil
(Concord) is a proprietary, prescription-only preparation of the (*non-depolarizing*) SKELETAL MUSCLE RELAXANT gallamine triethiodide. It can be used to induce muscle paralysis during surgery, and is available in a form for injection.
✚▲ Side-effects/warnings: See GALLAMINE TRIETHIODIDE.

flecainide acetate
is an ANTI-ARRHYTHMIC which is used to regularize the heartbeat in certain specific conditions. Administration is normally in hospital and is either oral or by slow intravenous injection.
✚ Side-effects: Dizziness; disturbed vision and cornea disturbances; nausea and vomiting; jaundice; liver changes, mental changes (eg memory loss and confusion) and others.
▲ Warnings: Administer with caution to patients with certain heart, kidney or liver disorders, jaundice, or who are pregnant or breast-feeding. Treatment will be initiated in hospital.
✪ Related entry: Tambocor.

Fleet Phospho-soda
(De Witt) is a proprietary, non-prescription compound preparation of the (*osmotic*) LAXATIVE sodium phosphates (sodium dihydrogen phosphate dihydrate, disodium phosphate dodecahydrate). It can be used as a bowel-cleansing solution to ensure that the bowel is free of solid contents prior to, for example, colonic surgery, radiological examination or colonoscopy. It is available in the form of an oral solution.
✚▲ Side-effects/warnings: See SODIUM ACID PHOSPHATE.

Fleet Ready-to-use Enema
(De Witt) is a proprietary, non-prescription compound preparation of the (*osmotic*) LAXATIVE sodium phosphate and sodium acid phosphate. It can be used to relieve constipation and to evacuate the rectum prior to abdominal procedures.
✚▲ Side-effects/warnings: See SODIUM ACID PHOSPHATE.

Fletchers' Arachis Oil Retention Enema
(Pharmax) is a proprietary, non-prescription preparation of arachis (peanut) oil, which can be used as a (*faecal softener*) LAXATIVE. It is not normally given to children, except on medical advice.
✚▲ Side-effects/warnings: See ARACHIS OIL.

Fletchers' Enemette
(Pharmax) is a proprietary, non-prescription preparation of the (*stimulant*) LAXATIVE docusate sodium and glycerol. It can be used to relieve constipation and to evacuate the rectum prior to abdominal procedures.

+▲ Side-effects/warnings: See DOCUSATE SODIUM; GLYCEROL.

Fletchers' Phosphate Enema

(Pharmax) is a proprietary, non-prescription compound preparation of the (*osmotic*) LAXATIVE sodium phosphate and sodium acid phosphate. It can be used to relieve constipation and to evacuate the rectum prior to abdominal procedures.
+▲ Side-effects/warnings: See SODIUM ACID PHOSPHATE.

Flexin Continus

(Napp) is a proprietary, prescription-only preparation of the (NSAID) NON-NARCOTIC ANALGESIC and ANTIRHEUMATIC indometacin (indomethacin). It can be used to treat the pain and inflammation of rheumatic and other acute, severe musculoskeletal disorders and period pain. It is available as modified-release tablets (in three strengths: *Flexin-25 Continus*; *Flexin-50 Continus*; *Flexin-75 Continus*).
+▲ Side-effects/warnings: See INDOMETACIN.

Flixonase

(A&H; GSK) is a proprietary, prescription-only preparation of the CORTICOSTEROID fluticasone propionate. It can be used to treat nasal rhinitis and hay fever, and is available as a nasal spray and nasal drops (called *Flixonase Nasule*; for nasal polyps).
+▲ Side-effects/warnings: See FLUTICASONE PROPIONATE.

Flixotide

(A&H; GSK) is a proprietary, prescription-only preparation of the CORTICOSTEROID fluticasone propionate. It can be used for the prevention and treatment of allergic and vasomotor rhinitis, and is available in a range of forms for aerosol inhalation, including an *Evohaler* aerosol and as a dry powder for inhalation with an *Accuhaler* or *Diskhaler* device.
+▲ Side-effects/warnings: See FLUTICASONE PROPIONATE.

Flolan

(GlaxoWellcome; GSK) is a proprietary, prescription-only preparation of the ANTIPLATELET aggregation drug epoprostenol. It can be used to prevent formation of clots, for example, in conjunction with HEPARIN in kidney dialysis, and is available in a form for intravenous infusion.
+▲ Side-effects/warnings: See EPOPROSTENOL.

Flomax MR

(Yamanouchi) is a proprietary, prescription-only preparation of the ALPHA-ADRENOCEPTOR BLOCKER tamsulosin hydrochloride. It can be used to treat urinary retention (eg in benign prostatic hyperplasia), and is available as capsules.
+▲ Side-effects/warnings: See TAMSULOSIN HYDROCHLORIDE.

Florinef

(Squibb; Bristol-Myers Squibb) is a proprietary, prescription-only preparation of the CORTICOSTEROID fludrocortisone acetate, which can be used for its *mineralocorticoid* activity to treat adrenal gland insufficiency. It is available as tablets.
+▲ Side-effects/warnings: See FLUDROCORTISONE ACETATE.

Floxapen

(SmithKline Beecham; GSK) is a proprietary, prescription-only preparation of the ANTIBACTERIAL and (PENICILLIN) ANTIBIOTIC flucloxacillin. It can be used to treat a range of bacterial infections, and is available as capsules, a syrup and in a form for injection.
+▲ Side-effects/warnings: See FLUCLOXACILLIN.

Flu-Amp

(Generics) is a proprietary, prescription-only compound preparation of the broad-spectrum, penicillin-like ANTIBACTERIAL and ANTIBIOTIC ampicillin and the *penicillinase-resistant*, penicillin-like antibacterial and antibiotic flucloxacillin (called *co-fluampicil*). It can be used to treat severe mixed infections where penicillin-resistant bacterial infection is probable. It is available as capsules.
+▲ Side-effects/warnings: See AMPICILLIN; CO-FLUAMPICIL; FLUCLOXACILLIN.

Fluanxol

(Lundbeck) is a proprietary, prescription-only preparation of flupentixol (as dihydrochloride), which has ANTIPSYCHOTIC properties and also ANTIDEPRESSANT actions. It can be used in the

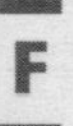

short-term treatment of depressive illness, and is available as tablets.
✚▲ Side-effects/warnings: See FLUPENTIXOL.

Fluarix

(SmithKline Beecham; GSK) is a proprietary, prescription-only preparation of influenza VACCINE (split virion vaccine; Flu/Vac/Split). It can be used as immunization for the prevention of influenza, and is available in a form for injection.
✚▲ Side-effects/warnings: See INFLUENZA VACCINE.

Fluclomix

(Ashbourne) is a proprietary, prescription-only preparation of the ANTIBACTERIAL and (PENICILLIN) ANTIBIOTIC flucloxacillin. It can be used to treat bacterial infections, particularly staphylococcal infections that prove to be resistant to penicillin, and is available as capsules.
✚▲ Side-effects/warnings: See FLUCLOXACILLIN.

flucloxacillin

is an ANTIBACTERIAL and ANTIBIOTIC drug of the PENICILLIN family. It can be used to treat bacterial infections, particularly those resistant to penicillin (eg penicillinase-producing staphylococcal infections, including MRSA) and in the treatment of ear infections, pneumonia, impetigo, cellulitis and staphylococcal endocarditis. Administration is either oral or by injection.
✚▲ Side-effects/warnings: See BENZYLPENICILLIN. Administer with caution to patients with porphyria. There have been reports of hepatic (liver) and cholestatic jaundice.
✪ **Related entries: co-fluampicil; Floxapen; Flu-Amp; Fluclomix; Galfloxin; Ladropen; Magnapen.**

fluconazole

is an (AZOLE) ANTIFUNGAL drug which can be used in the treatment of many fungal infections of the mucous membranes, of the vagina (candidiasis) or mouth, oesophagitis, athlete's foot and cryptococcal meningitis. It can also be used to prevent fungal infections in immunocompromised patients following chemotherapy or radiotherapy. Administration is either oral or by injection.
✚ Side-effects: Nausea, abdominal discomfort and flatulence, diarrhoea, headaches, rash, angioedema, anaphylaxis and alteration in liver enzymes.
▲ Warnings: It should be administered with care to patients with certain kidney disorders or who are pregnant or breast-feeding.
✪ **Related entries: Diflucan; Diflucan One.**

flucytosine

is a synthetic ANTIFUNGAL drug which can be used to treat especially serious systemic infections by yeasts and fungi, such as systemic candidiasis. Administration is either oral or by intravenous infusion.
✚ Side-effects: There may be diarrhoea with nausea and vomiting; rashes may occur, and there may be confusion, hallucinations, headaches, vertigo, sedation, blood and liver problems, and others.
▲ Warnings: It should be administered with caution to patients who suffer from certain kidney or liver disorders, blood disorders; or who are pregnant or breast-feeding. During treatment, there should be regular blood counts and liver-function tests.
✪ **Related entry: Ancotil.**

Fludara

(Schering Health) is a proprietary, prescription-only preparation of the ANTICANCER drug fludarabine phosphate. It can be used in the treatment of leukaemia, and is available in a form for injection.
✚▲ Side-effects/warnings: See FLUDARABINE PHOSPHATE.

fludarabine phosphate

is an (*antimetabolite*) CYTOTOXIC drug which can be used as an ANTICANCER treatment primarily of certain leukaemias (B-cell chronic lymphatic leukaemia). Administration is by injection.
✚▲ Side-effects/warnings: See CYTOTOXIC.
✪ **Related entry: Fludara.**

fludrocortisone acetate

is a CORTICOSTEROID which is used for its *mineralocorticoid* activity to correct a deficiency of HORMONE from the adrenal gland, and is used to treat the resulting salt-and-water imbalance in the body. It is also used in neuropathetic postural hypotension. Administration is oral.
✚▲ Side-effects/warnings: See CORTICOSTEROID.
✪ **Related entry: Florinef.**

fludroxycortide

(flurandrenolone) is a CORTICOSTEROID with ANTI-INFLAMMATORY properties. It is used in the treatment of inflammatory skin disorders, such as eczema. Administration is by topical application.
✚▲ Side-effects/warnings: See CORTICOSTEROID; though serious systemic effects are unlikely with topical application, but there may be local skin reactions.
✪ **Related entry: Haelan.**

flumazenil

is a specialist drug, a BENZODIAZEPINE antagonist which can be used to reverse the sedative effects of benzodiazepine drugs on the central nervous system induced during anaesthesia, in intensive care or for diagnostic procedures. Administration is by intravenous infusion or injection.
✚▲ Side-effects/warnings: This is a specialist drug used under hospital conditions.
✪ **Related entry: Anexate.**

flumetasone pivalate

(flumethasone pivalate) is a CORTICOSTEROID with ANTI-INFLAMMATORY properties. It is used in the treatment of inflammatory skin disorders, particularly eczema of the outer ear. Administration is by topical application.
✚▲ Side-effects/warnings: See CORTICOSTEROID. There may be local sensitivity reactions; avoid prolonged use. Serious systemic effects are rare with topical application. Do not use in untreated infection.
✪ **Related entry: Locorten-Vioform.**

flumethasone pivalate

see FLUMETASONE PIVALATE.

flunisolide

is an ANTI-ALLERGIC and CORTICOSTEROID drug which is used to prevent and treat allergic nasal rhinitis, such as hay fever. Administration is by nasal spray.
✚▲ Side-effects/warnings: See CORTICOSTEROID. When applied topically to the nose, serious side-effects are rare. It may cause local side-effects such as irritation and dryness of the nose and throat, nose-bleeds and ulceration.
✪ **Related entry: Syntaris.**

flunitrazepam

is a BENZODIAZEPINE which is used as a HYPNOTIC in the short-term treatment of insomnia in cases where some degree of sedation during the daytime is acceptable. Administration is oral.
✚▲ Side-effects/warnings: See BENZODIAZEPINE. More subject to habituation and misuse than some others of the class, preparations of it are on the Controlled Drugs list.
✪ **Related entry: Rohypnol.**

fluocinolone acetonide

is a CORTICOSTEROID with ANTI-INFLAMMATORY properties. It is used in the treatment of inflammatory skin disorders, such as eczema and psoriasis. Administration is by topical application. It is also a constituent in several compound preparations that contain ANTIBACTERIAL or ANTIMICROBIAL drugs.
✚▲ Side-effects/warnings: See CORTICOSTEROID; though systemic effects are unlikely with topical application, but there may be local skin reactions.
✪ **Related entries: Synalar; Synalar C; Synalar N.**

fluocinonide

is a CORTICOSTEROID with ANTI-INFLAMMATORY properties. It is used in the treatment of severe, inflammatory skin disorders, such as eczema and psoriasis, that are unresponsive to less powerful corticosteroids. Administration is by topical application.
✚▲ Side-effects/warnings: See CORTICOSTEROID; though serious systemic effects are unlikely with topical application, but there may be local skin reactions.
✪ **Related entry: Metosyn.**

fluocortolone

is a CORTICOSTEROID with ANTI-INFLAMMATORY properties. It is used in the treatment of severe, inflammatory skin disorders, such as eczema and psoriasis, that are unresponsive to less powerful corticosteroids. Administration is by topical application.
✚▲ Side-effects/warnings: See CORTICOSTEROID; though serious systemic effects are unlikely with topical application, but there may be local skin reactions.
✪ **Related entries: Ultralanum Plain; Ultraproct.**

Fluor-a-day

(Dental Health) is a proprietary, non-prescription preparation of sodium fluoride that can be used in children for protection against

F

dental caries in areas where water is not fluoridated. It is available as tablets for taking by mouth.
✚▲ Side-effects/warnings: see FLUORIDE.

fluorescein sodium

is a dye that is used on the surface of an eye in ophthalmic diagnostic procedures. Administration is topical as eye-drops (sometimes with a local anaesthetic).
✚▲ Side-effects/warnings: It is regarded as safe in normal topical use.
✪ **Related entries: Minims Fluorescein Sodium; Minims Lignocaine and Fluorescein; Minims Proxymetacaine and Fluorescein.**

fluoride

is a halogen element necessary to the body and is ingested as a trace element in a well-balanced diet. It is now considered to be necessary for strong bones and good teeth enamel, and is most effective if absorbed in children when these are still growing. Because a balanced level of fluoride leads to growth of dental enamel with considerably increased resistance to bacteria-induced decay (dental caries), fluoride is added to the household drinking water in most areas of the UK (if it is not already naturally present). Additionally, there is good evidence that topical fluoride solutions applied to the teeth also increase the strength of enamel, and for this reason fluoride-containing compounds (eg sodium fluoride, stannous fluoride, sodium monofluorophosphate) are added to many toothpastes. Fluoride (usually SODIUM FLUORIDE) is also available as topical mouthwashes or gels, or for taking orally.
✚ Side-effects: There may be occasional white flecks on teeth with recommended doses; if recommended doses are exceeded there may be yellowish-brown discolouration of the teeth.
▲ Warnings: Fluoride supplements are not normally used in areas where drinking water is naturally or artificially fluoridated.
✪ **Related entries: Duraphat; Endekay; Endekay Fluodrops; Fluor-a-day; FluoriGard.**

FluoriGard

(Colgate-Palmolive) is a proprietary, non-prescription preparation of sodium fluoride that can be used in children for protection against dental caries in areas where water is not fluoridated. It is available as tablets (in two strengths) for taking by mouth; as a topical daily mouthwash, also as a topical daily gel (*Gel-Kam*; as stannous fluoride in glycerol basis).
✚▲ Side-effects/warnings: see FLUORIDE.

fluorometholone

is a CORTICOSTEROID with ANTI-INFLAMMATORY properties which is used as a short-term treatment of inflammatory eye conditions. Administration is by eye-drops.
✚▲ Side-effects/warnings: See CORTICOSTEROID; though serious systemic effects are unlikely with topical application, but there may be local skin reactions.
✪ **Related entry: FML.**

fluoroquinolone

see QUINOLONE.

fluorouracil

is an (*antimetabolite*) CYTOTOXIC drug which is used as an ANTICANCER treatment primarily of solid tumours (eg of the colon and breast) and malignant skin lesions. It works by preventing the cancer cells from replicating and so prevents the growth of the cancer. It is sometimes given with FOLINIC ACID (in advanced colorectal cancer). Administration can be oral, topical or by injection.
✚▲ Side-effects/warnings: See CYTOTOXIC.
✪ **Related entry: Efudix.**

fluoxetine

is an ANTIDEPRESSANT of the SSRI group which are used to treat depressive illness, having the advantage over some earlier antidepressants because it has relatively less SEDATIVE and ANTICHOLINERGIC (ANTIMUSCARINIC) side-effects. It has more recently also been used for bulimia nervosa and obsessive-compulsive disorders. The onset of action may take some weeks to reach full effect and offset on discontinuation is also slow. Administration is oral.
✚ Side-effects: See SSRI: also possible changes in blood sugar, fever, neuroleptic malignant syndrome-like symptoms (raised body temperature, fluctuating level of consciousness, muscle rigidity, pallor, cardiovascular effects, sweating, and urinary incontinence), possible blood and liver changes. Important

hypersensitivity reactions (skin reactions including angioedema and urticaria, muscle pain, and other allergic reactions including anaphylaxis; discontinue if rash occurs), inflammation of the respiratory tract; other possible hypersensitivity signs reported.
▲ Warnings: See SSRI: it should be given with caution to patients with liver, kidney or heart disorders and those who have a history of mania, epilepsy, diabetes or who are pregnant or breast-feeding. It should not be administered during a manic phase. May impair driving ability.
✪ **Related entry: Prozac.**

flupenthixol
see FLUPENTIXOL.

flupenthixol deconoate
see FLUPENTIXOL.

flupentixol
(flupenthixol) is chemically one of the *thioxanthenes*, which have properties similar to the PHENOTHIAZINE group. It is used as an ANTIPSYCHOTIC in the treatment of schizophrenia and other psychoses, particularly where there is apathy and withdrawal, but not for mania or psychomotor hyperactivity. It is also used (at a lower dose) as an ANTIDEPRESSANT in the short-term treatment of depressive illness. Administration is oral. It is also used as flupenthixol decanoate administered as a deep intramuscular depot injection (the drug is slowly released) for maintenance of patients suffering from schizophrenia and other psychotic disorders.
✚▲ Side-effects/warnings: These depend on the route of administration and use. See CHLORPROMAZINE HYDROCHLORIDE; but it is less sedating and extrapyramidal symptoms are more common; it should be avoided in senile, overactive or excitable patients and in those with porphyria. There may be pain, redness and swelling at the injection site.
✪ **Related entries: Depixol; Depixol Conc.; Depixol Low Volume; Fluanxol.**

fluphenazine
is a powerful ANTIPSYCHOTIC which is chemically one of the PHENOTHIAZINE group. It is used in the treatment of psychoses, such as schizophrenia and with other drugs (adjunctive management) for the short-term control of other behavioural states. It can also be used as an ANXIOLYTIC for the short-term treatment of severe anxiety. It is used in two forms, and administration of the hydrochloride form is oral and the decanoate form by depot deep intramuscular injection, and is available in a compound preparation with the ANTIDEPRESSANT drug NORTRIPTYLINE HYDROCHLORIDE.
✚▲ Side-effects/warnings: These depend on route of administration, and use. See CHLORPROMAZINE HYDROCHLORIDE; but with less sedation, fewer anticholinergic and hypotensive side-effects, but there are extrapyramidal symptoms (muscle tremor and rigidity, and also dystonic and akinesic motor movements).
✪ **Related entries: Modecate; Moditen; Motipress; Motival.**

flurandrenolone
see FLUDROXYCORTIDE.

flurazepam
is a BENZODIAZEPINE which is used as a HYPNOTIC to treat insomnia in cases where some degree of sedation during the daytime is acceptable. Administration is oral.
✚▲ Side-effects/warnings: See BENZODIAZEPINE.
✪ **Related entry: Dalmane.**

flurbiprofen
is a (NSAID) NON-NARCOTIC ANALGESIC and ANTIRHEUMATIC with effects similar to those of aspirin. It is used particularly in the treatment of pain and inflammation in musculoskeletal disorders, period pain and postoperative pain. It can also be used topically for relief of sore throat. Administration can be either oral or topical (including suppositories).
✚▲ Side-effects/warnings: See NSAID. May cause irritation when used for relief of sore throat (as lozenges); there may be mouth ulcers and taste disturbances.
✪ **Related entries: Froben; Ocufen; Strefen.**

flutamide
is a HORMONE ANTAGONIST (an ANTI-ANDROGEN) which is used as an ANTICANCER drug for the treatment of prostate cancer. Administration is oral.
✚ Side-effects: There may be gynaecomastia

F

(growth of breasts) and milk secretion, diarrhoea, nausea and vomiting, increased appetite, tiredness and sleep disturbances, decreased libido, gastrointestinal and chest pain, blurred vision, oedema, rashes, blood disturbances, headache, dizziness, thirst, rash, blood and liver disorders.
▲ Warnings: Administer with caution to patients suffering certain heart or liver disorders. Liver function should be monitored.
✪ **Related entries: Chimax; Drogenil.**

fluticasone propionate

is a very potent CORTICOSTEROID which is used as an ANTI-INFLAMMATORY treatment for skin disorders, including dermatitis and eczemas that are unresponsive to less potent corticosteroids; also as an ANTI-ASTHMATIC to prevent attacks (used by inhalation by a variety of methods). Topical administration is as a cream. As an ANTI-ALLERGIC treatment and for prophylaxis of allergic hay fever and vasomotor rhinitis, and nasal polyps it is administered by a nasal spray or nasal drops (for polyps).
✚▲ Side-effects/warnings: See CORTICOSTEROID. When used topically there are few serious side-effects, but there may be local reactions. It is used for short-term treatment only.
✪ **Related entries: Cutivate; Flixonase; Flixotide; Seretide.**

fluvastatin

is a (*statin*) LIPID-REGULATING DRUG used in hyperlipidaemia to reduce the levels, or change the proportions, of various lipids in the bloodstream (particularly where there is heart disease, or a risk of heart attacks or stroke). It is usually administered only to those patients in whom a strict and regular dietary regime, alone, is not having the desired effect. Administration is oral.
✚▲ Side-effects/warnings: See SIMVASTATIN. It should not be used in severe kidney impairment. Patients should report any muscle weakness, pain or tenderness to their doctor.
✪ **Related entry: Lescol; Lescol XL.**

Fluvirin

(Evans Vaccines) is a proprietary, prescription-only preparation of influenza (inactivated surface antigen; Flu/Vac/SA) VACCINE. It can be used as immunization for the prevention of influenza, and is available in a form for injection.
✚▲ Side-effects/warnings: See INFLUENZA VACCINE.

fluvoxamine maleate

is an ANTIDEPRESSANT of the SSRI group. It is used to treat depressive illness and obsessive-compulsive disorders. It has the advantage over some other earlier antidepressants because it has fewer SEDATIVE and ANTICHOLINERGIC (ANTIMUSCARINIC) side-effects. Administration is oral.
✚▲ Side-effects/warnings: See SSRI. Also, there may be effects on the heart; rarely postural hypotension, confusion and hallucinations, unsteady gait, rarely abnormal liver function; hypersensitivity reactions (rash, itching, muscle pain, photosensitivity, anaphylactic type reactions), milk secretion.
✪ **Related entry: Faverin.**

FML

(Allergan) is a proprietary, prescription-only preparation of the CORTICOSTEROID and ANTI-INFLAMMATORY fluorometholone. It can be used for the short-term treatment of inflammatory eye conditions, and is available as eye-drops.
✚▲ Side-effects/warnings: See FLUOROMETHOLONE.

folic acid

is a vitamin of the B complex and is also known as pteroylglutamic acid. It has an important role in the synthesis of nucleic acids (DNA and RNA). Good food sources of folic acid include liver and vegetables and its consumption is particularly necessary during the first few months of pregnancy. The Department of Health recommends taking folic acid supplements to help prevent neural tube defects when taken before and during pregnancy. There are also certain forms of anaemia (eg megaloblastic anaemia) that can be treated with folic acid (as well as with supplements of CYANOCOBALAMIN). Administration is oral. Sometimes it is incorporated into preparations containing iron salts for preventing deficiency (eg in pregnancy).
▲ Warnings: Except when taking folic acid during pregnancy to prevent neural tube defects in babies, treatment with folic acid generally also indicates parallel treatment with cyanocobalamin (vitamin B_{12}).

✪ **Related entries: Fefol; Ferfolic SV; Ferrograd Folic; Folicare; Galfer FA; Lexpec; Lexpec with Iron; Lexpec with Iron-M; Pregaday; Slow-Fe Folic.**

Folicare

(Rosemont) is a non-prescription preparation of folic acid. It can be used as a VITAMIN supplement, for example, during pregnancy or to treat a deficiency. Available as a oral solution.
✚▲ Side-effects/warnings: See FOLIC ACID.

folinic acid

see CALCIUM FOLINATE.

follicle-stimulating hormone

(FSH) is a HORMONE secreted by the anterior pituitary gland and the chorionic tissue of the placenta. It is one of the gonadotrophin (gonadotropin) hormones, along with LUTEINISING HORMONE (LH). In women (in conjunction with LH), it causes the monthly ripening in one ovary of a follicle and stimulates ovulation. In men, it stimulates the production of sperm in the testes. It may be injected therapeutically in infertility treatment to stimulate ovulation. It is available in combination with LH, as human menopausal gonadotrophin (see HUMAN MENOPAUSAL GONADOTROPHINS); MENOTROPHIN. It is now available in recombinant (synthetic) forms called FOLLITROPIN ALPHA and FOLLITROPIN BETA. See also CHORIONIC GONADOTROPHIN.

follitropin alpha

is a recombinant (synthetic) form of human FOLLICLE-STIMULATING HORMONE. FSH is secreted by the anterior pituitary gland and the chorionic tissue of the placenta. It is one of the gonadotrophin (gonadotropin) hormones (along with LUTEINISING HORMONE; LH). In women (in conjunction with LH), it causes the monthly ripening in one ovary of a follicle and stimulates ovulation. In men, it stimulates the production of sperm in the testes. It can be injected in infertility treatment to stimulate ovulation. It is available, in combination with LH, as human menopausal gonadotrophin. See also CHORIONIC GONADOTROPHIN.
✚▲ Side-effects/warnings: See HUMAN MENOPAUSAL GONADOTROPHINS.
✪ **Related entry: Gonal-F.**

follitropin beta

is a recombinant (synthetic) form of FOLLICLE-STIMULATING HORMONE (FSH), which is a HORMONE secreted by the anterior pituitary gland and the chorionic tissue of the placenta. FSH is one of the gonadotrophin (gonadotropin) hormones (along with LUTEINISING HORMONE; LH). In women, in conjunction with LH, it causes the monthly ripening in one ovary of a follicle and stimulates ovulation. In men, it stimulates the production of sperm in the testes. Follitropin beta can be injected in infertility treatment to stimulate ovulation. It is available in combination with LH as human menopausal gonadotrophin. See also CHORIONIC GONADOTROPHIN.
✚▲ Side-effects/warnings: See HUMAN MENOPAUSAL GONADOTROPHINS.
✪ **Related entry: Puregon.**

fomepizole

is an ENZYME INHIBITOR drug which is used as an ANTIDOTE to poisoning by ethylene glycol (antifreeze). Administration is by intravenous infusion.
✚▲ Side-effects/warnings: Pain in the abdomen, vomiting, hypotension, headache, vertigo, rash, blood changes, seizures, pain at injection site.

fomivirsen sodium

is an ANTIVIRAL drug which is used specifically for local treatment of cytomegalovirus retinitis in patients with AIDS when other therapies are not effective or suitable. It is given by injection into the posterior chamber of the eye (intravitreal).
✚ Side-effects: There may be many effects on the eye including irritation and inflammation, conjunctival haemorrhage, visual disturbances, cataract, intraocular pressure increase, various retinal and vitreous disorders. Less commonly, fomivirsen treatment may cause conjunctivitis, keratitis, oedema of the cornea, cystoid macular oedema, HIV ocular microangiopathy, photophobia, lens pigment deposits, orbital cellulitis and photopsia (sensation of flashes of light). It is a specialist drug and all possible side-effects will be explained prior to treatment.
▲ Warnings: Intraocular pressure and visual field will be monitored throughout treatment.
✪ **Related entry: Vitravene.**

Foradil

(Novartis) is a proprietary, prescription-only

F

preparation of the BETA-RECEPTOR STIMULANT formoterol fumarate (eformoterol fumarate). It can be used as a BRONCHODILATOR in reversible obstructive airways disease and as an ANTI-ASTHMATIC treatment, and has a prolonged action. It is available as a powder for inhalation.
✚▲ Side-effects/warnings: See FORMOTEROL FUMARATE. This drug should not be used to relieve acute attacks and existing corticosteroid treatment must be continued. The stated dose must not be exceeded, and if a previously effective dose fails to relieve symptoms, consult your doctor.
✪ **Related entries: Foradil; Oxis; Symbicort.**

Forcaltonin
(Strakan) is a proprietary, prescription-only preparation of the PARATHYROID HORMONE calcitonin, in the form of salcatonin (*calcitonin (salmon)*). It can be used to lower blood levels of calcium when they are abnormally high (hypercalcaemia). It is available in a form for subcutaneous, intramuscular or intravenous injection.
✚▲ Side-effects/warnings: See SALCATONIN.

formaldehyde
is a powerful KERATOLYTIC agent which is used in mild solution to dissolve away layers of toughened or warty skin, especially in the treatment of verrucas (plantar warts) on the soles of the feet. It is used topically.
✚▲ Side-effects/warnings: See SALICYLIC ACID.
✪ **Related entry: Veracur.**

formoterol fumarate
(eformoterol fumarate) is a SYMPATHOMIMETIC and BETA-RECEPTOR STIMULANT β_2-receptor selectivity. It is mainly used as a BRONCHODILATOR in reversible obstructive airways disease and as an ANTI-ASTHMATIC treatment, for example, for nocturnal asthma and to prevent exercise-induced bronchospasm, in those who require long-term therapy. It is similar to SALMETEROL.
✚▲ Side-effects/warnings: See SALBUTAMOL. Also, taste disturbances, rash and other skin reactions, insomnia, nausea and effects on the eye. It is used with care in patients who are pregnant or breast-feeding. (Users will be cautioned not to exceed the stated dose and if a previously effective dose fails to relieve symptoms, they should consult their doctor.) It should not be used for immediate relief of attacks.

Fortipine LA 40
(Goldshield) is a proprietary, prescription-only preparation of the CALCIUM-CHANNEL BLOCKER nifedipine. It can be used as an ANTI-ANGINA treatment in the prevention of attacks and as an ANTIHYPERTENSIVE. It is available as modified-release tablets.
✚▲ Side-effects/warnings: See NIFEDIPINE.

Fortovase
(Roche) is a proprietary, prescription-only preparation of the ANTIVIRAL saquinavir. It can be used in the treatment of HIV infection, and is available as capsules.
✚▲ Side-effects/warnings: See SAQUINAVIR.

Fortral
(Sanofi-Synthelabo) is a proprietary, prescription-only preparation of the (OPIOID) NARCOTIC ANALGESIC pentazocine. It can be used to relieve pain, and is available as capsules, tablets, suppositories and in a form for injection. (It is on the Controlled Drugs list.)
✚▲ Side-effects/warnings: See PENTAZOCINE.

Fortum
(GlaxoWellcome; GSK) is a proprietary, prescription-only preparation of the ANTIBACTERIAL and (CEPHALOSPORIN) ANTIBIOTIC ceftazidime. It can be used to treat a range of infections, and is available in a form for intravenous injection or infusion.
✚▲ Side-effects/warnings: See CEFTAZIDIME.

Fosamax
(MSD) is a proprietary, prescription-only preparation of alendronic acid. It can be used to treat postmenopausal osteoporosis, and is available as tablets.
✚▲ Side-effects/warnings: See ALENDRONIC ACID.

Fosamax Once Weekly
(MSD) is a recently introduced, proprietary, prescription-only preparation of alendronic acid. It can be used to prevent and treat osteoporosis, including postmenopausal and corticosteroid-induced osteporosis , and is available as tablets (taken once a week).
✚▲ Side-effects/warnings: See ALENDRONIC ACID.

foscarnet sodium

is an ANTIVIRAL drug which can be used to treat cytomegaloviral (CMV) retinitis in patients with AIDS infection, also for (mucocutaneous) herpes simplex infection. Administration is by intravenous infusion.

✚ Side-effects: These include various blood-cell deficiencies, effects on the functioning of the kidney and liver, gastrointestinal disturbances, nausea, vomiting, rash and fatigue, anorexia, headache.

▲ Warnings: It is a specialist drug, and there will be full assessment and patient monitoring throughout treatment. It is not administered to patients who are pregnant or breast-feeding. Use with extreme care in those with kidney impairment.

✪ **Related entry: Foscavir.**

Foscavir

(AstraZeneca) is a proprietary, prescription-only preparation of the ANTIVIRAL drug foscarnet sodium. It can be used to treat viral infections, especially of the eye (cytomegaloviral retinitis) in patients with AIDS infection, and is available in a form for intravenous infusion.

✚▲ Side-effects/warnings: See FOSCARNET SODIUM.

fosfestrol tetrasodium

is a drug that is converted in the body to DIETHYLSTILBESTROL, which is a drug with sex hormone activity as an OESTROGEN. It is used in men as an ANTICANCER treatment for cancer of the prostate gland. Administration is oral or by injection.

✚▲ Side-effects/warnings: See DIETHYLSTILBESTROL.

✪ **Related entry: Honvan.**

fosinopril

is an ACE INHIBITOR and acts as a VASODILATOR. It can be used as an ANTIHYPERTENSIVE and as a congestive HEART FAILURE TREATMENT often when other treatments cannot be used. It is frequently administered in conjunction with other classes of drug, particularly (THIAZIDE) DIURETIC drugs. Administration is oral.

✚ Side-effects: See ACE INHIBITOR. Also, chest and muscle pains.

▲ Warnings: See ACE INHIBITOR.

✪ **Related entry: Staril.**

fosphenytoin sodium

is a ANTICONVULSANT and ANTI-EPILEPTIC drug, which in fact is a pro-drug of phenytoin, and has the advantage over the older drug in that it can be given more rapidly and when given intravenously causes fewer reactions at the injection site. It can be used in the emergency treatment of status epilepticus and convulsive seizures during neurosurgical operations or head injury. It is available in a form for injection.

✚▲ Side-effects/warnings: See PHENYTOIN.

✪ **Related entry: Pro-Epanutin**

Fragmin

(Pharmacia) is a proprietary, prescription-only preparation of the ANTICOAGULANT dalteparin sodium, which is a low molecular weight version of heparin. It can be used for long-duration prevention of venous thrombo-embolism, particularly in orthopaedic use. It is available in a number of forms for injection.

✚▲ Side-effects/warnings: See DALTEPARIN SODIUM.

framycetin sulphate

is a broad-spectrum ANTIBACTERIAL and ANTIBIOTIC drug of the AMINOGLYCOSIDE family. As with all aminoglycoside antibiotics, framycetin is active against some Gram-positive and many Gram-negative bacteria, and is used to treat infections of the eye, ear and open wounds (when it is used in a gauze dressing). Administration is largely restricted to topical application because of its toxicity.

✚▲ Side-effects/warnings: See GENTAMICIN; but topical application limits its toxic side-effects.

✪ **Related entries: Sofradex; Soframycin.**

Frisium

(Hoechst Marion Roussel; Aventis Pharma) is a proprietary, prescription-only preparation of the (BENZODIAZEPINE) ANXIOLYTIC clobazam. It can be used in the short-term treatment of anxiety and, in conjunction with other drugs, in ANTI-EPILEPTIC therapy. It is available as tablets.

✚▲ Side-effects/warnings: See CLOBAZAM.

Froben

(Knoll) is a proprietary, prescription-only preparation of the (NSAID) NON-NARCOTIC ANALGESIC and ANTIRHEUMATIC flurbiprofen. It can be used to treat arthritic and rheumatic pain

and inflammation, other musculoskeletal disorders, migraine, period pain and pain after surgical operations. It is available as tablets, as modified-release capsules (*Froben SR*) for rheumatic disease and as suppositories.
✚▲ Side-effects/warnings: See FLURBIPROFEN.

Froop

(Ashbourne) is a proprietary, prescription only preparation of the (*loop*) DIURETIC furosemide (frusemide). It can be used to treat oedema, and low urine production due to kidney failure (oliguria). It is available as tablets.
✚▲ Side-effects/warnings: See FUROSEMIDE.

Froop-Co

(Ashbourne) is a proprietary, prescription-only compound preparation of the (*potassium-sparing*) DIURETIC amiloride hydrochloride and the (*loop*) diuretic furosemide (frusemide) (a combination called co-amilofruse 5/40). It can be used to treat oedema, and is available as tablets.
✚▲ Side-effects/warnings: See AMILORIDE HYDROCHLORIDE; FUROSEMIDE.

Fru-Co

(IVAX) is a proprietary, prescription-only compound preparation of the (*potassium-sparing*) DIURETIC amiloride hydrochloride and the (*loop*) diuretic furosemide (frusemide) (a combination called co-amilofruse 5/40). It can be used to treat oedema, and is available as tablets.
✚▲ Side-effects/warnings: See AMILORIDE HYDROCHLORIDE; FUROSEMIDE.

fructose

(laevulose; fruit sugar) is a simple sugar (a monosaccharide). Fructose and GLUCOSE make up the *disaccharide* sucrose when chemically combined, which is the sugar found naturally in cane sugar and sugar-beet and is a major source of carbohydrate and energy. In the body, sucrose is metabolized into the simple sugars. The glucose level in the blood is closely regulated by the two hormones, INSULIN and GLUCAGON. Fructose, as part of a normal diet, can therefore be used as a source of energy and is a constituent of honey and in certain fruits (such as figs). It offers no particular advantage in normal individuals, but medically may be recommended for use, without prescription, by patients who suffer from glucose or galactose intolerance.

Frumil

(Helios) is a proprietary, prescription-only compound preparation of the (*potassium-sparing*) DIURETIC amiloride hydrochloride and the (*loop*) diuretic furosemide (frusemide) (a combination called co-amilofruse 5/40). It can be used to treat oedema, and is available as tablets.
✚▲ Side-effects/warnings: See AMILORIDE HYDROCHLORIDE; FUROSEMIDE.

Frumil Forte

(Helios) is a proprietary, prescription-only compound preparation of the (*potassium-sparing*) DIURETIC amiloride hydrochloride and the (*loop*) diuretic furosemide (frusemide) (a combination called co-amilofruse 10/80). It can be used to treat oedema, and is available as tablets.
✚▲ Side-effects/warnings: See AMILORIDE HYDROCHLORIDE; FUROSEMIDE.

Frumil LS

(Helios) is a proprietary, prescription-only compound preparation of the (*potassium-sparing*) DIURETIC amiloride hydrochloride and the (*loop*) diuretic furosemide (frusemide) (a combination called co-amilofruse 2.5/20). It can be used to treat oedema, and is available as tablets.
✚▲ Side-effects/warnings: See AMILORIDE HYDROCHLORIDE; FUROSEMIDE.

frusemide

see FUROSEMIDE.

Frusene

(Orion) is a proprietary, prescription-only compound preparation of the (*potassium-sparing*) DIURETIC triamterene and the (*loop*) diuretic furosemide (frusemide). It can be used to treat oedema, and is available as tablets.
✚▲ Side-effects/warnings: See FUROSEMIDE; TRIAMTERENE. Urine may appear blue.

FSH

see FOLLICLE-STIMULATING HORMONE.

Fucibet

(Leo) is a proprietary, prescription-only compound preparation of the CORTICOSTEROID betamethasone and the ANTIBACTERIAL and ANTIBIOTIC fusidic acid. It can be used to treat skin disorders, such as psoriasis and eczema, in

which bacterial infection is present. Available as a cream.
✚▲ Side-effects/warnings: See BETAMETHASONE; FUSIDIC ACID.

Fucidin
(Leo) is a proprietary, prescription-only preparation of the narrow-spectrum ANTIBACTERIAL and ANTIBIOTIC fusidic acid. It can be used against staphylococcal infections, especially infections of the skin and bone and also abscesses, that prove to be resistant to penicillin. It is available in many forms: for topical application as a gel, as a cream, as an ointment; for oral administration as tablets or suspension; and in a form for intravenous injection (all contain as their active constituent either fusidic acid or one of its salts).
✚▲ Side-effects/warnings: See FUSIDIC ACID.

Fucidin H
(Leo) is a proprietary, prescription-only compound preparation of the narrow-spectrum ANTIBACTERIAL and ANTIBIOTIC fusidic acid and the ANTI-INFLAMMATORY and CORTICOSTEROID hydrocortisone (as acetate). It can be used to treat skin inflammation where there is bacterial infection, such as eczema. It is available for topical application as a cream and ointment (as sodium fusidate).
✚▲ Side-effects/warnings: See FUSIDIC ACID; HYDROCORTISONE.

Fucithalmic
(Leo) is a proprietary, prescription-only preparation of the narrow-spectrum ANTIBACTERIAL and ANTIBIOTIC fusidic acid. It can be used against infections of the eye, and is available as eye-drops.
✚▲ Side-effects/warnings: See FUSIDIC ACID.

Full Marks Liquid
(SSL) is a proprietary, non-prescription preparation of the PEDICULICIDAL phenothrin. It can be used for the treatment of head lice infestation, and is available as a water-based liquid emulsion. It is not normally given to infants under six months, except on medical advice.
✚▲ Side-effects/warnings: See PHENOTHRIN.

Full Marks Lotion
(SSL) is a proprietary, non-prescription preparation of the PEDICULICIDAL phenothrin. It can be used for the treatment of head lice and pubic lice, and is available as a lotion. It is not normally given to infants under six months, except on medical advice.
✚▲ Side-effects/warnings: See PHENOTHRIN.

Full Marks Mousse
(SSL) is a proprietary, non-prescription preparation of the PEDICULICIDAL phenothrin. It can be used for the treatment of head lice, and is available as scalp mousse. It is not normally given to infants under six months, except on medical advice.
✚▲ Side-effects/warnings: See PHENOTHRIN.

fungicidal
see ANTIFUNGAL.

Fungilin
(Squibb; Bristol-Myers Squibb) is a proprietary, prescription-only preparation of the ANTIFUNGAL and ANTIBIOTIC amphotericin. It can be used to treat fungal infections, especially candidiasis (thrush) of the mouth and gastrointestinal tract. It is available as tablets, a liquid oral suspension and as lozenges.
✚▲ Side-effects/warnings: See AMPHOTERICIN.

Fungizone
(Squibb; Bristol-Myers Squibb) is a proprietary, prescription-only preparation of the ANTIFUNGAL amphotericin in a formulation as sodium deoxycholate complex. that is intended to minimize toxicity. It can be used to treat systemic fungal infections, and is available in a form for intravenous infusion.
✚▲ Side-effects/warnings: See AMPHOTERICIN.

Furadantin
(Goldshield) is a proprietary, prescription-only preparation of the ANTIBACTERIAL nitrofurantoin. It can be used to treat urinary tract infections, and is available as tablets.
✚▲ Side-effects/warnings: See NITROFURANTOIN.

furosemide
(frusemide) is a powerful DIURETIC of the *loop* class. It can be used to treat oedema, and low urine production due to kidney failure (oliguria). Administration can be oral or by injection or intravenous infusion.

F

✚ Side-effects: There may be lowered blood levels of potassium, sodium, magnesium and chloride. There may be an abnormally low blood pressure (hypotension), gastrointestinal disturbances, raised levels of urea in the blood, gout; raised blood glucose, changes in fats in the blood, tinnitus and deafness. There may be skin rashes, photosensitivity, effects on bone marrow, blood changes, pancreatitis. Many of these effects are only seen with high or prolonged dosage.
▲ Warnings: It should be administered with care to patients with certain kidney disorders, who are pregnant or breast-feeding, who have gout, diabetes, an enlarged prostate gland or liver failure or porphyria.
✪ **Related entries: Aridil; co-amilofruse 10/80; co-amilozide 2.5/25; co-amilofruse 5/40; Diumide-K Continus; Froop; Froop-Co; Fru-Co; Frumil; Frumil Forte; Frumil LS; Frusene; Lasikal; Lasilactone; Lasix; Lasoride; Min-I-Jet Frusemide; Rusyde.**

fusafungine

is an ANTIBIOTIC drug with ANTIBACTERIAL and ANTIFUNGAL properties, which is used in a proprietary preparation to treat infection and inflammation in the nose and throat. Administration is by topical application.
✪ **Related entry: Locabiotal.**

fusidic acid

(sodium fusidate) is a narrow-spectrum ANTIBACTERIAL and ANTIBIOTIC drug. It is commonly used in combination with other antibiotics to treat staphylococcal infections, especially infections of the skin, infections of the lining of the heart, infections of the bone (osteomyelitis) and the eye, that prove to be resistant to PENICILLIN. The drug works by inhibiting protein synthesis at the ribosome level in sensitive organisms (Gram-positive bacteria). Administration can be oral, by intravenous infusion or by topical application. It is also used in the form of its salt sodium fusidate and as diethanolamine fusidate.
✚ Side-effects: Depending on route of administration, there may be nausea and vomiting; rash; jaundice; hypersensitivity reactions on topical application.
▲ Warnings: Regular monitoring of liver function during treatment is essential.
✪ **Related entries: Fucibet; Fucidin; Fucidin H; Fucithalmic.**

Fybogel Mebeverine

(Reckitt & Colman; Reckitt Benckiser) is a proprietary, non-prescription compound preparation of the ANTISPASMODIC mebeverine hydrochloride and the LAXATIVE ispaghula husk. It can be used to relieve the symptoms of abdominal pain and bowel problems associated with gastrointestinal disorders such as irritable bowel syndrome. It is available as oral granules which are stirred into water. It is not given to children under 12 years, except on medical advice.
✚▲ Side-effects/warnings: See ISPAGHULA HUSK; MEBEVERINE HYDROCHLORIDE.

Fybogel Orange

(Reckitt Benckiser Healthcare) is a proprietary, non-prescription preparation of the (*bulking-agent*) LAXATIVE ispaghula husk. It can be used to treat a number of gastrointestinal disorders, and is available as effervescent granules (also as *Fybogel Orange*). It is not normally given to children under six years, except on medical advice.
✚▲ Side-effects/warnings: See ISPAGHULA HUSK.

Fybozest Orange

(Reckitt Benckiser Health) is a proprietary, non-prescription preparation of the (*bulking-agent*) LAXATIVE ispaghula husk. It can also be used in intestinal atony and to reduce cholesterol uptake in patients with hypercholesteraemia as part of a lipid-lowering diet. It is available as effervescent granules. It is not normally given to children, except on medical advice.
✚▲ Side-effects/warnings: See ISPAGHULA HUSK.

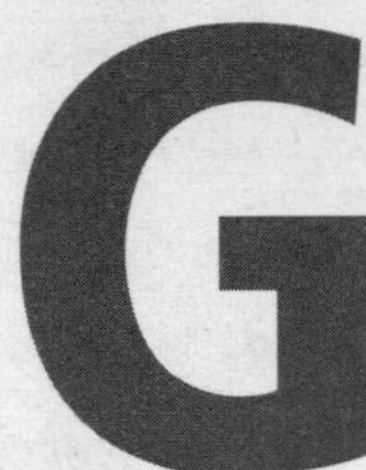

gabapentin

is an ANTICONVULSANT and ANTI-EPILEPTIC drug. It can be used as an adjunct to assist in the control of partial seizures that have not responded to other anti-epileptic drugs. Administration is oral.

✚ Side-effects: These include; fatigue, sleepiness, dizziness, unsteady gait, eye-flicker and double vision, headache, tremor, nausea and vomiting, rhinitis, weight gain, convulsions, dyspepsia, cough, aches, pains and tingling.

▲ Warnings: It should be administered with care in certain seizures, to patients with certain kidney disorders, or who are pregnant or breast-feeding. Withdrawal of treatment should be gradual.

✪ **Related entry: Neurontin.**

Gabitril

(Sanofi-Synthelabo) is a proprietary, prescription-only preparation of the ANTICONVULSANT and ANTI-EPILEPTIC tiagabine (as hydrochloride). It can be used to assist in the control of partial seizures, and is available as tablets.

✚▲ Side-effects/warnings: See TIAGABINE.

Galake

(Galen) is a proprietary, prescription-only compound analgesic preparation of the (OPIOID) ANTITUSSIVE dihydrocodeine tartrate and the NON-NARCOTIC ANALGESIC and ANTIPYRETIC paracetamol (in the ratio 500:10(mg) – a combination known as co-dydramol). It can be used to treat pain, and is available as tablets.

✚▲ Side-effects/warnings: See DIHYDROCODEINE TARTRATE; PARACETAMOL.

galantamine

is an ANTICHOLINESTERASE recently introduced for the symptomatic treatment of mild to moderate dementia of Alzheimer's disease. It is thought only to slow the rate of cognitive deterioration in about half of patients treated. Authorities have identified those patients that may benefit by assessing what is known as a mini mental-state examination (MMSE) score. Diagnosis and treatment is initiated by specialists with assessment throughout treatment. It is available in a form for oral administration.

✚ Side-effects: Gastrointestinal effects such as nausea and vomiting, diarrhoea, abdominal pain and dyspepsia; anorexia and weight loss, fatigue, drowsiness and dizziness, headache; sometimes insomnia, confusion, rhinitis, urinary tract infection; tremor; fainting and severe bradycardia.

▲ Warnings: Galantamine should not be given to people with have severely impaired kidney function, who are breast-feeding, have certain metabolic disorders (of galactose metabolism), or with urinary retention or gastrointestinal obstruction. It is used with caution in women who are pregnant, by people with impaired liver function, various heart disorders or who have a susceptibility to peptic ulcers, asthma or other chronic obstructive pulmonary disease.

✪ **Related entry: Reminyl.**

Galcodine

(Galen) is a proprietary, prescription-only preparation of the (OPIOID) ANTITUSSIVE codeine phosphate. It can be used to relieve a dry, painful cough, and is available as a sugar-free linctus.

✚▲ Side-effects/warnings: See CODEINE PHOSPHATE.

Galcodine Paediatric

(Galen) is a proprietary, prescription-only preparation of the (OPIOID) ANTITUSSIVE codeine phosphate. It can be used to relieve a dry, painful cough, and is available as a linctus.

✚▲ Side-effects/warnings: See CODEINE PHOSPHATE.

Galenamet

(Galen) is a proprietary, prescription-only preparation of the H_2-ANTAGONIST cimetidine. It can be used as an ULCER-HEALING DRUG for benign peptic ulcers (in the stomach or duodenum), gastro-oesophageal reflux and dyspepsia and associated conditions. It is available as tablets.

✚▲ Side-effects/warnings: See CIMETIDINE.

G

Galenamox
(Galen) is a proprietary, prescription-only preparation of the broad-spectrum ANTIBACTERIAL and (PENICILLIN) ANTIBIOTIC amoxicillin. It can be used to treat systemic bacterial infections, and is available as capsules and an oral suspension.
✚▲ Side-effects/warnings: See AMOXICILLIN.

Galenphol Linctus
(Galen) is a proprietary, non-prescription preparation of the (OPIOID) ANTITUSSIVE pholcodine. It can be used for a dry, painful cough, and is available as a sugar-free linctus.
✚▲ Side-effects/warnings: See PHOLCODINE.

Galenphol Paediatric Linctus
(Galen) is a proprietary, non-prescription preparation of the (OPIOID) ANTITUSSIVE pholcodine. It can be used for a dry, painful cough, and is available as a sugar-free linctus. It is not normally given to children under one year, except on medical advice.
✚▲ Side-effects/warnings: See PHOLCODINE.

Galfer
(Galen) is a proprietary, non-prescription preparation of ferrous fumarate. It can be used as an IRON supplement in iron-deficiency ANAEMIA TREATMENT, and is available as capsules and a syrup.
✚▲ Side-effects/warnings: See FERROUS FUMARATE.

Galfer FA
(Galen) is a proprietary, non-prescription compound preparation of ferrous fumarate and folic acid. It can be used as an IRON and folic acid supplement during pregnancy. Available as capsules.
✚▲ Side-effects/warnings: See FERROUS FUMARATE; FOLIC ACID.

Galfloxin
(Galen) is a proprietary, prescription-only preparation of the ANTIBACTERIAL and (PENICILLIN) ANTIBIOTIC flucloxacillin. It can be used to treat bacterial infections, especially staphylococcal infections that prove to be resistant to penicillin. It is available as capsules.
✚▲ Side-effects/warnings: See FLUCLOXACILLIN.

gallamine triethiodide
is a *non-depolarizing* SKELETAL MUSCLE RELAXANT which is used to induce muscle paralysis during surgery. Administration is by injection.
✚▲ Side-effects/warnings: It is a specialist drug used by anaesthetists in hospital.
○ Related entry: Flaxedil.

Galloway's Cough Syrup
(Warner Lambert Consumer Healthcare; Pfizer) is a proprietary, non-prescription preparation of the EXPECTORANT ipecacuaha with squill vinegar. It can be used for the relief of coughs and hoarseness, and is available as a syrup.
✚▲ Side-effects/warnings: See IPECACUANHA.

Galpseud
(Galen) is a proprietary, non-prescription preparation of the SYMPATHOMIMETIC pseudoephedrine hydrochloride. It can be used as a NASAL DECONGESTANT, and is available as tablets or as a linctus for dilution. It is not normally given to children under two years, except on medical advice.
✚▲ Side-effects/warnings: See PSEUDOEPHEDRINE HYDROCHLORIDE.

Gamanil
(Merck) is a proprietary, prescription-only preparation of the (TRICYCLIC) ANTIDEPRESSANT lofepramine (as hydrochloride). It can be used to treat depressive illness, and is available as tablets.
✚▲ Side-effects/warnings: See LOFEPRAMINE.

Gammabulin
(Hyland Immuno) is a proprietary, prescription-only preparation of human NORMAL IMMUNOGLOBULIN. It can be used to confer immediate *passive immunity* against infection by viruses, including hepatitis A virus, rubeola (measles) and rubella (German measles). It is available in a form for intramuscular injection.
✚▲ Side-effects/warnings: See NORMAL IMMUNOGLOBULIN.

gamma globulin
see NORMAL IMMUNOGLOBULIN.

gamolenic acid
is used in preparations that are taken by mouth to relieve atopic eczema and breast pain (mastalgia).
✚ Side-effects: There may be nausea, headache, indigestion, rarely skin disorders and abdominal pain.

G

▲ Warnings: It is used with caution in patients who are pregnant or epileptics.
✪ **Related entries: Efamast; Epogam.**

ganciclovir

is an ANTIVIRAL drug related to ACICLOVIR (acyclovir), but although more active against certain viral infections (cytomegalovirus) it is more toxic. Its use is therefore restricted to the treatment of life-threatening or sight-threatening cytomegalovirus (CMV) infections in immunocompromised patients, and to prevent cytomegalovirus disease during immunosuppressive therapy following organ transplant operations. Administration is oral, by intravenous infusion, or ocular implants.
✚ Side-effects: There are many side-effects; various blood cell deficiencies; sore throat and swelling of the face; fever and rash; effects on liver function, gastrointestinal disturbances; and a number of other reactions.
▲ Warnings: It is a specialist drug, and there will be full assessment and patient monitoring throughout treatment. It is not be given to patients who are pregnant or breast-feeding. Blood monitoring is necessary. An adequate fluid intake must be maintained.
✪ **Related entries: Cymevene; Virgan; Vitrasert.**

Ganda

(Chauvin) is a proprietary, prescription-only compound preparation of the ADRENERGIC-NEURONE BLOCKER guanethidine monosulphate and the SYMPATHOMIMETIC adrenaline acid tartrate (epinephrine). It can be used as a GLAUCOMA TREATMENT, and is available as eye-drops (in two strengths).
✚▲ Side-effects/warnings: See ADRENALINE ACID TARTRATE; GUANETHIDINE MONOSULPHATE.

ganglion-blocker

drugs are from a class of agents that block transmission in the peripheral autonomic nervous system at the nervous junction called ganglia. These drugs work by preventing the actions of ACETYLCHOLINE, which is the neurotransmitter at these junctions and so, in effect, ganglion-blockers are a type of ANTICHOLINERGIC drug. The cholinergic receptors at which ganglion-blockers act are called nicotinic receptors (since NICOTINE is a strong stimulant at such receptors) and these are similar, but not identical, to the cholinergic receptors of the same name that are found at the skeletal neuromuscular junction. One result of this is that some of the SKELETAL MUSCLE RELAXANT drugs (eg GALLAMINE TRIETHIODIDE) have some ganglion-blocking side-effects and *vice versa*. The ganglion-blockers were introduced as ANTIHYPERTENSIVE drugs (and are very effective as such), but their actions and side-effects are so widespread that they are now rarely used in medicine. However, TRIMETAPHAN CAMSILATE is still in use because it reduces blood pressure by reducing vascular tone normally induced by the sympathetic nervous system, and as it is short-acting it makes a useful HYPOTENSIVE for controlling blood pressure during surgery.

A quite different group of anticholinergic drugs, the ANTIMUSCARINIC, have very extensive uses in medicine. For this reason, the term 'anticholinergic' is commonly used synonymously with antimuscarinic, though this is not really correct. (Examples of drugs that block the actions of acetylcholine at muscarinic receptors are ATROPINE SULPHATE, BENZHEXOL HYDROCHLORIDE and HYOSCINE HYDROBROMIDE.)

ganirelix

is an analogue of gonadorelin (gonadothropin-releasing hormone; GnRH), which is a hypothalamic HORMONE. Short-term it stimulates pituitary gland's secretion of gonadotrophin, but on prolonged administration it acts as an indirect HORMONE ANTAGONIST in that it reduces gonadotrophin output. It is used in the treatment of infertility by assisted reproductive techniques (IVF) under specialist supervision. Administration is by injection.
✚ Side-effects: Headache and nausea, reactions at the site of the injection; dizziness and malaise.
▲ Warnings: Ganirelix is not to be used in women who are already pregnant or breast-feeding, or who have impaired liver or kidney function.
✪ **Related entry: Orgalutran.**

Garamycin

(Schering-Plough) is a proprietary, prescription-only preparation of the ANTIBACTERIAL and (AMINOGLYCOSIDE) ANTIBIOTIC gentamicin (as sulphate). It can be used to treat many forms of infection, and is available as eye- and ear-drops.
✚▲ Side-effects/warnings: See GENTAMICIN.

G

Gardenal Sodium

(Concord) is a proprietary, prescription-only preparation of the BARBITURATE phenobarbital (as sodium) and is on the Controlled Drugs list. It can be used as an ANTICONVULSANT and ANTI-EPILEPTIC to treat most forms of epilepsy, and is available in a form for injection.
✚▲ Side-effects/warnings: See PHENOBARBITAL.

Gastrobid Continus

(Napp) is a proprietary, prescription-only preparation of the ANTI-EMETIC and ANTINAUSEANT metoclopramide hydrochloride. It can be used to treat nausea and vomiting, particularly in gastrointestinal disorders and after treatment with radiation or cytotoxic drugs. It also has gastric MOTILITY STIMULANT actions and can be used in the treatment of non-ulcer dyspepsia, gastric stasis and for the prevention of reflux oesophagitis. It is available as modified-release tablets.
✚▲ Side-effects/warnings: See METOCLOPRAMIDE HYDROCHLORIDE.

Gastrocote Liquid

(SSL) is a proprietary, non-prescription compound preparation of the ANTACID agents aluminium hydroxide, sodium bicarbonate and magnesium trisilicate and the DEMULCENT alginic acid (as sodium alginate). It can be used for the symptomatic relief of acid indigestion, and is available as a liquid.
✚▲ Side-effects/warnings: See ALGINIC ACID; ALUMINIUM HYDROXIDE; MAGNESIUM TRISILICATE; SODIUM BICARBONATE.

Gastrocote Tablets

(SSL) is a proprietary, non-prescription compound preparation of the ANTACID agents aluminium hydroxide, sodium bicarbonate and magnesium trisilicate and the DEMULCENT alginic acid. It can be used for the symptomatic relief of acid indigestion, and is available as chewable tablets. It is not normally given to children under six years, except on medical advice.
✚▲ Side-effects/warnings: See ALGINIC ACID; ALUMINIUM HYDROXIDE; MAGNESIUM TRISILICATE; SODIUM BICARBONATE.

Gastroflux

(Ashbourne) is a proprietary, prescription-only preparation of the ANTI-EMETIC and ANTINAUSEANT metoclopramide hydrochloride. It can be used to treat nausea and vomiting, particularly of gastrointestinal disorders and after treatment with radiation or cytotoxic drugs. It also has gastric MOTILITY STIMULANT actions and can be used in the treatment of non-ulcer dyspepsia, gastric stasis and for the prevention of reflux oesophagitis. It is available as tablets.
✚▲ Side-effects/warnings: See METOCLOPRAMIDE HYDROCHLORIDE.

Gaviscon 250

(Reckitt Benckiser Healthcare) is a proprietary, non-prescription compound preparation of the ANTACID agents aluminium hydroxide, sodium bicarbonate and magnesium trisilicate, and the DEMULCENT alginic acid. It can be used for the symptomatic relief of indigestion and heartburn, and is available as tablets. It is not normally given to children.
✚▲ Side-effects/warnings: See ALGINIC ACID; ALUMINIUM HYDROXIDE; MAGNESIUM TRISILICATE; SODIUM BICARBONATE.

Gaviscon 500 Lemon Flavour Tablets

(Reckitt Benckiser Healthcare) is a proprietary, non-prescription compound preparation of the ANTACID agents aluminium hydroxide, sodium bicarbonate and magnesium trisilicate, and the DEMULCENT alginic acid. It can be used for the symptomatic relief of indigestion and heartburn, and is available as tablets. It is not normally given to children.
✚▲ Side-effects/warnings: See ALGINIC ACID; ALUMINIUM HYDROXIDE; MAGNESIUM TRISILICATE; SODIUM BICARBONATE.

Gaviscon Advance

(Reckitt Benckiser Healthcare) is a proprietary, non-prescription compound preparation of the ANTACID potassium bicarbonate, and the DEMULCENT alginic acid (as sodium alginate). It can be used for the symptomatic relief of heartburn and indigestion, and is available as an oral suspension. It is not normally given to children, except on medical advice.
✚▲ Side-effects/warnings: See ALGINIC ACID; POTASSIUM BICARBONATE.

Gaviscon Infant

(Reckitt Benckiser Healthcare) is a proprietary, non-prescription preparation of the DEMULCENT

alginic acid (as sodium alginate and magnesium alginate). It can be used for the treatment of regurgitation, and is available as a powder. It is for infants and is not normally given to children, except under medical direction.
✚▲ Side-effects/warnings: See ALGINIC ACID.

GelTears

(Chauvin) is a proprietary, non-prescription preparation of carbomer. It can be used as artificial tears where there is dryness of the eye due to disease (eg keratoconjunctivitis sicca). It is available as a gel for application to the eye.
✚▲ Side-effects/warnings: See CARBOMER.

gemcitabine

is an (*antimetabolite*) CYTOTOXIC drug which is used as an ANTICANCER treatment of locally advanced or metastatic non-small cell lung cancer, also advanced metastatic adenocarcinoma of the pancreas, and, when given with cisplatin, advanced bladder cancer. Administration is by injection.
✚▲ Side-effects/warnings: See CYTOTOXIC.
✪ **Related entry: Gemzar.**

Gemeprost

(Beacon) is a proprietary, prescription-only preparation of the PROSTAGLANDIN analogue gemeprost. It is available as a pessary.
✚▲ Side-effects/warnings: See GEMEPROST.

gemeprost

is a PROSTAGLANDIN (an analogue of prostaglandin E_1), which is a LOCAL HORMONE naturally involved in the control of uterine motility, that is used in early pregnancy in operative procedures. It is administered to the cervix by pessary to cause softening and dilation. It is also used as an ABORTIFACIENT to cause therapeutic abortion and to remove the fetus following intra-uterine death.
✚ Side-effects: Vaginal bleeding and uterine pain; nausea, vomiting, flushing and shivering, headache and dizziness, a raised temperature and diarrhoea, muscle weakness, chills, backache, chest pain and breathing difficulties. Uterine rupture has been reported.
▲ Warnings: It is administered with care to patients who have vaginal or cervical infections, or cardiovascular insufficiency, asthma or glaucoma.
✪ **Related entry: Gemeprost.**

gemfibrozil

is a (*fibrate*) LIPID-REGULATING DRUG used in hyperlipidaemia to reduce the levels, or change the proportions, of various lipids (eg to lower triglycerides and lower LDL-cholesterol and raise LDL-cholesterol) in the bloodstream. Generally, it is administered only to patients in whom a strict and regular dietary regime, alone, is not having the desired effect. Administration is oral.
✚ Side-effects: These include dizziness, blurred vision, headache, gastrointestinal disturbances, skin disorders, pain in the extremities, muscle pain and impotence.
▲ Warnings: It is not to be given to alcoholics, patients with liver damage, gallstones or who are pregnant or breast-feeding. Blood and liver function should be monitored and eyes tested. Patients should report any muscle weakness, pain or tenderness to their doctor.
✪ **Related entries: Emfib; Lopid.**

Gemzar

(Lilly) is a proprietary, prescription-only preparation of the ANTICANCER drug gemcitabine (as hydrochloride). It is available in a form for injection.
✚▲ Side-effects/warnings: See GEMCITABINE.

general anaesthetic

drugs reduce sensation in the whole body with a loss of consciousness, and are used for surgical procedures. LOCAL ANAESTHETIC drugs, in contrast, affect sensation in a specific, local area without the loss of consciousness. The general anaesthetic that is used to initially induce anaesthesia is often different from the drug, or drugs, administered to maintain the anaesthesia. For induction, short-acting general anaesthetics that can be injected are convenient (eg thiopental sodium, etomidate, propofol), but for maintenance during long operations, inhalation anaesthetics are commonly used (eg halothane, desflurane, diethyl ether, isoflurane and enflurane). In order to minimize the depth of anaesthesia necessary for a surgical procedure, premedication with, or concurrent use of, other drugs is usually necessary. Another injection anaesthetic is ketamine, used for atypical situations and sometimes for children. A range of ancillary drugs is also valuable, including TRANQUILLIZER or SEDATIVE drugs (eg the BENZODIAZEPINE group), ANALGESIC drugs (eg

G

MORPHINE SULPHATE), SKELETAL MUSCLE RELAXANT drugs (eg GALLAMINE TRIETHIODIDE) and concurrent use of local anaesthetics (eg LIDOCAINE HYDROCHLORIDE).

Genotropin

(Pharmacia) is a proprietary, prescription-only preparation of somatropin, which is the biosynthetic form of human growth hormone. It is used to treat growth hormone deficiency and associated symptoms (in particular, short stature). It is available in several forms for injection, including a powder for reconstitution, in cartridges.
✚▲ Side-effects/warnings: See SOMATROPIN.

gentamicin

is a broad-spectrum ANTIBACTERIAL and ANTIBIOTIC drug, which is the most widely used of the AMINOGLYCOSIDE family. Although it does have activity against Gram-positive bacteria, it is used primarily against serious infections caused by Gram-negative bacteria. It is not orally absorbed and is therefore given by intravenous injection or infusion for the treatment of, for example, septicaemia, meningitis, infections of the heart (usually in conjunction with PENICILLIN), the biliary tract, prostate gland, eye and ear and skin infections, and pneumonia in hospital patients. Because of its potential toxicity to the ear (ototoxicity), which could result in deafness, and its toxicity to the kidney (nephrotoxicity), treatment should be short term. It is also available in the form of drops, creams and ointments for topical application.
✚ Side-effects: Depending on the route of administration; prolonged or high dosage may be damaging to the ear, and cause deafness and balance disorders – treatment must be discontinued if this occurs; there may also be reversible kidney damage. Various tests will be necessary to monitor progress. Avoid prolonged use. There may be local sensitivity reactions when used topically.
▲ Warnings: Again, these depend on the route of administration. But it should not be administered to patients who are pregnant or breast-feeding, or who suffer from myasthenia gravis or impaired kidney function. Kidney and neuronal function and gentamicin blood concentrations must be monitored.
✪ Related entries: Cidomycin; Garamycin; Genticin; Gentisone HC; Isotonic Gentamicin Injection; Minims Gentamicin.

gentian violet

see CRYSTAL VIOLET.

Genticin

(Roche) is a proprietary, prescription-only preparation of the ANTIBACTERIAL and (AMINOGLYCOSIDE) ANTIBIOTIC gentamicin (as sulphate). It can be used to treat many forms of infection, and is available in a form for injection and as eye- and ear-drops.
✚▲ Side-effects/warnings: See GENTAMICIN.

Gentisone HC

(Roche) is a proprietary, prescription-only compound preparation of the ANTIBACTERIAL and (AMINOGLYCOSIDE) ANTIBIOTIC gentamicin (as sulphate) and the ANTI-INFLAMMATORY and CORTICOSTEROID hydrocortisone (as acetate). It can be used to treat bacterial infections of the middle ear, and is available as ear-drops.
✚▲ Side-effects/warnings: See GENTAMICIN; HYDROCORTISONE.

Geref 50

(Serono) is a proprietary, prescription-only preparation of sermorelin. It is used to test the release of GROWTH HORMONE, and is available in a form for injection.
✚▲ Side-effects/warnings: See SERMORELIN.

Germolene Cream

(Bayer) is a proprietary, non-prescription compound preparation of the ANTISEPTIC chlorhexidine (as gluconate) and phenol. It can be used for cleaning all types of lesions, ranging from minor skin disorders or blisters to minor burns and small wounds, and preventing them from becoming infected. It is available as a cream.
✚▲ Side-effects/warnings: See CHLORHEXIDINE; PHENOL.

Germolene Ointment

(Bayer) is a proprietary, non-prescription compound preparation of the ASTRINGENT zinc oxide , the ANTISEPTIC phenol, the EMOLLIENT paraffin, and the COUNTER-IRRITANT, or RUBEFACIENT, methyl salicylate, with lanolin, starch and octaphonium chloride. It can be used for cleaning many types of lesions, ranging from

minor skin disorders or blisters to minor burns and small wounds, and preventing them from becoming infected. It is available as an ointment.
✚▲ Side-effects/warnings: See LANOLIN; LIQUID PARAFFIN; METHYL SALICYLATE; PHENOL; ZINC OXIDE.

Germoloids Cream

(Bayer) is a proprietary, non-prescription compound preparation of the LOCAL ANAESTHETIC lidocaine hydrochloride and the ASTRINGENT agent zinc oxide. It can be used for the symptomatic relief of the pain and itching of haemorrhoids and pruritus ani. It is available as a cream, and is not normally given to children, except on medical advice.
✚▲ Side-effects/warnings: See LIDOCAINE HYDROCHLORIDE; ZINC OXIDE.

Germoloids Ointment

(Bayer) is a proprietary, non-prescription compound preparation of the LOCAL ANAESTHETIC lidocaine hydrochloride and the ASTRINGENT agent zinc oxide. Used for the symptomatic relief of the pain and itching of haemorrhoids and pruritus ani. Available as an ointment. It is not normally given to children, except on medical advice.
✚▲ Side-effects/warnings: See LIDOCAINE HYDROCHLORIDE; ZINC OXIDE.

Germoloids Suppositories

(Bayer) is a proprietary, non-prescription compound preparation of the LOCAL ANAESTHETIC lidocaine hydrochloride and the ASTRINGENT agent zinc oxide. It can be used for the symptomatic relief of the pain and itching of haemorrhoids and pruritus ani. It is available as suppositories, and is not normally given to children, except on medical advice.
✚▲ Side-effects/warnings: See LIDOCAINE HYDROCHLORIDE; ZINC OXIDE.

gestodene

is a PROGESTOGEN which is used as a constituent of the combined ORAL CONTRACEPTIVE preparations that contain OESTROGEN and a progestogen. Administration is oral.
✚▲ Side-effects/warnings: See PROGESTOGEN.
✪ Related entries: Femodene; Femodene ED; Femodette; Minulet; Tri-Minulet; Triadene.

Gestone

(Ferring) is a proprietary, prescription-only preparation of the PROGESTOGEN progesterone. It can be used to treat many hormonal deficiency disorders in women, abnormal bleeding from the uterus and for maintenance of early pregnancy in recurrent miscarriage. It is available in a form for injection.
✚▲ Side-effects/warnings: See PROGESTERONE.

gestonorone caproate

(gestronol hexanoate) is a synthetic form of PROGESTOGEN which is used in women as an ANTICANCER treatment for cancer of the uterine lining (endometrium), and benign prostatic hyperplasia (BPH) in men. Administration is by intramuscular injection.
✚▲ Side-effects/warnings: See PROGESTOGEN.

gestrinone

is a drug that inhibits output of GONADOTROPHIN hormones (it has general actions similar to DANAZOL). It can be used to treat endometriosis (the presence of areas of uterus-lining, endometrium, outside the uterus). Administration is oral.
✚ Side-effects: Oily skin, spots, acne, fluid retention, body weight gain, growth of hair, voice changes; liver changes; headache; gastrointestinal upsets; change in libido, flushing, breast size decrease; depression, nervousness, appetite changes; muscle cramps.
▲ Warnings: It is not used for those who are pregnant or breast-feeding; have severe liver, kidney or heart impairment; or problems associated with previous sex hormone treatment. It is used with care in moderate heart or kidney impairment.
✪ Related entry: Dimetriose.

Givitol

(Galen) is a proprietary, non-prescription preparation of ferrous fumarate (with vitamins B group and C). It can be used as an IRON supplement in iron-deficiency ANAEMIA TREATMENT, and is available as capsules.
✚▲ Side-effects/warnings: See FERROUS FUMARATE.

Glandosane

(Fresenius Kabi) is a proprietary, non-prescription compound preparation of CARMELLOSE SODIUM, SORBITOL, POTASSIUM CHLORIDE, sodium chloride and other salts. It can

G

be used as a form of ARTIFICIAL SALIVA for application to the mouth and throat in conditions that make the mouth abnormally dry (eg Sicca syndrome or following radiotherapy). It is available as an aerosol spray.
✚▲ Side-effects/warnings: See CARMELLOSE SODIUM; POTASSIUM CHLORIDE; SODIUM CHLORIDE; SORBITOL.

glatiramer acetate

is a recently introduced IMMUNOMODULATOR drug comprised of synthetic polypeptides (small proteins). It has been used for the reduction of frequency of relapses in ambulatory patients with relapsing-remitting multiple sclerosis. It is administered by injection and treatment is initiated by a specialist.
✚ Side-effects: Flushing, chest pain, effects on the heart (palpitations and tachycardia) and shortness of breath may occur shortly after injection. There may be nausea, peripheral swelling and swelling of the face, fainting, asthenia, headache, tremor, sweating, lymphatic system disorders, increased muscle tone, joint pains, rash; convulsions, hypersensitivity reactions (including anaphylaxis, bronchospasm and urticaria) reported rarely. There may be reactions at the injection site.
▲ Warnings: Glatiramer acetate must be used with caution in those with heart conditions; impaired kidney function; who are pregnant or breast-feeding.
✪ Related entry: Copaxone.

glaucoma treatment 🅱

involves the use of drugs to lower the raised intraocular pressure (pressure in the eyeball) that usually is a characteristic of the group of eye conditions called glaucoma. It can lead to damage to the optic nerve and consequently vision can be affected. A number of types of drug help reduce this pressure (which has nothing directly to do with blood pressure). It is usually due to reduced outflow of fluid (aqueous humour) from the eye, so drugs often work by increasing this outflow. Which one is used depends on what sort of glaucoma is being treated (eg simple, open-angle, closed-angle, etc.). BETA-BLOCKER drugs are effective in most cases (eg BETAXOLOL HYDROCHLORIDE, CARTEOLOL HYDROCHLORIDE, LEVOBUNOLOL HYDROCHLORIDE and METIPRANOLOL), some SYMPATHOMIMETIC drugs (eg APRACLONIDINE, BRIMONIDINE TARTRATE and DIPIVEFRINE HYDROCHLORIDE) and certain cholinergic drugs (eg CARBACHOL and PILOCARPINE). Also, CARBONIC-ANHYDRASE INHIBITOR drugs (ACETAZOLAMIDE; DORZOLAMIDE) are used because they reduce the formation of aqueous humour in the eye. LATANOPROST and TRAVOPROST (PROSTAGLANDIN analogues) are now used to treat open-angle glaucoma and ocular hypertension when other drugs are inappropriate. It is important to note that certain classes of drugs, such as the CORTICOSTEROID and ANTICHOLINERGIC (ANTIMUSCARINIC, eg ATROPINE SULPHATE) classes, cause a rise in intraocular pressure and if administered to people predisposed to glaucoma may precipitate an acute attack.

Glau-opt

(Opus; Trinity) is a proprietary, prescription-only preparation of the BETA-BLOCKER timolol maleate. It can be used for GLAUCOMA TREATMENT, and is available as eye-drops.
✚▲ Side-effects/warnings: See TIMOLOL MALEATE.

glibenclamide

is a SULPHONYLUREA and is used in DIABETIC TREATMENT of Type II diabetes (non-insulin-dependent diabetes mellitus; NIDDM; maturity-onset diabetes). It works by augmenting what remains of INSULIN production in the pancreas. Administration is oral.
✚ Side-effects: These are generally minor and rare, but there may be some sensitivity reactions, such as a rash and also blood disorders. There may be headache and gastrointestinal upsets, weight gain.
▲ Warnings: It should not be administered to patients with certain liver, kidney or endocrine disorders, or who are pregnant or breast-feeding. There may be weight gain so diet should be controlled. It is used with caution in kidney or liver impairment, or in the elderly because of possible hypoglycaemia. Several drugs increase the hypoglycaemic effect of sulphanylureas (eg ETHANOL, MAOI antidepressants, PHENYLBUTAZONE), and some that depress them (eg *loop-class* diuretics; corticosteroid).
✪ Related entries: Daonil; Diabetamide; Euglucon; Gliken; Semi-Daonil.

G

Glibenese

(Pfizer) is a proprietary, prescription-only preparation of the SULPHONYLUREA glipizide. It can be used in DIABETIC TREATMENT of Type II diabetes (non-insulin-dependent diabetes mellitus; NIDDM; maturity-onset diabetes), and is available as tablets.
✚▲ Side-effects/warnings: See GLIPIZIDE.

gliclazide

is one of the SULPHONYLUREA and is used in DIABETIC TREATMENT of Type II diabetes (non-insulin-dependent diabetes mellitus; NIDDM; maturity-onset diabetes). It works by augmenting what remains of INSULIN production in the pancreas. Administration is oral.
✚▲ Side-effects/warnings: See GLIBENCLAMIDE; however, it may be chosen for patients with renal impairment and the elderly because it is shorter-acting.
✪ **Related entries: DIAGLYK; Diamicron; Diamicron MR.**

Gliken

(Kent) is a proprietary, prescription-only preparation of the SULPHONYLUREA glibenclamide. It is used in DIABETIC TREATMENT of Type II diabetes (non-insulin-dependent diabetes mellitus; NIDDM; maturity-onset diabetes), and is available as tablets.
✚▲ Side-effects/warnings: See GLIBENCLAMIDE.

glimepiride

is one of the SULPHONYLUREA and is used in DIABETIC TREATMENT of Type II diabetes (non-insulin-dependent diabetes mellitus; NIDDM; maturity-onset diabetes). It works by augmenting what remains of INSULIN production in the pancreas. Administration is oral.
✚▲ Side-effects/warnings: See GLIBENCLAMIDE. Hypersensitivity reactions are more common. There may be changes in liver function, so tests may need to be carried out. It is avoided in women who are pregnant or breast-feeding. If changing from another oral hypoglycaemic, a 'washout' period may be necessary (to avoid hypoglycaemia).
✪ **Related entry: Amaryl.**

glipizide

is one of the SULPHONYLUREA and is used in DIABETIC TREATMENT of Type II diabetes (non-insulin-dependent diabetes mellitus; NIDDM; maturity-onset diabetes). It works by augmenting what remains of INSULIN production in the pancreas. Administration is oral.
✚▲ Side-effects/warnings: See GLIBENCLAMIDE. Also drowsiness and dizziness.
✪ **Related entries: Glibenese; Minodiab.**

gliquidone

is one of the SULPHONYLUREA and is used in DIABETIC TREATMENT of Type II diabetes (non-insulin-dependent diabetes mellitus; NIDDM; maturity-onset diabetes). It works by augmenting what remains of INSULIN production in the pancreas. Administration is oral.
✚▲ Side-effects/warnings: See GLIBENCLAMIDE; however, it is more suitable for patients with kidney impairment.
✪ **Related entry: Glurenorm.**

Glivec

(Novartis) is a recently introduced proprietary, prescription-only preparation of the ANTICANCER drug imatinib (as mesilate). It can be used to treat myeloid leukaemia, and is available as capsules.
✚▲ Side-effects/warnings: See IMATINIB.

GlucaGen HypoKit

(Novo Nordisk) is a proprietary, prescription-only preparation of the HORMONE glucagon. It can be used in emergency for patients with low blood sugar levels, and as a diagnostic aid to test blood glucose control mechanisms. Administration is by injection (with *GlucaGen HypoKit*).
✚▲ Side-effects/warnings: See GLUCAGON.

glucagon

is a HORMONE produced and secreted by the pancreas in order to cause an increase in blood sugar levels, that is, it is a hyperglycaemic agent. It is normally part of a balancing mechanism with INSULIN, which has the opposite effect (see HYPOGLYCAEMIC). Therapeutically, glucagon can be administered to patients with low blood sugar levels (hypoglycaemia) in an emergency, but it is mainly used for diagnostic purposes. Administration is by injection.
✚ Side-effects: Diarrhoea, nausea; vomiting; occasionally hypersensitivity reactions.
▲ Warnings: It is not to be administered to patients with phaeochromocytoma, and with care for those with glucagonoma or insulinoma.

G

✪ **Related entry: GlucaGen HypoKit.**

Glucamet

(Opus; Trinity) is a proprietary, prescription-only preparation of the BIGUANIDE metformin hydrochloride. It is used in DIABETIC TREATMENT of Type II diabetes (non-insulin-dependent diabetes mellitus; NIDDM; maturity-onset diabetes), and is available as tablets.

✚▲ Side-effects/warnings: See METFORMIN HYDROCHLORIDE.

Glucobay

(Bayer) is a proprietary, prescription-only preparation of acarbose. It is used in DIABETIC TREATMENT, and is available as tablets.

✚▲ Side-effects/warnings: See ACARBOSE.

Glucophage

(Lipha) is a proprietary, prescription-only preparation of the BIGUANIDE metformin hydrochloride. It is used in DIABETIC TREATMENT of Type II diabetes (non-insulin-dependent diabetes mellitus; NIDDM; maturity-onset diabetes), and is available as tablets.

✚▲ Side-effects/warnings: See METFORMIN HYDROCHLORIDE.

glucose

or dextrose, is a simple sugar and is an important source of energy for the body – and the main source of energy for the brain. Once digested, it is stored in tissues including the liver and muscles in the form of glycogen and its break down in the muscles back into glucose produces energy. The level of glucose in the blood is critical and harmful symptoms can occur if the level is too high or too low. Therapeutically, it may be administered as a dietary supplement in conditions of low blood sugar level, to treat abnormally high acidity of body fluids (acidosis) or to increase glucose levels in the liver following liver damage. Diabetics on certain HYPOGLYCAEMIC drugs need to carry glucose to deal with possible hypotensive crises. Administration is either oral or by intravenous infusion.

✪ **Related entries: Beechams Veno's Expectorant; Dioralyte Natural; Dioralyte Tablets Raspberry Flavour; Topal.**

Glurenorm

(Sanofi-Synthelabo) is a proprietary, prescription-only preparation of the SULPHONYLUREA gliquidone. It is used in DIABETIC TREATMENT of Type II diabetes (non-insulin-dependent diabetes mellitus; NIDDM; maturity-onset diabetes), and is available as tablets.

✚▲ Side-effects/warnings: See GLIQUIDONE.

glutaraldehyde

is a DISINFECTANT, or ANTISEPTIC, which is similar to formaldehyde, but is stronger and faster-acting. It is mostly used to sterilize medical and surgical equipment. Therapeutically, it can be used in solution for warts (particularly verrucas) and as a KERATOLYTIC to remove hard, dead skin.

✚▲ Side-effects/warnings: See SALICYLIC ACID. Its effects as a treatment are not always predictable; skin treated may become irritated or sensitized. There may be rashes. It stains the skin brown.

✪ **Related entry: Glutarol.**

Glutarol

(Dermal) is a proprietary, non-prescription preparation of the KERATOLYTIC agent glutaraldehyde. It can be used to treat warts, and is available as a solution for topical application.

✚▲ Side-effects/warnings: See GLUTARALDEHYDE.

glycerin(e)

see GLYCEROL.

glycerol

or glycerin(e), is a colourless, sweet viscous liquid that is chemically an alcohol. It is used therapeutically as a constituent in many EMOLLIENT skin preparations, as a sweetening agent for medications and as a LAXATIVE in the form of anal suppositories. Taken orally, glycerol can be used for short-term GLAUCOMA TREATMENT.

✚▲ Side-effects/warnings: It is regarded as safe in normal topical use.

✪ **Related entries: Care Glycerin Suppositories for Adults; Compound Thymol Glycerin, BP; Care Glycerin Suppositories for Children; Care Glycerin Suppositories for Infants; Decubal Clinic; Earex Plus Ear Drops; Exterol Ear Drops; Earex Plus Ear Drops; Fletchers' Enemette; Lemsip Cough + Cold Dry Cough; Lockets Medicated Linctus; Micolette**

G

Micro-enema; Micralax Micro-enema; Neutrogena Dermatological Cream; Otex Ear Drops; Relaxit Micro-enema; Tixylix Baby Syrup.

glyceryl trinitrate

is a short-acting VASODILATOR and ANTI-ANGINA drug. It is used to prevent attacks of angina pectoris (ischaemic heart pain), for instance when taken before exercise, for symptomatic relief during an acute attack and in HEART FAILURE TREATMENT. It works by dilating the blood vessels returning blood to the heart and so reducing the workload of the heart. It is short-acting, but its effect can be extended through use of modified-release sublingual tablets (kept under the tongue) and buccal tablets (kept behind the upper lip). It is also administered by aerosol spray (which is sprayed under the tongue from where it is absorbed into the systemic circulation), by intravenous injection or in ointments and dressings placed on the surface of the chest so that it can be absorbed through the skin.

✚ Side-effects: There may be a throbbing headache, flushing, dizziness; some patients experience an increase in heart rate and postural hypotension (fall in blood pressure on standing); when given by injection, there may be additional side-effects.

▲ Warnings: It can be administered with caution to patients who suffer from hypothermia, malnutrition and certain cardiovascular disorders, and those with severe liver, kidney or thyroid impairment. It should not be used in individuals with hypersensitivity to nitrates; hypotensive conditions and hypovolaemia; various heart and cardiovascular conditions; marked anaemia, head trauma, cerebral haemorrhage, closed-angle glaucoma.

✪ **Related entries: Coro-Nitro Pump Spray; Deponit; Glytrin Spray; GTN 300 mcg; Minitran; Nitro-Dur; Nitrocine; Nitrolingual Pumpspray; Nitromin; Nitronal; Percutol; Suscard; Sustac; Transiderm-Nitro.**

glycol salicylate

is a NSAID (non-steroidal anti-inflammatory drug) that has COUNTER-IRRITANT, or RUBEFACIENT, actions and can be applied to the skin for symptomatic relief of pain in underlying organs, for instance in rheumatic and other musculoskeletal disorders. Administration is topical. See also SALICYLATE; SALICYLIC ACID.

✚▲ Side-effects/warnings: See NSAID; though normally little is absorbed into the circulation and local side-effects are limited to mild irritation. It should not be used on broken skin or mucous membranes.

✪ **Related entries: Algipan Rub; Ralgex Cream; Ralgex Freeze Spray; Ralgex Heat Spray; Ralgex Stick.**

glycopyrronium bromide

is an ANTICHOLINERGIC (ANTIMUSCARINIC) drug which is used in preoperative medication for drying up saliva and other secretions. Administration is by injection.

✚▲ Side-effects/warnings: See ATROPINE SULPHATE.

✪ **Related entries: Robinul; Robinul-Neostigmine.**

Glypressin

(Ferring) is a proprietary preparation of terlipressin, an analogue of the pituitary HORMONE antidiuretic hormone (ADH, or vasopressin). It is used as a VASOCONSTRICTOR to treat bleeding from varices (varicose veins) in the oesophagus, and is available in a form for injection.

✚▲ Side-effects/warnings: See TERLIPRESSIN.

Glytrin Spray

(Sanofi-Synthelabo) is a proprietary, non-prescription preparation of the VASODILATOR and ANTI-ANGINA drug glyceryl trinitrate. It can be used to treat and prevent angina pectoris, and is available as a sublingual aerosol spray in metered doses.

✚▲ Side-effects/warnings: See GLYCERYL TRINITRATE.

GnRH

see GONADORELIN.

Goddard's Embrocation

(LRC) is a proprietary, non-prescription preparation of TURPENTINE OIL (with ammonia and acetic acid), which has COUNTER-IRRITANT, or RUBEFACIENT, action. It can be applied to the skin for symptomatic relief of underlying muscle or joint pain, and is available as an embrocation for topical application.

▲ Warnings: See TURPENTINE OIL. Do not use on inflamed or broken skin, or on mucous membranes.

gold

in the form of the chemical compounds sodium aurothiomalate and auranofin is used

therapeutically as an ANTIRHEUMATIC treatment for rheumatoid arthritis and juvenile arthritis. Gold compounds work very slowly and it may take several months of treatment before full beneficial effects. Administration is by injection.
✚▲ Side-effects/warnings: See AURANOFIN; SODIUM AUROTHIOMALATE.

Golden Eye Ointment

(Typharm) is a proprietary, non-prescription preparation of the ANTIBACTERIAL dibrompropamidine isethionate. It can be used to treat eye infections. Available as an eye ointment.
✚▲ Side-effects/warnings: See DIBROMPROPAMIDINE ISETHIONATE.

gonadorelin

(gonadotrophin-releasing hormone; GnRH; LH-RH) is the hypothalamic HORMONE that acts on the pituitary gland to release the GONADOTROPHIN hormones (luteinising hormone; LH, and follicle-stimulating hormone; FSH). It is therefore also known as luteinising hormone-releasing hormone, LH-RH, or more correctly LH-FSH-RH. Gonadorelin is in fact the synthetic version of naturally occurring gonadotrophin-releasing hormone and is used for diagnostic purposes (to assess pituitary function). It has been used for treatment, but now synthetic analogues of gonadorelin (BUSERELIN, GOSERELIN, LEUPRORELIN ACETATE, TRIPTORELIN and NAFARELIN) are instead used to treat endometriosis, infertility and breast and prostate cancer. Administration is by injection.
✚ Side-effects: Rarely, there may be headache, abdominal pain and nausea; increased menstrual bleeding, the site of infusion may become painful.
▲ Warnings: Caution in pituitary adenoma.
✪ Related entry: HRF.

gonadotrophin 🅴

is the name of a group of hormones (see HORMONE) that are produced and secreted by the anterior pituitary gland (when stimulated by GONADOTROPHIN-RELEASING HORMONE from the hypothalamus); as well as, in pregnancy, in large amounts by the placenta. They act on the ovary in women, and on the testes in men, to promote the production in turn of other SEX HORMONES and of ova (eggs) or sperm, respectively. The major gonadotrophins are FOLLICLE-STIMULATING HORMONE (FSH) and LUTEINISING HORMONE (LH). The similar hormones released by the chorionic tissue of the placenta in pregnancy are called CHORIONIC GONADOTROPHIN and evidence in the urine for the presence of this is the basis of many pregnancy tests. These hormones are used as an infertility treatment where infertility is due to lack of ovulation.

gonadotrophin-releasing hormone

see GONADORELIN.

gonadotropin

see GONADOTROPHIN.

Gonal-F

(Serono) is a proprietary, prescription-only HORMONE preparation of follitropin alpha, which is a synthetic form of FOLLICLE-STIMULATING HORMONE (FSH). It can be used to treat infertility in women, and is available in a form for injection.
✚▲ Side-effects/warnings: See FOLLITROPIN ALPHA.

Gopten

(Knoll) is a proprietary, prescription-only preparation of the ACE INHIBITOR trandolapril. It can be used as an ANTIHYPERTENSIVE, often in conjunction with other classes of drug, and is available as capsules.
✚▲ Side-effects/warnings: See TRANDOLAPRIL.

goserelin

is an analogue of GONADORELIN (gonadothrophin-releasing hormone; GnRH), which is a hypothalamic HORMONE. On prolonged administration it acts as an indirect HORMONE ANTAGONIST in that it reduces the pituitary gland's secretion of gonadotrophin (after an initial surge), which results in reduced secretion of SEX HORMONES by the ovaries or testes. It is used to treat endometriosis, and as an ANTICANCER drug for breast cancer and cancer of the prostate gland, and is used in infertility treatment. Administration is by subcutaneous injection.
✚▲ Side-effects/warnings: See BUSERELIN. Additionally, there may be rashes and possibly bruises at the site of injection.
✪ Related entries: Zoladex; Zoladex LA.

gramicidin

is an ANTIBIOTIC drug with ANTIBACTERIAL properties which is incorporated into a number of eye- and ear-drop preparations along with

NEOMYCIN SULPHATE, NYSTATIN and TRIAMCINOLONE.
✚▲ Side-effects/warnings: It is regarded as safe in normal topical use.
✪ **Related entries: Graneodin; Neosporin; Sofradex; Tri-Adcortyl; Tri-Adcortyl Otic.**

Graneodin

(Squibb; Bristol-Myers Squibb) is a proprietary, prescription-only preparation of the ANTIBACTERIAL and (AMINOGLYCOSIDE) ANTIBIOTIC neomycin sulphate with the antibiotic gramicidin. It can be used to treat bacterial infections of the skin and to prevent infection. It is available as an ointment for topical application.
✚▲ Side-effects/warnings: See GRAMICIDIN; NEOMYCIN SULPHATE.

granisetron

is an ANTI-EMETIC and ANTINAUSEANT which gives relief from nausea and vomiting, especially in patients receiving cytotoxic radiotherapy or chemotherapy, or after operations. It acts as a serotonin receptor antagonist blocking the action of the natural mediator SEROTONIN. Administration is either oral or by intravenous injection or infusion.
✚ Side-effects: Headache, rash, constipation and change in liver function.
▲ Warnings: Administer with care to patients who are pregnant or breast-feeding.
✪ **Related entry: Kytril.**

Granocyte

(Chugai) is a proprietary, prescription-only preparation of the specialist drug lenograstim, used to treat neutropenia during chemotherapy in ANTICANCER treatment. It is available in a form for intravenous infusion.
✚▲ Side-effects/warnings: see LENOGRASTIM.

Gregoderm

(Unigreg) is a proprietary, prescription-only compound preparation of the ANTI-INFLAMMATORY and CORTICOSTEROID hydrocortisone, the ANTIBACTERIAL and (AMINOGLYCOSIDE) ANTIBIOTIC neomycin sulphate, the antibacterial and (POLYMYXIN) antibiotic polymyxin B sulphate and the ANTIFUNGAL and antibiotic nystatin. It can be used to treat inflammation of the skin in which infection is also present, and is available as an ointment for topical application.
✚▲ Side-effects/warnings: See HYDROCORTISONE; NEOMYCIN SULPHATE; NYSTATIN; POLYMYXIN B SULPHATE.

griseofulvin

is a powerful ANTIFUNGAL and ANTIBIOTIC drug. It is most commonly used for large-scale skin infections, especially those that prove resistant to other drugs. During treatment, which may be prolonged, it is deposited selectively in the skin, hair and nails and so prevents further fungal invasion. Administration is oral.
✚ Side-effects: There may be headache with nausea and vomiting; some patients experience sensitivity to light, rash, dizziness, fatigue, confusion, co-ordination problems and blood disorders.
▲ Warnings: It should not be administered to patients who suffer from severe liver problems, porphyria, who are pregnant, or have systemic lupus erythematosus. It should be administered with caution to patients who are breast-feeding. Men should not father children until six months after treatment. Avoid alcohol because its effects are enhanced. It can impair driving ability.
✪ **Related entry: Grisovin.**

Grisovin

(GlaxoWellcome; GSK) is a proprietary, prescription-only preparation of the ANTIFUNGAL and ANTIBIOTIC griseofulvin. It can be used to treat fungal infections of the scalp, skin and nails, and is available as tablets.
✚▲ Side-effects/warnings: See GRISEOFULVIN.

growth factors 🅴

are proteins produced normally in tiny quantities by cells in the body, acting as a sort of local hormone to promote cell growth and have complex effects on cells. One of these, human *platelet-derived growth factor* (PDGF), manufactured by recombinant technology in a form known as BECAPLERMIN, is used as a topical preparation in the treatment of neuropathic diabetic ulcers.

growth hormone

see SOMATOTROPIN; SOMATROPIN.

GTN 300 mcg

(Martindale) is a proprietary, non-prescription preparation of the VASODILATOR and ANTI-

ANGINA drug glyceryl trinitrate. It can be used to treat and prevent angina pectoris, and is available as short-acting sublingual tablets.
✚▲ Side-effects/warnings: See GLYCERYL TRINITRATE.

guaiacol

is found in plant oils and is incorporated into proprietary preparations as an EXPECTORANT, though evidence of its efficacy is lacking. Administration is oral.
✚▲ Side-effects/warnings: It is regarded as safe in normal use at high dilution. Little is known about it, but at higher concentration is causes a burning sensation in the mouth and is irritant.
✪ Related entry: Pulmo Bailly.

guaifenesin

(guaiphenesin) is incorporated into a number of proprietary preparations as an EXPECTORANT, though good evidence of its efficacy is lacking. Administration is oral.
✚▲ Side-effects/warnings: It is regarded as safe in normal use: however, some authorities believe it best avoided in early pregnancy or in certain respiratory problems.
✪ Related entries: Actifed Expectorant; Adult Meltus Expectorant for Chesty Coughs and Catarrh; Adult Meltus Expectorant with Decongestant; Beechams All-In-One; Beechams Veno's Expectorant; Benylin Chesty Coughs (Non-Drowsy); Benylin Children's Chesty Coughs;Dimotane Expectorant; Honey and Lemon Meltus Expectorant; Jackson's All Fours; Jackson's Bronchial Balsam; Junior Meltus Expectorant for Chesty Coughs and Catarrh; Junior Meltus Sugar and Colour Free Expectorant; Lemsip Cough + Cold Chesty Cough; Liqufruta Garlic Cough Medicine; Robitussin Chesty Cough Medicine; Robitussin Chesty Cough with Congestion; Sudafed Expectorant; Tixylix Chesty Cough; Vicks Vaposyrup for Chesty Coughs.

guaiphenesin

see GUAIFENESIN.

guanethidine monosulphate

is an ADRENERGIC-NEURONE BLOCKER, which is an ANTISYMPATHETIC class of drug that prevents release of NORADRENALINE (also called norepinephrine) from sympathetic nerves. It can be used as an ANTIHYPERTENSIVE mainly for hypertensive crisis. Administration is either oral or by injection.
✚ Side-effects: Postural hypotension; fluid retention; nasal congestion; diarrhoea, failure to ejaculate; drowsiness.
▲ Warnings: It should not be administered to patients with certain renal or heart disorders or phaeochromocytoma; it should be administered with caution to those who are elderly, pregnant or have peptic ulcers, asthma or coronary or cerebral arteriosclerosis.
✪ Related entries: Ganda; Ismelin.

Guarem

(Rybar; Shire) is a proprietary, non-prescription preparation of guar gum, which is a form of DIABETIC TREATMENT. It is available as sachets of granules that are dissolved in fluid and drunk before a meal or sprinkled onto food.
✚▲ Side-effects/warnings: See GUAR GUM.

guar gum

is a form of DIABETIC TREATMENT in as much that if it is taken in sufficient quantities it reduces the rise in blood glucose which occurs after meals, probably by delaying absorption of carbohydrate foodstuffs. It may also be used to relieve the symptoms of Dumping Syndrome. Taken orally.
✚ Side-effects: Flatulence, distension of the intestine with possible obstruction.
▲ Warnings: Do not use when there is pre-existing intestinal obstruction. Fluid intake should be maintained. Gum preparations should usually be taken with plenty of water and not last thing at night.
✪ Related entry: Guarem.

Gyno-Daktarin

(Janssen-Cilag) is a proprietary, prescription-only range of preparations of the ANTIFUNGAL drug miconazole (as nitrate). The various preparations can be used to treat fungal infections of the vagina or vulva (eg candidiasis; thrush). They are available as an intravaginal cream (with its own applicator), vaginal inserts (pessaries), an *Ovule* (a vaginal capsule) called *Gyno-Daktarin 1* and a *Combipack* that combines the cream and the pessaries.
✚▲ Side-effects/warnings: See MICONAZOLE.

Gynol II

(Janssen-Cilag) is a proprietary, non-prescription SPERMICIDAL CONTRACEPTIVE for use in

combination with barrier methods of contraception (such as a condom). It is available as a jelly containing nonoxinol.
✚▲ Side-effects/warnings: See NONOXINOL.

Gyno-Pevaryl

(Janssen-Cilag) is a proprietary, non-prescription range of preparations of the ANTIFUNGAL drug econazole nitrate. The various preparations can be used to treat fungal infections of the vagina or vulva (eg candidiasis; thrush). They are available as a cream for topical application as vaginal inserts (pessaries) in two formulations with one under the name *Gyno-Pevaryl 1*, *Combipacks* and *CP packs* that contain the cream and pessaries.
✚▲ Side-effects/warnings: See ECONAZOLE NITRATE.

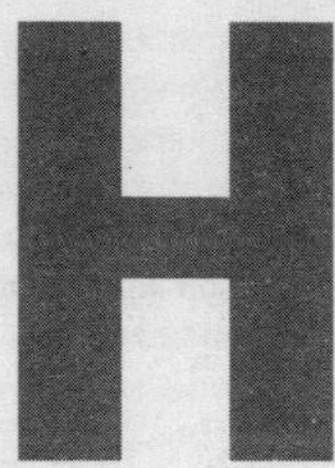

H_2-antagonist

drugs act to block the actions of histamine at a class of histamine receptor called H_2, which is found in the gastric mucosa (stomach lining) and promotes secretion of gastric acid (hydrochloric or peptic acid). The over-production of peptic acid may be involved in ulceration of the gastric (stomach) and duodenal (first part of small intestine) linings, or be the cause of pain in reflux oesophagitis (regurgitation of acid and enzymes into the oesophagus). H_2-antagonists are commonly used as ulcer-healing drugs (see ULCER-HEALING DRUG) and for a wide variety of dyspepsia and other peptic acid complaints. They promote healing of peptic ulcers. Technically, these drugs are ANTIHISTAMINE agents, but somewhat confusingly this term is not applied to them because it is reserved for the much earlier class of drugs that act at H_1 receptors and which have quite different actions (they are used, among other purposes, to treat allergic reactions). See CIMETIDINE; FAMOTIDINE; NIZATIDINE; RANITIDINE.

✚ Side-effects: May include diarrhoea and other gastrointestinal disturbances, liver function changes; headache, dizziness and tiredness; rash. Less common side-effects include pancreatitis, heart function changes, confusion, depression, hallucinations (particularly in the elderly or ill); also hypersensitivity reactions (including fever, muscle pain, anaphylaxis), blood disorders and effects on the heart. There have been occasional reports with some H_2-antagonists of impotence and the growth of breasts in men.

▲ Warnings: Caution in liver or kidney impairment; pregnancy or breast-feeding. They may mask symptoms of gastric cancer; and this possibility must be excluded before treatment particularly the middle-aged or over.

Haelan

(Typharm) is a proprietary, prescription-only preparation of the CORTICOSTEROID and ANTI-INFLAMMATORY drug fludroxycortide. It can be used to treat inflammatory skin disorders, such as eczema, and is available as a cream, ointment and adhesive tape for topical application.

✚▲ Side-effects/warnings: See FLUDROXYCORTIDE.

Haemophilus influenzae type B vaccine

(Hib) for IMMUNIZATION prevents *Haemophilus influenzae* infection (bacteria that cause respiratory infection and meningitis). It is given as a routine childhood preventive vaccination, and is administered by injection.

✚▲ Side-effects/warnings: See VACCINE.

✪ Related entries: ACT-HIB DTP dc; Act-HIB; Hiberix; HibTITER; Infanrix-HIB.

haemostatic

drugs include a wide range of drugs that enhance the process of haemostasis in the body; that is, act to slow or prevent bleeding (haemorrhage). They are used mostly to treat disorders in which bleeding is prolonged and potentially dangerous (eg haemophilia). They can act in a variety of ways. Several are VASOCONSTRICTOR drugs that work directly by constricting small blood vessels so reducing bleeding (eg TERLIPRESSIN and VASOPRESSIN). Others cause inhibition of proteolytic enzymes that normally dissolve blood clots (eg APROTININ). Others again work by an uncertain mechanism to reduce the fragility of the wall of capillary blood vessels (eg ETAMSYLATE, OXERUTINS). Where excessive bleeding is due to a chronic deficiencies of necessary blood factors, the situation may be corrected by injecting vitamin K (MENADIOL SODIUM PHOSPHATE) or some of the blood factors themselves (factors VII, VIII, IX) and protein C concentrate.

Halciderm Topical

(Squibb; Bristol-Myers Squibb) is a proprietary, prescription-only preparation of the CORTICOSTEROID and ANTI-INFLAMMATORY halcinonide. It can be used to treat inflammatory skin disorders, such as eczema, and is available as a cream for topical application.

✚▲ Side-effects/warnings: See HALCINONIDE.

halcinonide

is a CORTICOSTEROID with ANTI-INFLAMMATORY

properties. It is used to treat severe inflammatory skin disorders, psoriasis and recalcitrant eczema, that are unresponsive to less potent corticosteroids. Administration is by topical application.

✚▲ Side-effects/warnings: See CORTICOSTEROID; though serious systemic effects are unlikely with topical application, but there may be local skin reactions.

✪ **Related entry: Halciderm Topical.**

Haldol

(Janssen-Cilag) is a proprietary, prescription-only preparation of the ANTIPSYCHOTIC haloperidol. It can be used to treat psychotic disorders, such as schizophrenia. It can also be used for the short-term treatment of severe anxiety and of some involuntary motor (movement) disturbances. Additionally, it can be used for intractable hiccups. It is available as a liquid, tablets and in a form for injection and depot deep intramuscular injection (as the decanoate).

✚▲ Side-effects/warnings: See HALOPERIDOL.

Half-Beta-Prograne

(Tillomed) is a proprietary, prescription-only preparation of the BETA-BLOCKER propranolol hydrochloride. It can be used as an ANTIHYPERTENSIVE for raised blood pressure, as an ANTI-ANGINA treatment to relieve symptoms and improve exercise tolerance and as an ANTI-ARRHYTHMIC to regularize heartbeat and to treat myocardial infarction. It can also be used as an ANTITHYROID drug for short-term treatment of thyrotoxicosis, as an ANTIMIGRAINE treatment to prevent attacks, as an ANXIOLYTIC, particularly for symptomatic relief of tremor and palpitations, and, with an ALPHA-ADRENOCEPTOR BLOCKER, in the acute treatment of phaeochromocytoma. It is available as modified-release capsules.

✚▲ Side-effects/warnings: See PROPRANOLOL HYDROCHLORIDE.

Half-Inderal LA

(AstraZeneca) is a proprietary, prescription-only preparation of the BETA-BLOCKER propranolol hydrochloride. It can be used as an ANTIHYPERTENSIVE for raised blood pressure, as an ANTI-ANGINA treatment to relieve symptoms and improve exercise tolerance and as an ANTI-ARRHYTHMIC to regularize heartbeat and to treat myocardial infarction. It can also be used as an ANTITHYROID drug for short-term treatment of thyrotoxicosis, as an ANTIMIGRAINE treatment to prevent attacks, as an ANXIOLYTIC, particularly for symptomatic relief of tremor and palpitations, and, with an ALPHA-ADRENOCEPTOR BLOCKER, in the acute treatment of phaeochromocytoma. It is available as modified-release capsules.

✚▲ Side-effects/warnings: See PROPRANOLOL HYDROCHLORIDE.

Half Securon SR

(Knoll) is a proprietary, prescription-only preparation of the CALCIUM-CHANNEL BLOCKER verapamil hydrochloride. It can be used as an ANTIHYPERTENSIVE and ANTI-ANGINA treatment in the prevention of attacks and after myocardial infarction. It is available as modified-release tablets.

✚▲ Side-effects/warnings: See VERAPAMIL HYDROCHLORIDE.

Half Sinemet CR

(DuPont; Bristol-Myers Squibb) is a proprietary, prescription-only compound preparation of carbidopa and levodopa (carbidopa/levodopa ratio of 25:100 mg), which is a combination called co-careldopa. It can be used to treat parkinsonism, but not the parkinsonian symptoms induced by drugs (see ANTIPARKINSONISM), and is available as modified-release tablets.

✚▲ Side-effects/warnings: See LEVODOPA.

halibut-liver oil

is an excellent source of retinol (vitamin A) and also contains VITAMIN D. A non-proprietary preparation is available in the form of capsules, but it should not be taken without initial medical diagnosis. Retinol deficiency is rare and if any treatment should be required it must be under medical supervision in order to avoid the potentially unpleasant side-effects of excess vitamin A in the body. Administration is oral.

✚▲ Side-effects/warnings: See RETINOL.

haloperidol

is a powerful ANTIPSYCHOTIC drug of the butyrophenone group. It is used to treat and tranquillize patients with psychotic disorders

H

(such as schizophrenia) and as an ANXIOLYTIC for other behavioural disturbance, especially for emergency control. It can also be used in the short-term treatment of severe anxiety. Quite separately from the previous uses, it can be administered to treat other conditions that may cause tremor, tics, involuntary movements or involuntary utterances (eg Gilles de la Tourette syndrome). It can also be used to treat intractable hiccup, and as an ANTINAUSEANT and ANTI-EMETIC to treat nausea and vomiting. Administration is either oral or by injection or depot deep intramuscular injection (in the form of the undecanoate salt).
✚▲ Side-effects/warnings: These depend on route of administration, and use. See CHLORPROMAZINE HYDROCHLORIDE; but with fewer sedative effects, fewer anticholinergic and hypotensive symptoms and photosensitivity and skin pigmentation are rare. However, extrapyramidal symptoms are more frequent and there may be weight loss.
✪ **Related entries: Dozic; Haldol; Serenace.**

halquinol
is a mild ANTIFUNGAL and ANTIBACTERIAL agent (actually a variable mix of two chemicals, one being *chloroxine*) which can be used in preparations primarily in the topical treatment of infections caused by (bacterial) seborrhoeic dermatitis and dandruff, and for (fungal) tinea species infection (eg athlete's foot). Administration is by topical application.
✚▲ Side-effects/warnings: It is considered safe used as directed, but sensitivity reactions have been reported.
✪ **Related entry: Valpeda Foot Cream.**

Halycitrol
(LAB) is a proprietary, non-prescription compound preparation of retinol (VITAMIN A) and VITAMIN D and can be used in vitamin deficiency. It is available in an oral emulsion.
✚▲ Side-effects/warnings: See RETINOL.

Harmogen
(Pharmacia) is a proprietary, prescription-only preparation of the OESTROGEN estropipate (piperazine estrone sulphate). It can be used in HRT and osteoporosis prophylaxis, and is available as tablets.
✚▲ Side-effects/warnings: See ESTROPIPATE.

HAV
see HEPATITIS A VACCINE.

Havrix Monodose
(SmithKline Beecham; GSK) is a proprietary, prescription-only VACCINE preparation of the hepatitis A vaccine. It can be used to protect people at risk from infection with hepatitis A, and is available in a form for injection.
✚▲ Side-effects/warnings: See HEPATITIS A VACCINE.

Hay-Crom Aqueous
(IVAX) is a proprietary, prescription-only preparation of the ANTI-ALLERGIC drug sodium cromoglicate. It can be used to treat allergic conjunctivitis, and is available as eye-drops.
✚▲ Side-effects/warnings: See SODIUM CROMOGLICATE.

Hay-Crom Hay Fever Eye Drops
(IVAX) is a proprietary, non-prescription preparation of the ANTI-ALLERGIC drug sodium cromoglicate. It can be used to treat allergic and vernal conjunctivitis, and is available as eye-drops.
✚▲ Side-effects/warnings: See SODIUM CROMOGLICATE.

Haymine
(Pharmax) is a proprietary, non-prescription compound preparation of the ANTIHISTAMINE chlorphenamine maleate (chlorpheniramine maleate) and the SYMPATHOMIMETIC ephedrine hydrochloride. It can be used as a NASAL DECONGESTANT for the symptomatic relief of the allergic symptoms of hay fever and allergic rhinitis, and is available as tablets. Not normally given to children, except on medical advice.
✚▲ Side-effects/warnings: See CHLORPHENAMINE MALEATE; EPHEDRINE HYDROCHLORIDE.

HBIG
see HEPATITIS B IMMUNOGLOBULIN (HBIG).

HB-Vax II
(Aventis Pasteur) is a proprietary, prescription-only VACCINE preparation of hepatitis B vaccine. It can be used to give protection from hepatitis B in people at risk, and is available in a form for injection.

✚▲ Side-effects/warnings: See HEPATITIS B VACCINE.

HBvaxPRO

(Aventis Pasteur) is a proprietary, prescription-only VACCINE preparation of hepatitis B vaccine. It can be used to protect people at risk from infection with hepatitis B, and is available in a form for injection.

✚▲ Side-effects/warnings: See HEPATITIS B VACCINE.

Hc45 Hydrocortisone Cream

(Crookes) is a proprietary, non-prescription cream preparation of the (ANTI-INFLAMMATORY) CORTICOSTEROID hydrocortisone. It can be used to treat allergic contact dermatitis, irritant contact dermatitis, allergic insect bite reactions, and mild to moderate eczema. It is not normally given to children under ten years, except on medical advice.

✚▲ Side-effects/warnings: See HYDROCORTISONE.

HCG

see CHORIONIC GONADOTROPHIN.

heart failure treatment

is used to rectify the functioning of a failing heart. It can involve the administration of a number of different drug types. Heart failure is a term used for the condition in which the amount of blood pumped by the heart is not sufficient to meet the oxygen and metabolic needs of the body either during work or at rest. The causes of heart failure include disease within the heart (mainly ischaemia – an inadequate supply of blood to the muscle that can also cause angina pain) or an excessive load imposed on the heart by arterial and other forms of hypertension. CARDIAC GLYCOSIDE drugs increase the force of contraction and have been widely used in heart failure treatment, though nowadays they are usually used in conjunction with other drugs. ANTIHYPERTENSIVE drugs are often used, and here drugs which cause blood vessels to dilate and therefore reduce the workload of the heart may be valuable (eg an ACE INHIBITOR such as CAPTOPRIL or ENALAPRIL MALEATE). Some of the DIURETIC drugs (eg CHLORTALIDONE, BUMETANIDE and FUROSEMIDE (frusemide)) have a vasodilating action; also because heart failure can lead to fluid retention (oedema; especially of the lungs, legs, ankles and feet), diuretics may be used in treating this. Alternatively, other VASODILATOR drugs can be used, such as the NITRATE drugs (eg GLYCERYL TRINITRATE, ISOSORBIDE DINITRATE, ISOSORBIDE MONONITRATE) or HYDRALAZINE HYDROCHLORIDE, to relax vascular smooth muscle, especially if there is ischaemic pain. Lastly, the CARDIAC STIMULANT class, such as the SYMPATHOMIMETIC drugs DOPEXAMINE HYDROCHLORIDE and DOBUTAMINE HYDROCHLORIDE, are usually reserved for emergencies.

Hedex Extra Tablets

(GSK Consumer Healthcare) is a proprietary, non-prescription compound analgesic preparation of the NON-NARCOTIC ANALGESIC and ANTIPYRETIC paracetamol and the STIMULANT caffeine. It can be used for the pain of headache (including migraine), neuralgia, period pain and to relieve cold symptoms. It is available as tablets and is not normally given to children, except on medical advice.

✚▲ Side-effects/warnings: See CAFFEINE; PARACETAMOL.

Hedex Ibuprofen Tablets

(GSK Consumer Healthcare) is a proprietary, non-prescription preparation of the NON-NARCOTIC ANALGESIC and ANTIPYRETIC ibuprofen. It can be used for the pain of headache (including migraine), tension headaches, backache, period pain and to relieve cold and flu symptoms. It is available as tablets, and is not given to children, except on medical advice.

✚▲ Side-effects/warnings: See IBUPROFEN.

Hedex Tablets

(GSK Consumer Healthcare) is a proprietary, non-prescription preparation of the NON-NARCOTIC ANALGESIC and ANTIPYRETIC paracetamol. It can be used for the pain of headache (including migraine and tension headaches), backache, period pain and to relieve cold and flu symptoms. It is available as tablets, and is not normally given to children under six years, except on medical advice.

✚▲ Side-effects/warnings: See PARACETAMOL.

HeliClear

(Wyeth) is a proprietary, prescription-only

compound preparation of the PROTON-PUMP INHIBITOR lansoprazole together with the ANTIBIOTIC drugs clarithromycin and amoxicillin (as trihydrate). It can be used as an ULCER-HEALING DRUG for the eradication of *Helicobacter pylori* in patients with duodenal ulcer. It is available in a triple pack containing appropriate capsules and tablets.

✚▲ Side-effects/warnings: See AMOXICILLIN; CLARITHROMYCIN; LANSOPRAZOLE.

HeliMet

(Wyeth) is a proprietary, prescription-only compound preparation of the PROTON-PUMP INHIBITOR lansoprazole (as ZOTON) together with the antibacterial agents clarithromycin (as KLARICID) and metronidazole. It can be used as an ULCER-HEALING DRUG for the eradication of *Helicobacter pylori* in patients with duodenal ulcer. It is available in a triple pack containing appropriate capsules and tablets.

✚▲ Side-effects/warnings: See CLARITHROMYCIN; LANSOPRAZOLE; METRONIDAZOLE.

Hemabate

(Pharmacia) is a proprietary, prescription-only preparation of the PROSTAGLANDIN analogue carboprost. It can be used to treat haemorrhage following childbirth, especially where other drugs have proved to be ineffective, and is available in a form for injection.

✚▲ Side-effects/warnings: See CARBOPROST.

Heminevrin

(AstraZeneca) is a proprietary, prescription-only preparation of clomethiazole (as base or edisylate). It can be used as a HYPNOTIC for treating severe insomnia (especially in the elderly), as an ANTICONVULSANT and ANTI-EPILEPTIC for treating status epilepticus, eclampsia, the symptoms caused by withdrawal from alcohol. It is available as capsules and a syrup.

✚▲ Side-effects/warnings: See CLOMETHIAZOLE.

heparin

is a natural ANTICOAGULANT in the body, which is produced by the liver, leukocytes (white blood cells) and found in some other sites including mast cells. It inhibits the action of the enzyme thrombin, which is needed for the final stages of blood coagulation. For therapeutic use, it is purified after extraction from bovine lungs and porcine intestinal mucosa. It is available in several forms, including low molecular-weight forms CERTOPARIN, DALTEPARIN SODIUM, ENOXAPARIN, REVIPARIN SODIUM and TINZAPARIN SODIUM. Also there are heparinoid forms (DANAPAROID SODIUM). Administration is generally by injection (eg during surgery) to prevent or treat thrombosis (eg deep vein thrombosis or pulmonary embolism) and similar conditions. It is also used, together with FIBRINOLYTIC (thrombolytic) drugs, in the management of myocardial infarction (heart attack). Its effect does not last long and treatment may have to be repeated frequently, or it can be given by constant intravenous infusion.

✚ Side-effects: Should haemorrhage occur, it may be difficult to stop the bleeding for a time – although, because heparin is so short-acting, merely discontinuing treatment is usually effective fairly quickly. There may be sensitivity reactions. Prolonged use may cause a loss of calcium from the bones and of hair from the head. There may be skin reactions.

▲ Warnings: It should not be administered to patients with haemophilia, thrombocytopenia, peptic ulcer, hypertension, severe kidney or liver disorders, or who have recently undergone major trauma or surgery, especially to the eye or nervous system. It should be administered with caution to those who are pregnant or who have kidney disorders.

✪ Related entries: Calciparine; Minihep; Monoparin; Monoparin Calcium; Multiparin.

heparinoids

are compounds chemically similar to the HEPARIN-type of ANTICOAGULANT. The version called DANAPAROID SODIUM is thought to have some advantages over heparin as an anticoagulant and is used to prevent deep vein thrombosis, particularly in orthopaedic surgery, and may be used in some patients who are hypersensitive to heparin. Other heparinoids are used topically to improve circulation in the skin in the treatment of conditions such as bruising, chilblains, thrombophlebitis, varicose veins and also haemorrhoids, though it is not entirely clear how they work. They are used by injection or topically.

✚▲ Side-effects/warnings: See HEPARIN for intravenous use; by topical application it is relatively free of side-effects.

✪ **Related entries: Anacal Rectal Ointment; Anacal Suppositories; danaparoid sodium; Hirudoid; Lasonil; Movelat Relief Cream; Movelat Relief Gel; Orgaran.**

hepatitis A vaccine

consists of a VACCINE, used for IMMUNIZATION, that is prepared from biosynthetic inactivated hepatitis A virus (HAV). It is an alternative to human NORMAL IMMUNOGLOBULIN for frequent travellers to moderate to high risk areas, and for high-risk laboratory staff including those who work with the virus. Administration is by intramuscular injection.

✚▲ Side-effects/warnings: See VACCINE.

✪ **Related entries: Avaxim; Epaxal; Havrix Monodose; Hepatyrix; Twinrix; ViATIM.**

Hepatitis B Immunoglobulin

(Public Health Laboratory Service; BPL; SNBTS) (Antihepatatis B Immunoglobulin) is a non-proprietary, prescription-only preparation of hepatitis B immunoglobulin, which is a SPECIFIC IMMUNOGLOBULIN used to give immediate immunity against infection by the hepatitis B virus. It is available in a form for intramuscular injection (or intravenously on a named-patient basis).

✚▲ Side-effects/warnings: See IMMUNIZATION.

hepatitis B immunoglobulin (HBIG)

is a SPECIFIC IMMUNOGLOBULIN that is used for IMMUNIZATION to give immediate *passive immunity* against infection by the hepatitis B virus. It is used specifically to immunize personnel in medical laboratories and hospitals who may be infected and to treat babies of mothers infected by the virus during pregnancy. Administration is by intramuscular injection. See HEPATITIS B VACCINE.

✚▲ Side-effects/warnings: See IMMUNIZATION.

✪ **Related entry: Hepatitis B Immunoglobulin.**

hepatitis B vaccine

consists of a VACCINE, used for IMMUNIZATION, that is prepared from biosynthetic inactivated (prepared by DNA technology from yeast cells) hepatitis B virus surface antigen (HBsAg). It is given to patients with a high risk of infection from the hepatitis B virus mostly through contact with a carrier (eg intravenous-injecting drug abusers, and healthcare workers who handle blood samples). Administration is by intramuscular injection.

✚▲ Side-effects/warnings: See VACCINE.

✪ **Related entries: Engerix B; HB-Vax II; HBvaxPRO; Twinrix.**

Hepatyrix

(SmithKline Beecham; GSK) is a proprietary, prescription-only VACCINE preparation of hepatitis A vaccine combined with typhoid vaccine. It can be used to for immunization against hepatitis A infection and typhoid fever in patients aged over 15 years. It is available in a form for injection.

✚▲ Side-effects/warnings: See HEPATITIS A VACCINE; TYPHOID VACCINE.

Herceptin

(Roche) is a recently introduced proprietary preparation of the ANTICANCER drug trastuzumab. It can be used in the treatment of a particular type of breast cancer, and is administered by intravenous infusion.

✚▲ Side-effects/warnings: See TRASTUZUMAB.

heroin

is the common term for the (OPIOID) NARCOTIC ANALGESIC drug DIAMORPHINE HYDROCHLORIDE.

Herpid

(Yamanouchi) is a proprietary, prescription-only preparation of the ANTIVIRAL idoxuridine (in dimethyl sulfoxide). It can be used to treat infections of the skin by herpes simplex or herpes zoster, and is available in a form for topical application with its own applicator.

✚▲ Side-effects/warnings: See IDOXURIDINE.

Hetrazan

(Lederle; Wyeth) is a proprietary preparation of the ANTHELMINTIC drug diethylcarbamazine, which is effective against microfilarial tropical diseases. Administration is oral.

✚▲ Side-effects/warnings: See DIETHYLCARBAMAZINE.

Hewletts Cream

(Kestrel) is a proprietary, non-prescription preparation of zinc oxide in hydrous wool fat, soft white paraffin and arachis oil with oleic acid. It can be used for minor abrasions and burns, and is available as a cream for topical application to the skin for nursing hygiene and chapped hands.

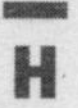

✚▲ Side-effects/warnings: See ARACHIS OIL; LIQUID PARAFFIN; WOOL FAT; ZINC OXIDE.

hexachlorophane

(hexachlorophene) is an ANTISEPTIC agent. It can be used on the skin for many purposes, including to prevent staphylococcal infections of the skin in newborn babies and to treat recurrent boils. Administration is topical. It is incorporated into various preparations used in operating theatres and surgeries.
✚ Side-effects: Rarely, there may be sensitivity reactions and increased sensitivity to light.
▲ Warnings: It should not be used on areas of raw or badly burned skin. It is not for use by pregnant women.
✪ **Related entry: Ster-Zac Powder.**

hexachlorophene

see HEXACHLOROPHANE.

Hexalen

(Ipsen) is a proprietary, prescription-only preparation of the ANTICANCER drug altretamine, used in the treatment of ovarian cancer. It is available as capsules.
✚▲ Side-effects/warnings: See ALTRETAMINE.

hexamine hippurate

see METHENAMINE HIPPURATE.

hexetidine

is an ANTISEPTIC mouthwash or gargle which is used for routine oral hygiene and to cleanse and freshen the mouth and for minor infections.
✚▲ Side-effects/warnings: Reasonably safe in normal topical use at recommended amounts.
✪ **Related entry: Oraldene.**

Hexopal

(Sanofi-Synthelabo) is a proprietary, non-prescription preparation of the VASODILATOR inositol nicotinate. It can be used to help improve blood circulation to the hands and feet when this is impaired, for instance, in peripheral vascular disease (Raynaud's phenomenon). It is available as tablets (a stronger one called *Tablets Forte*) and an oral suspension.
✚▲ Side-effects/warnings: See INOSITOL NICOTINATE.

hexylresorcinol

is an ANTISEPTIC used for routine oral hygiene and to cleanse and freshen the mouth.
✚▲ Side-effects/warnings: Reasonably safe in normal topical use at recommended concentrations.
✪ **Related entries: Beechams Throat-Plus Blackcurrant Lozenges;Beechams Throat-Plus Lemon Lozenges; Lemsip Sore Throat Anti-bacterial Citrus Fruits Lozenge; Lemsip Sore Throat Anti-bacterial Lozenge; Strepsils Extra; TCP Sore Throat Lozenges.**

Hib

is an abbreviation for HAEMOPHILUS INFLUENZAE TYPE B VACCINE.

Hiberix

(SmithKline Beecham; GSK) is a proprietary, prescription-only VACCINE preparation for *Haemophilus influenzae* type B infection, and is available in a form for injection.
✚▲ Side-effects/warnings: See HAEMOPHILUS INFLUENZAE TYPE B VACCINE;

Hibicet Hospital Concentrate

(SSL) is a proprietary, non-prescription compound preparation of the ANTISEPTIC chlorhexidine (as gluconate) and cetrimide. Can be used, after dilution, for cleaning, disinfecting and swabbing wounds, and is available as a solution.
✚▲ Side-effects/warnings: See CETRIMIDE; CHLORHEXIDINE.

Hibisol

(SSL) is a proprietary, non-prescription preparation of the ANTISEPTIC chlorhexidine (as gluconate). It can be used for disinfecting the skin and hands, and is available as a solution.
✚▲ Side-effects/warnings: See CHLORHEXIDINE.

Hibitane

(SSL) is the name of a range of proprietary, non-prescription ANTISEPTIC preparations that are based on solutions of chlorhexidine.
✚▲ Side-effects/warnings: See CHLORHEXIDINE.

HibTITER

(Wyeth; and from Health Authorities or Farillon, as part of immunization) is a proprietary, prescription-only VACCINE preparation which is used to provide protection against *Haemophilus influenzae* infection. It is available in a form for injection.

✚▲ Side-effects/warnings: See HAEMOPHILUS INFLUENZAE TYPE B VACCINE.

Hill's Balsam Chesty Cough Liquid for Children

(Boehringer Ingelheim) is a proprietary, non-prescription preparation of the EXPECTORANT agent ipecacuanha (with citric acid). It can be used to relieve chesty coughs and bronchial catarrh, and is available as a liquid.
✚▲ Side-effects/warnings: See IPECACUANHA.

Hill's Balsam Chesty Cough Pastilles

(Boehringer Ingelheim) is a proprietary, non-prescription preparation of the EXPECTORANT agent ipecacuanha with menthol, peppermint and benzoic tincture compound. It can be used to relieve chesty coughs, colds and catarrh, and is available as pastilles. It is not normally given to children, except on medical advice.
✚▲ Side-effects/warnings: See IPECACUANHA; MENTHOL.

Hill's Balsam Dry Cough Liquid

(Boehringer Ingelheim) is a proprietary, non-prescription preparation of the OPIOID and ANTITUSSIVE pholcodine. It can be used to relieve dry tickly and unproductive coughs, and is available as a liquid. It is not normally given to children, except on medical advice.
✚▲ Side-effects/warnings: See PHOLCODINE.

Hioxyl Cream

(Quinoderm) is a proprietary, non-prescription preparation of the ANTISEPTIC agent HYDROGEN PEROXIDE. It can be used to treat bedsores, leg ulcers and pressure sores, and is available as a cream for topical application.
✚▲ Side-effects/warnings: See HYDROGEN PEROXIDE.

Hiprex

(3M) is a proprietary, non-prescription preparation of the ANTIBACTERIAL methenamine hippurate. It can be used to treat or prevent infections of the urinary tract. It is available as tablets.
✚▲ Side-effects/warnings: See METHENAMINE HIPPURATE.

Hirudoid

(Sankyo Pharma) is a proprietary, non-prescription preparation of heparinoid. It can be used to improve circulation in conditions such as bruising, haematoma and superficial thrombophlebitis. It is available as a cream and a gel, and is not recommended for children under five years.
✚▲ Side-effects/warnings: See HEPARINOIDS.

Histalix Syrup

(Wallace) is a proprietary, non-prescription compound preparation of the ANTIHISTAMINE diphenhydramine hydrochloride, the EXPECTORANT ammonium chloride and menthol. It can be used to relieve troublesome cough where there is respiratory chest congestion. It is available as a syrup and is not normally given to children under one years, except on medical advice.
✚▲ Side-effects/warnings: See AMMONIUM CHLORIDE; DIPHENHYDRAMINE HYDROCHLORIDE; MENTHOL.

Histergan Cream

(Wallace) is a proprietary, non-prescription preparation of the ANTIHISTAMINE diphenhydramine hydrochloride. It can be used as a topical cream to relieve skin irritation associated with allergic rash and itching, minor skin afflictions and insect bites. It is not normally given to children under six years, except on medical advice.
✚▲ Side-effects/warnings: See DIPHENHYDRAMINE HYDROCHLORIDE.

Histergan Syrup

(Wallace) is a proprietary, non-prescription preparation of the ANTIHISTAMINE diphenhydramine hydrochloride. It can be used for the relief of allergic conditions such as allergic rashes and itching, hay fever and insect bites and stings. It is available as a syrup.
✚▲ Side-effects/warnings: See DIPHENHYDRAMINE HYDROCHLORIDE.

Hivid

(Roche) is a proprietary, prescription-only preparation of zalcitabine (DDC). It can be used as an ANTIVIRAL drug in the treatment of HIV infection, and is available as tablets.
✚▲ Side-effects/warnings: See ZALCITABINE.

HNIG

see NORMAL IMMUNOGLOBULIN.

H

homatropine hydrobromide
is an ANTICHOLINERGIC (ANTIMUSCARINIC) drug which can be used to dilate the pupil and paralyse the focusing of the eye for ophthalmic examination, and to treat anterior segment inflammation. Administration is by topical application.
+▲ Side-effects/warnings: See ATROPINE SULPHATE. When applied locally it has few side-effects, but it should not be used in patients with raised intraocular pressure (it may precipitate glaucoma).
✪ **Related entry: Minims Homatropine Hydrobromide.**

Honey and Lemon Meltus Expectorant
(SSL) is a proprietary, non-prescription preparation of the EXPECTORANT agent guaifenesin (guaiphenesin). It can be used for the symptomatic relief of chesty coughs and to soothe the throat. It is available as a syrup and is not normally given to children under two years, except on medical advice.
+▲ Side-effects/warnings: See GUAIFENESIN.

Honvan
(ASTA Medica) is a proprietary, prescription-only preparation of fosfestrol tetrasodium, which is converted in the body to DIETHYLSTILBESTROL (which has OESTROGEN activity as a sex hormone). It can be used in men as an ANTICANCER treatment for cancer of the prostate gland, and is available as tablets and in a form for injection.
+▲ Side-effects/warnings: See FOSFESTROL TETRASODIUM.

hormone
is the term used to describe a substance produced and secreted by a gland. In the case of endocrine hormones they are carried by the bloodstream to the organs on which they have their effect. Hormones can be divided into several families. The *adrenal hormones* are secreted by the adrenal glands (a small paired-gland just above the kidneys), of which there are two distinct types: adrenal cortical hormones and adrenal medullary hormones. The adrenocortical hormones come from the cortical (outer) region of the adrenal gland (eg CORTICOSTEROID hormones, which are steroids (see STEROID) with glucocorticoid or mineralocorticoid activity). The adrenomedullary hormones come from the medullary (inner) region of the adrenal gland (eg ADRENALINE and NORADRENALINE).

The THYROID HORMONES and the *parathyroid hormones* come from the thyroid and parathyroid glands at the base of the neck (eg CALCITONIN, parathormone, THYROXINE and TRIIODOTHYRONINE). The *glucose-regulatory hormones* are produced by the pancreas (eg GLUCAGON and INSULIN). The SEX HORMONES come mainly from the ovaries or the testes (eg the androgens (see ANDROGEN), such as TESTOSTERONE; the oestrogens (see OESTROGEN), such as ESTRADIOL and ESTRIOL; and the progestogens (see PROGESTOGEN), such as PROGESTERONE.

The *pituitary gland*, situated at the base of the skull, is an important producer of several vital hormones. There are two distinct classes of pituitary hormones: the posterior pituitary hormones OXYTOCIN and VASOPRESSIN (antidiuretic hormone; ADH); and the anterior pituitary hormones, which include CORTICOTROPHIN (adrenocorticotrophic hormone; ACTH), SOMATOTROPIN (growth hormone; GH); PROLACTIN and THYROTROPHIN (thyroid-stimulating hormone; TSH); or the GONADOTROPHIN hormones – FOLLICLE-STIMULATING HORMONE (FSH) and LUTEINISING HORMONE (LH)(also produced by the chorionic tissue of the placenta).

The release of anterior pituitary hormones is controlled, in turn, by factors that travel, in a specialized system of portal blood vessels, the short distance from the hypothalamus (an adjacent brain area). These *hypothalamic hormones* include corticotrophin-releasing hormone (CRH; or corticotrophin-releasing factor, CRF); GONADORELIN (gonadotrophin-releasing hormone, GnRH; or gonadotropin-releasing factor, GRF; LH-RH); growth hormone-releasing hormone (GHRH, or growth hormone-releasing factor, GRF); growth hormone release-inhibiting hormone (GHRIH; somatostatin, or growth hormone-release-inhibiting factor, GHRIF); and PROTIRELIN (thyrotrophin-releasing hormone; TRH). Many of these hormones can be administered therapeutically to people with a hormonal deficiency, sometimes in synthetic form. Synthetic HORMONE ANTAGONIST drugs have

H

been developed either to reduce the release of hormones (eg in cancers of endocrine glands) or, with sex hormones, to reduce normal release or the effects of normal levels of hormone, for example, where this inhibition benefits cancers of certain organs such as the prostate gland, the endometrium of the uterus or of the breast (eg TAMOXIFEN).

hormone antagonist

drugs prevent the action of hormones (see HORMONE). Some act directly at the hormone receptors (special recognition sites on cells) where they compete and prevent activation of these sites of the hormone (eg TAMOXIFEN at oestrogen receptors). Others which act indirectly are also sometimes called hormone antagonists, and work by interfering with the production, or the release, of the hormone (eg OCTREOTIDE inhibits the release of hormones from cancerous cells).

hormone replacement therapy

see HRT.

Hormonin

(Shire) is a proprietary, prescription-only compound preparation of the natural, OESTROGEN SEX HORMONES estradiol and estriol. It can be used in HRT and for osteoporosis prevention, and is available as tablets.

✚▲ Side-effects/warnings: See ESTRADIOL; ESTRIOL.

HRF

(Intrapharm) is a proprietary, prescription-only preparation of the HORMONE gonadorelin (gonadotrophin-releasing hormone, GnRH). It can be used as a diagnostic aid in assessing the functioning of the pituitary gland, and is available in a form for intravenous injection or infusion.

✚▲ Side-effects/warnings: See GONADORELIN.

HRT

(hormone replacement therapy) is a term commonly applied to drug treatment for women to supplement the diminished production of OESTROGEN, a major sex hormone (see SEX HORMONES), by the body during the menopause (whether natural or surgically induced). In a more general sense the term refers to the use of any synthetic or natural hormone to supplement a deficiency in the body (eg THYROID HORMONES, GROWTH HORMONE, ANTIDIURETIC HORMONE and INSULIN).

HRT in women is essentially *oestrogen replacement therapy*, and consists of the administration of small amounts of usually natural or sometimes synthetic oestrogens (eg CONJUGATED OESTROGENS, MESTRANOL, ESTRADIOL, ESTROPIPATE, DIETHYLSTILBESTROL), which are used to alleviate menopausal vasomotor symptoms (eg flushing), night sweats and vaginitis (thinning and drying of the vagina), palpitations, tingling, mood changes and other symptoms in women whose lives are inconvenienced by these conditions. Additionally, there is good evidence that HRT will reduce post-menopausal osteoporosis (brittle bones) and often is beneficial in reducing the risk of atherosclerosis, myocardial infarction and stroke; possibly also a delayed onset or reduced incidence of Alzheimer's disease. However, a number of risk factors need to be taken into account (particularly a possible increase in blood clotting) according to the individual's medical background (including previous drug treatments, familial and genetic traits, history of stroke or hypertension, smoking habits, exercise and body weight, likelihood of breast cancer), so expert counselling is necessary. In those at risk of osteoporosis, treatment may be advised to start prior to the menopause. In women who have had a hysterectomy, long-term treatment with oestrogen alone may be used, but otherwise a PROGESTOGEN (eg DYDROGESTERONE, LEVONORGESTREL, NORETHISTERONE, NORGESTREL) may also be prescribed (to reduce the risk of endometrial cystic hyperplasia and possible cancer of the uterus). Administration of HRT drugs, often cyclically, can be oral as tablets, by topical application (eg vaginal cream, skin gels or skin patches) or implants. Possible side-effects are given under OESTROGEN or PROGESTOGEN entries.

HT Defix

(SNBTS) is a proprietary, prescription-only (heat-treated) preparation of factor IX fraction, dried, which is prepared from human blood plasma. It can be used in treating patients with a deficiency in factor IX (haemophilia B), and is available in a form for intravenous infusion.

✚▲ Side-effects/warnings: See FACTOR IX FRACTION, DRIED.

HTIG

see TETANUS IMMUNOGLOBULIN.

Humalog

(Lilly) is a proprietary, prescription-only preparation of INSULIN LISPRO, which is a recombinant human insulin analogue. It is used to treat and maintain diabetic patients, and is available in vials for injection.
✚▲ Side-effects/warnings: See INSULIN.

Humalog Mix25

(Lilly) is a proprietary, prescription-only preparation of BIPHASIC INSULIN LISPRO which is a recombinant human insulin analogue (containing mixed insulin lispro and insulin lispro protamine) and is of intermediate-acting. It is used to treat and maintain diabetic patients, and is available in cartridges for injection.
✚▲ Side-effects/warnings: See INSULIN.

Humalog Mix50

(Lilly) is a proprietary, prescription-only preparation of recombinant human insulin analogue (insulin lispro with insulin lispro protamine). It is used to treat and maintain diabetic patients, and is available in prefilled disposable injection devices.
✚▲ Side-effects/warnings: See INSULIN.

human antihaemophilic fraction, dried

see FACTOR VIII FRACTION (DRIED).

Human Actrapid

(Novo Nordisk) is a proprietary, prescription-only preparation of synthesized neutral SOLUBLE INSULIN. It is used in DIABETIC TREATMENT to treat and maintain diabetic patients. It is available in vials for injection, in cartridges (*Penfil*) for use with *NovoPen* injectors and as prefilled disposable injectors (*Actrapid*). It has a short duration of action.
✚▲ Side-effects/warnings: See INSULIN.

human chorionic gonadotrophin

see CHORIONIC GONADOTROPHIN.

human growth hormone

see SOMATOTROPIN; SOMATROPIN.

Human Insulatard ge

(Novo Nordisk) is a proprietary, prescription-only preparation of human ISOPHANE INSULIN. It is used in DIABETIC TREATMENT to maintain diabetic patients, and is available in vials for injection and as cartridges (*Penfill*) for *Autopen*, *Inovo* or *Novopen* injection devices and as *Insulatard InnoLet* prefilled disposable injection devices. It has an intermediate duration of action.
✚▲ Side-effects/warnings: See INSULIN.

human menopausal gonadotrophins

is a HORMONE preparation, and is a collective name for combinations of the gonadotrophins (gonadotropins) FOLLICLE-STIMULATING HORMONE (FSH) and LUTEINISING HORMONE (LH) (one form of which is called MENOTROPHIN). In pregnancy these hormones are produced in large amounts by the chorionic tissue of the placenta (but are similar to those normally produced by the pituitary gland). The preparation is extracted from the urine of postmenopausal women and has various uses, including as an infertility treatment for women with proven hypopituitarism, or who do not respond to the drug CLOMIPHENE CITRATE (another drug commonly used to treat infertility) and in superovulation treatment in assisted conception (as with *in vitro* fertilization; IVF). Administration is by injection.
✚ Side-effects: Hyperstimulation of the ovaries, multiple pregnancy, local reactions at the injection site.
▲ Warnings: It should be given with caution to women with ovarian cysts, thyroid, adrenal or pituitary gland tumours or certain other disorders. A full assessment will be carried out.
✪ Related entries: Menogon; Menopur.

Human Mixtard 10

(Novo Nordisk) is a proprietary, prescription-only preparation of BIPHASIC ISOPHANE INSULIN (human) containing both ISOPHANE INSULIN and SOLUBLE INSULIN (in a proportion of 90% to 10% respectively). It is used to treat and maintain diabetic patients, has an intermediate duration of action, and is available in vials for injection.
✚▲ Side-effects/warnings: See INSULIN.

Human Mixtard 20

(Novo Nordisk) is a proprietary, prescription-only preparation of BIPHASIC ISOPHANE INSULIN (human) containing both ISOPHANE INSULIN and SOLUBLE INSULIN (in a proportion of 80% to 20% respectively). It is used to treat and maintain diabetic patients, has an intermediate duration of

action, and is available in vials for injection.
✚▲ Side-effects/warnings: See INSULIN.

Human Mixtard 30

(Novo Nordisk) is a proprietary, prescription-only preparation of BIPHASIC ISOPHANE INSULIN (human) containing both ISOPHANE INSULIN and SOLUBLE INSULIN (in a proportion of 70% to 30% respectively). It is used to treat and maintain diabetic patients, has an intermediate duration of action, and is available in a number of forms for injection, including prefilled injection devices (eg *Mixtard 30 InnoLet*, *Innovo* and *Novopen*) and *Penfill* cartridges (for *Autopen*).
✚▲ Side-effects/warnings: See INSULIN.

Human Mixtard 30 ge

(Novo Nordisk) is a proprietary, prescription-only preparation of BIPHASIC ISOPHANE INSULIN (human) containing both ISOPHANE INSULIN and SOLUBLE INSULIN (in a proportion of 70% to 30% respectively). It is used to treat and maintain diabetic patients, has an intermediate duration of action, and is available in vials for injection.
✚▲ Side-effects/warnings: See INSULIN.

Human Mixtard 40

(Novo Nordisk) is a proprietary, prescription-only preparation of BIPHASIC ISOPHANE INSULIN (human) containing both ISOPHANE INSULIN and SOLUBLE INSULIN (in a proportion of 60% to 40% respectively). It is used to treat and maintain diabetic patients, has an intermediate duration of action, and is available in vials for injection.
✚▲ Side-effects/warnings: See INSULIN.

Human Mixtard 50

(Novo Nordisk) is a proprietary, prescription-only preparation of BIPHASIC ISOPHANE INSULIN (human) containing both ISOPHANE INSULIN and SOLUBLE INSULIN (in a proportion of 50% to 50% respectively). It is used to treat and maintain diabetic patients, has an intermediate duration of action, and is available in vials for injection.
✚▲ Side-effects/warnings: See INSULIN.

Human Monotard

(Novo Nordisk) is a proprietary, prescription-only preparation of human INSULIN ZINC SUSPENSION. It is used in DIABETIC TREATMENT to treat and maintain diabetic patients, and is available in vials for injection and has a long duration of action.
✚▲ Side-effects/warnings: See INSULIN.

human normal immunoglobulin

see NORMAL IMMUNOGLOBULIN.

Human Ultratard

(Novo Nordisk) is a proprietary, prescription-only preparation of human INSULIN ZINC SUSPENSION (CRYSTALLINE). It is used in DIABETIC TREATMENT to treat and maintain diabetic patients, and is available in vials for injection and has a long duration of action.
✚▲ Side-effects/warnings: See INSULIN.

Human Velosulin

(Novo Nordisk) is a proprietary, prescription-only preparation of human SOLUBLE INSULIN. It is used in DIABETIC TREATMENT to treat and maintain diabetic patients, and is available in vials for injection and has a short duration of action.
✚▲ Side-effects/warnings: See INSULIN.

Humatrope

(Lilly) is a proprietary, prescription-only preparation of somatropin, which is the biosynthetic form of the pituitary HORMONE human growth hormone. Can be used to treat hormonal deficiency and associated symptoms (in particular, short stature). Available in a form for injection.
✚▲ Side-effects/warnings: See SOMATROPIN.

Humulin I

(Lilly) is a proprietary, prescription-only preparation of human ISOPHANE INSULIN. It is used in DIABETIC TREATMENT to maintain diabetic patients, and is available in vials for injection and as cartridges (*B-D Pen*) for *B-D Pen* injection devices. It has an intermediate duration of action.
✚▲ Side-effects/warnings: See INSULIN.

Humulin Lente

(Lilly) is a proprietary, prescription-only preparation of human INSULIN ZINC SUSPENSION. It is used in DIABETIC TREATMENT to treat and maintain diabetic patients, and is available in vials for injection. It has a long duration of action.
✚▲ Side-effects/warnings: See INSULIN.

Humulin M2

(Lilly) is a proprietary, prescription-only

preparation of BIPHASIC ISOPHANE INSULIN, human insulins. It is used in DIABETIC TREATMENT to treat and maintain diabetic patients and contains both ISOPHANE INSULIN and SOLUBLE INSULIN in a proportion of 80% to 20% respectively. It is available in vials for injection or as cartridges for the *B-D pen* or *Humapen* device and has an intermediate duration of action.
✚▲ Side-effects/warnings: See INSULIN.

Humulin M3
(Lilly) is a proprietary, prescription-only preparation of BIPHASIC ISOPHANE INSULIN, human insulins. It is used in DIABETIC TREATMENT to treat and maintain diabetic patients and contains both ISOPHANE INSULIN and SOLUBLE INSULIN in a proportion of 70% to 30% respectively. It is available in vials for injection or as cartridges for the *B-D pen* or *Humapen* device and has an intermediate duration of action.
✚▲ Side-effects/warnings: See INSULIN.

Humulin M5
(Lilly) is a proprietary, prescription-only preparation of BIPHASIC ISOPHANE INSULIN, mixed human insulins. It is used in DIABETIC TREATMENT to treat and maintain diabetic patients and contains both ISOPHANE INSULIN and SOLUBLE INSULIN in a proportion of 50% to 50% respectively. It is available in vials for injection or as cartridges for the *B-D pen* or *Humapen* device and has an intermediate duration of action.
✚▲ Side-effects/warnings: See INSULIN.

Humulin S
(Lilly) is a proprietary, prescription-only preparation of human synthesized neutral SOLUBLE INSULIN. It is used in DIABETIC TREATMENT to treat and maintain diabetic patients, and is available in vials for injection or as cartridges for the *B-D pen* or *Humapen* device. It has a short duration of action.
✚▲ Side-effects/warnings: See INSULIN.

Humulin Zn
(Lilly) is a proprietary, prescription-only preparation of human INSULIN ZINC SUSPENSION (CRYSTALLINE). It is used in DIABETIC TREATMENT to treat and maintain diabetic patients, and is available in vials for injection. It has a long duration of action.
✚▲ Side-effects/warnings: See INSULIN.

Hyalase
(CP) is a non-proprietary, prescription-only preparation of the enzyme (see ENZYMES) hyaluronidase. It can be used to increase the permeability of soft tissues to injected drugs, and is available in a form for injection.
✚▲ Side-effects/warnings: See HYALURONIDASE.

hyaluronidase
is an enzyme which can be used to increase the permeability of soft tissues to injected drugs, and to facilitate reabsorption of excess blood and fluids. Administration is by injection.
✚ Side-effects: Sometimes there are allergic sensitivity reactions.
▲ Warnings: It is used under hospital conditions, and a full assessment of patient suitability will be carried out.
✪ Related entries: Hyalase; Lasonil.

Hyate C
(Speywood) is a porcine, prescription-only preparation of factor VIII inhibitor bypassing fraction, and is used in patients with factor VIII inhibitors. It is available in a form for injection.
✚▲ Side-effects/warnings: See FACTOR VIII INHIBITOR BYPASSING FRACTION.

Hycamtin
(Merck) is proprietary, prescription-only preparation of the ANTICANCER drug topotecan (as hydrochloride) and can be used in the treatment of ovarian cancer. It is available in a form for intravenous infusion.
✚▲ Side-effects/warnings: See TOPOTECAN.

Hydergine
(Novartis) is a proprietary, prescription-only preparation of the mixture of drugs known as co-dergocrine mesilate, which has ALPHA-ADRENOCEPTOR BLOCKER properties, and is a VASODILATOR of blood vessels in the brain. Used primarily to assist in the management of elderly patients with mild to moderate dementia. Available as tablets.
✚▲ Side-effects/warnings: See CO-DERGOCRINE MESILATE.

hydralazine hydrochloride
is a VASODILATOR drug which is used to treat

acute and chronic cardiovascular disorders, such as in HEART FAILURE TREATMENT, in hypertensive crisis, and as an ANTIHYPERTENSIVE for long-term control of high blood pressure (where it is often administered with other drugs).
Administration is either oral or by intravenous injection or infusion.
✚ Side-effects: Effects on heart beat, hypotension, fluid retention, flushing, headache, dizziness, gastrointestinal upsets, lupus erythematosus with prolonged usage, blood disorders, and a number of others (eg on skin, nerves and muscle).
▲ Warnings: Special care is taken when used with certain other cardiovascular disorders, in pregnancy and when breast-feeding. It is not used for those with porphyria, some types of systemic lupus, and certain other cardiovascular disorders.
✪ Related entry: Apresoline.

hydrating agent 🅱

is the term used to describe any of a number of substances soothe and soften the skin. They are incorporated into ointments and skin creams that are used to treat conditions where the skin is dry or flaky (eg eczema). They are usually fats or oils, such as LANOLIN and LIQUID PARAFFIN and can be combined with other hydrating agents such as UREA. In conditions where there is a skin infection, hydrating agents can be combined with ANTIMICROBIAL or ANTIFUNGAL drugs, and ANTI-INFLAMMATORY and CORTICOSTEROID drugs can be added where there is inflammation.

Hydrea

(Squibb; Bristol-Myers Squibb) is a proprietary, prescription-only preparation of the ANTICANCER drug hydroxycarbamide (hydroxyurea). It can be used to treat leukaemia, and is available as capsules.
✚▲ Side-effects/warnings: See HYDROXYCARBAMIDE.

Hydrex

(Adams) is a proprietary, non-prescription preparation of the ANTISEPTIC chlorhexidine (as gluconate). It can be used to treat minor wounds and burns on the skin and hands, and is available as a solution and surgical rub.
✚▲ Side-effects/warnings: See CHLORHEXIDINE.

hydrochloric acid

is a strong acid that, within the body (as gastric acid), is part of the gastric juice secreted from special cells within the mucosal lining of the stomach. It provides the acid environment that is essential for the working of the enzyme pepsin, which begins the process of digestion that then continues within the small intestine. Over-production of acid (hyperacidity) can cause the symptoms of dyspepsia (indigestion) and this can be exacerbated by alcohol and NSAID drugs.
ANTACID drugs give symptomatic relief of acute dyspepsia and gastritis. But for chronic problems associated with peptic ulcers (gastric or duodenal ulcers) and oesophagitis ulcer-healing drugs are required (see ULCER-HEALING DRUG, H_2-ANTAGONIST and PROTON-PUMP INHIBITOR).
Under-production of acid (hypochlorhydria and achlorhydria) can also be a problem.

hydrochlorothiazide

is a DIURETIC of the THIAZIDE class. It can be used as an ANTIHYPERTENSIVE, either alone or in conjunction with other drugs, and in the treatment of oedema. Administration is oral.
✚▲ Side-effects/warnings: See BENDROFLUMETHIAZIDE.
✪ Related entries: Accuretic; Acezide; Amil-Co; Amilmaxco 5/50; Capozide; Capto-co; Carace Plus; co-amilozide 2.5/25; co-amilozide 5/50; CoAprovel; Co-Betaloc; Co-Betaloc SA; co-triamterzide 50/25; co-zidocapt; Cozaar-Comp; Dyazide; Innozide; Kalten; Moducren; Moduret 25; Moduretic; Monozide 10; Secadrex; Triam-Co; Zestoretic.

hydrocortisone

is a CORTICOSTEROID with ANTI-INFLAMMATORY properties, which can be administered therapeutically (sometimes in compound preparations with ANTIBACTERIAL, ANTIBIOTIC or ANTIFUNGAL drugs) to treat many kinds of inflammation, including rheumatic disease, to treat allergic conditions, shock, inflammatory bowel disease, haemorrhoids, eye and skin inflammation and hypersensitivity reactions, adrenocortical insufficiency. It can be administered in a number of forms: hydrocortisone, hydrocortisone acetate, hydrocortisone butyrate, hydrocortisone sodium phosphate or hydrocortisone sodium succinate; and by several different routes, including by topical application as a lotion, ointment, eye ointment, cream, lozenge, gel, suppositories,

H

spray, foam, ear-drops or scalp lotion, or as tablets or by injection.

✚▲ Side-effects/warnings: See CORTICOSTEROID. Side-effects depend on the route of administration, but serious systemic effects are unlikely with topical application, though there may be local reactions.

✪ **Related entries: Actinac; Alphaderm; Alphosyl HC; Anugesic-HC; Anusol-HC; Calmurid HC; Canesten Hydrocortisone; Canesten-HC; Colifoam; Corlan; Daktacort; Dermacort Cream; Dioderm; Econacort; Efcortelan; Efcortesol; Eurax-Hydrocortisone; Fucidin H; Gentisone HC; Gregoderm; Hc45 Hydrocortisone Cream; Hydrocortistab; Hydrocortone; Lanacort Ointment; Locoid; Locoid C; Mildison; Neo-Cortef; Nystaform-HC; Otosporin; Perinal; Proctosedyl; Quinocort; Solu-Cortef; Terra-Cortril; Terra-Cortril Nystatin; Timodine; Uniroid-HC; Vioform-Hydrocortisone; Xyloproct.**

hydrocortisone acetate

see HYDROCORTISONE.

hydrocortisone butyrate

see HYDROCORTISONE.

hydrocortisone sodium phosphate

see HYDROCORTISONE.

hydrocortisone sodium succinate

see HYDROCORTISONE.

Hydrocortistab

(Sovereign) is a proprietary, prescription-only preparation of the CORTICOSTEROID and ANTI-INFLAMMATORY hydrocortisone (as acetate). It can be used to treat local inflammation in joints and soft tissues, and is available in a form for injection.

✚▲ Side-effects/warnings: See HYDROCORTISONE.

Hydrocortone

(MSD) is a proprietary, prescription-only preparation of the CORTICOSTEROID and ANTI-INFLAMMATORY hydrocortisone. It can be used to make up hormonal deficiency and to treat inflammation, shock and certain allergic conditions. It is available as tablets.

✚▲ Side-effects/warnings: See HYDROCORTISONE.

hydroflumethiazide

is a DIURETIC of the THIAZIDE class. It can be used, usually in conjunction with other drugs in congestive HEART FAILURE TREATMENT. Administration is oral.

✚▲ Side-effects/warnings: See BENDROFLUMETHIAZIDE.

✪ **Related entries: Aldactide 25; Aldactide 50; co-flumactone 25/25; co-flumactone 50/50.**

hydrogen peroxide

is a general ANTISEPTIC which can be used for a wide range of purposes and is available in several forms: in solution and as a cream to cleanse and deodorize wounds and ulcers; as drops to clean ears; and as a mouthwash and gargle for oral hygiene.

✚▲ Side-effects/warnings: Reasonably safe in topical use at recommended concentrations. However, in strong solution it can badly damage tissues.

✪ **Related entries: Exterol Ear Drops; Hioxyl Cream; Otex Ear Drops.**

Hydromol Emollient

(Adams Healthcare) is a proprietary, non-prescription preparation of the EMOLLIENT liquid paraffin and isopropyl myristate. It is available as a bath additive for treating dry skin conditions such as senile pruritis and eczema.

✚▲ Side-effects/warnings: See LIQUID PARAFFIN.

hydromorphone hydrochloride

is a powerful (OPIOID) NARCOTIC ANALGESIC. It can be used in the treatment of severe pain, such as in cancer. Its use quickly tends to tolerance and then dependence (addiction). Administration is oral. All preparations are on the Controlled Drugs list.

✚▲ Side-effects/warnings: See OPIOID.

✪ **Related entry: Palladone.**

Hydrotalcite

(Peckforton) is a proprietary, non-prescription preparation of the ANTACID hydrotalcite. It can be used to relieve dyspepsia, and is available as an oral suspension. It is not normally given to children under six, except on medical advice.

✚▲ Side-effects/warnings: See HYDROTALCITE.

hydrotalcite

is an ANTACID that comprises a chemical mixture

H

of basic salts of aluminium and magnesium (actually it is aluminium magnesium carbonate hydroxide hydrate). It is incorporated into preparations to relieve hyperacidity and dyspepsia. It is taken orally.
✚▲ Side-effects/warnings: Treatment with carbonates as an antacid may cause belching (due to carbon dioxide). Aluminium-containing antacids are not used in people with hypophosphataemia (low blood phosphates); and are used with caution in those with porphyria. They may decrease the absorption of a number of other drugs, including ANTIBIOTIC (particularly TETRACYCLINES), ANTIFUNGAL and ACE INHIBITOR drugs. Since magnesium-containing antacids tend to be laxative whereas aluminium-containing antacids may be constipating, a mixture of the two is considered sometimes to be an advantage.
✪ Related entries: Actal Pastils; Altacite Plus; Hydrotalcite.

hydroxocobalamin

is the form of vitamin B_{12} that is now used therapeutically, having replaced CYANOCOBALAMIN in the treatment of megaloblastic anaemia (including pernicious anaemia), being retained longer in the body so reducing the frequency of administration. Supplements of hydroxocobalamin are administered only by injection, because vitamin B_{12} deficiency is usually caused by malabsorption, which renders oral administration ineffective.
✚▲ Side-effects/warnings: There may be skin itching in overdose; also fever, chills, hot flushes, dizziness, allergic reactions.
✪ Related entries: Cobalin-H; Neo-Cytamen.

hydroxycarbamide

(hydroxyurea) is a CYTOTOXIC drug which is used as an ANTICANCER treatment for chronic myeloid leukaemia and sometimes for polycythaemia. Administration is oral.
✚▲ Side-effects/warnings: See CYTOTOXIC.
✪ Related entry: Hydrea.

hydroxychloroquine sulphate

is a drug that has ANTI-INFLAMMATORY and ANTIRHEUMATIC properties. It can be used primarily to treat rheumatoid arthritis (including juvenile arthritis), and also for systemic and discoid lupus erythematosus, and is usually used when other, more common treatments (eg with NSAIDs) are unsuccessful. Its effects may not be seen for four to six months. Administration is oral.
✚▲ Side-effects/warnings: See CHLOROQUINE. (Although it is not used for malaria, it is a similar chemical and has similar side-effects and warnings.)
✪ Related entry: Plaquenil.

hydroxyethylcellulose

is a constituent of a preparation that is used as artificial tears and which is given to patients with dry eyes (tear deficiency) due to disease (eg Sjörgren's syndrome). Administration is topical.
✚▲ Side-effects/warnings: It is regarded as safe in normal topical use.
✪ Related entry: Minims Artificial Tears.

hydroxyprogesterone caproate

(hydroxyprogesterone hexanoate) is a PROGESTOGEN which can be used to treat recurrent miscarriage. Administration is by long-lasting, intramuscular depot injection.
✚▲ Side-effects/warnings: See PROGESTOGEN. Also laboured breathing, coughing.
✪ Related entry: Proluton Depot.

hydroxyprogesterone hexanoate

see HYDROXYPROGESTERONE CAPROATE.

hydroxyurea

see HYDROXYCARBAMIDE.

hydroxyzine hydrochloride

is an ANTIHISTAMINE with some additional ANXIOLYTIC properties. It can be used to relieve allergic symptoms, such as pruritus (itching and rash) and for short-term treatment of anxiety. Administration is oral.
✚▲ Side-effects/warnings: See ANTIHISTAMINE. Because of its sedative side-effects, the performance of skilled tasks, such as driving, may be impaired. It is not used in pregnancy or breast-feeding, and is used with caution in kidney impairment.
✪ Related entries: Atarax; Ucerax.

Hygroton

(Alliance) is a proprietary, prescription-only preparation of the (THIAZIDE-like) DIURETIC chlortalidone. It can be used, either alone or in

conjunction with other drugs, in the treatment of oedema, HEART FAILURE and as an ANTIHYPERTENSIVE. It is available as tablets.
✚▲ Side-effects/warnings: See CHLORTALIDONE.

hyoscine butylbromide

is an ANTICHOLINERGIC (ANTIMUSCARINIC) drug which can be used as an ANTISPASMODIC for the symptomatic relief of smooth muscle spasm in the gastrointestinal tract and genitourinary tract. Administration is either oral or by injection.
✚▲ Side-effects/warnings: See ATROPINE SULPHATE; but with fewer actions on the central nervous system. Avoid in porphyria.
✪ **Related entry: Buscopan; Buscopan Tablets**

hyoscine hydrobromide

(known as scopolamine hydrobromide in the USA) is a BELLADONNA ALKALOID derived from plants of the belladonna family and is a powerful ANTICHOLINERGIC (ANTIMUSCARINIC) drug. It is an effective SEDATIVE. It also has ANTINAUSEANT properties and can be used to prevent motion sickness, and to prevent and treat vertigo and nausea associated with Ménière's disease and middle-ear surgery. In a solution, it can be used in ophthalmic treatments to paralyse the muscles of the pupil either for surgery or to rest the eye following surgery. It is used as premedication prior to surgery because of its anti-emetic, sedative, secretion-drying and amnesia properties. Administration is either topical or by injection. See HYOSCINE BUTYLBROMIDE for use of hyoscine as an ANTISPASMODIC. It is also present in some compound preparations on sale to the public to relieve period pain.
✚ Side-effects: Depending on the type of administration and use, there may be drowsiness, dry mouth, dizziness, blurred vision and difficulty in urination; in doses for premedication and obstetrics it may cause confusion, hallucinations, behavioural disturbances, amnesia, ataxia, occasionally excitement and slowing of the heartbeat (especially in the elderly).
▲ Warnings: It is not to be given to patients with porphyria or closed-angle glaucoma. It should be administered with caution to those who are pregnant or breast-feeding, elderly or have urinary retention, cardiovascular disease, or liver or kidney impairment. Because it has sedative properties, the performance of skilled tasks, such as driving, may be impaired.
✪ **Related entries: Feminax; Joy-Rides; Junior Kwells; Kwells Tablets; Scopoderm TTS.**

hyoscyamine

see ATROPINE SULPHATE.

hypnotic 🅱

drugs induce sleep by an action on the brain. They are used mainly to treat insomnia and to sedate patients who are mentally ill, but can also be used for the short-term treatment of insomnia due to jet lag, shift work, emotional problems or serious illness. The best-known and most-used hypnotics are the BENZODIAZEPINE drugs (which can also be used as ANXIOLYTIC drugs) such as DIAZEPAM, NITRAZEPAM, FLUNITRAZEPAM and FLURAZEPAM, which have a relatively long duration of action and may cause drowsiness the next day. There are some benzodiazepines that have a comparatively short duration of action and cause less drowsiness, eg LOPRAZOLAM, LORMETAZEPAM and TEMAZEPAM. Other types of drug that are used as hypnotics include CHLORAL HYDRATE, TRICLOFOS SODIUM and CLOMETHIAZOLE (chlormethiazole); also ZOLPIDEM TARTRATE and ZOPICLONE, which are not chemically benzodiazepines, but work on the same RECEPTORS. Members of the BARBITURATE group (eg AMOBARBITAL) are now rarely used, because they can readily cause dependence and are extremely dangerous in overdose.
▲ Warnings: Some herbal remedies (eg St John's wort, valerian, kava kava) have the potential to interfere with the effects of hypnotic drugs, and can increase or decrease their efficacy or cause adverse reactions.

Hypnovel

(Roche) is a proprietary, prescription-only preparation of the BENZODIAZEPINE midazolam. It can be used as an ANXIOLYTIC and SEDATIVE, where its ability to cause amnesia is useful in preoperative medication, dental surgery and local anaesthesia, because the patient forgets the unpleasant procedure. It is available in a form for injection.
✚▲ Side-effects/warnings: See MIDAZOLAM.

hypoglycaemic 🅱

drugs reduce the levels of glucose (sugar) in the bloodstream. They are used mainly in the treatment of diabetes mellitus. The ORAL

HYPOGLYCAEMIC drugs are primarily used to treat Type II diabetes (non-insulin-dependent diabetes mellitus; NIDDM; maturity-onset diabetes), for example, the SULPHONYLUREA drugs (eg CHLORPROPAMIDE and GLIBENCLAMIDE), the BIGUANIDE drug METFORMIN HYDROCHLORIDE and ACARBOSE and GUAR GUM. Administration of INSULIN, which is mainly used in Type I diabetes (insulin-dependent diabetes mellitus; IDDM; juvenile-onset diabetes), is by injection.

Hypolar Retard 20

(Lagap) is a proprietary, prescription-only preparation of the CALCIUM-CHANNEL BLOCKER nifedipine. It can be used as an ANTI-ANGINA treatment in the prevention of attacks and as an ANTIHYPERTENSIVE. It is available as modified-release tablets.

✚▲ Side-effects/warnings: See NIFEDIPINE.

Hypotears

(Novartis Ophthalmics) is a proprietary, non-prescription preparation of polyvinyl alcohol. It can be used as artificial tears in conditions where there is dryness of the eye due to tear deficiency. It is available as eye-drops.

✚▲ Side-effects/warnings: See POLYVINYL ALCOHOL.

hypotensive

drugs lower blood pressure and there are many drugs that have such an action. Some drugs do so on acute (short-term) administration as a deliberate part of their medical use. For instance, NITRATE drugs, which are used to treat angina attacks, have an immediate and powerful VASODILATOR action which redistributes blood flow in the body and beneficially reduces the workload of the heart. In a hypertensive crisis the aim is an immediate fall in blood pressure and this can be achieved by the injection of vasodilators, such as SODIUM NITROPRUSSIDE, GLYCERYL TRINITRATE or LABETALOL HYDROCHLORIDE. However, other types of drug may cause an unwanted fall in blood pressure to below normal levels as one of their side-effects, which may limit their usefulness in susceptible patients. This undesirable side-effect usually occurs as postural hypotension (a fall in blood pressure on standing quickly, where the brain is starved of blood, causing the patient to feel dizzy or faint) and can be minimized, or avoided, by taking the drug in question on retiring to bed. Also, this side-effect often becomes less of a problem if the drug is taken as part of a chronic (long-term) treatment.

The term ANTIHYPERTENSIVE is, by convention, commonly used in medicine to describe drugs that are used to lower abnormally high blood pressure (hypertension) and which are usually administered on a long-term basis. Such drugs are not necessarily hypotensive in normal (normotensive) individuals.

Hypovase

(Invicta; Pfizer) is a proprietary, prescription-only preparation of the ALPHA-ADRENOCEPTOR BLOCKER prazosin hydrochloride. It can be used as an ANTIHYPERTENSIVE, in peripheral vascular disease; also to treat benign prostatic hyperplasia (BPH). It is available as tablets.

✚▲ Side-effects/warnings: See PRAZOSIN HYDROCHLORIDE.

hypromellose

is a constituent of artificial tears, which are used to treat extremely dry eyes due to certain disorders. It is available as eye-drops and often in combination with a variety of drugs.

✚▲ Side-effects/warnings: It is regarded as safe in normal topical use.

✪ Related entries: Artelac SDU; Ilube; Isopto Alkaline; Isopto Atropine; Isopto Carbachol; Isopto Frin; Isopto Plain; Maxidex; Maxitrol; Moisture-eyes; Tears Naturale.

Hypurin Bovine Isophane

(CP) is a proprietary, prescription-only preparation of highly purified bovine ISOPHANE INSULIN. It is used in DIABETIC TREATMENT to treat and maintain diabetic patients, and is available in vials for injection. It has an intermediate duration of action.

✚▲ Side-effects/warnings: See INSULIN.

Hypurin Bovine Lente

(CP) is a proprietary, prescription-only preparation of highly purified bovine INSULIN ZINC SUSPENSION. It is used in DIABETIC TREATMENT to treat and maintain diabetic patients, and is available in vials for injection. It has a relatively long duration of action.

✚▲ Side-effects/warnings: See INSULIN.

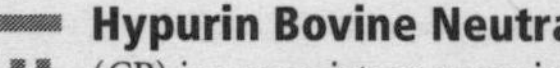

Hypurin Bovine Neutral

(CP) is a proprietary, prescription-only preparation of highly purified bovine SOLUBLE INSULIN. It is used in DIABETIC TREATMENT to treat and maintain diabetic patients, and is available in vials for injection. It has a relatively short duration of action.

✚▲ Side-effects/warnings: See INSULIN.

Hypurin Bovine Protamine Zinc

(CP) is a proprietary, prescription-only preparation of highly purified bovine PROTAMINE ZINC INSULIN. It is used in DIABETIC TREATMENT to treat and maintain diabetic patients, and is available in vials for injection. It has a long duration of action.

✚▲ Side-effects/warnings: See INSULIN.

Hypurin Porcine Biphasic Isophane 30/70 Mix

(CP) is a proprietary, prescription-only preparation of BIPHASIC ISOPHANE INSULIN (porcine) containing both ISOPHANE INSULIN and SOLUBLE INSULIN (in a proportion of 70% to 30% respectively). It is used to treat and maintain diabetic patients, has an intermediate duration of action, and is available in vials for injection.

✚▲ Side-effects/warnings: See INSULIN.

Hypurin Porcine Isophane

(CP) is a proprietary, prescription-only preparation of highly purified porcine ISOPHANE INSULIN It is used in DIABETIC TREATMENT to treat and maintain diabetic patients, and is available in vials for injection. It has an intermediate duration of action.

✚▲ Side-effects/warnings: See INSULIN.

Hypurin Porcine Neutral

(CP) is a proprietary, prescription-only preparation of highly purified porcine SOLUBLE INSULIN. It is used in DIABETIC TREATMENT to treat and maintain diabetic patients, and is available in vials for injection. It has a relatively short duration of action.

✚▲ Side-effects/warnings: See INSULIN.

Hytrin

(Abbott) is a proprietary, prescription-only preparation of the ALPHA-ADRENOCEPTOR BLOCKER terazosin (as terazosin hydrochloride). It can be used as an ANTIHYPERTENSIVE, and is available as tablets.

✚▲ Side-effects/warnings: See TERAZOSIN.

Hytrin BPH

(Abbott) is a proprietary, prescription-only preparation of the ALPHA-ADRENOCEPTOR BLOCKER terazosin (as terazosin hydrochloride). It can be used to treat urinary retention (eg in benign prostatic hyperplasia; BPH), and is available as tablets.

✚▲ Side-effects/warnings: See TERAZOSIN.

Ibugel

(Dermal) is a proprietary, non-prescription preparation of the (NSAID) NON-NARCOTIC ANALGESIC and ANTIRHEUMATIC ibuprofen, which has COUNTER-IRRITANT, or RUBEFACIENT, actions. It can be applied to the skin for symptomatic relief of underlying rheumatic and muscular pain and sprains. It is available as a gel for topical application to the skin and is not normally used for children, except on medical advice.

✚▲ Side-effects/warnings: See IBUPROFEN; but adverse effects on topical application are limited.

Ibuleve Gel

(DDD) is a proprietary, non-prescription preparation of the (NSAID) NON-NARCOTIC ANALGESIC and ANTIRHEUMATIC ibuprofen, which has COUNTER-IRRITANT, or RUBEFACIENT, actions. It can be used for the symptomatic relief of rheumatic and muscular pain, backache, arthritic pain, sprains, strains and to reduce swelling and inflammation. It is available as a gel for massage into the affected area. It is also available in a stronger form called *Ibuleve Maximum Strength Gel.* It is not normally given to children under 12 years, except on medical advice.

✚▲ Side-effects/warnings: See IBUPROFEN; but adverse effects on topical application are limited.

Ibuleve Mousse

(DDD) is a proprietary, non-prescription preparation of the (NSAID) NON-NARCOTIC ANALGESIC and ANTIRHEUMATIC ibuprofen, which has COUNTER-IRRITANT, or RUBEFACIENT, actions. It can be used for the symptomatic relief of muscular aches, arthritic pain, sprains and strains and to reduce swelling and inflammation. It is available as a mousse for massage into the affected area, and is not normally used for children under 12 years, except on medical advice.

✚▲ Side-effects/warnings: See IBUPROFEN but adverse effects on topical application are limited.

Ibuleve Spray

(DDD) is a proprietary, non-prescription preparation of the (NSAID) NON-NARCOTIC ANALGESIC and ANTIRHEUMATIC ibuprofen, which has COUNTER-IRRITANT, or RUBEFACIENT, actions. It can be used for the symptomatic relief of rheumatic and muscular pain, arthritic pain, backache, sprains and strains. It is available as a spray for the affected area and is not normally used for children under 12 years, except on medical advice.

✚▲ Side-effects/warnings: See IBUPROFEN but adverse effects on topical application are limited.

Ibumousse

(Dermal) is a proprietary, non-prescription preparation of the (NSAID) NON-NARCOTIC ANALGESIC and ANTIRHEUMATIC ibuprofen, which has COUNTER-IRRITANT, or RUBEFACIENT, actions. It can be applied to the skin for symptomatic relief of underlying rheumatic and muscular pain and sprains. It is available as a foam for topical application to the skin and is not normally used for children, except on medical advice.

✚▲ Side-effects/warnings: See IBUPROFEN; but adverse effects on topical application are limited.

ibuprofen

is a (NSAID) NON-NARCOTIC ANALGESIC and ANTIRHEUMATIC drug. It is used primarily to treat the pain of rheumatism and other musculoskeletal disorders, moderate pain of inflammatory origin and postoperative pain. Although its anti-inflammatory property is not as powerful as a number of other NSAIDs, it has fewer side-effects and so tends to be relatively well tolerated, so higher dosage may be used to compensate. Accordingly, it was the first and only modern NSAID for oral use licensed for non-prescription, over-the-counter sale in the UK. It has extensive use both in its own right and as the major active constituent in compound analgesic preparations for the treatment of minor to moderate pain, including headache, migraine, period pain, toothache and muscle ache. Its ANTIPYRETIC action helps symptomatic relief of the fever associated with colds and flu. It is also available for use in babies and children (including juvenile arthritis), and is usually considered safe to take also during breast-feeding. Administration can be oral or by topical application.

✚▲ Side-effects/warnings: See NSAID; but ibuprofen is better tolerated and causes fewer gastrointestinal disturbances than the majority of its class.

✪ **Related entries: Advil Tablets; Advil Tablets Extra Strength; Anadin Ibuprofen; Anadin Ultra; Arthrofen; Boots Ibuprofen Gel; Brufen; Brufen Retard; Care Extra Strength Ibuprofen Tablets 400mg; Care Extra Strength Long Lasting Pain Relief; Care Ibuprofen Gel; Care Ibuprofen Tablets 200mg; Codafen Continus; Cuprofen Ibuprofen Tablets; Cuprofen Tablets Maximum Strength; Deep Relief; Ebufac; Fenbid; Fenbid Forte Gel; Hedex Ibuprofen Tablets; Ibugel; Ibuleve Gel; Ibuleve Mousse; Ibuleve Spray; Ibumousse; Ibuspray; Ibutop Cuprofen Ibuprofen Gel; Ibutop Ralgex Ibuprofen Gel; Lemsip Pharmacy Powercaps; Lidifen; Mentholatum Ibuprofen Gel; Motrin; Nurofen; Nurofen Advance; Nurofen Caplets; Nurofen Cold & Flu; Nurofen for Children Sugar Free; Nurofen Long Lasting; Nurofen Liquid Capsules; Nurofen Meltlets; Nurofen Muscular Pain Relief Gel; Nurofen Plus; Pacifene; Pacifene Maximum Strength; Proflex Pain Relief; Proflex Sustained Relief Capsules; Radian B Ibuprofen Gel; Rimafen; Solpaflex Tablets.**

Ibuspray

(Dermal) is a proprietary, prescription-only preparation of the (NSAID) NON-NARCOTIC ANALGESIC and ANTIRHEUMATIC ibuprofen, which has COUNTER-IRRITANT, or RUBEFACIENT, actions. It can be used for the symptomatic relief of underlying rheumatic and muscular pain, sprains and neuralgia. It is available as a spray for topical application to the skin and is not normally used for children, except on medical advice.

✚▲ Side-effects/warnings: See IBUPROFEN; but adverse effects on topical application are limited.

Ibutop Cuprofen Ibuprofen Gel

(SSL) is a proprietary, non-prescription preparation of the (NSAID) NON-NARCOTIC ANALGESIC and ANTIRHEUMATIC ibuprofen. It can be used to treat all kinds of pain and inflammation, especially pain from arthritis and rheumatism, strains, sprains, sports injuries and other musculoskeletal disorders, and is available as a gel for topical application. It is not normally given to children, except on medical advice.

✚▲ Side-effects/warnings: See IBUPROFEN; but adverse effects on topical application are limited.

Ibutop Ralgex Ibuprofen Gel

(SSL) is a proprietary, non-prescription preparation of the (NSAID) NON-NARCOTIC ANALGESIC and ANTIRHEUMATIC ibuprofen. It can be used to treat all kinds of pain and inflammation, especially pain from arthritis and rheumatism, strains, sprains, sports injuries and other musculoskeletal disorders, and is available as a gel for topical application. It is not normally given to children, except on medical advice.

✚▲ Side-effects/warnings: See IBUPROFEN; but adverse effects on topical application are limited.

ichthammol

is a thick, dark brown liquid derived from bituminous oils. It is used in ointments or in glycerol solution for the topical treatment of ulcers and inflammation of the skin. It is milder than COAL TAR and is useful in treating the less-severe forms of eczema. A common mode of administration is as an impregnated bandage with ZINC PASTE.

✚▲ Side-effects/warnings: See COAL TAR. Some patients may experience skin irritation; the skin may become sensitized. It must not be placed in contact with broken skin surfaces.

idarubicin hydrochloride

is a CYTOTOXIC drug (of ANTIBIOTIC origin) with properties similar to doxorubicin hydrochloride, and which is used as an ANTICANCER drug, particularly for acute leukaemias and breast cancer. Administration can be oral or by injection.

✚▲ Side-effects/warnings: See CYTOTOXIC.

✪ **Related entry: Zavedos.**

idoxuridine

is an ANTIVIRAL drug which can be used in solution to treat infections caused by herpes viruses in and around the mouth or eye, on external genitalia and the skin. It has rather weak and variable results. It works by stopping the virus multiplying by interfering with DNA

synthesis. Administration is by topical application only.
✚ Side-effects: It may cause initial irritation and/or stinging on application; changes in taste; overuse may cause softening of the skin.
▲ Warnings: Avoid contact with the eyes and mucous membranes. It should not be used in pregnancy and caution when breast-feeding. It will damage fabrics. Do not use in the mouth.
✪ **Related entry: Herpid.**

ifosfamide

is an (*alkylating agent*) CYTOTOXIC drug which is used in ANTICANCER treatment. It works by interfering with cellular DNA and so inhibits cell replication. Administration is by intravenous injection, and often simultaneously with the synthetic drug MESNA which reduces the toxic side-effects.
✚▲ Side-effects/warnings: See CYTOTOXIC.
✪ **Related entry: Mitoxana.**

Ikorel

(Rhône-Poulenc Rorer; Aventis Pharma) is a proprietary, prescription-only preparation of the POTASSIUM-CHANNEL ACTIVATOR and VASODILATOR nicorandil. It can be used as an ANTI-ANGINA drug to prevent and treat angina pectoris, and is available as tablets.
✚▲ Side-effects/warnings: See NICORANDIL.

Ilube

(Alcon) is a proprietary, prescription-only preparation of the MUCOLYTIC acetylcysteine and a small proportion of the synthetic tear fluid hypromellose. It can be used to treat a deficiency of tears in the eyes, and is available as eye-drops.
✚▲ Side-effects/warnings: See ACETYLCYSTEINE; HYPROMELLOSE.

imatinib

is a recently introduced (protein-tyrosine kinase inhibitor) CYTOTOXIC drug, which is used as an ANTICANCER treatment for myeloid leukaemia. It works by interference with the action of an abnormal form of an enzyme (called tyrosine kinase) in the body that can cause this condition. Administration is oral.
✚ Side-effects: It may cause vomiting, nausea, diarrhoea, muscle pain, oedema and headache. It is a new drug and so all side-effects are not yet known.
▲ Warnings: Imatinib should not be used when breast-feeding, and used with caution during pregnancy.
✪ **Related entry: Glivec.**

Imazin XL

(Napp) is a proprietary, non-prescription compound preparation of the VASODILATOR drug isosorbide mononitrate and the ANTIPLATELET drug aspirin. It can be used as an ANTI-ANGINA drug for secondary prevention of myocardial infarction. It is available as tablets in two strengths (the stronger called *Forte Tablets*).
✚▲ Side-effects/warnings: See ASPIRIN; ISOSORBIDE MONONITRATE.

Imdur

(AstraZeneca) is a proprietary, non-prescription preparation of the VASODILATOR drug isosorbide mononitrate, which can be used as an ANTI-ANGINA drug. It is available as modified-release tablets (*Durules*).
✚▲ Side-effects/warnings: See ISOSORBIDE MONONITRATE.

imidapril hydrochloride

is an ACE INHIBITOR and acts as a VASODILATOR. It can be used as an ANTIHYPERTENSIVE and often in conjunction with other classes of drug, particularly (THIAZIDE) DIURETIC drugs. Administration is oral.
✚ Side-effects: See ACE INHIBITOR. Also dry mouth, tongue inflammation, abdominal pain, ileus; bronchitis, laboured breathing; sleep disturbances, confusion, depression, blurred vision, ringing in the ears, impotence.
▲ Warnings: See ACE INHIBITOR.
✪ **Related entry: Tanatril.**

imidazoles

see AZOLE.

imiglucerase

is an enzyme (see ENZYMES) made by recombinant DNA technology, which is used as a replacement in the specialist METABOLIC DISORDER TREATMENT of Gaucher's disease (a genetically determined enzyme deficiency disease affecting the spleen, liver, bone marrow and lymph nodes). Administration is by intravenous infusion.
✚ Side-effects: Itching, pain, swelling or abscess

at injection site; hypersensitivity reactions; also nausea and vomiting, diarrhoea and abdominal pain, fatigue, headache, dizziness, rash, fever.
▲ Warnings: It is a specialist drug, and assessment will be made of patient suitability. It is administered with care to patients who are pregnant or breast-feeding.
✪ **Related entry: Cerezyme.**

Imigran

(GlaxoWellcome; GSK) is a proprietary, prescription-only preparation of the ANTIMIGRAINE drug sumatriptan. It can be used to treat acute migraine attacks and cluster headaches, and is available as tablets, in a form for self-injection and as a nasal spray (it is absorbed into the circulation from the nasal mucosa).
✚▲ Side-effects/warnings: See SUMATRIPTAN.

imipenem with cilastatin

is an ANTIBACTERIAL and ANTIBIOTIC drug pair, with the two drugs always used together. Imipenem is a new sort of BETA-LACTAM with a broad-spectrum of activity against many Gram-positive and Gram-negative bacteria. However, it is partly degraded by an enzyme in the kidney and is therefore combined with CILASTATIN, which is an ENZYME INHIBITOR. It can be used to treat infections in the periphery, such as the urethra and cervix, and to prevent infection during surgery. Administration is by intravenous injection or infusion.
✚ Side-effects: Vomiting and nausea, diarrhoea and abdominal pain; altered taste and mouth ulcers; skin rashes; convulsions, blood disorders; pain at site of injection; brain and nerve disturbances. The urine may be coloured red.
▲ Warnings: Administer with caution to those who have impaired kidney function, who are pregnant or have brain disorders, such as epilepsy (it can cause seizures). It should not be used by breast-feeding women.
✪ **Related entry: Primaxin.**

imipramine hydrochloride

is an ANTIDEPRESSANT of the TRICYCLIC class, but which has fewer SEDATIVE properties than many other tricyclics. It is therefore more suited for the treatment of withdrawn and apathetic patients, rather than those who are agitated and restless. As is the case with other such drugs, it can also be used to treat bed-wetting at night by children. Administration is oral.
✚▲ Side-effects/warnings: See AMITRIPTYLINE HYDROCHLORIDE.
✪ **Related entry: Tofranil.**

imiquimod

is a KERATOLYTIC agent which can be used to treat and dissolve warts of the external genital and perianal areas. It is applied topically.
✚▲ Side-effects/warnings: Local reactions including pain, itching, reddening, erosion and removal of surface skin, oedema; rarely local ulceration and scabs.
▲ Warnings: Avoid normal skin, inflamed skin and open wounds; not suitable for treating internal genital warts. It is used carefully in uncircumcised men (as there is a risk of damaging the foreskin). The cream should be washed off before sexual contact. Care should be taken in pregnancy or breast-feeding.
✪ **Related entry: Aldara.**

ImmuCyst

(Cambridge) is a recently introduced proprietary, prescription-only preparation of BCG vaccine (Connaught strain), and is available in a form for bladder instillation for the treatment of primary or recurrent bladder carcinoma *in situ* and for the prevention of recurrence following surgery.
✚▲ Side-effects/warnings: See BCG VACCINE.

Immukin

(Boehringer Ingelheim) is a proprietary, prescription-only preparation of the IMMUNOMODULATOR interferon gamma (in the form of gamma-1b). It can be used in conjunction with ANTIMICROBIAL and ANTIBIOTIC drugs to reduce the frequency of serious infections in patients with chronic granulomatous disease. It is available in a form for injection.
✚▲ Side-effects/warnings: See INTERFERON.

immunization 🅔

agents are used in the immunization procedure, which can be used to prevent an individual from contracting specific infections, or help treat existing infection. This is achieved by using one of two methods, providing *active* or *passive* immunity.

Active immunity is conferred by vaccination (that is, administering a VACCINE), which involves the injection or administration of bacterial or viral agents that are live (but weakened, 'attenuated'), dead or *toxoids* (chemically-modified microbial toxins; also called *detoxified exotoxins*). These agents act as *antigens* to trigger the body's own defence mechanisms to manufacture antibodies. This method gives long-lasting, but not necessarily permanent, protection.

Passive immunity is conferred by the injection of a quantity of prepared blood serum already containing mixed antibodies (NORMAL IMMUNOGLOBULIN) or of selected antibodies (SPECIFIC IMMUNOGLOBULIN), and so helps to prevent the person contracting the infection or helps to treat an already existing infection. This method gives immediate protection but is short-lived (lasting several weeks). Injection of antitoxins (agents that neutralize the toxins that are produced by the disease-causing organism) is another way of imparting a form of passive immunity. See ANTISERUM; ANTITOXIN; IMMUNOGLOBULIN.

✚▲ Side-effects/warnings: These vary greatly depending on the particular vaccine or immunoglobulin and the individual. However, all involve administering foreign protein and so some sort of sensitivity reaction is usual. Commonly, there is malaise, fever and chills. There may be a reaction at the injection site. Expert advice is required.

immunoglobulin

is a term used to describe any of several classes of proteins of the immune system that naturally act as antibodies in the bloodstream. They are produced by B-lymphocytes in response to the presence of a specific *antigen* (any substance the body regards as foreign or dangerous) and circulate within the blood. Immunoglobulin deficiencies are often associated with increased risk of infection. They can be administered therapeutically, by injection or infusion, to confer immediate immunity, commonly known as *passive immunity*, against certain diseases. To minimize the risk of allergic reactions, the immunoglobulins that are used therapeutically are normally of human origin rather than from an animal (when they are usually referred to as *antiserum* or *antisera*). Two classes of human immunoglobulins are used to protect either patients suffering from infection or individuals exposed to infection: NORMAL IMMUNOGLOBULIN and SPECIFIC IMMUNOGLOBULIN. Normal immunoglobulin is prepared from the pooled serum of at least 1000 donors who have antibodies to viruses prevalent in a normal population (including for hepatitis A, measles and rubella). *Specific immunoglobulin* is prepared in a similar way, except that the pooled blood plasma used to obtain the immunoglobulins is from donors with high levels of the particular antibody that is required (eg for hepatitis B, rabies, tetanus or varicella-zoster). See ANTISERUM; IMMUNIZATION.

✪ Related entries: anti-D (Rh0) immunoglobulin; hepatitis B immunoglobulin (HBIG); Rabies Immunoglobulin; tetanus immunoglobulin; Varicella-Zoster Immunoglobulin.

immunomodulator

agents (biological response modifiers or immune response modifiers) are used to modify the activity of the body's immune system, usually with the intent of improving defence against infection (especially as ANTIVIRAL agents) and possibly in ANTICANCER therapy of malignant growths. These terms are not used in an exact sense, and some very different types of drug are commonly referred to as biological response modifiers. In practice, the meaning somewhat overlaps the terms IMMUNOSTIMULANT and IMMUNOSUPPRESSANT (eg CORTICOSTEROID drugs). The best-known immunomodulators are the INTERFERON and interleukin (eg ALDESLEUKIN) cytokines. Newly introduced agents working through modifying the immune response include GLATIRAMER ACETATE, which has immunosuppressant or immunomodulator action and is used in MS treatment, and a form of BCG VACCINE used by bladder instillation which acts as an immunostimulant or immunomodulator in the treatment of bladder carcinoma.

Immunoprin

(Ashbourne) is a proprietary, prescription-only preparation of the (*cytotoxic*) IMMUNOSUPPRESSANT azathioprine. It can be used to treat a variety of autoimmune and inflammatory diseases and also tissue rejection in transplant patients, and is available as tablets.

✚▲ Side-effects/warnings: See AZATHIOPRINE.

immunostimulant

agents are used to boost the efficiency of the

body's immune system, and thus improve defence against infections and possibly malignant growths. In the recent past, preparations of inactivated bacteria, *Corynebacterium parvum* (Coparvax), for example, were injected into the pleural cavity of the chest or the abdominal peritoneal cavity to treat the collection of fluids (effusion) there, with the intention of increasing the local activity of the natural immune system. This particular therapy did not prove to be very successful and has largely been discontinued, though a number of similar agents are currently being evaluated or are licensed in other countries (some for use against certain forms of cancer). VACCINE preparations are used for systemic long-term immunostimulation against specific bacterial or viral organisms, through administration of live but weakened (attenuated) organisms, dead but immunogenic organisms or live non-pathogenic organisms closely related to the invading microbe. Many vaccines are administered with *immunoadjuvant* drugs (eg aluminium phosphate) to enhance their immunostimulant actions. Interferons (see INTERFERON) and interleukins are discussed under IMMUNOMODULATOR.

immunosuppressant 🅱

drugs impair immune responses, that is, the body's resistance to the presence of infection, foreign bodies or what the body considers to be foreign bodies or chemicals. Because of this property, such drugs can be used to prevent tissue rejection following donor grafting or transplant surgery (although there is then the risk of unopposed infection). They are also commonly used to treat autoimmune diseases (when the immune system is triggered into acting against part of the body itself; that is, it incorrectly considers a part of itself to be 'foreign body'). Immunosuppressant drugs can also be used to treat chronic inflammatory diseases, such as rheumatoid arthritis, lupus erythematosus and collagen disorders (some of which may have an autoimmune component). The best-known and most-used immunosuppressants are the CORTICOSTEROID drugs (eg PREDNISOLONE), the non-steroid drugs AZATHIOPRINE, CHLORAMBUCIL, CYCLOPHOSPHAMIDE and CICLOSPORIN, and some specialist drugs: BASILIXIMAB, DACLIZUMAB, LEFLUMOMIDE, MYCOPHENOLATE MOFETIL and RITUXIMAB.

Imodium Capsules

(Johnson & Johnson • MSD) is a proprietary, non-prescription preparation of the (OPIOID) ANTIDIARRHOEAL loperamide hydrochloride. It can be used for the symptomatic relief of acute diarrhoea and its associated discomfort, and is available as capsules. It is not given to children, except on medical advice.

✚▲ Side-effects/warnings: See LOPERAMIDE HYDROCHLORIDE.

Imodium Liquid

(Janssen-Cilag) is a proprietary, non-prescription preparation of the (OPIOID) ANTIDIARRHOEAL loperamide hydrochloride. It can be used for the symptomatic relief of acute diarrhoea and its associated discomfort, and is available as a liquid. It is not given to children, except on medical advice.

✚▲ Side-effects/warnings: See LOPERAMIDE HYDROCHLORIDE.

Imodium Plus

(Johnson & Johnson • MSD) is a proprietary, non-prescription compound preparation of the (OPIOID) ANTIDIARRHOEAL loperamide hydrochloride and the ANTIFOAMING AGENT dimeticone (as simeticone or simethicone). It can be used for the symptomatic relief of acute diarrhoea, and is available as liquid. It is not given to children, except on medical advice.

✚▲ Side-effects/warnings: See DIMETICONE; LOPERAMIDE HYDROCHLORIDE.

Implanton

(Organon) is a proprietary, prescription-only preparation of the PROGESTOGEN etonogestrel, which is used as an ORAL CONTRACEPTIVE in the form of an implant (a single flexible rod into the arm, lasting up to three years).

✚▲ Side-effects/warnings: See ETONOGESTREL.

impotence treatment 🅱

drugs are given to men to treat erectile dysfunction. They are VASODILATOR drugs that act on intracavernosal vessels in the penis to cause engorgement with blood, and consequently erection. The agents used formerly were given by direct intracavernosal injection into the penis (eg ALPROSTADIL, PAPAVERINE, PHENTOLAMINE MESILATE, MOXISYLYTE). The drug SILDENAFIL (Viagra) is taken by mouth.

Imuderm

(Goldshield) is a proprietary, non-prescription compound preparation of light liquid paraffin and almond oil, which have EMOLLIENT properties. It can be used for dry skin conditions, including dermatitis, eczema, pruritus of the elderly and ichthyosis, and is available as a bath oil.

✚▲ Side-effects/warnings: See LIQUID PARAFFIN.

Imunovir

(Ardern) is a proprietary, prescription-only preparation of the ANTIVIRAL drug inosine pranobex. It can be used to treat herpes simplex infections and warts in mucous membranes and adjacent skin (eg genital warts). It is available as tablets.

✚▲ Side-effects/warnings: See INOSINE PRANOBEX.

Imuran

(GlaxoWellcome; GSK) is a proprietary, prescription-only preparation of the (*cytotoxic*) IMMUNOSUPPRESSANT azathioprine. It can be used to treat a variety of autoimmune and inflammatory diseases and tissue rejection in transplant patients. It is available as tablets and in a form for injection.

✚▲ Side-effects/warnings: See AZATHIOPRINE.

Inactivated Influenza Vaccine (Split Virion)

(Aventis Pasteur) is a proprietary, prescription-only preparation of influenza VACCINE (split virion vaccine; Flu/Vac/Split). It can be used as immunization for the prevention of influenza, and is available in a form for injection.

✚▲ Side-effects/warnings: See INFLUENZA VACCINE.

indapamide

is a DIURETIC of the THIAZIDE-like class which can be used as an ANTIHYPERTENSIVE, either alone or in conjunction with other drugs. Administration is oral.

✚ Side-effects: These may include headache, dizziness, fatigue; nausea and anorexia; muscle cramps; gastrointestinal upsets; skin rashes and other disorders; hypotension.

▲ Warnings: It is not to be used after recent stroke, or where there is severe liver impairment; care will be taken when administering to patients with certain kidney disorders, parathyroid disease (blood electrolytes must be measured), or who are pregnant or breast-feeding.

✪ **Related entries: Natrilix; Nindaxa 2.5.**

Inderal

(AstraZeneca) is a proprietary, prescription-only preparation of the BETA-BLOCKER propranolol hydrochloride. It can be used as an ANTIHYPERTENSIVE for raised blood pressure, as an ANTI-ANGINA treatment to relieve symptoms and improve exercise tolerance and as an ANTI-ARRHYTHMIC to regularize heartbeat and to treat myocardial infarction. It can also be used as an ANTITHYROID drug for short-term treatment of thyrotoxicosis, as an ANTIMIGRAINE treatment to prevent attacks, as an ANXIOLYTIC, particularly for symptomatic relief of tremor and palpitations, and, with an ALPHA-ADRENOCEPTOR BLOCKER, in the acute treatment of phaeochromocytoma. It is available as tablets and in a form for injection.

✚▲ Side-effects/warnings: See PROPRANOLOL HYDROCHLORIDE.

Inderal-LA

(AstraZeneca) is a proprietary, prescription-only preparation of the BETA-BLOCKER propranolol hydrochloride. It can be used as an ANTIHYPERTENSIVE for raised blood pressure, as an ANTI-ANGINA treatment to relieve symptoms and improve exercise tolerance and as an ANTI-ARRHYTHMIC to regularize heartbeat and to treat myocardial infarction. It can also be used as an ANTITHYROID drug for short-term treatment of thyrotoxicosis, as an ANTIMIGRAINE treatment to prevent attacks, as an ANXIOLYTIC, particularly for symptomatic relief of tremor and palpitations, and, with an ALPHA-ADRENOCEPTOR BLOCKER, in the acute treatment of phaeochromocytoma. It is available as modified-release capsules.

✚▲ Side-effects/warnings: See PROPRANOLOL HYDROCHLORIDE.

Inderetic

(AstraZeneca) is a proprietary, prescription-only compound preparation of the BETA-BLOCKER propranolol hydrochloride and the (THIAZIDE) DIURETIC bendroflumethiazide. It can be used as an ANTIHYPERTENSIVE for raised blood pressure, and is available as capsules.

✚▲ Side-effects/warnings: See BENDROFLUMETHIAZIDE; PROPRANOLOL HYDROCHLORIDE.

Inderex

(AstraZeneca) is a proprietary, prescription-only compound preparation of the BETA-BLOCKER propranolol hydrochloride and the (THIAZIDE) DIURETIC bendroflumethiazide. It can be used as an ANTIHYPERTENSIVE for raised blood pressure, and is available as capsules.
✚▲ Side-effects/warnings: See BENDROFLUMETHIAZIDE; PROPRANOLOL HYDROCHLORIDE.

indinavir

is a (*protease inhibitor*) ANTIVIRAL drug which is often used together with (*reverse transcriptase*) antivirals. It can be used in the treatment of HIV infection. Administration is oral.
✚ Side-effects: It is a specialist drug, and there will be full assessment of patient suitability, with an explanation of possible side-effects. There may be nausea, vomiting, diarrhoea, abdominal discomfort; taste disturbance and dry mouth; headache, insomnia, dizziness, muscle pain and loss of sensation in the extremities; dry skin, pruritus, rash; changes in kidney function, blood changes, blood in the urine, vision disturbances and other effects.
▲ Warnings: It should not be given to patients who are breast-feeding. Administer with caution where there is impaired liver function, certain kidney disturbances, haemophilia or pregnancy.
✪ **Related entry: Crixivan.**

Indivina

(Orion) is a proprietary, prescription-only compound preparation of the female SEX HORMONES estradiol (as valerate; an OESTROGEN) and medroxyprogesterone acetate (a PROGESTOGEN). It can be used to treat menopausal problems and osteoporosis in HRT, and is available as tablets in three forms.
✚▲ Side-effects/warnings: See ESTRADIOL; MEDROXYPROGESTERONE ACETATE.

Indocid

(MSD) is a proprietary, prescription-only preparation of the (NSAID) NON-NARCOTIC ANALGESIC and ANTIRHEUMATIC indometacin (indomethacin). It can be used to treat the pain such as that of rheumatic disease and other musculoskeletal disorders, period pain or acute gout. It is available as capsules, as suppositories and as a sugar-free suspension.
✚▲ Side-effects/warnings: See INDOMETACIN.

Indocid PDA

(MSD) is a proprietary, prescription-only preparation of the (NSAID) NON-NARCOTIC ANALGESIC and ANTIRHEUMATIC indometacin (indomethacin). It can be used (in this preparation only) for specialist, emergency, short-term treatment of premature infants with a heart defect (patent ductus arteriosus), while preparations are being made for surgery. It is available in a form for intravenous infusion.
✚▲ Side-effects/warnings: See INDOMETACIN.

Indocid-R

(MSD) is a proprietary, prescription-only preparation of the (NSAID) NON-NARCOTIC ANALGESIC and ANTIRHEUMATIC indometacin (indomethacin). It can be used to treat the pain of rheumatic disease and other musculoskeletal disorders, period pain or acute gout. It is available as modified-release capsules.
✚▲ Side-effects/warnings: See INDOMETACIN.

Indolar SR

(Lagap) is a proprietary, prescription-only preparation of the (NSAID) NON-NARCOTIC ANALGESIC and ANTIRHEUMATIC indometacin (indomethacin). It can be used to relieve the pain of rheumatic disease, gout and other inflammatory musculoskeletal disorders and period pain, and is available as modified-release capsules.
✚▲ Side-effects/warnings: See INDOMETACIN.

Indomax

(Ashbourne) is a proprietary, prescription-only preparation of the (NSAID) NON-NARCOTIC ANALGESIC and ANTIRHEUMATIC indometacin (indomethacin). It can be used to relieve the pain of rheumatic disease and other musculoskeletal disorders, period pain and acute gout, and is available as capsules.
✚▲ Side-effects/warnings: See INDOMETACIN.

Indomax 75 SR

(Ashbourne) is a proprietary, prescription-only preparation of the (NSAID) NON-NARCOTIC ANALGESIC and ANTIRHEUMATIC indometacin (indomethacin). It can be used to relieve the pain

of rheumatic disease and other musculoskeletal disorders, period pain and acute gout, and is available as modified-release capsules.
✚▲ Side-effects/warnings: See INDOMETACIN.

indometacin

(indomethacin) is a (NSAID) NON-NARCOTIC ANALGESIC and ANTIRHEUMATIC drug which can be used to treat rheumatic and muscular pain caused by inflammation. It can also be used to treat period pain and acute gout. Administration is mainly oral as tablets, capsules, modified-release capsules or a liquid; but its use in suppositories is especially effective for the relief of overnight pain and stiffness in the morning. Most of its proprietary preparations are not normally given to children, but one form is used (under specialist supervision with extensive monitoring) in premature babies who have patent ductus arteriosus (failure of this connecting vessel between the pulmonary artery and aorta to close after birth).
✚▲ Side-effects/warnings: See NSAID; there may also be pronounced intestinal disturbances; headaches, dizziness and, though rare, drowsiness, confusion, insomnia, depression, convulsions, blood disorders, blurred vision, blood pressure changes and other side-effects. It is not to be used in people who have blood coagulation defects, or kidney, epilepsy or certain other disorders. Dizziness may affect performance of skilled tasks such as driving.
✪ Related entries: Flexin Continus; Indocid; Indocid PDA; Indocid-R; Indolar SR; Indomax; Indomax 75 SR; Indomod; Pardelprin; Rheumacin LA; Rimacid.

indomethacin

see INDOMETACIN.

Indomod

(Pharmacia) is a proprietary, prescription-only preparation of the (NSAID) NON-NARCOTIC ANALGESIC and ANTIRHEUMATIC indometacin (indomethacin). It can be used to treat the pain of rheumatic disease and other musculoskeletal disorders, period pain and acute gout, and is available as modified-release capsules.
✚▲ Side-effects/warnings: See INDOMETACIN.

indoramin

is a selective ALPHA-ADRENOCEPTOR BLOCKER drug. It is used as an ANTIHYPERTENSIVE treatment, often in conjunction with other classes of drug (eg BETA-BLOCKER or DIURETIC drugs), and can be used to treat urinary retention in benign prostatic hyperplasia (BPH). Administration is oral.
✚▲ Side-effects/warnings: See ALPHA-ADRENOCEPTOR BLOCKER; also nasal congestion, weight gain, (extrapyramidal) movement problems, and failure to ejaculate. Also, avoid alcohol since it enhances its effect. It must be used carefully in patients with liver or kidney impairment; in elderly patients or those with Parkinson's disease, epilepsy or depression. Should not be used in patients receiving MAOIs or in those who have heart failure.
✪ Related entries: Baratol; Doralese.

Infacol

(Pharmax) is a proprietary, non-prescription preparation of the ANTIFOAMING AGENT dimeticone (as simeticone (simethicone)). It can be used to relieve infant colic and griping pain, and is available as an oral liquid.
✚▲ Side-effects/warnings: See DIMETICONE.

Infanrix

(SmithKline Beecham; GSK) is a proprietary, prescription-only preparation of the VACCINE, a *triple vaccine*, that contains diphtheria vaccine (see DIPHTHERIA VACCINE), TETANUS VACCINE and PERTUSSIS VACCINE used as a booster dose in children (up to six years of age) who have received a primary course. It is available in a form for injection.
✚▲ Side-effects/warnings: See DIPHTHERIA VACCINE; PERTUSSIS VACCINE; TETANUS VACCINE.

Infanrix-HIB

(SmithKline Beecham; GSK) is a proprietary, prescription-only preparation of the VACCINE, a *quadruple vaccine*, used to prevent *Haemophilus influenzae* infection that also contains diphtheria vaccine (see DIPHTHERIA VACCINE), TETANUS VACCINE and PERTUSSIS VACCINE and may be used as part of childhood immunization programme. It is available in a form for injection.
✚▲ Side-effects/warnings: see HAEMOPHILUS INFLUENZAE TYPE B VACCINE; DIPHTHERIA VACCINE; PERTUSSIS VACCINE; TETANUS VACCINE.

influenza vaccine
for IMMUNIZATION helps protect people from catching influenza. It is recommended only for persons at high risk of catching known strains of influenza; such as the elderly, asthmatics, diabetics, and those with chronic heart or kidney disease. This is because, unlike some viruses, the influenza viruses A and B are constantly changing in physical form and antibodies manufactured in the body to deal with one strain at one time will not necessarily be effective on the same strain at another time. Administration is by injection.
✚▲ Side-effects/warnings: See VACCINE. Because these vaccines are prepared from virus strains grown in chicken embryos, they are not used in individuals known to be sensitive to eggs.
✪ **Related entries: Agrippal; Begrivac; Fluarix; Fluvirin; Inactivated Influenza Vaccine (Split Virion); Influvac Sub-unit.**

Influvac Sub-unit
(Solvay) is a proprietary, prescription-only preparation of influenza (inactivated surface antigen; Flu/Vac/SA) VACCINE. It can be used as immunization for the prevention of influenza, and is available in a form for injection.
✚▲ Side-effects/warnings: See INFLUENZA VACCINE.

Innohep
(Leo) is a proprietary, prescription-only preparation of the ANTICOAGULANT tinzaparin sodium, which is a low molecular weight version of heparin. It can be used for long-duration prevention of venous thrombo-embolism, particularly in orthopaedic use, and is available in forms for injection.
✚▲ Side-effects/warnings: See TINZAPARIN SODIUM.

Innovace
(MSD) is a proprietary, prescription-only preparation of the ACE INHIBITOR enalapril maleate. It can be used as an ANTIHYPERTENSIVE and in congestive HEART FAILURE TREATMENT, and is available as tablets.
✚▲ Side-effects/warnings: See ENALAPRIL MALEATE.

Innozide
(MSD) is a proprietary, prescription-only compound preparation of the ACE INHIBITOR enalapril maleate and the (THIAZIDE) DIURETIC hydrochlorothiazide. It can be used as an ANTIHYPERTENSIVE, and is available as tablets.
✚▲ Side-effects/warnings: See ENALAPRIL MALEATE; HYDROCHLOROTHIAZIDE.

inosine pranobex
is an ANTIVIRAL drug which is used to treat herpes simplex infections in mucous membranes and adjacent skin (eg genital warts). Administration is oral.
✚ Side-effects: Increased uric acid levels in the blood and urine.
▲ Warnings: It should not be administered to patients with impaired kidney function or high blood levels of uric acid (for instance in gout).
✪ **Related entry: Imunovir.**

inositol nicotinate
is a VASODILATOR which can be used orally to help improve blood circulation to the hands and feet when this is impaired, for example, in peripheral vascular disease (Raynaud's phenomenon). Administration is oral.
✚▲ Side-effects/warnings: See NICOTINIC ACID.
✪ **Related entry: Hexopal.**

Instillagel
(CliniMed) is a proprietary, non-prescription compound preparation of the ANTISEPTIC chlorhexidine (as gluconate) and the LOCAL ANAESTHETIC lidocaine hydrochloride. It can be used to treat painful inflammation of the urethra, and is available as a gel in disposable syringes.
✚▲ Side-effects/warnings: See CHLORHEXIDINE; LIDOCAINE HYDROCHLORIDE.

insulin
is a protein HORMONE produced and secreted by the Islets of Langerhans within the pancreas. It has the effect of reducing the level of glucose (blood sugar) in the bloodstream and is part of a balancing mechanism with the opposing hormone GLUCAGON (which increases blood sugars). Its deficiency, or lack of effect (in the disorder called diabetes mellitus) results in high levels of blood sugar, which can rapidly lead to severe symptoms and potentially coma and death. Patients suffering from diabetes can be divided into two main groups, which largely determines the nature of their treatment. Those who have Type I diabetes (insulin-dependent

diabetes mellitus; IDDM; juvenile-onset diabetes) are generally maintained for life on one or other of the insulin preparations. Those who develop Type II diabetes (non-insulin-dependent diabetes mellitus; NIDDM; maturity-onset diabetes) can usually be managed by treatment with ORAL HYPOGLYCAEMIC drugs or by diet alone and less commonly require insulin injections. Most diabetics take some form of insulin on a regular (daily) basis, generally by subcutaneous injection. Modern genetic engineering has enabled the production of quantities of the human form of insulin, which is now replacing the former insulins extracted from cows (bovine insulin) or pigs (porcine insulin). There are marked differences in absorption time between the various human types – which dictates both the rate of onset (ie how fast it acts) and duration of action – between insulin preparations. This depends on their pH (acidity) and whether preparations are solutions, suspensions or complexes with other chemicals such as zinc or protamine. Consequently, forms are available that are short-acting (eg SOLUBLE INSULIN) or intermediate-acting (eg insulin zinc suspension (amorphous)), or long-acting (eg INSULIN ZINC SUSPENSION (CRYSTALLINE)). Many diabetic patients use more than one type of insulin in proportions appropriate to their own specific needs. Insulin is usually administered by patients themselves, by subcutaneous injection into the thigh, buttock, upper arm or abdomen. Insulin preparations cannot be given by the oral route because insulin is a protein and so is destroyed in the gastrointestinal tract.

✚ Side-effects: Hypoglycaemia in overdose. Local reactions at injection site.

▲ Warnings: Expert counselling, initial training and blood-glucose monitoring is required because patients must maintain a stable blood-glucose level over long periods. Choice of suitable preparations, or combination of preparations, for injection may take some time to establish. Patients should be warned of possible hazards in driving over long periods and should only drive if *hypoglycaemic aware*. It is used with care in patients who have kidney impairment. Patients should be careful when also taking a BETA-BLOCKER, since these can blunt hypoglycaemic awareness.

✪ **Related entries: Insulin preparations all fall into one or other of the following generic insulin groups (divided with regard both to chemical content and duration of action): biphasic insulin lispro; insulin aspart; insulin zinc suspension; insulin zinc suspension (crystalline); isophane insulin; protamine zinc insulin.**

insulin aspart

is a recombinant (biosynthetic) human insulin analogue, which is used in DIABETIC TREATMENT to maintain diabetic patients. It has a faster rate of onset and offset of action than soluble insulin. Administration is by injection.

✚▲ Side-effects/warnings: See INSULIN.

✪ **Related entry: NovoRapid.**

insulin injection

see SOLUBLE INSULIN.

insulin lispro

(recombinant human insulin analogue) is a recombinant (biosynthetic) human insulin analogue, which is used in DIABETIC TREATMENT to maintain diabetic patients. It is relatively short-acting. Administration is by injection.

✚▲ Side-effects/warnings: See INSULIN. There may be local allergic reactions.

✪ **Related entry: Humalog**

insulin zinc suspension

(Insulin Zinc Suspension (Mixed, I.Z.S.) is a form of highly purified bovine and/or porcine insulin or human insulin, prepared as a sterile neutral complex with zinc salts, which is used in DIABETIC TREATMENT to maintain diabetic patients. Administration is by injection and it has a long duration of action.

✚▲ Side-effects/warnings: See INSULIN.

✪ **Related entries: Human Monotard; Humulin Lente; Hypurin Bovine Lente.**

insulin zinc suspension (crystalline)

(Cryst.I.Z.S.) is a form of highly purified bovine or human insulin, prepared as a sterile complex with zinc salts, which is used in DIABETIC TREATMENT to maintain diabetic patients. It is available in vials for injection and has a long duration of action.

✚▲ Side-effects/warnings: See INSULIN.

✪ **Related entries: Human Ultratard; Humulin Zn.**

Intal

(Rhône-Poulenc Rorer; Aventis Pharma) is a

proprietary, prescription-only preparation of sodium cromoglicate (sodium cromoglycate). It can be used as a prophylactic (preventive) ANTI-ASTHMATIC treatment. It is available as a liquid in aerosol units (available with a spacer device, *Syncroner* and large volume inhaler, *Fisonair*), as a nebulizer solution or as a powder for inhalation in *Spincaps* (which can be used with the *Spinhaler Insufflator*).

✚▲ Side-effects/warnings: See SODIUM CROMOGLICATE.

Integrilin

(Schering-Plough) is a proprietary, prescription-only preparation of the ANTIPLATELET drug eptifibatide. It can be used, in conjunction with other drugs, to prevent thrombosis in myocardial infarction (under hospital specialist supervision). It is available in a form for intravenous injection or infusion.

✚▲ Side-effects/warnings: See EPTIFIBATIDE.

interferon

agents are inducible proteins synthesized by mammalian cells in tiny quantities, though they can now be produced artificially by recombinant technology (at great expense). There are three or more types; alpha- , beta- and gamma-interferons. They can modify the host response by inducing production of enzymes, for instance, that inhibit translocation of viral mRNA into viral protein, and thus have an ANTIVIRAL action through preventing virus reproduction. They are administered by injection in the treatment of HIV infection, for multiple sclerosis and in ANTICANCER treatment and for other chemotherapy. The interleukin mediators (eg ALDESLEUKIN) are similar (they all form part of the *cytokine* family of mediators) and can help in anticancer therapy. Interferons have complex effects on cells, cell function and immunity, and their toxicity (and cost) has limited their use. The main forms used in medical treatments are from four main groups, alpha-interferon, beta-interferon and interferon gamma-1b (immune interferon), and recombinant interleukin-2 (aldesleukin).

Interferon alpha (forms interferon alfa-2a and interferon alfa-2b) is used as an anticancer treatment for particular cancers, particularly lymphomas (eg AIDS-related Kaposi's sarcoma), certain cancers of the kidney, some solid tumours and other conditions, including chronic active hepatitis B and C.

A recently introduced derivative form called peginterferon alfa (peginterferon alpha-2b, rbe) can be used combined with RIBAVIRIN for chronic hepatitis C. Pegylation prolongs the persistence of the interferon in the blood.

Interferon beta (interferon beta-1a and interferon beta-1b) can be used to treat relapsing-remitting multiple sclerosis.

Interferon gamma is used in conjunction with ANTIMICROBIAL and ANTIBIOTIC drugs to reduce the frequency of serious infection in patients with chronic granulatomatous disease. Interferon gamma (interferon gamma-1b) is used together with ANTIBACTERIAL drugs to reduce frequency of serious infection in patients with chronic granulomatous disease.

Recombinant interleukin-2 (aldesleukin), is used as an anticancer drug, mainly for treating metastatic kidney cell carcinoma.

✚▲ Side-effects/warnings: Interferons are only used in specialist clinics after full evaluation. There are many conditions that preclude the use of interferons. Side-effects depend on the interferon used, however, there may be severe flu-like symptoms; chills, muscle pains, fever, headache, lethargy and depression, confusion, vomiting, rashes and injection-site reactions have been reported. The blood-producing capacity of the bone marrow may be reduced, there may be thyroid abnormalities, some people experience high or low blood pressure and heartbeat irregularities. Liver toxicity has been reported.

✪ **Related entries: Avonex; Betaferon; Immukin; Intron A; PegIntron; Proleukin; Rebif; Roferon-A; Viraferon; ViraferonPeg.**

interferon alpha

see INTERFERON.

interferon beta

see INTERFERON.

interferon gamma

see INTERFERON.

Intralgin

(3M) is a proprietary, non-prescription compound preparation of the LOCAL ANAESTHETIC benzocaine with SALICYLAMIDE, which has a COUNTER-IRRITANT, or RUBEFACIENT,

action. It can be applied to the skin for symptomatic relief of underlying muscle or joint pain, and is available as a gel, and is not normally given to children, except on medical advice.
+▲ Side-effects/warnings: See BENZOCAINE; SALICYLAMIDE; but adverse effects are minimal on topical application.

Intron A

(Schering-Plough) is a proprietary, prescription-only preparation of the IMMUNOMODULATOR interferon (in the form alpha-2b, rbe). It can be used as an ANTICANCER treatment mainly for hairy cell leukaemia, follicular lymphoma, chronic myelogenous leukaemia, lymph or liver metastases of carcinoid tumour, as an adjunct to surgery in malignant melanoma and maintenance of remission in multiple myeloma, and also as an ANTIVIRAL for chronic hepatitis B and C. It is available in forms for injection.
+▲ Side-effects/warnings: See INTERFERON.

Invirase

(Roche) is a proprietary, prescription-only preparation of the ANTIVIRAL saquinavir (as mesilate). It can be used in the treatment of HIV infection, and is available as capsules.
+▲ Side-effects/warnings: See SAQUINAVIR.

iodine

is a non-metallic element which is accumulated by the body in the thyroid gland (situated at the base of the neck) and is used by the cells of this gland to synthesize the thyroid hormones THYROXINE and TRIIODOTHYRONINE, which control a number of normal metabolic processes and growth. Nutritional sources of iodine include seafood, vegetables grown in soil containing iodine and iodinated table salt. A deficiency is one of the possible causes of goitre, where the thyroid gland becomes enlarged. Therapeutically, iodine (as Aqueous Iodine Oral Solution) can be used in thyrotoxicosis prior to surgery; also iodine is used in solution as an ANTISEPTIC. Some herbal remedies, such as kelp, should not be taken in excess as they contain high levels of iodine, in particular they can interfere with thyroid medications.
✪ Related entries: Aqueous Iodine Oral Solution; TCP Antiseptic Ointment.

Ionax Scrub

(Galderma) is a proprietary, non-prescription preparation of the ANTISEPTIC benzalkonium chloride with abrasive polyethylene granules within a foaming aqueous-alcohol base. It can be used in the treatment of acne.
+▲ Side-effects/warnings: See BENZALKONIUM CHLORIDE.

Ionil T

(Galderma) is a proprietary, non-prescription compound preparation of the ANTISEPTIC benzalkonium chloride, the KERATOLYTIC salicylic acid and coal tar. It can be used as a treatment for scalp psoriasis and seborrhoeic dermatitis with dandruff, and is available as a shampoo. It is not normally given to children, except on medical advice.
+▲ Side-effects/warnings: See BENZALKONIUM CHLORIDE; COAL TAR; SALICYLIC ACID.

Iopidine

(Alcon) is a proprietary, prescription-only preparation of the SYMPATHOMIMETIC apraclonidine. It can be used to control or prevent postoperative elevation of intraocular pressure (pressure of the eyeball) after laser surgery and to treat glaucoma, and is available as eye-drops.
+▲ Side-effects/warnings: See APRACLONIDINE.

ipecac

see IPECACUANHA.

ipecacuanha

is an extract from the ipecac plant. It contains two ALKALOID (emetine and cephaeline) that have an irritant action on the gastrointestinal tract and is therefore a powerful EMETIC. It can be used to clear the stomach in certain cases of non-corrosive poisoning when the patient is conscious (particularly in children). In smaller doses it can also be used as an EXPECTORANT in mixtures and tinctures and syrups. Emetine (and certain derivatives) has been used as an AMOEBICIDAL.
+ Side-effects: Depending on use, there may be excessive vomiting, effects on the heart (if absorbed), damage to epithelium (surface tissues) of the gastrointestinal tract. In high dosage it can cause severe gastric upset. It is considered safe when used as an expectorant.
✪ Related entries: Ammonia and Ipecacuanha Mixture, BP; Buttercup Infant Cough Syrup; Galloway's Cough Syrup; Fennings Little Healers;

Hill's Balsam Chesty Cough Liquid for Children; Hill's Balsam Chesty Cough Pastilles; Jackson's Troublesome Coughs; Lockets Medicated Linctus.

ipratropium bromide

is an ANTICHOLINERGIC (ANTIMUSCARINIC) drug with BRONCHODILATOR properties. It can be used to treat obstructive airways disease, where it is more often used for chronic bronchitis than as an ANTI-ASTHMATIC treatment. For this treatment it is administered by inhalation from an aerosol or a nebulizer. It is also used, in the form of a nasal spray, as a NASAL DECONGESTANT to treat watery rhinitis.

✚ Side-effects: There may be dryness of mouth; rarely, there is urinary retention and/or constipation.

▲ Warnings: It is administered with caution to patients with glaucoma (it can precipitate an attack) or enlargement of the prostate gland, or who are pregnant. Protect eyes when using the nebulizer. It is important not to exceed the prescribed dose.

✪ **Related entries: Atrovent; Combivent; Duovent; Respontin; Rinatec; Ipratropium Steri-Neb.**

Ipratropium Steri-Neb

(IVAX) is a proprietary, prescription-only preparation of the ANTICHOLINERGIC and BRONCHODILATOR ipratropium bromide. It can be used to treat the symptoms of chronic bronchitis, and is available as a nebulizer solution unit.

✚▲ Side-effects/warnings: See IPRATROPIUM BROMIDE.

irbesartan

is an ANGIOTENSIN-RECEPTOR BLOCKER, which is a class of drugs that work by blocking angiotensin receptors. Angiotensin II is a circulating HORMONE that is a powerful VASOCONSTRICTOR and so blocking its effects leads to a fall in blood pressure. Therefore irbesartan can be used as an ANTIHYPERTENSIVE. Administration is oral.

✚▲ Side-effects/warnings: See LOSARTAN POTASSIUM. Also, flushing and increase in certain blood enzymes reported. Should not be used in those who have certain heart valve disorders or who are breast-feeding.

✪ **Related entry: Aprovel; CoAprovel.**

irinotecan hydrochloride

is a CYTOTOXIC drug, one of a new group of drugs termed *topoisomerase I inhibitors*, and can be used as an ANTICANCER drug in the treatment of colorectal cancer. Administration is by intravenous infusion.

✚▲ Side-effects/warnings: See CYTOTOXIC.

✪ **Related entry: Campto**

iron

is a metallic element essential to the body in several ways, particularly its role as the red blood cell constituent haemoglobin, as the transporter of oxygen around the body and in a similar form in muscle to accept the oxygen, and for certain enzymes to function. Iron deficiency due to disease states that prevent its proper absorption, or because of its deficiency in the diet, lead to forms of anaemia (*iron-deficiency anaemia*). It is used therapeutically usually to treat anaemia caused by dietary deficiency and sometimes to prevent deficiency in susceptible people. Supplements can be administered orally (in the form of FERROUS FUMARATE, FERROUS GLUCONATE, FERROUS GLYCINE SULPHATE, FERROUS SULPHATE and other salts) or by injection or intravenous infusion (in the form of iron sucrose and other preparations). Ascorbic acid is sometimes added to aid absorption from the intestine. There are numerous iron-and-vitamin supplements available, which can be useful during pregnancy if required. Excellent food sources of iron include meat and liver. Iron is dangerously toxic even in small overdose. In the event of poisoning, an ANTIDOTE in the form of DESFERRIOXAMINE MESILATE can be used to treat an overload of iron in the tissues.

✚▲ Side-effects/warnings: See FERROUS SULPHATE. Severe toxic effects can occur if large amounts are ingested. Zinc, which is present in some mineral supplements, may reduce the absorption of iron.

iron sorbital

is a colloidal complex of iron, sorbitol and citric acid (with dextrin) that is rich in IRON and which is used in iron-deficiency ANAEMIA TREATMENT to restore iron to the body. Administration is by injection.

✚ Side-effects: Nausea and vomiting, diarrhoea, blood in the urine, taste disturbances, dizziness, flushing, muscle pains; hypersensitivity (allergic) reactions (including urticaria and effects on the cardiovascular system; rarely anaphylactoid

reactions; there may be reaction at the injection site).
▲ Warnings: Not used in patients with liver or kidney disease; in untreated urinary-tract infections; or in early pregnancy; and is best avoided in patients with heart problems. It is used with care in those with known allergic disorders (including asthma), in the elderly, debilitated or those who are underweight.
✪ Related entry: Jectofer.

iron sucrose
is a complex of ferric hydroxide with sucrose that is rich in IRON and which is used in iron-deficiency ANAEMIA TREATMENT to restore iron to the body. Administration is by injection or intravenous infusion.
✚ Side-effects: Nausea and vomiting, taste disturbances, headache, hypotension; less frequently, tingling in the extremities, abdominal disorders, muscle pain, fever, flushing, urticaria, peripheral oedema; rarely serious allergic reactions, There may be reactions at the injection site.
▲ Warnings: Not used in patients with liver disease; or who are pregnant, have a history of allergic disorders (including asthma, eczema and anaphylaxis); infection. This is a drug given when resuscitation facilities are available; oral iron therapy should not be taken until five days after the last injection.
✪ Related entry: Venofer.

Isib 60XL
(Ashbourne) is a proprietary, non-prescription preparation of the VASODILATOR drug isosorbide mononitrate, which can be used as an ANTI-ANGINA drug. It is available as modified-release tablets.
✚▲ Side-effects/warnings: See ISOSORBIDE MONONITRATE.

Ismelin
(Alliance) is a proprietary, prescription-only preparation of the ADRENERGIC-NEURONE BLOCKER guanethidine monosulphate. It can be used as an ANTIHYPERTENSIVE for moderate to severe high blood pressure, and is available in a form for injection.
✚▲ Side-effects/warnings: See GUANETHIDINE MONOSULPHATE.

Ismo
(Roche) is a proprietary, non-prescription preparation of the VASODILATOR drug isosorbide mononitrate, which can be used as an ANTI-ANGINA drug. It is available as tablets (in three strengths).
✚▲ Side-effects/warnings: See ISOSORBIDE MONONITRATE.

Ismo Retard
(Roche) is a proprietary, non-prescription preparation of the VASODILATOR drug isosorbide mononitrate, which can be used as an ANTI-ANGINA drug. It is available as modified-release tablets.
✚▲ Side-effects/warnings: See ISOSORBIDE MONONITRATE.

isocarboxazid
is an ANTIDEPRESSANT of the MONOAMINE-OXIDASE INHIBITOR (MAOI) class. It can be used to treat depressive illness. Administration is oral.
✚▲ Side-effects/warnings: See PHENELZINE; but it has a more stimulant action.

Isocard
(Eastern) is a proprietary, non-prescription preparation of the VASODILATOR drug isosorbide dinitrate, which can be used as an ANTI-ANGINA drug. It is available as transdermal spray for application to clean dry skin on the chest wall from where it is absorbed.
✚▲ Side-effects/warnings: See ISOSORBIDE DINITRATE.

Isogel
(Warner Lambert Consumer Healthcare; Pfizer) is a proprietary, non-prescription preparation of the (*bulking-agent*) LAXATIVE ispaghula husk. It can be used to treat a number of gastrointestinal disorders, including irritable bowel syndrome, and is available as granules.
✚▲ Side-effects/warnings: See ISPAGHULA HUSK.

Isoket
(Schwarz) is a proprietary, prescription-only preparation of the VASODILATOR drug isosorbide dinitrate, which can be used as an ANTI-ANGINA drug. It is available in a form for injection.
✚▲ Side-effects/warnings: See ISOSORBIDE DINITRATE.

Isoket Retard
(Schwarz) is a proprietary, non-prescription

preparation of the VASODILATOR drug isosorbide dinitrate, which can be used as an ANTI-ANGINA drug. It is available in a form for injection.
✚▲ Side-effects/warnings: See ISOSORBIDE DINITRATE.

isometheptene mucate

is a SYMPATHOMIMETIC drug which is used as an ANTIMIGRAINE treatment for acute attacks. Administration is oral.
✚ Side-effects: Dizziness, peripheral blood circulation and blood disturbances and rashes have been reported.
▲ Warnings: It should be administered with caution to patients with cardiovascular disease, diabetes or hyperthyroidism; do not administer to those with glaucoma, hypertension, severe heart, liver or kidney disorders, porphyria, or who are pregnant or breast-feeding.
✪ **Related entry: Midrid.**

Isomide CR

(Tillomed) is a proprietary, prescription-only preparation of the ANTI-ARRHYTHMIC disopyramide (as disopyramide phosphate), and is available as capsules.
✚▲ Side-effects/warnings: See DISOPYRAMIDE.

isoniazid

is an ANTIBACTERIAL drug which is used, in combination with other drugs, as an ANTITUBERCULAR treatment. It can also be administered to prevent the contraction of tuberculosis by close associates of an infected patient. Administration is either oral or by injection (alone or in combination with RIFAMPICIN).
✚ Side-effects: These include nausea and vomiting; sensitivity reactions, including rash and fever and peripheral neuritis (which may be prevented by taking vitamin B_6), convulsions and/or psychotic episodes, blood disorders and other complications.
▲ Warnings: It is not to be administered to patients with liver disease induced by drug treatment; administer with caution to patients with impaired kidney or liver function, epilepsy, alcoholism, who are pregnant or breast-feeding or who have porphyria. (Patients with abnormal metabolism (slow acetylators) are known to need the dose to be adjusted to avoid unacceptable side-effects.)
✪ **Related entries: Rifater; Rifinah; Rimactazid.**

isophane insulin

(isophane insulin injection; isophane protamine insulin injection, isophane insulin (NHP)) is a form of purified bovine, porcine or human insulin, prepared as a sterile complex with protamine, which is used in DIABETIC TREATMENT to maintain diabetic patients. It is available in vials for injection and has an intermediate duration of action.
✚▲ Side-effects/warnings: See INSULIN.
✪ **Related entries: Human Insulatard ge; Human Mixtard 10; Human Mixtard 20; Human Mixtard 30; Human Mixtard 30 ge; Human Mixtard 40; Human Mixtard 50; Humulin I; Humulin M2; Humulin M3; Humulin M5; Hypurin Bovine Isophane; Pork Insulatard; Hypurin Porcine Biphasic Isophane 30/70 Mix; Hypurin Porcine Isophane; Pork Insulatard; Pork Mixtard 30.**

isophane insulin injection

see ISOPHANE INSULIN.

isophane insulin (NHP)

see ISOPHANE INSULIN.

isophane protamine insulin injection

see ISOPHANE INSULIN.

isoprenaline

is a synthetic SYMPATHOMIMETIC substance similar to ADRENALINE which stimulates the heart, so it may be used as a CARDIAC STIMULANT to produce an increased rate and force of contraction (eg in heart block or severe bradycardia), when it is administered (as isoprenaline hydrochloride) by injection.
✚▲ Side-effects/warnings: There may be headache, tremor, sweating, increased heart rate and heartbeat irregularities and a decrease in blood pressure. It should be administered with caution to patients with certain heart diseases or excessive secretion of thyroid hormones (hyperthyroidism), or who are diabetic.
✪ **Related entries: Min-I-Jet Isoprenaline; Saventrine IV.**

Isopto Alkaline

(Alcon) is a proprietary, non-prescription preparation of HYPROMELLOSE. It can be used as

artificial tears to treat dryness of the eyes due to disease, and is available as eye-drops.
✚▲ Side-effects/warnings: HYPROMELLOSE.

Isopto Atropine

(Alcon) is a proprietary, prescription-only preparation of the ANTICHOLINERGIC drug atropine sulphate (with hypromellose). It can be used to dilate the pupil and to facilitate inspection of the eye and for refraction procedures in young children, and for the treatment of anterior uveitis. It is available as eye-drops.
✚▲ Side-effects/warnings: See ATROPINE SULPHATE; HYPROMELLOSE.

Isopto Carbachol

(Alcon) is a proprietary, prescription-only preparation of the PARASYMPATHOMIMETIC drug carbachol with hypromellose. It can be used in GLAUCOMA TREATMENT because it lowers intraocular pressure (pressure in the eyeball) and constricts the pupil. It is available as eye-drops.
✚▲ Side-effects/warnings: See CARBACHOL; HYPROMELLOSE.

Isopto Frin

(Alcon) is a proprietary, non-prescription preparation of the SYMPATHOMIMETIC phenylephrine hydrochloride and hypromellose. It can be used to give temporary relief of redness caused by minor irritations, and is available as eye-drops.
✚▲ Side-effects/warnings: See HYPROMELLOSE; PHENYLEPHRINE HYDROCHLORIDE.

Isopto Plain

(Alcon) is a proprietary, non-prescription preparation of HYPROMELLOSE. It can be used as artificial tears to treat dryness of the eyes due to disease, and is available as eye-drops.
✚▲ Side-effects/warnings: See HYPROMELLOSE.

Isordil

(Shire) is a proprietary, non-prescription preparation of the VASODILATOR drug isosorbide dinitrate, which can be used as an ANTI-ANGINA. It is available as short-acting oral and sublingual tablets.
✚▲ Side-effects/warnings: See ISOSORBIDE DINITRATE.

isosorbide dinitrate

is a short-acting VASODILATOR and ANTI-ANGINA drug. It is used to prevent attacks of angina pectoris (ischaemic heart pain), for instance when taken before exercise for symptomatic relief during an acute attack, and as an adjunct (to aid and assist) in left ventricular HEART FAILURE TREATMENT. It works by dilating the blood vessels returning blood to the heart and so reducing the heart's workload. It is short-acting, but its effect can be extended through the use of modified-release tablets kept under the tongue (sublingual tablets). Administration can be oral as tablets (for swallowing, chewing or holding under the tongue), as modified-release capsules, as a spray or aerosol (applied under the tongue) or in a form for intravenous injection or infusion.
✚▲ Side-effects/warnings: See GLYCERYL TRINITRATE.
✪ Related entries: Angitak; Cedocard-Retard; Isocard; Isoket; Isoket Retard; Isordil.

isosorbide mononitrate

is a short-acting VASODILATOR and ANTI-ANGINA drug. It is used to prevent attacks of angina pectoris (ischaemic heart pain) when taken before exercise, during an acute attack and as an adjunct (to aid and assist) in HEART FAILURE TREATMENT. It works by dilating the blood vessels returning blood to the heart and so reducing the heart's workload. It is short-acting, but its effect can be extended through the use of modified-release tablets. Administration is oral. Also available is a form combined with aspirin, for both angina treatment and prevention of myocardial infarction.
✚▲ Side-effects/warnings: See GLYCERYL TRINITRATE.
✪ Related entries: Angeze; Angeze SR; Chemydur 60XL; Dynamin; Elantan; Elantan LA; Imazin XL; Imdur; Isib 60XL; Ismo; Ismo Retard; Isotard; Isotrate; Modisal XL; Monit; Monit SR; Mono-Cedocard Retard-50; Monomax SR; Monosorb XL 60.

Isotard

(Galen) is a proprietary, non-prescription preparation of the VASODILATOR drug isosorbide mononitrate, which can be used as an ANTI-ANGINA drug. It is available as capsules and tablets with a range of strengths: *Isotard 25XL*, *Isotard 40XL*, *Isotard 50XL* and *Isotard 60XL*.
✚▲ Side-effects/warnings: See ISOSORBIDE MONONITRATE.

Isotonic Gentamicin Injection

(Baxter) is a proprietary, prescription-only preparation of the ANTIBACTERIAL and (AMINOGLYCOSIDE) ANTIBIOTIC gentamicin (as sulphate). It can be used to treat many forms of infection, particularly serious infections by Gram-negative bacteria, and is available in a form for intravenous infusion.
✚▲ Side-effects/warnings: See GENTAMICIN.

Isotrate

(Bioglan) is a proprietary, non-prescription preparation of the VASODILATOR drug isosorbide mononitrate, which can be used as an ANTI-ANGINA drug. It is available as tablets.
✚▲ Side-effects/warnings: See ISOSORBIDE MONONITRATE.

isotretinoin

is chemically a RETINOID (a derivative of RETINOL, or vitamin A) and has a marked effect on the cells that make up the skin epithelium (surface tissues). Actually, it is a chemical form of TRETINOIN (an isomer). It can be used for the long-term, systemic treatment of severe acne. Administration is either oral or by topical application.
✚▲ Side-effects/warnings: See TRETINOIN for the side-effects of topical application. There are many side-effects with oral administration, including effects on the skin, mucous membranes (eg nasal mucosa), visual disturbances and other effects on the eyes, hair thinning, headache, nausea, drowsiness, sweating, muscle and joint pain, effects on the liver and blood function.
▲ Warnings: See TRETINOIN for topical application. For oral administration, do not use when pregnant (or one month before or after treatment), when breast-feeding or in certain liver or kidney disorders.
✪ **Related entries: Isotrex; Isotrexin; Retinova; Roaccutane.**

Isotrex

(Stiefel) is a proprietary, prescription-only preparation of isotretinoin (a RETINOID). It can be used for the long-term treatment of severe acne, and is available as tablets and a gel.
✚▲ Side-effects/warnings: See ISOTRETINOIN.

Isotrexin

(Stiefel) is a proprietary, prescription-only compound preparation of the RETINOID isotretinoin together with the ANTIBACTERIAL and (MACROLIDE) ANTIBIOTIC drug erythromycin. It can be used to treat unresponsive acne. It is available as a gel for topical application.
✚▲ Side-effects/warnings: see ERYTHROMYCIN; ISOTRETINOIN.

Isovorin

(Wyeth) is a proprietary, prescription-only preparation of calcium levofolinate, which can be used to counteract the toxic effects of certain anticancer drugs, especially METHOTREXATE. It is available in a form for injection.
✚▲ Side-effects/warnings: See CALCIUM LEVOFOLINATE.

Ispagel

(Richmond) is a proprietary, non-prescription preparation of the (*bulking-agent*) LAXATIVE ispaghula husk. It can be used to treat a number of gastrointestinal disorders that require a high-fibre diet, including irritable bowel syndrome and diverticular disease. It is available as sachets of a powder for solution in water. It is not normally given to children under six years, except on medical advice.
✚▲ Side-effects/warnings: See ISPAGHULA HUSK.

ispaghula husk

is a *bulking-agent* LAXATIVE which works by increasing the overall mass of faeces (and retaining a lot of water) and so stimulating bowel movement (the full effect may not be achieved for days). It can be used for treating a range of bowel conditions, including diverticular disease and irritable bowel syndrome, and in patients who cannot tolerate bran. It also can be used as a LIPID-REGULATING DRUG to help reduce blood lipid levels in those people with moderate hypercholesterolaemia. Administration is oral as granules or a powder for dissolving in water.
✚ Side-effects: There may be flatulence, abdominal distension.
▲ Warnings: Preparations of ispaghula husk should not be administered to patients who have difficulty swallowing, with obstruction of the intestines, lack of tone in the colon or faecal impaction. Fluid intake during treatment should be higher than usual. Preparations containing ispaghula husk swell on contact with liquids and

should be carefully swallowed with water, and should not be taken last thing at night.
✪ **Related entries: Fybogel Orange; Fybogel Mebeverine; Fybozest Orange; Ispagel; Isogel; Konsyl; Manevac; Regulan Lemon & Lime.**

isradipine

is a CALCIUM-CHANNEL BLOCKER which is used as an ANTIHYPERTENSIVE. Administration is oral.
✚ Side-effects: These include flushing, headache; dizziness, increased heart rate and palpitations; rashes and itching; rarely, increased body weight, oedema, fatigue, abdominal discomfort.
▲ Warnings: Care is required in liver or kidney disorders, or in pregnancy. It is given with caution to patients with some types of heart problems. Grapefruit juice should be avoided since it affects metabolism of the drug.
✪ **Related entry: Prescal.**

Istin

(Pfizer) is a proprietary, prescription-only preparation of the CALCIUM-CHANNEL BLOCKER amlodipine besilate. It can be used as an ANTIHYPERTENSIVE and as an ANTI-ANGINA drug in the prevention of attacks. It is available as tablets.
✚▲ Side-effects/warnings: See AMLODIPINE BESILATE.

itraconazole

is a broad-spectrum (AZOLE) ANTIFUNGAL drug which can be used to treat resistant forms of candidiasis (thrush) of the vagina, vulva or oropharyngeal region, infections of the skin and mucous membranes and infections of the fingernails by tinea organisms, including ringworm and athlete's foot; also as prophylaxis in AIDS patients to prevent relapse into fungal infections. Administration is oral.
✚ Side-effects: Nausea and gastrointestinal disturbances, abdominal pains, dyspepsia, skin disorders, headaches and liver disorders.
▲ Warnings: It should not be administered to patients with certain liver or kidney disorders, or who are pregnant or breast-feeding. Because of rare reports of heart failure, authorities advise that doctors take special care when they prescribe this drug for people at risk of heart failure, especially to those who have pre-existing heart disease, older people, those treated at high doses or for long periods, and those being treated with other drugs such calcium-channel blockers that depress the strength of the heart beat.
✪ **Related entry: Sporanox.**

ivermectin

is an ANTHELMINTIC drug which is very effective in the treatment of the tropical disease onchocerciasis (infestation by the filarial worm-parasite *Onchocerca volvulus*); also for strongyloidiasis (nematode *Strongyloides* infection). Although it is not available in the UK, it is an important drug that may be met by the traveller. The destruction of the worms, however, may cause an allergic response. It is now the drug of choice because a single treatment produces a large reduction in the level of parasites, though more than one course of treatment with ivermectin may be necessary to eradicate the infestation. Administration is oral (on a named-patient basis).
✚▲ Side-effects/warnings: This is a specialist drug in the UK, requiring careful medical supervision during treatment.
✪ **Related entry: Mectizan.**

Jaaps Health Salts

(Roche Consumer Health) is a proprietary, non-prescription compound preparation of the ANTACID and (*osmotic*) LAXATIVE sodium bicarbonate with sodium potassium tartrate and tartaric acid. It can be used for the symptomatic relief of indigestion and heartburn, and as a mild laxative for the relief of constipation. It is available as an effervescent powder.
✚▲ Side-effects/warnings: See SODIUM BICARBONATE.

Jackson's All Fours

(Anglian Pharma) is a proprietary, non-prescription preparation of the EXPECTORANT agent guaifenesin (guaiphenesin). It can be used for the symptomatic relief of chesty coughs, and is available as a syrup. It is not normally given to children under 12 years, except on medical advice.
✚▲ Side-effects/warnings: See GUAIFENESIN.

Jackson's Bronchial Balsam

(Anglian Pharma) is a proprietary, non-prescription preparation of the EXPECTORANT guaifenesin which can be used for the symptomatic relief of bronchial catarrh and night-time ticklish coughs. It is available as a liquid and is not normally given to children, except on medical advice.
✚▲ Side-effects/warnings: See GUAIFENESIN.

Jackson's Febrifuge

(Anglian Pharma) is a proprietary, non-prescription preparation of the (NSAID) NON-NARCOTIC ANALGESIC and ANTIRHEUMATIC sodium salicylate. It can be used for the symptomatic relief of flu, sore throat, feverish colds and muscle pains. It is available as a liquid and is not normally given to children under 12 years, except on medical advice.
✚▲ Side-effects/warnings: See SODIUM SALICYLATE.

Jackson's Herbal Laxative

(Anglian Pharma) is a proprietary, non-prescription compound preparation of the (*stimulant*) LAXATIVE drugs senna, rhubarb and cascara. It can be used to relieve constipation. Available as an oral liquid, it is not normally given to children under seven years, except on medical advice.
✚▲ Side-effects/warnings: See RHUBARB; SENNA.

Jackson's Indian Brandee

(Anglian Pharma) is a proprietary, non-prescription preparation of capsicum tincture (with cardamum). It is a traditional herbal remedy and can be used to produce a feeling of warmth for the symptomatic relief of digestive discomfort and flatulence, and is available as an oral liquid. It is not normally given to children, except on medical advice.
✚▲ Side-effects/warnings: See CAPSICUM OLEORESIN.

Jackson's Troublesome Coughs

(Anglian Pharma) is a proprietary, non-prescription preparation of the EXPECTORANT ipecacuaha with glycerol and purified honey. It can be used for relief of troublesome coughs, and is available as a syrup.
✚▲ Side-effects/warnings: See IPECACUANHA.

J Collis Browne's Mixture

(SSL) is a proprietary, non-prescription preparation of the (OPIOID) ANTIDIARRHOEAL and ANTITUSSIVE drug morphine anhydrous and peppermint oil. It can be used for the symptomatic relief of occasional diarrhoea and its associated pain and discomfort, and coughs. It is available as a liquid. It is not normally given to children under six years, except on medical advice.
✚▲ Side-effects/warnings: See MORPHINE HYDROCHLORIDE; PEPPERMINT OIL.

J Collis Browne's Tablets

(SSL) is a proprietary, non-prescription preparation of the (OPIOID) ANTIDIARRHOEAL morphine (as hydrochloride), kaolin and calcium carbonate. It can be used for the symptomatic relief of occasional diarrhoea and its associated

pain and discomfort, and is available as tablets. It is not normally given to children under six years, except on medical advice.
✚▲ Side-effects/warnings: See CALCIUM CARBONATE; KAOLIN; MORPHINE SULPHATE.

Jectofer

(AstraZeneca) is a proprietary, non-prescription preparation of a complex of iron sorbitol that can be used as an IRON supplement in iron-deficiency ANAEMIA TREATMENT, and is available in a form for injection.
✚▲ Side-effects/warnings: See IRON SORBITAL.

Jomethid XL

(Alpharma) is a proprietary, prescription-only preparation of the (NSAID) NON-NARCOTIC ANALGESIC and ANTIRHEUMATIC ketoprofen. It can be used to relieve the pain of arthritis and rheumatism and other musculoskeletal disorders, and is available as modified-release capsules.
✚▲ Side-effects/warnings: See KETOPROFEN.

Joy-Rides

(Stafford-Miller; GSK) is a proprietary, non-prescription preparation of the ANTICHOLINERGIC drug hyoscine hydrobromide. It can be used as an ANTINAUSEANT to prevent motion sickness, and is available as chewable tablets. It is not normally given to children under three years, except on medical advice.
✚▲ Side-effects/warnings: See HYOSCINE HYDROBROMIDE.

Junior Kwells

(Roche Consumer Health) is a proprietary, non-prescription preparation of the ANTICHOLINERGIC hyoscine hydrobromide. It can be used as an ANTINAUSEANT to prevent motion sickness, and is available as melt-in-the-mouth tablets. It is not normally given to children under four years, except on medical advice.
✚▲ Side-effects/warnings: See HYOSCINE HYDROBROMIDE.

Junior Meltus Expectorant for Chesty Coughs and Catarrh

(SSL) is a proprietary, non-prescription preparation of the EXPECTORANT agent guaifenesin (guaiphenesin), the ANTISEPTIC agent CETYLPYRIDINIUM CHLORIDE, sucrose and honey. It can be used for the symptomatic relief of coughs and catarrh associated with flu, colds and mild throat infections. It is available as a liquid and is not normally given to children under one year, except on medical advice.
✚▲ Side-effects/warnings: See CETYLPYRIDINIUM CHLORIDE; GUAIFENESIN.

Junior Meltus for Dry Tickly Coughs and Catarrh

(SSL) is a proprietary, non-prescription compound preparation of the SYMPATHOMIMETIC and DECONGESTANT pseudoephedrine hydrochloride and the OPIOID and ANTITUSSIVE dextromethorphan hydrobromide. It can be used for the symptomatic relief of unproductive coughs and congestion of the upper airways. It is available as a liquid and is not normally given to children under two years, except on medical advice.
✚▲ Side-effects/warnings: See DEXTROMETHORPHAN HYDROBROMIDE; PSEUDOEPHEDRINE HYDROCHLORIDE.

Junior Meltus Night Time

(SSL) is a proprietary, non-prescription preparation of the ANTIHISTAMINE diphenhydramine hydrochloride with sodium citrate. It can be used for the relief of irritating coughs and to soothe a sore throat. It is available as a syrup and is not normally given to children under one year, except on medical advice.
✚▲ Side-effects/warnings: See DIPHENHYDRAMINE HYDROCHLORIDE.

Junior Meltus Sugar and Colour Free Expectorant

(SSL) is a proprietary, non-prescription preparation of the EXPECTORANT agent guaifenesin (guaiphenesin), the ANTISEPTIC agent CETYLPYRIDINIUM CHLORIDE. It can be used for the symptomatic relief of coughs and catarrh associated with flu, colds and throat infections. It is available as a liquid, and is not normally given to children under one year, except on medical advice.
✚▲ Side-effects/warnings: See CETYLPYRIDINIUM CHLORIDE; GUAIFENESIN.

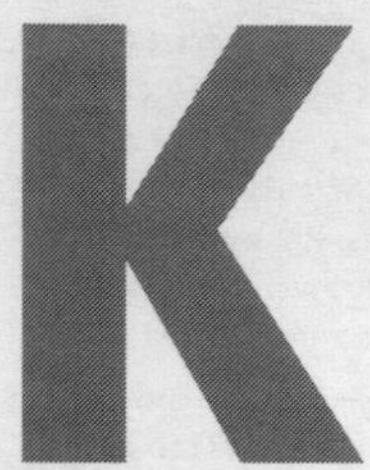

Kabiglobulin

(Pharmacia) is a proprietary, prescription-only preparation of human NORMAL IMMUNO-GLOBULIN. It can be used in IMMUNIZATION to confer immediate *passive immunity* to infection by viruses such as hepatitis A virus, rubeola (measles) and rubella (German measles). It is available in a form for intramuscular injection.
✚▲ Side-effects/warnings: See NORMAL IMMUNOGLOBULIN.

Kaletra

(Abbott) is a proprietary, prescription-only compound preparation of the (*protease inhibitor*) ANTIVIRAL drugs ritonavir and lopinavir. Can be used in the treatment of HIV infection in combination with other drugs, and is available as an oral solution and capsules.
✚▲ Side-effects/warnings: See LOPINAVIR WITH RITONAVIR.

Kalspare

(Dominion) is a proprietary, prescription-only compound preparation of the (THIAZIDE-related) DIURETIC chlortalidone and the (*potassium-sparing*) diuretic triamterene. It can be used for oedema and as an ANTIHYPERTENSIVE, and is available as tablets.
✚▲ Side-effects/warnings: See CHLORTALIDONE; TRIAMTERENE.

Kalten

(AstraZeneca) is a proprietary, prescription-only compound preparation of the BETA-BLOCKER atenolol and the DIURETIC drugs hydrochlorothiazide and amiloride hydrochloride. It can be used as an ANTIHYPERTENSIVE for raised blood pressure, and is available as capsules.
✚▲ Side-effects/warnings: See AMILORIDE HYDROCHLORIDE; ATENOLOL; HYDROCHLOROTHIAZIDE.

Kamillosan

(Goldshield) is a proprietary, non-prescription compound preparation of wool fat (and camomile extract). It can be used as an EMOLLIENT to treat and soothe nappy rash, sore nipples and chapped hands. It is available as an ointment.
✚▲ Side-effects/warnings: See WOOL FAT.

Kaodene

(Sovereign) is a proprietary, prescription-only preparation of the (OPIOID) ANTIDIARRHOEAL codeine phosphate together with the absorbent and antidiarrhoeal drug kaolin. It is used only for short-term treatment of diarrhoea, and is available as a suspension.
✚▲ Side-effects/warnings: See CODEINE PHOSPHATE; KAOLIN.

Kaolin and Morphine Mixture, BP

is a non-proprietary, non-prescription compound preparation that combines KAOLIN, the white clay (china clay), and the ANTIDIARRHOEAL and antimotility drug tincture of morphine. It is available as a suspension.
✚▲ Side-effects/warnings: See KAOLIN; MORPHINE SULPHATE.

kaolin

is a purified and sometimes powdered white clay (china clay) which is used as an adsorbent, particularly in ANTIDIARRHOEAL preparations (with or without OPIOID, such as CODEINE PHOSPHATE OF MORPHINE SULPHATE), and also to treat food poisoning and some digestive disorders when it is given orally. Additionally, it can be used in some poultices and dusting powders.
✚▲ Side-effects/warnings: Applied topically or taken by mouth, it is normally free of adverse reactions.
✪ Related entries: Enterosan; J Collis Browne's Tablets; Kaodene; Kaolin and Morphine Mixture, BP.

Kapake

(Galen) is a proprietary, prescription-only compound preparation of the (OPIOID) NARCOTIC ANALGESIC codeine phosphate and the NON-NARCOTIC ANALGESIC paracetamol (a combination known as co-codamol 30/500). It can be used as a painkiller, and is available as tablets, capsules and sachets (called *Kapake Insts*

in two strengths, one a higher-dose 60/1000 version).
✚▲ Side-effects/warnings: See CODEINE PHOSPHATE; PARACETAMOL.

Kaplon
(Berk; APS) is a proprietary, prescription-only preparation of the ACE INHIBITOR captopril. It can be used as an ANTIHYPERTENSIVE and in HEART FAILURE TREATMENT, usually in conjunction with other classes of drug. It is available as tablets.
✚▲ Side-effects/warnings: See CAPTOPRIL.

Karvol Decongestant Capsules
(Crookes) is a proprietary, non-prescription preparation of levomenthol (menthol), chlorbutol (chlorobutanol) and thymol (with aromatic oils). It can be used as a NASAL DECONGESTANT for the symptomatic relief of colds. It is available as capsules which are sprinkled over bedding or added to hot water for the essences to be inhaled. It is not normally given to children under three months, except on medical advice.
✚▲ Side-effects/warnings: See CHLORBUTOL; MENTHOL; THYMOL.

Karvol Decongestant Drops
(Crookes) is a proprietary, non-prescription preparation of levomenthol (menthol), chlorbutol (chlorobutanol) and thymol (with aromatic oils). It can be used as a NASAL DECONGESTANT for the symptomatic relief of colds. It is available as a liquid for inhalation of vapours after sprinkling drops onto a tissue, bedding or into hot water.
✚▲ Side-effects/warnings: See CHLORBUTOL; MENTHOL; THYMOL.

Kefadim
(Lilly) is a proprietary, prescription-only preparation of the ANTIBACTERIAL and (CEPHALOSPORIN) ANTIBIOTIC ceftazidime. It can be used particularly to treat a range of infections, and is available in a form for intravenous injection or infusion.
✚▲ Side-effects/warnings: See CEFTAZIDIME.

Kefadol
(Dista; Lilly) is a proprietary, prescription-only preparation of the ANTIBACTERIAL and (CEPHALOSPORIN) ANTIBIOTIC cefamandole. It can be used to treat a range of infections, and is available in a form for intravenous injection or infusion.
✚▲ Side-effects/warnings: See CEFAMANDOLE.

Keflex
(Lilly) is a proprietary, prescription-only preparation of the ANTIBACTERIAL and (CEPHALOSPORIN) ANTIBIOTIC cefalexin. It can be used to treat many forms of infection, including of the urogenital tract, and is available as capsules, tablets and an oral suspension.
✚▲ Side-effects/warnings: See CEFALEXIN.

Keftid
(Galen) is a proprietary, prescription-only preparation of the ANTIBACTERIAL and (CEPHALOSPORIN) ANTIBIOTIC cefaclor (as monohydrate). It can be used to treat a wide range of bacterial infections, particularly of the urinary tract. It is available as capsules and an oral suspension.
✚▲ Side-effects/warnings: See CEFACLOR.

Kefzol
(Lilly) is a proprietary, prescription-only preparation of the ANTIBACTERIAL and (CEPHALOSPORIN) ANTIBIOTIC cefazolin. It can be used to treat bacterial infections, and is available in a form for intravenous injection or infusion.
✚▲ Side-effects/warnings: See CEFAZOLIN.

Kelfizine W
(Pharmacia) is a proprietary, prescription-only preparation of the (SULPHONAMIDE) ANTIBACTERIAL sulfametopyrazine. It can be used primarily to treat chronic bronchitis and infections of the urinary tract, and is available as tablets.
✚▲ Side-effects/warnings: See SULFAMETOPYRAZINE.

Kemadrin
(GlaxoWellcome; GSK) is a proprietary, prescription-only preparation of the ANTICHOLINERGIC procyclidine hydrochloride. It can be used in the treatment of parkinsonism, and is available as tablets and in a form for injection.
✚▲ Side-effects/warnings: See PROCYCLIDINE HYDROCHLORIDE.

K

Kemicetine

(Pharmacia) is a proprietary, prescription-only preparation of the broad-spectrum ANTIBACTERIAL and ANTIBIOTIC chloramphenicol. It can be used to treat life-threatening infections, and is available in a form for injection.

✚▲ Side-effects/warnings: See CHLORAMPHENICOL.

Kenalog

(Squibb; Bristol-Myers Squibb) is a proprietary, prescription-only preparation of the CORTICOSTEROID and ANTI-INFLAMMATORY triamcinolone (in the form of acetonide). It can be used to treat inflammation and allergic conditions, and is available in a form for injection.

✚▲ Side-effects/warnings: See TRIAMCINOLONE.

Kenalog Intra-articular/ Intramuscular

(Squibb; Bristol-Myers Squibb) is a proprietary, prescription-only preparation of the CORTICOSTEROID and ANTI-INFLAMMATORY triamcinolone (in the form of acetonide). It can be used to treat inflammation of the joints and the soft tissues, and is available in a form for injection.

✚▲ Side-effects/warnings: See TRIAMCINOLONE.

Kentene

(Kent) is a proprietary, prescription-only preparation of the (NSAID) NON-NARCOTIC ANALGESIC and ANTIRHEUMATIC piroxicam. It can be used to treat acute gout, arthritic and rheumatic pain and other musculoskeletal disorders. It is available as capsules.

✚▲ Side-effects/warnings: See PIROXICAM.

Keppra

(UCB Pharma) is a recently introduced proprietary, prescription-only preparation of the ANTICONVULSANT and ANTI-EPILEPTIC levetiracetam. It can be used to assist in the control of partial seizures with or without secondary generalization that have not responded to other drugs, and is available as tablets.

✚▲ Side-effects/warnings: See LEVETIRACETAM.

Keral

(Menarini) is a proprietary, prescription-only preparation of the (NSAID) NON-NARCOTIC ANALGESIC and ANTIRHEUMATIC dexketoprofen (as trometamol), which can be used in the short-term treatment of mild to moderate pain including period pain. It is available as tablets.

✚▲ Side-effects/warnings: See DEXKETOPROFEN.

keratolytic 🅴

agents (or desquamating agents) are used to clear the skin of hyperkeratoses (thickened and horny patches) and scaly areas that occur in some forms of eczema, ichthyosis and psoriasis, and also in the treatment of acne. The standard keratolytic is SALICYLIC ACID, but there are others such as BENZOIC ACID, COAL TAR, DITHRANOL, ICHTHAMMOL and ZINC PASTE (several of which can usefully be applied in the form of a paste inside an impregnated bandage).

Keri

(Bristol-Myers-Squibb) is a proprietary, non-prescription compound preparation of liquid paraffin and lanolin oil. It can be used as an EMOLLIENT to soften dry skin, relieve itching and to treat nappy rash. It is available as a lotion.

✚▲ Side-effects/warnings: See LANOLIN; LIQUID PARAFFIN.

Kerlone

(Sanofi-Synthelabo) is a proprietary, prescription-only preparation of the BETA-BLOCKER betaxolol hydrochloride. It can be used as an ANTIHYPERTENSIVE for raised blood pressure. It is available as tablets.

✚▲ Side-effects/warnings: See BETAXOLOL HYDROCHLORIDE.

Ketil CR

(Tillomed) is a proprietary, prescription-only preparation of the (NSAID) NON-NARCOTIC ANALGESIC and ANTIRHEUMATIC ketoprofen. It can be used to relieve the pain of arthritis and rheumatism and other musculoskeletal disorders, and is available as modified-release capsules.

✚▲ Side-effects/warnings: See KETOPROFEN.

Ketocid

(Trinity) is a proprietary, prescription-only preparation of the (NSAID) NON-NARCOTIC ANALGESIC and ANTIRHEUMATIC ketoprofen. It can be used to relieve the pain of arthritis and rheumatism and other musculoskeletal disorders,

and is available as modified-release capsules.
+▲ Side-effects/warnings: See KETOPROFEN.

ketoconazole

is an (AZOLE) ANTIFUNGAL drug which can be used to treat deep-seated, serious fungal infections (mycoses) and to prevent infection in immunosuppressed patients. In particular, it is used to treat resistant candidiasis (thrush), gastrointestinal infections and other infections including seborrhoeic dermatitis and pityriasis versicolor. Administration is oral or topical.
+ Side-effects: Depending on the route of administration, serious liver damage may occur, there may be an itching skin rash, nausea and vomiting, headache, abdominal pain, blood disorders and breast enlargement in men.
▲ Warnings: Depending on route of administration, it should not be administered to patients who have impaired liver function or porphyria, or who are pregnant. Because it may cause serious liver toxicity, it should not be used for minor fungal infections. Liver function should be monitored.
✪ Related entries: Daktarin Gold Cream; Nizoral; Nizoral Dandruff Shampoo.

ketoprofen

is a (NSAID) NON-NARCOTIC ANALGESIC and ANTIRHEUMATIC drug which can be used to treat rheumatic and muscular pain caused by inflammation, pain after eg orthopaedic surgery, acute gout and period pain. Administration is either oral or by injection. Also in topical preparations for relief of pain in musculoskeletal conditions.
+▲ Side-effects/warnings: See NSAID. There may be pain at the site of injection, or irritation with suppositories.
✪ Related entries: Fenoket; Jomethid XL; Ketil CR; Ketocid; Ketotard 200XL; Ketovail; Ketozip XL; Larafen CR; Orudis; Oruvail; Oruvail Gel; Powergel.

ketorolac trometamol

is a (NSAID) NON-NARCOTIC ANALGESIC which is used in the short-term management of moderate to severe, acute postoperative pain and to prevent and reduce inflammation following eye surgery. Administration can be oral, by topical application or injection.
+▲ Side-effects/warnings: See NSAID; but it is used with care, because it is a recently introduced drug and its side-effects have not been thoroughly established.
✪ Related entries: Acular; Toradol.

Ketotard 200XL

(Galen) is a proprietary, prescription-only preparation of the (NSAID) NON-NARCOTIC ANALGESIC and ANTIRHEUMATIC ketoprofen. It can be used to relieve the pain of arthritis and rheumatism and other musculoskeletal disorders, and is available as modified-release capsules.
+▲ Side-effects/warnings: See KETOPROFEN.

ketotifen

is an ANTIHISTAMINE which has additional ANTI-ALLERGIC properties somewhat like those of SODIUM CROMOGLICATE, and can be used as an ANTI-ASTHMATIC drug to prevent asthmatic attacks. Administration is oral.
+ Side-effects: It may cause drowsiness with dryness in the mouth; dizziness and weight gain.
▲ Warnings: Because it may cause drowsiness, it may impair the performance of skilled tasks, such as driving; effects of alcohol are enhanced. Care is required in pregnancy and breast-feeding.
✪ Related entry: Zaditen.

Ketovail

(APS) is a proprietary, prescription-only preparation of the (NSAID) NON-NARCOTIC ANALGESIC and ANTIRHEUMATIC ketoprofen. It can be used to relieve the pain of arthritis and rheumatism and other musculoskeletal disorders and period pain, and is available as modified-release capsules.
+▲ Side-effects/warnings: See KETOPROFEN.

Ketozip XL

(Ashbourne) is a proprietary, prescription-only preparation of the (NSAID) NON-NARCOTIC ANALGESIC and ANTIRHEUMATIC ketoprofen. It can be used to relieve the pain of arthritis and rheumatism and other musculoskeletal disorders, and is available as modified-release capsules.
+▲ Side-effects/warnings: See KETOPROFEN.

Kiflone

(Berk; APS) is a proprietary, prescription-only preparation of the ANTIBACTERIAL and (CEPHALOSPORIN) ANTIBIOTIC cefalexin. It can be used to treat many forms of infection, including of the urogenital tract, and is available as capsules

and tablets.
✚▲ Side-effects/warnings: See CEFALEXIN.

Kinidin Durules

(AstraZeneca) is a proprietary, prescription-only preparation of the ANTI-ARRHYTHMIC drug quinidine (as quinidine bisulphate). It can be used to treat heartbeat irregularities, and is available as modified-release tablets.
✚▲ Side-effects/warnings: See QUINIDINE.

Klaricid

(Abbott) is a proprietary, prescription-only preparation of the ANTIBACTERIAL and (MACROLIDE) ANTIBIOTIC clarithromycin. It can be used to treat and prevent many forms of infection, and is available in a form for intravenous infusion. It is available as tablets, granules and a paediatric suspension. There is a stronger form called 'Klaricid XL'.
✚▲ Side-effects/warnings: See CLARITHROMYCIN.

Kliofem

(Novo Nordisk) is a proprietary, prescription-only preparation of the OESTROGEN estradiol and the PROGESTOGEN norethisterone. It can be used to treat menopausal symptoms (including osteoporosis prophylaxis) as HRT, and is available as tablets.
✚▲ Side-effects/warnings: See ESTRADIOL; NORETHISTERONE.

Kliovance

(Novo Nordisk) is a proprietary, prescription-only calendar pack containing tablets of the OESTROGEN estradiol and tablets of the PROGESTOGEN norethisterone. It can be used in HRT.
✚▲ Side-effects/warnings: See ESTRADIOL; NORETHISTERONE.

Kogenate

(Bayer) is a proprietary, prescription-only preparation of factor VIII fraction (octocog alfa), which acts as a HAEMOSTATIC to reduce or stop bleeding in the treatment of disorders in which bleeding is prolonged and potentially dangerous (mainly haemophilia A). It is available in a form for intravenous injection or infusion.
✚▲ Side-effects/warnings: See FACTOR VIII FRACTION (DRIED).

Kolanticon Gel

(Peckforton) is a proprietary, non-prescription compound preparation of the ANTACID agents aluminium hydroxide and magnesium oxide, the ANTICHOLINERGIC dicycloverine hydrochloride (dicyclomine hydrochloride) and the ANTIFOAMING AGENT dimeticone. It can be used to treat gastrointestinal disorders where there is spasm. It is available as an oral gel.
✚▲ Side-effects/warnings: See ALUMINIUM HYDROXIDE; DICYCLOVERINE HYDROCHLORIDE; DIMETICONE.

Konakion

(Roche) is a proprietary, prescription-only preparation of vitamin K_1 (phytomenadione). It can be used to treat deficiency of vitamin K and is available as tablets.
✚▲ Side-effects/warnings: See VITAMIN K.

Konakion MM

(Roche) is a proprietary, prescription-only preparation of vitamin K_1 (phytomenadione). It can be used, as a colloidal formulation, to treat deficiency of vitamin K and is available in a form for injection.
✚▲ Side-effects/warnings: See VITAMIN K.

Konakion MM Paediatric

(Roche) is a proprietary, prescription-only preparation of vitamin K_1 (phytomenadione). It can be used, as a colloidal formulation, in newborn babies to prevent vitamin-K deficiency bleeding (haemorrhagic disease of the newborn). It is available in forms for injection or for giving by mouth.
✚▲ Side-effects/warnings: See VITAMIN K.

Konkion Neonatal Injection

(Roche) is a proprietary, prescription-only preparation of vitamin K_1 (phytomenadione). It can be used to treat deficiency of vitamin K and is available in a form for intramuscular injection for healthy newborns of over 36 weeks gestation.
✚▲ Side-effects/warnings: See VITAMIN K.

Konsyl

(Eastern) is a proprietary, non-prescription preparation of the (*bulking-agent*) LAXATIVE ispaghula husk. It can be used to treat constipation and other disorders (including some types of diarrhoea), and is available as powder (in different

strengths and flavours). It is not normally given to children under six years, except on medical advice.
✚▲ Side-effects/warnings: See ISPAGHULA HUSK.

Kwells Tablets

(Roche Consumer Health) is a proprietary, non-prescription preparation of the ANTICHOLINERGIC hyoscine hydrobromide. It can be used as an ANTINAUSEANT to prevent motion sickness, and is available as melt-in-the-mouth tablets. It is not normally given to children under ten years, except on medical advice.
✚▲ Side-effects/warnings: See HYOSCINE HYDROBROMIDE.

Kytril

(Roche) is a proprietary, prescription-only preparation of the ANTI-EMETIC and ANTINAUSEANT granisetron. It can be used to give relief from nausea and vomiting, especially in patients receiving radiotherapy or chemotherapy. It is available as tablets, paediatric liquid and in a form for intravenous injection or infusion.
✚▲ Side-effects/warnings: See GRANISETRON.

labetalol hydrochloride

is an unusual drug that combines both BETA-BLOCKER and ALPHA-ADRENOCEPTOR BLOCKER properties. It is a VASODILATOR and can be used as an ANTIHYPERTENSIVE to reduce high blood pressure, including in pregnancy, after myocardial infarction, in angina and during surgery, and in phaeochromocytoma. Administration is either oral or by intravenous injection or infusion.

✚ Side-effects: There may be tiredness, weakness, headache, and/or tingling of the scalp, nausea and vomiting; rashes may occur; there may be liver damage; pain in the upper body; difficulty in urinating. There may be postural hypotension.

▲ Warnings: See PROPRANOLOL HYDROCHLORIDE. It should not be given to patients who are pregnant, breast-feeding or with certain liver disorders. It may cause liver problems, so symptoms of this should be looked out for. Withdrawal should be gradual.

✪ Related entry: Trandate.

Labosept Pastilles

(LAB) is a proprietary, non-prescription preparation of the ANTISEPTIC dequalinium chloride which can be used to treat sore throats. It is available as pastilles.

✚▲ Side-effects/warnings: See: DEQUALINIUM CHLORIDE.

lacidipine

is a CALCIUM-CHANNEL BLOCKER which is used as an ANTIHYPERTENSIVE. Administration is oral.

✚ Side-effects: Include flushing, headache; oedema, dizziness, weakness, muscle cramps, palpitations; rashes and itching; gastrointestinal upsets and increased production of urine; chest pains (this may require stopping taking the drug), mood disturbances. There may be an excessive growth of the gums.

▲ Warnings: Administer with caution to patients with certain heart and liver disorders. Do not use in pregnancy or breast-feeding. Grapefruit juice should be avoided since it affects the metabolism of the drug.

✪ Related entry: Motens.

Lacri-Lube

(Allergan) is a proprietary, non-prescription compound preparation of liquid paraffin and white soft paraffin (and lanolin alcohols). It can be used as an eye lubricant for people with dry eye conditions, and is available as an eye ointment.

✚▲ Side-effects/warnings: See LIQUID PARAFFIN; WHITE SOFT PARAFFIN.

Lactitol

(Novartis Consumer Health) is a non-proprietary, non-prescription preparation of the (*osmotic*) LAXATIVE lactitol which can be used to relieve constipation. It is available as a powder. It is not given to children less that one year old, and to older children only with medical advice.

✚▲ Side-effects/warnings: See LACTITOL.

lactitol

is an *osmotic* LAXATIVE and is a sugar-like compound, a derivative of lactulose. It can be used to relieve constipation and works by retaining fluid in the intestine and may take up to 48 hours to have full effect. It can also be used to treat hepatic encephalopathy. Administration is oral.

✚▲ Side-effects/warnings: see LACTULOSE.

✪ Related entry: Lactitol.

Lacto-Calamine Lotion

(Schering Plough Consumer Health) is a proprietary, non-prescription compound preparation of zinc oxide, zinc carbonate and phenol with hamamelis water as a topical lotion, which can be used for relief of skin irritation and burns, and insect bites and stings.

✚▲ Side-effects/warnings: See PHENOL; ZINC OXIDE.

lactulose

is an *osmotic* LAXATIVE and is a sugar-like compound. It can be used to relieve constipation and works by retaining fluid in the intestine and may take up to 48 hours to have full effect. It can also be used to treat hepatic encephalopathy. Administration is oral.

✚ Side-effects: Some patients may experience

flatulence, intestinal cramps or abdominal discomfort.
▲ Warnings: It should not be administered to patients with any form of intestinal obstruction. Because lactulose is itself a form of sugar, patients who have blood sugar abnormalities should seek medical advice before using it.
✪ **Related entries: Duphalac Solution; Regulose.**

Ladropen
(Berk; APS) is a proprietary, prescription-only preparation of the ANTIBACTERIAL and (PENICILLIN) ANTIBIOTIC flucloxacillin. It can be used to treat a range of bacterial infections, and is available as capsules, an oral solution and in a form for injection.
✚▲ Side-effects/warnings: See FLUCLOXACILLIN.

Lamictal
(GlaxoWellcome; GSK) is a proprietary, prescription-only preparation of the ANTICONVULSANT and ANTI-EPILEPTIC lamotrigine. It can be used to treat epilepsy including partial and tonic-clonic seizures. It is available as tablets and dispersible tablets.
✚▲ Side-effects/warnings: See LAMOTRIGINE.

Lamisil
(Novartis) is a proprietary, prescription-only preparation of the ANTIFUNGAL terbinafine. It can be used to treat fungal infections, for instance of the nails and ringworm, and is available as tablets and a cream.
✚▲ Side-effects/warnings: See TERBINAFINE.

lamivudine
(3TC) is a (*reverse transcriptase*) ANTIVIRAL drug which can be used in the treatment of HIV infection, normally in combination with other antiviral drugs; also in chronic hepatitis B infection. Administration is oral.
✚ Side-effects: Nausea and vomiting, diarrhoea, abdominal pain; headache, cough, malaise, insomnia; muscular pain, nasal symptoms; also reports of peripheral neuropathy, rarely pancreatitis, blood disturbances or changes in liver enzymes.
▲ Warnings: It is a specialist drug, and there will be full assessment and patient monitoring throughout treatment. It is not to be used by those who are breast-feeding. It should be administered with caution in kidney impairment, where there is a history of pancreatitis or in pregnancy.
✪ **Related entries: Combivir; Epivir; Trizivir; Zeffix.**

lamotrigine
is an ANTICONVULSANT and ANTI-EPILEPTIC drug. It is used, sometimes in conjunction with other drugs, to treat epilepsy, including partial and tonic-clonic seizures. Administration is oral.
✚ Side-effects: These are many and may include rashes, fever, malaise, flu-like symptoms, drowsiness; rarely, liver dysfunction, blood changes, blurred vision, headache, gastrointestinal upsets and nausea, movement and mood changes.
▲ Warnings: It is not administered to patients with liver impairment. It should be administered with caution to those who are pregnant or breast-feeding. All the body functions known to be influenced by the drug should be monitored.
✪ **Related entry: Lamictal.**

Lamprene
(Alliance) is a proprietary, prescription-only preparation of the ANTIBACTERIAL drug clofazimine. It can be used, in combination with other drugs, in the treatment of the major form of leprosy, and is available as capsules.
✚▲ Side-effects/warnings: See CLOFAZIMINE.

Lanacane Cream
(Combe International) is a proprietary, non-prescription preparation of the LOCAL ANAESTHETIC benzocaine. It can be used to treat local pain and skin irritation, and is available as a cream. It is not normally given to children, except on medical advice.
✚▲ Side-effects/warnings: See BENZOCAINE.

Lanacort Creme
(Combe International) is a proprietary, non-prescription preparation of the CORTICOSTEROID and ANTI-INFLAMMATORY hydrocortisone. It can be used to treat mild inflammation of the skin, such as eczema, and is available as a cream for topical application. It is not normally used for children under ten years, except on medical advice.
✚▲ Side-effects/warnings: See HYDROCORTISONE.

Lanacort Ointment
(Combe International) is a proprietary, non-prescription preparation of the CORTICOSTEROID and ANTI-INFLAMMATORY hydrocortisone. It can

be used to treat mild inflammation of the skin, such as eczema, and is available as an ointment for topical application. It is not normally used for children under ten years, except on medical advice.
✚▲ Side-effects/warnings: See HYDROCORTISONE.

lanolin

is a constituent of WOOL FAT and is incorporated into several EMOLLIENT preparations. It can be used on cracked, dry or scaling skin, where it encourages hydration and is commonly combined with LIQUID PARAFFIN.
✚▲ Side-effects/warnings: Some people are sensitive to wool fat preparations; there may be an eczematous rash.
✪ Related entries: E45; Keri; Sudocrem Antiseptic Cream; Sudocream Antiseptic Healing Cream.

Lanoxin

(GlaxoWellcome; GSK) is a proprietary, prescription-only preparation of the CARDIAC GLYCOSIDE digoxin. It can be used as a CARDIAC STIMULANT in HEART FAILURE TREATMENT and as an ANTI-ARRHYTHMIC to treat heartbeat irregularities. It is available as tablets and a form for injection or intravenous infusion.
✚▲ Side-effects/warnings: See DIGOXIN.

Lanoxin-PG

(GlaxoWellcome; GSK) is a proprietary, prescription-only preparation of the CARDIAC GLYCOSIDE digoxin. It can be used as a CARDIAC STIMULANT in HEART FAILURE TREATMENT and as an ANTI-ARRHYTHMIC to treat heartbeat irregularities. Available as tablets and an elixir.
✚▲ Side-effects/warnings: See DIGOXIN.

lanreotide

is a newly introduced drug with properties similar to octreotide. They are long-lasting analogues of the hypothalamic HORMONE somatostatin (hypothalamic release-inhibiting hormone) and they reduce the release of a number of other hormones from the pituitary gland and some other sites. It is used as an ANTICANCER drug to relieve symptoms caused by the release of hormones from carcinoid and non-carcinoid (*neuroendocrine*) tumours of the endocrine system (including VIPomas and glucagonomas), and for the short-term treatment of acromegaly. Administration is by intramuscular injection.
✚▲ Side-effects/warnings: See OCTREOTIDE.
✪ Related entries: Somatuline Autogel; Somatuline LA.

lansoprazole

is an ULCER-HEALING DRUG. It works as an inhibitor of gastric acid secretion in the parietal (acid-producing) cells of the stomach lining by acting as a PROTON-PUMP INHIBITOR. It is used for the treatment of benign gastric and duodenal ulcers (including those complicating NSAID therapy), dyspepsia, Zollinger-Ellison syndrome and reflux oesophagitis. It can also be used in conjunction with antibiotics to treat gastric *Helicobacter pylori* infection. Administration is oral.
✚▲ Side-effects/warnings: See PROTON-PUMP INHIBITOR. Also reported: dyspepsia, urticaria and various skin disorders, alopecia, photosensitivity, angioedema, tingling in the extremities, kidney problems, anaphylaxis, liver dysfunction, hair loss, various blood changes, bruising, peripheral oedema, fatigue, malaise, taste disturbance, vertigo, hallucinations, mental confusion, rarely growth of breasts in men, impotence.
✪ Related entries: HeliClear; HeliMet; Zoton.

Lanvis

(GlaxoWellcome; GSK) is a proprietary, prescription-only preparation of the ANTICANCER drug tioguanine. It can be used in the treatment of leukaemia, and is available as tablets.
✚▲ Side-effects/warnings: See TIOGUANINE.

Larafen CR

(Lagap) is a proprietary, prescription-only preparation of the (NSAID) NON-NARCOTIC ANALGESIC and ANTIRHEUMATIC ketoprofen. It can be used to relieve arthritic and rheumatic pain and to treat other musculoskeletal disorders and period pain. It is available as modified-release capsules.
✚▲ Side-effects/warnings: See KETOPROFEN.

Largactil

(Hawgreen) is a proprietary, prescription-only preparation of the (PHENOTHIAZINE) ANTIPSYCHOTIC chlorpromazine hydrochloride. It can be used to treat patients undergoing serious behavioural disturbances, who are psychotic (especially schizophrenics), or with severe anxiety where a degree of sedation is useful. It can also be used as an ANTINAUSEANT and ANTI-EMETIC to

relieve nausea and vomiting, particularly in terminal illness, and for intractable hiccup. It is available as tablets, a syrup, a suspension and in a form for injection.
✚▲ Side-effects/warnings: See CHLORPROMAZINE HYDROCHLORIDE.

Lariam

(Roche) is a proprietary, prescription-only preparation the ANTIMALARIAL drug mefloquine. It can be used to prevent or treat malaria, and is available as tablets.
✚▲ Side-effects/warnings: See MEFLOQUINE.

Lasikal

(Borg) is a proprietary, prescription-only compound preparation of the (*loop*) DIURETIC furosemide (frusemide) and the potassium supplement POTASSIUM CHLORIDE. It can be used to treat oedema, and is available as modified-release tablets.
✚▲ Side-effects/warnings: See FUROSEMIDE; POTASSIUM CHLORIDE. Swallow tablets whole with plenty of water when in an upright position.

Lasilactone

(Borg) is a proprietary, prescription-only compound preparation of the (*aldosterone-antagonist* and *potassium-sparing*) DIURETIC spironolactone and the (*loop*) diuretic furosemide (frusemide). It can be used to treat resistant oedema, and is available as capsules.
✚▲ Side-effects/warnings: See FUROSEMIDE; SPIRONOLACTONE.

Lasix

(Borg) is a proprietary, prescription-only preparation of the (loop) DIURETIC furosemide (frusemide). It can be used to treat oedema, and low urine production due to kidney failure (oliguria). It is available as tablets, a paediatric liquid and in a form for intravenous injection or infusion.
✚▲ Side-effects/warnings: See FUROSEMIDE.

Lasonil

(Bayer) is a proprietary, non-prescription compound preparation of a heparinoid and the enzyme (see ENZYMES) hyaluronidase, which helps it to reach the affected area. It can be used in treating superficial soft-tissue injuries, such as bruising and sprains. It is available as an ointment.
✚▲ Side-effects/warnings: See HEPARINOIDS; HYALURONIDASE.

Lasoride

(Borg) is a proprietary, prescription-only compound preparation of the (*potassium-sparing*) DIURETIC amiloride hydrochloride and the (*loop*) diuretic furosemide (frusemide) (a combination called co-amilofruse 5/40). It can be used to treat oedema, and is available as tablets.
✚▲ Side-effects/warnings: See AMILORIDE HYDROCHLORIDE; FUROSEMIDE.

latanoprost

is a PROSTAGLANDIN analogue which is used as a novel GLAUCOMA TREATMENT for open-angle glaucoma and ocular hypertension in patients for whom other drugs are not suitable. Administration is topical in the form of eye-drops.
✚ Side-effects: Brown pigmentation of the iris, irritation of the eye, changes to the eyelashes, hyperaemia or other effects on the eye.
▲ Warnings: Patients should be advised of possible iris colouration; administer with care in patients with asthma. It should be avoided by those who are pregnant or breast-feeding.
✪ Related entries: Xalacom; Xalatan.

laxative

agents and other purgatives are preparations that promote defecation and so relieve constipation. They can be divided into several different types. The *faecal softener* laxatives (eg LIQUID PARAFFIN) soften the faeces for easier evacuation. The *bulking-agent* laxatives increase the overall volume of the faeces, which then stimulates bowel movement. Bulking agents are usually some form of fibre, eg BRAN, ISPAGHULA HUSK, METHYLCELLULOSE and STERCULIA. The *stimulant* laxatives act on the intestinal muscles to increase motility. Many traditional remedies for constipation are stimulants, such as cascara, CASTOR OIL, SENNA and elixir of figs. However, there are modern variants with less of a stimulant action and which also have other properties, eg BISACODYL, DANTRON, DOCUSATE SODIUM (dioctyl sodium sulphosuccinate) and SODIUM PICOSULFATE (sodium picosulphate). Finally, the *osmotic* laxatives, which are chemical salts that work by retaining water in the intestine so increasing overall liquidity, eg LACTULOSE,

LACTITOL, MAGNESIUM HYDROXIDE and MAGNESIUM SULPHATE (note that magnesium salts are also used as an ANTACID). Suppositories and enemas also aid in promoting defecation. Laxatives are also used to treat constipation which results as a side-effect of another drug, to clear the alimentary tract before radiological or surgical procedures, and to help expel parasites after ANTHELMINTIC treatment.
✚▲ Side-effects/warnings: It is important not to overuse laxatives. This can lead to low blood potassium (hypokalaemia) and damage to the colon (atonic and non-functioning colon). Use in children on medical advice only. See individual entries.

Laxoberal
(Boerhinger Ingelheim) is a proprietary, non-prescription preparation of the (*stimulant*) LAXATIVE sodium picosulfate. It can be used to relieve constipation, and is available as an elixir. It is not normally given to children under four years, except on medical advice.
✚▲ Side-effects/warnings: See SODIUM PICOSULFATE.

Ledclair
(Sinclair) is a proprietary, prescription-only preparation of sodium calcium edetate, used as an ANTIDOTE to treat poisoning by heavy metals, especially lead. Administration is by injection.
✚▲ Side-effects/warnings: see SODIUM CALCIUM EDETATE.

Lederfen
(Lederle; Wyeth) is a proprietary, prescription-only preparation of the (NSAID) NON-NARCOTIC ANALGESIC and ANTIRHEUMATIC fenbufen. It can be used to relieve pain, particularly rheumatic and arthritic pain and inflammation, and to treat other musculoskeletal disorders. It is available as tablets and capsules.
✚▲ Side-effects/warnings: See FENBUFEN.

Lederfolin
(Lederle; Wyeth) is a proprietary, prescription-only preparation of calcium folinate, which can be used to counteract some of the toxic effects of certain anticancer drugs, especially METHOTREXATE. It is available in a form for injection.
✚▲ Side-effects/warnings: See CALCIUM FOLINATE.

Ledermycin
(Lederle; Wyeth) is a proprietary, prescription-only preparation of the ANTIBACTERIAL and (TETRACYCLINES) ANTIBIOTIC demeclocycline hydrochloride. It can be used to treat a wide range of infections, and is available as capsules.
✚▲ Side-effects/warnings: See DEMECLOCYCLINE HYDROCHLORIDE.

leflumomide
is an IMMUNOSUPPRESSANT drug used as a disease-modifying ANTIRHEUMATIC to treat active episodes. The beneficial effect does not develop until after several weeks and takes a long time to wear off. Its use is confined to specialist centres. Administration is oral.
✚ Side-effects: This is a new drug and possible side-effects and warnings are extensive – the drug is only used under specialist supervision.
▲ Warnings: Immunosuppressant drugs damp-down the immune system and there is bone-marrow depression, so there is a risk of infections. It is not used in those who are pregnant or with liver impairment.
✪ **Related entry: Arava.**

Lemsip Cold + Flu Breathe Easy
(Reckitt Benckiser Healthcare) is a proprietary, non-prescription preparation of the NON-NARCOTIC ANALGESIC and ANTIPYRETIC paracetamol and the SYMPATHOMIMETIC and DECONGESTANT phenylephrine hydrochloride (and vitamin C (ascorbic acid)). It can be used to relieve cold and flu symptoms, nasal congestion and to reduce raised body temperature. It is available as sachets of powder for making up in hot water, and is not normally given to children, except on medical advice.
✚▲ Side-effects/warnings: See ASCORBIC ACID; PARACETAMOL; PHENYLEPHRINE HYDROCHLORIDE.

Lemsip Cold + Flu Combined Relief Capsules
(Reckitt Benckiser Healthcare) is a proprietary, non-prescription preparation of the NON-NARCOTIC ANALGESIC and ANTIPYRETIC paracetamol, the SYMPATHOMIMETIC and DECONGESTANT phenylephrine hydrochloride and the STIMULANT caffeine. It can be used to relieve cold and flu symptoms, and is available as capsules. Not normally given to children under 12, except on medical advice.
✚▲ Side-effects/warnings: See CAFFEINE; PARACETAMOL; PHENYLEPHRINE HYDROCHLORIDE.

Lemsip Cold + Flu Max Strength

(Reckitt Benckiser Healthcare) is a proprietary, non-prescription preparation of the NON-NARCOTIC ANALGESIC and ANTIPYRETIC paracetamol, the SYMPATHOMIMETIC and DECONGESTANT phenylephrine hydrochloride (and vitamin C (ascorbic acid)). It can be used to relieve cold and flu symptoms, and nasal congestion. It is available as sachets of powder for making up in hot water, and is not normally given to children, except on medical advice.
✚▲ Side-effects/warnings: See ASCORBIC ACID; PARACETAMOL; PHENYLEPHRINE HYDROCHLORIDE.

Lemsip Cold + Flu Max Strength Capsules

(Reckitt Benckiser Healthcare) is a proprietary, non-prescription preparation of the NON-NARCOTIC ANALGESIC and ANTIPYRETIC paracetamol and the SYMPATHOMIMETIC and DECONGESTANT phenylephrine hydrochloride and caffeine. It can be used to relieve cold and flu symptoms and nasal congestion. It is available as capsules, and is not normally given to children, except on medical advice.
✚▲ Side-effects/warnings: See CAFFEINE; PARACETAMOL; PHENYLEPHRINE HYDROCHLORIDE.

Lemsip Cold + Flu Original Lemon

(Reckitt Benckiser Healthcare) is a proprietary, non-prescription preparation of the NON-NARCOTIC ANALGESIC and ANTIPYRETIC paracetamol and the SYMPATHOMIMETIC and DECONGESTANT phenylephrine hydrochloride (and vitamin C (ascorbic acid)). It can be used to relieve cold and flu symptoms, and is available as sachets of powder for making up in hot water. It is not normally given to children, except on medical advice.
✚▲ Side-effects/warnings: See ASCORBIC ACID; PARACETAMOL; PHENYLEPHRINE HYDROCHLORIDE.

Lemsip Cough + Cold Chesty Cough

(Reckitt Benckiser Healthcare) is a proprietary, non-prescription preparation of the EXPECTORANT agent guaifenesin (guaiphenesin). It can be used to relieve sore throats and deep chesty coughs. It is available as a linctus and is not normally given to children under two years, except on medical advice.
✚▲ Side-effects/warnings: See GUAIFENESIN.

Lemsip Cough + Cold Dry Cough

(Reckitt Benckiser Healthcare) is a proprietary, non-prescription preparation of a linctus containing lemon oil, honey, citric acid and glycerol, and is taken for the symptomatic relief of dry tickly coughs and sore throats.
✚▲ Side-effects/warnings: See GLYCEROL.

Lemsip Pharmacy Flu Strength

(Reckitt Benckiser Healthcare) is a proprietary, non-prescription preparation of the NON-NARCOTIC ANALGESIC and ANTIPYRETIC paracetamol and the SYMPATHOMIMETIC and DECONGESTANT pseudoephedrine hydrochloride (and vitamin C (ascorbic acid)). It can be used to relieve flu and cold symptoms, including aches and pains, nasal congestion and fever. It is available as sachets for making up in hot water, and is not normally given to children, except under medical advice.
✚▲ Side-effects/warnings: See ASCORBIC ACID; PARACETAMOL; PSEUDOEPHEDRINE HYDROCHLORIDE.

Lemsip Pharmacy Powercaps

(Reckitt Benckiser Healthcare) is a proprietary, non-prescription preparation of the NON-NARCOTIC ANALGESIC and ANTIPYRETIC drug ibuprofen and the SYMPATHOMIMETIC and DECONGESTANT pseudoephedrine hydrochloride. It can be used to relieve heavy cold and flu symptoms and nasal congestion. It is available as sachets of powder for making up in hot water, and is not normally given to children, except on medical advice.
✚▲ Side-effects/warnings: See IBUPROFEN; PSEUDOEPHEDRINE HYDROCHLORIDE.

Lemsip Sore Throat Anti-bacterial Citrus Fruits Lozenge

(Reckitt Benckiser Healthcare) is a proprietary, non-prescription compound preparation of the ANTISEPTIC hexylresorcinol with vitamin C (ascorbic acid). It can be used to relieve painful sore throat and is available as lozenges. Not normally given to children under six, except on medical advice.
✚▲ Side-effects/warnings: See HEXYLRESORCINOL; ASCORBIC ACID.

Lemsip Sore Throat Anti-bacterial Lozenge

(Reckitt Benckiser Healthcare) is a proprietary,

non-prescription compound preparation of the ANTISEPTIC hexylresorcinol. It can be used to relieve painful sore throat and is available as lozenges. It is not normally given to children under six years, except on medical advice.
✚▲ Side-effects/warnings: See HEXYLRESORCINOL.

lenograstim

(recombinant human granulocyte-colony stimulating factor, rHuG-CSF) is a specialist drug used to reduce neutropenia (a shortage of neutrophil white blood-cells in the circulation) by stimulating neutrophil production when this has been reduced during chemotherapy in ANTICANCER treatment, and this may reduce the incidence of associated sepsis. Administration is by intravenous infusion.
✚▲ Side-effects/warnings: These are many. This is a specialist drug used only after full evaluation under hospital conditions.
✪ **Related entry: Granocyte.**

Lentizol

(Parke-Davis; Pfizer) is a proprietary, prescription-only preparation of the (TRICYCLIC) ANTIDEPRESSANT amitriptyline hydrochloride. It can be used to treat depressive illness, particularly in cases where some degree of sedation is required, and is available as modified-release capsules.
✚▲ Side-effects/warnings: See AMITRIPTYLINE HYDROCHLORIDE.

lepirudin

is an ANTICOAGULANT, and is a synthetic (recombinant process) version of natural hirudin from the salivary glands of the medicinal leech. It is a *parenteral* anticoagulant (not active by mouth, and must be injected), and can be used for anticoagulation in those patients requiring parenteral antithrombotic treatment but who show adverse reactions to heparin (eg thrombocytopenia). The dose of lepirudin is adjusted according to laboratory blood tests. Administration is by intravenous injection/ infusion at least once a day.
✚ Side-effects: Signs of bleeding; reduced haemoglobin concentration; fever, hypersensitivity reactions (such as rash); reactions at injection site.
▲ Warnings: Should not be used in pregnancy or breast-feeding. Use with care in kidney or liver impairment; recent bleeding or risk of bleeding, stroke or cerebrovascular accident, recent surgery, severe hypertension, bacterial endocarditis. Regular blood tests are required to check effect of doses.
✪ **Related entry: Refludan.**

lercanidipine hydrochloride

is a CALCIUM-CHANNEL BLOCKER which can be used as an ANTIHYPERTENSIVE to treat mild to moderate hypertension. Administration is oral.
✚ Side-effects: Flushing, palpitations / tachycardia, headache, dizziness, weakness, peripheral oedema; also gastrointestinal disturbances, drowsiness, hypotension, muscle pains, rash, excessive production of urine.
▲ Warnings: It is not used in people with certain heart and cardiovascular problems, or in pregnancy or breast-feeding. Care in cases of kidney or liver impairment; certain other heart problems; avoid grapefruit juice (which may affect metabolism of the drug).
✪ **Related entry: Zanidip.**

Lescol

(Novartis) is a proprietary, prescription-only preparation of the LIPID-REGULATING DRUG fluvastatin. It can be used in hyperlipidaemia to change the proportions of various lipids in the bloodstream. It is available as capsules.
✚▲ Side-effects/warnings: See FLUVASTATIN.

Lescol XL

(Novartis) is a proprietary, prescription-only preparation of the LIPID-REGULATING DRUG fluvastatin. It can be used in hyperlipidaemia to change the proportions of various lipids in the bloodstream. It is available as modified-release tablets.
✚▲ Side-effects/warnings: See FLUVASTATIN.

letrozole

is an ANTICANCER drug which is used to treat advanced breast cancer in postmenopausal women. It is a non-steroidal compound, an ENZYME INHIBITOR (an *aromatase inhibitor*) that works as an indirect HORMONE ANTAGONIST by inhibiting the conversion of the male sex hormone ANDROGEN to the female sex hormone OESTROGEN. Administration is oral.
✚ Side-effects: Hot flushes; nausea and vomiting; dyspepsia, diarrhoea, constipation, abdominal pain, anorexia; chest pain, shortness of breath,

coughing; dizziness, fatigue, headache; infection; muscle pain, oedema, weight gain, rash and pruritus.
▲ Warnings: It should not be used in premenopausal women or in those who are pregnant or breast-feeding, or with severely impaired liver function, and should be used with care in impaired kidney function.
✪ **Related entry: Femara.**

Leucomax

(Novartis, Schering-Plough) is a proprietary, prescription-only preparation of the specialist drug molgramostim used to treat neutropenia during chemotherapy in ANTICANCER treatment. It is available in a form for intravenous infusion.
✚▲ Side-effects/warnings: see MOLGRAMOSTIM.

Leukeran

(GlaxoWellcome; GSK) is a proprietary, prescription-only preparation of the IMMUNOSUPPRESSANT and CYTOTOXIC (ANTICANCER) drug chlorambucil. It can be used to treat various forms of cancer (eg ovarian cancer and Hodgkin's disease), and is available as tablets.
✚▲ Side-effects/warnings: See CHLORAMBUCIL.

leukotriene-receptor antagonist

drugs work as ANTI-ALLERGIC agents by blocking the actions of leukotrienes, which are natural inflammatory mediators released in most tissues and organs including the lungs. Montelukast is used in ANTI-ASTHMATIC treatment as a form of add-on therapy for individuals not adequately controlled by inhaled CORTICOSTEROID and short-acting BETA-RECEPTOR STIMULANT drugs to prevent mild to moderate asthma attacks (including exercise-induced bronchospasm). A further example is ZAFIRLUKAST.

leuprorelin acetate

is an analogue of GONADORELIN (gonadothrophin-releasing hormone; GnRH), which is a hypothalamic HORMONE. On prolonged administration it acts as an indirect HORMONE ANTAGONIST in that it reduces the pituitary gland's secretion of gonadotrophin (after an initial surge), which results in reduced secretion of SEX HORMONES by the ovaries or testes. It can be used to treat endometriosis (a growth of the lining of the uterus) and is also used as an ANTICANCER drug for cancer of the prostate gland. Administration is by injection.
✚▲ Side-effects/warnings: See BUSERELIN. There may also be fatigue, peripheral oedema, nausea, effect on the blood, and irritation at the injection site.
✪ **Related entries: Prostap 3; Prostap SR.**

Leustat

(Janssen-Cilag) is a proprietary, prescription-only preparation of the ANTICANCER drug cladribine. It can be used to treat leukaemia, and is available in a form for intravenous infusion.
✚▲ Side-effects/warnings: See CLADRIBINE.

levamisole

is an ANTHELMINTIC drug which is the drug of choice in treating infestation by roundworms (*Ascaris lumbricoides*) and is well tolerated with rarely any side-effects. Administration is oral. It is available only on a named-patient basis in the UK.
✚▲ Side-effects/warnings: Rarely, mild nausea, vomiting.

levetiracetam

is a recently introduced ANTICONVULSANT and ANTI-EPILEPTIC drug. It can be used as an adjunct to assist in the control of partial seizures that have not responded to other anti-epileptic drugs. Administration is oral.
✚ Side-effects: Drowsiness, asthenia, dizziness; less commonly, appetite loss, gastrointestinal effects such as diarrhoea, dyspepsia and nausea; also memory loss, ataxia, depression, emotional lability, aggression, insomnia, nervousness, tremor, vertigo, headache, double vision, rash.
▲ Warnings: Levetiracetam should be used with caution in those with liver or kidney impairment; who are pregnant or breast-feeding. Sudden withdrawal of levetiracetam should be avoided.
✪ **Related entry: Keppra.**

levobunolol hydrochloride

is a BETA-BLOCKER which can be used as a GLAUCOMA TREATMENT for chronic simple glaucoma. It is thought to work by slowing the rate of production of the aqueous humour in the eye. Administration is as eye-drops.
✚ Side-effects: There may be some systemic absorption after using eye-drops, so some of the side-effects listed under PROPRANOLOL HYDROCHLORIDE may be seen. Dry eyes, stinging, redness, pain and some local allergic reactions,

including conjunctivitis may also occur.
▲ Warnings: In view of possible absorption, some side-effects should be borne in mind, particularly bronchospasm in asthmatics and interactions with some calcium-channel blockers.
✪ **Related entry: Betagan.**

levobupivacaine hydrochloride

is a LOCAL ANAESTHETIC with a long duration of action. It is an amide derivative of lignocaine hydrochloride and one chemical form (an isomer) of bupivacaine hydrochloride, and is particularly long-lasting. It can be used for spinal anaesthesia, including epidural injection (but not in obstetrics), and also for nerve block and by local infiltration. Administration is by injection.
✚▲ Side-effects/warnings: See LIGNOCAINE HYDROCHLORIDE.
✪ **Related entry: Chirocaine.**

levocabastine

is an ANTIHISTAMINE which can be used for the symptomatic relief of allergic rhinitis and allergic conjunctivitis. Administration is topical.
✚▲ Side-effects/warnings: See ANTIHISTAMINE; but any adverse effects are less severe when given locally. Local application to the nasal mucosa may cause irritation and taste disturbances; to the eye it may cause blurred vision and irritation. There may be headache, drowsiness, oedema, skin rash, breathlessness. It may be used with care in people with impaired kidney function.
✪ **Related entry: Livostin.**

levocetirizine hydrochloride

is a recently developed ANTIHISTAMINE, a form (isomer) of CETIRIZINE HYDROCHLORIDE, with less side-effects (for example, it causes less sedation) than some of the older types of antihistamine. It can be used for the symptomatic relief of allergic symptoms such as hay fever and urticaria. Administration is oral.
✚▲ Side-effects/warnings: See ANTIHISTAMINE, but it doesn't often cause sedation or anticholinergic side-effects. It should be administered with caution in pregnancy or breast-feeding. It should not be used by people who have severely impaired kidney function.
✪ **Related entry: Xyzal.**

levodopa

is a powerful ANTIPARKINSONISM drug which is used to treat parkinsonism, but not the symptoms of parkinsonism induced by drugs. Levodopa is converted into the neurotransmitter DOPAMINE within the brain and works by replenishing dopamine levels in the part of the brain (striatum) where there is depletion in Parkinson's disease. It is effective in reducing the slowness of movement and rigidity associated with parkinsonism, but is not as successful in controlling the tremor. Administration is oral. It is often combined with other types of drug (eg the ENZYME INHIBITOR, CARBIDOPA) that inhibit the conversion of levodopa to dopamine outside the brain, therefore enabling as much levodopa as possible to reach the brain before it is converted and so maximizing its effect, and so that a lower dose can be used, with a consequent reduction in side-effects. It is the presence of such an inhibitor that may produce involuntary movements.
✚ Side-effects: Anorexia, nausea, vomiting, insomnia, agitation, postural hypotension (or sometimes short-lived hypertension), dizziness, heart rate changes, red discolouration of the urine and other fluids, rarely sensitivity reactions, abnormal involuntary muscle movements, psychiatric changes, depression, drowsiness, headache, rashes, flushing, sweating, gastrointestinal bleeding, and peripheral nerve disturbances.
▲ Warnings: It is not to be administered to patients with closed-angle glaucoma; it should be administered with caution to those with lung disease, peptic ulcers, cardiovascular disease, diabetes, certain bone disorders, open-angle glaucoma, skin melanoma or psychiatric disorders; or who are pregnant or breast-feeding. Monitoring of heart, blood, liver and kidney functions may be necessary during prolonged treatment. Iron and the vitamin pyridoxine (present in some multivitamin preparations) can reduce the effectiveness of levodopa.
✪ **Related entries: co-beneldopa; co-careldopa; Half Sinemet CR; Madopar; Sinemet; Sinemet CR.**

levofloxacin

is a (QUINOLONE) ANTIBIOTIC-like ANTIBACTERIAL that is active against both Gram-positive and Gram-negative organisms. It can be used to treat numerous infections, including chronic bronchitis, community-acquired pneumonia, urinary-tract infections, skin and soft tissue infections. It is given orally or by intravenous infusion.

✚▲ Side-effects/warnings: See QUINOLONE. It should be used with caution in kidney impairment. May impair performance of skilled tasks (eg driving). Other side-effects include weakness, rarely tremor, anxiety, hypotension, speeding of the heart, hypoglycaemia, liver and kidney complications; local reactions with infusion.
✪ **Related entry: Tavanic.**

levomenthol
see MENTHOL.

levomepromazine
(methotrimeprazine) is chemically a PHENOTHIAZINE. It is used as an ANTIPSYCHOTIC drug to tranquillize patients suffering from psychotic disorders, such as schizophrenia, and also to calm and soothe patients with a terminal illness. Administration can be either oral or by injection.
✚▲ Side-effects/warnings: See CHLORPROMAZINE HYDROCHLORIDE; but there is more of a sedative effect and a risk of postural hypotension.
✪ **Related entry: Nozinan.**

Levonelle-2
(Schering Health) is a proprietary, prescription-only ORAL CONTRACEPTIVE (also known as the 'morning-after pill') that contains a PROGESTOGEN, levonorgestrel. It can be used up to 72 hours after sexual intercourse has taken place.
✚▲ Side-effects/warnings: See LEVONORGESTREL.

levonorgestrel
is a PROGESTOGEN which is used as a constituent of the *combined* ORAL CONTRACEPTIVE preparations that contain OESTROGEN with a progesterone and also in progesterone-only pills. It is also used (in combination with oestrogens) in HRT and as an emergency 'morning-after pill'. Administration is oral as tablets, as capsules for implanting, or an intra-uterine system (and some discontinued implant systems may be in place until about 2004, eg Norplant).
✚▲ Side-effects/warnings: See PROGESTOGEN.
✪ **Related entries: Eugynon 30; Levonelle-2; Logynon; Logynon ED; Microgynon 30; Microgynon 30 ED; Microval; Mirena; Norgeston; Nuvelle; Nuvelle TS; Ovran; Ovran 30; Ovranette; Trinordiol.**

levothyroxine sodium
is the name now used for the form used in therapeutics of THYROXINE (actually it is sodium L-thyroxine; T_4), one of the two natural THYROID HORMONES. It is used clinically to make up a hormonal deficiency on a regular maintenance basis and to treat associated symptoms. It may also be used in the treatment of goitre and thyroid cancer. Administration is oral.
✚ Side-effects: There may be heartbeat irregularities and increased heart rate, angina pain; headache, muscle cramp, flushing, sweating and fever, diarrhoea, vomiting, tremors, restlessness, insomnia.
▲ Warnings: It is prescribed with caution to patients with certain cardiovascular or hormonal disorders, or who are pregnant or breast-feeding. Iron can reduce the effects of levothyroxine.
✪ **Related entry: Eltroxin.**

Lexpec
(Hillcross; Rosemont) is a proprietary, prescription-only preparation of folic acid. It can be used as a VITAMIN supplement, for example, during pregnancy or to treat a deficiency, and is available as a syrup.
✚▲ Side-effects/warnings: See FOLIC ACID.

Lexpec with Iron
(Rosemont) is a proprietary, prescription-only compound preparation of ferric ammonium citrate and folic acid. It can be used as an IRON and folic acid supplement during pregnancy, and is available as a syrup.
✚▲ Side-effects/warnings: See FERRIC AMMONIUM CITRATE; FOLIC ACID.

Lexpec with Iron-M
(Rosemont) is a proprietary, prescription-only compound preparation of ferric ammonium citrate and folic acid. It can be used as an IRON and folic acid supplement during pregnancy, and is available as a syrup.
✚▲ Side-effects/warnings: See FERRIC AMMONIUM CITRATE; FOLIC ACID.

LH
see LUTEINISING HORMONE.

LH-RH
see GONADORELIN.

Liberate
(SNBTS) is a proprietary, prescription-only

preparation of dried human factor VIII fraction (High Potency Factor VIII Concentrate). It acts as a HAEMOSTATIC to reduce or stop bleeding in the treatment of disorders in which bleeding is prolonged and potentially dangerous (mainly haemophilia A). It is available in a form for intravenous injection or infusion.

✚▲ Side-effects/warnings: See FACTOR VIII FRACTION (DRIED).

Librium

(ICN) is a proprietary, prescription-only preparation of the (BENZODIAZEPINE) ANXIOLYTIC chlordiazepoxide. It can be used in the short-term treatment of anxiety and, with other drugs, for acute alcohol withdrawal symptoms, and is available as capsules.

✚▲ Side-effects/warnings: See CHLORDIAZEPOXIDE.

Lidifen

(Berk; APS) is a proprietary, prescription-only preparation of the (NSAID) NON-NARCOTIC ANALGESIC and ANTIRHEUMATIC ibuprofen. It can be used to relieve pain and inflammation, particularly the pain of rheumatic disease and other musculoskeletal disorders, and is available as tablets.

✚▲ Side-effects/warnings: See IBUPROFEN.

lidocaine hydrochloride

(lignocaine hydrochloride) is the most commonly used of all the LOCAL ANAESTHETIC drugs. It can be administered by a number of routes and always close to its site of action. When administered by injection or infiltration, it can be used for dental and minor surgery (such as sutures). By epidural injection (into a space surrounding the nerves of the spinal cord), it can be used in childbirth or major surgery (sometimes in combination with a GENERAL ANAESTHETIC). When injected into a vascular region, it is co-injected with ADRENALINE ACID TARTRATE which acts as a VASOCONSTRICTOR and so limits the rate at which the lignocaine is washed away. When applied topically, it is well absorbed from mucous membranes and abraded skin and can be used to treat discomfort at many sites, such as in teething gel for babies. It is also used in eye-drops as an anaesthetic for minor surgery on the eye. Additionally, lidocaine is used as an ANTI-ARRHYTHMIC (particularly in the emergency treatment of arrhythmias and fibrillation following heart attack), when it is administered by intravenous injection. It is available in forms suitable for infiltration, intravenous injection or infusion, or topically as a gel, ointment, spray, lotion, lozenges or eye-drops.

✚ Side-effects: These depend on what it is being used for and the route of administration. There may be a slowing of the heartbeat, a fall in blood pressure, drowsiness, and depression of respiration. There may be allergic hypersensitivity reactions, tingling in the extremities, dizziness and confusion.

▲ Warnings: Depending on the route of administration, it should not be administered to patients with certain heart disorders or porphyria. It should be used with caution in those with liver or respiratory impairment, or epilepsy. Excessive use in babies (eg as a teething gel) should be avoided.

✪ Related entries: Anbesol Adult Strength Gel; Anbesol Liquid; Anbesol Teething Gel; Anodesyn Ointment; Anodesyn Suppositories; Betnovate; Bradosol Plus (Sugar Free); Calgel Teething Gel; Dentinox Teething Gel; Depo-Medrone with Lidocaine; Emla; Germoloids Cream; Germoloids Ointment; Germoloids Suppositories; Instillagel; Lypsyl Cold Sore Gel; Medijel Gel; Medijel Pastels; Min-I-Jet Lignocaine; Minims Lignocaine and Fluorescein; Perinal; Rinstead Teething Gel; Solarcaine Gel; Strepsils Pain Relief Plus; Strepsils Pain Relief Spray; Vagisil Medicated Creme; Woodward's Teething Gel; Xylocaine; Xyloproct.

lignocaine hydrochloride

see LIDOCAINE HYDROCHLORIDE.

Li-Liquid

(Rosemont) is a proprietary, prescription-only preparation of the ANTIMANIA drug lithium (as lithium citrate). It can be used to prevent and treat mania, manic-depressive bouts and recurrent depression, and is available as an oral solution.

✚▲ Side-effects/warnings: See LITHIUM.

Limclair

(Sinclair) is a proprietary, prescription-only preparation of trisodium edetate. It can be used to treat the symptoms of hypercalcaemia (excess calcium in the blood) and calcification of the

cornea, or lime burns, of the eyeball. It is available in a form for injection, or for the eye, as a solution.
✚▲ Side-effects/warnings: See TRISODIUM EDETATE.

linezolid
is a recently introduced (oxazolidinone) ANTIBACTERIAL which is active against Gram-positive bacteria, including methicillin-resistant *Staphylococcus aureus* (MRSA), although resistance to linezolid can develop with prolonged treatment or if the dose is less than optimal. It is only used for people who have infections that are resistant to other antibacterials or when other antibacterials are not tolerated well. It is used particularly for pneumonia and some skin and soft-tissue infections.
✚ Side-effects: Nausea and vomiting, diarrhoea, taste disturbances and headache. Less frequently, there may be effects on the mouth and gastrointestinal system, such as dryness, glossitis, stomatitis, tongue discoloration, constipation, abdominal pain, dyspepsia, gastritis and pancreatitis; also, thirst, high blood pressure, fever, fatigue, dizziness, insomnia, paraesthesia, tinnitus, excessive production of urine, rash, pruritus and urticaria, sweating, blurred vision and effects on the blood such as anaemia, white blood-cell disturbances and electrolyte disturbances. There may be reactions at the injection site.
▲ Warnings: Linezolid should not be used when breast-feeding, and used with caution by those with liver or kidney impairment, or who are pregnant. There should be monitoring of blood counts, particularly as myelosupression is a particular risk. Because linezolid is a monoamine-oxidase inhibitor (MAOI), concomitant treatment with another MAOI (such as a MONOAMINE-OXIDASE INHIBITOR antidepressant) or within two weeks of stopping another MAOI must be avoided. Close observation and blood-pressure monitoring is necessary, especially in people with uncontrolled hypertension, phaeochromocytoma, carcinoid tumour, thyrotoxicosis, manic-depression or schizophrenia, acute confusional states, or in those receiving SSRI or tricyclic antidepressants, directly and indirectly acting sympathomimetics or vasopressive or dopaminergic drugs. Buspirone or pethidine and its use may need to be avoided in these people. People prescribed linezolid should avoid consuming large amounts of tyramine-rich foods (such as mature cheese, yeast extracts, certain alcoholic beverages, also fermented soya bean products). Herbal medicines that are known to interact with MAOI treatment are best avoided (eg St John's wort).
✪ **Related entry: Zyvox.**

Lioresal
(Novartis) is a proprietary, prescription-only preparation of the SKELETAL MUSCLE RELAXANT baclofen. It can be used to treat muscle spasm caused by an injury to or a disease of the central nervous system. It is available as tablets and as an oral liquid.
✚▲ Side-effects/warnings: See BACLOFEN.

liothyronine sodium
is the name now used for the form used in therapeutics of TRIIODOTHYRONINE (actually it is L-tri-iodothyronine; T_3), one of the two natural THYROID HORMONES. It is used clinically to make up hormonal deficiency (hypothyroidism) and to treat associated symptoms (myxoedema).
✚▲ Side-effects/warnings: See LEVOTHYROXINE SODIUM.
✪ **Related entries: Tertroxin; Triiodothyronine.**

Lipantil
(Fournier) is a proprietary, prescription-only preparation of the LIPID-REGULATING DRUG fenofibrate. It can be used in hyperlipidaemia to modify the proportions of various lipids in the bloodstream. It is available as capsules (in three strengths, *Micro 67*, *Micro 200* and *Micro 267*).
✚▲ Side-effects/warnings: See FENOFIBRATE.

lipid-regulating drug
(lipid-lowering drug) is the term used to describe any of a class of drugs used in clinical conditions of hyperlipidaemia, where the blood plasma contains very high levels of certain of the lipids cholesterol and/or triglycerides (natural fats of the body). Current medical opinion suggests that if diet, or drugs, can be used to lower levels of LDL-cholesterol (low-density lipoprotein) while raising HDL-cholesterol (high-density lipoprotein), then there may be a regression of the progress of coronary atherosclerosis (a diseased state of the arteries of the heart where plaques of lipid material narrow blood vessels, which contributes to angina pectoris attacks and the formation of abnormal clots that go on to

cause heart attacks and strokes). Because the drugs lower some lipid levels whilst raising others, this group of drugs is now referred to as *lipid-regulating* rather than *lipid-lowering* drugs. Currently, lipid-regulating drugs are used with priority where there is a family history of hyperlipidaemia, or clinical signs (eg cardiovascular disorders, or those with the highest plasma concentrations of cholesterol) indicating the need for intervention. In most individuals, an appropriate low-fat diet can adequately do what is required. Also some can be used in ANTI-ANGINA and HEART FAILURE TREATMENT through lowering of atheromatous disease.

Lipid-lowering drugs work in a number of ways: CHOLESTYRAMINE and COLESTIPOL HYDROCHLORIDE are ion-exchange resins that reduces bile salt reabsorption from the gut, so changing cholesterol metabolism, lowering LDL-cholesterol production (though triglycerides levels may rise). The *fibrate group* of drugs (BEZAFIBRATE, CIPROFIBRATE, CLOFIBRATE, FENOFIBRATE and GEMFIBROZIL) reduce, in particular triglycerides, but also increase LDL-cholesterol and raise HDL-cholesterol. The (*statin*) drugs (ATORVASTATIN, FLUVASTATIN, PRAVASTATIN SODIUM and SIMVASTATIN) are ENZYME INHIBITOR drugs which inhibit an enzyme which synthesizes cholesterol in the liver with the main effect that LDL-cholesterol is lowered. The *nicotinic acid group* (ACIPIMOX and NICOTINIC ACID) can lower cholesterol and triglyceride levels by an action on enzymes in the liver. The *fish oils* (eg OMEGA-3 MARINE TRIGLYCERIDES) are dietary supplements that may be useful in treating high triglyceride levels (hypertriglyceridaemia).

▲ Warnings: It has been reported that forms of NICOTINIC ACID (niacin) if taken with drugs of the statin group (eg lovastatin) may result in toxic effects (myopathy and rhabdomyolysis) and so are best avoided. See individual drug entries for more information.

Lipitor

(Parke-Davis; Pfizer) is a proprietary, prescription-only preparation of the LIPID-REGULATING DRUG atorvastatin. It can be used in hyperlipidaemia to change the proportions of various lipids in the bloodstream. It is available as tablets.

✚▲ Side-effects/warnings: See ATORVASTATIN.

Lipostat

(Squibb; Bristol-Myers Squibb) is a proprietary, prescription-only preparation of the LIPID-REGULATING DRUG pravastatin sodium. It can be used in hyperlipidaemia to change the proportions of various lipids in the bloodstream. It is available as tablets.

✚▲ Side-effects/warnings: See PRAVASTATIN SODIUM.

Liqufruta Garlic Cough Medicine

(Warner Lambert Consumer Healthcare; Pfizer) is a proprietary, non-prescription preparation of the EXPECTORANT agent guaifenesin (guaiphenesin). It can be used to relieve chesty coughs, hoarseness and sore throats when there is an infection of the respiratory tract. It is available as an oral liquid.

✚▲ Side-effects/warnings: See GUAIFENESIN.

Liqui-Char

(Oxford) is a proprietary, non-prescription preparation of activated charcoal. It can be used to treat patients suffering from poisoning or a drug overdose. It is available as an oral suspension.

✚▲ Side-effects/warnings: See ACTIVATED CHARCOAL.

Liquid Gaviscon

(Reckitt Benckiser Healthcare) is a proprietary, non-prescription compound preparation of the ANTACID agents sodium bicarbonate and calcium carbonate, and the DEMULCENT alginic acid (as sodium alginate). It can be used for the symptomatic relief of heartburn and indigestion due to acid reflux, and is available as a liquid suspension. It is not normally given to children under two years, except on medical advice.

✚▲ Side-effects/warnings: See ALGINIC ACID; CALCIUM CARBONATE; SODIUM BICARBONATE.

liquid paraffin

is a traditional (*faecal-softener*) LAXATIVE which can be used to relieve constipation. It is a constituent of a number of proprietary laxatives and some non-proprietary preparations. It is also incorporated into many skin treatment preparations as an EMOLLIENT.

✚ Side-effects: Because only a little of the paraffin

is absorbed in the intestines, seepage may occur from the anus causing local irritation. Prolonged use may interfere with the absorption of fat-soluble vitamins and other problems.
▲ Warnings: Prolonged or continuous use of liquid paraffin as a laxative is to be avoided. It should not be taken immediately before going to bed.
✪ Related entries: Alcoderm; Care Aqueous Cream; Cetraben Emollient Cream; Dermol 200 Shower Emollient; Dermalo; Dermol 500 Lotion; Diprobath; Doublebase; E45; Emulsiderm Emollient; Emulsifying Ointment, BP; Hewletts Cream; Hydromol Emollient; Imuderm; Keri; Lacri-Lube; Lubri-Tears; Mil-Par; Oilatum Bath Formula; Oilatum Junior; Oilatum Junior Flare-Up; Polytar Emmollient; Simple Eye Ointment; Sprilon; Unguentum M.

Liquifilm Tears

(Allergan) is a proprietary, non-prescription preparation of polyvinyl alcohol. It can be used as artificial tears where there is dryness of the eyes, and is available as eye-drops (with or without povidone).
✚▲ Side-effects/warnings: See POLYVINYL ALCOHOL; POVIDONE.

liquorice

is an extract from a leguminous plant. It has a strong flavour and can be used in medicines with unpleasant tastes. Liquorice extract also has a weak EXPECTORANT activity and is therefore incorporated into a number of cough remedies. There are certain preparations of liquorice that have been used to treat peptic ulcers, some are prepared from 'deglycyrrhizinised liquorice' and others are a synthetic chemical derivative of glycyrrhizinic acid (CARBENOXOLONE SODIUM).
✚ Side-effects: In high doses, glycyrrhizinic acid, a constituent of liquorice, commonly causes sodium and water retention, and occasionally hypokalaemia.
▲ Warnings: Glycyrrhizinic acid may cause or exacerbate hypertension, oedema, cardiac failure and muscle weakness.
✪ Related entry: Ammonia and Ipecacuanha Mixture, BP.

lisinopril

is an ACE INHIBITOR and acts as a VASODILATOR. It can be used as an ANTIHYPERTENSIVE and congestive HEART FAILURE TREATMENT, often used in conjunction with other classes of drug, particularly (THIAZIDE) DIURETIC drugs; also in diabetic neuropathy and after myocardial infarction. Administration is oral.
✚▲ Side-effects/warnings: See ACE INHIBITOR. Also speeding of the heart, cerebrovascular accident, myocardial infarction; dry mouth, confusion and mood changes, muscle weakness, sweating, impotence and hair loss.
✪ Related entries: Carace; Carace Plus; Zestoretic; Zestril.

Liskonum

(SmithKline Beecham; GSK) is a proprietary, prescription-only preparation of the ANTIMANIA drug lithium (as lithium carbonate). It can be used to prevent and treat mania, manic-depressive bouts and recurrent depression, and is available as tablets.
✚▲ Side-effects/warnings: See LITHIUM.

lisuride maleate

(lysuride maleate) is an ANTIPARKINSONISM drug that is an ERGOT ALKALOID derivative and which works as a DOPAMINE-RECEPTOR STIMULANT, acting particularly on DOPAMINE receptors in the brain.

It has actions that are similar to those of BROMOCRIPTINE and is particularly useful in patients who cannot tolerate levodopa. Administration is oral.
✚ Side-effects: Headache, nausea and vomiting, dizziness, lethargy, malaise, psychotic reactions (including hallucinations), drowsiness, hypotensive reactions, rashes, constipation and abdominal pain.
▲ Warnings: It should be administered with caution to patients with a history of psychosis, porphyria, who have had a pituitary tumour; or are pregnant. It should not be given to patients with certain, severe cardiovascular disorders. It may impair the performance of skilled tasks, such as driving.

lithium

in the form of lithium carbonate or lithium citrate is singularly effective as an ANTIMANIA drug to control or prevent the hyperactive manic episodes in manic-depressive illness, and can be used to prevent depression in recurrent depressive illness and other behavioural problems. It may also reduce the frequency and severity of depressive episodes. How it works remains imperfectly understood, but its use is so successful that the side-effects (caused by its toxicity) are deemed to be justified. Administration, following specialist advice, is oral.

See also, topically, LITHIUM SUCCINATE (with different pharmacology) which is used as an ANTISEBORRHOEIC.

✚ Side-effects: Lithium for oral use is prescribed following specialist advice and full evaluation. Many long-term patients experience nausea, thirst and excessive urination, gastrointestinal disturbance including vomiting and diarrhoea, weakness and tremor. There may be fluid retention and consequent weight gain. Visual disturbances, worsening gastric problems, vomiting, muscle weakness, twitching, tremor and lack of co-ordination (and eventually convulsions and coma) indicate lithium intoxication.

▲ Warnings: Lithium should not be administered to patients with certain heart or kidney disorders, or imperfect sodium balance in the bloodstream. It should be administered with caution to those who are pregnant or breast-feeding, who are elderly, taking diuretics or have myasthenia gravis. Prolonged treatment may cause serious kidney damage and thyroid gland dysfunction; prolonged overdosage eventually causes serious effects on the brain. Consequently, blood levels of lithium must be regularly checked for toxicity, thyroid function must be monitored and there must be adequate intake of fluids and sodium. Dietary changes that might change sodium intake should be avoided. Diuretic drugs, SSRI antidepressant drugs, sodium salts (eg SODIUM BICARBONATE) and NSAIDS, may decrease lithium excretion and increase its effects and CNS toxicity. Withdrawal must be gradual.

✪ Related entries: Camcolit; Efalith; Li-Liquid; Liskonum; Priadel.

lithium carbonate

see LITHIUM.

lithium citrate

see LITHIUM.

lithium succinate

is used as an ANTISEBORRHOEIC for seborrhoeic dermatitis. Administration is topical.

✚▲ Side-effects/warnings: Occasionally there may be skin irritation. Avoid mucous membranes and eyes.

✪ Related entry: Efalith.

Livial

(Organon) is a proprietary, prescription-only preparation of the drug tibolone, which has both OESTROGEN and PROGESTOGEN activity. It can be used in HRT, and is available as tablets.

✚▲ Side-effects/warnings: See TIBOLONE.

Livostin

(Novartis Ophthalmics) is proprietary, prescription-only preparation of the ANTIHISTAMINE levocabastine. It can be used for the symptomatic relief of allergic rhinitis and allergic conjunctivitis, and is available as a nasal spray and as eye-drops. A version available without a prescription is called *Livostin direct*.

✚▲ Side-effects/warnings: See LEVOCABASTINE.

Lloyd's Cream

(SSL) is a proprietary, non-prescription preparation of diethylamine salicylate, which has a COUNTER-IRRITANT, OR RUBEFACIENT, action. It can be applied to the skin for the symptomatic relief of musculoskeletal rheumatic and inflammatory pains, and is available as a cream. It is not normally given to children under six years, except on medical advice.

✚▲ Side-effects/warnings: See DIETHYLAMINE SALICYLATE.

Locabiotal

(Servier) is a proprietary, prescription-only preparation of the ANTI-INFLAMMATORY and ANTIBIOTIC drug fusafungine. It can be used to treat infection, for instance in the nose and throat, and is available as an aerosol with a nose and mouth adapter.

✚▲ Side-effects/warnings: See FUSAFUNGINE.

local anaesthetic 🅱

drugs are used to reduce sensation (especially pain) in a specific, local area of the body and without loss of consciousness. GENERAL ANAESTHETIC drugs, in contrast, decrease sensation only because of a loss of consciousness. Local anaesthetics work by reversibly blocking the transmission of impulses in nerves. They can be administered by a number of routes and always close to their site of action. By local injection or infiltration, they can be used for dental and minor surgery (such as sutures) and vasectomy. A more extensive loss of sensation with nerve block (eg injected near to the nerve supplying a limb) or with spinal anaesthesia (eg epidural injection in childbirth) or intrathecal block (for extensive procedures) produces a loss of sensation in whole areas of the body sufficient to allow major surgery (though with some, quickly reversible paralysis). Local anaesthetics are particularly valuable where the use of a general anaesthetic carries a high risk, or when the co-operation of the patient is required. When administered into a vascular region, ADRENALINE is co-injected and acts as a VASOCONSTRICTOR to limit the rate at which the anaesthetic is washed away. When applied topically, certain local anaesthetics are well absorbed from mucous membranes and abraded skin and can be used to treat discomfort at many sites. See BENZOCAINE; BUPIVACAINE HYDROCHLORIDE; CINCHOCAINE; COCAINE; LIDOCAINE HYDROCHLORIDE; OXETHAZAINE; OXYBUPROCAINE HYDROCHLORIDE; PRILOCAINE HYDROCHLORIDE; PROCAINAMIDE HYDROCHLORIDE; PROCAINE; PROXYMETACAINE; TETRACAINE.

local hormone 🅱

is the term used to describe mediators that are released within the body to act at a site local to their point of release. In this respect, as mediators of body signals, they differ from blood-borne (*endocrine*) hormones (see HORMONE), which are released from specific glands and generally act remote to the point of release, and neurotransmitters, which are released only from nerves and act very close to the point of release. Local hormones have many functions in the body.

One of their best-understood functions is their role in inflammation. It is known that local hormones are often released as a result of an injury to tissues or because of an allergic reaction and mediate responses in the body that are pro-inflammatory (cause inflammation). Reactions such as these are generally intended to protect the body, but if too extreme or inappropriate they can cause adverse effects on health and need to be controlled with drugs. Many of the ANTI-INFLAMMATORY and ANTI-ALLERGIC drugs in common medical use work by preventing the formation, release or actions of local hormones. Examples of pro-inflammatory local hormones are histamine and the members of the PROSTAGLANDIN family. ANTIHISTAMINE drugs inhibit the effects in the body of the local hormone histamine by blocking its RECEPTORS, whereas the NSAID drugs (eg ASPIRIN and IBUPROFEN) work by preventing the formation, and hence release, of the prostaglandin local hormones. CORTICOSTEROID and SODIUM CROMOGLICATE-related drugs are also of value in treating allergic conditions where local hormones are released; for example, for asthma and skin conditions such as eczema and psoriasis.

By no means all actions of local hormones are undesirable and many are part of normal body function. For instance, the prostaglandins play a part in controlling the blood flow in the mucosal lining of the stomach and intestine and act as CYTOPROTECTANT and ulcer-healing drugs (see ULCER-HEALING DRUG). Prostaglandins may also have a role in controlling motility and other functions of the intestine and uterus. The latter actions are used in obstetrics by the administration of synthetic preparations of the naturally occurring members of the prostaglandin family, such as prostaglandin E_2 (DINOPROSTONE) or prostacyclin (EPOPROSTENOL), or synthetic analogues (eg MISOPROSTOL), which mimic the actions where prostaglandins are potent in contraction of the uterus, softening and dilation of the cervix and dilation of blood vessels. These actions can be used for abortion and in aiding labour and after childbirth.

Loceryl

(Galderma) is a proprietary, prescription-only preparation of the ANTIFUNGAL drug amorolfine. It can be used topically to treat fungal skin infections, and is available as a cream and a nail lacquer.

✚▲ Side-effects/warnings: See AMOROLFINE.

Lockets Medicated Linctus

(Thornton & Ross) is a proprietary, non-prescription compound preparation of the EXPECTORANT ipecacuanha with glycerol and purified honey. It can be used to relieve cough and sore throat. Available as an oral liquid. Not normally given to children, except on medical advice.

✚▲ Side-effects/warnings: See GLYCEROL; IPECACUANHA.

Locoid

(Yamanouchi) is a proprietary, prescription-only preparation of the CORTICOSTEROID hydrocortisone (as butyrate). It can be used for serious inflammatory skin conditions, such as eczema and psoriasis, and is available as a cream (*Lipocream*), an ointment and a scalp lotion, and a lotion for topical application (*Locoid Crelo*).
✚▲ Side-effects/warnings: See HYDROCORTISONE.

Locoid C

(Yamanouchi) is a proprietary, prescription-only compound preparation of the CORTICOSTEROID hydrocortisone (as butyrate) and the ANTIMICROBIAL chlorquinaldol. It can be used to treat inflammatory skin conditions, such as eczema, and is available as a cream and an ointment.
✚▲ Side-effects/warnings: See CHLORQUINALDOL; HYDROCORTISONE.

Locorten-Vioform

(Novartis Consumer Health) is a proprietary, prescription-only compound preparation of the CORTICOSTEROID flumetasone pivalate and the ANTIMICROBIAL clioquinol. It can be used to treat eczematous inflammation of the outer ear, and is available as ear-drops.
✚▲ Side-effects/warnings: See CLIOQUINOL; FLUMETASONE PIVALATE.

Lodine SR

(Shire) is a proprietary, prescription-only preparation of the (NSAID) NON-NARCOTIC ANALGESIC and ANTIRHEUMATIC etodolac. It can be used to treat the pain of osteoarthritis and rheumatoid arthritis, and is available as tablets.
✚▲ Side-effects/warnings: See ETODOLAC.

lodoxamide

is an ANTI-INFLAMMATORY drug introduced for seasonal allergic conjunctivitis. Administration is as eye-drops.
✚ Side-effects: Short-lived mild burning and stinging, itching and excess tear formation; also, flushing and dizziness.
✪ **Related entry: Alomide.**

Loestrin 20

(Parke-Davis; Pfizer) is a proprietary, prescription-only compound preparation that can be used as a (*monophasic*) ORAL CONTRACEPTIVE of the *COC* (low strength) type that combines an OESTROGEN and a PROGESTOGEN, in this case ethinylestradiol and norethisterone. It is available as tablets in a calendar pack.
✚▲ Side-effects/warnings: See ETHINYLESTRADIOL; NORETHISTERONE.

Loestrin 30

(Parke-Davis; Pfizer) is a proprietary, prescription-only compound preparation that can be used as a (*monophasic*) ORAL CONTRACEPTIVE of the *COC* (standard strength) type that combines an OESTROGEN and a PROGESTOGEN, in this case ethinylestradiol and norethisterone. It is available as tablets in a calendar pack.
✚▲ Side-effects/warnings: See ETHINYLESTRADIOL; NORETHISTERONE.

Lofensaid

(Trinity) is a prescription-only, proprietary version of the (NSAID) NON-NARCOTIC ANALGESIC and ANTIRHEUMATIC diclofenac sodium. It can be used to treat arthritic and rheumatic pain and inflammation and other musculoskeletal disorders. It is available as tablets.
✚▲ Side-effects/warnings: See DICLOFENAC SODIUM.

lofepramine

is an ANTIDEPRESSANT of the TRICYCLIC group. It has less SEDATIVE properties than other antidepressants and is therefore more suitable for the treatment of withdrawn and apathetic patients, rather than those who are agitated and restless. Administration is oral.
✚▲ Side-effects/warnings: See AMITRIPTYLINE HYDROCHLORIDE; but is less sedating. It should not be prescribed to patients with severe liver or kidney damage.
✪ **Related entries: Gamanil; Lomont.**

lofexidine hydrochloride

is a drug that is used to alleviate OPIOID withdrawal symptoms. It appears to have actions on sympathetic neurones in the brain in a similar way to CLONIDINE HYDROCHLORIDE. Administration is oral.
✚ Side-effects: Drowsiness, dry mouth, throat

and nose, hypotension, slowing of the heart and hypertension on withdrawal.
▲ Warnings: Use with caution in patients with certain heart and vascular disorders, kidney impairment, a history of depression or who are pregnant or breast-feeding.
✪ **Related entry: BritLofex.**

Logynon
(Schering Health) is a proprietary, prescription-only compound preparation that can be used as a (*triphasic*) ORAL CONTRACEPTIVE of the *COC* (standard strength) type that combines an OESTROGEN and a PROGESTOGEN, in this case ethinylestradiol and levonorgestrel. It is available as tablets in a calendar pack.
✚▲ Side-effects/warnings: See ETHINYLESTRADIOL; LEVONORGESTREL.

Logynon ED
(Schering Health) is a proprietary, prescription-only compound preparation that can be used as a (*triphasic*) ORAL CONTRACEPTIVE (and also for certain menstrual problems) of the (standard strength) *COC* type that combines an OESTROGEN and a PROGESTOGEN, in this case ethinylestradiol and levonorgestrel. It is available as tablets in a calendar pack.
✚▲ Side-effects/warnings: See ETHINYLESTRADIOL; LEVONORGESTREL.

lomefloxacin
is a broad-spectrum (QUINOLONE) ANTIBIOTIC-like ANTIBACTERIAL. It can be used to treat infections of the eye. Administration is in the from of eye-drops.
✚▲ Side-effects/warnings: See QUINOLONE. Given topically, there are few side-effects, but there may be local irritation (and rarely hypersensitivity reactions). Caution in pregnancy and breast-feeding.
✪ **Related entry: Okacyn.**

Lomexin
(Akita) is a proprietary, prescription-only preparation of the ANTIFUNGAL drug fenticonazole nitrate. It can be used to treat vaginal candidiasis (thrush), and is available as vaginal pessaries.
✚▲ Side-effects/warnings: See FENTICONAZOLE NITRATE.

Lomont
(Rosemont) is a proprietary, prescription-only preparation of the (TRICYCLIC) ANTIDEPRESSANT lofepramine (as hydrochloride). It can be used to treat depressive illness, and is available as an oral suspension.
✚▲ Side-effects/warnings: See LOFEPRAMINE.

Lomotil
(Goldshield) is a proprietary, prescription-only compound preparation of the ANTICHOLINERGIC drug atropine sulphate and the (OPIOID) ANTIDIARRHOEAL diphenoxylate hydrochloride, which is a combination called co-phenotrope. It can be used to treat chronic diarrhoea (eg in mild chronic ulcerative colitis), and is available as tablets.
✚▲ Side-effects/warnings: See ATROPINE SULPHATE; DIPHENOXYLATE HYDROCHLORIDE.

Lomustine
(Medac) is a non-proprietary, prescription-only preparation of the ANTICANCER drug lomustine. It can be used in the treatment of a number of cancers, and is available as capsules.
✚▲ Side-effects/warnings: See LOMUSTINE.

lomustine
is an (*alkylating agent*) CYTOTOXIC drug which is used as an ANTICANCER treatment, particularly for Hodgkin's disease (a type of cancer of the lymphatic tissues) and some solid tumours. It works by disrupting cellular DNA and so inhibiting cell replication. Administration is oral.
✚▲ Side-effects/warnings: See CYTOTOXIC. Nausea and vomiting can be quite severe.
✪ **Related entry: Lomustine**

Loniten
(Pharmacia) is a proprietary, prescription-only preparation of the VASODILATOR minoxidil. It can be used as an ANTIHYPERTENSIVE to treat severe acute hypertension (usually in combination with a DIURETIC OF BETA-BLOCKER), and is available as tablets.
✚▲ Side-effects/warnings: See MINOXIDIL.

LoperaGen
(Norgine) is a proprietary, prescription-only preparation of the (OPIOID) ANTIDIARRHOEAL loperamide hydrochloride. Can be used for the symptomatic relief of diarrhoea. Available as capsules.
✚▲ Side-effects/warnings: See LOPERAMIDE HYDROCHLORIDE.

L

loperamide hydrochloride

is an (OPIOID) ANTIDIARRHOEAL drug which acts on the nerves of the intestine to inhibit peristalsis (the waves of muscular activity that move along the contents of the intestines), so reducing motility, and also decreases fluid secretion in the intestines. Administration is oral. (Preparations containing loperamide hydrochloride are available without prescription for the treatment of acute diarrhoea only.)

✚▲ Side-effects/warnings: See OPIOID; but when used to treat acute diarrhoea there is little or no risk of dependence and it is less sedative. It is used with care in liver disease and pregnancy.

✪ **Related entries: Arret; Boots Diareze; Care Loperamide Hydrochloride Capsules 2 mg; Diah-Limit; Diasorb; Diocalm Ultra; Diocaps; Imodium Capsules; Imodium Liquid; Imodium Plus; LoperaGen; Norimode.**

Lopid

(Parke-Davis; Pfizer) is a proprietary, prescription-only preparation of the LIPID-REGULATING DRUG gemfibrozil. It can be used in hyperlipidaemia to modify the proportions of various lipids in the bloodstream. It is available as capsules (*Lopid 300*) and tablets (*Lopid 600*).

✚▲ Side-effects/warnings: See GEMFIBROZIL.

lopinavir

is a (*protease inhibitor*) ANTIVIRAL drug, available only in combination with the (*protease inhibitor*) ritonavir, and is used (in combination with other antiretrovirals) in the treatment of HIV infection. Administration is oral.

✚▲ Side-effects/warnings: See LOPINAVIR WITH RITONAVIR.

lopinavir with ritonavir

is a combination of two (*protease inhibitor*) ANTIVIRAL drugs, available only in combination, and is used (in combination with other antiretrovirals) in the treatment of HIV infection. Administration is oral.

✚ Side-effects: There are many, including diarrhoea, nausea and vomiting, abdominal discomfort and colitis, asthenia, insomnia, headache and rash. There may also be other less common effects.

▲ Warnings: It is not to be given to breast-feeding women, and with caution to those with liver or kidney impairment, or who are pregnant. The oral solution contains propylene glycol but there is increased susceptibility to propylene glycol toxicity in slow metabolizers, haemophiliacs, the pregnant and diabetics.

✪ **Related entry: Kaletra.**

Lopranol-LA

(Opus; Trinity) is a proprietary, prescription-only preparation of the BETA-BLOCKER propranolol hydrochloride. It can be used as an ANTIHYPERTENSIVE for raised blood pressure, as an ANTI-ANGINA treatment to relieve symptoms and improve exercise tolerance and as an ANTI-ARRHYTHMIC to regularize heartbeat and to treat myocardial infarction. It can also be used as an ANTITHYROID drug for short-term treatment of thyrotoxicosis, as an ANTIMIGRAINE treatment to prevent attacks, as an ANXIOLYTIC, particularly for symptomatic relief of tremor and palpitations, and, with an ALPHA-ADRENOCEPTOR BLOCKER, in the acute treatment of phaeochromocytoma. It is available as modified-release capsules.

✚▲ Side-effects/warnings: See PROPRANOLOL HYDROCHLORIDE.

Loprazolam

(Hoechst Marion Roussel; Aventis Pharma) is a non-proprietary, prescription-only preparation of the BENZODIAZEPINE loprazolam. It can be used as a relatively short-acting HYPNOTIC for the short-term treatment of insomnia, and is available as tablets.

✚▲ Side-effects/warnings: See LOPRAZOLAM.

loprazolam

is a BENZODIAZEPINE which is used as a relatively short-acting HYPNOTIC for the short-term treatment of insomnia. Administration is oral.

✚▲ Side-effects/warnings: See BENZODIAZEPINE.

✪ **Related entry: Loprazolam.**

Lopresor

(Novartis) is a proprietary, prescription-only preparation of the BETA-BLOCKER metoprolol tartrate. It can be used as an ANTIHYPERTENSIVE for raised blood pressure, as an ANTI-ANGINA treatment to relieve symptoms and improve exercise tolerance and as an ANTI-ARRHYTHMIC to regularize heartbeat and to treat myocardial infarction. It can also be used as an ANTITHYROID drug for short-term treatment of thyrotoxicosis and as an ANTIMIGRAINE treatment to prevent attacks. It is available as tablets (the modified-release version is called *Lopresor SR*).

✚▲ Side-effects/warnings: See METOPROLOL TARTRATE.

Lopresor SR

(Novartis) is a proprietary, prescription-only preparation of the BETA-BLOCKER metoprolol tartrate. It can be used as an ANTIHYPERTENSIVE for raised blood pressure. It is available as modified-release tablets.

✚▲ Side-effects/warnings: See METOPROLOL TARTRATE.

loratadine

is a recently developed ANTIHISTAMINE which has less sedative side-effects than some older members of its class and can be used for the symptomatic relief of allergic symptoms, such as hay fever and urticaria. Administration is oral.

✚▲ Side-effects/warnings: See ANTIHISTAMINE. But the incidence of sedative and anticholinergic effects is low; nevertheless, it may impair the performance of skilled tasks, such as driving. It should not be given to patients who are pregnant or breast-feeding.

✪ **Related entries: Clarityn; Clarityn Allergy Syrup; Clarityn Allergy Tablets.**

lorazepam

is a BENZODIAZEPINE with a number of applications. It is used as an ANXIOLYTIC in the short-term treatment of anxiety, as a HYPNOTIC for insomnia, as an ANTI-EPILEPTIC in status epilepticus and as a SEDATIVE in preoperative medication, because its ability to cause amnesia means that the patient forgets the unpleasant procedure. Administration is either oral or by injection.

✚▲ Side-effects/warnings: See BENZODIAZEPINE.

✪ **Related entry: Ativan.**

lormetazepam

is a BENZODIAZEPINE which is used as a relatively short-acting HYPNOTIC for the short-term treatment of insomnia. Administration is oral.

✚▲ Side-effects/warnings: See BENZODIAZEPINE.

lornoxicam

is a recently introduced (NSAID) NON-NARCOTIC ANALGESIC and ANTIRHEUMATIC drug, which can be used to treat pain and inflammation in rheumatoid arthritis, osteoarthritis and acute lumbo-sciatica, and pain after, for example, orthopaedic surgery. Administration is oral or by injection.

✚▲ Side-effects/warnings: See NSAID. There may also be flatulence, dry mouth, inflammation of the lining of the mouth, changes in taste and appetite, weight changes, speeding of the heart, agitation and tremor, a feeling of being unwell, paraesthesia, urination difficulties, muscle pain, sweating, hair loss, and reactions at the injection site. This drug is not used for patients with a range of conditions including heart and kidney conditions, and bleeding disorders.

✪ **Related entry: Xefo.**

Loron

(Roche) is a proprietary, prescription-only preparation of the CALCIUM METABOLISM MODIFIER sodium clodronate. It can be used to treat high calcium levels associated with malignant tumours and bone lesions. It is available as capsules (*Loron capsules*) and as tablets (*Loron 520*).

✚▲ Side-effects/warnings: See SODIUM CLODRONATE.

losartan potassium

is the first of the ANGIOTENSIN-RECEPTOR BLOCKER drugs, which work by blocking angiotensin receptors. Angiotensin II is a circulating HORMONE that is a powerful VASOCONSTRICTOR and blocking its effects leads to a fall in blood pressure. Losartan potassium can therefore be used as an ANTIHYPERTENSIVE. Administration is oral.

✚ Side-effects: Angiotensin-receptor antagonists in general cause postural hypotension (particularly in those on diuretics), raised blood potassium and angioedema. Losartan has caused taste disturbance, dizziness and changes in liver function, diarrhoea, muscle aches, rash, itching.

▲ Warnings: Angiotensin-receptor antagonists in general should be avoided in pregnancy and breast-feeding. It should be administered with care to those who have liver or kidney impairment or renal stenosis.

✪ **Related entries: Cozaar; Cozaar-Comp.**

Losec

(AstraZeneca) is a proprietary, prescription-only

preparation of the PROTON-PUMP INHIBITOR omeprazole. It can be used as an ULCER-HEALING DRUG and it is used for the treatment of benign gastric and duodenal ulcers (including those that complicate NSAID therapy), acid-related dyspepsia, Zollinger-Ellison syndrome and reflux oesophagitis (inflammation of the oesophagus caused by regurgitation of acid and enzymes), and acid reflux disease. It can also be used in conjunction with antibiotics to treat gastric *Helicobacter pylori* infection. It is available as capsules, dispersible tablets (*MUPS*) and a form for intravenous infusion.
✚▲ Side-effects/warnings: See OMEPRAZOLE.

Lotriderm
(Dominion) is a proprietary, prescription-only compound preparation of the CORTICOSTEROID betamethasone (as dipropionate) and the ANTIFUNGAL clotrimazole. It can be used to treat fungal infections, particularly those associated with inflammation, and is available as a cream for topical application.
✚▲ Side-effects/warnings: See BETAMETHASONE; CLOTRIMAZOLE.

low molecular weight heparin 🅱
is a form of ANTICOAGULANT of the HEPARIN type which has a smaller chemical size but has certain advantages over heparin. They are several examples and all are effective in the prevention of venous thrombo-embolism, particularly in orthopaedic practice. They have a longer duration of action than unfractionated heparin. Some low molecular weight heparins can be used in the treatment of deep-vein thrombosis and for the prevention of clotting in extracorporeal circuits, and for unstable angina. See CERTOPARIN; DALTEPARIN SODIUM; ENOXAPARIN; TINZAPARIN SODIUM.

Loxapac
(Lederle; Wyeth) is a proprietary, prescription-only preparation of the ANTIPSYCHOTIC drug loxapine. It can be used to treat acute and chronic psychoses, and is available as capsules.
✚▲ Side-effects/warnings: See LOXAPINE.

loxapine
is an ANTIPSYCHOTIC drug which is used to treat acute and chronic psychoses. Administration is oral.
✚▲ Side-effects/warnings: See CHLORPROMAZINE HYDROCHLORIDE; but there may be nausea and vomiting, changes in weight, shortness of breath, drooping of the eyelids, raised body temperature, tingling sensation in the extremities, flushing and headache. It is not used in people with porphyria.
✪ **Related entry: Loxapac.**

Luborant
(Antigen) is a proprietary, non-prescription compound preparation of carmellose sodium, potassium chloride, sorbitol and other salts. It can be used as a form of ARTIFICIAL SALIVA for application to the mouth and throat in conditions (eg certain drug treatments, diseases and radiotherapy) that make the mouth abnormally dry. It is available as an oral spray.
✚▲ Side-effects/warnings: See CARMELLOSE SODIUM; POTASSIUM CHLORIDE; SODIUM CHLORIDE; SORBITOL.

Lubri-Tears
(Alcon) is a proprietary, non-prescription compound preparation of liquid paraffin and white soft paraffin and wool fat. It can be used as an eye lubricant for dry eye conditions, and is available as an eye ointment.
✚▲ Side-effects/warnings: See LIQUID PARAFFIN; WHITE SOFT PARAFFIN; WOOL FAT.

Ludiomil
(Novartis) is a proprietary, prescription-only preparation of the TRICYCLIC-related ANTIDEPRESSANT maprotiline hydrochloride. It can be used to treat depressive illness, especially in cases where sedation is required, and is available as tablets.
✚▲ Side-effects/warnings: See MAPROTILINE HYDROCHLORIDE.

Lugol's solution
see AQUEOUS IODINE ORAL SOLUTION.

Lustral
(Pfizer) is a proprietary, prescription-only preparation of the (SSRI) ANTIDEPRESSANT sertraline; and is also used for obsessive-compulsive disorders. It is available as tablets.
✚▲ Side-effects/warnings: See SERTRALINE.

luteinising hormone
(LH) is a HORMONE secreted by the anterior pituitary gland and (along with FOLLICLE-

STIMULATING HORMONE; FSH) is a gonadotrophin (gonadotropin) hormone. In women, in conjunction with FSH, it causes the monthly ripening in one ovary of a follicle and stimulates ovulation. In men, it facilitates the production of sperm in the testes (hence its alternative name interstitial cell-stimulating hormone; ICSH). It may be injected therapeutically, along with FSH, in infertility treatment to stimulate ovulation. It is available, in combination with FSH, as human menopausal gonadotrophin (see HUMAN MENOPAUSAL GONADOTROPHINS); MENOTROPHIN. See also CHORIONIC GONADOTROPHIN and MENOTROPHIN.
✪ **Related entry: Menogon.**

lutropin alpha

is a recently introduced recombinant (synthetic) form of a gonadotrophin (gonadotropin) HORMONE, LUTEINISING HORMONE (LH). LH is normally secreted by the anterior pituitary gland and (along with FOLLICLE-STIMULATING HORMONE). In women, LH in conjunction with FSH causes the monthly ripening in one ovary of a follicle and stimulates ovulation. In men, it facilitates the production of sperm in the testes (its alternative name is interstitial cell-stimulating hormone; ICSH). It may be injected therapeutically, along with FSH, in infertility treatment to stimulate ovulation. It is given by injection.
✚ Side-effects: Nausea and vomiting, pain in the pelvis and abdomen, sleepiness, over-stimulation of the ovary and ovarian cyst, breast pain, thromboembolism and others. Its use can cause ectopic pregnancies. There may be reactions at the site where it is injected.
▲ Warnings: Lutropin alpha is not used in women with ovarian enlargement or cysts, tumours of pituitary and hypothalamus, undiagnosed vaginal bleeding, breast, uterus or ovarian cancer. Before it is prescribed, the doctor will exclude certain causes of infertility to assess its suitability.
✪ **Related entry: Luveris.**

Luveris

(Serono) is a proprietary, prescription-only HORMONE preparation of lutropin alpha, which is a synthetic form of LUTEINISING HORMONE (LH). It can be used to treat infertility in women and is available in a form for injection.
✚▲ Side-effects/warnings: See LUTROPIN ALPHA.

Lyclear Creme Rinse

(Warner Lambert Consumer Healthcare; Pfizer) is a proprietary, non-prescription preparation of the SCABICIDAL and PEDICULICIDAL drug permethrin. It can be used for the treatment of head-louse infestation, and is available as a cream rinse. It is not normally used on infants under six months, except on medical advice.
✚▲ Side-effects/warnings: See PERMETHRIN.

Lyclear Dermal Creme

(Kestrel) is a proprietary, non-prescription preparation of the SCABICIDAL and PEDICULICIDAL drug permethrin. It can be used for the treatment of scabies and for crab lice in adults (over 18 years). It is available as a skin cream.
✚▲ Side-effects/warnings: See PERMETHRIN.

lymecycline

is a broad-spectrum ANTIBACTERIAL and (TETRACYCLINES) ANTIBIOTIC which can be used to treat infections of many kinds. Administration is oral.
✚▲ Side-effects/warnings: See TETRACYCLINE.
✪ **Related entry: Tetralysal 300.**

Lypsyl Cold Sore Gel

(Novartis Consumer Health) is a proprietary, non-prescription compound preparation of the LOCAL ANAESTHETIC lidocaine hydrochloride, the ANTISEPTIC cetrimide, and the ASTRINGENT zinc sulphate. It can be used for the symptomatic relief of painful cold sores, and is available as a gel for topical application. It is not normally given to children, except on medical advice.
✚▲ Side-effects/warnings: See CETRIMIDE; LIDOCAINE HYDROCHLORIDE; ZINC SULPHATE.

lysuride maleate

see LISURIDE MALEATE.

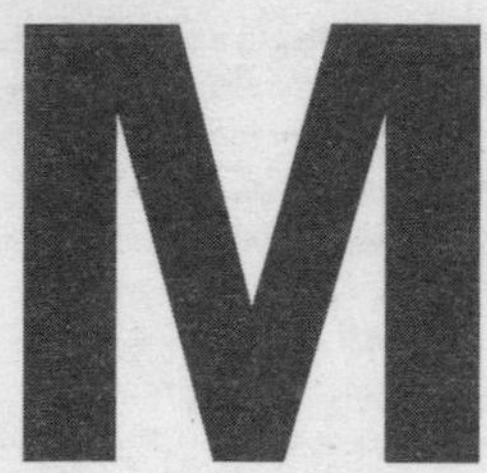

Maalox Plus

(Rhône-Poulenc Rorer; Aventis Pharma) is a proprietary, non-prescription compound preparation of the ANTACID agents magnesium hydroxide and aluminium hydroxide together with the ANTIFOAMING AGENT activated dimeticone. It can be used for the symptomatic relief of dyspepsia, gastric hyperacidity and gastritis. It is available as a suspension and as tablets.

✚▲ Side-effects/warnings: See ALUMINIUM HYDROXIDE; DIMETICONE; MAGNESIUM HYDROXIDE.

Maalox TC Tablets and Suspension

(Rhône-Poulenc Rorer; Aventis Pharma) is a proprietary, non-prescription compound preparation of the ANTACID agents magnesium hydroxide and aluminium hydroxide (in a combination called *co-magaldrox*). It can be used for the symptomatic relief of dyspepsia, and is available as a tablets.

✚▲ Side-effects/warnings: See ALUMINIUM HYDROXIDE; MAGNESIUM HYDROXIDE.

MabCampath

(Schering Health) is a proprietary, prescription-only preparation of alemtuzumab, which is a (CYTOTOXIC) IMMUNOSUPPRESSANT. It has recently been introduced for ANTICANCER treatment in individuals who have chronic lymphocytic leukaemia. It is available in a form for intravenous infusion.

✚▲ Side-effects/warnings: See ALEMTUZUMAB.

MabThera

(Roche) is a proprietary, prescription-only preparation of the drug rituximab, a (CYTOTOXIC) IMMUNOSUPPRESSANT. It has recently been introduced for ANTICANCER treatment in individuals who have chemotherapy-resistant advanced follicular lymphoma. It is available in a form for intravenous infusion.

✚▲ Side-effects/warnings: See RITUXIMAB.

Macrobid

(Goldshield) is a proprietary, prescription-only preparation of the ANTIBACTERIAL nitrofurantoin. It can be used to treat urinary tract infections and before surgery, and is available as capsules.

✚▲ Side-effects/warnings: See NITROFURANTOIN.

Macrodantin

(Goldshield) is a proprietary, prescription-only preparation of the ANTIBACTERIAL nitrofurantoin. It can be used to treat urinary tract infections, and is available as capsules.

✚▲ Side-effects/warnings: See NITROFURANTOIN.

macrolide 🅱

drugs are a chemical class of antibiotics (see ANTIBIOTIC) which are used for their ANTIBACTERIAL action. They have a similar spectrum of action to PENICILLIN, but act in a different way; they work by inhibiting microbial protein synthesis (they are *bacteriostatic* or *bacteriocidal* depending on concentration and circumstances). Their principal use is as an alternative antibiotic in patients who are allergic to penicillin. The original and best-known member of the group is ERYTHROMYCIN, which is effective against many bacteria, including streptococci (which can cause soft tissue and respiratory tract infections), Legionella (legionnaires' disease) and chlamydia (urethritis), and is also used in the treatment of acne, chronic prostatitis, diphtheria and whooping cough. The macrolides are relatively non-toxic (eg nausea, vomiting, diarrhoea) and serious side-effects are rare. See also AZITHROMYCIN; CLARITHROMYCIN.

Madopar

(Roche) is a proprietary, prescription-only compound preparation of levodopa and BENSERAZIDE HYDROCHLORIDE, which is a combination called co-beneldopa. It can be used to treat parkinsonism, but not the parkinsonian symptoms induced by drugs (see

ANTIPARKINSONISM). It is available as tablets, capsules (both in several preparations of different strengths) and modified-release capsules called *Madopar CR*.
✚▲ Side-effects/warnings: See LEVODOPA.

Magnapen

(CP) is a proprietary, prescription-only compound preparation of the broad-spectrum, penicillin-like ANTIBACTERIAL and ANTIBIOTIC ampicillin and the *penicillinase-resistant*, penicillin-like antibacterial and antibiotic flucloxacillin (a combination called *co-fluampicil*). It can be used to treat severe mixed infections where penicillin-resistant bacterial infection is probable. It is available as capsules, a syrup and in a form for injection.
✚▲ Side-effects/warnings: See AMPICILLIN; CO-FLUAMPICIL; FLUCLOXACILLIN.

magnesium

is a metallic element necessary to the body and is ingested as a trace element in a well-balanced diet (a good source is leafy green vegetables). It is essential to the bones and important for the proper functioning of nerves and muscles. It is essential in the regulation of several enzymes. Therapeutically, magnesium is used in the form of its salts: MAGNESIUM CARBONATE, MAGNESIUM HYDROXIDE, magnesium oxide (magnesia) and MAGNESIUM TRISILICATE are ANTACID; MAGNESIUM SULPHATE (Epsom salt/salts) is a LAXATIVE. Magnesium deficiency is usually treated with supplements of MAGNESIUM CHLORIDE.

magnesium carbonate

is an ANTACID that also has LAXATIVE properties. It is a mild antacid but fairly long-acting and is a constituent of many proprietary preparations that are used to relieve hyperacidity and dyspepsia and for the symptomatic relief of heartburn or a peptic ulcer. Administration is oral.
✚ Side-effects: There may be belching due to the internal liberation of carbon dioxide; and diarrhoea.
▲ Warnings: It should be administered with caution to patients with impaired function of the kidneys, or who are taking certain other drugs. It is not to be taken by those with low phosphate levels.
✪ Related entries: Actonorm Powder; Aludrox Tablets; Andrews Antacid; Bisodol Extra Strong Mint; Bisodol Indigestion Relief Powder; Bisodol Indigestion Relief Tablets; Bisodol Wind Relief; Citramag; Digestif Rennie Peppermint Flavour; Dijex Tablets; Rennie Deflatine; Rennie Duo; Topal.

magnesium chloride

is the form of MAGNESIUM that can be used to make up a magnesium deficiency in the body, which may result from either prolonged diarrhoea or vomiting or due to alcoholism. It is also incorporated into saline for eyewashes.
✚▲ Side-effects/warnings: It is regarded as safe in normal topical use.

magnesium hydroxide

or hydrated magnesium oxide (*magnesia*), is an ANTACID that also has LAXATIVE properties. As an antacid it is comparatively weak but fairly long-acting and is a constituent of many proprietary preparations that are used to relieve hyperacidity and dyspepsia and for the symptomatic relief of heartburn or a peptic ulcer. It can also be used to treat constipation. Administration is oral.
✚ Side-effects: There may be diarrhoea.
▲ Warnings: It should be administered with caution to patients with impaired function of the kidneys, certain gastrointestinal conditions or who are taking certain other drugs.
✪ Related entries: Actonorm Gel; Aludrox Tablets; Dijex Suspension; Maalox Plus; Maalox TC Tablets and Suspension; Mil-Par; Mucaine; Mucogel Suspension; Phillips' Milk of Magnesia; Phillips' Milk of Magnesia Tablets.

magnesium sulphate

(Epsom salt(s)) is an *osmotic* LAXATIVE. It works by preventing the reabsorption of water within the intestines and can be used to facilitate rapid bowel evacuation. Occasionally, it can also be used as a MAGNESIUM supplement in magnesium deficiency, in the emergency treatment of heart arrhythmias and for patients thought to have suffered myocardial infarction and in eclampsia (by injection or intravenous infusion). Applied topically as a paste with GLYCEROL it can be used to treat boils and carbuncles.
✚ Side-effects: When taken orally, there may be colic and diarrhoea, and after excess doses (orally or by injection), there may be nausea, vomiting,

M

thirst, flushing, effects on heart and blood pressure, depression, confusion, drowsiness, and other effects. Topical application is considered safe.
▲ Warnings: When administered orally, care must be taken in patients with renal or liver impairment and do not use in severe gastrointestinal impairment.
✪ **Related entry: Original Andrews Salts.**

magnesium trisilicate

is used as an ANTACID and has a long duration of action. It is a constituent of many proprietary preparations that are used to relieve hyperacidity and dyspepsia and for the symptomatic relief of heartburn or a peptic ulcer. Administration is oral.
✚ Side-effects: It may cause diarrhoea.
▲ Warnings: It should be administered with caution to patients with impaired function of the kidneys, or who are taking certain other drugs.
✪ **Related entries: Asilone Heartburn Liquid; Asilone Heartburn Tablets; Gastrocote Liquid; Gastrocote Tablets; Gaviscon 250; Gaviscon 500 Lemon Flavour Tablets; Pyrogastrone.**

major tranquillizer 🅔

see ANTIPSYCHOTIC.

Malarone

(GlaxoWellcome; GSK) is a proprietary, prescription-only compound preparation of the ANTIMALARIAL proguanil hydrochloride together with the ANTIPROTOZOAL atovaquone. It can be used in the prevention of malaria, and is available as tablets.
✚▲ Side-effects/warnings: See ATOVAQUONE; PROGUANIL HYDROCHLORIDE.

malathion

is an insecticidal drug which is used as a PEDICULICIDAL to treat infestations by head and pubic ('crab') lice, or as a SCABICIDAL to treat skin infestation by mites (scabies). Administration is topical.
✚ Side-effects: Skin irritation.
▲ Warnings: Avoid contact with the eyes and do not use on broken or infected skin. Some preparations (eg those in an alcohol base) are not suitable for asthmatics or those with eczema. Repeated application is not recommended.
✪ **Related entries: Derbac-M Liquid; Prioderm Cream Shampoo; Prioderm Lotion; Quellada-M Cream Shampoo; Quellada-M Liquid; Suleo-M Lotion.**

malic acid

is a weak organic acid found in apples and some fruits. It is incorporated into some medicinal preparations, such as ARTIFICIAL SALIVA and skin treatments, to adjust their acidity.
✚▲ Side-effects/warnings: It is regarded as safe in normal topical use.
✪ **Related entries: Aserbine; Salivix.**

Maloprim

(GlaxoWellcome; GSK) is a proprietary, prescription-only compound preparation of the ANTIBACTERIAL and ANTIMALARIAL dapsone and the antimalarial pyrimethamine. It can be used to prevent visitors to tropical regions from contracting malaria, and is available as tablets.
✚▲ Side-effects/warnings: See DAPSONE; PYRIMETHAMINE.

Manerix

(Roche) is a proprietary, prescription-only preparation of the MONOAMINE-OXIDASE INHIBITOR (MAOI) ANTIDEPRESSANT moclobemide, and can be used to treat major depressive illness and social phobia. It is available as tablets.
✚▲ Side-effects/warnings: See MOCLOBEMIDE.

Manevac

(Galen) is a proprietary, non-prescription compound preparation of the (*bulking-agent*) LAXATIVE ispaghula husk and the (*stimulant*) laxative senna. It can be used to treat constipation, and is available as granules. It is not normally given to children, except on medical advice.
✚▲ Side-effects/warnings: See ISPAGHULA HUSK; SENNA.

mannitol

is one of the *osmotic* class of DIURETIC drugs. It consists of substances secreted into the kidney proximal tubules, which are not resorbed and so carry water and mineral salts into the urine, therefore increasing the volume produced. Therapeutically, it is used primarily to treat oedema, particularly cerebral (brain) oedema. It may also be used in GLAUCOMA TREATMENT to

decrease pressure within the eyeball in acute attacks. Administration is by intravenous infusion.
✚ Side-effects: There may be chills and fever.
▲ Warnings: It is not to be administered to patients with congestive heart failure or fluid on the lungs (pulmonary oedema). An escape of mannitol into the tissues from the site of infusion (vein) can cause inflammation and death of the surrounding tissue.

MAOI

see MONOAMINE-OXIDASE INHIBITOR.

maprotiline hydrochloride

is a TRICYCLIC-related ANTIDEPRESSANT drug which is used to treat depressive illness, particularly in cases where some degree of sedation is called for. Administration is oral.
✚▲ Side-effects/warnings: See AMITRIPTYLINE HYDROCHLORIDE; but some ANTICHOLINERGIC actions are less marked; however, rashes are common and there is a danger of convulsions and precipitated epileptic episodes; it is therefore not recommended for epileptics.
✪ Related entry: Ludiomil.

Marcain

(AstraZeneca) is a proprietary, prescription-only preparation of the LOCAL ANAESTHETIC bupivacaine hydrochloride, usually injected close to nerves. It is available in several forms for injection, for example, *Marcain Heavy*.
✚▲ Side-effects/warnings: See BUPIVACAINE HYDROCHLORIDE.

Marcain with Adrenaline

(AstraZeneca) is a proprietary, prescription-only compound preparation of the LOCAL ANAESTHETIC bupivacaine hydrochloride and the VASOCONSTRICTOR adrenaline acid tartrate (epinephrine), which prolongs its duration of action. It is available in a range of forms for injection.
✚▲ Side-effects/warnings: See ADRENALINE ACID TARTRATE; BUPIVACAINE HYDROCHLORIDE.

Marevan

(AstraZeneca) is a proprietary, prescription-only preparation of the synthetic ANTICOAGULANT warfarin sodium. It can be used to prevent clot formation in heart disease, following heart surgery (especially following implantation of prosthetic heart valves), to prevent venous thrombosis and pulmonary embolism. It is available as tablets.
✚▲ Side-effects/warnings: See WARFARIN SODIUM.

Marvelon

(Organon) is a proprietary, prescription-only compound preparation that can be used as a (*monophasic*) ORAL CONTRACEPTIVE of the *COC* (standard strength) type that combines an OESTROGEN and a PROGESTOGEN, in this case ethinylestradiol and desogestrel. It is available as tablets.
✚▲ Side-effects/warnings: See DESOGESTREL; ETHINYLESTRADIOL.

Maxalt

(MSD) is a proprietary, prescription-only preparation of the ANTIMIGRAINE drug rizatriptan. It can be used to treat acute migraine attacks. It is available as tablets and *melt wafers* that are placed on the tongue.
✚▲ Side-effects/warnings: See RIZATRIPTAN.

Maxepa

(Seven Seas) is a proprietary, prescription-only preparation of the LIPID-REGULATING DRUG omega-3 marine triglycerides. It can be used in hyperlipidaemia to change the proportions of various lipids. It is available as capsules and a liquid.
✚▲ Side-effects/warnings: See OMEGA-3 MARINE TRIGLYCERIDES.

Maxidex

(Alcon) is a proprietary, prescription-only compound preparation of the CORTICOSTEROID and ANTI-INFLAMMATORY dexamethasone. It can be used to treat inflammation of the eye, and is available as eye-drops.
✚▲ Side-effects/warnings: See DEXAMETHASONE.

Maximum Strength Aspro Clear

(Roche Consumer Health) is a proprietary, non-prescription preparation of the (NSAID) NON-NARCOTIC ANALGESIC, ANTIRHEUMATIC and ANTIPYRETIC aspirin. It can be used to relieve pain, including headache, neuralgia, period and dental pain, to relieve cold and flu symptoms and sore throats, to reduce raised body temperature

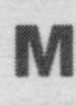

and to treat musculoskeletal pain. It is available as effervescent tablets and is not normally given to children, except on medical advice.
✚▲ Side-effects/warnings: See ASPIRIN.

Maxitrol

(Alcon) is a proprietary, prescription-only compound preparation of the ANTI-INFLAMMATORY and CORTICOSTEROID dexamethasone, the ANTIBACTERIAL and (AMINOGLYCOSIDE) ANTIBIOTIC neomycin sulphate and the antibacterial and (POLYMYXIN) antibiotic polymyxin B sulphate and hypromellose ('artificial tears'). It can be used to treat inflammation of the eye when infection is also present, and is available as eye-drops and eye-ointment.
✚▲ Side-effects/warnings: See DEXAMETHASONE; HYPROMELLOSE; NEOMYCIN SULPHATE; POLYMYXIN B SULPHATE.

Maxivent

(Ashbourne) is a proprietary, prescription-only preparation of the BETA-RECEPTOR STIMULANT salbutamol. It can be used as a BRONCHODILATOR in reversible obstructive airways disease such as in ANTI-ASTHMATIC treatment. It is available in an aerosol inhalant (solution as *Maxivent Steripoules*).
✚▲ Side-effects/warnings: See SALBUTAMOL.

Maxolon

(Shire) is a proprietary, prescription-only preparation of the ANTI-EMETIC and ANTINAUSEANT metoclopramide hydrochloride. It can be used for the treatment of nausea and vomiting, particularly when associated with gastrointestinal disorders and after treatment with radiation or cytotoxic drugs or gastric disorders. It is available as tablets, a syrup, a liquid form (*Maxolon Paediatric Liquid*), as modified-release capsules (*Maxolon SR*) and in several forms for injection (eg *Maxolon High Dose*).
✚▲ Side-effects/warnings: See METOCLOPRAMIDE HYDROCHLORIDE.

Maxtrex

(Pharmacia) is a proprietary, prescription-only preparation of the IMMUNOSUPPRESSANT and (CYTOTOXIC) ANTICANCER drug methotrexate. It can be used to treat rheumatoid arthritis and lymphoblastic leukaemia, other lymphomas and solid tumours, also severe resistant psoriasis. It is available as tablets.
✚▲ Side-effects/warnings: See METHOTREXATE.

MCR-50

see MONO-CEDOCARD RETARD-50.

mebendazole

is an (AZOLE) ANTHELMINTIC drug which can be used in the treatment of infestation by roundworm, threadworm, whipworm and hookworm. Administration is oral.
✚ Side-effects: These are rare, but there may be diarrhoea and abdominal pain; hypersensitivity reactions (rash, urticaria and angioedema).
▲ Warnings: It should be administered with caution to those who are pregnant or breast-feeding.
✪ Related entries: Ovex Tablets; Pripsen Mebendazole Tablets; Vermox.

mebeverine hydrochloride

is an ANTISPASMODIC drug which is used to treat muscle spasm in the gastrointestinal tract, which causes abdominal pain and constipation, eg irritable bowel syndrome. Administration is oral.
✚▲ Side-effects/warnings: It should not be taken by patients with paralytic ileus. Avoid in porphyria.
✪ Related entries: Colofac; Colofac 100; Colofac IBS; Colofac MR; Equilon; Fybogel Mebeverine.

meclozine hydrochloride

is a sedating ANTIHISTAMINE which is used primarily as an ANTINAUSEANT in the treatment or prevention of motion sickness and vomiting. Administration is oral.
✚▲ Side-effects/warnings: See CYCLIZINE.
✪ Related entry: Sea-Legs.

Mectizan

(MSD) is a proprietary preparation of the ANTHELMINTIC drug ivermectin, which is effective in treating chronic *Strongyloides* infection. Administration is oral.
✚▲ Side-effects/warnings: See IVERMECTIN.

mecysteine hydrochloride

(methyl cysteine hydrochloride) is a MUCOLYTIC drug used to reduce the viscosity of sputum and so acts as an EXPECTORANT in patients with disorders of the upper respiratory tract (eg chronic asthma or bronchitis).

Administration is oral.
✪ Related entry: Visclair.

Medicoal

(Concord) is a proprietary, non-prescription preparation of activated charcoal. It can be used to treat patients suffering from poisoning or a drug overdose. It is available as granules.
✚▲ Side-effects/warnings: See ACTIVATED CHARCOAL.

Medijel Gel

(DDD) is a proprietary, non-prescription compound preparation of the LOCAL ANAESTHETIC lidocaine hydrochloride (lignocaine) and the ANTISEPTIC aminacrine hydrochloride. It can be used for the temporary relief of pain caused by mouth ulcers, denture rubbing and sore gums, and is available as a gel for topical application.
✚▲ Side-effects/warnings: See AMINACRINE HYDROCHLORIDE; LIDOCAINE HYDROCHLORIDE.

Medijel Pastels

(DDD) is a proprietary, non-prescription compound preparation of the LOCAL ANAESTHETIC lidocaine hydrochloride and the ANTISEPTIC aminacrine hydrochloride. It can be used for the temporary relief of pain caused by mouth ulcers, denture rubbing and sore gums, and is available as pastels.
✚▲ Side-effects/warnings: See AMINACRINE HYDROCHLORIDE; LIDOCAINE HYDROCHLORIDE.

Medinol Over 6 Paracetamol Oral Suspension

(SSL) is a proprietary, non-prescription preparation of the NON-NARCOTIC ANALGESIC paracetamol. It can be used for relieving the symptoms of pain and feverish conditions, and is available as an oral suspension. It is not normally given to children under six years.
✚▲ Side-effects/warnings: See PARACETAMOL.

Medinol Under 6 Paracetamol Oral Suspension

(SSL) is a proprietary, non-prescription preparation of the NON-NARCOTIC ANALGESIC paracetamol. It can be used for relieving the symptoms of pain and feverish conditions, and is available as an oral suspension. It is not normally given to children under three months (except to treat fever after immunizations at two months), except on medical advice.
✚▲ Side-effects/warnings: See PARACETAMOL.

Medised

(SSL) is a proprietary, non-prescription compound preparation of the NON-NARCOTIC ANALGESIC paracetamol and the SEDATIVE and ANTIHISTAMINE drug promethazine hydrochloride. It can be used for reducing temperature and relieving the symptoms of painful or feverish conditions, such as toothache, headache, sore throats, chickenpox, colds and flu and to help restful sleep. It is available as a suspension and is not normally given to children under one year, except on medical advice.
✚▲ Side-effects/warnings: See PARACETAMOL; PROMETHAZINE HYDROCHLORIDE.

Medised Infant

(SSL) is a proprietary, non-prescription compound preparation of the NON-NARCOTIC ANALGESIC paracetamol and the SEDATIVE and ANTIHISTAMINE drug diphenhydramine hydrochloride. It can be used for reducing temperature and relieving the symptoms of painful or feverish conditions, such as toothache, headache, sore throats, chickenpox, colds and flu. It also helps restful sleep. It is available as a liquid suspension, and is not normally given to children under three months, except on medical advice.
✚▲ Side-effects/warnings: See PARACETAMOL; DIPHENHYDRAMINE HYDROCHLORIDE.

Medised Sugar Free Colour Free

(SSL) is a proprietary, non-prescription compound preparation of the NON-NARCOTIC ANALGESIC paracetamol and the SEDATIVE and ANTIHISTAMINE drug promethazine hydrochloride. It can be used for reducing temperature and relieving the symptoms of painful or feverish conditions, such as toothache, headache, sore throats, colds and flu and nasal irritation. It is available as a suspension and is not normally given to children under one year, except on medical advice.
✚▲ Side-effects/warnings: See PARACETAMOL; PROMETHAZINE HYDROCHLORIDE.

Medrone

(Pharmacia) is a proprietary, prescription-only preparation of the CORTICOSTEROID and ANTI-

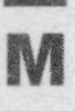

INFLAMMATORY drug methylprednisolone. It can be used to treat allergic disorders and cerebral oedema, and is available as tablets.
✚▲ Side-effects/warnings: See METHYLPREDNISOLONE.

medroxyprogesterone acetate

is a synthetic PROGESTOGEN. One of its uses is as an ORAL CONTRACEPTIVE, alternatively given by deep intramuscular injection every three months. Another is as part of HRT (hormone replacement therapy). It can also be used as a hormonal supplement in women whose progestogen level requires boosting. Additionally, it can be used in the treatment of cancer of the kidney, breast, uterine endometrium and, less commonly, of the prostate gland in men. Administration is either oral or by injection.
✚▲ Side-effects/warnings: See PROGESTOGEN.
✪ Related entries: Adgyn Medro; Depo-Provera; Farlutal; Indivina; Premique; Provera; Tridestra.

mefenamic acid

is a (NSAID) NON-NARCOTIC ANALGESIC and ANTIRHEUMATIC drug which is used primarily to treat mild to moderate pain and inflammation in rheumatoid arthritis, osteoarthritis and other musculoskeletal disorders, including juvenile arthritis. It is also used to treat period pain and menorrhagia (heavy bleeding). Administration is oral.
✚▲ Side-effects/warnings: See NSAID. It has weaker anti-inflammatory properties than most drugs of this class and a higher incidence of diarrhoea. There may be blood disturbances (haemolytic anaemia) and treatment may need to be discontinued. It is not used in people with inflammatory bowel disease or porphyria. There may be drowsiness, and skin reactions (relatively common with NSAIDs).
✪ Related entries: Dysman 250; Ponstan.

mefloquine

is an (*4-aminoquinoline*) ANTIMALARIAL drug which is used to prevent and treat malaria infection, including uncomplicated falciparum malaria and chloroquine-resistant vivax malaria. Administration is oral.
✚ Side-effects: There are many and include nausea and vomiting, visual disturbances, rash and itching; diarrhoea, abdominal pain and disturbances of the gastrointestinal tract and liver, dizziness, loss of balance, headache, sleep disorders. Susceptible patients may undergo psychotic episodes and neuropsychiatric reactions (including motor and sensory neuropathies, anxiety, panic attacks, depression, hallucinations, overt psychosis and convulsions), tinnitus and vestibular disorders and visual disturbances. Also circulatory disorders (hypotension and hypertension), bradycardia, tachycardia, heart disorders, muscle weakness, myalgia, arthralgia, urticaria, pruritus, alopecia, disturbances in liver function, asthenia, malaise, fatigue, fever, loss of appetite, disturbed blood counts and AV block and encephalopathy, and others. The performance of skilled tasks, such as driving, may be impaired. Patients must consult their doctor if adverse symptoms are experienced after discontinuation of treatment. Driving skills and other skilled tasks may be affected by dizziness and disturbed balance up to three weeks after treatment.
▲ Warnings: These depend on whether it is used to prevent or to treat malaria. It should not be used in patients with certain kidney, liver or heart disorders. It should not be given to those who are breast-feeding or pregnant (and avoid getting pregnant for three months after treatment with mefloquine), or to those with a history of convulsions. There may be serious psychiatric disorders, or hypersensitivity to quinine.
✪ Related entry: Lariam.

Mefoxin

(MSD) is a proprietary, prescription-only preparation of the ANTIBACTERIAL and (CEPHALOSPORIN) ANTIBIOTIC cefoxitin. It can be used to treat a range of bacterial infections, and is available in a form for intravenous injection or infusion.
✚▲ Side-effects/warnings: See CEFOXITIN.

Megace

(Bristol-Myers Squibb) is a proprietary, prescription-only preparation of the PROGESTOGEN megestrol acetate. It can be used as an ANTICANCER treatment for cancer of the endometrium of the uterus and breast. It is available as tablets.
✚▲ Side-effects/warnings: See MEGESTROL ACETATE.

megestrol acetate

is a PROGESTOGEN, a female sex hormone (see SEX

HORMONES), which is used primarily as an ANTICANCER treatment when the presence of OESTROGEN is significant (eg breast cancer or cancer of the endometrium of the uterus). Administration is oral.

+▲ Side-effects/warnings: See PROGESTOGEN.

✪ **Related entry: Megace.**

Meggezones

(Schering-Plough Consumer Health) is a proprietary, non-prescription compound preparation of menthol. It can be used for the relief of a sore throat, coughs, colds and nasal congestion. It is available as pastilles.

+▲ Side-effects/warnings: See MENTHOL.

Melleril

(Novartis) is a proprietary, prescription-only preparation of the ANTIPSYCHOTIC thioridazine. It can be used to treat and tranquillize patients with psychotic disorders (such as schizophrenia) and other behavioural disturbance, and also in the short-term treatment of anxiety. It is available as tablets, a suspension and a syrup.

+▲ Side-effects/warnings: See THIORIDAZINE.

meloxicam

is a (NSAID) NON-NARCOTIC ANALGESIC and ANTIRHEUMATIC drug which is used to treat pain and inflammation in rheumatoid arthritis and ankylosing spondylitis, and for short-term treatment of osteoarthritis. Administration is either oral or by suppositories.

+▲ Side-effects/warnings: See NSAID. Avoid suppositories if there are haemorrhoids or proctitis, and it is used with caution in those with impaired kidneys. There is a relatively high risk of gastric bleeding.

✪ **Related entry: Mobic.**

melphalan

is an (*alkylating agent*) CYTOTOXIC drug which is used as an ANTICANCER treatment of various forms of cancers, myelomas, some solid tumours and lymphomas. It works by a direct action on the DNA of the cancer cells and so prevents cell replication. Administration is either oral or by injection.

+▲ Side-effects/warnings: See CYTOTOXIC.

✪ **Related entry: Alkeran.**

menadiol sodium phosphate

(vitamin K_3) is a synthetic form of VITAMIN K. It is sometimes used in medicine in preference to vitamins K_1 and K_2, because these natural forms are only fat-soluble, whereas vitamin K_3 is water-soluble and is therefore effective when taken by mouth to treat vitamin deficiency caused by fat malabsorption syndromes (eg due to obstruction of the bile ducts or in liver disease). In malabsorption syndromes it is important to make up a deficiency on a regular basis, because vitamin K is essential for maintaining the clotting factors in the blood and for calcification of bone. Administration is oral.

+▲ Side-effects/warnings: See VITAMIN K.

Mengivac (A+C)

(SmithKline Beecham; GSK) is a proprietary, prescription-only preparation of a VACCINE that is used to give protection against the organism meningococcus (*Neisseria meningitidis* groups A and C), which can cause serious infections such as meningitis. It is available in a form for injection.

+▲ Side-effects/warnings: See MENINGOCOCCAL POLYSACCHARIDE VACCINE.

Meningitec

(Wyeth) is a proprietary, prescription-only VACCINE preparation. It can be used to give protection against the organism meningococcus (*Neisseria meningitidis* group C), which can cause serious infection such as meningitis. It is available in a form for injection.

+▲ Side-effects/warnings: See MENINGOCOCCAL POLYSACCHARIDE VACCINE.

meningitis vaccine

see MENINGOCOCCAL POLYSACCHARIDE VACCINE.

meningococcal polysaccharide vaccine

is a VACCINE that is used for IMMUNIZATION against infection from the organism meningococcus (*Neisseria meningitidis*), which can cause serious infections, such as meningitis. It may be given to those intending to travel 'rough' through parts of the world where the risk of meningococcal infection is much higher than in the UK and in a 'catch-up' programme targeting those groups at highest risk in the UK (teenagers, students, schoolchildren).

There are three different groups or types of vaccines. Meningococcal Group C conjugate vaccine provides protection in the long-term

against infection by serogroup C of *Neisseria meningitidis* in children from two months old, and it is now a component of the primary course of childhood immunization (usually in three doses for children aged two to four months). This vaccine protects against Group C diseases only, so anyone travelling abroad to risk areas (eg much of the Indian subcontinent, Saudi Arabia/Mecca and much of Africa) should be immunized with a subcutaneous or intramuscular injection of combined meningococcal polysaccharide A and C vaccine (even if they have earlier received meningococcal group C conjugate vaccine). Recently, a meningococcal polysaccharide vaccine active against meningococci of groups *A, C, W135 and Y* has been introduced, and is officially recommended for travellers to areas which have a high prevalance of the disease (including Saudi Arabia during the annual pilgrimages). Also, this vaccine may be used to protect those with impaired immunity such as people without spleens.
✚▲ Side-effects/warnings: See VACCINE.
✪ **Related entries: AC Vax; ACWY Vax; Mengivac (A+C); Meningitec; Menjugate; Neis Vac-C.**

Menjugate
(Chiron / Farillon) is a proprietary, prescription-only VACCINE preparation. It can be used to give protection against the organism meningococcus (*Neisseria meningitidis* group C), which can cause serious infections, such as meningitis. It is available in a form for injection.
✚▲ Side-effects/warnings: See MENINGOCOCCAL POLYSACCHARIDE VACCINE.

Menogon
(Ferring) is a proprietary, prescription-only preparation of human menopausal chorionic gonadotrophins (gonadotropins) in a form called MENOTROPHIN. It can be used primarily to treat women suffering from specific hormonal deficiencies in infertility treatment and in assisted conception. It is available in a form for injection.
✚▲ Side-effects/warnings: See HUMAN MENOPAUSAL GONADOTROPHINS.

Menopur
(Ferring) is a proprietary, prescription-only preparation of human menopausal chorionic gonadotrophins (gonadotropins) in a form called MENOTROPHIN. It can be used primarily to treat women suffering from specific hormonal deficiencies in infertility treatment and in assisted conception. It is available in a form for injection.
✚▲ Side-effects/warnings: See HUMAN MENOPAUSAL GONADOTROPHINS.

Menorest
(Novartis) is a proprietary, prescription-only preparation of the OESTROGEN estradiol. It can be used in HRT and in osteoporosis prevention, and is available as skin patches in different strengths.
✚▲ Side-effects/warnings: See ESTRADIOL.

Menoring-50
(Galen) is a proprietary, prescription-only preparation of the female sex hormone (an OESTROGEN) estradiol. It can be used in HRT to treat urogenital complaints in postmenopausal women, and is available as a vaginal ring.
✚▲ Side-effects/warnings: See ESTRADIOL.

menotrophin
(menotropins) is a HORMONE preparation and is a collective name for combinations of the GONADOTROPHIN hormones – FOLLICLE-STIMULATING HORMONE (FSH) and LUTEINISING HORMONE (LH) – in a particular ratio (1:1). It is largely equivalent to HUMAN MENOPAUSAL GONADOTROPHINS.
✚▲ Side-effects/warnings: See HUMAN MENOPAUSAL GONADOTROPHINS.
✪ **Related entry: Menogon.**

menotropins
see MENOTROPHIN.

menthol
is a white, crystalline substance derived from peppermint oil (an essential oil extracted from a plant of the mint family) and is chemically a TERPENE. It is available in several specific chemical forms, of which levomenthol is one of the preferred isomers. It is commonly used, with or without the volatile substance eucalyptus oil, in inhalations intended to clear the nasal or catarrhal congestion associated with colds, rhinitis (inflammation of the nasal mucous membrane) or sinusitis. It has mild local anaesthetic actions, and is included in some COUNTER-IRRITANT, OR RUBEFACIENT, preparations that are rubbed into the skin to relieve muscle or joint pain, and is incorporated

into preparations used to treat gallstones or kidney stones.

✚▲ Side-effects/warnings: It is regarded as safe in normal topical use, but avoid using it on cuts or abraded skin.

✪ **Related entries: Balmosa Cream; Benylin Chesty Coughs (Non-Drowsy); Benylin Chesty Coughs (Original); Benylin Children's Coughs and Colds; Benylin Children's Night Coughs; Benylin Cough and Congestion;Benylin Dry Coughs (Original); Benylin with Codeine; Boots Medicated Pain Relief Plaster; Buttercup Infant Cough Syrup; Cabdriver's Adult Cough Linctus; Covonia Bronchial Balsam; Deep Freeze Cold Gel; Deep Freeze Spray; Deep Heat Massage Liniment; Deep Heat Maximum Strength; Deep Heat Rub; Deep Relief; Dubam Cream; Hill's Balsam Chesty Cough Pastilles; Histalix Syrup; Karvol Decongestant Capsules; Karvol Decongestant Drops; Meggezones; Mentholatum Antiseptic Lozenges; Mentholatum Vapour Rub; Merocets Plus Lozenges; Radian B Heat Spray; Radian B Muscle Lotion; Radian B Muscle Rub; Ralgex Stick; Rinstead Sugar Free Pastilles; Rowachol; Strepsils Menthol and Eucalyptus; Tiger Balm Red (Extra Strength); Tiger Balm White (Regular Strength); Tixycolds Cold and Hayfever Inhalant Capsules; Vicks Inhaler; Vicks Vaporub; Vicks Vaposyrup for Tickly Coughs;Woodward's Baby Chest Rub.**

Mentholatum Antiseptic Lozenges

(Mentholatum) is a proprietary, non-prescription preparation of the ANTISEPTIC amylmetacresol with menthol and eucalyptus oil. It can be used for symptomatic relief of coughs, colds, congestion and sore throat, and is available in a form of lozenges. It is not normally given to children under three years, except on medical advice.

✚▲ Side-effects/warnings: See AMYLMETACRESOL; MENTHOL.

Mentholatum Ibuprofen Gel

(Mentholatum) is a proprietary, non-prescription preparation of the (NSAID) NON-NARCOTIC ANALGESIC and ANTIRHEUMATIC ibuprofen. It can be used to relieve superficial musculoskeletal disorders such as rheumatic and muscular pains, backache, sprains and strains, and is available as a gel for topical application. It is not given to children under 14 years, except on medicial advice.

✚▲ Side-effects/warnings: See IBUPROFEN; but adverse effects on topical application are limited.

Mentholatum Vapour Rub

(Mentholatum) is a proprietary, non-prescription compound preparation of camphor, menthol and methyl salicylate, which have COUNTER-IRRITANT, or RUBEFACIENT, actions. It can be applied to the skin for symptomatic relief of muscular rheumatism, fibrosis, lumbago and sciatica, for pain associated with unbroken chilblains, colds, catarrh, hay fever and insect bites. It is available as an ointment. It is not normally given to children under one year, except on medical advice.

✚▲ Side-effects/warnings: See CAMPHOR; MENTHOL; METHYL SALICYLATE.

mepacrine hydrochloride

has ANTIPROTOZOAL properties and is used primarily to treat infection of the small intestine by the intestinal protozoan *Giardia lamblia*. Giardiasis (lambliasis) occurs throughout the world, particularly in children, and is contracted by eating contaminated food. However, mepacrine has largely been superseded by METRONIDAZOLE, which is now the drug of choice. Administration is oral.

✚ Side-effects: Gastrointestinal disturbances, nausea and vomiting; headache and dizziness; stimulation of the central nervous system and psychoses; discolouration of the skin and dermatitis (with prolonged use); blood disturbances; discolouration of nails, palate and cornea (with vision disturbances).

▲ Warnings: Mepacrine hydrochloride should not be administered to patients with psoriasis; and should be administered with care to those with liver impairment or psychosis.

meprobamate

is an ANXIOLYTIC which is sometimes used in the short-term treatment of anxiety. It is also used in a compound analgesic preparation. It is potentially more hazardous than the BENZODIAZEPINE in overdose and can cause dependence (addiction). Administration is oral. Preparations containing meprobamate are on the Controlled Drugs list.

✚ Side-effects: See BENZODIAZEPINE; but they are more common and there are also gastrointestinal disturbances, hypotension, tingling in the

extremities, weakness, headache, disturbances of vision and blood changes. Drowsiness is a very common side-effect and may affect driving. The effects of alcohol are enhanced.
▲ Warnings: It should not be administered to patients with porphyria, who have certain lung and breathing disorders or who are breast-feeding. It should be administered with caution to those with respiratory difficulties, epilepsy, impaired liver or kidney function, drug or alcohol abuse, personality disorders or who are pregnant. Withdrawal of treatment must be gradual otherwise convulsions may occur.
✪ **Related entry: Equagesic.**

meptazinol

is a powerful, synthetic (OPIOID) NARCOTIC ANALGESIC which is used to treat moderate to severe pain, including pain in childbirth, renal colic, or during or following surgery. Administration can be either oral or by injection.
✚▲ Side-effects/warnings: See OPIOID; but less respiratory depression.
✪ **Related entry: Meptid.**

Meptid

(Shire) is a proprietary, prescription-only preparation of the (OPIOID) NARCOTIC ANALGESIC meptazinol (as hydrochloride). It can be used to treat moderate to severe pain, particularly during or following surgical procedures and also in childbirth. It is available as tablets and in a form for injection.
✚▲ Side-effects/warnings: See MEPTAZINOL.

mepyramine maleate

is an ANTIHISTAMINE which can be used for the symptomatic relief of allergic symptoms such as skin reactions. Administration is topical.
✚▲ Side-effects/warnings: See ANTIHISTAMINE. It has marked sedative properties, but normally not enough will be absorbed from unabraded skin to have systemic effects.
✪ **Related entries: Anthisan Bite and Sting Cream; Anthisan Plus Sting Relief Spray; Wasp-Eze Spray.**

Merbentyl

(Florizel) is a proprietary, prescription-only preparation of the ANTICHOLINERGIC drug dicyloverine hydrochloride (dicyclomine hydrochloride). It can be used as an ANTISPASMODIC for the symptomatic relief of smooth muscle spasm in the gastrointestinal tract, and is available as tablets and a syrup. (There are preparations available without prescription, but they are subject to amount limitations.)
✚▲ Side-effects/warnings: See DICYLOVERINE HYDROCHLORIDE.

Merbentyl 20

(Florizel) is a proprietary, prescription-only preparation of the ANTICHOLINERGIC drug dicyloverine hydrochloride (dicyclomine hydrochloride). It can be used as an ANTISPASMODIC for the symptomatic relief of muscle spasm in the gastrointestinal tract, and is available as tablets.
✚▲ Side-effects/warnings: See DICYLOVERINE HYDROCHLORIDE.

mercapatamine

(cysteamine) is an amino acid used as a METABOLIC DISORDER TREATMENT for a disease, nephropathic cystinosis, where there is deposition of cystine in the kidneys. It is given orally.
✚ Side-effects: Nausea and vomiting, diarrhoea, anorexia, breath and body odour, lethargy, fever, rash; also dehydration, hypertension, abdominal discomfort and gastroenteritis, drowsiness, headache, nervousness, depression; blood and liver disorders, rarely gastrointestinal ulceration and bleeding, hallucinations, seizures, urticaria, kidney disorders.
▲ Warnings: Not to be used in pregnancy or breast-feeding. Blood monitoring will be carried out. The form used can be sprinkled on food (at a temperature suitable for eating); but not acidic drinks (eg orange juice).
✪ **Related entry: Cystagon.**

mercaptopurine

is an (*antimetabolite*) CYTOTOXIC drug which is used as an ANTICANCER treatment of acute leukaemias. It works by preventing cell replication. Administration is oral.
✚▲ Side-effects/warnings: See CYTOTOXIC. Avoid its use in patients with porphyria.
✪ **Related entry: Puri-Nethol.**

Mercilon

(Organon) is a proprietary, prescription-only compound preparation that can be used as a

(*monophasic*) ORAL CONTRACEPTIVE of the *COC* (low strength) type that combines an OESTROGEN and a PROGESTOGEN, in this case ethinylestradiol and desogestrel. It is available as tablets.
✚▲ Side-effects/warnings: See DESOGESTREL; ETHINYLESTRADIOL.

Merocaine Lozenges

(SSL) is a proprietary, non-prescription compound preparation of the ANTISEPTIC agent CETYLPYRIDINIUM CHLORIDE and the LOCAL ANAESTHETIC benzocaine in the form of lozenges. It can be used for the temporary relief of the pain and discomfort of a sore throat and superficial, minor mouth infections. It is available as lozenges, and is not normally given to children under 12 years, except on medical advice.
✚▲ Side-effects/warnings: See BENZOCAINE; CETYLPYRIDINIUM CHLORIDE.

Merocet Gargle/Mouthwash

(SSL) is a proprietary, non-prescription preparation of the ANTISEPTIC agent cetylpyridinium chloride. It can be used for the symptomatic relief of sore throat and minor irritations of the throat and mouth. It is available as an oral solution for use as a gargle or mouthwash. It is not normally given to children under six years, except on medical advice.
✚▲ Side-effects/warnings: See CETYLPYRIDINIUM CHLORIDE.

Merocets Lozenges

(SSL) is a proprietary, non-prescription preparation of the ANTISEPTIC agent CETYLPYRIDINIUM CHLORIDE. It can be used for the symptomatic relief of sore throat and minor irritations of the throat and mouth, and is available as lozenges. It is not normally given to children under six, except on medical advice.
✚▲ Side-effects/warnings: See CETYLPYRIDINIUM CHLORIDE.

Merocets Plus Lozenges

(SSL) is a proprietary, non-prescription compound preparation of menthol with the ANTISEPTIC cetylpridinium chloride with eucalyptus oil. It can be used for the relief of a sore throat, nasal congestion and minor mouth and throat irritations. It is available as lozenges.
✚▲ Side-effects/warnings: See MENTHOL; CETYLPYRIDINIUM CHLORIDE.

Meronem

(AstraZeneca) is a proprietary, prescription-only compound preparation of the ANTIBACTERIAL and (BETA-LACTAM) ANTIBIOTIC meropenem. It can be used to treat a range of infections, and is available in a form for injection or intravenous infusion.
✚▲ Side-effects/warnings: See MEROPENEM.

meropenem

is an ANTIBACTERIAL and ANTIBIOTIC drug. It is a new sort of BETA-LACTAM (a carbapenem) with a broad-spectrum of activity against many Gram-positive and Gram-negative bacteria. Unlike the earlier similar drug IMIPENEM WITH CILASTATIN, it is not degraded by an enzyme in the kidney. It can be used to treat meningitis, infections in the periphery, such as the urethra and cervix, and for infections acquired in hospitals. Administration is by injection.
✚ Side-effects: Nausea, vomiting, diarrhoea, abdominal pain, liver disorders, blood disorders, headache, weakness, rash, pruritus and urticaria, convulsions have been reported, and there may be local reactions, including pain, at the injection site.
▲ Warnings: Administer with caution to patients with liver or kidney impairment, or who are pregnant or breast-feeding. It is administered with care to those with hypersensitivity to penicillins and other beta-lactams.
✪ **Related entry: Meronem.**

mesalazine

is an AMINOSALICYLATE which can be used in the treatment of ulcerative colitis, particularly in patients sensitive to the SULPHONAMIDE content of SULFASALAZINE. Administration can be either oral or by suppositories or a foam enema.
✚ Side-effects: Nausea, diarrhoea, abdominal pain, headache, exacerbated colitis symptoms, kidney, liver and pancreas problems and blood disorders. Patients should tell their doctor if they have any unexplained bruising, bleeding, sore throat, fever or malaise, because of possible effects on the blood requiring treatment to be stopped.
▲ Warnings: It should not be administered to patients who have severe kidney or liver impairment, blood-clotting problems, or who are allergic to aspirin or other salicylates; it should be administered with caution to those who are

pregnant or breast-feeding.
✪ **Related entries: Asacol; Pentasa; Salofalk.**

mesna
is a synthetic drug which has the property of combating the haemorrhagic cystitis that is a toxic complication caused by CYTOTOXIC drugs (eg CYCLOPHOSPHAMIDE and IFOSFAMIDE). It works by reacting with a toxic metabolite (a breakdown product called acrolein) produced by the cytotoxic drugs and which is the cause of the haemorrhagic cystitis. Mesna is therefore used as an adjunct in the treatment of certain forms of cancer. Administration is oral or by injection.
✚ Side-effects: If dosage is high, it may cause gastrointestinal disturbances, headache, tiredness, pain in the limbs and joints, depression, irritability, rash and lack of energy, heart effects, hypersensitivity reactions.
✪ **Related entry: Uromitexan.**

mesterolone
is an ANDROGEN, which promotes the development of the secondary male sexual characteristics. Therapeutically, it may be administered to treat hormonal deficiency, for instance, for delayed puberty in boys and infertility in men. Administration is oral.
✚▲ Side-effects/warnings: See ANDROGEN; but there is no effect on sperm production.
✪ **Related entry: Pro-Viron.**

Mestinon
(ICN) is a proprietary, prescription-only preparation of the ANTICHOLINESTERASE and PARASYMPATHOMIMETIC pyridostigmine (as bromide). It can be used to treat myasthenia gravis, and is available as tablets.
✚▲ Side-effects/warnings: See PYRIDOSTIGMINE.

mestranol
is a synthetic OESTROGEN which is a constituent in several *combined* ORAL CONTRACEPTIVE preparations and is also used in HRT. Administration is oral as tablets in a calendar pack.
✚▲ Side-effects/warnings: See OESTROGEN.
✪ **Related entry: Norinyl-1.**

metabolic disorder treatment
drugs or dietary supplements can be used to correct defects in the body's metabolism, some of them due to inborn errors of metabolism usually caused by an inherited defective enzyme. Some of these drugs are chelating agents (see CHELATING AGENT) that work by chemically binding to certain metallic ions and other substances, making them less toxic and allowing their excretion (eg of copper in Wilson's disease; PENICILLAMINE or TRIENTINE DIHYDROCHLORIDE). In most of the 200 or so known cases of inborn errors of metabolism, such enzyme deficiencies may lead to a shortage in the body of an amino acid (eg carnitine deficiency; treated with a dietary supplement of CARNITINE), too high levels for instance in phenylketonuria (where failure of conversion of phenylalanine into tyrosine leads to a build up of excess of the former; treated by a special diet containing low levels of phenylalanine), nephropathic cystinosis (where levels of the amino acid cystine are too high, which is corrected by treatment with another amino acid, MERCAPATAMINE added to the diet) or too high levels of a toxic metabolite (eg for urea cycle disorders where there is a build-up of ammonia in the body, corrected by giving sodium phenylbutyrate to give an alternative route for nitrogen excretion).

Metalyse
(Boehringer Ingelheim) is a proprietary, prescription-only preparation of the FIBRINOLYTIC tenecteplase. It can be used to treat myocardial infarction, and is available in a form for injection.
✚▲ Side-effects/warnings: See TENECTEPLASE.

Metanium
(Roche Consumer Health) is a proprietary, non-prescription preparation of TITANIUM DIOXIDE (and other titanium salts) in an ointment base and can be used to treat nappy rash.
✚▲ Side-effects/warnings: TITANIUM DIOXIDE.

metaraminol
is an ALPHA-ADRENOCEPTOR STIMULANT, a SYMPATHOMIMETIC and VASOCONSTRICTOR drug which can be used to treat cases of acute hypotension, particularly in emergency situations. Administration is by intravenous injection or infusion.
✚▲ Side-effects/warnings: See NORADRENALINE ACID TARTRATE. It is a specialist drug used under hospital conditions.
✪ **Related entry: Aramine.**

Metenix 5

(Borg) is a proprietary, prescription-only preparation of the (THIAZIDE-like) DIURETIC metolazone. It can be used, either alone or in conjunction with other drugs, in the treatment of oedema and as an ANTIHYPERTENSIVE. It is available as tablets.

✚▲ Side-effects/warnings: See METOLAZONE.

metformin hydrochloride

is a BIGUANIDE drug which is used in DIABETIC TREATMENT of Type II diabetes (non-insulin-dependent diabetes mellitus; NIDDM; maturity-onset diabetes), particularly in patients whose diabetes is not well controlled by diet or other drugs. It works by increasing the utilization and decreasing the formation of glucose, to make up for the reduction in insulin available from the pancreas. It does not usually cause a body weight gain (unlike many other diabetes treatments), so is used especially in obese individuals. Administration is oral.

✚ Side-effects: Gastrointestinal side-effects are common at first and may continue. There may be nausea and vomiting, with diarrhoea and weight loss. Body uptake of CYANOCOBALAMIN (vitamin B_{12}) or its analogues may be reduced.

▲ Warnings: It should not be administered to patients with certain heart, liver or kidney impairment, who are dehydrated, alcoholics, have severe infection, trauma or are pregnant or breast-feeding.

✪ **Related entries: Glucamet; Glucophage.**

methadone hydrochloride

is a NARCOTIC ANALGESIC drug (an OPIOID) and on the Controlled Drugs list. It is used primarily to relieve severe pain, but is less effective and less SEDATIVE than morphine but acts for a longer time. It is used in a linctus as an ANTITUSSIVE for cough in terminal disease and is also used (in an oral preparation) as a substitute for more powerful addictive opioids in detoxification therapy. Administration can be either oral or by injection.

✚▲ Side-effects/warnings: See OPIOID.

✪ **Related entries: Methadose; Physeptone.**

Methadose

(Rosemont) is a proprietary, prescription-only preparation of the (OPIOID) NARCOTIC ANALGESIC methadone hydrochloride, which is on the Controlled Drugs list. It is used for drug-dependent persons in detox therapy, and is available as an oral solution diluted with a special diluent.

✚▲ Side-effects/warnings: See METHADONE HYDROCHLORIDE.

methenamine hippurate

(hexamine hippurate) is an ANTIBACTERIAL drug which is used to treat recurrent infections of the urinary tract. Administration is oral.

✚ Side-effects: Gastrointestinal upsets, rash and bladder irritation.

▲ Warnings: It should not be used in patients with severe kidney impairment, dehydration and metabolic acidosis; it should be administered with care to those who are pregnant.

✪ **Related entry: Hiprex.**

methionine

is a natural amino acid that can be used as an ANTIDOTE to poisoning caused by an overdose of the NON-NARCOTIC ANALGESIC paracetamol. The initial symptoms of poisoning usually settle within 24 hours, but are followed by a serious toxic effect on the liver that takes several days to develop. The purpose of treatment is to prevent these latter effects and must start as soon as possible after the overdose has been taken (it works if taken within twelve hours of paracetamol ingestion). Methionine is used until the drug ACETYLCYSTEINE can be given by intravenous infusion. Administration is oral.

✚▲ Side-effects/warnings: It is regarded as safe in normal topical use, though when incorporated into paracetamol preparations it may make the tablets smell of ammonia.

✪ **Related entries: co-methiamol; Methionine Tablets; Paradote.**

Methionine Tablets

(Celltech) is a proprietary, prescription-only preparation of the ANTIDOTE methionine. It can be used for emergency treatment of overdose poisoning by the NON-NARCOTIC ANALGESIC paracetamol, and is available as tablets.

✚▲ Side-effects/warnings: See METHIONINE.

methocarbamol

is a SKELETAL MUSCLE RELAXANT which is used for the symptomatic relief of muscle spasm and works by an action on the central nervous system.

Administration is either oral or by injection.
✚ Side-effects: Light-headedness, lassitude, dizziness, confusion, restlessness, anxiety, drowsiness, nausea, rash, angioedema and convulsions.
▲ Warnings: It should not be administered to patients with brain damage, epilepsy or myasthenia gravis. It should be administered with care to those with impaired liver or kidney function. Drowsiness may impair the performance of skilled tasks, such as driving; avoid alcohol as its effects are enhanced.
✪ **Related entry: Robaxin.**

methotrexate

is an (*antimetabolite*) CYTOTOXIC drug which is used primarily as an ANTICANCER treatment of childhood acute lymphoblastic leukaemia, but also to treat non-Hodgkin's lymphomas, choriocarcinoma and some solid tumours. It works by inhibiting the activity of an enzyme essential to the DNA metabolism in cells. It is also used as an IMMUNOSUPPRESSANT to treat rheumatoid arthritis and (under specialist supervision) severe resistant psoriasis. Administration is either oral or by injection.
✚▲ Side-effects/warnings: See CYTOTOXIC. It should not be given to patients with severe kidney impairment; and avoid its use in those with porphyria.
✪ **Related entry: Maxtrex.**

methotrimeprazine

see LEVOMEPROMAZINE.

methoxamine hydrochloride

is an ALPHA-ADRENOCEPTOR STIMULANT, SYMPATHOMIMETIC and VASOCONSTRICTOR drug which is used primarily to raise lowered blood pressure, eg when caused by the induction of anaesthesia. Administration is by intravenous injection or infusion.
✚▲ Side-effects/warnings: See NORADRENALINE ACID TARTRATE. There may be hypertension. It is a specialist drug used under hospital conditions.
✪ **Related entry: Vasoxine.**

methylcellulose

is a (*bulking-agent*) LAXATIVE which works by increasing the overall mass of faeces and also retaining a lot of water and so stimulating bowel movement. However, the full effect may not be achieved for many hours. It can be used in patients who cannot tolerate bran when treating a range of bowel conditions, including diverticular disease and irritable bowel syndrome. Separately, it may be used as part of obesity treatment to reduce intake, since it may act as an APPETITE SUPPRESSANT through giving a feeling of satiety. Administration is oral.
✚ Side-effects: Flatulence and abdominal distension, intestinal obstruction. Preparations that swell in contact with liquid must be carefully swallowed with water and should not be taken just before going to bed at night.
▲ Warnings: It should not be used when there is gastrointestinal obstruction. It is important to maintain adequate fluid intake.
✪ **Related entry: Celevac.**

methyl cysteine hydrochloride

see MECYSTEINE HYDROCHLORIDE.

methyldopa

is an ANTISYMPATHETIC drug which acts in the brain to reduce the activity of the sympathetic nervous system. It can be used as an ANTIHYPERTENSIVE (commonly in combination with other drugs) of moderate to severe hypertension, and in hypertensive crisis. Administration is either oral or by intravenous injection or infusion.
✚ Side-effects: There are many side-effects including: dry mouth, gastrointestinal disturbances, drowsiness, fluid retention, diarrhoea; sedation, sleep disturbances, depression, headache, dizziness, aches and pains, tingling in the extremities, disturbances of sexual function, impaired liver function, skin and blood disorders and nasal stuffiness; parkinsonian symptoms.
▲ Warnings: It should not be administered to patients with certain blood or liver disorders, phaeochromocytoma or a history of depression. It should be administered with care to those with kidney damage. Regular blood counts and tests on liver function are necessary during treatment. The drug may cause drowsiness and impair the ability to drive or operate machinery; and the effects of alcohol may be enhanced. Although methydopa is safe in asthmatics, there are sulphites in ampoules that may cause hypersensitivity reactions (eg bronchospasm and shock). Iron can reduce the hypertensive effects of methyldopa.
✪ **Related entry: Aldomet.**

methyldopate hydrochloride
is the form of the ANTIHYPERTENSIVE drug methyldopa that is used for injection.
✚▲ Side-effects/warnings: See METHYLDOPA.

methyl nicotinate
is a VASODILATOR which can be used to help improve blood circulation. It can be used with other constituents in compound preparations for topical use in the mouth or ears to relieve the pain of teething, ulcers or minor scratches. Administration is by topical application.
✚▲ Side-effects/warnings: It is regarded as safe in normal topical use at appropriate dosage.
✪ **Related entries: Algipan Rub; Deep Heat Spray; Ralgex Cream; Ralgex Heat Spray; Transvasin Heat Spray.**

methylphenidate hydrochloride
is a drug that is used to treat hyperkinesis (hyperactivity) or attention-deficit hyperactivity disorder in children. (In contrast, in adults it acts as a weak stimulant, but is not used therapeutically.) Administration is oral. Preparations of methylphenidate are on the Controlled Drugs list.
✚▲ Side-effects/warnings: See DEXAMFETAMINE SULPHATE; also, rash, urticaria and dermatitis, hair loss, fever and blood changes (requiring monitoring).
✪ **Related entry: Ritalin.**

methylprednisolone
is a CORTICOSTEROID with ANTI-INFLAMMATORY properties. It is used to relieve the inflammation of allergic reaction, to treat cerebral oedema (fluid retention in the brain) and rheumatic disease. Administration (as methylprednisolone, methylprednisolone acetate or methylprednisolone sodium succinate) can be oral, or by injection or intravenous infusion.
✚▲ Side-effects/warnings: See CORTICOSTEROID.
✪ **Related entries: Depo-Medrone; Depo-Medrone with Lidocaine; Medrone; Solu-Medrone.**

methylrosanilium chloride
see CRYSTAL VIOLET.

methyl salicylate
is a NSAID (non-steroidal anti-inflammatory drug) that has COUNTER-IRRITANT, or RUBEFACIENT, actions and can be applied to the skin for symptomatic relief of pain in underlying organs, for instance in rheumatic and other musculoskeletal disorders. It is administered topically to the skin, and is available as a liniment and ointment and in several proprietary preparations as a cream or a balsam. See also SALICYLATE; SALICYLIC ACID.
✚▲ Side-effects/warnings: See NSAID; though normally little is absorbed into the circulation and local side-effects are limited to mild irritation. It can cause sensitivity to bright sunlight; systemic effects may occur with prolonged or excessive use. It should not be used on broken skin or mucous membranes.
✪ **Related entries: Balmosa Cream; Boots Medicated Pain Relief Plaster; Chymol Emollient Balm; Deep Heat Massage Liniment; Deep Heat Maximum Strength; Deep Heat Rub; Deep Heat Spray; Dubam Cream; Germolene Ointment; Mentholatum Vapour Rub; Monphytol; PR Heat Spray; Radian B Heat Spray; Radian B Muscle Rub; Ralgex Stick; TCP Antiseptic Ointment.**

methyl violet
see CRYSTAL VIOLET.

methysergide
is a potentially dangerous drug that is used, under strict medical supervision in hospital, as an ANTIMIGRAINE treatment to prevent severe recurrent attacks and similar headaches in patients for whom other forms of treatment have failed. (It is also sometimes used in carcinoid syndrome.) It works as an antimigraine drug mainly as a VASOCONSTRICTOR by acting as a serotonin receptor antagonist. Administration is oral.
✚ Side-effects: This is a specialist drug used under supervised conditions. There are many side-effects and these include: nausea, vomiting, abdominal discomfort, heartburn, insomnia, weight gain, rashes, mental disturbances, hair loss, cramps, effects on the cardiovascular system, oedema, drowsiness and dizziness.
▲ Warnings: It is not to be used in patients with certain kidney, lung, liver or cardiovascular disorders; severe hypertension, urinary tract disorders, collagen disease or cellulitis; or who are pregnant or breast-feeding. It is used with caution in those with peptic ulcer.
✪ **Related entry: Deseril.**

M

metipranolol

is a BETA-BLOCKER which can be used as a GLAUCOMA TREATMENT for chronic simple glaucoma. It is thought to work by slowing the rate of production of the aqueous humour in the eye. Administration is topical.

✚ Side-effects: There may be some systemic absorption after using eye-drops, so some of the side-effects listed under PROPRANOLOL HYDROCHLORIDE may be seen. Dry eyes, stinging, redness, pain and some local allergic reactions, including conjunctivitis may also occur. Its preparation does not contain the preservative benzalkonium chloride, found in several eye-drops for glaucoma, so it can be used by patients who are allergic to this preservative and those wearing soft contact lenses. It may cause granulomatous anterior uveitis, if so treatment should be discontinued.

▲ Warnings: In view of possible absorption, dangerous side-effects should be borne in mind, particularly the danger of bronchospasm in asthmatics and interactions with some calcium-channel blockers. As eye-drops, not all warnings apply, but it should not be used (except when there is no option) for people with uncontrolled heart failure, bradycardia and certain other heart complaints.

✪ Related entry: Minims Metipranolol.

metirosine

is an ANTISYMPATHETIC drug which inhibits one of the enzymes (tyrosine hydroxylase) that produce NORADRENALINE (norepinephrine) and is used (on a named-patient basis only) in the preoperative treatment of phaeochromocytoma (sometimes with an ALPHA-ADRENOCEPTOR BLOCKER). Administration is oral.

✚ Side-effects: Sedation, severe diarrhoea, sensitivity reactions and extrapyramidal movement symptoms.

▲ Warnings: Increased fluid intake during treatment is essential. Regular checks on overall blood volume may be carried out. Because it causes sedation, it may affect the ability to drive or operate machinery.

✪ Related entry: Demser.

metoclopramide hydrochloride

is an effective ANTI-EMETIC and ANTINAUSEANT drug with useful MOTILITY STIMULANT properties. It can be used to prevent vomiting caused by gastrointestinal disorders or by chemotherapy or radiotherapy (in the treatment of cancer). It works both by a direct action on the vomiting centre of the brain (where it is an ANTAGONIST of dopamine) and by actions within the intestine. It enhances the strength of oesophageal sphincter contraction (preventing the passage of stomach contents up into the gullet), stimulates emptying of the stomach and increases the rate at which food is moved along the intestine. These last actions lead to its use in non-ulcer dyspepsia, for gastric stasis and to prevent reflux oesophagitis. It is also used during intestine examination to speed up the movement of barium through the intestine following a barium meal. It can also be used to relieve the nausea associated with migraine attacks. Administration is either oral or by injection.

✚ Side-effects: There may be extrapyramidal effects (dystonic reactions, especially facial), particularly in the young and elderly; tardive dyskinesia (involuntary motor movements). Drowsiness, restlessness, depression and diarrhoea. Dopamine antagonists raised levels of the hormone PROLACTIN in the blood, which can lead to growth of breasts and secretion of milk.

▲ Warnings: It should be administered with caution to those with impaired kidney or liver function or porphyria, or who are pregnant, breast-feeding or under 20 years old.

✪ Related entries: Gastrobid Continus; Gastroflux; Maxolon; MigraMax; Paramax; Primperan.

metolazone

is a THIAZIDE-like DIURETIC. It can be used as an ANTIHYPERTENSIVE, either alone or in conjunction with other types of drugs, and also in the treatment of oedema. Administration is oral.

✚▲ Side-effects/warnings: See BENDROFLUMETHIAZIDE. There can be marked diuresis (urine production) when given with frusemide.

✪ Related entry: Metenix 5.

Metopirone

(Alliance) is a proprietary, prescription-only preparation of the ENZYME INHIBITOR metyrapone. It can be used to treat conditions that result from the excessive secretion of corticosteroids into the bloodstream (eg Cushing's syndrome). It is available as capsules.

✚▲ Side-effects/warnings: See METYRAPONE.

metoprolol tartrate

is a BETA-BLOCKER which can be used as an ANTIHYPERTENSIVE for raised blood pressure, as an ANTI-ANGINA treatment to relieve symptoms and improve exercise tolerance, as an ANTI-ARRHYTHMIC to regularize heartbeat and to treat myocardial infarction, as an ANTIMIGRAINE treatment to prevent migraine attacks, and can also be used as an ANTITHYROID drug for short-term treatment of thyrotoxicosis. Administration is either oral or by injection. It is also available for use as an antihypertensive treatment in the form of compound preparations with DIURETIC drugs.

✚▲ Side-effects/warnings: See PROPRANOLOL HYDROCHLORIDE.

✪ **Related entries: Betaloc; Betaloc-SA; Co-Betaloc; Co-Betaloc SA; Lopresor; Lopresor SR.**

Metosyn

(Bioglan) is a proprietary, prescription-only preparation of the CORTICOSTEROID and ANTI-INFLAMMATORY fluocinonide. It can be used to treat severe, inflammatory skin disorders, such as eczema, that are unresponsive to less powerful drugs and also psoriasis. It is available as a cream (*FAPG cream*) and ointment.

✚▲ Side-effects/warnings: See FLUOCINONIDE.

Metrodin High Purity

(Serono) is a proprietary, prescription-only preparation of urofollitropin, which is a form of the pituitary HORMONE, follicle-stimulating hormone (FSH), and is prepared from human menopausal urine that contains FSH. It can be used primarily to treat women suffering from specific hormonal deficiencies in infertility treatment and in assisted conception. It is available in a form for injection.

✚▲ Side-effects/warnings: See UROFOLLITROPIN.

Metrogel

(Novartis) is a proprietary, prescription-only preparation of the ANTIMICROBIAL metronidazole, which has ANTIBACTERIAL and ANTIPROTOZOAL actions. It can be applied topically as a gel to treat acute acne rosacea outbreaks.

✚▲ Side-effects/warnings: See METRONIDAZOLE.

Metrolyl

(Lagap) is a proprietary, prescription-only preparation of the ANTIMICROBIAL metronidazole, which has ANTIBACTERIAL and ANTIPROTOZOAL actions. It can be used to treat a wide range of infections. It is available in a form for intravenous infusion.

✚▲ Side-effects/warnings: See METRONIDAZOLE.

metronidazole

is an (AZOLE) ANTIMICROBIAL drug with ANTIBACTERIAL and ANTIPROTOZOAL actions. As an antibacterial agent its spectrum is narrow, being limited to activity against anaerobic bacteria, including bacterial vaginal infections caused by *Gardnerella vaginalis*, dental infections, leg ulcers, pressure sores and during surgery. It has a place in eradication regimes against *Helicobacter pylori*, an organism that causes peptic ulcers. It acts by interfering with bacterial DNA replication. As an antiprotozoal it is specifically active against the protozoa *Entamoeba histolytica* (which causes dysentery), *Giardia lamblia* (giardiasis; an infection of the small intestine) and *Trichomonas vaginalis* (vaginitis). It is also used to treat outbreaks of acne rosacea and to deodorize fungating, malodorous tumours. Additionally, it has been used to treat guinea worms (*Dracunculus medinensis*). Administration can be oral as tablets or a suspension (as metronidazole benzoate), topical in the form of anal suppositories or vaginal pessaries, skin gel or cream, or by intravenous injection or infusion.

✚ Side-effects: Depending on route of administration, these may include nausea and vomiting with drowsiness, headache, dizziness, ataxia, rashes and itching, furred tongue and unpleasant taste, aches and pains, blood reactions, hypersensitivity reactions, and others. Some patients experience a discolouration of the urine. Prolonged treatment may eventually cause neuromuscular disorders or seizures. When given intravaginally there may be local irritation, abnormal discharge, increased pelvic pressure, candiasis. When applied topically to the skin, there may be local irritation; avoid strong sunlight.

▲ Warnings: It should be administered with caution to patients with impaired liver function or who are pregnant or breast-feeding. During treatment patients must avoid alcohol, which would cause very unpleasant side-effects.

✪ **Related entries: Anabact; Elyzol; Flagyl; Flagyl**

Compak; Flagyl S; HeliMet; Metrogel; Metrolyl; Metrotop; Noritate; Rozex; Vaginyl; Zidoval; Zyomet.

Metrotop

(SSL) is a proprietary, prescription-only preparation of the ANTIMICROBIAL metronidazole, which has both ANTIPROTOZOAL and ANTIBACTERIAL properties. It can be used to deodorize and treat fungating, malodorous tumours, and is available as a gel for topical application.
✚▲ Side-effects/warnings: See METRONIDAZOLE.

metyrapone

is an ENZYME INHIBITOR that inhibits the production of both *glucocorticoid* and *mineralocorticoid* CORTICOSTEROID by the adrenal glands. It can therefore be used to treat conditions that result from the excessive secretion of corticosteroids into the bloodstream (such as Cushing's syndrome). It is also used to test the function of the anterior pituitary gland. Administration is oral.
✚ Side-effects: Occasional nausea and vomiting, dizziness, headache, hypotension and allergic reactions.
▲ Warnings: It is a specialist drug and so full assessment of patient suitability will be carried out. It should not be used by those who are pregnant or breast-feeding. Drowsiness may impair driving ability.
✪ Related entry: Metopirone.

mexiletine hydrochloride

is an ANTI-ARRHYTHMIC drug which is used to reduce heartbeat irregularities (ventricular arrhythmias) particularly after a heart attack (myocardial infarction). Administration is either oral or by intravenous injection or infusion.
✚ Side-effects: Nausea and vomiting; constipation; tremor, eye-twitch, confusion; jaundice and hepatitis; blood disorders, effects on the heart and blood pressure.
▲ Warnings: It should not be administered to patients who have certain heart conditions; and use with care in those with certain liver disorders.
✪ Related entries: Mexitil; Mexitil PL.

Mexitil

(Boehringer Ingelheim) is a proprietary, prescription-only preparation of the ANTI-ARRHYTHMIC drug mexiletine hydrochloride. It can be used to treat irregularities of the heartbeat, and is available as capsules and in a form for intravenous injection or infusion.
✚▲ Side-effects/warnings: See MEXILETINE HYDROCHLORIDE.

Mexitil PL

(Boehringer Ingelheim) is a proprietary, prescription-only preparation of the ANTI-ARRHYTHMIC drug mexiletine hydrochloride. It can be used to treat irregularities of the heartbeat, and is available as modified-release capsules (*Perlongets*).
✚▲ Side-effects/warnings: See MEXILETINE HYDROCHLORIDE.

Miacalcic

(Novartis) is a proprietary, prescription-only preparation of the thyroid hormone (see THYROID HORMONES) calcitonin, in the form of salcatonin (*calcitonin (salmon)*). It can be used to lower blood levels of calcium when they are abnormally high (hypercalcaemia). It is available in a form for subcutaneous, intramuscular or intravenous injection.
✚▲ Side-effects/warnings: See SALCATONIN.

mianserin hydrochloride

is a TRICYCLIC-related ANTIDEPRESSANT which is used to treat depressive illness, especially in cases where a degree of sedation may be useful. Administration is oral.
✚▲ Side-effects/warnings: See AMITRIPTYLINE HYDROCHLORIDE; but potentially serious blood disorders may occur (a regular full blood count is necessary if there is fever, sore throat or other signs of infection). Flu-like symptoms may occur with fever, painful joints and jaundice, also some cardiovascular effects.

Micanol

(Bioglan) is a proprietary, non-prescription preparation of dithranol. It can be used to treat subacute and chronic psoriasis, and is available as a cream (a stronger version is available only on prescription).
✚▲ Side-effects/warnings: See DITHRANOL.

Micardis

(Boehringer Ingelheim) is a proprietary, prescription-only preparation of the

ANGIOTENSIN-RECEPTOR BLOCKER telmisartan. It can be used as an ANTIHYPERTENSIVE, and is available as tablets.
✚▲ Side-effects/warnings: See TELMISARTAN.

Micolette Micro-enema

(Dexcel) is a proprietary, non-prescription preparation of sodium citrate, glycerol, the SURFACTANT sodium lauryl sulphoacetate; also potassium sorbate and sorbitol. It can be used as a LAXATIVE, and is used as an enema for adults and children over three years.
✚▲ Side-effects/warnings: See GLYCEROL; SODIUM CITRATE; SODIUM LAURYL SULPHATE; SORBITOL.

miconazole

is an (AZOLE) ANTIFUNGAL drug which can be used to treat and prevent many forms of fungal infection, oropharyngeal infections such as candidiasis, and skin infections including acne. Administration can be by topical application, commonly as an oral gel.
✚ Side-effects: Nausea and vomiting, diarrhoea, allergic reactions.
▲ Warnings: It is not to be used in patients with porphyria or liver impairment; it is administered with care to those who are pregnant or breast-feeding. When used topically as an oral gel there may be systemic absorption and this may lead to serious drug interactions (eg with terfendine).
✪ Related entries: Daktacort; Daktarin; Daktarin Cream; Daktarin Dual Action Cream; Daktarin Dual Action Powder; Daktarin Dual Action Spray Powder; Daktarin Oral Gel; Daktarin Powder; Gyno-Daktarin.

Micralax Micro-enema

(Celltech) is a proprietary, non-prescription preparation of sodium citrate, glycerol, the SURFACTANT sodium lauryl sulphoacetate (mixed sodium alkylsulphoacetates) with glycerol (also sorbic acid). It can be used as a LAXATIVE, and is used as an enema for adults and children over three years.
✚▲ Side-effects/warnings: See GLYCEROL; SODIUM CITRATE; SODIUM LAURYL SULPHATE.

Microgynon 30

(Schering Health) is a proprietary, prescription-only compound preparation which can be used as a (*monophasic*) ORAL CONTRACEPTIVE of the *COC* (standard strength) type that combines an OESTROGEN and a PROGESTOGEN, in this case ethinylestradiol and levonorgestrel. It is available as tablets in a calendar pack.
✚▲ Side-effects/warnings: See ETHINYLESTRADIOL; LEVONORGESTREL.

Microgynon 30 ED

(Schering Health) is a proprietary, prescription-only compound preparation which can be used as a (*monophasic*) ORAL CONTRACEPTIVE of the *COC* (standard strength) type that combines an OESTROGEN and a PROGESTOGEN, in this case ethinylestradiol and levonorgestrel. It is available as tablets in a calendar pack.
✚▲ Side-effects/warnings: See ETHINYLESTRADIOL; LEVONORGESTREL.

Micronor

(Janssen-Cilag) is a proprietary, prescription-only preparation which can be used as an ORAL CONTRACEPTIVE of the PROGESTOGEN-only pill (*POP*) type and contains norethisterone. It is available as tablets in a calendar pack.
✚▲ Side-effects/warnings: See NORETHISTERONE.

Micronor HRT

(Janssen-Cilag) is a proprietary, prescription-only preparation of the PROGESTOGEN norethisterone. It can be used in HRT, and is available as tablets.
✚▲ Side-effects/warnings: See NORETHISTERONE.

Microval

(Wyeth) is a proprietary, prescription-only preparation which can be used as an ORAL CONTRACEPTIVE of the PROGESTOGEN-only pill (*POP*) type and contains levonorgestrel. It is available as tablets in a calendar pack.
✚▲ Side-effects/warnings: See LEVONORGESTREL.

Mictral

(Sanofi-Synthelabo) is a proprietary, prescription-only preparation of the (QUINOLONE) ANTIBIOTIC-like ANTIBACTERIAL nalidixic acid. It can be used to treat infections, particularly of the urinary tract, and is available as granules.
✚▲ Side-effects/warnings: See NALIDIXIC ACID.

M

midazolam
is a BENZODIAZEPINE which can be used as an ANXIOLYTIC and SEDATIVE in preoperative medication, because its ability to cause amnesia means that the patient forgets the unpleasant procedure. Administration is by injection.
✚▲ Side-effects/warnings: It is a specialist drug used under controlled conditions.
✪ **Related entry: Hypnovel.**

Midrid
(Manx) is a proprietary, non-prescription preparation of the NON-NARCOTIC ANALGESIC paracetamol and the SYMPATHOMIMETIC and ANTIMIGRAINE drug isometheptene mucate. It can be used to relieve migraine and throbbing headaches, and is available as capsules. It is not given to children, except on medical advice.
✚▲ Side-effects/warnings: See ISOMETHEPTENE MUCATE; PARACETAMOL.

Mifegyne
(Exelgyn) is a proprietary, prescription-only preparation of the uterine stimulant mifepristone. It is used as an ABORTIFACIENT for termination of pregnancy, and is available as tablets.
✚▲ Side-effects/warnings: See MIFEPRISTONE.

mifepristone
is a PROGESTOGEN HORMONE ANTAGONIST which is used as an ABORTIFACIENT for termination of uterine pregnancy. It is taken by mouth under medical supervision with monitoring or another method of termination, sometimes a PROSTAGLANDIN (eg GEMEPROST).
✚ Side-effects: Vaginal bleeding (which can be severe), uterine pain, nausea and vomiting, faintness, hypotension, rashes; infections of the uterus and urinary tract.
▲ Warnings: It is a specialist drug, and a full assessment will be made of patient suitability, with counselling. Smoking and alcohol must be avoided for two days before and on the day of treatment with mifepristone. It is not given to people with porphyria.
✪ **Related entry: Mifegyne.**

Migraleve
(Warner Lambert Consumer Healthcare; Pfizer) is a proprietary, non-prescription ANTIMIGRAINE treatment, a compound preparation which is used only for acute migraine attacks not for preventing them. It is available in the form of different coloured tablets: pink, containing the ANTIHISTAMINE buclizine hydrochloride, the NON-NARCOTIC ANALGESIC paracetamol and the (OPIOID) NARCOTIC ANALGESIC codeine phosphate; and yellow, without buclizine hydrochloride. The preparations are not normally given to children under ten years, except on medical advice.
✚▲ Side-effects/warnings: See BUCLIZINE HYDROCHLORIDE; CODEINE PHOSPHATE; PARACETAMOL.

Migraleve Pink
(Warner Lambert Consumer Healthcare; Pfizer) is a proprietary, non-prescription ANTIMIGRAINE treatment. It is used for treating symptoms of migraine headache, nausea and vomiting, but is not for preventing migraine attacks. It is a compound preparation of the ANTIHISTAMINE buclizine hydrochloride, the NON-NARCOTIC ANALGESIC paracetamol and the (OPIOID) NARCOTIC ANALGESIC codeine phosphate. It is available in the form of pink tablets taken as soon as it is known that a migraine attack is imminent, and is not normally given to children under ten years, except on medical advice.
✚▲ Side-effects/warnings: See BUCLIZINE HYDROCHLORIDE; CODEINE PHOSPHATE; PARACETAMOL.

Migraleve Yellow
(Warner Lambert Consumer Healthcare; Pfizer) is a proprietary, non-prescription ANTIMIGRAINE treatment. It is used for treating the symptoms of migraine headache that persist in the later stages of an attack (following treatment with *Migraleve Pink*), but is not for preventing migraine attacks. It is a compound preparation of the the NON-NARCOTIC ANALGESIC paracetamol and the (OPIOID) NARCOTIC ANALGESIC codeine phosphate. It is available in the form of yellow tablets, and is not normally given to children under ten years, except on medical advice.
✚▲ Side-effects/warnings: See CODEINE PHOSPHATE; PARACETAMOL.

MigraMax
(Elan) is a proprietary, prescription-only compound preparation of the ANTI-EMETIC and ANTINAUSEANT metoclopramide hydrochloride

and the NON-NARCOTIC ANALGESIC aspirin (as lysine acetylsalicylate). It can be used as an ANTIMIGRAINE treatment for acute migraine attacks, and is available as an oral powder (for dissolving in water at onset of attack).

✚▲ Side-effects/warnings: See ASPIRIN; METOCLOPRAMIDE HYDROCHLORIDE. Note the side-effects in young people.

Migril

(CP) is a proprietary, prescription-only compound preparation of the ergot VASOCONSTRICTOR ergotamine tartrate, the ANTINAUSEANT cyclizine (as hydrochloride) and the STIMULANT caffeine (as hydrate). It can be used as an ANTIMIGRAINE treatment and also for some other vascular headaches, and is available as tablets.

✚▲ Side-effects/warnings: See CAFFEINE; CYCLIZINE; ERGOTAMINE TARTRATE.

Mildison

(Yamanouchi) is a proprietary, prescription-only preparation of the CORTICOSTEROID and ANTI-INFLAMMATORY hydrocortisone. It can be used to treat mild inflammatory skin conditions, such as eczema, and is available as a cream (called *Lipocream*).

✚▲ Side-effects/warnings: See HYDROCORTISONE.

Mil-Par

(Merck Consumer Health; Seven Seas) is a proprietary, non-prescription compound preparation of the ANTACID magnesium hydroxide and the LAXATIVE liquid paraffin. It can be used for the temporary relief of constipation. It is available as a liquid. It is not normally given to children under three, except on medical advice.

✚▲ Side-effects/warnings: See LIQUID PARAFFIN; MAGNESIUM HYDROXIDE.

milrinone

is a PHOSPHODIESTERASE INHIBITOR which is used, in the short term, in congestive HEART FAILURE TREATMENT (especially where other drugs have been unsuccessful) and in acute heart failure. Administration is by intravenous injection or infusion.

✚▲ Side-effects/warnings: See ENOXIMONE. Blood potassium should be controlled and kidney function monitored. It may cause chest pain.

✪ Related entry: Primacor.

mineral supplement 🅴

refers to formulations of some of the salts of essential (required in the diet) dietary minerals, which may be taken, usually by mouth, to make up deficiencies in the diet, or where there are problems with absorption of the minerals into the body from normal foodstuffs. Examples include: calcium, IRON, FLUORIDE, MAGNESIUM, ZINC, phosphorus, sodium and potassium. Sometimes the deficiency is due to drug action, and needs to be continually rectified (eg some DIURETIC drugs cause a large loss of potassium from the body, and this must be made good on a continuous basis with POTASSIUM CHLORIDE).

Minihep

(Leo) is a proprietary, prescription-only preparation of the ANTICOAGULANT heparin (as heparin sodium). Used to treat various forms of thrombosis. Available in a form for injection.

✚▲ Side-effects/warnings: See HEPARIN.

Min-I-Jet Adrenaline

(Celltech) is a proprietary, prescription-only preparation of the natural HORMONE adrenaline acid tartrate (epinephrine). It is used as a SYMPATHOMIMETIC drug to treat acute and severe bronchial asthma attacks, in the emergency treatment of acute allergic reactions and for angioedema and cardiopulmonary resuscitation. It is available in a form for intramuscular, subcutaneous or intravenous injection.

✚▲ Side-effects/warnings: See ADRENALINE ACID TARTRATE.

Min-I-Jet Aminophylline

(Celltech) is a proprietary, prescription-only preparation of the BRONCHODILATOR aminophylline. It can be used to treat severe acute asthma attacks, and is available in a form for intravenous injection or intravenous infusion.

✚▲ Side-effects/warnings: See AMINOPHYLLINE.

Min-I-Jet Bretylate Tosylate

(Celltech) is a proprietary, prescription-only preparation of bretylium tosilate. It can be used in resuscitation and as an ANTI-ARRHYTHMIC treatment of ventricular arrhythmias where other treatments have not been successful. It is available in a form for injection.

✚▲ Side-effects/warnings: See BRETYLIUM TOSILATE.

Min-I-Jet Frusemide
(Celltech) is a proprietary, prescription-only preparation of the (*loop*) DIURETIC furosemide (frusemide). It can be used to treat oedema, and low urine production due to kidney failure (oliguria). It is available in a form for intravenous injection or infusion.
✚▲ Side-effects/warnings: See FUROSEMIDE.

Min-I-Jet Isoprenaline
(Celltech) is a proprietary, prescription-only preparation of the BETA-RECEPTOR STIMULANT and SYMPATHOMIMETIC isoprenaline (as isoprenaline hydrochloride). It can be used as a CARDIAC STIMULANT to treat acute heart block and severe bradycardia, and is available in a form for intravenous injection.
✚▲ Side-effects/warnings: See ISOPRENALINE.

Min-I-Jet Lignocaine
(Celltech) is a proprietary, prescription-only preparation of the LOCAL ANAESTHETIC lidocaine hydrochloride. It can be used as an ANTI-ARRHYTHMIC drug to treat irregularities in the heartbeat, especially after a heart attack, and is available in a form for injection.
✚▲ Side-effects/warnings: See LIDOCAINE HYDROCHLORIDE.

Min-I-Jet Naloxone
(Celltech) is a proprietary, prescription-only preparation of the OPIOID ANTAGONIST naloxone hydrochloride. It can be used to treat overdosage with opioids and postoperative respiratory depression (caused by opioid analgesia during operations), and is available in syringes ready for use.
✚▲ Side-effects/warnings: See NALOXONE HYDROCHLORIDE.

Min-I-Jet Sodium Bicarbonate
(Celltech) is a proprietary, prescription-only preparation of sodium bicarbonate. It can be used to treat metabolic acidosis, and is available in a form for injection.
✚▲ Side-effects/warnings: See SODIUM BICARBONATE.

Minims Amethocaine Hydrochloride
(Chauvin) is a proprietary, prescription-only preparation of the LOCAL ANAESTHETIC tetracaine (as hydrochloride). It can be used by topical application for ophthalmic procedures, and is available as eye-drops.
✚▲ Side-effects/warnings: See TETRACAINE.

Minims Artificial Tears
(Chauvin) is a proprietary, non-prescription preparation of HYDROXYETHYLCELLULOSE. It is used as artificial tears where there is dryness of the eyes due to disease, and is available as eye-drops.
✚▲ Side-effects/warnings: See HYDROXYETHYLCELLULOSE.

Minims Atropine Sulphate
(Chauvin) is a proprietary, prescription-only preparation of the ANTICHOLINERGIC drug atropine sulphate. It can be used to dilate the pupil and to facilitate inspection of the eye and for refraction procedures in young children, and for the treatment of anterior uveitis. It is available as eye-drops.
✚▲ Side-effects/warnings: See ATROPINE SULPHATE.

Minims Benoxinate (Oxybuprocaine) Hydrochloride
(Chauvin) is a proprietary, prescription-only preparation of the LOCAL ANAESTHETIC oxybuprocaine hydrochloride. It can be used by topical application for ophthalmic procedures, and is available as eye-drops.
✚▲ Side-effects/warnings: See OXYBUPROCAINE HYDROCHLORIDE.

Minims Chloramphenicol
(Chauvin) is a proprietary, prescription-only preparation of the ANTIBACTERIAL and ANTIBIOTIC chloramphenicol. It can be used to treat bacterial infections in the eye, and is available as eye-drops.
✚▲ Side-effects/warnings: See CHLORAMPHENICOL.

Minims Cyclopentolate
(Chauvin) is a proprietary, prescription-only preparation of the ANTICHOLINERGIC drug cyclopentolate hydrochloride. It can be used to dilate the pupil and paralyse focusing and so facilitate inspection of the eyes, and is available as eye-drops.
✚▲ Side-effects/warnings: See CYCLOPENTOLATE HYDROCHLORIDE.

Minims Dexamethasone
(Chauvin) is a proprietary, prescription-only preparation of the ANTI-INFLAMMATORY and CORTICOSTEROID dexamethasone. It can be used to treat inflammation of the eye when infection is also present, and is available as eye-drops.
✚▲ Side-effects/warnings: See DEXAMETHASONE.

Minims Fluorescein Sodium
(Chauvin) is a proprietary, non-prescription preparation of the dye FLUORESCEIN SODIUM. It can be used on the surface of the eye in ophthalmic diagnostic procedures to detect foreign bodies and lesions, and is available as eye-drops.
✚▲ Side-effects/warnings: See FLUORESCEIN SODIUM.

Minims Gentamicin
(Chauvin) is a proprietary, prescription-only preparation of the ANTIBACTERIAL and (AMINOGLYCOSIDE) ANTIBIOTIC gentamicin (as sulphate). It can be used to treat many forms of infection, and is available as an eye ointment.
✚▲ Side-effects/warnings: See GENTAMICIN.

Minims Homatropine Hydrobromide
(Chauvin) is a proprietary, prescription-only preparation of the ANTICHOLINERGIC drug homatropine hydrobromide. It can be used to dilate the pupils and paralyse certain eye muscles to allow ophthalmic examination, and in the treatment of anterior segment inflammation. It is available as eye-drops.
✚▲ Side-effects/warnings: See HOMATROPINE HYDROBROMIDE.

Minims Lignocaine and Fluorescein
(Chauvin) is a proprietary, prescription-only preparation of the LOCAL ANAESTHETIC lidocaine hydrochloride (with the diagnostic dye fluorescein sodium). It is used in ophthalmic procedures, and is available as eye-drops.
✚▲ Side-effects/warnings: See FLUORESCEIN SODIUM; LIDOCAINE HYDROCHLORIDE.

Minims Metipranolol
(Chauvin) is a proprietary, prescription-only preparation of the BETA-BLOCKER metipranolol. It can be used for GLAUCOMA TREATMENT, and is available as eye-drops.
✚▲ Side-effects/warnings: See METIPRANOLOL. It is used by patients allergic to the preservative benzalkonium chloride, which is found in several other similar eye-drops, and can be used by those wearing soft contact lenses.

Minims Neomycin Sulphate
(Chauvin) is a proprietary, prescription-only preparation of the ANTIBACTERIAL and (AMINOGLYCOSIDE) ANTIBIOTIC neomycin sulphate. It can be used to treat bacterial infections in the eye, and is available as eye-drops.
✚▲ Side-effects/warnings: See NEOMYCIN SULPHATE.

Minims Phenylephrine Hydrochloride
(Chauvin) is a proprietary, non-prescription preparation of the SYMPATHOMIMETIC drug phenylephrine hydrochloride. It can be used to dilate the pupils for ophthalmic examination, and is available as eye-drops.
✚▲ Side-effects/warnings: See PHENYLEPHRINE HYDROCHLORIDE.

Minims Pilocarpine Nitrate
(Chauvin) is a proprietary, prescription-only preparation of the PARASYMPATHOMIMETIC pilocarpine. It can be used to constrict the pupil and in GLAUCOMA TREATMENT. Available as eye-drops.
✚▲ Side-effects/warnings: See PILOCARPINE.

Minims Prednisolone
(Chauvin) is a proprietary, prescription-only preparation of the CORTICOSTEROID and ANTI-INFLAMMATORY prednisolone (as sodium phosphate). It can be used to treat conditions in and around the eye, and is available as eye-drops.
✚▲ Side-effects/warnings: See PREDNISOLONE.

Minims Proxymetacaine and Fluorescein
(Chauvin) is a proprietary, prescription-only compound preparation of the dye fluorescein sodium and the LOCAL ANAESTHETIC proxymetacaine hydrochloride. It can be used on the surface of the eye in ophthalmic procedures and is available as eye-drops.
✚▲ Side-effects/warnings: see FLUORESCEIN SODIUM; PROXYMETACAINE.

Minims Proxymetacaine Hydrochloride
(Chauvin) is a proprietary, prescription-only

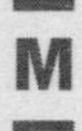

preparation of the LOCAL ANAESTHETIC proxymetacaine (as hydrochloride). It can be used during ophthalmic procedures, and is available as eye-drops.
✚▲ Side-effects/warnings: See PROXYMETACAINE.

Minims Rose Bengal
(Chauvin) is a proprietary, non-prescription preparation of the dye ROSE BENGAL. It can be used on the surface of the eye for ophthalmic diagnostic procedures to detect foreign bodies and lesions, and is available as eye-drops.
✚▲ Side-effects/warnings: See ROSE BENGAL.

Minims Saline
(Chauvin) is a proprietary, non-prescription preparation of saline solution (sodium chloride). It can be used for the irrigation of the eyes and to facilitate the removal of harmful substances, and is available as eye-drops.
✚▲ Side-effects/warnings: See SODIUM CHLORIDE.

Minims Tropicamide
(Chauvin) is a proprietary, prescription-only preparation of tropicamide. It can be used to dilate the pupils to facilitate inspection of the eyes, and is available as eye-drops.
✚▲ Side-effects/warnings: See TROPICAMIDE.

Minitran
(3M) is a proprietary, non-prescription preparation of the VASODILATOR and ANTI-ANGINA drug glyceryl trinitrate. It can be used to treat and prevent angina pectoris. It is available as a self-adhesive dressing (patch) from which, when placed on the chest wall or upper arm, it is absorbed through the skin and helps to give lasting relief.
✚▲ Side-effects/warnings: See GLYCERYL TRINITRATE.

Minocin
(Lederle; Wyeth) is a proprietary, prescription-only preparation of the ANTIBACTERIAL and (TETRACYCLINES) ANTIBIOTIC minocycline. It can be used to treat a wide range of infections, and is available as tablets.
✚▲ Side-effects/warnings: See MINOCYCLINE.

Minocin MR
(Lederle; Wyeth) is a proprietary, prescription-only preparation of the ANTIBACTERIAL and (TETRACYCLINES) ANTIBIOTIC minocycline. It can be used to treat a wide range of infections (including acne), and is available as capsules.
✚▲ Side-effects/warnings: See MINOCYCLINE.

minocycline
is a broad-spectrum ANTIBACTERIAL and (TETRACYCLINES) ANTIBIOTIC. It has a wider range of actions than most other tetracyclines, because it is also effective in preventing certain forms of meningitis (caused by *Neisseria meningitidis*). Administration is oral.
✚▲ Side-effects/warnings: See TETRACYCLINE. It may cause dizziness and vertigo, rashes and pigmentation. There have been reports of liver damage and systemic lupus erythematosus. It can be used in patients with impaired kidney function.
✪ Related entries: Aknemin; Blemix; Dentomycin; Minocin; Minocin MR.

Minodiab
(Pharmacia) is a proprietary, prescription-only preparation of the SULPHONYLUREA glipizide. It is used in DIABETIC TREATMENT of Type II diabetes (non-insulin-dependent diabetes mellitus; NIDDM; maturity-onset diabetes), and is available as tablets.
✚▲ Side-effects/warnings: See GLIPIZIDE.

minor tranquillizer 🄴
see ANXIOLYTIC.

minoxidil
is a VASODILATOR which can be used as an ANTIHYPERTENSIVE (often combined with a DIURETIC or BETA-BLOCKER). Administration is oral. It can also be used, as a lotion, to treat male-pattern baldness (in men and women).
✚ Side-effects: There are gastrointestinal disturbances and weight gain; there may also be fluid retention, a rise in the heart rate and breast tenderness. When used topically to the scalp, there may be itching and dermatitis. It can increase hair growth which may be a problem when it is used for hypertension.
▲ Warnings: It should not be administered to patients with phaeochromocytoma. Administer with care to those who are pregnant or have certain heart disorders or porphyria. When used as a lotion, avoid contact with the eyes and

mucous membranes.
✪ Related entries: Loniten; Regaine Extra Strength; Regaine Regular Strength.

Mintec

(Shire) is a proprietary, non-prescription preparation of the ANTISPASMODIC peppermint oil. It can be used to relieve the discomfort of abdominal colic and distension, particularly in irritable bowel syndrome, and is available as capsules. It is not recommended for children.
✚▲ Side-effects/warnings: See PEPPERMINT OIL.

Mintezol

(IDIS) is a proprietary, prescription-only preparation of the ANTHELMINTIC drug tiabendazole. It can be used to treat intestinal infestations, especially by the *Strongyloides* species, and to assist in the treatment of resistant infections by hookworm, whipworm and roundworm. It is available as chewable tablets.
✚▲ Side-effects/warnings: See TIABENDAZOLE.

Minulet

(Wyeth) is a proprietary, prescription-only compound preparation which can be used as a (*monophasic*) ORAL CONTRACEPTIVE of the *COC* (standard strength) type that combines an OESTROGEN and a PROGESTOGEN, in this case ethinylestradiol and gestodene. It is available as tablets in a calendar pack.
✚▲ Side-effects/warnings: See ETHINYLESTRADIOL; GESTODENE.

Miochol-E

(Novartis Ophthalmics) is a proprietary, prescription-only preparation of the PARASYMPATHOMIMETIC acetylcholine chloride. It is used mainly to contract the pupils prior to surgery on the iris, the cornea or other sections of the eye. It is available as a solution for intraocular irrigation.
✚▲ Side-effects/warnings: See ACETYLCHOLINE CHLORIDE.

Mirapexin

(Pharmacia) is a prescription-only preparation of the ANTIPARKINSONISM drug pramipexole (as hydrochloride). It is available in as tablets.
✚▲ Side-effects/warnings: See PRAMIPEXOLE.

Mirena

(Schering Health) is a proprietary, prescription-only CONTRACEPTIVE device that releases the PROGESTOGEN levonorgestrel. It is available in the form of an intrauterine system, a T-shaped plastic frame with a drug reservoir and threads attached to the base (fitted by a doctor).
✚▲ Side-effects/warnings: See LEVONORGESTREL.

mirtazapine

is an 'atypical' ANTIDEPRESSANT that works by increasing brain neurotransmission by NORADRENALINE and SEROTONIN (5-HT). It has few ANTICHOLINERGIC (antimuscarinic) side-effects, but causes sedation during initial treatment. It can be used to treat depressive illness and administration is oral.
✚ Side-effects: Sedation, increased appetite and weight gain; less commonly changed liver enzymes or jaundice (treatment should be stopped); rarely oedema, postural hypotension, tremor and other side-effects.
▲ Warnings: Should be used with caution in severe liver or kidney impairment, epilepsy, heart disorders, low blood pressure, in pregnancy or breast-feeding; in urinary retention, glaucoma, diabetes mellitus, psychoses, manic-depression. Patients are advised to report any fever, sore throat or other signs of infection during treatment. Blood studies should be made if blood changes are suspected. Symptoms such as sore throat and inflammation of the mouth, fever and other signs of infection should be reported. Withdrawal of the drug should be gradual.
✪ Related entry: Zispin.

misoprostol

is a synthetic analogue of the PROSTAGLANDIN E_1 (ALPROSTADIL). It can be used as an ULCER-HEALING DRUG, because it inhibits acid secretion and promotes protective blood flow to the mucosal layer of the intestine. It cannot be used to treat dyspepsia, but can be very useful in protecting against ulcers caused by non-steroidal anti-inflammatory drugs (NSAIDS) and for this reason it is now also available in combination with some (NSAID) NON-NARCOTIC ANALGESIC and ANTIRHEUMATIC drugs (eg *Arthrotec* and *Napratec*) in the treatment of rheumatic disease. Administration is oral.
✚ Side-effects: Diarrhoea (which may be severe), nausea, flatulence and vomiting, abdominal pain, dyspepsia, abnormal vaginal bleeding,

M

dizziness and rashes.
▲ Warnings: It should not be administered to women who are pregnant or planning pregnancy since risks are involved if taken when the woman is pregnant; and used with caution in patients with certain cardiovascular problems.
✪ **Related entries: Arthrotec; Cytotec; Napratec.**

Mistamine
(Galderma) is a proprietary, prescription-only preparation of the ANTIHISTAMINE mizolastine . It can be used to treat the symptoms of allergic disorders, such as hay fever and urticaria, and is available as modified-release tablets.
✚▲ Side-effects/warnings: See MIZOLASTINE.

mitomycin
is a CYTOTOXIC drug (of ANTIBIOTIC origin), which is used as an ANTICANCER treatment of cancers of the upper gastrointestinal tract, bladder tumours and breast tumours. Administration is by injection or bladder instillation.
✚▲ Side-effects/warnings: See CYTOTOXIC. It can cause lung fibrosis and kidney damage.
✪ **Related entry: Mitomycin C Kyowa.**

Mitomycin C Kyowa
(Kyowa Hakko) is a proprietary, prescription-only preparation of the (CYTOTOXIC) ANTICANCER drug mitomycin. It can be used in the treatment of upper gastrointestinal cancer, breast cancer and some superficial bladder tumours. It is available in forms for injection.
✚▲ Side-effects/warnings: See MITOMYCIN.

Mitoxana
(ASTA Medica) is a proprietary, prescription-only preparation of the ANTICANCER drug ifosfamide, which can be used in the treatment of cancer. It is available in a form for injection.
✚▲ Side-effects/warnings: See IFOSFAMIDE.

mitoxantrone
(mitozantrone) is a CYTOTOXIC drug (of ANTIBIOTIC origin) that is chemically related to doxorubicin. It is used as an ANTICANCER treatment for several types of cancer, for example, breast cancer. Administration is by intravenous infusion.
✚▲ Side-effects/warnings: See CYTOTOXIC; there are also effects on the heart.
✪ **Related entries: Novantrone; Onkotrone.**

mitozantrone
see MITOXANTRONE.

Mivacron
(GlaxoWellcome; GSK) is a proprietary, prescription-only preparation of the (*non-depolarizing*) SKELETAL MUSCLE RELAXANT mivacurium chloride. It can be used to induce muscle paralysis during surgery, and is available in a form for injection.
✚▲ Side-effects/warnings: See MIVACURIUM CHLORIDE.

mivacurium chloride
is a (*non-depolarizing*) SKELETAL MUSCLE RELAXANT which is used to induce muscle paralysis during surgery. Administration is by injection.
✚▲ Side-effects/warnings: It is a specialist drug used by anaesthetists in hospital.
✪ **Related entry: Mivacron.**

mizolastine
is an ANTIHISTAMINE which has only recently been developed and has fewer sedative side-effects than some of the older antihistamines. It can be used for the symptomatic relief of allergic conditions, such as hay fever and urticaria. Administration is oral.
✚▲ Side-effects/warnings: See ANTIHISTAMINE; but the incidence of sedative and anticholinergic effects is low, though it may impair driving. May cause weight gain. Not used in cardiac disease, low blood potassium, pregnancy or breast-feeding.
✪ **Related entries: Mistamine; Mizollen.**

Mizollen
(Sanofi-Synthelabo) is a proprietary, prescription-only preparation of the ANTIHISTAMINE mizolastine. It can be used to treat the symptoms of allergic disorders, such as hay fever and urticaria, and is available as modified-release tablets.
✚▲ Side-effects/warnings: See MIZOLASTINE.

MMR II
(Aventis Pasteur) is a proprietary, prescription-only preparation of a VACCINE (MMR vaccine) that can be used for the prevention of measles,

mumps and rubella (German measles) in children. It is available in a form for injection.
✚▲ Side-effects/warnings: See MMR VACCINE.

MMR vaccine

is a combined VACCINE used for IMMUNIZATION against measles, mumps and rubella. It uses live but weakened (attenuated) strains of the viruses and was introduced with the objective of eliminating rubella (German measles), mumps and measles, through universal vaccination of children before they began school. The first dose is given to children at 12-15 months, with a booster at age 3-5 years. It is also given in the control of outbreaks of measles, and to susceptible children within three days of exposure to infection (measles only). The vaccine is available from District Health Authorities or manufacturers under a number of names.
✚▲ Side-effects/warnings: See VACCINE. There may be fever, malaise and/or rash about a week after administration; there may be a swelling of the parotid gland (salivary gland in the jaw) after two to three weeks.
✪ **Related entries: MMR II; Priorix.**

Mobic

(Boehringer Ingelheim) is a proprietary, prescription-only preparation of the (NSAID) NON-NARCOTIC ANALGESIC and ANTIRHEUMATIC meloxicam. It can be used to treat pain and inflammation in rheumatoid arthritis, for ankylosing spondylitis, and for short-term treatment of osteoarthritis. It is available as tablets and suppositories.
✚▲ Side-effects/warnings: See MELOXICAM.

Mobiflex

(Roche) is a proprietary, prescription-only preparation of the (NSAID) NON-NARCOTIC ANALGESIC and ANTIRHEUMATIC tenoxicam. It can be used to treat the pain and inflammation of rheumatism and other musculoskeletal disorders. It is available as tablets or in a form for injection.
✚▲ Side-effects/warnings: See TENOXICAM.

moclobemide

is a type of MONOAMINE-OXIDASE INHIBITOR (MAOI) ANTIDEPRESSANT which is used to treat major depressive illness. It is a reversible inhibitor of the monoamine oxidase type A (therefore termed RIMA) and reported to show less potentiation of dangerous side-effects of tyramine found in foodstuffs (a common side-effect of other MAOIs), though large quantities of these (eg ripe cheese, yeast extract) should still be avoided. Interactions with other medicines are also claimed to be less. It should not be used in conjunction with conventional MAO inhibitors, but in view of its short duration of action the switch to other forms of antidepressant may be quicker than is usual (though a five-week gap is still required before moving to FLUOXETINE). However, there may be a more STIMULANT action than with most other MAOIs, making it less suitable for agitated patients. It can also be used to treat social phobia. Administration is oral.
✚ Side-effects: There is some stimulation resulting in restlessness, agitation, dry mouth, oedema, milk production, sleep disturbances; also dizziness, nausea, visual and gastrointestinal disorders, confusion, skin reactions, changes in liver enzymes and lowered blood sodium.
▲ Warnings: It should not be used in those who are acutely confused or who have phaeochromocytoma. Care in those who are agitated or excited, have severe liver impairment, a thyroid imbalance or who are pregnant or breast-feeding. It may bring on manic-depressive behaviour.
✪ **Related entry: Manerix.**

modafinil

is a drug that works directly on the brain as a CNS STIMULANT and can be used to treat narcolepsy (a condition involving irresistible attacks of sleep during the daytime). Administration is oral.
✚ Side-effects: Anorexia, abdominal pain, headache, personality disorder, insomnia, excitation, euphoria, nervousness, palpitations, increased heart rate, hypertension, tremor; also dry mouth, gastrointestinal disturbances (including nausea, stomach discomfort); rashes and itching.
▲ Warnings: It is not be administered to people who are pregnant, breast-feeding; who have hypertension or certain heart disorders or chest pain. It is used with caution in those with liver or kidney impairment. There is a possibility of patients becoming drug dependent.
✪ **Related entry: Provigil.**

Modalim

(Sanofi-Synthelabo) is a proprietary,

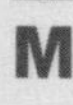

prescription-only preparation of the LIPID-REGULATING DRUG ciprofibrate. It can be used in hyperlipidaemia to modify the proportions of various lipids in the bloodstream. It is available as tablets.
✚▲ Side-effects/warnings: See CIPROFIBRATE.

Modecate
(Sanofi-Synthelabo) is a proprietary, prescription-only preparation of the ANTIPSYCHOTIC drug fluphenazine (as decanoate). It is available in two strengths for depot deep intramuscular injection; the stronger preparation is called *Modecate Concentrate*.
✚▲ Side-effects/warnings: See FLUPHENAZINE.

Modisal XL
(Lagap) is a proprietary, non-prescription preparation of the VASODILATOR and ANTI-ANGINA drug isosorbide mononitrate. It can be used to treat and prevent angina pectoris, and is available as modified-release tablets.
✚▲ Side-effects/warnings: See ISOSORBIDE MONONITRATE.

Moditen
(Sanofi-Synthelabo) is a proprietary, prescription-only preparation of the ANTIPSYCHOTIC drug fluphenazine. It is available as tablets (as fluphenazine hydrochloride).
✚▲ Side-effects/warnings: See FLUPHENAZINE.

Modrasone
(Dominion) is a proprietary, prescription-only preparation of the CORTICOSTEROID and ANTI-INFLAMMATORY alclometasone dipropionate. It can be used to treat inflammatory skin conditions, such as eczema, and is available as a cream and an ointment for topical application.
✚▲ Side-effects/warnings: See ALCLOMETASONE DIPROPIONATE.

Modrenal
(Wanskerne) is a proprietary, prescription-only preparation of the ENZYME INHIBITOR trilostane. It can be used to treat conditions that result from the excessive secretion of corticosteroids into the bloodstream (eg Cushing's syndrome); also primary hyperaldosterism. It can also be used in the ANTICANCER treatment of postmenopausal breast cancer. It is available as capsules.
✚▲ Side-effects/warnings: See TRILOSTANE.

Moducren
(MSD) is a proprietary, prescription-only compound preparation of the BETA-BLOCKER timolol maleate and the DIURETIC hydrochlorothiazide and amiloride hydrochloride (*co-amilozide*). It can be used as an ANTIHYPERTENSIVE for raised blood pressure, and is available as tablets.
✚▲ Side-effects/warnings: See AMILORIDE HYDROCHLORIDE; HYDROCHLOROTHIAZIDE; TIMOLOL MALEATE.

Moduret 25
(DuPont; Bristol-Myers Squibb) is a proprietary, prescription-only compound preparation of the (*potassium-sparing*) DIURETIC amiloride hydrochloride and the (THIAZIDE) diuretic hydrochlorothiazide (a combination called co-amilozide 2.5/25). It can be used to treat oedema and congestive heart failure, and as an ANTIHYPERTENSIVE. It is available as tablets.
✚▲ Side-effects/warnings: See AMILORIDE HYDROCHLORIDE; HYDROCHLOROTHIAZIDE.

Moduretic
(DuPont; Bristol-Myers Squibb) is a proprietary, prescription-only compound preparation of the (*potassium-sparing*) DIURETIC amiloride hydrochloride and the THIAZIDE diuretic hydrochlorothiazide (a combination called co-amilozide 5/50). It can be used to treat oedema and as an ANTIHYPERTENSIVE. It is available as tablets.
✚▲ Side-effects/warnings: See AMILORIDE HYDROCHLORIDE; HYDROCHLOROTHIAZIDE.

moexipril hydrochloride
is an ACE INHIBITOR and acts as a VASODILATOR. It can be used as an ANTIHYPERTENSIVE, often in conjunction with other classes of drugs, particularly (THIAZIDE) DIURETIC drugs. Administration is oral.
✚ Side-effects: See ACE INHIBITOR. Also heart arrhythmias, angina and chest pain, fainting, cerebrovascular accident, myocardial infarction; appetite and weight changes; dry mouth, photosensitivity, flushing, nervousness and mood changes, anxiety, drowsiness, sleep disturbance, tinnitus, influenza-like symptoms, sweating and laboured breathing.
▲ Warnings: See ACE INHIBITOR.
✪ **Related entry: Perdix.**

Mogadon

(ICN) is a proprietary, prescription-only preparation of the BENZODIAZEPINE nitrazepam. It can be used as a relatively long-acting HYPNOTIC for the short-term treatment of insomnia, where a degree of sedation during the daytime is acceptable. It is available as tablets.
✚▲ Side-effects/warnings: See NITRAZEPAM.

Moisture-eyes

(Co-Pharma) is a proprietary, non-prescription preparation of HYPROMELLOSE. It can be used as artificial tears to treat dryness of the eyes due to disease, and is available as eye-drops.
✚▲ Side-effects/warnings: See HYPROMELLOSE.

Molcer Ear Drops

(Wallace) is a proprietary, non-prescription preparation of dioctyl sodium sulphosuccinate. It can be used to dissolve earwax prior to its removal by syringing, and is available as ear-drops.
✚▲ Side-effects/warnings: See DIOCTYL SODIUM SULPHOSUCCINATE.

molgramostim

(recombinant human granulocyte macrophage-colony stimulating factor, GM-CSF) is a specialist drug used to reduce neutropenia (a shortage of neutrophil white blood-cells in the circulation) by stimulating white cell production (all granulocytes and monocytes) when this has been reduced during chemotherapy in ANTICANCER treatment, and this may reduce the incidence of associated sepsis. Administration is by intravenous infusion.
✚▲ Side-effects/warnings: These are many. This is a specialist drug used only after full evaluation under hospital conditions.
✪ **Related entry: Leucomax.**

Molipaxin

(Hoechst Marion Roussel; Aventis Pharma) is a proprietary, prescription-only preparation of the (TRICYCLIC-related) ANTIDEPRESSANT trazodone hydrochloride. It can be used to relieve the symptoms of depressive illness. It is available as capsules, a liquid and tablets.
✚▲ Side-effects/warnings: See TRAZODONE HYDROCHLORIDE.

mometasone furoate

is a CORTICOSTEROID with ANTI-INFLAMMATORY and ANTI-ALLERGIC properties. It is used to treat severe inflammatory skin disorders such as psoriasis and eczemas unresponsive to less potent corticosteroids; also for allergic rhinitis. Administration is by topical application.
✚▲ Side-effects/warnings: See CORTICOSTEROID. Serious systemic effects are unlikely with topical application, though there may be local reactions.
✪ **Related entries: Elocon; Nasonex.**

Monit

(Sanofi-Synthelabo) is a proprietary, non-prescription preparation of the VASODILATOR drug isosorbide mononitrate. It can be used as an ANTI-ANGINA drug, and is available as tablets and *LS* tablets.
✚▲ Side-effects/warnings: See ISOSORBIDE MONONITRATE.

Monit SR

(Sanofi-Synthelabo) is a proprietary, non-prescription preparation of the VASODILATOR drug isosorbide mononitrate. It can be used as an ANTI-ANGINA drug, and is available as modified-release tablets.
✚▲ Side-effects/warnings: See ISOSORBIDE MONONITRATE.

monoamine-oxidase inhibitor

drugs, or MAOIs, are ENZYME INHIBITOR drugs and constitute one of the three major classes of ANTIDEPRESSANT drugs that are used to relieve the symptoms of depressive illness. Chemically, they are usually hydrazine derivatives and include ISOCARBOXAZID and PHENELZINE. Although they are well established, having been used for many years, they are nowadays used much less often than the TRICYCLIC antidepressants, largely because of the dangers of potentially serious interactions with foodstuffs and with other drugs. Also, they have side-effects including tremors, excitement, weight gain and hypotension. However, they may be used when other classes of antidepressant have not proved useful, or for some reason cannot be used. Their action is said to be better suited for use in patients with hypochondria, phobias or hysterical episodes. Treatment often takes some weeks to show maximal beneficial effects. If a monoamine-oxidase inhibitor is used after certain other antidepressants, including tricyclics and SSRIS (or *vice versa*), a suitably long wash-out period must be allowed for to minimize interactions. MAOIs work by inhibiting the enzyme that metabolizes monoamines (including noradrenaline and serotonin), which, in the brain, results in a change in mood. However, this same enzyme detoxifies the amine tyramine in the body, so when certain foodstuffs that contain this amine (eg cheese, fermented soya bean products, meat or yeast extracts and some alcoholic beverages) are ingested, or medicines that contain sympathomimetic amines are taken (eg cough and cold 'cures' that contain ephedrine hydrochloride or pseudoephedrine hydrochloride) the outcome may be a hypertensive crisis. A patient-guidance treatment card is provided that should be carried at all times. As well as the foodstuffs mentioned, there are some herbal remedies (such as black cohosh) and nutritional supplements (such as brewer's yeast) that should also be avoided by people taking monoamine-oxidase inhibitors because of the risk of potentially dangerous interactions. Many drugs should not be taken within several weeks of taking MAOIs. See PHENELZINE for principal actions and side-effects.

Another type of MAO, represented by MOCLOBEMIDE, are reversible inhibitors of the monoamine oxidase type A (therefore termed RIMA) and are reported to show less potentiation of dangerous side-effects of tyramine found in foodstuffs, and interactions with other medicines are claimed to be less. Drugs of the amfetamine (amphetamine) class have serious hypertensive interactions with MAOIs.

Mono-Cedocard Retard-50 (MCR-50)

(Pharmacia) is a proprietary, non-prescription preparation of the VASODILATOR drug isosorbide mononitrate, which can be used as an ANTI-ANGINA drug. It is available as capsules.

✚▲ Side-effects/warnings: See ISOSORBIDE MONONITRATE.

Monoclate-P

(Aventis Behring) is a proprietary, prescription-only preparation of dried human factor VIII fraction, which acts as a HAEMOSTATIC drug to reduce or stop bleeding in the treatment of disorders in which bleeding is prolonged and potentially dangerous (mainly haemophilia A). It is available in a form for intravenous injection or infusion.

✚▲ Side-effects/warnings: See FACTOR VIII FRACTION (DRIED).

Monocor

(Lederle; Wyeth) is a proprietary, prescription-only preparation of the BETA-BLOCKER bisoprolol fumarate. It can be used as an ANTIHYPERTENSIVE for raised blood pressure and as an ANTI-ANGINA treatment to relieve symptoms and improve exercise tolerance. It is available as tablets.

✚▲ Side-effects/warnings: See BISOPROLOL FUMARATE.

monoethanolamine oleate

see ETHANOLAMINE OLEATE.

Monomax SR

(Trinity) is a proprietary, prescription-only preparation of the VASODILATOR drug isosorbide mononitrate. It can be used as an ANTI-ANGINA drug, and is available as modified-release capsules.

✚▲ Side-effects/warnings: See ISOSORBIDE MONONITRATE.

Mononine

(Aventis Behring) is a proprietary, prescription-only preparation of factor IX fraction, dried, prepared from human blood plasma. It can be used to treat patients with a deficiency in factor IX (haemophilia B), and is available in a form for intravenous infusion.

✚▲ Side-effects/warnings: See FACTOR IX FRACTION, DRIED.

Monoparin

(CP) is a proprietary, prescription-only preparation of the ANTICOAGULANT heparin (as heparin sodium). It can be used to treat various forms of thrombosis, and is available in a form for injection.

✚▲ Side-effects/warnings: See HEPARIN.

Monoparin Calcium

(CP) is a proprietary, prescription-only preparation of the ANTICOAGULANT heparin (as heparin calcium). It can be used to treat various forms of thrombosis, and is available in a form for injection.

✚▲ Side-effects/warnings: See HEPARIN.

Monosorb XL 60

(Dexcel) is a proprietary, prescription-only

preparation of the VASODILATOR drug isosorbide mononitrate. It can be used as an ANTI-ANGINA drug, and is available as modified-release tablets.
✚▲ Side-effects/warnings: See ISOSORBIDE MONONITRATE.

Monotrim

(Solvay) is a proprietary, prescription-only preparation of the SULPHONAMIDE-like ANTIBACTERIAL trimethoprim. It can be used to treat infections, and is available as tablets, a sugar-free suspension and in a form for injection.
✚▲ Side-effects/warnings: See TRIMETHOPRIM.

Monovent

(Lagap) is a proprietary, prescription-only preparation of the BETA-RECEPTOR STIMULANT terbutaline sulphate. It can be used as a BRONCHODILATOR in reversible obstructive airways disease, such as in ANTI-ASTHMATIC treatment. It may also be used to prevent premature labour. It is available as a syrup.
✚▲ Side-effects/warnings: See TERBUTALINE SULPHATE.

Monozide 10

(Lederle; Wyeth) is a proprietary, prescription-only compound preparation of the BETA-BLOCKER bisoprolol fumarate and the (THIAZIDE) DIURETIC hydrochlorothiazide. It can be used as an ANTIHYPERTENSIVE for raised blood pressure, and is available as tablets.
✚▲ Side-effects/warnings: See BISOPROLOL FUMARATE; HYDROCHLOROTHIAZIDE.

Monphytol

(LAB) is a proprietary, non-prescription compound preparation of a number of ANTISEPTIC and KERATOLYTIC agents, including methyl undecenoate, methyl salicylate, salicylic acid, propyl salicylate and chlorbutol (chlorobutanol). It can be used to treat the skin infection athlete's foot. It is available as a paint for topical application. It is not normally given to children, except on medical advice.
✚▲ Side-effects/warnings: See CHLORBUTOL; METHYL SALICYLATE; SALICYLIC ACID.

montelukast

is an ANTI-ASTHMATIC drug. It can be used as an add-on therapy for individuals not adequately controlled by inhaled CORTICOSTEROID and short-acting BETA-RECEPTOR STIMULANT drugs to prevent mild to moderate asthma attacks (including exercise-induced bronchospasm, but not to treat acute attacks). It represents a new drug class called LEUKOTRIENE-RECEPTOR ANTAGONIST drugs which work as ANTI-ALLERGIC agents by blocking the actions of leukotrienes, which are natural inflammatory mediators released in the lungs. Administration is oral.
✚ Side-effects: It may cause gastrointestinal problems, headache; respiratory-tract infection, dizziness, gastrointestinal problems, dry mouth, skin reactions, fever, muscle and joint pains.
▲ Warnings: Use with caution in pregnancy and breast-feeding. Unusual symptoms need to be reported to the doctor because of current concern about development of the so-called Churg-Strauss syndrome.
✪ **Related entry: Singulair.**

moracizine hydrochloride

is a specialist ANTI-ARRHYTHMIC drug which can be used (on a named-patient basis only) to prevent and treat certain serious heartbeat irregularities (ventricular arrhythmias), particularly after a heart attack. Administration is oral.
✚ Side-effects: Gastrointestinal disturbances; headache, fatigue, palpitations; heart failure; jaundice; blood disorders, dizziness, chest pain and changes in liver function.
▲ Warnings: It should be used with caution in people who are pregnant or breast-feeding, and avoided in people with a wide variety of heart disturbances, or in patients with certain kidney or liver disorders. It is a specialist drug used on a named-patient basis.
✪ **Related entry: Ethmozine.**

Moraxen

(Schwarz) is a proprietary, prescription-only preparation of the (OPIOID) NARCOTIC ANALGESIC morphine sulphate and is on the Controlled Drugs list. It can be used to treat severe pain, for example in the terminally ill, and is available in the form of rectal tampons (non-dissolving suppositories).
✚▲ Side-effects/warnings: See MORPHINE SULPHATE.

Morcap SR

(Sanofi-Synthelabo) is a proprietary,

prescription-only preparation of the (OPIOID) NARCOTIC ANALGESIC morphine sulphate, and is on the Controlled Drugs list. It can be used primarily to relieve pain following surgery and the pain experienced during the final stages of a terminal malignant disease. It is available as modified-release capsules.
✚▲ Side-effects/warnings: See MORPHINE SULPHATE.

Morhulin Ointment

(SSL) is a proprietary, non-prescription compound preparation of zinc oxide and cod-liver oil. It can be used as an EMOLLIENT for minor wounds, pressure sores, skin ulcers, eczema and nappy rash, and is available as an ointment.
✚▲ Side-effects/warnings: See COD-LIVER OIL; ZINC OXIDE.

morphine hydrochloride

see MORPHINE SULPHATE.

morphine sulphate

is a powerful (OPIOID) NARCOTIC ANALGESIC and is the principal alkaloid of opium. It is widely used to treat severe pain and to relieve the associated stress and anxiety since it induces a state of mental detachment and euphoria. It is used during operations as an analgesic and to enhance the actions of GENERAL ANAESTHETIC drugs; to relieve cough in the terminally ill as an ANTITUSSIVE (though it may cause nausea and vomiting); and for reducing secretion and peristalsis in the intestine, so it has a powerful ANTIDIARRHOEAL and antimotility action and is used in some antidiarrhoeal mixtures. Tolerance occurs extremely readily and dependence (addiction) may follow. Administration may be oral, by suppositories, or by injection or infusion (morphine is more active when given by injection). Proprietary preparations that contain morphine (in the form of morphine tartrate, hydrochloride or sulphate) are all on the Controlled Drugs list. It is also available as a compound preparation with atropine (when used in general anaesthesia) and with an ANTI-EMETIC, such as CYCLIZINE.
✚▲ Side-effects/warnings: See OPIOID. It may also cause itching and a rash.
✪ Related entries: Cyclimorph; Diocalm; Enterosan; J Collis Browne's Mixture; J Collis Browne's Tablets; Kaolin and Morphine Mixture, BP; Moraxen; Morcap SR; MST Continus; MXL; Oramorph; papaveretum; Sevredol; Zomorph.

Motens

(Boehringer Ingelheim) is a proprietary, prescription-only preparation of the CALCIUM-CHANNEL BLOCKER lacidipine. It can be used as an ANTIHYPERTENSIVE, and is available as tablets.
✚▲ Side-effects/warnings: See LACIDIPINE.

Motifene 75 mg

(Sankyo) is a proprietary, prescription-only preparation of the (NSAID) NON-NARCOTIC ANALGESIC and ANTIRHEUMATIC diclofenac sodium. It can be used to treat the pain and inflammation of arthritis and rheumatism and other musculoskeletal disorders, including juvenile arthritis. It is available as modified-release capsules.
✚▲ Side-effects/warnings: See DICLOFENAC SODIUM.

motility stimulant 🅱

drugs increase gut motility, that is, they stimulate stomach emptying and the rate of passage of food along the intestine. They can also enhance closure of the oesophageal sphincter, thereby reducing reflux passage of stomach contents up into the oesophagus and may have ANTI-EMETIC properties. Older drugs of this class (eg METOCLOPRAMIDE HYDROCHLORIDE) have undesirable effects on the brain. Some more recently introduced motility stimulants do not have this action and are thought to work by acting at receptors for 5-HT (serotonin) to cause release of acetylcholine (see neurotransmitter) from nerves within the gut wall. DOMPERIDONE increases gastrointestinal motility by a poorly understood mechanism, and can be used in disorders of gastric (stomach) emptying and chronic gastric reflux.

Motilium

(Sanofi-Synthelabo) is a proprietary, prescription-only preparation of the ANTINAUSEANT and ANTI-EMETIC domperidone. It can be used to treat drug-induced nausea and vomiting, especially during treatment with cytotoxic drugs, and for drug-treatment in Parkinson's disease. It is available as tablets, a sugar-free suspension and as suppositories.
✚▲ Side-effects/warnings: See DOMPERIDONE.

Motilium 10

(Johnson & Johnson • MSD) is a proprietary, non-prescription preparation of the ANTINAUSEANT and ANTI-EMETIC domperidone. In this form sold to the public in certain limited amounts, it can be used to relieve symptoms (stomach discomfort) such as excess fullness and epigastric bloating, nausea, belching accompanied by epigastric discomfort and heartburn that occur after a meal. It is available as tablets. It is not normally given to children under 16 years, except on medical advice

✚▲ Side-effects/warnings: See DOMPERIDONE.

Motipress

(Sanofi-Synthelabo) is a proprietary, prescription-only compound preparation of the ANTIPSYCHOTIC drug fluphenazine (as hydrochloride) and the (TRICYCLIC) ANTIDEPRESSANT nortriptyline hydrochloride; in the ratio 1:20. It is available as tablets.

✚▲ Side-effects/warnings: See FLUPHENAZINE; NORTRIPTYLINE HYDROCHLORIDE.

Motival

(Sanofi-Synthelabo) is a proprietary, prescription-only compound preparation of the ANTIPSYCHOTIC drug fluphenazine (as hydrochloride) and the (TRICYCLIC) ANTIDEPRESSANT nortriptyline hydrochloride; in the ratio 1:20. It can be used to treat depressive illness with anxiety, and is available as tablets.

✚▲ Side-effects/warnings: See FLUPHENAZINE; NORTRIPTYLINE HYDROCHLORIDE.

Motrin

(Pharmacia) is a proprietary, prescription-only preparation of the (NSAID) NON-NARCOTIC ANALGESIC and ANTIRHEUMATIC ibuprofen. It can be used to relieve pain, particularly the pain and inflammation of rheumatic disease and other musculoskeletal disorders, and is available as tablets.

✚▲ Side-effects/warnings: See IBUPROFEN.

Movelat Relief Cream

(Sankyo Pharma) is a proprietary, non-prescription compound preparation of salicylic acid and heparinoid (mucopolysaccharide polysulphate), which both have COUNTER-IRRITANT, OF RUBEFACIENT, actions. It can be applied to the skin for symptomatic relief of underlying muscle or joint pain, such as sprains, strains and rheumatic conditions. It is available as a cream and is not normally used for children, except on medical advice.

✚▲ Side-effects/warnings: See HEPARINOIDS; SALICYLIC ACID; but adverse effects are minimal on topical application.

Movelat Relief Gel

(Sankyo Pharma) is a proprietary, non-prescription compound preparation of salicylic acid and heparinoid (mucopolysaccharide polysulphate), which both have COUNTER-IRRITANT, OF RUBEFACIENT, actions. It can be applied to the skin for symptomatic relief of underlying muscle or joint pain, such as sprains, strains and rheumatic conditions. It is available as a gel and is not normally used for children, except on medical advice.

✚▲ Side-effects/warnings: See HEPARINOIDS; SALICYLIC ACID; but adverse effects are minimal on topical application.

moxisylyte

(thymoxamine) is an ALPHA-ADRENOCEPTOR BLOCKER which can be used, because of its VASODILATOR properties, in the treatment of peripheral vascular disease (Raynaud's phenomenon), and in IMPOTENCE TREATMENT for erectile dysfunction. Administration is oral.

✚ Side-effects: Diarrhoea, nausea, flushing, headache, dizziness; reports of liver reactions including cholestatic jaundice and hepatitis.

▲ Warnings: It should not be administered to patients with certain liver disorders. Given with caution to patients with diabetes.

✪ Related entry: Opilon.

moxonidine

is an ANTIHYPERTENSIVE which can be used to treat mild to moderate essential hypertension. It has a site of action within the central nervous system. Administration is oral.

✚ Side-effects: Dry mouth; tiredness, headache, sedation, dizziness, nausea, sleep disturbances.

▲ Warnings: It should not be used in those with a history of angioedema; various heart disorders; severe coronary artery disease, unstable angina; severe liver disease or severe renal impairment; also possibly a number of other disorders; or in pregnancy and breast-feeding. It should be administered with care to those with kidney impairment.

Withdrawal of treatment should be gradual.
✪ Related entry: Physiotens.

MST Continus

(Napp) is a proprietary, prescription-only preparation of the (OPIOID) NARCOTIC ANALGESIC morphine sulphate and is on the Controlled Drugs list. It is available as modified-release tablets and as an oral suspension.
✚▲ Side-effects/warnings: See MORPHINE SULPHATE.

Mucaine

(Wyeth) is a proprietary, prescription-only compound preparation of the ANTACID agents aluminium hydroxide and magnesium hydroxide and the LOCAL ANAESTHETIC drug oxetacaine. It can be used to relieve reflux oesophagitis and hiatus hernia, and is available as an oral suspension.
✚▲ Side-effects/warnings: See ALUMINIUM HYDROXIDE; MAGNESIUM HYDROXIDE; OXETACAINE.

Mucodyne

(Rhône-Poulenc Rorer; Aventis Pharma) is a proprietary, prescription-only preparation of the MUCOLYTIC and EXPECTORANT carbocisteine. It can be used to reduce the viscosity of sputum and thus facilitate expectoration in patients with chronic asthma or bronchitis. It is available as capsules and a syrup.
✚▲ Side-effects/warnings: See CARBOCISTEINE.

Mucogel Suspension

(Pharmax) is a proprietary, non-prescription compound preparation of the ANTACID agents aluminium hydroxide and magnesium hydroxide (a combination called *co-magaldrox*). It can be used to relieve dyspepsia, and is available as an oral suspension. It is not normally given to children, except on medical advice.
✚▲ Side-effects/warnings: See ALUMINIUM HYDROXIDE; MAGNESIUM HYDROXIDE.

mucolytic 🄴

drugs dissolve, or help break down, mucus. They are generally used in an effort to reduce the viscosity of sputum in the upper airways and thus facilitate expectoration (coughing up sputum) and so they may also be regarded as EXPECTORANT. It is not clear how they work, though mucolytic agents are commonly used to treat such conditions as asthma and chronic bronchitis. They can also be used to increase tear secretion (lacrimation) in chronic conditions where this is reduced, causing sore, dry eyes. The best-known and most-used mucolytics are ACETYLCYSTEINE, CARBOCISTEINE and MECYSTEINE HYDROCHLORIDE (methyl cysteine hydrochloride).

mucopolysaccharide polysulphate

see HEPARINOIDS.

Multiparin

(CP) is a proprietary, prescription-only preparation of the ANTICOAGULANT heparin (as heparin sodium). It can be used to treat various forms of thrombosis, and is available in a form for injection.
✚▲ Side-effects/warnings: See HEPARIN.

multivitamin 🄴

preparations contain a selection of various VITAMINS. There are a large number of such preparations available and are mostly used as dietary supplements and for making up vitamin deficiencies. The choice of a particular multivitamin depends on its content. They are not normally available through the National Health Service, except to prevent or treat deficiency or when used in infusion solutions. However, *Mothers' and Children's Vitamin Drops* (vitamins A, C and D) is recommended by the Department of Health for routine supplement to the diet of pregnant women and young children, and is available without prescription direct to families under the Welfare Food Scheme.
✪ Related entry: Vitamin Tablets (with Calcium and Iodine) for Nursing Mothers.

mupirocin

is an ANTIBACTERIAL and ANTIBIOTIC drug which is unrelated to any other antibiotic. It can be used to treat bacterial skin infection and is of value in treating infections caused by bacteria resistant to other antibacterials, for instance which is carried in and around the nostrils (eg methoxycillin-resistant *Staphylococcus aureus*; MRSA). Administration is by topical application.
✚ Side-effects: It may sting at the site of application.
▲ Warnings: It is not to be used on patients with

known hypersensitivity to mupirocin (or any of the constituents of the ointment preparation). Care in kidney impairment.
✪ Related entries: Bactroban; Bactroban Nasal.

MUSE
(Astra) is a PROSTAGLANDIN, alprostadil (PGE_1). It is a prescription-only IMPOTENCE TREATMENT for men to manage penile erectile dysfunction. It is used by direct urethral application.
✚▲ Side-effects/warnings: See ALPROSTADIL.

mustine hydrochloride
see CHLORMETHINE HYDROCHLORIDE.

MXL
(Napp) is a proprietary, prescription-only preparation of the (OPIOID) NARCOTIC ANALGESIC morphine sulphate, and is on the Controlled Drugs list. It is available as modified-release capsules.
✚▲ Side-effects/warnings: See MORPHINE SULPHATE.

Mycil Athlete's Foot Spray
(Crookes) is a proprietary, non-prescription preparation of the ANTIFUNGAL drug tolnaftate. It can be used to treat fungal infections responsible for athlete's foot (tinea pedis), dhobie itch (tinea cruris) and prickly heat (miliaria). It is available as a spray for topical application.
✚▲ Side-effects/warnings: See TOLNAFTATE.

Mycil Ointment
(Crookes) is a proprietary, non-prescription compound preparation of the ANTIFUNGAL drug tolnaftate and the ANTISEPTIC benzalkonium chloride. It can be used to treat fungal infections responsible for athlete's foot (tinea pedis), dhobie itch (tinea cruris) and prickly heat (miliaria). It is available as an ointment for topical application.
✚▲ Side-effects/warnings: See BENZALKONIUM CHLORIDE; TOLNAFTATE.

Mycil Powder
(Crookes) is a proprietary, non-prescription compound preparation of the ANTIFUNGAL drug tolnaftate and the ANTISEPTIC chlorhexidine (as hydrochloride). It can be used to treat fungal infections responsible for athlete's foot (tinea pedis), dhobie itch (tinea cruris) and prickly heat (miliaria). It is available as a powder for topical application.
✚▲ Side-effects/warnings: See CHLORHEXIDINE; TOLNAFTATE.

Mycobutin
(Pharmacia) is a proprietary, prescription-only preparation of the ANTIBACTERIAL, ANTITUBERCULAR and ANTIBIOTIC rifabutin. It can be used in the prevention of treatment of certain infections, and is available as capsules.
✚▲ Side-effects/warnings: See RIFABUTIN.

mycophenolate mofetil
is a newly introduced (CYTOTOXIC) IMMUNOSUPPRESSANT drug. It is mainly used to reduce tissue rejection in transplant patients as prophylaxis of acute kidney or heart transplant rejection (in combination with CORTICOSTEROID and CICLOSPORIN) in specialist use.
Administration is oral or by intravenous infusion.
✚ Side-effects: These are many and include nausea and vomiting, diarrhoea or constipation, abdominal pain; hypertension, oedema, chest pain; shortness of breath, cough; insomnia, headache, dizziness and tremor; susceptibility to a range of infections; various blood effects, hyperglycaemia, and a number of others.
▲ Warnings: It is not to be given to patients who are, or plan shortly to become, pregnant or are breast-feeding; monitoring is required throughout treatment with blood count check; used with care in serious gastrointestinal disease (risk of haemorrhage).
✪ Related entry: CellCept.

Mycota Cream
(SSL) is a proprietary, non-prescription, preparation of the ANTIFUNGAL agents zinc undecenoate and undecenoic acid. It can be used to treat athlete's foot, and is available as a cream for topical application.
✚▲ Side-effects/warnings: See UNDECENOIC ACID.

Mycota Powder
(SSL) is a proprietary, non-prescription preparation of the ANTIFUNGAL agents zinc undecenoate and UNDECENOIC ACID. It can be used to treat athlete's foot, and is available as a dusting powder for topical application.
✚▲ Side-effects/warnings: See UNDECENOIC ACID.

Mycota Spray
(SSL) is a proprietary, non-prescription

M

preparation of the ANTIFUNGAL agents undecenoic acid and dichlorophen. It can be used to treat athlete's foot, and is available as a spray for topical application.
✚▲ Side-effects/warnings: See DICHLOROPHEN; UNDECENOIC ACID.

Mydriacyl

(Alcon) is a proprietary, prescription-only preparation of the ANTICHOLINERGIC drug tropicamide. It can be used to dilate the pupil to facilitate inspection of the eyes, and is available as eye-drops.
✚▲ Side-effects/warnings: See TROPICAMIDE.

Mydrilate

(Intrapharm) is a proprietary, prescription-only preparation of the ANTICHOLINERGIC drug cyclopentolate hydrochloride. It can be used to dilate the pupils and paralyse focusing of the eye to allow ophthalmic examination, and is available as eye-drops.
✚▲ Side-effects/warnings: See CYCLOPENTOLATE HYDROCHLORIDE.

Myleran

(GSK) is a proprietary, prescription-only preparation of the (CYTOTOXIC) ANTICANCER drug busulfan. It can be used in the treatment of chronic myeloid leukaemias, and is available as tablets.
✚▲ Side-effects/warnings: See BUSULFAN.

Myocet

(Elan) is a proprietary, prescription-only preparation of the ANTICANCER drug doxorubicin hydrochloride. It is used with cyclophosphamide to treat metastatic breast cancer. It is available in a form (encapsulated in liposomes) for injection.
✚▲ Side-effects/warnings: See DOXORUBICIN HYDROCHLORIDE.

Myocrisin

(JHC) is a proprietary, prescription-only preparation of the ANTI-INFLAMMATORY and ANTIRHEUMATIC sodium aurothiomalate. It can be used to treat rheumatoid arthritis and juvenile arthritis, and is available in a form for injection.
✚▲ Side-effects/warnings: See SODIUM AUROTHIOMALATE.

Myotonine

(Glenwood) is a proprietary, prescription-only preparation of the PARASYMPATHOMIMETIC bethanechol chloride. It can be used to treat urinary retention, particularly following surgery, and is available as tablets.
✚▲ Side-effects/warnings: See BETHANECHOL CHLORIDE.

Mysoline

(AstraZeneca) is a proprietary, prescription-only preparation of the ANTICONVULSANT and ANTI-EPILEPTIC primidone. It can be used in the treatment of all forms of epilepsy (except absence seizures) and of essential tremor. It is available as tablets and an oral suspension.
✚▲ Side-effects/warnings: See PRIMIDONE.

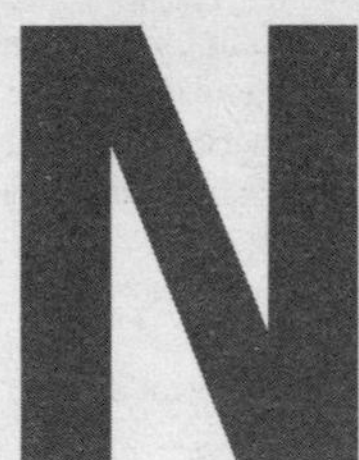

nabilone

is a synthetic cannabinoid (a drug derived from cannabis). It is used as an ANTI-EMETIC and ANTINAUSEANT to relieve toxic side-effects, particularly the nausea and vomiting associated with chemotherapy. However, it too has significant side-effects. Administration is oral.

✚ Side-effects: Euphoria, dizziness, drowsiness, vertigo, dry mouth, visual and sleep disturbances, difficulty in concentrating, nausea, headache, confusion, psychosis, depression, movement disorders, loss of appetite and abdominal pain.

▲ Warnings: It is administered with care to patients with heart disease, hypertension or psychiatric disorders. It is not used in people who are pregnant, breast-feeding or who have certain liver disorders. The effects of alcohol may be enhanced and it may impair the performance of skilled tasks, such as driving.

nabumetone

is a (NSAID) NON-NARCOTIC ANALGESIC and ANTIRHEUMATIC drug. It is used primarily to relieve pain and inflammation, particularly in osteoarthritis and rheumatoid arthritis. Administration is oral.

✚▲ Side-effects/warnings: See NSAID.

✪ **Related entry: Relifex.**

nadolol

is a BETA-BLOCKER which can be used as an ANTIHYPERTENSIVE for raised blood pressure, as an ANTI-ANGINA treatment to relieve symptoms and improve exercise tolerance and as an ANTI-ARRHYTHMIC to regularize heartbeat. It can also be used as an ANTITHYROID drug for short-term treatment of thyrotoxicosis and as an ANTIMIGRAINE treatment to prevent attacks. Administration is oral. It is also available, as an antihypertensive treatment, in the form of compound preparations with DIURETIC drugs.

✚▲ Side-effects/warnings: See PROPRANOLOL HYDROCHLORIDE.

✪ **Related entries: Corgard; Corgaretic 40; Corgaretic 80.**

nafarelin

is an analogue of the hypothalamic hormone GONADORELIN (gonadothrophin-releasing hormone; GnRH). Given long-term, it acts as an *indirect* HORMONE ANTAGONIST with ANTI-ANDROGEN and ANTI-OESTROGEN activity. It reduces the secretion of gonadotrophin by the pituitary gland, which results in the reduced secretion of SEX HORMONES by the ovaries. It is used to treat endometriosis (a growth of the lining of the uterus at inappropriate sites) and for pituitary desensitization before induction of ovulation for *in vitro* fertilization. Administration is by topical application as a nasal spray (it is absorbed into the systemic circulation from the nasal mucosa).

✚▲ Side-effects/warnings: See BUSERELIN. Also, side-effects include muscle pain, acne, palpitations and effects on liver function.

✪ **Related entry: Synarel.**

naftidrofuryl oxalate

is a VASODILATOR which dilates the blood vessels of the extremities and so can be used to treat peripheral vascular disease (Raynaud's phenomenon). Administration is either oral or by intravenous infusion.

✚▲ Side-effects/warnings: There may be nausea and pain in the abdomen, rash, effects on the liver.

✪ **Related entries: Praxilene; Stimlor.**

nalbuphine hydrochloride

is a NARCOTIC ANALGESIC, an OPIOID, that is very similar to morphine in relieving pain, but with fewer side-effects. Like morphine, it is used primarily to relieve moderate to severe pain, especially during or after surgery and in myocardial infarction. Administration is by injection.

✚▲ Side-effects/warnings: See OPIOID; it is reported to cause less nausea and vomiting than morphine.

✪ **Related entry: Nubain.**

Nalcrom

(Pantheon) is a proprietary, prescription-only

N

preparation of the ANTI-ALLERGIC drug sodium cromoglicate. It can be used to treat allergy to certain foodstuffs, and is available as capsules.
✚▲ Side-effects/warnings: See SODIUM CROMOGLICATE.

nalidixic acid

is a (QUINOLONE) ANTIBIOTIC-like ANTIBACTERIAL, one of the original members of the quinolone family. It is used primarily to treat infections of the urinary tract. Administration is oral.
✚▲ Side-effects/warnings: See QUINOLONE. It is not to be used by patients with porphyria or a history of convulsive disorders. Avoid strong sunlight. Additional side-effects include certain psychoses, weakness.
✪ **Related entries: Mictral; Negram; Uriben.**

Nalorex

(DuPont; Bristol-Myers Squibb) is a proprietary, prescription-only preparation of the OPIOID ANTAGONIST naltrexone hydrochloride. It can be used to reverse the effects of (OPIOID) NARCOTIC ANALGESIC drugs. Pharmacologically, it is an opioid and is used in detoxification therapy for formerly opioid-dependent individuals to help prevent relapse. It is available as tablets.
✚▲ Side-effects/warnings: See NALTREXONE HYDROCHLORIDE.

naloxone hydrochloride

is a powerful OPIOID ANTAGONIST which is used primarily as an ANTIDOTE to an overdose of (OPIOID) NARCOTIC ANALGESICS. It is quick but short-acting and effectively reverses the respiratory depression, coma or convulsions that follow overdosage of opioids. Administration is by intramuscular or intravenous injection and may be repeated at short intervals until there is some response. It is also used at the end of operations to reverse respiratory depression caused by (opioid) narcotic analgesics, and in newborn babies where mothers have been administered large amounts of opioid (such as pethidine) for pain-relief during labour. Administration is by injection or infusion.
▲ Warnings: It should not be administered to patients who are physically dependent on narcotics.
✪ **Related entries: Min-I-Jet Naloxone; Narcan.**

naltrexone hydrochloride

is an OPIOID ANTAGONIST of (OPIOID) NARCOTIC ANALGESIC. It is used in detoxification treatment for formerly opioid-dependent individuals to help prevent relapse. Since it is an antagonist of dependence-causing opioids (such as heroin), it will precipitate withdrawal symptoms in those already taking opioids. During naltrexone treatment, the euphoric effects of habit-forming opioids are blocked, so helping prevent re-addiction. Treatment is started in specialist clinics. (For overdose with opioids the related drug naloxone is normally used.) Administration is oral.
✚ Side-effects: There may be nausea, vomiting, abdominal pain, anxiety, nervousness, difficulty in sleeping, headache and pain in the joints and muscles. There may also be diarrhoea or constipation, thirst, sweating, increased tear production, dizziness, chills, irritability, rash, lethargy and decreased sexual potency. There have been reports of liver and blood abnormalities.
▲ Warnings: It should be administered with care to patients with certain kidney or liver disorders. Opioid-dependent patients should not try to overcome the effects of naltrexone (by taking more opioid) as this can cause dangerous intoxication.
✪ **Related entry: Nalorex.**

nandrolone

is an ANABOLIC STEROID which has similar actions to the male sex hormone TESTOSTERONE (though it has far fewer masculinizing effects). It can be used to treat aplastic anaemia and sometimes osteoporosis in postmenopausal women. Administration (in the form of nandrolone decanoate) is by injection.
✚ Side-effects: Acne, sodium retention with oedema, virilization (voice changes in women, loss of menstrual periods), inhibition of sperm production, effects on the bones and liver function, liver tumours reported occasionally on prolonged treatment.
▲ Warnings: It is not to be administered to patients with severe liver function disorders, cancer of the prostate gland, male breast cancer or porphyria; or who are pregnant or breast-feeding. Administer with caution to those with impaired heart or kidney or liver function, hypertension, diabetes, epilepsy or migraine. When used by young patients, bone growth should be monitored.
✪ **Related entry: Deca-Durabolin.**

N

naphazoline hydrochloride

is an ALPHA-ADRENOCEPTOR STIMULANT, a SYMPATHOMIMETIC, which is generally used for its VASOCONSTRICTOR properties so it has been used as a NASAL DECONGESTANT and is currently used as a conjunctival decongestant for symptomatic relief of conjunctivitis when applied to the eye as drops.
✚▲ Side-effects/warnings: See EPHEDRINE HYDROCHLORIDE.
✪ **Related entry: Optrex Clear Eyes Eye Drops.**

Napratec

(Searle; Pharmacia) is a proprietary, prescription-only compound preparation of the powerful (NSAID) NON-NARCOTIC ANALGESIC and ANTIRHEUMATIC naproxen and the ULCER-HEALING DRUG the PROSTAGLANDIN misoprostol. It is used to treat the pain and inflammation of rheumatoid arthritis, osteoarthritis and ankylosing spondylitis. This combination represents a novel approach to minimizing the gastrointestinal side-effects of the NSAID by supplementing the local hormone whose production has been inhibited and which is necessary for unimpaired blood circulation in the gastrointestinal lining. It is available as tablets (in a combination pack containing tablets of each constituent).
✚▲ Side-effects/warnings: See MISOPROSTOL; NAPROXEN.

Naprosyn

(Roche) is a proprietary, prescription-only preparation of the (NSAID) NON-NARCOTIC ANALGESIC and ANTIRHEUMATIC naproxen. It can be used to relieve pain and inflammation, particularly rheumatic and arthritic pain and other musculoskeletal disorders, also period pain and acute gout. It is available as tablets, enteric-coated tablets (*Naprosyn EC*), modified-release tablets (*Naprosyn S/R*), an oral suspension, granules for oral solution and as suppositories.
✚▲ Side-effects/warnings: See NAPROXEN.

naproxen

is a (NSAID) NON-NARCOTIC ANALGESIC and ANTIRHEUMATIC drug. It is used to relieve pain and inflammation, particularly of rheumatic disease, acute gout, juvenile arthritis and other musculoskeletal disorders and period pain. Administration (as naproxen or naproxen sodium) can be either oral or by suppositories.
✚▲ Side-effects/warnings: See NSAID. The risk of gastrointestinal side-effects is intermediate for this group. Suppositories may cause rectal irritation and bleeding.
✪ **Related entries: Arthrosin; Arthroxen; Napratec; Naprosyn; Nycopren; Synflex; Timpron.**

Naramig

(GlaxoWellcome; GSK) is a proprietary, prescription-only preparation of the (TRIPTAN) ANTIMIGRAINE drug naratriptan (as hydrochloride). It can be used to treat acute migraine attacks. It is available as tablets.
✚▲ Side-effects/warnings: see NARATRIPTAN.

naratriptan

is a (TRIPTAN) ANTIMIGRAINE drug which is used to treat acute migraine attacks (but not to prevent attacks). It works as a VASOCONSTRICTOR (through acting as a serotonin receptor stimulant selective for SEROTONIN 5-HT_1 receptors), producing a rapid constriction of blood vessels surrounding the brain. Administration is oral.
✚ Side-effects: See SUMATRIPTAN for general side-effects of drugs of this class. Naratriptan may cause speeding or slowing of the heart; visual disturbances.
▲ Warnings: See SUMATRIPTAN for general warnings for drugs of this class. It is not used in patients with peripheral vascular disease, care in patients with kidney impairment. Drowsiness may impair the performance of skilled tasks, such as driving.
✪ **Related entry: Naramig.**

Narcan

(DuPont; Bristol-Myers Squibb) is a proprietary, prescription-only preparation of the OPIOID ANTAGONIST naloxone hydrochloride, which is used to treat acute overdosage of (OPIOID) NARCOTIC ANALGESICS, such as morphine. It is available in ampoules for injection and as a weaker form (*Narcan Neonatal*) for the treatment of respiratory depression in babies born to mothers who have been given narcotic analgesics during labour, who are drug addicts, or to reverse opioid-induced respiratory depression (after operations).
✚▲ Side-effects/warnings: See NALOXONE HYDROCHLORIDE.

narcotic

agents induce stupor and insensibility.

N

Commonly, the term is applied to the OPIOID drugs (such as MORPHINE SULPHATE and DIAMORPHINE HYDROCHLORIDE), but it can also be used to describe SEDATIVE and HYPNOTIC drugs and ETHANOL, which act directly on the brain centres to depress their functioning. In law, certainly in the USA, the term tends to be used to describe any *addictive* drug that is used illegally and is the subject of abuse, even if it is a stimulant (eg cocaine or amfetamine (amphetamine)). See also NARCOTIC ANALGESIC.

narcotic analgesic

drugs are OPIOID drugs, such as MORPHINE SULPHATE, and have powerful actions on the central nervous system and alter the perception of pain. Because of their numerous possible side-effects, the most important of which is drug dependence (habituation, or addiction), this class is usually used under strict medical supervision and normally the drugs are only available on prescription. Other notable side-effects include depression of respiration, nausea and vomiting, sometimes hypotension, constipation (therefore they can be used as ANTIDIARRHOEAL drugs), inhibition of coughing (ANTITUSSIVE) and constriction of the pupils (miosis). Other narcotic analgesics are CODEINE PHOSPHATE, DIAMORPHINE HYDROCHLORIDE (heroin), METHADONE HYDROCHLORIDE, PENTAZOCINE and PETHIDINE HYDROCHLORIDE. Narcotic analgesics are used for different types and severities of pain. For example, pethidine is used during labour, since it produces prompt, short-lasting analgesia and causes less respiratory depression to the baby than some other narcotic analgesics. It is now recognized that the characteristic pharmacology of the narcotic analgesics follows from their acting as mimics of natural opioid neurotransmitters (enkephalins, endorphins, dynorphins) in the brain. Most effects of the opioid narcotic analgesics (eg respiratory depression) may be reversed with an OPIOID ANTAGONIST (eg naloxone hydrochloride). See also NON-NARCOTIC ANALGESIC; NSAID.

narcotic antagonist

see OPIOID ANTAGONIST.

Nardil

(Hansam) is a proprietary, prescription-only preparation of the (MONOAMINE-OXIDASE INHIBITOR) ANTIDEPRESSANT phenelzine. It can be used to treat depressive illness, and is available as tablets.

+▲ Side-effects/warnings: See PHENELZINE.

Narphen

(Napp) is a proprietary, prescription-only preparation of the (OPIOID) NARCOTIC ANALGESIC phenazocine hydrobromide, and is on the Controlled Drugs list. It can be used to relieve severe pain, and is available as tablets.

+▲ Side-effects/warnings: See PHENAZOCINE HYDROBROMIDE.

Nasacort

(Rhône-Poulenc Rorer; Aventis Pharma) is a proprietary, prescription-only preparation of the CORTICOSTEROID drug triamcinolone (in the form of acetonide). It can be used to prevent and treat allergic nasal rhinitis. It is available as a nasal spray.

+▲ Side-effects/warnings: See TRIAMCINOLONE.

nasal decongestant

drugs relieve or reduce the symptoms of congestion of the nose. They are generally, and most safely, administered in the form of nose-drops or as a nasal spray, which avoids the tendency of such drugs to cause side-effects like raised blood pressure, though some are administered orally. However, by the nasal route, there may be 'rebound' congestion after an initial decongestant phase. Most nasal decongestants are SYMPATHOMIMETIC drugs with ALPHA-ADRENOCEPTOR STIMULANT properties, which work by constricting blood vessels in general, including those within the mucous membranes of the nasal cavity, so reducing the thickness of the membranes, improving drainage and possibly also decreasing mucous and fluid secretions. However, rhinitis (inflammation of the mucous membrane of the nose), especially when caused by allergy (eg hay fever), is usually dealt with by using ANTIHISTAMINE, which inhibits the detrimental and congestive effects of histamine released by the allergic response, or by drugs which inhibit the allergic response itself, and so effectively reduce inflammation (eg CORTICOSTEROID drugs and SODIUM CROMOGLICATE). Nasal decongestants are often included in compound preparations intended to

relieve cold symptoms.
▲ Warnings: There can be serious reactions if nasal decongestants containing sympathomimetic drugs are taken with other drugs such as MAOIs or some herbal remedies.

Naseptin

(Alliance) is a proprietary, prescription-only compound preparation of the ANTIBACTERIAL and (AMINOGLYCOSIDE) ANTIBIOTIC neomycin sulphate and the ANTISEPTIC chlorhexidine (as hydrochloride). It can be used to treat staphylococcal infections in and around the nostrils, and is available as a cream for topical application.
✚▲ Side-effects/warnings: See CHLORHEXIDINE; NEOMYCIN SULPHATE.

Nasobec Hayfever

(IVAX) is a proprietary, non-prescription preparation of the CORTICOSTEROID and ANTI-INFLAMMATORY beclometasone dipropionate. It can be used to relieve the symptoms of conditions such as hay fever and allergic and other types of rhinitis. It is available as a nasal spray.
✚▲ Side-effects/warnings: See BECLOMETASONE DIPROPIONATE.

Nasonex

(Schering-Plough) is a proprietary, prescription-only preparation of the CORTICOSTEROID drug mometasone furoate. It can be used to treat allergic nasal rhinitis. It is available as a nasal spray.
✚▲ Side-effects/warnings: See MOMETASONE FUROATE

nateglinide

is a newly introduced drug which is used in DIABETIC TREATMENT of Type II diabetes (non-insulin-dependent diabetes mellitus; NIDDM; maturity-onset diabetes), particularly in patients who are not totally dependent on additional supplies of INSULIN. It works by stimulating insulin release from the pancreas, and can be used together with another diabetic drug, METFORMIN HYDROCHLORIDE. Administration is oral.
✚ Side-effects: Taking nateglinide can result in low blood sugar levels and it may cause hypersensitivity reactions, including rashes, pruritus and urticaria.
▲ Warnings: It should not be used by pregnant or breast-feeding women, or by people with diabetic ketoacidosis. It is prescribed with caution in people who are debilitated and malnourished or who have impaired liver function.
✪ **Related entry: Starlix.**

Natrilix

(Servier) is a proprietary, prescription-only preparation of the (THIAZIDE-like) DIURETIC indapamide. It can be used as an ANTIHYPERTENSIVE, and is available as tablets (also in a modified-release version called *Natrilix SR*).
✚▲ Side-effects/warnings: See INDAPAMIDE.

Navelbine

(Fabre) is a proprietary, prescription-only preparation of the ANTICANCER drug vinorelbine (as tartrate). It can be used to treat breast and some lung cancers. It is available in a form for injection.
✚▲ Side-effects/warnings: See VINORELBINE.

Navidrex

(Alliance) is a proprietary, prescription-only preparation of the (THIAZIDE) DIURETIC cyclopenthiazide. It can be used to treat oedema and as an ANTIHYPERTENSIVE, and is available as tablets.
✚▲ Side-effects/warnings: See CYCLOPENTHIAZIDE.

Navispare

(Novartis) is a proprietary, prescription-only compound preparation of the (*potassium-sparing*) DIURETIC amiloride hydrochloride and the (THIAZIDE) diuretic cyclopenthiazide. It can be used as an ANTIHYPERTENSIVE, and is available as tablets.
✚▲ Side-effects/warnings: See AMILORIDE HYDROCHLORIDE; CYCLOPENTHIAZIDE.

Navoban

(Novartis) is a proprietary, prescription-only preparation of the ANTI-EMETIC and ANTINAUSEANT tropisetron. It can be used to give relief from nausea and vomiting, especially in patients receiving chemotherapy. It is available as capsules or in a form for injection.
✚▲ Side-effects/warnings: See TROPISETRON.

Nebcin

(Lilly) is a proprietary, prescription-only

preparation of the ANTIBACTERIAL and (AMINOGLYCOSIDE) ANTIBIOTIC tobramycin. It can be used to treat a range of serious bacterial infections, and is available in a form for injection.
✚▲ Side-effects/warnings: See TOBRAMYCIN.

Nebilet
(Menarini) is a proprietary, prescription-only preparation of the BETA-BLOCKER nebivolol (as hydrochloride). It can be used as an ANTIHYPERTENSIVE for raised blood pressure. It is available as tablets.
✚▲ Side-effects/warnings: See NEBIVOLOL.

nebivolol
is a BETA-BLOCKER which is a VASODILATOR and can be used as an ANTIHYPERTENSIVE for raised blood pressure. Administration is oral.
✚▲ Side-effects/warnings: See PROPRANOLOL HYDROCHLORIDE. Also oedema, headache, depression, disturbances of vision, tingling in the extremities, impotence. It is not used in people with liver impairment.
✪ **Related entry: Nebilet.**

nedocromil sodium
is used as an ANTI-ALLERGIC drug to prevent recurrent attacks of asthma and allergic rhinitis (hay fever), or when applied topically for allergic conjunctivitis and vernal keratoconjunctivitis in the eye. Administration is by inhalation from an aerosol, or as eye-drops.
✚ Side-effects: If absorbed, there may be nausea, headache, vomiting, dyspepsia and abdominal pain. With eye-drops there may be transient stinging and burning; also bitter taste reported. After inhalation, there may be coughing and throat irritation.
✪ **Related entries: Rapitil; Tilade.**

nefazodone
is an ANTIDEPRESSANT that chemically is dissimilar to members of the major groups, but like the SSRI and TRICYCLIC groups inhibits re-uptake of 5-HT, but also blocks 5-HT receptors. It is used to treat depressive illness and has the advantage over the tricyclics in that it has relatively less SEDATIVE and ANTICHOLINERGIC (ANTIMUSCARINIC) side-effects. Administration (as hydrochloride) is oral.
✚ Side-effects: Muscle weakness, dry mouth, nausea, sleepiness, dizziness; less often, chills, fever, hypotension on standing (and rarely fainting), constipation, light-headedness, tingling in the extremities, confusion, unsteady gait and minor visual disturbances.
▲ Warnings: It is not to be used by patients who are breast-feeding. It is administered with care to those with epilepsy, a history of mania, who are elderly, with liver and kidney impairment, or who are pregnant. It may impair performance of skilled tasks, such as driving.
✪ **Related entry: Dutonin.**

nefopam hydrochloride
is a NON-NARCOTIC ANALGESIC which is used to treat moderate pain. Administration is either oral or by injection.
✚ Side-effects: There may be nausea, nervous agitation, dizziness, light-headedness, headache, insomnia or drowsiness; dry mouth, difficulty in urination, blurred vision, increased heart rate and sweating. Confusion and hallucinations have been reported and it may colour the urine pink.
▲ Warnings: It should not be administered to patients who suffer from convulsive disorders. Given with care in liver and kidney disorders, urinary retention, pregnancy and breast-feeding.
✪ **Related entry: Acupan.**

Negram
(Sanofi-Synthelabo) is a proprietary, prescription-only preparation of the (QUINOLONE) ANTIBIOTIC-like ANTIBACTERIAL nalidixic acid. It can be used to treat various infections, particularly those of the urinary tract, and is available as tablets and an oral suspension.
✚▲ Side-effects/warnings: See NALIDIXIC ACID.

Neis Vac-C
(Baxter / Farillon) is a proprietary, prescription-only VACCINE preparation. It can be used to give protection against the organism meningococcus (*Neisseria meningitidis* group C), which can cause serious infections, such as meningitis. It is available in a form for injection.
✚▲ Side-effects/warnings: See MENINGOCOCCAL POLYSACCHARIDE VACCINE.

nelfinavir
is a (*protease inhibitor*) ANTIVIRAL drug which is often used together with (*reverse transcriptase*) antivirals. It can be used in the treatment of progressive or advanced HIV infection.

Administration is oral.

✚ Side-effects: Nausea, diarrhoea and flatulence; rash, hepatitis, changes in blood counts and enzymes.

▲ Warnings: It is a specialist drug, and there will be full assessment and patient monitoring throughout treatment. It should not be given to patients who are breast-feeding, and is administered with caution where there is diabetes, impaired liver or kidney function, haemophilia or pregnancy.

✪ **Related entry: Viracept.**

Neo Baby Cream

(Wallace) is a proprietary, non-prescription compound preparation of the ANTISEPTIC benzalkonium chloride and cetrimide. It can be used to treat nappy rash, sweat rash and other skin irritations, and is available as a cream.

✚▲ Side-effects/warnings: See BENZALKONIUM CHLORIDE; CETRIMIDE.

Neoclarityn

(Schering-Plough) is a proprietary, non-prescription preparation of the ANTIHISTAMINE desloratadine. It can be used to treat the symptoms of allergic disorders, such as for symptomatic relief of hay fever, and is available as tablets.

✚▲ Side-effects/warnings: See DESLORATADINE.

Neo-Cortef

(Dominion) is a proprietary, prescription-only compound preparation of the ANTI-INFLAMMATORY and CORTICOSTEROID drug hydrocortisone (as acetate) and the ANTIBACTERIAL and (AMINOGLYCOSIDE) ANTIBIOTIC neomycin sulphate. It can be used to treat bacterial infections in the outer ear and inflammation in the eye, and is available as ear-drops, eye-drops and an ointment.

✚▲ Side-effects/warnings: See HYDROCORTISONE; NEOMYCIN SULPHATE.

Neo-Cytamen

(Celltech) is a proprietary, prescription-only preparation of the VITAMIN hydroxocobalamin. It can be used to correct diagnosed clinical deficiency of vitamin B_{12}, including pernicious anaemia, and is available in a form for injection.

✚▲ Side-effects/warnings: See HYDROXOCOBALAMIN.

Neogest

(Schering) is a proprietary, prescription-only preparation which can be used as an ORAL CONTRACEPTIVE of the PROGESTOGEN-only pill (*POP*) type and contains norgestrel. It is available as tablets in a calendar pack.

✚▲ Side-effects/warnings: See NORGESTREL.

Neo Gripe Mixture

(Wallace) is a proprietary, non-prescription preparation of the ANTACID sodium bicarbonate with dill seed oil and ginger tincture. It can be used to relieve wind and related pain, and is available as a liquid.

✚▲ Side-effects/warnings: See SODIUM BICARBONATE.

Neo-Mercazole

(Roche) is a proprietary, prescription-only preparation of carbimazole. It can be used to treat the effects of an excess of thyroid hormones (thyrotoxicosis), and is available as tablets.

✚▲ Side-effects/warnings: See CARBIMAZOLE.

neomycin sulphate

is a broad-spectrum ANTIBACTERIAL and ANTIBIOTIC drug, and an original member of the AMINOGLYCOSIDE family. It is effective in treating some superficial bacterial infections and has quite a widespread use when used topically (in the eyes, ears or on the skin). However, it is too toxic to be administered by intravenous or intramuscular injection. It is occasionally taken by mouth to reduce the levels of bacteria in the colon prior to intestinal surgery or examination, or in liver failure. When administered orally it is not absorbed from the gastrointestinal tract. Administration can be either oral or topical

✚▲ Side-effects/warnings: See GENTAMICIN. Prolonged or widespread topical application may eventually lead to sensitivity reactions.

✪ **Related entries: Audicort; Betnesol-N; Betnovate-N; Cicatrin; Dermovate-NN; Graneodin; Gregoderm; Maxitrol; Minims Neomycin Sulphate; Naseptin; Neo-Cortef; Neosporin; Nivemycin; Otomize; Otosporin; Predsol-N; Synalar N; Tri-Adcortyl; Tri-Adcortyl Otic; Vista-Methasone-N.**

Neo-NaClex

(Goldshield) is a proprietary, prescription-only preparation of the (THIAZIDE) DIURETIC

bendroflumethiazide. It can be used as an ANTIHYPERTENSIVE and to treat oedema. It is available as tablets.
✚▲ Side-effects/warnings: See BENDROFLUMETHIAZIDE.

Neo-NaClex-K

(Goldshield) is a proprietary, prescription-only compound preparation of the (THIAZIDE) DIURETIC bendroflumethiazide and the potassium supplement POTASSIUM CHLORIDE. It can be used in as an ANTIHYPERTENSIVE and to treat oedema. It is available as tablets, which should be swallowed whole with plenty of fluid at mealtimes or when in an upright position.
✚▲ Side-effects/warnings: See BENDROFLUMETHIAZIDE; POTASSIUM CHLORIDE.

Neoral

(Novartis) is a proprietary, prescription-only preparation of the IMMUNOSUPPRESSANT ciclosporin. It can be used to prevent tissue rejection in transplant patients, to treat severe, active rheumatoid arthritis and certain severe, resistant skin conditions (under specialist supervision). It is available as capsules and an oral solution.
✚▲ Side-effects/warnings: See CICLOSPORIN.

NeoRecormon

(Roche) is a proprietary, prescription-only preparation of epoetin beta (synthesized human erythropoietin beta). It can be used in ANAEMIA TREATMENT for conditions such as those known to be associated with chronic renal failure. It is available in a number of forms for injection.
✚▲ Side-effects/warnings: See EPOETIN.

Neosporin

(Dominion) is a proprietary, prescription-only compound preparation of the ANTIBACTERIAL and ANTIBIOTIC neomycin sulphate, the antibacterial and (*polymyxin*) antibiotic polymyxin B sulphate and gramicidin. It can be used to treat infections of the eye, and is available as eye-drops.
✚▲ Side-effects/warnings: See GRAMICIDIN; NEOMYCIN SULPHATE; POLYMYXIN B SULPHATE.

neostigmine

is an ANTICHOLINESTERASE drug which enhances the effects of the neurotransmitter acetylcholine (and of certain cholinergic drugs). Because of this property, it has PARASYMPATHOMIMETIC actions and can be used to stimulate the bladder to treat urinary retention. It can also be used to treat the neuromuscular transmission disorder myasthenia gravis. Administration is either oral (as neostigmine bromide) or by injection (as neostigmine methylsulphate).
✚ Side-effects: Nausea and vomiting, increased salivation, diarrhoea and abdominal cramps.
▲ Warnings: It should not be administered to patients with intestinal or urinary blockage; it should be administered with caution to those with asthma, epilepsy, in those who have suffered myocardial infarction, peptic ulcer, parkinsonism, hypotension, slow heart rate, kidney impairment or who are pregnant or breast-feeding.
✪ **Related entry: Robinul-Neostigmine.**

Neotigason

(Roche) is a proprietary, prescription-only preparation of acitretin. It can be used as a systemic treatment of long-term, severe psoriasis and certain other skin disorders, and is available as oral capsules.
✚▲ Side-effects/warnings: See ACITRETIN.

Nephril

(Pfizer) is a proprietary, prescription-only preparation of the (THIAZIDE) DIURETIC polythiazide. It can be used in the treatment of oedema and as an ANTIHYPERTENSIVE. It is available as tablets.
✚▲ Side-effects/warnings: See POLYTHIAZIDE.

Nerisone

(Schering Health) is a proprietary, prescription-only preparation of the CORTICOSTEROID and ANTI-INFLAMMATORY diflucortolone valerate. It can be used to treat severe, inflammatory skin disorders, such as eczema and psoriasis. It is available as creams and an ointment for topical application (a stronger preparation, *Nerisone Forte*, is also available).
✚▲ Side-effects/warnings: See DIFLUCORTOLONE VALERATE.

Netillin

(Schering-Plough) is a proprietary, prescription-only preparation of the ANTIBACTERIAL and (AMINOGLYCOSIDE) ANTIBIOTIC netilmicin (as

sulphate). It can be used to treat a range of serious bacterial infections, and is available in a form for injection.
✚▲ Side-effects/warnings: See NETILMICIN.

netilmicin
is a broad-spectrum (AMINOGLYCOSIDE) ANTIBIOTIC which can be used, alone or in combination with other antibiotics, to treat serious bacterial infections caused by Gram-negative bacteria. Administration is by injection.
✚▲ Side-effects/warnings: See GENTAMICIN. It may cause ototoxicity.
✪ Related entry: Netillin.

Neulactil
(JHC) is a proprietary, prescription-only preparation of the ANTIPSYCHOTIC drug pericyazine. It can be used to treat psychotic disorders, such as schizophrenia, and also severe anxiety in the short term. It is available as tablets and a syrup.
✚▲ Side-effects/warnings: See PERICYAZINE.

Neupogen
(Amgen) is a proprietary, prescription-only preparation of the specialist drug filgrastim used to treat neutropenia during chemotherapy in ANTICANCER treatment. It is available in a form for injection or intravenous infusion.
✚▲ Side-effects/warnings: See FILGRASTIM.

NeuroBloc
(Elan) is a proprietary, prescription-only preparation of botulinum B toxin, which is used to treat conditions characterized by abnormal muscle tone, spasmodic torticollis (cervical dystonia). It is available in a form for injection.
✚▲ Side-effects/warnings: See BOTULINUM TOXIN.

neuroleptic 🅴
see ANTIPSYCHOTIC.

Neurontin
(Parke-Davis; Pfizer) is a proprietary, prescription-only preparation of the ANTICONVULSANT and ANTI-EPILEPTIC gabapentin. It can be used to assist in the control of seizures that have not responded to other drugs, and is available as capsules.
✚▲ Side-effects/warnings: See GABAPENTIN.

neutral insulin
see SOLUBLE INSULIN.

Neutrexin
(Ipsen) is a proprietary, prescription-only preparation of the ANTIPROTOZOAL trimetrexate. It can be used to treat pneumonia caused by the protozoan micro-organism *Pneumocystis carinii* in patients whose immune system has been suppressed, for instance, in HIV infection. It is available in a form for injection.
✚▲ Side-effects/warnings: See TRIMETREXATE.

Neutrogena Dermatological Cream
(Johnson & Johnson) is a proprietary, non-prescription EMOLLIENT preparation of glycerol. It can be used for dry skin, and is available as a cream.
✚▲ Side-effects/warnings: See GLYCEROL.

nevirapine
is a (*non-nucleoside* group of *reverse transcriptase inhibitor*) ANTIVIRAL drug which can be used in the treatment of HIV infection, in combination with other antiviral drugs. Administration is oral.
✚ Side-effects: Rash; skin disorders, jaundice and liver toxicity (can be serious), nausea and vomiting, diarrhoea and abdominal pain, headache, drowsiness and fatigue; fever, muscle pains, hypersensitivity reactions and a number of other side-effects.
▲ Warnings: It is a specialist drug, and there will be full assessment and patient monitoring throughout treatment. It is used with caution in liver or kidney impairment, or pregnancy. It is not used in breast-feeding.
✪ Related entry: Viramune.

Nexium
(AstraZeneca) is a newly introduced proprietary, prescription-only preparation of the PROTON-PUMP INHIBITOR esomeprazole (as magnesium trihydrate). It can be used as an ULCER-HEALING DRUG and for associated conditions, such as gastro-oesophageal reflux. Available as tablets.
✚▲ Side-effects/warnings: See ESOMEPRAZOLE.

niacin
is another name for NICOTINIC ACID, which is one of VITAMIN B group.

nicardipine hydrochloride
is a CALCIUM-CHANNEL BLOCKER which can be

used as an ANTI-ANGINA drug to prevent attacks and also as an ANTIHYPERTENSIVE. Administration is oral.
✚ Side-effects: There may be nausea and headache; dizziness, flushing, palpitations; drowsiness or insomnia; hypotension, oedema, gastrointestinal disturbances; increased salivation; rashes; increased frequency of urination; tingling in the extremities, depression, ringing in the ears, shortness of breath, and impotence.
▲ Warnings: Administer with care to those with certain heart, aortic, kidney or liver disorders, and who are elderly. Do not use in pregnancy, breast-feeding and cardiovascular problems. Treatment may have to be stopped if ischaemic heart pain occurs. Grapefruit juice should be avoided since it affects metabolism of the drug.
✪ Related entries: Cardene; Cardene SR.

Nicef

(Galen) is a proprietary, prescription-only preparation of the ANTIBACTERIAL and (CEPHALOSPORIN) ANTIBIOTIC cefradine. It can be used to treat a range of bacterial infections, and is available as capsules.
✚▲ Side-effects/warnings: See CEFRADINE.

niclosamide

is a synthetic ANTHELMINTIC drug which is used (on a named-patient basis only) to treat infestation by tapeworms. Administration is oral.
✚ Side-effects: There may be gastrointestinal disturbances (nausea, retching and abdominal pain), light-headedness and itchy skin.

nicorandil

is a POTASSIUM-CHANNEL ACTIVATOR and VASODILATOR drug which can be used as an ANTI-ANGINA treatment to prevent and treat angina pectoris. Administration is oral.
✚ Side-effects: Headache (especially on first taking the drug, but usually transitory); cutaneous (skin) vasodilatation with flushing; nausea, vomiting, dizziness and weakness have also been reported. At high dosage, there may be effects on heart rate and blood pressure.
▲ Warnings: It should not be used in patients with hypotension or certain heart disorders. Administer with care to those who are pregnant or breast-feeding, with low blood pressure, pulmonary oedema or certain types of myocardial infarction. It may impair the performance of skilled tasks, such as driving and operating machinery.
✪ Related entry: Ikorel.

Nicorette Chewing Gum

(Pharmacia) is a proprietary, non-prescription preparation of nicotine. It can be used to alleviate the withdrawal symptoms experienced when giving up smoking tobacco products. It is available as a chewing gum in two strengths (2mg and 4mg). The nicotine is absorbed from the mucosal lining of the mouth. It should be used only by people over 18 years and must be kept out of the reach of children.
✚▲ Side-effects/warnings: See NICOTINE.

Nicorette Inhalor

(Pharmacia) is a proprietary, non-prescription preparation of nicotine. It can be used to alleviate the withdrawal symptoms experienced when giving up smoking tobacco products. It is available in the form of an inhalation cartridge. It should be used only by people over 18 years and must be kept out of the reach of children.
✚▲ Side-effects/warnings: See NICOTINE.

Nicorette Microtab

(Pharmacia) is a proprietary, non-prescription preparation of nicotine. It can be used to alleviate the withdrawal symptoms experienced when giving up smoking tobacco products. It is available as sublingual tablets (the nicotine is absorbed from the mucosal lining of the mouth). It should be used only by people over 18 years and must be kept out of the reach of children.
✚▲ Side-effects/warnings: See NICOTINE.

Nicorette Nasal Spray

(Pharmacia) is a proprietary, prescription-only preparation of nicotine. It can be used to alleviate the withdrawal symptoms experienced when giving up smoking tobacco products. It is available in the form of a nasal spray.
✚▲ Side-effects/warnings: See NICOTINE.

Nicorette Patch

(Pharmacia) is a proprietary, non-prescription preparation of nicotine. It can be used to alleviate the withdrawal symptoms experienced when giving up smoking tobacco products. It is available (in strengths of 5mg, 10mg and 15mg) in the form of a skin patch for transdermal delivery (the nicotine is absorbed through the skin). It should be used only by people over 18 years and must be kept out of the reach of children.

✚▲ Side-effects/warnings: See NICOTINE.

nicotinamide

is a derivative (the amide) of the B-complex vitamin NICOTINIC ACID. It is used primarily as a constituent in vitamin supplements, especially in cases where a large dose is required, because it does not have as great a VASODILATOR effect as nicotinic acid. It is also used in some topical skin preparations for the treatment of acne (when it is used as a gel).

✚ Side-effects: When used topically, dryness of skin; also pruritus, redness, burning and irritation.

▲ Warnings: When used topically, avoid contact with eyes and mucous membranes (including nose and mouth); if it causes excessive dryness, irritation or peeling use it less often or in smaller amounts.

✪ **Related entry: Papulex.**

nicotine

is an ALKALOID found in tobacco products and is absorbed into the body whether the tobacco is smoked or chewed. It causes a SYMPATHOMIMETIC effect on the cardiovascular system with a rise in blood pressure and heart rate and stimulation of the central nervous system. Like many habituating drugs there is tolerance to its action, so bigger doses are required on continued usage and there is a marked psychological and physical withdrawal syndrome if an individual abruptly stops using it, in other words drug-dependence becomes established. It is available in various replacement forms to help those trying to give it up, including as chewing gum (it is absorbed into the systemic circulation from the lining of the mouth) and skin patches for transdermal delivery (absorbed through the skin). The drug bupropion (amfebutamone) is now available to help the psychological state of those withdrawing from nicotine. Combining drug therapy and behavioural support is more successful than either treatment alone.

✚ Side-effects: Cold and flu-like symptoms, with headache, nausea, dizziness, insomnia, dreaming, muscle ache, swelling of tongue, palpitations, anxiety, acid stomach and skin reaction (with patches), and others.

▲ Warnings: Do not use when pregnant or breast-feeding; use with care if there is cardiovascular disease, hyperthyroidism, diabetes, liver or kidney impairment, phaeochromocytoma, gastric ulcers or skin disorders (with patches). Patients should not smoke or use other nicotine products while receiving treatment of this kind. Treatment should be carried out for 10-12 weeks.

✪ **Related entries: Nicorette Chewing Gum; Nicorette Inhalor; Nicorette Microtab; Nicorette Nasal Spray; Nicorette Patch; Nicotinell Mint 1mg Lozenges; Nicotinell Mint Chewing Gum 4mg; Nicotinell Original Fruit 2mg Chewing Gum; Nicotinell TTS; NiQuitin CQ; NiQuitin CQ Clear 21mg, 14mg, 7mg.**

Nicotinell Mint 1mg Lozenges

(Novartis Consumer Health) is a proprietary, non-prescription preparation of nicotine. It can be used to alleviate the withdrawal symptoms experienced when giving up smoking tobacco products. It is available as lozenges. It is not given to those under 18 years, except under medical supervision, and must be kept out of the reach of children.

✚▲ Side-effects/warnings: See NICOTINE.

Nicotinell Mint Chewing Gum 4mg

(Novartis Consumer Health) is a proprietary, non-prescription preparation of nicotine. It can be used to alleviate the withdrawal symptoms experienced when giving up smoking tobacco products, especially for people who suffer severe withdrawal symptoms. It is available as chewing gum and is also available in 2mg strength. It is not given to those under 18 years, except under medical supervision, and must be kept out of the reach of children.

✚▲ Side-effects/warnings: See NICOTINE.

Nicotinell Original Fruit 2mg Chewing Gum

(Novartis Consumer Health) is a proprietary, non-prescription preparation of nicotine. It can be used to alleviate the withdrawal symptoms experienced when giving up smoking tobacco products. It is available in the form of chewing gum (2mg) and the nicotine is absorbed into the systemic circulation from the mucosal lining of the mouth.

It should be used only by people over 18 years and must be kept out of the reach of children.
✚▲ Side-effects/warnings: See NICOTINE.

Nicotinell TTS

(Novartis Consumer Health) is a proprietary, non-prescription preparation of nicotine. It can be used to alleviate the withdrawal symptoms experienced when giving up smoking tobacco products. It is available in the form of a skin patch for transdermal delivery (absorbed through the skin). It should be used only by people over 18 years and must be kept out of the reach of children.
✚▲ Side-effects/warnings: See NICOTINE.

nicotinic acid

or niacin is a B-complex VITAMIN. It is a derivative of pyridine and is required in the diet, but is also synthesized in the body to a small degree from the amino acid tryptophan. Dietary deficiency results in the disease pellagra, but deficiency is rare. Good food sources include meat, cereals and yeast extract. Nicotinic acid may be administered therapeutically as a vitamin supplement (as tablets), but its effect as a VASODILATOR precludes high dosage. It is, indeed, commonly used as a vasodilator, especially in symptomatic relief of peripheral vascular disease (Raynaud's phenomenon). It is also used as a LIPID-REGULATING DRUG because it beneficially modifies blood levels of various lipids (HDL and LDL) by inhibiting the synthesis and secretion of lipids in the liver. Derivatives are mainly used for their vasodilator actions, including INOSITOL NICOTINATE (and formally nicotinyl alcohol) by oral administration, and METHYL NICOTINATE topically. The derivative NICOTINAMIDE (as tablets) is used for vitamin actions (even though it is also has vasodilator actions).
✚ Side-effects: There may be nausea and vomiting, flushing, dizziness and headache; palpitations. Itching, rashes and some other side-effects may be reduced by taking with food. Sensitivity reactions and actions on the liver may occur.
▲ Warnings: It should not be administered to patients who are pregnant or breast-feeding; and administered with caution to those with diabetes, certain liver disorders, peptic ulcers or gout.
✪ Related entry: Crampex Tablets.

nicoumalone

see ACENOCOUMAROL.

nifedipine

is a CALCIUM-CHANNEL BLOCKER which is used as an ANTI-ANGINA drug to prevent attacks, and as an ANTIHYPERTENSIVE. It is also used in peripheral vascular disease (Raynaud's syndrome). Administration is oral as capsules or tablets (several in modified-release formulations – necessary in treating hypertension).
✚ Side-effects: These include nausea and headache; dizziness, flushing, palpitations and increased heart rate, lethargy and insomnia; hypotension, oedema; gastrointestinal disturbances; rashes; increased frequency of urination; blood upsets; impotence, depression and excessive growth of gums, effects on the eye and liver.
▲ Warnings: It should be administered with care to those with certain heart, cardiovascular, kidney or liver disorders, or who are breast-feeding. It is not used in patients who have porphyria. Treatment may have to be stopped if heart pain occurs. Grapefruit juice should be avoided since it affects metabolism of the drug. There are many different formulations of nifedipine, some of which are not suitable for people with other disorders or conditions.
✪ Related entries: Adalat; Adalat LA; Adalat Retard; Adipine MR; Angiopine; Angiopine MR; Beta-Adalat; Calanif; Cardilate MR; Coracten SR; Coracten XL; Coroday MR; Fortipine LA 40; Hypolar Retard 20; Nifedipress MR; Nifopress Retard; Nimodrel MR; Nifopress Retard; Slofedipine; Slofedipine XL; Tenif; Tensipine MR.

Nifedipress MR

(Dexel) is a proprietary, prescription-only preparation of the CALCIUM-CHANNEL BLOCKER nifedipine. It can be used as an ANTI-ANGINA drug in the prevention of attacks and as an ANTIHYPERTENSIVE. It is available as modified-release tablets.
✚▲ Side-effects/warnings: See NIFEDIPINE.

Niferex

(Tillomed) is a proprietary, non-prescription preparation of polysaccharide-iron complex. It can be used as an IRON supplement in iron-deficiency ANAEMIA TREATMENT, and is available also as an elixir that can be used, at appropriate

dosage, for infants and children.
✚▲ Side-effects/warnings: See POLYSACCHARIDE-IRON COMPLEX.

Nifopress Retard

(Goldshield) is a proprietary, prescription-only preparation of the CALCIUM-CHANNEL BLOCKER nifedipine. It can be used as an ANTI-ANGINA treatment in the prevention of attacks, as an ANTIHYPERTENSIVE for moderate hypertension, and peripheral vascular disease (Raynaud's phenomenon). It is available as modified-release tablets.
✚▲ Side-effects/warnings: See NIFEDIPINE.

Night Nurse Capsules

(GSK Consumer Healthcare) is a proprietary, non-prescription compound preparation of the NON-NARCOTIC ANALGESIC and ANTIPYRETIC paracetamol, the ANTITUSSIVE dextromethorphan hydrobromide and the SEDATIVE and ANTIHISTAMINE promethazine hydrochloride. It can be used for the symptomatic relief of colds, chills and flu at night. It is available as capsules and is not normally given to children, except on medical advice.
✚▲ Side-effects/warnings: See DEXTROMETHORPHAN HYDROBROMIDE; PARACETAMOL; PROMETHAZINE HYDROCHLORIDE.

Night Nurse Liquid

(GSK Consumer Healthcare) is a proprietary, non-prescription compound preparation of the NON-NARCOTIC ANALGESIC and ANTIPYRETIC paracetamol, the ANTITUSSIVE dextromethorphan hydrobromide and the SEDATIVE and ANTIHISTAMINE promethazine hydrochloride. It can be used for the symptomatic relief of colds, chills and flu during the night, and is available as a liquid. It is not normally given to children, except on medical advice.
✚▲ Side-effects/warnings: See DEXTROMETHORPHAN HYDROBROMIDE; PARACETAMOL; PROMETHAZINE HYDROCHLORIDE.

Nimbex

(GSK) is a proprietary, prescription-only preparation of the (*non-depolarizing*) SKELETAL MUSCLE RELAXANT cisatracurium (as besilate). It can be used to induce muscle paralysis of medium duration during surgery, and is available in a form for injection (and also in a form called *Nimbex Forte*).
✚▲ Side-effects/warnings: See CISATRACURIUM.

nimodipine

is a CALCIUM-CHANNEL BLOCKER which is used to treat and prevent ischaemic damage (neurological deficits) following subarachnoid haemorrhage (a relatively rare form of stroke), by reducing the risk of cerebrovascular vasospasm. Administration is either oral or by intravenous infusion.
✚ Side-effects: Changes in heart rate; hypotension, headaches, gastrointestinal disorders, flushes, nausea, feeling of warmth, blood disorders and changes in liver enzymes.
▲ Warnings: It can be administered with care because of cerebral oedema and greatly raised intracranial pressure; and with caution to patients with impaired kidney function or who are pregnant. Grapefruit juice should be avoided since it affects metabolism of the drug.
✪ **Related entry: Nimotop.**

Nimodrel MR

(Opus; Trinity) is a proprietary, prescription-only preparation of the CALCIUM-CHANNEL BLOCKER nifedipine. It can be used as an ANTI-ANGINA treatment in the prevention of attacks, and as an ANTIHYPERTENSIVE. It is available as modified release tablets.
✚▲ Side-effects/warnings: See NIFEDIPINE.

Nimotop

(Bayer) is a proprietary, prescription-only preparation of the CALCIUM-CHANNEL BLOCKER nimodipine. It can be used to treat and prevent ischaemic damage following subarachnoid haemorrhage, and is available as tablets and in a form for intravenous infusion.
✚▲ Side-effects/warnings: See NIMODIPINE.

Nindaxa 2.5

(Ashbourne) is a proprietary, prescription-only preparation of the (THIAZIDE-like) DIURETIC indapamide. It can be used as an ANTIHYPERTENSIVE, and is available as tablets.
✚▲ Side-effects/warnings: SeeINDAPAMIDE.

Nipent

(Lederle; Wyeth) is a proprietary, prescription-

only preparation of the ANTICANCER drug pentostatin. It can be used to treat hairy cell leukaemia, and is available in a form for intravenous infusion.
✚▲ Side-effects/warnings: See PENTOSTATIN.

NiQuitin CQ Clear 21mg, 14mg, 7mg

(GSK) is a proprietary, non-prescription preparation of nicotine. It can be used to alleviate the withdrawal symptoms experienced when giving up smoking tobacco products. It is available as clear transdermal patches in three strengths (and sizes). It is used by people aged from 12 to 18 years only under medical supervision. It must not be given to children and must be kept out of their reach.
✚▲ Side-effects/warnings: See NICOTINE.

NiQuitin CQ

(GSK Consumer Healthcare) is a proprietary, non-prescription preparation of nicotine. It can be used to alleviate the withdrawal symptoms experienced when giving up smoking tobacco products. It is available in the form of pinkish and clear (*NiQuitin CQ Clear*) skin patches (in several different strengths) for transdermal delivery (absorbed through the skin) and as lozenges.
✚▲ Side-effects/warnings: See NICOTINE.

nisoldipine

is a CALCIUM-CHANNEL BLOCKER which can be used as an ANTI-ANGINA drug to prevent attacks and as an ANTIHYPERTENSIVE. Administration is oral.
✚ Side-effects: These may include oedema in the lower extremities; headache; dizziness, flushing, weakness, hypotension, gastrointestinal disturbances, nausea, constipation, allergic skin reactions; increased frequency of urination, muscle pains, shortness of breath, low blood pressure (hypotension) and others.
▲ Warnings: Administer with care to those with certain heart, aortic, kidney or liver disorders, and who are elderly. It is not used in pregnancy or breast-feeding, or if there are certain heart and cardiovascular problems. Avoid eating grapefruit or drinking grapefruit juice, as this may affect the metabolism of the drug.
✪ **Related entry: Syscor MR.**

nitrate

drugs are powerful SMOOTH MUSCLE RELAXANT drugs. They are mainly used as VASODILATOR drugs to relax the walls of blood vessels in the treatment or prevention of angina pectoris (ischaemic heart pain) and in HEART FAILURE TREATMENT. The best-known and most-used nitrates include GLYCERYL TRINITRATE, ISOSORBIDE DINITRATE and ISOSORBIDE MONONITRATE. Administration is commonly as tablets to be held under the tongue (sublingual) until dissolved; buccal tablets (for between the upper lip and gum) and aerosol sprays (directed into the mouth) are also used. Other preparations available are modified-release tablets, capsules, impregnated dressings (for placing on the upper body), ointment for topical application on the chest and in a form for injection.

nitrazepam

is a BENZODIAZEPINE which is used as a relatively long-acting HYPNOTIC to treat insomnia in the short-term for cases where some degree of sedation during the daytime is acceptable. Administration is oral.
✚▲ Side-effects/warnings: See BENZODIAZEPINE.
✪ **Related entries: Mogadon; Remnos; Somnite.**

Nitrocine

(Schwarz) is a proprietary, prescription-only preparation of the VASODILATOR and ANTI-ANGINA drug glyceryl trinitrate. It can be used to treat and prevent angina pectoris, and is available in a form for injection.
✚▲ Side-effects/warnings: See GLYCERYL TRINITRATE.

Nitro-Dur

(Schering-Plough) is a proprietary, non-prescription preparation of the VASODILATOR and ANTI-ANGINA drug glyceryl trinitrate. It can be used prevent angina pectoris. It is available on a self-adhesive dressing (patch) and, when placed on the chest wall or upper arm, is absorbed through the skin and helps to give lasting relief.
✚▲ Side-effects/warnings: See GLYCERYL TRINITRATE.

nitrofurantoin

is an ANTIBACTERIAL drug which is used, in particular, to treat infections of the urinary tract and to prevent infection during surgery on the genitourinary tract. Administration is oral.
✚ Side-effects: There may be loss of appetite,

nausea, vomiting and diarrhoea; impaired lung function; peripheral neuropathy, causing tingling and other sensory disorders in the fingers and toes. Rarely, there is liver damage, allergic skin reactions and blood disorders.
▲ Warnings: It should not be administered to patients with impaired kidney function, porphyria or with G6PD deficiency. Administer with caution to those with diabetes, anaemia and certain lung and kidney disorders. Lung, liver, kidney and peripheral nerve function should be monitored in long-term treatment. Urine may be coloured yellow or brown. Magnesium salts, such as MAGNESIUM TRISILICATE, may reduce the effectiveness of nitrofurantoin.
✪ Related entries: Furadantin; Macrobid; Macrodantin.

Nitrolingual Pumpspray

(Lipha) is a proprietary, non-prescription preparation of the VASODILATOR drug isosorbide mononitrate, which can be used as an ANTI-ANGINA drug to treat and prevent angina pectoris. It is available as an aerosol spray used in metered doses under the tongue.
✚▲ Side-effects/warnings: See GLYCERYL TRINITRATE.

Nitromin

(Servier) is a proprietary, non-prescription preparation of the VASODILATOR and ANTI-ANGINA drug glyceryl trinitrate. It can be used to treat and prevent angina pectoris. It is available in the form of a sublingual aerosol spray in metered doses.
✚▲ Side-effects/warnings: See GLYCERYL TRINITRATE.

Nitronal

(Lipha) is a proprietary, prescription-only preparation of the VASODILATOR and ANTI-ANGINA drug glyceryl trinitrate. It can be used to treat and prevent angina pectoris, and is available in a form for injection.
✚▲ Side-effects/warnings: See GLYCERYL TRINITRATE.

nitrous oxide

is a gas that is used as an inhalant GENERAL ANAESTHETIC used for both induction and general anaesthesia. It is also an ANALGESIC and at subanaesthetic concentrations is used, for instance, in childbirth. Administration is by inhalation.
✚▲ Side-effects/warnings: Nausea and vomiting, and effects on the blood.

Nivaquine

(Rhône-Poulenc Rorer; Aventis Pharma) is a proprietary, prescription-only preparation of the ANTIMALARIAL drug chloroquine (as sulphate). It can be used to prevent or suppress certain forms of malaria and also as an ANTIRHEUMATIC to treat rheumatoid arthritis and lupus erythematosus. It is available as tablets, a syrup and in a form for injection. (This product also appears in a non-prescription preparation, as tablets or a syrup, labelled for use in the prevention of malaria.)
✚▲ Side-effects/warnings: See CHLOROQUINE.

Nivemycin

(Sovereign) is a proprietary, prescription-only preparation of the ANTIBACTERIAL and (AMINOGLYCOSIDE) ANTIBIOTIC neomycin sulphate. It can be used to reduce bacterial levels in the intestines before surgery, and is available as tablets.
✚▲ Side-effects/warnings: See NEOMYCIN SULPHATE.

nizatidine

is an H_2-ANTAGONIST and ULCER-HEALING DRUG. It can be used to assist in the treatment of benign peptic (gastric and duodenal) ulcers, to relieve heartburn in cases of reflux oesophagitis (caused by regurgitation of acid and enzymes into the oesophagus), also NSAID-associated ulceration, and a variety of conditions where reduction of acidity is beneficial. It works by reducing the secretion of gastric acid (by acting as a histamine receptor H_2-receptor antagonist), so reducing erosion and bleeding from peptic ulcers and allowing them a chance to heal. However, nizatidine should not be used until a full diagnosis of gastric bleeding or serious pain has been made, because its action in restricting gastric secretions may possibly mask the presence of stomach cancer. Administration is either oral or by intravenous injection or infusion. (Although it is a prescription-only drug when used for the treatment of ulcers and related conditions, it can be sold over-the-counter in limited quantities and dosage for occasional indigestion and heartburn for people over 16.)

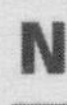

+▲ Side-effects/warnings: see H_2-ANTAGONIST. Also, there may be sweating, inflammation of blood vessels (vasculitis; with associated skin changes), other skin symptoms, raised uric acid levels in the blood. It is not used in those with liver impairment.

✪ **Related entries: Axid; Zinga.**

Nizoral

(Janssen-Cilag) is a proprietary, prescription-only preparation of the (AZOLE) ANTIFUNGAL drug ketoconazole. It can be used to treat serious systemic and skin-surface fungal infections, and is available as tablets and a cream for topical application. It is also available as a prescription-only shampoo used for scalp conditions, seborrhoeic dermatitis and dandruff. There are also brand variations on sale to the public with certain restrictions (on concentration and amount).

+▲ Side-effects/warnings: See KETOCONAZOLE.

Nizoral Dandruff Shampoo

(Johnson & Johnson MSD) is a proprietary, non-prescription compound preparation of the ANTIFUNGAL ketoconazole. It can be used for scalp conditions, dandruff and sebhorrhoeic dermatitis, and is available as a shampoo.

+▲ Side-effects/warnings: KETOCONAZOLE.

Nocutil

(Norgine) is a proprietary, prescription-only preparation of desmopressin, which is an analogue of the pituitary HORMONE vasopressin (ADH). It is administered in pituitary-originated DIABETES INSIPIDUS TREATMENT. It can be used in some diagnostic tests, and to prevent bed-wetting. It is available as a nasal spray (it is absorbed into the systemic circulation from the nasal mucosa).

+▲ Side-effects/warnings: See DESMOPRESSIN.

Nolvadex

(AstraZeneca) is a proprietary, prescription-only preparation of the sex HORMONE ANTAGONIST tamoxifen, which, because it inhibits the effect of OESTROGEN, is used primarily as an ANTICANCER treatment for cancers that depend on the presence of oestrogen in women, particularly breast cancer. It can also be used to treat certain conditions of infertility. It is available as tablets in three strengths (the stronger ones under the trade names *Nolvadex-D* and *Nolvadex-Forte*).

+▲ Side-effects/warnings: See TAMOXIFEN.

non-narcotic analgesic 🅱

drugs relieve pain. The term non-narcotic distinguishes them from the NARCOTIC ANALGESIC class, though they are referred to by many names, including *weak analgesics* and, in medical circles, a very large number are referred to as *non-steroidal anti-inflammatory drugs* or NSAIDS. The latter term refers to the valuable ANTI-INFLAMMATORY action of some members of the class. Non-narcotic analgesics are drugs that have no tendency to produce dependence (addiction), but are by no means free of side-effects. For example, ASPIRIN-like drugs can cause gastrointestinal upsets ranging from dyspepsia to serious haemorrhage. However, they can be used for a wide variety of purposes, from mild aches and pains (at a lower range of dosage) to the treatment of inflammatory joint disease (at higher dosages: see ANTIRHEUMATIC). PARACETAMOL does not have strong anti-inflammatory actions, but is non-narcotic and, along with other non-narcotic analgesics, has valuable ANTIPYRETIC action. These drugs work by altering the synthesis of prostaglandins (natural local hormones within the body) that cause pain. Often drugs in this class are used in combination with other ANALGESIC drugs (eg codeine) or with drugs of other classes (eg caffeine). See also IBUPROFEN and INDOMETACIN (indomethacin).

nonoxinol

is a SPERMICIDAL CONTRACEPTIVE drug which is used to assist barrier methods of contraception (such as the condom). Administration is by topical application as a jelly.

+▲ Side-effects/warnings: Regarded as safe when used as directed.

✪ **Related entries: Delfen; Duragel; Gynol II; Ortho-Creme; Orthoforms.**

non-steroidal anti-inflammatory drug 🅱

see NSAID.

nootropic agent 🅱

is the term used to describe a cognition enhancer (a memory enhancer or *smart drug*) that allegedly enhances mental performance. No drugs have been absolutely proved to have this action, but the term was coined to define drugs chemically resembling PIRACETAM (*Nootropil*), which were reported to improve mental function in tests. The main putative use for such drugs would be in the treatment of Alzheimer's disease (presenile dementia) and similar neurodegenerative diseases, though drug trials do not so far offer much encouragement. Several ways have been proposed for how these may work. Cerebral vasodilators are believed to increase blood supply to areas of the brain that are supposed to have a defective blood supply. Such drugs include PAPAVERINE, BETA-ADRENOCEPTOR STIMULANT drugs (eg isoxsuprine), CALCIUM-CHANNEL BLOCKER drugs (eg NIMODIPINE) and certain ERGOT ALKALOID with alpha-adrenoceptor blocking actions (see ALPHA-ADRENOCEPTOR BLOCKER: eg CO-DERGOCRINE MESILATE).

The defective function of neurones (cholinergic neurones) in the central nervous system that release the neurotransmitter ACETYLCHOLINE has long been thought to have a role in Alzheimer's disease, so ANTICHOLINESTERASE drugs (eg DONEPEZIL and RIVASTIGMINE) have been used to enhance cholinergic nerve function (though at the price of extensive side-effects).

Nootropil

(UCB Pharma) is a proprietary, prescription-only preparation of the ANTI-EPILEPTIC drug piracetam. It can be used in the treatment of cortical myoclonus (involuntary spasmic contractions of muscles of the body), and is available as tablets and an oral solution.

✚▲ Side-effects/warnings: See PIRACETAM.

noradrenaline

(norepinephrine) is both a HORMONE and a neurotransmitter and is chemically a catecholamine. It is produced and secreted (along with the closely related substance ADRENALINE) as a hormone into the bloodstream by the adrenal gland (from the region called the medulla, which is the central core of the adrenal gland – hence the term *adrenomedullary hormone*). The adrenal gland constitutes an important part of the sympathetic nervous system. Noradrenaline also acts as a neurotransmitter. It is released from nerve endings by electrical signals travelling from the central nervous system via nerves in the body, in order to activate or inhibit a wide variety of muscles, glands and metabolic processes. The responses of the body to stimulation of the sympathetic nervous system are primarily concerned with reactions to stress. In the face of stress, or the need for exertion, the body uses adrenaline and noradrenaline to cause constriction of some blood vessels while dilating others, with the net effect of the two catecholamines increasing blood flow to the skeletal muscles and heart. The heart rate is raised and there is relaxation of the smooth muscles of the intestine and bronchioles. There is also a rise in concentration of energy supplying glucose and free fatty-acids in the bloodstream. The actions of noradrenaline and adrenaline are similar, though noradrenaline causes a more marked rise in blood pressure, whereas adrenaline stimulates the heart more. In order to bring about one or more of these responses SYMPATHOMIMETIC drugs that mimic certain of these actions (eg adrenaline, ISOPRENALINE and PHENYLEPHRINE HYDROCHLORIDE) are administered therapeutically. Noradrenaline is not widely used because its actions are so widespread and there are many side-effects. As a drug, noradrenaline is used in the form of NORADRENALINE ACID TARTRATE.

noradrenaline acid tartrate

(norepinephrine bitartrate) is the chemical form of the naturally occurring NORADRENALINE that is used in medicine. Noradrenaline has both ALPHA-ADRENOCEPTOR STIMULANT and BETA-ADRENOCEPTOR STIMULANT properties, and is not widely used because its actions are so widespread. But in emergencies it may be used as a vasoconstrictor in acute hypotension and as a CARDIAC STIMULANT in cardiac arrest (when it is administered by injection).

✚▲ Side-effects/warnings: There may be palpitation of the heart with slowed and irregular heartbeat; peripheral ischaemia, hypertension and headache. It is a specialist drug used under hospital conditions.

Norcuron

(Organon) is a proprietary, prescription-only preparation of the (*non-depolarizing*) SKELETAL MUSCLE RELAXANT vecuronium bromide. It can be used to induce muscle paralysis during surgery, and is available in a form for injection.

✚▲ Side-effects/warnings: See VECURONIUM BROMIDE.

Norditropin

(Novo Nordisk) is a proprietary, prescription-only preparation of somatropin (the biosynthetic form of the pituitary HORMONE human growth hormone). It can be used to treat hormonal deficiency and associated symptoms (in particular, short stature). It is available in various forms for injection.

✚▲ Side-effects/warnings: See SOMATROPIN.

norepinephrine

see NORADRENALINE.

norepinephrine bitartrate

see NORADRENALINE ACID TARTRATE.

norethisterone

is a PROGESTOGEN. It is used primarily as a constituent in ORAL CONTRACEPTIVE preparations that combine an OESTROGEN with a progestogen, in PROGESTOGEN-only pill (*POP*) type, in implant contraception, in HRT (hormone replacement therapy), for menstrual problems (eg premenstrual syndrome) and endometriosis, and as an ANTICANCER drug to assist in the treatment of sex-hormone linked cancers (eg breast cancer). Administration is oral, topical as skin patches or by injection.

✚▲ Side-effects/warnings: See PROGESTOGEN.

✪ **Related entries: Adgyn Combi; BiNovum; Brevinor; Climagest; Climesse; Elleste-Duet; Estracombi; Estrapak 50; Evorel; Kliofem; Kliovance; Loestrin 20; Loestrin 30; Micronor; Micronor HRT; Noriday; Norimin; Norinyl-1; Noristerat; Nuvelle Continuous; Ovysmen; Primolut N; Synphase; TriNovum; Trisequens; Utovlan.**

norfloxacin

is a (QUINOLONE) ANTIBIOTIC-like ANTIBACTERIAL which can be used to treat infections especially of the urinary tract. Administration is oral.

✚▲ Side-effects/warnings: See QUINOLONE; but it may also include depression, anorexia and tinnitus, vasculitis, dermatitis, pancreatitis, kidney changes.

✪ **Related entry: Utinor.**

Norgalax Micro-enema

(Norgine) is a proprietary, non-prescription preparation of the (*stimulant*) LAXATIVE docusate sodium. It can be used to relieve constipation and also to evacuate the rectum prior to abdominal procedures. It is available as an enema. It is not normally given to children, except on medical advice.

✚▲ Side-effects/warnings: See DOCUSATE SODIUM.

norgestimate

is a PROGESTOGEN used as a constituent of the *combined* ORAL CONTRACEPTIVE preparations that contain an OESTROGEN and a PROGESTOGEN. Administration is oral.

✚▲ Side-effects/warnings: See PROGESTOGEN.

✪ **Related entry: Cilest.**

Norgeston

(Schering Health) is a proprietary, prescription-only preparation which can be used as an ORAL CONTRACEPTIVE of the PROGESTOGEN-only pill (*POP*) type and contains levonorgestrel. It is available as tablets in a calendar pack.

✚▲ Side-effects/warnings: See LEVONORGESTREL.

norgestrel

is a PROGESTOGEN, which is used in *progesterone-only* ORAL CONTRACEPTIVE preparations and also, in combination with OESTROGEN, in HRT (hormone replacement therapy). Administration is oral. (LEVONORGESTREL is a stronger form of norgestrel.)

✚▲ Side-effects/warnings: See PROGESTOGEN.

✪ **Related entries: Cyclo-Progynova; Neogest; Prempak-C.**

Noriday

(Pharmacia) is a proprietary, prescription-only preparation which can be used as an ORAL CONTRACEPTIVE of the PROGESTOGEN-only pill (*POP*) type and contains norethisterone. It is available as tablets in a calendar pack.

✚▲ Side-effects/warnings: See NORETHISTERONE.

Norimin

(Pharmacia) is a proprietary, prescription-only compound preparation which can be used as a (*monophasic*) ORAL CONTRACEPTIVE of the *COC* (standard strength) type that combines an OESTROGEN and a PROGESTOGEN, in this case

ethinylestradiol and norethisterone. It is available as tablets in a calendar pack.
✚▲ Side-effects/warnings: See ETHINYLESTRADIOL; NORETHISTERONE.

Norimode

(Tillomed) is a proprietary, prescription-only preparation of the (OPIOID) ANTIDIARRHOEAL loperamide hydrochloride. It can be used for the symptomatic relief of acute diarrhoea and its associated discomfort, and is available as capsules.
✚▲ Side-effects/warnings: See LOPERAMIDE HYDROCHLORIDE.

Norinyl-1

(Pharmacia) is a proprietary, prescription-only compound preparation which can be used as a (*monophasic*) ORAL CONTRACEPTIVE of the *COC* (standard strength) type that combines an OESTROGEN and a PROGESTOGEN, in this case mestranol and norethisterone. It is available as tablets in a calendar pack.
✚▲ Side-effects/warnings: See MESTRANOL; NORETHISTERONE.

Noristerat

(Schering Health) is a proprietary, prescription-only preparation which can be used as a parenteral CONTRACEPTIVE of the PROGESTOGEN-only (*POP*) pill type and contains norethisterone. It is available in a form for intramuscular depot implant injection.
✚▲ Side-effects/warnings: See NORETHISTERONE.

Noritate

(Kestrel) is a proprietary, prescription-only preparation of the ANTIMICROBIAL metronidazole, which has ANTIBACTERIAL and ANTIPROTOZOAL actions. It can be applied topically as a cream to treat acute acne rosacea outbreaks.
✚▲ Side-effects/warnings: See METRONIDAZOLE.

Normacol

(Norgine) is a proprietary, non-prescription preparation of the (*bulking-agent*) LAXATIVE sterculia. It can be used to relieve constipation, and is available as granules. It is not normally given to children under six years, except on medical advice.
✚▲ Side-effects/warnings: See STERCULIA.

Normacol Plus

(Norgine) is a proprietary, non-prescription preparation of the (*bulking-agent*) LAXATIVE sterculia (with added frangula bark). It can be used to relieve constipation, and is available as granules.
✚▲ Side-effects/warnings: See STERCULIA.

Normal Immunoglobulin

(Public Health Laboratories Services; BPL; SNBTS) is a proprietary, prescription-only preparation of human NORMAL IMMUNOGLOBULIN. It can be used in IMMUNIZATION to confer immediate *passive immunity* to infection by viruses such as hepatitis A virus, rubeola (measles) and rubella (German measles). It is available in a form for intramuscular injection. (Special forms given by intravenous infusion for replacement therapy are not detailed here.)
✚▲ Side-effects/warnings: See NORMAL IMMUNOGLOBULIN.

normal immunoglobulin

(gamma globulin; human normal immunoglobulin; HNIG) is used in IMMUNIZATION to give *passive immunity* by the injection of immunoglobulin (antibody) prepared from the pooled blood plasma donated by individuals with antibodies to viruses prevalent in the general population, including hepatitis A virus, rubeola (measles) and rubella (German measles). It is commonly given to patients at risk, such as infants who cannot tolerate vaccines that incorporate live (though weakened) viruses (*active immunity*), for rubella in pregnancy, and hepatitis A short-term protection for travellers in areas were the disease in endemic. Administration is normally by intramuscular injection, but there are also special forms for replacement therapy given by intravenous infusion, including formulations for patients undergoing a bone-marrow transplant, or patients with certain congenital blood component deficiencies, eg a gammaglobulinaemia, hypogammaglobulinaemia, idiopathic thrombocytopenic purpurea and Kawasaki syndrome; also sometimes used in the treatment of Guillain-Barré syndrome.)

N

✚▲ Side-effects/warnings: See IMMUNIZATION.
✪ **Related entries: Gammabulin; Kabiglobulin; Normal Immunoglobulin.**

Normax
(Celltech) is a proprietary, prescription-only preparation of co-danthramer 50/60, which is a (*stimulant*) LAXATIVE based on dantron and docusate sodium. It can be used to relieve constipation and to prepare patients for abdominal procedures. It is available as a suspension and capsules.
✚▲ Side-effects/warnings: See DANTRON; DOCUSATE SODIUM.

Norphyllin SR
(IVAX) is a proprietary, non-prescription preparation of the BRONCHODILATOR aminophylline. It can be used as an ANTI-ASTHMATIC, and is available as modified-release tablets.
✚▲ Side-effects/warnings: See AMINOPHYLLINE.

Norprolac
(Novartis) is a proprietary, prescription-only preparation of the DOPAMINE-RECEPTOR STIMULANT drug quinagolide. It can be used to treat HORMONE disorders (hyperprolactinaemia), and is available as tablets.
✚▲ Side-effects/warnings: See QUINAGOLIDE.

nortriptyline hydrochloride
is an ANTIDEPRESSANT of the TRICYCLIC group. It has fewer SEDATIVE properties than some of this type, and is used primarily to treat depressive illness and also some types of neuropathic pain, including diabetic neuropathy. Like several other drugs of its type, it may also be used to prevent bed-wetting by children. Administration is oral.
✚▲ Side-effects/warnings: See AMITRIPTYLINE HYDROCHLORIDE; but is less sedating.
✪ **Related entries: Allegron; Motipress; Motival.**

Norvir
(Abbott) is a proprietary, prescription-only preparation of the ANTIVIRAL drug ritonavir. It can be used in the treatment of HIV infection, and is available as an oral solution and capsules.
✚▲ Side-effects/warnings: See RITONAVIR.

Novantrone
(Lederle; Wyeth) is a proprietary, prescription-only preparation of the ANTICANCER drug mitoxantrone (mitozantrone). It can be used in the treatment of certain types of cancer, and is available in a form for intravenous infusion.
✚▲ Side-effects/warnings: See MITOXANTRONE.

NovoNorm
(Novo Nordisk) is a proprietary, prescription-only preparation of repaglinide. It can be used in DIABETIC TREATMENT of Type II diabetes (non-insulin-dependent diabetes mellitus; NIDDM; maturity-onset diabetes), and is available as tablets.
✚▲ Side-effects/warnings: See REPAGLINIDE.

NovoRapid
(Novo Nordisk) is a proprietary, prescription-only preparation of INSULIN ASPART, which is a recombinant human insulin analogue. It is used to treat and maintain diabetic patients, and is available in forms for injection.
✚▲ Side-effects/warnings: See INSULIN.

NovoSeven
(Novo Nordisk) is a proprietary, prescription-only preparation of recombinant human antihaemophilic factor VIIa, which acts as a HAEMOSTATIC drug to reduce or stop bleeding. It can be used in the treatment of disorders in which bleeding is prolonged and potentially dangerous, usually patients with inhibitors to factors VIII and IX. It is available in a form for intravenous injection or infusion.
✚▲ Side-effects/warnings: See FACTOR VIIA (RECOMBINANT).

Nozinan
(Link) is a proprietary, prescription-only preparation of the ANTIPSYCHOTIC drug levomepromazine (methotrimeprazine). It can be used to tranquillize patients with psychotic disorders, such as schizophrenia, and to calm and soothe those with terminal illness. It is available as tablets (as maleate) or in a form for injection (as hydrochloride).
✚▲ Side-effects/warnings: See LEVOMEPROMAZINE.

NSAID
is an abbreviation for *non-steroidal anti-inflammatory drug*, which is used to describe a large group of drugs, of which ASPIRIN is an

original member. Although they are all acidic compounds of different chemical structures, they have several important actions in common. They can be used as ANTI-INFLAMMATORY drugs (to the extent that some may be used as ANTIRHEUMATIC treatments), as NON-NARCOTIC ANALGESIC drugs (particularly when the pain is associated with inflammation) and as ANTIPYRETIC drugs (with the added advantage that they lower body temperature only when it is raised in fever). All these actions are thought to be due to the ability of NSAIDs to act as ENZYME INHIBITOR drugs (acting on the cyclo-oxygenase system; COX) to change the synthesis and metabolism of the natural LOCAL HORMONE mediators the PROSTAGLANDIN family, also thromboxanes. In practice, the side-effects of NSAIDs are so extensive that the use of individual members depends on the ability of individual patients to tolerate their side-effects, which is especially important when used for joint disease where generally high doses are taken for long periods of time. Some with the least side-effects are regarded as safe enough for non-prescription, over-the-counter sale, such as aspirin and IBUPROFEN. Although PARACETAMOL shares some of the NSAIDs' properties, it is only very weakly anti-inflammatory and is not always classified with them. See also ANALGESIC. Additionally, unrelated to any anti-inflammatory action (and working on a different form of COX), aspirin may be used as an ANTIPLATELET drug, because it can be used to beneficially reduce platelet aggregation.

Some newly developed NSAID drugs have more selectivity in inhibiting the COX-2 form of the enzyme (eg CELECOXIB, ETODOLAC, MELOXICAM and ROFECOXIB) and are thought to have fewer severe gastrointestinal side-effects. However, authorities have decided that they should not yet be routinely used in the management of patients with rheumatoid arthritis or osteoarthritis. For patients with a history of gastroduodenal ulcer or perforation or gastrointestinal bleeding. However, the use of COX-2 selective inhibitors may sometimes be considered.

✚ Side-effects: These vary in severity and in the frequency with which they occur depending on the NSAID used. Gastrointestinal upsets, dyspepsia, nausea, diarrhoea, bleeding and ulceration. There may be hypersensitivity reactions, including rash, bronchospasm, oedema, headache, blood disorders, ringing in the ears, dizziness and fluid retention. Reversible kidney failure, particularly in renal impairment. Liver damage is rare. The gastrointestinal upsets may be minimized by taking the drug with milk or food. There are other, less common, side-effects that have been reported. When NSAIDs are used topically (eg as gel or cream) most of these side-effects and warnings do not apply. However, hypersensitivity reactions (eg asthma-like symptoms) may occur in susceptible people if there is systemic absorption. Also, people using topical forms should avoid excess exposure to sunlight because of a photosensitizing action by NSAIDs.

▲ Warnings: Use with care in patients with allergic disorders (especially asthma and skin conditions), in the elderly and where there are certain liver or kidney disorders. They should not be used where there is a tendency to, or active, peptic ulceration; but different NSAIDs vary in the severity of their gastrointestinal side-effects (eg azapropazone is high-risk, whereas ibuprofen has a lower risk, and the remainder have an intermediate risk). NSAIDs should not be taken by those who are pregnant and some are to be avoided when breast-feeding (eg aspirin), or by those who have certain blood disorders. Many drugs can interact with NSAIDs and *vice versa*, including ANTICOAGULANT, ANTI-EPILEPTIC, CORTICOSTEROID and other drug groups. See ACECLOFENAC; ACEMETACIN; ALOXIPRIN; AMMONIUM SALICYLATE; ASPIRIN; AZAPROPAZONE; BENORILATE; CELECOXIB; CHOLINE SALICYLATE; DEXKETOPROFEN; DICLOFENAC SODIUM; DIETHYLAMINE SALICYLATE; DIFLUNISAL; ETHYL SALICYLATE; ETODOLAC; FELBINAC; FENBUFEN; FENOPROFEN; FLURBIPROFEN; GLYCOL SALICYLATE; IBUPROFEN; INDOMETHACIN; KETOPROFEN; KETOROLAC TROMETAMOL; LORNOXICAM; MEFENAMIC ACID; MELOXICAM; METHYL SALICYLATE; NABUMETONE; NAPROXEN; PHENYLBUTAZONE; PIROXICAM; ROFECOXIB; SODIUM SALICYLATE; SULINDAC; TENOXICAM; TIAPROFENIC ACID; TOLFENAMIC ACID.

Nubain

(DuPont; Bristol-Myers Squibb) is a proprietary, prescription-only preparation of the (OPIOID) NARCOTIC ANALGESIC nalbuphine hydrochloride.

It can be used to treat moderate to severe pain, particularly during or following surgical procedures or in myocardial infarction, and is available in a form for injection.
✚▲ Side-effects/warnings: See NALBUPHINE HYDROCHLORIDE.

Nuelin

(3M) is a proprietary, non-prescription preparation of the BRONCHODILATOR theophylline. It can be used as an ANTI-ASTHMATIC treatment. It is available as tablets and as a liquid.
✚▲ Side-effects/warnings: See THEOPHYLLINE.

Nuelin SA

(3M) is a proprietary, non-prescription preparation of the BRONCHODILATOR theophylline. It can be used as an ANTI-ASTHMATIC treatment. It is available as tablets and modified-release tablets (including *Nuelin SA 250*).
✚▲ Side-effects/warnings: See THEOPHYLLINE.

Nurofen

(Crookes Healthcare) is a proprietary, non-prescription preparation of the (NSAID) NON-NARCOTIC ANALGESIC, ANTIRHEUMATIC and ANTIPYRETIC ibuprofen. It can be used to relieve headache, period pain, muscular pain, dental pain and feverishness. It is available as tablets and is not normally given to children, except on medical advice.
✚▲ Side-effects/warnings: See IBUPROFEN.

Nurofen Advance

(Crookes Healthcare) is a proprietary, non-prescription preparation of the (NSAID) NON-NARCOTIC ANALGESIC, ANTIRHEUMATIC and ANTIPYRETIC ibuprofen. It can be used to relieve headache, period pain, muscular pain, dental pain and feverishness. It is available as tablets and is not normally given to children, except on medical advice.
✚▲ Side-effects/warnings: See IBUPROFEN.

Nurofen Caplets

(Crookes Healthcare) is a proprietary, non-prescription preparation of the (NSAID) NON-NARCOTIC ANALGESIC, ANTIRHEUMATIC and ANTIPYRETIC ibuprofen. It can be used to relieve headache, period pain, muscular pain, dental pain and feverishness. It is available as capsule-shaped tablets, and is not normally given to children, except on medical advice.
✚▲ Side-effects/warnings: See IBUPROFEN.

Nurofen Cold & Flu

(Crookes Healthcare) is a proprietary, non-prescription compound preparation of the (NSAID) NON-NARCOTIC ANALGESIC and ANTIRHEUMATIC ibuprofen, and the DECONGESTANT pseudoephedrine hydrochloride. It can be used to relieve symptoms of colds and flu, and is available as tablets. It is not normally given to children, except on medical advice.
✚▲ Side-effects/warnings: See IBUPROFEN; PSEUDOEPHEDRINE HYDROCHLORIDE.

Nurofen for Children Sugar Free

(Crookes Healthcare) is a proprietary, non-prescription preparation of the (NSAID) NON-NARCOTIC ANALGESIC, ANTIRHEUMATIC and ANTIPYRETIC ibuprofen. It can be used to relieve headache, pain and feverishness, including after vaccination. It is available as a suspension and given to infants and children from 6 months to 12 years.
✚▲ Side-effects/warnings: See IBUPROFEN.

Nurofen Liquid Capsules

(Crookes Healthcare) is a proprietary, non-prescription preparation of the (NSAID) NON-NARCOTIC ANALGESIC, ANTIRHEUMATIC and ANTIPYRETIC ibuprofen. It can be used for the relief of mild to moderate pain such as headache, period pain and feverishness. It is available as capsules, and is not given to children except on medical advice.
✚▲ Side-effects/warnings: See IBUPROFEN.

Nurofen Long Lasting

(Crookes Healthcare) is a proprietary, non-prescription preparation of the (NSAID) NON-NARCOTIC ANALGESIC and ANTIRHEUMATIC ibuprofen. It can be used for the long-lasting relief of backache, period pain, arthritic, rheumatic and muscular pains, headache and migraine. It is available as modified-release capsules, and is not given to children, except on medical advice.
✚▲ Side-effects/warnings: See IBUPROFEN.

Nurofen Meltlets

(Crookes Healthcare) is a proprietary, non-prescription compound preparation of the (NSAID) NON-NARCOTIC ANALGESIC, ANTIRHEUMATIC and ANTIPYRETIC ibuprofen. It can be used to relieve mild to moderate pain such as headache, backache, period pain, muscular and rheumatic pain, and for the symptoms of feverishness, colds and flu. It is available as self-dissolving tablets that dissolve on the tongue and are then swallowed. It is not given to children, except on medical advice.

✚▲ Side-effects/warnings: See IBUPROFEN.

Nurofen Muscular Pain Relief Gel

(Crookes) is a proprietary, non-prescription preparation of the (NSAID) NON-NARCOTIC ANALGESIC and ANTIRHEUMATIC ibuprofen. It can be used to treat pain and inflammation, especially rheumatic conditions, backache, sprains and strains. It is available as a gel for topical application. It is not given to children under 14 years, except on medicial advice.

✚▲ Side-effects/warnings: See IBUPROFEN; but adverse effects on topical application are limited.

Nurofen Plus

(Crookes Healthcare) is a proprietary, non-prescription compound preparation of the (NSAID) NON-NARCOTIC ANALGESIC, ANTIRHEUMATIC and ANTIPYRETIC ibuprofen and the (OPIOID) NARCOTIC ANALGESIC codeine. It can be used to relieve migraine, tension headache, period pain, dental pain, neuralgia, backache, sciatica and rheumatic pain. It is available as tablets and is not normally given to children, except on medical advice.

✚▲ Side-effects/warnings: See CODEINE PHOSPHATE; IBUPROFEN.

Nurse Harvey's Gripe Mixture

(Harvey-Scruton) is a proprietary, non-prescription preparation of the ANTACID sodium bicarbonate. It can be used to relieve wind, gripe and related pain and discomfort in infants over one month, and is available as a liquid.

✚▲ Side-effects/warnings: See SODIUM BICARBONATE.

Nurse Sykes Powders

(Anglian Pharma) is a proprietary, non-prescription compound preparation of the (NSAID) NON-NARCOTIC ANALGESIC and ANTIRHEUMATIC aspirin, the non-narcotic analgesic paracetamol and the STIMULANT caffeine. It can be used to relieve headaches, cold and flu symptoms, mild to moderate pain and aches and pains. It is available as a powder and is not normally given to children, except on medical advice.

✚▲ Side-effects/warnings: See ASPIRIN; CAFFEINE; PARACETAMOL.

Nu-Seals Aspirin

(Lilly) is a proprietary, prescription-only preparation of the (NSAID) NON-NARCOTIC ANALGESIC aspirin and can be used to treat as an ANTIPLATELET aggregation (antithrombotic) drug. It is available as tablets in two doses (75mg for antiplatelet use, also 300mg for analgesic use).

✚▲ Side-effects/warnings: See ASPIRIN.

Nutraplus

(Galderma) is a proprietary, non-prescription preparation of the HYDRATING AGENT urea. It can be used to treat dry, scaling and itching skin, and is available as a cream.

✚▲ Side-effects/warnings: See UREA.

nutritional preparation

(nutritional supplement) refers to preparations primarily used in medicine for the nutrition of patients who cannot tolerate normal foods for some reason. Their use is only seen as essential under certain circumstances, such as after major bowel surgery, serious stomach and intestinal disorders, for those allergic to certain food products, such as cows' milk or gluten (gluten-intolerance), FRUCTOSE for those unable to metabolize certain sugars or amino acids (eg for patients with phenylketonuria).

Nutrizym 10

(Merck) is a proprietary, non-prescription preparation of the digestive enzyme pancreatin. It can be used to compensate for deficiencies of digestive juices that are normally supplied by the pancreas. It is available as capsules.

✚▲ Side-effects/warnings: See PANCREATIN.

Nutrizym 22

(Merck) is a proprietary, prescription-only preparation of the digestive enzyme pancreatin. It can be used to compensate for deficiencies of digestive juices that are normally supplied by the pancreas. It is available as capsules containing

enteric-coated granules, which are at a higher strength than *Nutrizym 10*.
+▲ Side-effects/warnings: See PANCREATIN.

Nutrizym GR

(Merck) is a proprietary, non-prescription preparation of the digestive enzyme (see ENZYMES) pancreatin. It can be used to treat deficiencies of digestive juices that are normally supplied by the pancreas. It is available as capsules.
+▲ Side-effects/warnings: See PANCREATIN.

Nuvelle

(Schering Health) is a proprietary, prescription-only compound preparation of the OESTROGEN estradiol and the PROGESTOGEN levonorgestrel. It can be used to treat menopausal problems in HRT and in osteoporosis prevention, and is available as tablets (in various forms).
+▲ Side-effects/warnings: See LEVONORGESTREL; ESTRADIOL.

Nuvelle Continuous

(Schering Health) is a proprietary, prescription-only compound preparation of the OESTROGEN estradiol and the PROGESTOGEN norethisterone. It can be used to treat menopausal problems in HRT and osteoporosis prevention, and is available as tablets.
+▲ Side-effects/warnings: See NORETHISTERONE; ESTRADIOL.

Nuvelle TS

(Schering Health) is a proprietary, prescription-only compound preparation of the OESTROGEN estradiol, and the PROGESTOGEN levonorgestrel. It can be used to treat menopausal problems in HRT and is available in the form of self-adhesive patches (of two forms, called *TS Phase I* and *TS Phase II*).
+▲ Side-effects/warnings: See LEVONORGESTREL; ESTRADIOL.

Nycopren

(Ardern) is a proprietary, prescription-only preparation of the (NSAID) NON-NARCOTIC ANALGESIC and ANTIRHEUMATIC naproxen. It can be used to relieve pain and inflammation, particularly rheumatic and arthritic pain, acute gout and to treat other musculoskeletal disorders and period pain. It is available as tablets.
+▲ Side-effects/warnings: See NAPROXEN.

Nylax with Senna

(Crookes Healthcare) is a proprietary, non-prescription compound preparation of the (*stimulant*) LAXATIVE senna. It can be used for the short-term relief of constipation, and is available as tablets. It is not normally given to children under five years, except on medical advice.
+▲ Side-effects/warnings: See SENNA.

Nystaform

(Typharm) is a proprietary, prescription-only compound preparation of the ANTIFUNGAL and ANTIBIOTIC nystatin and the ANTISEPTIC chlorhexidine. It can be used to treat *Candida* fungal infections of the skin, and is available as a cream for topical application.
+▲ Side-effects/warnings: See CHLORHEXIDINE; NYSTATIN.

Nystaform-HC

(Typharm) is a proprietary, prescription-only compound preparation of the ANTIFUNGAL and ANTIBIOTIC nystatin, the ANTISEPTIC chlorhexidine (as hydrochloride), and the ANTI-INFLAMMATORY and CORTICOSTEROID hydrocortisone. It can be used to treat fungal infections with inflammation of the skin, such as eczema, and is available as a cream for topical application.
+▲ Side-effects/warnings: See CHLORHEXIDINE; HYDROCORTISONE; NYSTATIN.

Nystamont

(Rosemont) is a range of proprietary, prescription-only preparations of the ANTIFUNGAL and ANTIBIOTIC nystatin. They can be used to treat fungal infections (eg candidiasis; thrush) and are available as oral suspensions.
+▲ Side-effects/warnings: See NYSTATIN.

Nystan

(Squibb; Bristol-Myers Squibb) is a range of proprietary, prescription-only preparations of the ANTIFUNGAL and ANTIBIOTIC nystatin. They can be used to treat fungal infections (eg candidiasis; thrush) and are available in a variety of forms. Preparations for oral administration include tablets, a suspension, a gluten-, lactose- and sugar-free suspension, granules for solution and pastilles (for treating mouth infections). For

vaginal and vulval infections there is a vaginal cream and pessaries (vaginal inserts). A cream and an ointment are available for topical application.
✚▲ Side-effects/warnings: See NYSTATIN.

nystatin

is a *(polyene)* ANTIBIOTIC with ANTIFUNGAL properties. It is effective when administered topically or orally. When taken orally, it is not absorbed into the blood and its antifungal action is restricted to the mouth and gastrointestinal tract. Nystatin is primarily used to treat the yeast infection candidiasis (thrush) of the skin, mucous membranes, including vaginal infections, and intestinal tract, including around the mouth. Administration can be either oral or topical in a variety of forms.
✚ Side-effects: There may be nausea, vomiting or diarrhoea, local irritation, sensitization of the mouth and a rash.
✪ Related entries: Dermovate-NN; Flagyl Compak; Gregoderm; Nystaform; Nystaform-HC; Nystamont; Nystan; Terra-Cortril Nystatin; Timodine; Tinaderm-M; Tri-Adcortyl; Tri-Adcortyl Otic; Trimovate.

Nytol

(Stafford-Miller; GSK) is a proprietary, non-prescription preparation of the ANTIHISTAMINE diphenhydramine hydrochloride, which has marked SEDATIVE properties. It can be used to help induce sleep in the treatment of temporary sleep disturbances, and is available as caplets. It is not normally given to children under 16 years, except on medical advice.
✚▲ Side-effects/warnings: See DIPHENHYDRAMINE HYDROCHLORIDE.

Nytol One-a-Night

(Stafford-Miller; GSK) is a proprietary, non-prescription preparation of the ANTIHISTAMINE diphenhydramine hydrochloride, which has marked SEDATIVE properties. It can be used to help induce sleep in the treatment of temporary sleep disturbances, and is available as caplets. It is not normally given to children under 16 years, except on medical advice.
✚▲ Side-effects/warnings: See DIPHENHYDRAMINE HYDROCHLORIDE.

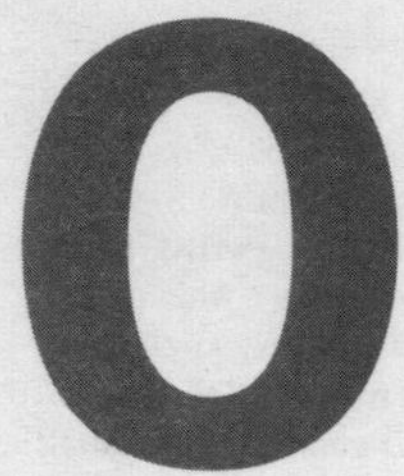

obesity treatment

drugs are used as an adjunct to (ie as well as) dietary changes to reduce body weight where this presents a medical risk. Most such drugs that have been used work as APPETITE SUPPRESSANT agents. Some of these act directly on the brain as STIMULANT agents, and are related to amfetamine (amphetamine), including phentermine, fenfluramine and dexfenfluramine, dexamfetamine and metamfetamine. However, all have now been withdrawn from mainstream medical practice in the UK because of concerns about harmful effects on the heart. A new and different type of drug that works on the brain to modify appetite, represented by the recently introduced agent SIBUTRAMINE, acts by inhibiting reuptake of noradrenaline, serotonin and dopamine in the central nervous system (a similar activity to certain ANTIDEPRESSANT drugs).

Another type works by bulking out the food eaten so that the body feels it has actually taken more than it has. The main bulking agent used medically is METHYLCELLULOSE, while others sometimes used are better known as (bulking-agent) LAXATIVE drugs, eg STERCULIA and ISPAGHULA HUSK. A recently introduced drug, ORLISTAT, works instead by reducing the absorption from the intestine of dietary fat.

All these drugs are intended to assist in the medical treatment of obesity, where the primary therapy is an appropriate diet.

Occlusal

(DermaPharm) is a proprietary, non-prescription preparation of the KERATOLYTIC agent salicylic acid. It can be used to remove warts and hard skin, and is available as a liquid paint.
✚▲ Side-effects/warnings: See SALICYLIC ACID.

octreotide

is a long-lasting analogue of the hypothalamic HORMONE somatostatin (hypothalamic release-inhibiting hormone). It reduces release of a number of other hormones from the pituitary gland and some other sites. It is used as an ANTICANCER drug for the relief of symptoms caused by the release of hormones from carcinoid and non-carcinoid tumours of the endocrine system, including VIPomas and glucagonomas, and for the short-term treatment of acromegaly. It can also be used to limit complications in pancreatic surgery. Administration is by subcutaneous or intravenous injection.
✚ Side-effects: Gastrointestinal upsets including nausea and vomiting, anorexia, bloating, pain, flatulence, fatty faeces and diarrhoea. Kidney dysfunction, blood sugar disturbances, gallstone formation, changes in liver function, and pain at injection site.
▲ Warnings: It should be used with caution in patients who are pregnant or breast-feeding or where kidney function is impaired. Regular gallbladder examination and thyroid monitoring is often recommended. Withdrawal of treatment should be gradual.
✪ **Related entries: Sandostatin; Sandostatin LAR.**

Ocufen

(Allergan) is a proprietary, prescription-only preparation of the (NSAID) NON-NARCOTIC ANALGESIC flurbiprofen (with polyvinyl alcohol). It can be used by topical application to inhibit constriction of the pupil during an operation on the eye and for other ophthalmological reasons (eg postoperative inflammation). Available as eye-drops.
✚▲ Side-effects/warnings: See FLURBIPROFEN; POLYVINYL ALCOHOL.

Oculotect

(Novartis Ophthalmics) is a proprietary, non-prescription preparation of POVIDONE. It is used in the management of tear deficiency in dry eye conditions, and is available as eye-drops.
✚▲ Side-effects/warnings: See POVIDONE.

Odrik

(Hoechst Marion Roussel; Aventis Pharma) is a proprietary, prescription-only preparation of the ACE INHIBITOR trandolapril. It can be used as an ANTIHYPERTENSIVE, and is available as capsules.
✚▲ Side-effects/warnings: See TRANDOLAPRIL.

oestradiol

see ESTRADIOL.

oestriol

see ESTRIOL.

Oestrogel

(Hoechst Marion Roussel; Aventis Pharma) is a proprietary, prescription-only preparation of the OESTROGEN estradiol. It can be used in HRT and in osteoporosis prevention. It is available in the form of a gel for topical application.

✚▲ Side-effects/warnings: See ESTRADIOL.

oestrogen

is the name given to any of a group of (STEROID) SEX HORMONES that promote the growth and functioning of the female sex organs and the development of female sexual characteristics. In their natural forms, they are produced and secreted mainly by the ovary (and to a small extent the placenta of pregnant women, the adrenal cortex in both sexes, and – in men – the testis). Natural (eg ESTRADIOL, ESTRIOL) and synthetic oestrogens are used therapeutically, sometimes in combination with progestogens (see PROGESTOGEN), to treat menstrual problems (eg absence of menstrual periods in primary amenorrhoria), menopausal problems (HRT; often with natural oestrogens) or other gynaecological problems, and as oral contraceptives (see ORAL CONTRACEPTIVE: in combination with progesterones). Some synthetic oestrogens are also used to treat certain cancers (eg prostate and breast cancer). The best-known and most-used oestrogens are the natural hormones estradiol and estriol, and the synthetic hormones ETHINYLESTRADIOL, MESTRANOL and DIETHYLSTILBESTROL.

✚ Side-effects: Depending on the dose, route of administration and the particular preparation used; there may be nausea, vomiting, weight gain and oedema, tender and enlarged breasts, premenstrual syndrome-like symptoms, headache, depression, dizziness, leg cramps; sometimes rash and changes in liver function.

▲ Warnings: They are not administered to patients with certain oestrogen-dependent cancers, a history of thrombosis, inflamed endometrial lining of the uterus or impaired liver function. Prolonged treatment (without progesterone) increases the risk of cancer of the endometrium. Depending on use, dose and route of administration, they may not be suitable for patients who are diabetic or epileptic, have certain cardiovascular or kidney disorders, multiple sclerosis, porphyria, who are pregnant or breast-feeding or who have hypertension or migraine.

ofloxacin

is a broad-spectrum (QUINOLONE) ANTIBIOTIC-like ANTIBACTERIAL. It can be used to treat infections of the genitourinary tract, including both gonorrhoea and non-gonorrhoeal infections, some respiratory infections, infections of the cervix and septicaemia. Administration can be either oral or by intravenous infusion, or topically (eye-drops).

✚▲ Side-effects/warnings: These depend on the route of administration. See QUINOLONE. Administer with caution to patients with a history of psychiatric illness. Other possible side-effects include inflamed tendons, anxiety, unsteady gait, tremor, psychotic reactions and effects on the blood and cardiovascular system, and others. As eye-drops, side-effects include local irritation, photophobia, dizziness, numbness, headache and nausea.

✪ Related entries: Exocin; Tarivid.

Oilatum Bath Formula

(Stiefel) is a proprietary, non-prescription preparation of the EMOLLIENT liquid paraffin. It can be used to soften skin and treat contact dermatitis, eczema and other dry skin conditions, and is available as a bath emulsion.

✚▲ Side-effects/warnings: See LIQUID PARAFFIN.

Oilatum Cream

(Stiefel) is a proprietary, non-prescription preparation of the EMOLLIENT arachis oil (peanut oil). It can be used to soften skin, and is available as a cream.

✚▲ Side-effects/warnings: See ARACHIS OIL.

Oilatum Junior

(Stiefel) is a proprietary, non-prescription preparation of the EMOLLIENT liquid paraffin. It can be used to treat contact and atopic dematitis and some other skin complaints, and is available as a bath additive.

✚▲ Side-effects/warnings: See LIQUID PARAFFIN.

Oilatum Junior Flare-Up

(Stiefel) is a proprietary, non-prescription preparation of the EMOLLIENT liquid paraffin

with the ANTISEPTIC triclosan and benzalkonium chloride. It can be used to treat eczema flare-ups, and is available as a bath additive. It can also be used for children and babies older than six months.
✚▲ Side-effects/warnings: See BENZALKONIUM CHLORIDE; LIQUID PARAFFIN; TRICLOSAN.

Okacyn
(Novartis Ophthalmics) is a prescription-only proprietary preparation of the broad-spectrum (QUINOLONE) ANTIBIOTIC-like ANTIBACTERIAL lomefloxacin. It can be used to treat infections of the eye in the form of eye-drops.
✚▲ Side-effects/warnings: See LOMEFLOXACIN.

olanzapine
is an ANTIPSYCHOTIC drug (one of a group sometimes termed 'atypical' antipsychotics) which can be used to tranquillize patients suffering from schizophrenia. Administration is oral.
✚ Side-effects: Atypical antipsychotics include weight gain, dizziness, postural hypotension, extrapyramidal symptoms (usually mild and transient, but occasionally tardive dyskinesia on long-term administration). Olanzapine may cause mild anticholinergic effects; drowsiness, increased appetite, oedema.
▲ Warnings: Atypical antipsychotics are used with caution in patients with cardiovascular disease, history of epilepsy and Parkinson's disease; may affect performance of skilled tasks, including driving. Also; use with caution in pregnancy, prostatic hypertrophy, paralytic ileus, diabetes, liver or kidney impairment, with certain heart or blood disorders. Not used in angle-closure glaucoma or breast-feeding.
✪ Related entry: Zyprexa.

Olbetam
(Pharmacia) is a proprietary, prescription-only preparation of the LIPID-REGULATING DRUG acipimox. It can be used in hyperlipidaemia to beneficially change the proportions of various lipids in the bloodstream. It is available as capsules.
✚▲ Side-effects/warnings: See ACIPIMOX.

olive oil
can be used therapeutically to soften earwax prior to syringing the ears, or to treat the yellow-brown, flaking skin that commonly appears on the heads of young infants (cradle cap) prior to shampooing.

olsalazine sodium
is an AMINOSALICYLATE which is used primarily to induce and maintain remission of the symptoms of ulcerative colitis – often in patients who are sensitive to the more commonly prescribed sulfasalazine. Administration is oral.
✚ Side-effects: Nausea, watery diarrhoea, abdominal cramps, headaches, dyspepsia, joint pain and rashes, and blood disorders. Patients should tell their doctor if they have any unexplained bruising, bleeding, sore throat, fever or malaise, because of possible effects on the blood requiring treatment to be stopped.
▲ Warnings: It should not be administered to patients who are allergic to aspirin or other salicylates, or where there is impaired kidney function; administer with caution to those who are pregnant or breast-feeding.
✪ Related entry: Dipentum.

omega-3 marine triglycerides
are derived from fish oils and used as lipid-regulating drugs (see LIPID-REGULATING DRUG) in hyperlipidaemia to reduce the levels of various lipids (mainly to reduce triglyceride levels) in the bloodstream (particularly in those at risk from ischaemic heart disease or pancreatitis). Administration is oral.
✚▲ Side-effects/warnings: There may be belching and nausea.
✪ Related entry: Maxepa.

omeprazole
is an ULCER-HEALING DRUG. It works by being a PROTON-PUMP INHIBITOR and so interferes with the secretion of gastric acid from the parietal (acid-producing) cells of the stomach lining. It is used for the treatment of benign gastric and duodenal ulcers (including those that complicate NSAID therapy), acid-related dyspepsia, Zollinger-Ellison syndrome and reflux oesophagitis (inflammation of the oesophagus caused by regurgitation of acid and enzymes), and acid reflux disease. It can also be used in conjunction with antibiotics to treat gastric *Helicobacter pylori* infection. Omeptazole may be useful in cases where there has been a poor response to conventional therapies, especially H_2-

ANTAGONIST drugs. Administration is oral or intravenous infusion.
✚ Side-effects: See PROTON-PUMP INHIBITOR. Also, reported urticaria and various other skin disorders, hair loss, anaphylaxis, fever, photosensitivity, tingling in the extremities, vertigo, kidney problems, hair loss, sleepiness, insomnia, increased sweating, development of breasts in men. Also, rarely, impotence, taste disturbance, inflammation of the mucous membrane of the mouth, Candida infection of the gut, liver dysfunction, various blood changes, peripheral oedema, malaise.
▲ Warnings: See PROTON-PUMP INHIBITOR.
✪ **Related entry: Losec.**

OncoTICE

(Organon) is a recently introduced non-proprietary, prescription-only preparation of BCG vaccine (TICE strain). It is available in a form for bladder instillation for the treatment of primary or recurrent bladder carcinoma *in situ* and for the prevention of recurrence following surgery.
✚▲ Side-effects/warnings: See BCG VACCINE.

Oncovin

(Lilly) is a proprietary, prescription-only preparation of the ANTICANCER drug vincristine sulphate. It can be used in the treatment of a range of cancers, and is available in a form for injection.
✚▲ Side-effects/warnings: See VINCRISTINE SULPHATE.

ondansetron

is an ANTI-EMETIC and ANTINAUSEANT which gives relief from nausea and vomiting, especially in patients receiving chemotherapy and where other drugs are ineffective. It acts as a serotonin receptor antagonist, blocking the action of the naturally occurring mediator SEROTONIN. Administration is oral, by suppositories or by intravenous injection or infusion.
✚ Side-effects: Constipation; headache, hiccups, sensation of warmth or flushing sensations; sometimes hypersensitivity reactions short-lasting visual disturbances and dizziness (after intravenous administration); involuntary movements, seizures, chest pain, heart slowing and rhythm changes, effects of the cardiovascular system, rectal irritation with suppositories.
▲ Warnings: It is administered with caution to patients with liver impairment, or who are pregnant or breast-feeding.
✪ **Related entry: Zofran.**

One-Alpha

(Leo) is a proprietary, prescription-only preparation of the VITAMIN D analogue alfacalcidol. It can be used to treat a deficiency of vitamin D, and is available as capsules, an oral solution and in a form for injection.
✚▲ Side-effects/warnings: See ALFACALCIDOL.

Onkotrone

(ASTA Medica) is a proprietary, prescription-only preparation of the ANTICANCER drug mitoxantrone (mitozantrone). It can be used in the treatment of certain types of cancer, and is available in a form for intravenous infusion.
✚▲ Side-effects/warnings: See MITOXANTRONE.

opiate 🄴

drugs are members of a class that are chemically alkaloids (see ALKALOID), and chemically are closely related to the natural constituents of opium (eg MORPHINE SULPHATE). They powerfully influence certain functions of the central nervous system, and because of this property they can be used as NARCOTIC ANALGESIC drugs to relieve pain. They also have two other actions: they can be used as ANTITUSSIVE drugs to reduce coughing; and, because of an antimotility action, as powerful ANTIDIARRHOEAL drugs. Therapeutically, the most important opiate is probably morphine. They are all potentially habituating (addictive), especially the synthetic derivative of heroin, DIAMORPHINE HYDROCHLORIDE. Today, the term OPIOID is increasingly used to embrace all drugs irrespective of chemical structure, as well as naturally occurring peptide neurotransmitters, that share this common pharmacology.

Opilon

(Hansam) is a proprietary, prescription-only preparation of the ALPHA-ADRENOCEPTOR BLOCKER moxisylyte (thymoxamine; as hydrochloride), which has VASODILATOR properties. It can be used to treat peripheral vascular disease (primary Raynaud's phenomenon), also erectile dysfunction (impotence). It is available as tablets.

+▲ Side-effects/warnings: See MOXISYLYTE.

opioid

is a term that has superseded OPIATE and includes agents similar in structure and pharmacology to morphine as well as agents with polypeptide structures. Opioids influence the central nervous system and can be used as NARCOTIC ANALGESIC drugs to relieve pain. They can also be used therapeutically for their ANTITUSSIVE and ANTIDIARRHOEAL, or antimotility, actions. It is now recognized that the characteristic actions of opioids are due to their ability to mimic natural neurotransmitters (enkephalins, endorphins, dynorphins) and because of this the term opioid is used for any chemical (synthetic or natural) that acts on opioid RECEPTORS.

All opioid drugs have similar pharmacological actions and potential side-effects. But the severity of these effects, and the strength of their analgesic and other therapeutic actions, varies with individual drugs, the dose and route of administration. The risk of habituation (addiction) is also much greater with the stronger drugs (eg morphine and diamorphine) than with the weaker ones (eg dextromethorphan, codeine and dihydrocodeine). See ALFENTANIL; BUPRENORPHINE; CO-CODAMOL; CO-DYDRAMOL; CO-PHENOTROPE; CO-PROXAMOL; CODEINE PHOSPHATE; DEXTROMETHORPHAN HYDROBROMIDE; DEXTROMORAMIDE; DEXTROPROPOXYPHENE HYDROCHLORIDE; DIAMORPHINE HYDROCHLORIDE; DIPIPANONE; FENTANYL; LOPERAMIDE HYDROCHLORIDE; MEPTAZINOL; METHADONE HYDROCHLORIDE; MORPHINE SULPHATE; NALBUPHINE HYDROCHLORIDE; NALOXONE HYDROCHLORIDE; NALTREXONE HYDROCHLORIDE; OXYCODONE; PAPAVERETUM; PENTAZOCINE; PETHIDINE HYDROCHLORIDE; PHENAZOCINE HYDROBROMIDE; PHOLCODINE; REMIFENTANIL; TRAMADOL HYDROCHLORIDE.

+ Side-effects: Depending on use, type and dose, there may be nausea and vomiting, drowsiness, loss of appetite, urinary retention and constipation. There is commonly sedation and euphoria, which may lead to a state of mental detachment or confusion. Also, there may be a dry mouth, flushing of the face, sweating, headache, palpitations, changes in heart rate, postural hypotension (a lowering of blood pressure on standing, causing dizziness), rashes, miosis (pupil constriction), mood change and hallucinations. Note that some opioids such as pholcodine are relatively free of side-effects.

▲ Warnings: Opioids (even the weaker ones) should not be administered to patients with seriously depressed breathing disorders, asthmatics, who have prostatic hypertrophy, convulsive disorders, have raised intracranial pressure or a head injury. Depending on use, type and dose, they should be administered with caution to those with hypotension, certain liver or kidney disorders, or hypothyroidism (under-activity of the thyroid gland); or who are pregnant or breast-feeding. Treatment by injection may cause pain and tissue damage at the site of the injection. Drowsiness may affect the performance of skilled tasks such as driving. Note that the effects of alcohol may be enhanced (including respiratory depression).

opioid antagonist

drugs oppose the actions of OPIOID drugs, which are used for a number of purposes, including as NARCOTIC ANALGESIC drugs for pain-relief, as ANTITUSSIVE drugs and as ANTIDIARRHOEAL or antimotility treatments. It is now recognized that opioids achieve their characteristic actions by mimicking naturally occurring peptide neurotransmitters (enkephalins, endorphins and dynorphins), so now the term opioid is used to describe any chemical, synthetic or natural, that acts on *opioid* RECEPTORS.

Opioid antagonists occupy these receptors without stimulating them and so can reverse the actions of a wide range of opioid drugs. This is a potentially beneficial action, because an opioid antagonist, such as NALOXONE HYDROCHLORIDE, can effectively reverse the respiratory depression, coma or convulsions that result from an overdose of opioids. Administration of naloxone hydrochloride is by intramuscular or intravenous injection and may be repeated at short intervals until there is some response. It is also used at the end of operations to reverse respiratory depression caused by narcotic analgesics, and in newborn babies where mothers have been given large amounts of opioid (such as pethidine) for pain-relief during labour. It is also very effective in reviving individuals who have overdosed on heroin.

NALTREXONE HYDROCHLORIDE, another opioid antagonist, is used in detoxification therapy to help prevent relapse of formerly opioid-dependent patients. It is able to do this because as an antagonist of dependence-forming opioids (such as heroin), it will precipitate withdrawal symptoms in those already taking opioids.

Oprisine

(Opus; Trinity) is a proprietary, prescription-only preparation of the (*cytotoxic*) IMMUNOSUPPRESSANT azathioprine. It can be used to treat tissue rejection in transplant patients and for a variety of autoimmune and inflammatory diseases. It is available as tablets.
✚▲ Side-effects/warnings: See AZATHIOPRINE.

Opticrom Allergy Eye Drops

(Rhône-Poulenc Rorer; Aventis Pharma) is a proprietary, non-prescription preparation of the ANTI-ALLERGIC sodium cromoglicate, used to treat allergic conjunctivitis. Available as eye-drops.
✚▲ Side-effects/warnings: See SODIUM CROMOGLICATE.

Opticrom Aqueous

(Rhône-Poulenc Rorer; Aventis Pharma) is a proprietary, prescription-only preparation of the ANTI-ALLERGIC drug sodium cromoglicate. It can be used to treat allergic conjunctivitis, and is available as eye-drops.
✚▲ Side-effects/warnings: See SODIUM CROMOGLICATE.

Optil

(Opus; Trinity) is a proprietary, prescription-only preparation of the CALCIUM-CHANNEL BLOCKER diltiazem hydrochloride. It can be used as an ANTIHYPERTENSIVE and as an ANTI-ANGINA drug. It is available as modified-release tablets.
✚▲ Side-effects/warnings: See DILTIAZEM HYDROCHLORIDE.

Optilast

(ASTA Medica) is proprietary, prescription-only preparation of the ANTIHISTAMINE azelastine hydrochloride. It can be used for the symptomatic relief of allergic conjunctivitis, and is available as eye-drops.
✚▲ Side-effects/warnings: See AZELASTINE HYDROCHLORIDE.

Optil SR

(Opus; Trinity) is a proprietary, prescription-only preparation of the CALCIUM-CHANNEL BLOCKER diltiazem hydrochloride. It can be used as an ANTIHYPERTENSIVE and as an ANTI-ANGINA drug. It is available as modified-release tablets.
✚▲ Side-effects/warnings: See DILTIAZEM HYDROCHLORIDE.

Optil XL

(Opus; Trinity) is a proprietary, prescription-only preparation of the CALCIUM-CHANNEL BLOCKER diltiazem hydrochloride. It can be used as an ANTIHYPERTENSIVE and as an ANTI-ANGINA drug. It is available as modified-release capsules.
✚▲ Side-effects/warnings: See DILTIAZEM HYDROCHLORIDE.

Optimax

(Merck) is a proprietary, prescription-only preparation of the ANTIDEPRESSANT tryptophan. It can be used by hospital specialists to treat long-standing depressive illness in cases where no other treatment is suitable. It is available as tablets.
✚▲ Side-effects/warnings: See TRYPTOPHAN.

Optimine

(Schering-Plough) is a proprietary, non-prescription preparation of azatadine maleate, an ANTIHISTAMINE which can be used for the symptomatic relief of allergic symptoms such as hay fever and urticaria, and is available in the form of a syrup. It is not recommended for children under one year.
✚▲ Side-effects/warnings: See AZATADINE MALEATE.

Optrex Allergy Eye Drops

(Crookes Healthcare) is a proprietary, non-prescription preparation of the ANTI-ALLERGIC drug sodium cromoglicate. It can be used to treat seasonal allergic conjunctivitis, and is available as eye-drops.
✚▲ Side-effects/warnings: See SODIUM CROMOGLICATE.

Optrex Clear Eyes Eye Drops

(Crookes Healthcare) is a proprietary, non-prescription preparation of the VASOCONSTRICTOR drug naphazoline hydrochloride (with witch hazel). It can be used to give relief of redness caused by minor eye irritations, and is available as eye-drops. It is not

recommended for children, except on medical advice.
✚▲ Side-effects/warnings: See NAPHAZOLINE HYDROCHLORIDE.

Orabase

(ConvaTec) is a proprietary, non-prescription preparation of CARMELLOSE SODIUM (with pectin and gelatin). It can be used for the mechanical protection of oral and perioral lesions, and is available as an oral paste.
✚▲ Side-effects/warnings: See CARMELLOSE SODIUM.

Orahesive

(ConvaTec) is a proprietary, non-prescription preparation of CARMELLOSE SODIUM (with pectin and gelatin). It can be used to protect oral and perioral lesions, and is available as a powder.
✚▲ Side-effects/warnings: See CARMELLOSE SODIUM.

oral contraceptive

refers to any of several prophylactic (preventive) sex hormone preparations (see SEX HORMONES), which are taken by women to prevent conception following sexual intercourse and are commonly referred to as the *Pill*. The majority of oral contraceptives contain both an OESTROGEN (usually ETHINYLESTRADIOL, sometimes MESTRANOL) and a PROGESTOGEN (eg NORETHISTERONE, GESTODENE, DESOGESTREL). The oestrogen inhibits the release of FOLLICLE-STIMULATING HORMONE (FSH) and prevents egg development; the progestogen inhibits release of LUTEINISING HORMONE (LH), prevents ovulation and makes the cervix mucus unsuitable for sperm. Their combined action is to alter the uterine lining (endometrium) and prevent any fertilized eggs from implanting. This type of preparation is known as the *combined oral contraceptive* (*COC*), or *combined pill*, and is taken daily for three weeks and stopped for one week during which menstruation occurs (*phased monophasic* form).

Two further forms of the combined pill (the phased formulations) are the biphasic and triphasic pills. In these the hormonal content varies according to the time of the month at which each pill is to be taken (and are produced in a 'calendar pack') and the dose is reduced to the bare minimum. Another type of pill is the progestogen-only pill (*POP*), where the progestogens used include norethisterone, etynodiol acetate, LEVONORGESTREL and this is thought to work by making the cervical mucus inhospitable to sperm and by preventing implantation. This form has the advantage that it can be used by breast-feeding women.

An alternative to the progesterone-only pill is to administer the progestogen not orally, but as an injection or an implant (which is renewed every three months). Post-coital contraception is also available in an emergency and involves the use of a high-dose combined preparation – the 'morning-after pill'. All the oral contraceptive preparations produce side-effects and a form that is suited to each patient requires expert advice. Various oral contraceptive preparations are also used in the treatment of certain menstrual problems.
✚▲ Side-effects/warnings: See OESTROGEN; PROGESTOGEN. Adverse effects are more pronounced with the combined pill; thrombo-embolism, weight gain, nausea, flushing, irritability, depression, dizziness, increased blood pressure, impaired liver function and glucose tolerance, amenorrhoea after coming off the pill. Slight changes in cervical and breast cancer rates (depending on dose and preparation). There is a small risk of venous thromboembolism (though less than that of pregnancy), and authorities recommend that women on the combined pill who are travelling for periods of over five hours should exercise during travel and consider using elastic hosiery.

The effectiveness of oral contraceptives may be altered, usually reduced, by a wide variety of drugs including ANTIBACTERIAL, ANTICOAGULANT, ANTIDEPRESSANT, ANTI-EPILEPTIC, ANTIFUNGAL and ANTIVIRAL agents, and also some nutritional supplements and herbal remedies, such as St John's wort.

Oraldene

(Warner Lambert Consumer Healthcare; PfizerS) is a proprietary, non-prescription preparation of the ANTISEPTIC hexetidine. It can be used to treat and prevent gingivitis, minor mouth infections, including thrush and sores and ulcers in the mouth. It is available as a mouthwash. It is not normally given to children under six years, except on medical advice.
✚▲ Side-effects/warnings: See HEXETIDINE.

oral hypoglycaemic

drugs are usually synthetic agents taken by mouth to reduce the levels of glucose (sugar) in the bloodstream and are used mainly in the treatment of Type II diabetes (non-insulin-dependent diabetes mellitus; NIDDM; maturity-onset diabetes) when there is some residual capacity in the pancreas to produce the HORMONE insulin. The main type of oral hypoglycaemic is the SULPHONYLUREA group (eg CHLORPROPAMIDE and GLIBENCLAMIDE), but the (BIGUANIDE) METFORMIN HYDROCHLORIDE and ACARBOSE are also effective. Additionally, GUAR GUM can be administered in the diet. Newer oral hypoglycaemic drugs include NATEGLINIDE, REPAGLINIDE, PIOGLITAZONE and ROSIGLITAZONE, which work in different ways and may be suitable for some people. However, INSULIN, which is mainly used in Type I diabetes (insulin-dependent diabetes mellitus; IDDM; juvenile-onset diabetes), can not be taken by mouth since it is destroyed by enzymes in the gastrointestinal tract (so is not an *oral* hypoglycaemic) and must be injected.

Oramorph

(Boehringer Ingelheim) is a proprietary, prescription-only preparation of the (OPIOID) NARCOTIC ANALGESIC morphine sulphate. It is available as oral solutions, oral unit-dose vials and as modified-release tablets called *Oramorph SR*. The more concentrated unit-dose vials and the SR tablets are on the Controlled Drugs list.
✚▲ Side-effects/warnings: See MORPHINE SULPHATE.

Orap

(Janssen-Cilag) is a proprietary, prescription-only preparation of the ANTIPSYCHOTIC drug pimozide. It can be used (with care) to treat and tranquillize patients with psychotic disorders, particularly those with schizophrenia, and also to treat Gilles de la Tourette syndrome. It is available as tablets.
✚▲ Side-effects/warnings: See PIMOZIDE.

orciprenaline sulphate

is a SYMPATHOMIMETIC and BETA-RECEPTOR STIMULANT which has some beta$_2$-receptor selectivity (though much less than SALBUTAMOL and is therefore more likely to cause side-effects). It is mainly used as a BRONCHODILATOR in reversible obstructive airways disease and as an ANTI-ASTHMATIC treatment. Administration is orally or by aerosol.
✚▲ Side-effects/warnings: See SALBUTAMOL; but it is more likely to cause heart problems such as arrhythmias.
✪ **Related entry: Alupent.**

Orelox

(Hoechst Marion Roussel; Aventis Pharma) is a proprietary, prescription-only preparation of the ANTIBACTERIAL and (CEPHALOSPORIN) ANTIBIOTICcefpodoxime. It can be used to treat a range of infections, and is available as tablets and an oral suspension.
✚▲ Side-effects/warnings: See CEFPODOXIME.

Orgalutran

(Organon) is a recently introduced proprietary, prescription-only preparation of ganirelix, which is a drug that affects the release of gonadotrophins and is used in the treatment of infertility by assisted reproductive techniques (IVF) under specialist supervision. It is available in a form for injection.
✚▲ Side-effects/warnings: See GANIRELIX.

Orgaran

(Durbin) is a proprietary, prescription-only preparation of the heparinoid, danaparoid sodium. It can be used as an ANTICOAGULANT for the prevention of deep vein thrombosis, and is available in a form for injection.
✚▲ Side-effects/warnings: See DANAPAROID SODIUM.

Original Andrews Salts

(GSK Consumer Healthcare) is a proprietary, non-prescription compound preparation of the ANTACID sodium bicarbonate and the LAXATIVE magnesium sulphate (and citric acid). It can be used to relieve upset stomach, indigestion, symptoms of overindulgence and constipation. It is available as an effervescent powder and is not normally used for children under three years, except on medical advice
✚▲ Side-effects/warnings: See SODIUM BICARBONATE; MAGNESIUM SULPHATE.

Orimeten

(Novartis) is a proprietary, prescription-only preparation of the sex HORMONE ANTAGONIST

aminoglutethimide. It can be used as an ANTICANCER treatment for breast and prostate cancer and Cushing's syndrome caused by cancer of the thyroid gland, and is available as tablets.
✚▲ Side-effects/warnings: See AMINOGLUTETHIMIDE.

Orlept

(CP) is a proprietary, prescription-only preparation of the ANTICONVULSANT and ANTI-EPILEPTIC sodium valproate. It can be used to treat epilepsy, and is available as tablets and a liquid.
✚▲ Side-effects/warnings: See SODIUM VALPROATE.

orlistat

is a drug that is used as an adjunct in OBESITY TREATMENT, but unlike other drugs used for obesity, it is not an APPETITE SUPPRESSANT. Instead it is an ENZYME INHIBITOR, blocking the normal action of the enzyme pancreatic lipase in the intestine, so less of the dietary fat is absorbed into the body from the intestine. Administration is oral.
✚ Side-effects: Liquid oily faeces, flatulence, an urgency to defecate. Less frequently, abdominal and rectal pain; headache; menstrual irregularities; fatigue and anxiety. The various gastrointestinal effects can be minimized by reducing the amount of fat in the diet.
▲ Warnings: It should not be given to anyone who is pregnant or breast-feeding, or with chronic malabsorption syndrome or cholestasis. It can be used with care in diabetes mellitus; it may impair absorption of fat-soluble vitamins. If a meal is missed or contains no fat, the dose should not be taken. NICE has made specific recommendations regarding who is suitable for treatment with orlistat and for how long.
✪ **Related entry: Xenical.**

orphenadrine hydrochloride

is an ANTICHOLINERGIC (ANTIMUSCARINIC) drug which is used in the treatment of some types of parkinsonism (see ANTIPARKINSONISM). It increases mobility and decreases rigidity and tremor, but has only a limited effect on bradykinesia, and also the tendency to produce an excess of saliva is reduced. It is thought to work by correcting the over-effectiveness of the neurotransmitter ACETYLCHOLINE (cholinergic excess), which is caused by the deficiency of dopamine that occurs in parkinsonism. It also has the capacity to treat these conditions, in some cases, where they are produced by drugs. Administration is oral.
✚▲ Side-effects/warnings: See BENZHEXOL HYDROCHLORIDE; but it is more euphoric and may cause insomnia. Its use is avoided in patients with porphyria.
✪ **Related entries: Biorphen; Disipal.**

Ortho-Creme

(Janssen-Cilag) is a proprietary, non-prescription SPERMICIDAL CONTRACEPTIVE for use in combination with barrier methods of contraception (such as a condom). It is available as a cream containing nonoxinol in a water-soluble basis.
✚▲ Side-effects/warnings: See NONOXINOL.

Orthoforms

(Janssen-Cilag) is a proprietary, non-prescription SPERMICIDAL CONTRACEPTIVE for use in combination with barrier methods of contraception (such as a condom). It is available as a pessary containing nonoxinol.
✚▲ Side-effects/warnings: See NONOXINOL.

Ortho-Gynest

(Janssen-Cilag) is a proprietary, prescription-only preparation of the OESTROGEN estriol, which can be used to treat infection and irritation of the membranous surface of the vagina, including vaginal atrophy in HRT (hormone replacement therapy). It is available as pessaries and an intravaginal cream.
✚▲ Side-effects/warnings: See ESTRIOL.

Orudis

(Hawgreen) is a proprietary, prescription-only preparation of the (NSAID) NON-NARCOTIC ANALGESIC and ANTIRHEUMATIC ketoprofen. It can be used to relieve arthritic and rheumatic pain and inflammation, to treat other musculoskeletal disorders, pain and inflammation following orthopaedic surgery and also period pain. It is available as capsules and suppositories.
✚▲ Side-effects/warnings: See KETOPROFEN.

Oruvail

(Hawgreen) is a proprietary, prescription-only

preparation of the (NSAID) NON-NARCOTIC ANALGESIC and ANTIRHEUMATIC ketoprofen. It can be used to relieve arthritic and rheumatic pain and inflammation, to treat other musculoskeletal disorders, and pain and inflammation following orthopaedic surgery. It is available as capsules and in a form for injection.
✚▲ Side-effects/warnings: See KETOPROFEN.

Oruvail Gel

(Rhône-Poulenc Rorer; Aventis Pharma) is a proprietary, prescription-only preparation of the (NSAID) NON-NARCOTIC ANALGESIC and ANTIRHEUMATIC ketoprofen, which also has COUNTER-IRRITANT, or RUBEFACIENT, actions. It can be applied to the skin for symptomatic relief of underlying muscle or joint pain. It is available as a gel for topical application to the skin.
✚▲ Side-effects/warnings: See KETOPROFEN; but adverse effects on topical application are limited.

Ossopan

(Sanofi-Synthelabo) is a proprietary, non-prescription preparation of calcium carbonate (as hydroxyapatite). It can be used as a MINERAL SUPPLEMENT for calcium in cases of calcium deficiency. It is available as tablets and granules to be taken by mouth.
✚▲ Side-effects/warnings: See CALCIUM CARBONATE.

Otex Ear Drops

(DDD) is a proprietary, non-prescription preparation of the ANTISEPTIC and ANTIFUNGAL agent hydrogen peroxide in a complex with urea. It can be used to dissolve and wash out ear wax, and is available as ear-drops.
✚▲ Side-effects/warnings: See HYDROGEN PEROXIDE; UREA.

Otomize

(Stafford-Miller; GSK) is a proprietary, prescription-only compound preparation of the CORTICOSTEROID dextamethasone and the ANTIBACTERIAL and (AMINOGLYCOSIDE) ANTIBIOTIC neomycin sulphate (and acetic acid). It can be used to treat bacterial infections in the outer ear, and is available as an ear-spray.
✚▲ Side-effects/warnings: See DEXAMETHASONE; NEOMYCIN SULPHATE.

Otosporin

(GlaxoWellcome; GSK) is a proprietary, prescription-only compound preparation of the CORTICOSTEROID hydrocortisone, the ANTIBACTERIAL and (AMINOGLYCOSIDE) ANTIBIOTIC neomycin sulphate and the antibacterial and (POLYMYXIN) antibiotic polymyxin B sulphate. It can be used to treat infections and inflammation in the outer ear, and is available as ear-drops.
✚▲ Side-effects/warnings: See HYDROCORTISONE; NEOMYCIN SULPHATE; POLYMYXIN B SULPHATE.

Otradrops Adult

(Manx) is a proprietary, non-prescription preparation of the SYMPATHOMIMETIC and VASOCONSTRICTOR xylometazoline hydrochloride. It can be used as a NASAL DECONGESTANT for the symptomatic relief of nasal congestion, perennial and allergic rhinitis (such as hay fever) and sinusitis. It is available as a nasal solution and is not normally given to children under 12 years, except on medical advice.
✚▲ Side-effects/warnings: See XYLOMETAZOLINE HYDROCHLORIDE.

Otradrops Paediatric

(Manx) is a proprietary, non-prescription preparation of the SYMPATHOMIMETIC and VASOCONSTRICTOR xylometazoline hydrochloride. It can be used as a NASAL DECONGESTANT for the symptomatic relief of nasal congestion, perennial and allergic rhinitis (such as hay fever) and sinusitis. It is available as a nasal solution for children aged two to 12 years.
✚▲ Side-effects/warnings: See XYLOMETAZOLINE HYDROCHLORIDE.

Otraspray

(Manx) is a proprietary, non-prescription preparation of the SYMPATHOMIMETIC and VASOCONSTRICTOR xylometazoline hydrochloride. It can be used as a NASAL DECONGESTANT for the symptomatic relief of nasal congestion, perennial and allergic rhinitis (such as hay fever) and sinusitis. It is available as a spray for adults and children over two years.
✚▲ Side-effects/warnings: See XYLOMETAZOLINE HYDROCHLORIDE.

Otrivine Adult Menthol Nasal Spray

(Novartis Consumer Health) is a proprietary, non-prescription preparation of the

SYMPATHOMIMETIC and VASOCONSTRICTOR xylometazoline hydrochloride. It can be used as a NASAL DECONGESTANT for the symptomatic relief of nasal congestion, perennial and allergic rhinitis (such as hay fever) and sinusitis. It is available as a nasal spray and is not given to children except on medical advice.
✚▲ Side-effects/warnings: See XYLOMETAZOLINE HYDROCHLORIDE.

Otrivine Adult Nasal Spray
(Novartis Consumer Health) is a proprietary, non-prescription preparation of the SYMPATHOMIMETIC and VASOCONSTRICTOR xylometazoline hydrochloride. It can be used as a NASAL DECONGESTANT for the symptomatic relief of nasal congestion, allergic and other forms of rhinitis (including hay fever) and sinusitis. It is available as a spray and is not normally given to children, except on medical advice.
✚▲ Side-effects/warnings: See XYLOMETAZOLINE HYDROCHLORIDE.

Otrivine-Antistin
(Novartis Ophthalmics) is a proprietary, non-prescription of the ANTIHISTAMINE antazoline (as sulphate) and the SYMPATHOMIMETIC and VASOCONSTRICTOR xylometazoline hydrochloride. It can be used as an eye treatment to relieve conjunctivitis, and is available as eye-drops. Not normally given to children, except on medical advice.
✚▲ Side-effects/warnings: See ANTAZOLINE; XYLOMETAZOLINE HYDROCHLORIDE. Systemic absorption may lead to side-effects. Not to be used in angle-closure glaucoma.

Otrivine Children's Nasal Drops
(Novartis Consumer Health) is a proprietary, non-prescription preparation of the SYMPATHOMIMETIC and VASOCONSTRICTOR xylometazoline hydrochloride. It can be used as a NASAL DECONGESTANT for the symptomatic relief of nasal congestion, allergic and other forms of rhinitis (including hay fever) and sinusitis. It is available as a spray and is not normally given to children under three months, except on medical advice.
✚▲ Side-effects/warnings: See XYLOMETAZOLINE HYDROCHLORIDE.

Otrivine Measured Dose Sinusitis Spray
(Novartis Consumer Health) is a proprietary, non-prescription preparation of the SYMPATHOMIMETIC and VASOCONSTRICTOR xylometazoline hydrochloride. It can be used as a NASAL DECONGESTANT for the symptomatic relief of nasal congestion, allergic and other forms of rhinitis (including hay fever) and sinusitis. It is available as a nasal spray and is not normally given to children under 12 years, except on medical advice.
✚▲ Side-effects/warnings: See XYLOMETAZOLINE HYDROCHLORIDE.

Ovestin
(Organon) is a proprietary, prescription-only preparation of the OESTROGEN estriol. It can be used in HRT. Available as tablets and an intravaginal cream.
✚▲ Side-effects/warnings: See ESTRIOL.

Ovex Tablets
(Johnson & Johnson • MSD) is a proprietary, non-prescription preparation of the ANTHELMINTIC mebendazole. It can be used to treat infestation by threadworms, and is available as chewable tablets. It is not normally given to children under two years, except on medical advice.
✚▲ Side-effects/warnings: See MEBENDAZOLE.

Ovitrelle
(Serono) is a proprietary, prescription-only preparation of the HORMONE human choriogonadotropin alpha (a form of human gonadotrophin alpha; HCG). It can be used to treat undescended testicles and delayed puberty in boys, and also women for infertility treatment who are suffering from specific hormonal deficiency. It is available in a form for injection.
✚▲ Side-effects/warnings: See CHORIOGONADOTROPIN ALPHA.

Ovran
(Wyeth) is a proprietary, prescription-only compound preparation which can be used as a (*monophasic*) ORAL CONTRACEPTIVE of the *COC* (high strength) type that combines an OESTROGEN and a PROGESTOGEN, in this case ethinylestradiol and levonorgestrel. It is available as tablets in a calendar pack.
✚▲ Side-effects/warnings: See ETHINYLESTRADIOL; LEVONORGESTREL.

Ovran 30
(Wyeth) is a proprietary, prescription-only

compound preparation which can be used as a (*monophasic*) ORAL CONTRACEPTIVE of the *COC* (standard strength) type that combines an OESTROGEN and a PROGESTOGEN, in this case ethinylestradiol and levonorgestrel. It is available as tablets in a calendar pack.
✚▲ Side-effects/warnings: See ETHINYLESTRADIOL; LEVONORGESTREL.

Ovranette

(Wyeth) is proprietary, prescription-only compound preparation which can be used as a (*monophasic*) ORAL CONTRACEPTIVE of the *COC* (standard strength) type that combines an OESTROGEN and a PROGESTOGEN, in this case ethinylestradiol and levonorgestrel. It is available as tablets in a calendar pack.
✚▲ Side-effects/warnings: See ETHINYLESTRADIOL; LEVONORGESTREL.

Ovysmen

(Janssen-Cilag) is a proprietary, prescription-only compound preparation which can be used as a (*monophasic*) ORAL CONTRACEPTIVE of the *COC* (standard strength) type that combines an OESTROGEN and a PROGESTOGEN, in this case ethinylestradiol and norethisterone. It is available as tablets in a calendar pack.
✚▲ Side-effects/warnings: See ETHINYLESTRADIOL; NORETHISTERONE.

oxaliplatin

is a platinum compound CYTOTOXIC drug (derived from cisplatin) which is used as an ANTICANCER treatment specifically for colorectal cancer (in combination with other drugs). Administration is by injection.
✚▲ Side-effects/warnings: See CYTOTOXIC.
✪ **Related entry: Eloxatin.**

oxazepam

is a BENZODIAZEPINE which is used as an ANXIOLYTIC in the short-term treatment of anxiety, also as a HYPNOTIC for insomnia associated with anxiety. Administration is oral.
✚▲ Side-effects/warnings: See BENZODIAZEPINE.

oxcarbazepine

is a newly introduced ANTICONVULSANT and ANTI-EPILEPTIC drug (chemically related to CARBAMAZEPINE) which is used in the preventive treatment of some forms of epilepsy (partial seizures with or without secondarily generalized tonic-clonic seizures absence seizures). Administration is oral.
✚ Side-effects: Oxocarbazepine may cause gastrointestinal side-effects such as nausea, vomiting, constipation, diarrhoea and also abdominal pain. There may be drowsiness or dizziness, headache, agitation, memory loss, weakness, tremor and psychological disturbances, including confusion, impaired concentration and depression. Other possible side-effects are many and include acne, hair loss, rash, vertigo and effects oon the eye and visual system such as nystagmus and diplopia. There may also be (though less commonly) urticaria, effects on the blood, heart arrhythmias and other reactions including some potentially serious allergic reactions.
▲ Warnings: It is used with caution in people who are hypersensitive to the anticonvulsant drug carbamazepine, who have impaired liver or kidney function, who are either pregnant or breast-feeding, elderly, or have low blood sodium, heart failure or heart conduction disorders. Patients and their carers will be advised on how to recognize signs of blood, liver or skin disorders, and told to seek immediate medical attention if symptoms such as lethargy, confusion, muscular twitching, fever, sore throat, rash, blistering, mouth ulcers, bruising or bleeding develop. Withdrawal of oxcarbazepine should be gradual.
✪ **Related entry: Trileptal.**

oxerutins

are mixtures of RUTOSIDES that are thought to reduce the fragility and the permeability of capillary blood vessels. They are used to treat disorders of the veins, for example, cramp in the legs, and for oedema. Administration is oral.
✚ Side-effects: Flushing, headache, rashes and gastrointestinal disturbances.
✪ **Related entry: Paroven.**

oxetacaine

(oxethazaine) is a LOCAL ANAESTHETIC which is used by topical application to relieve local pain. It is a constituent of a proprietary ANTACID which is administered as an oral suspension.
✚▲ Side-effects/warnings: It is regarded as safe in normal topical use.
✪ **Related entry: Mucaine.**

oxethazaine
see OXETACAINE.

Oxis
(AstraZeneca) is a proprietary, prescription-only preparation of the BETA-RECEPTOR STIMULANT formoterol fumarate (eformoterol fumarate). It can be used as a BRONCHODILATOR in reversible obstructive airways disease and as an ANTI-ASTHMATIC treatment, and has a prolonged action. It is available as a powder and inhaler ('Turbohaler').
✚▲ Side-effects/warnings: See FORMOTEROL FUMARATE.

oxitropium bromide
is an ANTICHOLINERGIC (ANTIMUSCARINIC) drug that has the properties of a BRONCHODILATOR. It is primarily used to treat chronic bronchitis, but it can also be used as an ANTI-ASTHMATIC. Administration is by aerosol.
✚▲ Side-effects/warnings: See IPRATROPIUM BROMIDE. There may be blurring of vision. It is important not to exceed the prescribed dose.
✪ **Related entry: Oxivent.**

Oxivent
(Boehringer Ingelheim) is a proprietary, prescription-only preparation of the ANTICHOLINERGIC drug oxitropium bromide, which also has BRONCHODILATOR properties. It can be used to treat chronic bronchitis and some other disorders of the upper respiratory tract. It is available as an aerosol spray taken from a breath-activated *Autohaler* and as a metered aerosol.
✚▲ Side-effects/warnings: See OXITROPIUM BROMIDE.

oxpentifylline
see PENTOXIFYLLINE.

oxprenolol hydrochloride
is a BETA-BLOCKER which can be used as an ANTIHYPERTENSIVE for raised blood pressure, as an ANTI-ANGINA treatment to relieve symptoms and improve exercise tolerance and as an ANTI-ARRHYTHMIC to regularize heartbeat. It can also be used as an ANXIOLYTIC, particularly for symptomatic relief of tremor and palpitations. Administration is oral. It is also available, as an antihypertensive, in the form of compound preparations with a DIURETIC.
✚▲ Side-effects/warnings: See PROPRANOLOL HYDROCHLORIDE. It has intrinsic sympathomimetic activity, so there is less bradycardia and less coldness of the extremities.
✪ **Related entries: Slow-Trasicor; Trasicor; Trasidrex.**

Oxy 5 Lotion
(GSK Consumer Healthcare) is a proprietary, non-prescription preparation of the KERATOLYTIC and ANTIMICROBIAL drug benzoyl peroxide (5%). It can be used for the treatment of acne and spots, and is available as a lotion for topical application. It is not normally given to children, except on medical advice.
✚▲ Side-effects/warnings: See BENZOYL PEROXIDE.

Oxy 10 Lotion
(GSK Consumer Healthcare) is a proprietary, non-prescription preparation of the KERATOLYTIC and ANTIMICROBIAL drug benzoyl peroxide (10%). It can be used for the treatment of acne and spots, and is available as a lotion for topical application. It is not normally given to children, except on medical advice.
✚▲ Side-effects/warnings: See BENZOYL PEROXIDE.

oxybuprocaine hydrochloride
(benoxinate) is a LOCAL ANAESTHETIC which is used by topical application in ophthalmic procedures. Administration is by topical application.
✚ Side-effects: There may be initial stinging on application.
✪ **Related entry: Minims Benoxinate (Oxybuprocaine) Hydrochloride.**

oxybutynin hydrochloride
is an ANTICHOLINERGIC (ANTIMUSCARINIC) drug which can be used as an ANTISPASMODIC to treat urinary frequency, incontinence, bed-wetting and bladder spasms. Administration is oral.
✚ Side-effects: These include dry mouth, blurred vision, constipation, nausea, abdominal discomfort, difficulty in urination, flushing of the face, headache, dizziness, diarrhoea, dry skin and heart irregularities, and others.
▲ Warnings: It should not be administered to patients with intestinal obstruction, severe ulcerative colitis, toxic megacolon, glaucoma,

myasthenia gravis, or bladder obstruction. Administer with care to those with certain heart, liver or kidney disorders, hyperthyroidism, prostatic hypertrophy, hiatus hernia with reflux oesophagitis or porphyria; or to those are pregnant or breast-feeding.
✪ **Related entries: Contimin; Cystrin; Ditropan; Ditropan XL.**

oxycodone

is a powerful (OPIOID) NARCOTIC ANALGESIC. It can be used in the treatment of severe pain, such as in cancer or postoperative pain. Administration is oral (suppositories are also sometimes used). All preparations are on the Controlled Drugs list.
✚▲ Side-effects/warnings: See OPIOID.
✪ **Related entries: OxyContin; OxyNorm.**

OxyContin

(Napp) is a proprietary, prescription-only preparation of the (OPIOID) NARCOTIC ANALGESIC oxycodone, which is on the Controlled Drugs list. It can be used primarily to relieve severe pain, such as in cancer or postoperative pain. It is available as modified release tablets.
✚▲ Side-effects/warnings: See OXYCODONE.

oxymetazoline hydrochloride

is an ALPHA-ADRENOCEPTOR STIMULANT, a SYMPATHOMIMETIC, which is generally used for its VASOCONSTRICTOR properties that make it an effective NASAL DECONGESTANT. It is applied topically to the nasal passages where it constricts the blood vessels of the nose, reducing congestion in the nasal mucous membranes and possibly also reducing secretions. Administration is in the form of nose-drops or a nasal spray.
✚▲ Side-effects/warnings: See EPHEDRINE HYDROCHLORIDE.
✪ **Related entries: Afrazine Nasal Spray; Dristan Nasal Spray; Vicks Sinex Decongestant Nasal Spray.**

Oxymycin

(DDSA) is a proprietary, prescription-only preparation of the ANTIBACTERIAL and (TETRACYCLINES) ANTIBIOTIC oxytetracycline. It can be used to treat a wide range of infections, and is available as tablets.
✚▲ Side-effects/warnings: See OXYTETRACYCLINE.

OxyNorm

(Napp) is a proprietary, prescription-only preparation of the (OPIOID) NARCOTIC ANALGESIC oxycodone, which is on the Controlled Drugs list. It can be used primarily to relieve severe pain, such as in cancer or postoperative pain. It is available as capsules, liquid and a concentrated oral solution.
✚▲ Side-effects/warnings: See OXYCODONE.

Oxy On-The-Spot

(GSK Consumer Healthcare) is a proprietary, non-prescription preparation of the KERATOLYTIC and ANTIMICROBIAL drug benzoyl peroxide (2.5%). It can be used for the treatment of acne and spots, and is available as a cream for topical application. It is not normally given to children under six years, except on medical advice.
✚▲ Side-effects/warnings: See BENZOYL PEROXIDE.

Oxypertine

(Sanofi-Synthelabo) is a proprietary, prescription-only preparation of the ANTIPSYCHOTIC drug oxypertine. It can be used to treat and tranquillize patients with psychotic disorders, such as schizophrenia. It may also be used in the short-term treatment of severe anxiety. It is available as tablets and capsules.
✚▲ Side-effects/warnings: See OXYPERTINE.

oxypertine

is an ANTIPSYCHOTIC drug, one of the *benzamides* chemical group, which is used to treat and tranquillize patients with psychotic disorders, such as schizophrenia and mania. It may also be used as an ANXIOLYTIC in the short-term treatment of severe anxiety. Administration is oral.
✚▲ Side-effects/warnings: See CHLORPROMAZINE HYDROCHLORIDE; but with less extrapyramidal symptoms and there may be photophobia. There may be excitation or sedation depending on dose.
✪ **Related entry: Oxypertine.**

oxytetracycline

is a broad-spectrum ANTIBACTERIAL and (TETRACYCLINES) ANTIBIOTIC which can be used to treat many serious infections, particularly those of the urogenital and respiratory tracts and of the skin (eg acne; in combination with other

drugs). Administration is oral.
✚▲ Side-effects/warnings: See TETRACYCLINE. It should not be administered in cases of porphyria.
✪ **Related entries: Oxymycin; Oxytetramix; Terra-Cortril; Terra-Cortril Nystatin; Terramycin; Trimovate.**

Oxytetramix

(Ashbourne) is a proprietary, prescription-only preparation of the ANTIBACTERIAL and (TETRACYCLINES) ANTIBIOTIC oxytetracycline. It can be used to treat a wide range of infections, and is available as tablets.
✚▲ Side-effects/warnings: See OXYTETRACYCLINE.

oxytocin

is a natural pituitary HORMONE produced and secreted by the posterior pituitary gland. It increases the contractions of the uterus during normal labour and stimulates milk production. Therapeutically, it may be administered by intravenous injection or infusion to induce or assist labour (or abortion), to speed up the third stage of labour (delivery of the placenta) and it is also used in conjunction with ERGOMETRINE MALEATE to help stop bleeding following childbirth and abortion. It is given by injection or infusion.
✚▲ Side-effects/warnings: It is a specialist drug used in hospital circumstances. There will be a full patient assessment and monitoring of side-effects. High doses may lead to violent contractions of the uterus, which may rupture the uterine wall and/or cause fetal distress.
✪ **Related entries: Syntocinon; Syntometrine.**

oxytocin-receptor antagonist 🅔

drugs are a recently introduced class of agents that work by blocking some actions of oxytocin, a natural HORMONE produced and secreted by the posterior pituitary gland. Oxytocin promotes the flow of breast milk following childbirth, and is the major natural oxytocic hormone, that is, it increases the contractions of the uterus during normal labour. Oxytocin-receptor antagonist drugs can be used to delay the latter action, and are licensed for the inhibition of uncomplicated premature labour between 24 and 33 weeks of gestation, mainly as an alternative when BETA-RECEPTOR STIMULANT drugs are not appropriate (eg in cardiac disease). See ATOSIBAN.

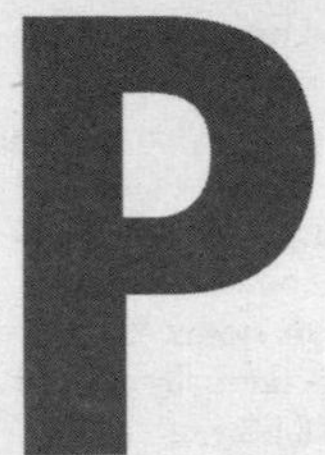

P2S

see PRALIDOXIME MESILATE.

Pacifene

(Sussex) is a proprietary, non-prescription preparation of the (NSAID) NON-NARCOTIC ANALGESIC, ANTIRHEUMATIC and ANTIPYRETIC ibuprofen. It can be used to relieve many types of pain, including headache, period pain, muscular pain, dental pain and feverishness, and also to relieve cold and flu symptoms. It is available as tablets and is not normally given to children, except on medical advice.

✚▲ Side-effects/warnings: See IBUPROFEN.

Pacifene Maximum Strength

(Sussex) is a proprietary, non-prescription preparation of the (NSAID) NON-NARCOTIC ANALGESIC, ANTIRHEUMATIC and ANTIPYRETIC ibuprofen. It can be used to relieve pain, including headache, period pain, muscular pain, dental pain and feverishness, and also to relieve cold and flu symptoms. It is available as tablets and is not normally given to children, except on medical advice.

✚▲ Side-effects/warnings: See IBUPROFEN.

paclitaxel

is a CYTOTOXIC drug, the first of a new group of drugs termed the *taxanes*. It is used as an ANTICANCER drug in the treatment of ovarian and breast cancer, and also non-small cell lung cancer. Administration is by intravenous infusion.

✚▲ Side-effects/warnings: See CYTOTOXIC.

✪ **Related entry: Taxol.**

Palfium

(Roche) is a proprietary, prescription-only preparation of the (OPIOID) NARCOTIC ANALGESIC dextromoramide, and is on the Controlled Drugs list. It can be used to relieve severe pain, and is available as tablets.

✚▲ Side-effects/warnings: See DEXTROMORAMIDE.

palivizumab

is an ANTIVIRAL drug, actually a monoclonal antibody (a form of pure antibody produced by a type of genetic molecular engineering), which can be used to treat respiratory tract infection by respiratory syncytial virus (RSV) in infants. It is administered by injection.

✚ Side-effects: Fever, nervousness, reactions at the injection site; less frequently, vomiting, diarrhoea, cough, wheeze, rhinitis, rash, pain, blood and liver changes.

▲ Warnings: It is a specialist drug, and there will be full assessment and patient monitoring throughout treatment. It is used with caution in severe infections, heart disease, blood disorders, febrile illness.

✪ **Related entry: Synagis.**

Palladone

(Napp) is a proprietary, prescription-only preparation of the (OPIOID) NARCOTIC ANALGESIC hydromorphone hydrochloride, which is on the Controlled Drugs list. It can be used primarily to relieve severe pain, such as in cancer. A modified-release form called *Palladone SR* is also available. Both are in the form of capsules.

✚▲ Side-effects/warnings: See HYDROMORPHONE HYDROCHLORIDE.

Paludrine

(AstraZeneca) is a proprietary, non-prescription preparation of the ANTIMALARIAL proguanil hydrochloride. It can be used in the prevention of malaria, and is available as tablets.

✚▲ Side-effects/warnings: See PROGUANIL HYDROCHLORIDE.

Paludrine/Avloclor

(AstraZeneca) is a proprietary, non-prescription *Travel Pack* containing the ANTIMALARIAL drugs chloroquine (as phosphate) and proguanil hydrochloride. It can be used to prevent or treat certain forms of malaria. It is available as tablets.

✚▲ Side-effects/warnings: See CHLOROQUINE; PROGUANIL HYDROCHLORIDE.

Pamergan P100

(Martindale) is a proprietary, prescription-only

compound preparation of the (OPIOID) NARCOTIC ANALGESIC pethidine hydrochloride and the SEDATIVE and HYPNOTIC (and ANTIHISTAMINE) promethazine hydrochloride (and is on the Controlled Drugs list). It can be used to relieve pain, especially during childbirth, and is available in a form for injection.
+▲ Side-effects/warnings: See PETHIDINE HYDROCHLORIDE; PROMETHAZINE HYDROCHLORIDE.

Panadeine Tablets

(Sterling Health; GSK Consumer Healthcare) is a proprietary, prescription-only compound analgesic preparation of the NON-NARCOTIC ANALGESIC and ANTIPYRETIC paracetamol and the NARCOTIC ANALGESIC codeine phosphate (a combination known as co-codamol 8/500). It can be used to treat pain, such as toothache, sore throat, period pain, arthritis and rheumatic pain, and to reduce high body temperature. It is available as tablets.
+▲ Side-effects/warnings: See CODEINE PHOSPHATE; PARACETAMOL.

Panadol Capsules

(GSK Consumer Healthcare) is a proprietary, non-prescription preparation of the NON-NARCOTIC ANALGESIC and ANTIPYRETIC paracetamol. It can be used to treat mild pain, such as musculoskeletal pain, toothache and period pain, to reduce high body temperature and to relieve cold and flu symptoms. It is available as capsules and is not normally given to children under 12 years, except on medical advice.
+▲ Side-effects/warnings: See PARACETAMOL.

Panadol Extra Soluble Tablets

(GSK Consumer Healthcare) is a proprietary, non-prescription compound preparation of the NON-NARCOTIC ANALGESIC and ANTIPYRETIC paracetamol and the STIMULANT caffeine. It can be used to treat mild pain, such as musculoskeletal pain, toothache and period pain, to reduce high body temperature and to relieve cold and flu symptoms. It is available as soluble tablets. Not normally given to children under 12, except on medical advice.
+▲ Side-effects/warnings: See CAFFEINE; PARACETAMOL.

Panadol Extra Tablets

(GSK Consumer Healthcare) is a proprietary, non-prescription compound preparation of the NON-NARCOTIC ANALGESIC and ANTIPYRETIC paracetamol and the STIMULANT caffeine. It can be used to treat mild pain, such as musculoskeletal pain, headache, toothache and period pain, to reduce high body temperature and to relieve cold and flu symptoms. It is available as tablets and is not normally given to children, except on medical advice.
+▲ Side-effects/warnings: See CAFFEINE; PARACETAMOL.

Panadol Night

(GSK Consumer Healthcare) is a proprietary, non-prescription compound preparation of the NON-NARCOTIC ANALGESIC and ANTIPYRETIC paracetamol and the ANTIHISTAMINE diphenhydramine hydrochloride. It can be used for the short-term treatment of pain at bedtime, for instance with toothache and where pain is causing difficulty in getting to sleep. It is available as tablets and is not to be given to children, except on medical advice.
+▲ Side-effects/warnings: See DIPHENHYDRAMINE HYDROCHLORIDE; PARACETAMOL.

Panadol Soluble

(GSK Consumer Healthcare) is a proprietary, non-prescription preparation of the NON-NARCOTIC ANALGESIC and ANTIPYRETIC paracetamol. It can be used to treat pain such as musculoskeletal pain, toothache and period pain, to reduce high body temperature and to relieve cold and flu symptoms. It is available as effervescent tablets and is not normally given to children under six years, except on medical advice.
+▲ Side-effects/warnings: See PARACETAMOL.

Panadol Tablets

(GSK Consumer Healthcare) is a proprietary, non-prescription preparation of the NON-NARCOTIC ANALGESIC and ANTIPYRETIC paracetamol. It can be used to treat pain, such as musculoskeletal pain, toothache and period pain, to reduce high body temperature and to relieve cold and flu symptoms. It is available as effervescent tablets and is not normally given to children under six years, except on medical advice.
+▲ Side-effects/warnings: See PARACETAMOL.

Panadol Ultra

(GSK Consumer Healthcare) is a proprietary, non-prescription compound preparation of the NON-NARCOTIC ANALGESIC and ANTIPYRETIC paracetamol and the (OPIOID) NARCOTIC ANALGESIC codeine phosphate (as hemihydrate). It can be used to treat pain, such as musculoskeletal pain, sciatica, strains, toothache and period pain, to reduce high body temperature and to relieve cold and flu symptoms and sore throat. It is available as tablets and is not to be given to children, except on medical advice.

✚▲ Side-effects/warnings: See CODEINE PHOSPHATE; PARACETAMOL.

Pancrease

(Janssen-Cilag) is a proprietary, non-prescription preparation of the digestive enzyme pancreatin. It can be used to compensate for a deficiency of the digestive juices that are normally supplied by the pancreas, and is available as capsules containing enteric-coated beads.

✚▲ Side-effects/warnings: See PANCREATIN.

Pancrease HL

(Janssen-Cilag) is a proprietary, prescription-only preparation of the digestive enzyme pancreatin. It can be used to compensate for a deficiency of the digestive juices that are normally supplied by the pancreas, and is available as capsules (at a higher strength than *Pancrease*).

✚▲ Side-effects/warnings: See PANCREATIN.

pancreatin

is the term used to describe extracts of the pancreas that contain pancreatic ENZYMES. It can be given by mouth to treat deficiencies due to impaired natural secretion by the pancreas, such as in cystic fibrosis, and also following operations involving removal of pancreatic tissue, such as panreatectomy and gastrectomy. The enzymes which help digest protein, starch and fat, are inactivated by the acid in the stomach and so preparations should be taken with food or with certain other drugs, such as H_2-ANTAGONIST drugs, that reduce acid secretion. Alternatively, pancreatin is available as enteric-coated tablets and capsules, which overcome some of these problems, but are destroyed by heat and should be mixed with food after its preparation. The majority of pancreatin preparations are of porcine origin and administered as capsules or granules.

✚ Side-effects: Irritation of the skin around the mouth and anus; there may be gastrointestinal upsets, including nausea, vomiting and abdominal discomfort; and at high dose there may be raised uric acid levels in the blood and urine.

▲ Warnings: There may be hypersensitivity reactions in those that handle the powder. There are particular problems (fibrotic structures in the bowel) that seem to be associated with high-dose preparations and these are only be taken with specialist advice.

✪ **Related entries: Creon; Creon 10 000; Creon 25 000; Nutrizym 10; Nutrizym 22; Nutrizym GR; Pancrease; Pancrease HL; Pancrex; Pancrex V.**

Pancrex

(Paines & Byrne) is a proprietary, non-prescription preparation of the digestive enzyme pancreatin. It can be used to compensate for a deficiency of the digestive juices that are normally supplied by the pancreas, and is available as granules.

✚▲ Side-effects/warnings: See PANCREATIN.

Pancrex V

(Paines & Byrne) is a proprietary, non-prescription preparation of the digestive enzyme pancreatin. It can be used to compensate for a deficiency of the digestive juices that are normally supplied by the pancreas, and is available in several strengths, some enteric-coated, as capsules (one preparation is called *Pancrex V 125*), tablets and a powder.

✚▲ Side-effects/warnings: See PANCREATIN.

pancuronium chloride

is a *non-depolarizing* SKELETAL MUSCLE RELAXANT which is used to induce muscle paralysis during surgery. Administration is by injection.

✚▲ Side-effects/warnings: It is a specialist drug used by anaesthetists in hospital.

✪ **Related entry: Pavulon.**

PanOxyl 5 Acnegel

(Stiefel) is a proprietary, non-prescription preparation of the KERATOLYTIC and ANTIMICROBIAL benzoyl peroxide (5%). It can be used to treat acne, and is available as a gel for topical application. It is not normally used on children, except on medical advice.

✚▲ Side-effects/warnings: See BENZOYL PEROXIDE.

P

PanOxyl 5 Cream
(Stiefel) is a proprietary, non-prescription preparation of the KERATOLYTIC and ANTIMICROBIAL benzoyl peroxide (5%). It can be used to treat acne, and is available as a cream for topical application.
✚▲ Side-effects/warnings: See BENZOYL PEROXIDE.

PanOxyl 5 Lotion
(Stiefel) is a proprietary, non-prescription preparation of the KERATOLYTIC and ANTIMICROBIAL benzoyl peroxide (5%). It can be used to treat acne, and is available as a lotion for topical application.
✚▲ Side-effects/warnings: See BENZOYL PEROXIDE.

PanOxyl 10 Acnegel
(Stiefel) is a proprietary, non-prescription preparation of the KERATOLYTIC and ANTIMICROBIAL benzoyl peroxide (10%). It can be used to treat acne, and is available as a gel for topical application. It is not normally used on children, except on medical advice.
✚▲ Side-effects/warnings: See BENZOYL PEROXIDE.

PanOxyl 10 Lotion
(Stiefel) is a proprietary, non-prescription preparation of the KERATOLYTIC and ANTIMICROBIAL benzoyl peroxide (10%). It can be used to treat acne, and is available as a lotion for topical application.
✚▲ Side-effects/warnings: See BENZOYL PEROXIDE.

PanOxyl Aquagel 2.5
(Stiefel) is a proprietary, non-prescription preparation of the KERATOLYTIC and ANTIMICROBIAL benzoyl peroxide (2.5%). It can be used to treat acne, and is available as a gel for topical application.
✚▲ Side-effects/warnings: See BENZOYL PEROXIDE.

PanOxyl Aquagel 5
(Stiefel) is a proprietary, non-prescription preparation of the KERATOLYTIC and ANTIMICROBIAL benzoyl peroxide (5%). It can be used to treat acne, and is available as a gel for topical application. It is not normally given to children, except on medical advice.
✚▲ Side-effects/warnings: See BENZOYL PEROXIDE.

PanOxyl Aquagel 10
(Stiefel) is a proprietary, non-prescription preparation of the KERATOLYTIC and ANTIMICROBIAL benzoyl peroxide (10%). It can be used to treat acne, and is available as a gel for topical application.
✚▲ Side-effects/warnings: See BENZOYL PEROXIDE.

PanOxyl Wash 10
(Stiefel) is a proprietary, non-prescription preparation of the KERATOLYTIC and ANTIMICROBIAL benzoyl peroxide (10%). It can be used to treat acne, and is available as a lotion for topical application. It is not normally used on children, except on medical advice.
✚▲ Side-effects/warnings: See BENZOYL PEROXIDE.

pantoprazole
is an ULCER-HEALING DRUG which works as an inhibitor of gastric acid secretion in the parietal (acid-producing) cells of the stomach lining by acting as a PROTON-PUMP INHIBITOR. It is administered for the treatment of benign gastric and duodenal ulcers, and also for reflux oesophagitis. Additionally, it can be used in conjunction with antibiotics to treat gastric *Helicobacter pylori* infection. Administration is oral or by injection.
✚▲ Side-effects/warnings: See PROTON-PUMP INHIBITOR. Also reported are fever, liver changes and blood lipid changes. Special care is necessary in kidney impairment.
✪ **Related entry: Protium.**

papaveretum
is a mixture of ALKALOID of opium in defined amounts, mostly being made up of morphine with the rest largely consisting of codeine and papaverine. It is used as an (OPIOID) NARCOTIC ANALGESIC primarily during or following surgery, but can also be used as a sedative prior to an operation. Administration is oral or by injection. Forms are available with HYOSCINE HYDROBROMIDE or ATROPINE SULPHATE.
✚▲ Side-effects/warnings: See MORPHINE SULPHATE.
✪ **Related entry: Aspav.**

papaverine
is a SMOOTH MUSCLE RELAXANT which is rarely used any more, though it is included in a proprietary pain remedy. There have been some recent trials of its use for IMPOTENCE TREATMENT by direct injection into the corpus cavernosum.

Administration is either oral or by injection.
✚ Side-effects: Local burning pain and haematoma (swelling) at the site of injection.
▲ Warnings: It should be administered with care to patients with certain cardiovascular disorders.

Papulex

(Manx) is a proprietary, non-prescription preparation of nicotinamide. It can be used to treat mild to moderate inflammatory acne, and is available as a gel.
✚▲ Side-effects/warnings: See NICOTINAMIDE.

paracetamol

(called acetaminophen in the USA) is a NON-NARCOTIC ANALGESIC which can be used to treat all forms of mild to moderate pain, especially headache (including migraine). It also has ANTIPYRETIC properties and can be used to reduce fever and raised body temperature, including following immunization in babies, and in brief febrile convulsions. In many ways it is similar to aspirin, except that it does not cause gastric irritation or relieve inflammation. Many proprietary preparations are compound analgesics that combine paracetamol and aspirin. Administration can be oral or as suppositories.
✚ Side-effects: There are few side-effects if dosage is low, though there may be rashes; after prolonged use, acute pancreatitis and blood disorders; high overdosage or prolonged use may result in liver or kidney dysfunction.
▲ Warnings: It should be administered with caution to patients with impaired liver or kidney function or who suffer from alcoholism (which causes liver damage).
✪ **Related entries: Alka-Seltzer XS; Alka XS Go; Anadin Extra; Anadin Cold Control Capsules; Anadin Cold Control Flu Strength Hot Lemon; Anadin Extra Soluble Tablets; Anadin Paracetamol Tablets; Beechams All-In-One; Beechams Cold and Flu Hot Blackcurrant; Beechams Cold and Flu Hot Lemon; Beechams Flu-Plus Caplets; Beechams Flu-Plus Hot Berry Fruits; Beechams Flu-Plus Hot Lemon; Beechams Powders Capsules; Benylin Day and Night; Benylin Four Flu Liquid; Benylin Four Flu Tablets; Boots Dental Pain Relief; Boots Tension Headache Relief; Calpol Infant Suspension; Calpol Infant Suspension Sachets; Calpol Six Plus Sugar Free/ Colour Free Suspension; Calpol Six Plus Suspension; Calpol Sugar-Free Infant Suspension; Calpol Sugar-Free Infant Suspension Sachets; co-codamol; co-dydramol; co-methiamol; co-proxamol; Cosalgesic; Day Nurse Capsules; Day Nurse Liquid; Disprin Extra; Disprol Paracetamol Suspension; Disprol Soluble Paracetamol Tablets; Distalgesic; Domperamol; Feminax; Fennings Children's Cooling Powders; Galake; Hedex Extra Tablets; Hedex Tablets; Kapake; Lemsip Cold + Flu Breathe Easy; Lemsip Cold + Flu Breathe Easy; Lemsip Cold + Flu Max Strength; Lemsip Cold + Flu Max Strength Capsules; Lemsip Cold + Flu Original Lemon; Lemsip Pharmacy Flu Strength; Medinol Over 6 Paracetamol Oral Suspension; Medinol Under 6 Paracetamol Oral Suspension; Medised; Medised Infant; Medised Sugar Free Colour Free; Midrid; Migraleve; Migraleve Pink; Migraleve Yellow; Night Nurse Capsules; Night Nurse Liquid; Nurse Sykes Powders; Panadeine Tablets; Panadol Capsules; Panadol Extra Soluble Tablets; Panadol Extra Tablets; Panadol Night; Panadol Soluble; Panadol Tablets; Panadol Ultra; Paracets Capsules; Paracets Cold Relief Powders; Paracets Plus Capsules; Paracets Tablets; Paracodol Capsules; Paracodol Tablets; Paradote; Parake; Paramax; Paramol Tablets; Propain Caplets; Remedeine; Resolve; Sinutab Tablets; Solpadeine Capsules; Solpadeine Max; Solpadeine Soluble Tablets; Solpadeine Tablets; Solpadol; Sudafed-Co Tablets; Syndol; Tixymol; Tylex; Veganin Tablets; Vicks Medinite.**

Paracets Capsules

(Sussex) is a proprietary, non-prescription preparation of the NON-NARCOTIC ANALGESIC and ANTIPYRETIC paracetamol. It can be used to treat mild to moderate pain, such as muscular and rheumatic pain, toothache and period pain, to reduce high body temperature and to relieve cold and flu symptoms. It is available as capsules and is not normally given to children under six years, except on medical advice.
✚▲ Side-effects/warnings: See PARACETAMOL.

Paracets Cold Relief Powders

(Sussex) is a proprietary, non-prescription compound preparation of the NON-NARCOTIC ANALGESIC and ANTIPYRETIC paracetamol and vitamin C (ascorbic acid). It can be used to relieve cold and flu symptoms. It is available as a powder and is not normally given to children.
✚▲ Side-effects/warnings: See ASCORBIC ACID; PARACETAMOL.

Paracets Plus Capsules

(Sussex) is a proprietary, non-prescription compound preparation of the NON-NARCOTIC ANALGESIC paracetamol, the SYMPATHOMIMETIC and DECONGESTANT phenylephrine hydrochloride and the STIMULANT caffeine. It can be used to relieve cold and flu symptoms, aches and pains and nasal congestion. It is available as capsules and is not normally given to children.

✚▲ Side-effects/warnings: See CAFFEINE; PARACETAMOL; PHENYLEPHRINE HYDROCHLORIDE.

Paracets Tablets

(Sussex) is a proprietary, non-prescription preparation of the NON-NARCOTIC ANALGESIC and ANTIPYRETIC paracetamol. It can be used to treat mild to moderate pain, such as toothache and period pain, to reduce high body temperature and to relieve cold and flu symptoms. It is available as tablets and is not normally given to children under six, except on medical advice.

✚▲ Side-effects/warnings: See PARACETAMOL.

Paracodol Capsules

(Roche Consumer Health) is a proprietary, non-prescription compound preparation of the NON-NARCOTIC ANALGESIC and ANTIPYRETIC paracetamol and the (OPIOID) NARCOTIC ANALGESIC codeine phosphate (a combination known as co-codamol 8/500). It can be used to treat mild to moderate pain, such as headache, muscular pain and rheumatic pain, and to relieve the symptoms of flu and feverish colds. It is available as tablets and is not normally given to children, except on medical advice.

✚▲ Side-effects/warnings: See CODEINE PHOSPHATE; PARACETAMOL.

Paracodol Tablets

(Roche Consumer Health) is a proprietary, non-prescription compound analgesic preparation of the NON-NARCOTIC ANALGESIC and ANTIPYRETIC paracetamol and the (OPIOID) NARCOTIC ANALGESIC codeine phosphate (a combination known as co-codamol 8/500). It can be used to relieve mild to moderate pain, such as headache, muscular aches and pains and sore throat. It is available as tablets and is not normally given to children under six, except on medical advice.

✚▲ Side-effects/warnings: See CODEINE PHOSPHATE; PARACETAMOL.

Paradote

(Penn) is a proprietary, non-prescription compound preparation of the (NSAID) NON-NARCOTIC ANALGESIC and ANTIPYRETIC paracetamol and the amino acid methionine (an ANTIDOTE to paracetamol overdose). It can be used to relieve painful and feverish conditions, such as period pain, toothache and cold and flu symptoms, and to reduce high body temperature (especially for patients likely to overdose). It is available as tablets and is not given to children, except on medical advice.

✚▲ Side-effects/warnings: See METHIONINE; PARACETAMOL.

paraffin

is a hydrocarbon derived from petroleum. Its main therapeutic use is as a base for ointments as either YELLOW SOFT PARAFFIN or WHITE SOFT PARAFFIN. As a mineral oil, LIQUID PARAFFIN is used as a LAXATIVE and is also incorporated into many preparations as an EMOLLIENT. See LIQUID PARAFFIN; WHITE SOFT PARAFFIN; YELLOW SOFT PARAFFIN.

Parake

(Galen) is a proprietary, non-prescription compound analgesic preparation of the NON-NARCOTIC ANALGESIC and ANTIPYRETIC paracetamol and the (OPIOID) NARCOTIC ANALGESIC codeine phosphate (a combination known as co-codamol 8/500). It can be used to relieve pain and to reduce high body temperature. It is available as tablets and is not normally given to children under six years, except on medical advice.

✚▲ Side-effects/warnings: See CODEINE PHOSPHATE; PARACETAMOL.

paraldehyde

is a drug that is used mainly as an ANTICONVULSANT and ANTI-EPILEPTIC in the treatment of status epilepticus (severe and continuous epileptic seizures). Administration is by injection or enema.

✚ Side-effects: Pain and abscess after injections; after enema, rectal irritation. There may be rashes.

▲ Warnings: It is administered with caution to patients with certain types of lung disease or impaired liver function, or who are pregnant or breast-feeding.

Paramax

(Sanofi-Synthelabo) is a proprietary, prescription-only compound preparation of the ANTI-EMETIC and ANTINAUSEANT metoclopramide hydrochloride and the NON-NARCOTIC ANALGESIC paracetamol. It can be used as an ANTIMIGRAINE treatment for acute migraine attacks, and is available as tablets and as sachets of effervescent powder.

+▲ Side-effects/warnings: See METOCLOPRAMIDE HYDROCHLORIDE; PARACETAMOL. Note the side-effects in young people.

Paramol Tablets

(SSL) is a proprietary, non-prescription compound analgesic preparation of the NON-NARCOTIC ANALGESIC paracetamol and the (OPIOID) ANTITUSSIVE and NARCOTIC ANALGESIC dihydrocodeine tartrate. It can be used for general pain relief and to reduce raised body temperature. It is available as tablets and is not normally given to children, except on medical advice.

+▲ Side-effects/warnings: See DIHYDROCODEINE TARTRATE; PARACETAMOL.

Paraplatin

(Bristol-Myers Squibb) is a proprietary, prescription-only preparation of the platinum compound (CYTOTOXIC) ANTICANCER drug carboplatin. It can be used specifically in the treatment of ovarian cancer, and is available in a form for injection.

+▲ Side-effects/warnings: See CARBOPLATIN.

parasympathomimetic 🅴

drugs have effects similar to those of the parasympathetic nervous system. They work by mimicking the actions of the natural neurotransmitter acetylcholine (eg CARBACHOL and PILOCARPINE). The ANTICHOLINESTERASE drugs are *indirect parasympathomimetics* because they prolong the duration of action of the naturally released acetylcholine (and can be used to treat myesthenia gravis; eg NEOSTIGMINE). *Direct parasympathomimetics* act at (so-called 'muscarinic') receptors for acetylcholine. Important parasympathomimetic actions include slowing of the heart, vasodilation, constriction of the bronchioles of the lung, stimulation of the muscles of the intestine and bladder (so can be used to treat urinary retention; eg BETHANECHOL CHLORIDE)and constriction of the pupil (so can be used in glaucoma treatment; eg pilocarpine), and altered focusing of the eye. ANTICHOLINERGIC (ANTIMUSCARINIC) drugs oppose some of these actions.

parathormone

see PARATHYROID HORMONE.

parathyrin

see PARATHYROID HORMONE.

parathyroid hormone 🅴

(parathormone; parathyrin; PTH) is secreted by the parathyroid glands which are situated in two pairs close to the thyroid gland at the base of the neck. It is concerned with regulation of calcium and phosphate metabolism, and to do this works in a complex interaction with VITAMIN D and one of the THYROID HORMONES, CALCITONIN (which is quite distinct in structure and function to THYROXINE and TRIIODOTHYRONINE). Its main action is to raise the calcium concentration in the blood while decreasing phosphate levels. The hormone itself is not currently used in therapeutics except sometimes as a diagnostic agent.

Pardelprin

(Alpharma) is a proprietary, prescription-only preparation of the (NSAID) NON-NARCOTIC ANALGESIC and ANTIRHEUMATIC indometacin (indomethacin). It can be used to treat the pain of rheumatic disease and other musculoskeletal disorders, period pains and acute gout. It is available as modified-release capsules.

+▲ Side-effects/warnings: See INDOMETACIN.

Pariet

(Eisai, Janssen-Cilag) is a newly introduced proprietary, prescription-only preparation of the PROTON-PUMP INHIBITOR rabeprazole sodium. It can be used as an ULCER-HEALING DRUG and for associated conditions, such as gastro-oesophageal reflux, and is available as tablets.

+▲ Side-effects/warnings: See RABEPRAZOLE SODIUM.

Parlodel

(Novartis) is a proprietary, prescription-only preparation of bromocriptine. It is used primarily to treat parkinsonism, but not the parkinsonian

symptoms caused by certain drug therapies (see ANTIPARKINSONISM). It can also be used to treat a number of other hormonal disorders, and is available as tablets and capsules.
✚▲ Side-effects/warnings: See BROMOCRIPTINE.

Parnate

(Goldshield) is a proprietary, prescription-only preparation of the MONOAMINE-OXIDASE INHIBITOR (MAOI) ANTIDEPRESSANT tranylcypromine. It is available as tablets.
✚▲ Side-effects/warnings: See TRANYLCYPROMINE.

Paroven

(Novartis) is a proprietary, non-prescription preparation of oxerutins. It can be used to treat cramp and other manifestations of poor circulation in the veins (venous insufficiency), such as oedema, and is available as capsules.
✚▲ Side-effects/warnings: See OXERUTINS.

paroxetine

is an ANTIDEPRESSANT of the recently developed SSRI group. It can be used to treat depressive illness, obsessive-compulsive disorder, panic disorder and social phobia. It has the advantage over some earlier antidepressants because it has less sedative and ANTICHOLINERGIC (ANTIMUSCARINIC) side-effects. Administration is oral.
✚▲ Side-effects/warnings: See SSRI. Also, postural hypotension reported, hypersensitivity reactions (rash and itching, urticaria, angioedema), effects on the liver. Facial twitches may occur. When it is being used to treat panic disorders, at first there may be a worsening of symptoms.
✪ **Related entry: Seroxat.**

Parvolex

(Celltech) is a proprietary, prescription-only preparation of the ANTIDOTE acetylcysteine. It can be used to treat overdose poisoning by the NON-NARCOTIC ANALGESIC paracetamol, and is available in a form for intravenous infusion.
✚▲ Side-effects/warnings: See ACETYLCYSTEINE.

Pavacol-D

(Boehringer Ingelheim) is a proprietary, non-prescription preparation of the (OPIOID) ANTITUSSIVE pholcodine. It can be used for troublesome dry or painful coughs, and is available as a syrup. It is not normally given to children under one year, except on medical advice.
✚▲ Side-effects/warnings: See PHOLCODINE.

Pavulon

(Organon) is a proprietary, prescription-only preparation of the (*non-depolarizing*) SKELETAL MUSCLE RELAXANT pancuronium bromide. It can be used to induce muscle paralysis during surgery, and is available in a form for injection.
✚▲ Side-effects/warnings: See PANCURONIUM CHLORIDE.

Paxidorm Syrup

(Wallace) is a proprietary, non-prescription preparation of the ANTIHISTAMINE diphenhydramine hydrochloride, which has marked SEDATIVE properties. It can be used to help induce sleep in the treatment of temporary sleep disturbances, and is available as a syrup. It is not normally given to children under 16 years, except on medical advice.
✚▲ Side-effects/warnings: See DIPHENHYDRAMINE HYDROCHLORIDE.

Paxidorm Tablets

(Wallace) is a proprietary, non-prescription preparation of the ANTIHISTAMINE diphenhydramine hydrochloride, which has marked sedative properties. It can be used to help induce sleep in the treatment of temporary sleep disturbances. It is available as tablets and is not normally given to children under 16 years, except on medical advice.
✚▲ Side-effects/warnings: See DIPHENHYDRAMINE HYDROCHLORIDE.

pediculicidal 🅱

drugs are used to kill lice of the genus *Pediculus*, which infest either the body (including pubic 'crab' lice) or the scalp, or both, and cause intense itching. Scratching tends to damage the skin surface and may eventually cause weeping lesions with bacterial infection as well. The best-known and most-used pediculicides include PERMETHRIN, PHENOTHRIN, MALATHION and CARBARYL. Lindane, which was once commonly administered, is now no longer used for lice on the scalp because resistant strains of lice have developed. Administration is topical, usually as a lotion or shampoo, but several repeated applications are not recommended because of side-effects.

PegIntron

(Schering-Plough) is a recently introduced proprietary, prescription-only preparation of the IMMUNOMODULATOR interferon (in the form peginterferon alpha-2b, rbe; produced by a type of molecular engineering). It can be used combined with ribavirin to treat chronic hepatitis C, or alone if treatment with ribavirin is not tolerated or is not suitable. It is available in a form for subcutaneous injection.
✚▲ Side-effects/warnings: See INTERFERON.

Penbritin

(SmithKline Beecham; GSK) is a proprietary, prescription-only preparation of the broad-spectrum ANTIBACTERIAL and (PENICILLIN) ANTIBIOTIC ampicillin. It can be used to treat systemic bacterial infections. It is available as capsules and in a form for injection.
✚▲ Side-effects/warnings: See AMPICILLIN.

penciclovir

is an ANTIVIRAL drug that is similar to ACICLOVIR (acyclovir). It is used to treat labial herpes simplex infection. Administration is topical.
✚▲ Side-effects/warnings: There may be stinging, burning and numbness. Avoid contact with mucous membranes and eyes.
✪ **Related entry: Vectavir.**

penicillamine

is a derivative of penicillin and is an extremely effective CHELATING AGENT. It binds various metal ions within the body, so facilitating their excretion (elimination from the body). It can be used as an ANTIDOTE to various types of metallic poisoning (eg copper and lead) and as a METABOLIC DISORDER TREATMENT to reduce copper levels in Wilson's disease; also sometimes for autoimmune hepatitis and cystinuria. It is also used in the long-term treatment of severe rheumatoid arthritis or juvenile chronic arthritis, where it has ANTI-INFLAMMATORY and ANTIRHEUMATIC actions. Administration is oral.
✚ Side-effects: These include nausea, anorexia, fever, rashes, taste impairment, blood and kidney disturbances, lupus-like syndrome or muscle weakness and others.
▲ Warnings: It should not be used in patients known to have sensitivity to penicillins or with lupus erythematosus. Administer with care to those with kidney impairment, who are pregnant and with known sensitivity to certain other drugs. Regular monitoring of blood, urine etc. is required. It may take several weeks before improvements are experienced. Tell your doctor if you develop sore throat, infection, fever, unexplained bruising, bleeding or purple patches, mouth ulcers, rashes, or non-specific illness. Zinc and iron, which can be used for medical purposes or in multivitamin preparations, can reduce the absorption of penicillamine and so diminish its effectiveness.
✪ **Related entry: Distamine.**

penicillin 🄴

refers to a family of ANTIBACTERIAL and ANTIBIOTIC drugs which work by interfering with the synthesis of bacterial cell walls (so killing growing bacteria – they are *bactericidal* – that is, they kill bacteria rather than simply inhibit their growth). The early penicillins were mainly effective against Gram-positive bacteria, though they could be used against the Gram-negative organisms and can be used to treat gonorrhoea and meningitis, as well as the organism causing syphilis. Later penicillins (eg AMPICILLIN and PIPERACILLIN) expanded the spectrum to include a greater range of organisms. They are absorbed rapidly by most (but not all; penetration to the cerebrospinal fluid is poor) body tissues and fluids and are excreted in the urine. One great disadvantage of penicillins is that many patients are allergic to them – allergy to one, means allergy to all of them – and may have reactions that range from a minor rash right up to anaphylactic shock, which occasionally can be fatal. Unfortunately, the occurrence of these, and other allergic reactions (eg vasculitis, intestinal nephritis) is unpredictable. Otherwise they are remarkably non-toxic. Rarely, very high dosage may cause convulsions, haemolytic anaemia or abnormally high levels of sodium or potassium in the body with consequent symptoms. Those taken orally tend to cause diarrhoea and there is also a risk with broad-spectrum penicillins of allowing a superinfection to develop.

A major problem in the therapeutic use of penicillins and some other beta-lactams has been the development of bacteria that are resistant to these antibiotics by virtue of producing an enzyme (*beta-lactamase; penicillinase*) that breaks down the drugs in the body, so limiting their action. These *penicillin-resistant* bacteria must be treated with more recently developed *penicillinase-resistant penicillins*, such as FLUCLOXACILLIN, or entirely different classes of antibiotics. Also, some antibiotic preparations combine a *penicillinase-sensitive* drug with an inhibitor of the penicillinase enzyme, which then artificially gives that antibiotic penicillinase-resistance (for example CLAVULANIC ACID and TAZOBACTAM are inhibitors of penicillinase (beta-lactamase).

The best-known and most-used penicillins include BENZYLPENICILLIN (penicillin G; the first of the penicillins), PHENOXYMETHYLPENICILLIN (penicillin V), FLUCLOXACILLIN, AMPICILLIN and AMOXICILLIN. See also PIVMECILLINAM HYDROCHLORIDE; TICARCILLIN.

penicillinase inhibitor

drugs are used to inhibit ENZYMES that are produced by certain (*penicillin-resistant*) bacteria, which break down some of the PENICILLIN class of ANTIBIOTICS, effectively rendering the latter useless. For example, staphylococci bacteria are commonly resistant to BENZYLPENICILLIN through developing an ability to produce penicillinase enzyme. Consequently, treatment of infections caused by such bacteria has normally necessitated the administration of either *penicillinase-resistant penicillins*, such as FLUCLOXACILLIN, or entirely different classes of antibiotic. However, some antibiotic preparations combine a *penicillinase-sensitive* drug with an inhibitor of the penicillinase enzyme, which then artificially gives that antibiotic penicillinase-resistance (for example CLAVULANIC ACID and TAZOBACTAM are inhibitors of penicillinase (beta-lactamase)).

penicillin G

see BENZYLPENICILLIN.

penicillin V

see PHENOXYMETHYLPENICILLIN.

Pennsaid

(Provalis) is a proprietary, prescription-only preparation of the (NSAID) NON-NARCOTIC ANALGESIC diclofenac sodium, which also has COUNTER-IRRITANT, or RUBEFACIENT, actions. It can be used for the symptomatic relief of underlying joint pain of osteoarthritis and is available as a solution for topical application to the skin.

✚▲ Side-effects/warnings: See DICLOFENAC SODIUM; but adverse effects on topical application are limited.

Pentacarinat

(JHC) is a proprietary, prescription-only preparation of the ANTIPROTOZOAL drug pentamidine isetionate. It can be used to treat protozoan pneumonia and other serious infections. It is available only for specialist use and is administered either by injection or inhalation.

✚▲ Side-effects/warnings: See PENTAMIDINE ISETIONATE.

pentamidine isethionate

see PENTAMIDINE ISETIONATE.

pentamidine isetionate

(pentamidine isethionate) is an ANTIPROTOZOAL drug which is used to treat pneumonia caused by the protozoan micro-organism *Pneumocystis carinii* in patients whose immune system has been suppressed (either following transplant surgery or because of a condition such as HIV infection). It has also been used as an antiprotozoal to treat forms of leishmaniasis and trypanosomiasis. It is available only for specialist use and is administered either by injection or inhalation.

✚▲ Side-effects/warnings: This is a specialist drug given after full assessment and with careful monitoring. It can cause severe hypotension while being administered or immediately after. There may also be serious pancreatitis, hypoglycaemia, arrhythmias, blood disorders, kidney failure and various other potentially serious side-effects. It is administered with care to patients with certain liver, kidney and blood disorders.

✪ **Related entry: Pentacarinat.**

Pentasa

(Ferring) is a proprietary, prescription-only preparation of the AMINOSALICYLATE mesalazine. It can be used to treat patients who suffer from ulcerative colitis, and is available as modified-release tablets, modified-release granules,

suppositories and as a retention enema.
✚▲ Side-effects/warnings: See MESALAZINE.

pentazocine

is a powerful NARCOTIC ANALGESIC which can be used to treat moderate to severe pain. It is an OPIOID and is like morphine sulphate in effect and action, but is less likely to cause dependence. However, it can precipitate withdrawal symptoms if used in patients dependent on opioids. Administration can be oral, sublingual, as suppositories, or by injection. The proprietary forms are on the Controlled Drugs list. It is also available as compound preparations in combination with PARACETAMOL.
✚▲ Side-effects/warnings: See OPIOID. Disturbances of thought and hallucinations are thought to occur. It is not suitable for use in patients with certain cardiovascular complications and should not be used by patients with porphyria.
✪ **Related entry: Fortral.**

Pentostam

(GlaxoWellcome; GSK) is a proprietary, prescription-only preparation of sodium stibogluconate, which has ANTIPROTOZOAL properties. It can be used to treat skin infections by protozoal micro-organisms of the genus *Leishmania* (eg leishmaniasis). It is available in a form for injection.
✚▲ Side-effects/warnings: See SODIUM STIBOGLUCONATE.

pentostatin

is a CYTOTOXIC drug (an antibiotic in origin) which is used as an ANTICANCER treatment for hairy cell leukaemia. Administration is by injection.
✚▲ Side-effects/warnings: See CYTOTOXIC.
✪ **Related entry: Nipent.**

pentoxifylline

(oxpentifylline) is a VASODILATOR drug which dilates the blood vessels of the extremities and can be used to treat peripheral vascular disease (Raynaud's phenomenon). Administration is oral.
✚ Side-effects: Gastrointestinal disturbances; agitation and sleep disturbances; headache, dizziness; sometimes flushing and other effects on the cardiovascular system and blood, hypersensitivity reactions.
▲ Warnings: It should not be used in porphyria, in people with certain cardiovascular problems, who are pregnant or breast-feeding. It should be used with care if there is liver or kidney problems.
✪ **Related entry: Trental.**

Pentrax

(DermaPharm) is a proprietary, non-prescription preparation of coal tar. It can be used to treat scaly scalp conditions, such as seborrhoeic dermatitis, dandruff and psoriasis of the scalp, and is available as a shampoo.
✚▲ Side-effects/warnings: See COAL TAR.

Pepcid

(MSD) is a proprietary, prescription-only preparation of the H_2-ANTAGONIST famotidine. It can be used as an ULCER-HEALING DRUG for benign peptic ulcers (in the stomach or duodenum), gastro-oesophageal reflux, dyspepsia, Zollinger-Ellison syndrome and associated conditions. It is available as tablets.
✚▲ Side-effects/warnings: See FAMOTIDINE.

Pepcid AC

(Johnson & Johnson • MSD) is a proprietary, non-prescription preparation of the H_2-ANTAGONIST famotidine. It is available without a prescription in a limited amount for short-term use for dyspepsia, heartburn, hyperacidity and associated conditions, and is available as tablets. It should not be given to children under 16 years, except on medical advice.
✚▲ Side-effects/warnings: See FAMOTIDINE.

peppermint oil

is used to relieve the discomfort of abdominal colic and distension, particularly in irritable bowel syndrome. It is thought to act as an ANTISPASMODIC by directly relaxing the smooth muscle of the intestinal walls. It is also incorporated into preparations to relieve catarrh and nasal congestion. Administration is oral.
✚ Side-effects: There may be heartburn and rarely allergic reactions, such as rash, headache, muscle tremor, slowing of the heart and unsteady gait, perianal irritation. When taken in capsule form, they should be swallowed whole since if they are broken, the peppermint oil might cause irritation of the mouth and oesophagus.
✪ **Related entries: Actonorm Powder; Califig**

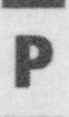

Herbal Laxative Tablets with Senna; Colpermin; Equilon Herbal; Hill's Balsam Chesty Cough Pastilles; J Collis Browne's Mixture; Mintec.

Peptac Liquid

(IVAX) is a proprietary, non-prescription compound preparation of the ANTACID agents calcium carbonate and sodium bicarbonate and the DEMULCENT alginic acid (as sodium alginate). It can be used for the symptomatic relief of heartburn and indigestion due to gastric reflux, and is available as a liquid. It is not normally given to children under six years, except on medical advice.
✚▲ Side-effects/warnings: See ALGINIC ACID; CALCIUM CARBONATE; SODIUM BICARBONATE.

Peptimax

(Ashbourne) is a proprietary, prescription-only preparation of the H_2-ANTAGONIST cimetidine. It can be used as an ULCER-HEALING DRUG for benign peptic ulcers (in the stomach or duodenum), gastro-oesophageal reflux, dyspepsia and associated conditions. It is available as tablets.
✚▲ Side-effects/warnings: See CIMETIDINE.

Pepto-Bismol

is a proprietary, non-prescription preparation of bismuth salicylate (bismuth subsalicylate), and can be used as an ANTACID and ANTIDIARRHOEAL agent in the treatment of stomach upsets, indigestion, nausea and diarrhoea. It is available as a liquid. It is not normally given to children under three years, except on medical advice.
✚▲ Side-effects/warnings: see BISMUTH SALICYLATE.

Percutol

(Dominion) is a proprietary, non-prescription preparation of the VASODILATOR and ANTI-ANGINA drug glyceryl trinitrate. It can be used to treat and prevent angina pectoris. It is available in the form of an ointment for use on a dressing secured to the skin surface (usually on the chest, arm or thigh).
✚▲ Side-effects/warnings: See GLYCERYL TRINITRATE.

Perdix

(Schwarz) is a proprietary, prescription-only preparation of the ACE INHIBITOR moexipril hydrochloride. It can be used as an ANTIHYPERTENSIVE, and is available as tablets.
✚▲ Side-effects/warnings: See MOEXIPRIL HYDROCHLORIDE.

Perfan

(Aventis Pharma) is a proprietary, prescription-only preparation of the PHOSPHODIESTERASE INHIBITOR enoximone. It can be used, in the short term, in congestive HEART FAILURE TREATMENT, especially where other drugs have not been successful. It is available in a form for intravenous injection or infusion.
✚▲ Side-effects/warnings: See ENOXIMONE.

pergolide

is an ANTIPARKINSONISM drug. It is an ERGOT ALKALOID derivative and works by stimulating the DOPAMINE receptors in the brain (a DOPAMINE-RECEPTOR STIMULANT). It is similar to BROMOCRIPTINE in that it is useful in reducing 'off' periods in the disease, and is usually given with LEVODOPA. Administration is oral.
✚ Side-effects: These include hallucinations, confusion, impaired muscle movements, somnolence, nausea and abdominal pain, dyspepsia, double vision, rhinitis, laboured breathing, insomnia, constipation or diarrhoea, hypotension and changes in heart rate or rhythm, effects on the lungs, and others.
▲ Warnings: Administer with care to patients with certain heart disorders, dyskinesias, history of confusion or hallucinations, porphyria; or who are pregnant or breast-feeding.
✪ **Related entry: Celance.**

Periactin

(MSD) is a proprietary, non-prescription preparation of cyproheptadine hydrochloride, which is a drug with ANTIHISTAMINE activity. It can be used for the symptomatic relief of allergic disorders, such as hay fever and urticaria, and also as an ANTIMIGRAINE treatment. It is available as tablets and a syrup.
✚▲ Side-effects/warnings: See CYPROHEPTADINE HYDROCHLORIDE.

periciazine

see PERICYAZINE.

pericyazine

(periciazine) is chemically a PHENOTHIAZINE and

is used as an ANTIPSYCHOTIC drug to treat patients suffering from schizophrenia and other psychoses and other behavioural disorders. It can also be used as an ANXIOLYTIC in the short-term treatment of severe anxiety. Administration is oral.
✚▲ Side-effects/warnings: See CHLORPROMAZINE HYDROCHLORIDE; but depend on use; it is more sedating and initially hypotension may occur.
✪ **Related entry: Neulactil.**

Perinal
(Dermal) is a proprietary, non-prescription compound preparation of the CORTICOSTEROID and ANTI-INFLAMMATORY hydrocortisone (as acetate) and the LOCAL ANAESTHETIC lidocaine hydrochloride. It can be used to treat haemorrhoids and inflammation in the anal region, and is available as a spray for topical application. It is not normally given to children under 14 years, except on medical advice.
✚▲ Side-effects/warnings: See HYDROCORTISONE; LIDOCAINE HYDROCHLORIDE.

perindopril
is an ACE INHIBITOR and acts as a VASODILATOR. It can be used as an ANTIHYPERTENSIVE and in congestive HEART FAILURE TREATMENT, and is often used in conjunction with other classes of drugs, particularly (THIAZIDE) DIURETIC drugs. Administration is oral.
✚ Side-effects: See ACE INHIBITOR. Also, muscle weakness, flushing, mood and sleep disturbances.
▲ Warnings: See ACE INHIBITOR.
✪ **Related entry: Coversyl.**

Periostat
(CollaGenex) is a proprietary, prescription-only preparation of the ANTIBACTERIAL and (TETRACYCLINES) ANTIBIOTIC doxycycline. It can be used to treat a wide range of infections, and also as an adjunct to scaling and root planing for the treatment of periodontitis. It is available as tablets.
✚▲ Side-effects/warnings: See DOXYCYCLINE.

permethrin
is a PEDICULICIDAL drug which can be used to treat infestations by lice and as a SCABICIDAL to treat skin infestation by mites (scabies). Administration is topical in the form of a cream rinse and a skin cream.
✚ Side-effects: Skin irritation, including itching, reddening and stinging; rarely, there may be swelling and rashes.
▲ Warnings: Avoid contact with the eyes and do not use on broken or infected skin. Administer with caution to patients who are pregnant or breast-feeding.
✪ **Related entries: Full Marks Lotion; Lyclear Creme Rinse; Lyclear Dermal Creme.**

Permitabs
(Bioglan) is a proprietary, non-prescription preparation of the ANTISEPTIC potassium permanganate. It can be used for cleaning and deodorizing suppurating eczematous reactions and wounds. It is available as tablets for dissolving in solution for topical application.
✚▲ Side-effects/warnings: See POTASSIUM PERMANGANATE.

perphenazine
is chemically a PHENOTHIAZINE. It is used as an ANTIPSYCHOTIC drug to treat schizophrenia and other severe psychoses, in the short-term treatment of severe anxiety in conjunction with other drugs (including a compound preparation with an ANTIDEPRESSANT), and as an ANTINAUSEANT and ANTI-EMETIC to relieve nausea and vomiting. Administration is oral.
✚▲ Side-effects/warnings: These depend on use, see CHLORPROMAZINE HYDROCHLORIDE; but is less sedating, but extrapyramidal symptoms (especially dystonia) are more likely.
✪ **Related entries: Fentazin; Triptafen.**

Persantin
(Boehringer Ingelheim) is a proprietary, prescription-only preparation of the ANTIPLATELET drug dipyridamole. It can be used to prevent thrombosis, and is available as tablets and in a form for injection. There is also a modified-release form called *Persantin Retard* in the form of capsules.
✚▲ Side-effects/warnings: See DIPYRIDAMOLE.

pertussis vaccine
(whooping-cough) is a VACCINE used for IMMUNIZATION and is a suspension of dead pertussis bacteria *Bordetella pertussis*. When injected, it causes the body's immune system to form antibodies against the bacteria and so

provide *active immunity*. Administration of the vaccine is normally by three injections one month apart and is combined with diphtheria and tetanus vaccine (*triple vaccine*) or adsorbed diphtheria, tetanus and pertussis vaccine (DTPer/Vac/Ads). It is given by injection.

✚▲ Side-effects/warnings: See VACCINE. Also, it is administered with particular care to children with a history of febrile convulsions, and with caution to children whose relatives have a history of seizures or who appear to have any form of neurological disorder.

✪ Related entries: ACT-HIB DTP dc; Adsorbed Diphtheria, Tetanus and Pertussis Vaccine; Adsorbed Diphtheria, Tetanus and [whole-cell] Pertussis Vaccine; Infanrix; Infanrix-HIB.

Per/Vac

is an abbreviation for PERTUSSIS VACCINE (whooping cough vaccine), which is usually administered in combination with diphtheria and tetanus vaccine (*triple vaccine*) as DTPer/Vac/Ads.

✚▲ Side-effects/warnings: See PERTUSSIS VACCINE.

pethidine hydrochloride

is an (OPIOID) NARCOTIC ANALGESIC which is used primarily for the relief of moderate to severe pain, especially during labour and operations. It is less effective than morphine and not suitable for relieving severe, chronic pain. Its effect is rapid and short-lasting, so its SEDATIVE properties are made use of only as a premedication prior to surgery, or to enhance the effects of anaesthetic drugs during or following surgery. Administration is either oral or by injection. All its proprietary and non-proprietary preparations are on the Controlled Drugs list.

✚▲ Side-effects/warnings: See OPIOID; but, compared to many opioids, it is less likely to cause constipation and there is less depression of respiration in the newborn when used to relieve pain during labour. It should not be used in patients with severe kidney damage. Overdose can cause convulsions.

✪ Related entry: Pamergan P100.

Pevaryl

(Janssen-Cilag) is a proprietary, non-prescription preparation of the ANTIFUNGAL drug econazole nitrate. It can be used to treat fungal infections on the skin, such as nail infections and in the genital areas, and is available as a cream.

✚▲ Side-effects/warnings: See ECONAZOLE NITRATE; but side-effects are limited with topical application.

Pharmalgen

(ALK-Abello) is a proprietary, prescription-only preparation of desensitizing vaccine. It is available in a version for bee venom or for wasp venom and can be used in diagnosing and desensitizing patients who are allergic to one or the other. It is available in a form for injection.

✚▲ Side-effects/warnings: See DESENSITIZING VACCINE.

Pharmorubicin Rapid Dissolution

(Pharmacia) is a proprietary, prescription-only preparation of the ANTICANCER drug epirubicin hydrochloride. It can be used to treat several types of cancer, and is available in a form for injection.

✚▲ Side-effects/warnings: See EPIRUBICIN HYDROCHLORIDE.

Pharmorubicin Solution for Injection

(Pharmacia) is a proprietary, prescription-only preparation of the ANTICANCER drug epirubicin hydrochloride. It can be used to treat several types of cancer, and is available in a form for injection.

✚▲ Side-effects/warnings: See EPIRUBICIN HYDROCHLORIDE.

phenazocine hydrobromide

is an (OPIOID) NARCOTIC ANALGESIC which is used primarily to relieve severe pain, and has less tendency to raise biliary pressure so can be used for pain arising from disorders of the bile ducts. Administration is oral. Its proprietary preparation is on the Controlled Drugs list.

✚▲ Side-effects/warnings: See OPIOID.

✪ Related entry: Narphen.

phenelzine

is an ANTIDEPRESSANT of the MONOAMINE-OXIDASE INHIBITOR (MAOI) group. It is used particularly when treatment with TRICYCLIC antidepressants (eg AMITRIPTYLINE HYDROCHLORIDE or IMIPRAMINE HYDROCHLORIDE) has failed, and is one of the safer, less STIMULANT MAO inhibitors. However, a suitably long wash-out period is necessary before switching between different groups of antidepressant. Administration (as phenelzine sulphate) is oral.

✚ Side-effects: These are many and may include; drowsiness, fatigue, headache; there may be weakness and dizziness, particularly on standing up from lying or sitting (postural hypotension). There may be dry mouth and blurred vision, difficulty in urinating, constipation, sweating, oedema, rash, nervousness and sexual disturbances. There may be changes in appetite and weight gain. Susceptible patients may experience agitation, confusion, hallucinations, tremor or even psychotic episodes. There are rare reports of jaundice and liver disorders, of severely lowered blood sodium and of peripheral nerve disease.

▲ Warnings: It should not be administered to patients with certain liver disorders, vascular disease of the brain or abnormal secretion of hormones by the adrenal glands (phaeochromocytoma). Administer with caution to patients with certain cardiovascular diseases, epilepsy, diabetes, blood disorders or who are agitated or elderly. Counselling, or supervision, over diet and taking any other medication is essential as serious adverse reactions can occur. Treatment with the drug requires a strict dietary regime (for example, a patient must avoid eating cheese, meat or yeast extracts, or drinking alcoholic beverages) and extreme care must be taken if using certain other forms of medication (eg 'cold-cures'). One symptom of (hypertensive) adverse effects from ripe foods and cheese is a throbbing headache. Withdrawal of treatment should be gradual. Driving skill is impaired.

✪ **Related entry: Nardil.**

Phenergan

(Rhône-Poulenc Rorer; Aventis Pharma) is a proprietary, non-prescription preparation of the ANTIHISTAMINE promethazine hydrochloride. It can be used for the symptomatic relief of allergic conditions of the upper respiratory tract and skin, including hay fever, allergic rhinitis, urticaria and for the treatment of anaphylactic reaction. It has marked SEDATIVE actions and can be used as a HYPNOTIC in treating temporary sleep disorders and as an ANTINAUSEANT to prevent motion sickness. It is available as tablets and an elixir. It is also available on a prescription-only basis in a form for injection.

✚▲ Side-effects/warnings: See PROMETHAZINE HYDROCHLORIDE.

phenindione

is a synthetic ANTICOAGULANT drug which is effective when taken orally (though it is not as commonly used as warfarin sodium) and is used in the treatment and prevention of thrombosis, such as after insertion of prosthetic heart valves. Administration is oral.

✚▲ Side-effects/warnings: See WARFARIN SODIUM. There may also be hypersensitivity reactions, including rashes and fever; blood disorders; diarrhoea; kidney and liver damage. Urine may be coloured pink or orange. Avoid when breast-feeding.

✪ **Related entry: Dindevan.**

pheniramine maleate

is an ANTIHISTAMINE which can be used for the symptomatic relief of allergic symptoms such as hay fever and urticaria. It is also a constituent of several cough and decongestant preparations. Administration is oral.

✚▲ Side-effects/warnings: See ANTIHISTAMINE. Because of its sedative property, the performance of skilled tasks, such as driving, may be impaired.

phenobarbital

(phenobarbitone) is a BARBITURATE which is used as an ANTICONVULSANT and ANTI-EPILEPTIC in the prevention of most types of recurrent epileptic seizures (except absence seizures) and for status epilepticus. Administration is either oral or by injection. Preparations containing phenobarbital are on the Controlled Drugs list.

✚▲ Side-effects/warnings: See BARBITURATE. It may cause megaloblastic anaemia.

✪ **Related entry: Gardenal Sodium.**

phenobarbitone

see PHENOBARBITAL.

phenol

or carbolic acid, is a DISINFECTANT and ANTISEPTIC which is used for cleaning wounds or inflammation (such as boils and abscesses), for mouth, throat or ear hygiene and to inject into haemorrhoids. Administration is topical.

✚ Side-effects: There may be skin irritation.

▲ Warnings: It is toxic and corrosive if swallowed in concentrated form.

✪ **Related entries: Blisteze; Germolene Cream; Germolene Ointment; Lacto-Calamine Lotion; TCP Antiseptic Ointment; TCP Liquid Antiseptic.**

phenolphthalein

is a *stimulant* LAXATIVE which works by having an irritant action on the gastrointestinal tract. It is now largely obsolete due to its side-effects and long-lasting action, which may continue for several days because the drug is recycled through the liver. Currently, there are no proprietary preparations that contain phenolphthalein.
✚▲ Side-effects/warnings: The laxative effects may continue for several days; there may be discolouration of the urine and skin rashes.

phenothiazine 🅱

drugs are a group of drugs with similar chemical structures. Many of them are used as ANTIPSYCHOTIC drugs (eg CHLORPROMAZINE HYDROCHLORIDE, FLUPHENAZINE, PROMAZINE HYDROCHLORIDE, THIORIDAZINE and TRIFLUOPERAZINE) and it is thought that their ability to block DOPAMINE receptors in the brain is the reason for their usefulness in treating psychoses (eg PERPHENAZINE and PROCHLORPERAZINE). There are other antipsychotic drugs that belong to yet other chemical groups, but in their actions tend to resemble some of the phenothiazines (including the *butyrophenones* (BENPERIDOL, HALOPERIDOL); *diphenylbutylpiperidines* (PIMOZIDE); *thioxanthenes* (FLUPENTIXOL, ZUCLOPENTHIXOL); *benzamides* (SULPIRIDE, OXYPERTINE, LOXAPINE). A number of phenothiazines have powerful ANTINAUSEANT or ANTI-EMETIC actions, and others (eg PIPERAZINE) are ANTHELMINTIC. See also LEVOMEPROMAZINE (methotrimeprazine); PERICYAZINE; PIPOTIAZINE PALMITATE; THIORIDAZINE.
▲ Warnings: Evening primrose oil, which some people take as a nutritional supplement, should be avoided when taking phenothiazines because it has been reported to increase the risk of epileptic side-effects.

phenothrin

is a PEDICULICIDAL drug which is used to treat infestations by head and pubic lice (crabs). Administration is topical.
✚ Side-effects: There may be skin irritation.
▲ Warnings: Avoid contact with the eyes and do not use on broken or infected skin. It may cause wheezing in asthmatics.
✪ **Related entries: Full Marks Lotion; Full Marks Mousse.**

phenoxybenzamine hydrochloride

is an ALPHA-ADRENOCEPTOR BLOCKER which is used, in combination with BETA-BLOCKER drugs, as a short-term ANTIHYPERTENSIVE and for severe hypertensive crises in phaeochromocytoma. It can also be used to manage severe shock that is unresponsive to conventional treatment. Administration is either oral, or by intravenous injection or infusion.
✚ Side-effects: The heart rate increases; there may be postural hypotension (dizziness, particularly on standing up from a lying or sitting position) and lethargy. There is sometimes nasal congestion and contraction of the pupils of the eye (miosis). There may be gastrointestinal disturbances or a failure to ejaculate.
▲ Warnings: It should be administered with caution to patients with certain heart and cardiovascular conditions, impaired kidney function or who are elderly.
✪ **Related entry: Dibenyline.**

phenoxymethylpenicillin

(penicillin V) is a widely used ANTIBACTERIAL and ANTIBIOTIC drug. It is particularly effective in treating tonsillitis, infection of the middle ear, certain skin infections and to prevent recurrent streptococcal throat infection, rheumatic fever or pneumococcal infection (eg following splenectomy or sickle cell anaemia). Administration is oral.
✚▲ Side-effects/warnings: See BENZYLPENICILLIN.
✪ **Related entries: Apsin; Tenkicin.**

Phensic Original

(Merck Consumer Health; Seven Seas) is a proprietary, non-prescription compound preparation of the (NSAID) NON-NARCOTIC ANALGESIC and ANTIRHEUMATIC aspirin and the STIMULANT caffeine. It can be used to treat mild to moderate pain and to relieve the symptoms of mild upper airways infections, such as colds and flu. It is available as capsule-shaped tablets and is not normally given to children, except on medical advice.
✚▲ Side-effects/warnings: See ASPIRIN; CAFFEINE.

phentolamine mesilate

(phentolamine mesylate) is an ALPHA-ADRENOCEPTOR BLOCKER which is used as an ANTIHYPERTENSIVE for hypertensive crises in phaeochromocytoma (it is also used in the diagnosis of this condition) and may have some use in IMPOTENCE TREATMENT for erectile dysfunction. Administration is by injection.
✚ Side-effects: Postural hypotension (fall in blood pressure on standing); dizziness; dry mouth and nasal congestion; chest pains and heart irregularities.
▲ Warnings: It should not be used in certain heart disorders or gastrointestinal disorders (ulcer). It should be administered with care to patients with kidney impairment, who are pregnant or have various vascular or blood disorders.
✪ Related entry: Rogitine.

phentolamine mesylate

see PHENTOLAMINE MESILATE.

phenylbutazone

is a (NSAID) NON-NARCOTIC ANALGESIC and ANTIRHEUMATIC which, because of its sometimes severe side-effects, is used solely in the treatment of ankylosing spondylitis under special conditions of medical supervision in hospitals. Even for that purpose it is used only when all other therapies have failed and treatment may then be prolonged. Administration is oral.
✚ Side-effects: There may be gastrointestinal disturbances, nausea, vomiting and allergic reactions, such as a rash. Less often there is inflammation of the salivary glands of the mouth, throat and neck; and visual disturbances. Rarely, there is severe fluid retention (which in susceptible patients may eventually precipitate heart failure) and serious and potentially dangerous blood disorders.
▲ Warnings: There are many; this is a specialist drug used under carefully monitored conditions.
✪ Related entry: Butacote.

phenylephrine hydrochloride

is an ALPHA-ADRENOCEPTOR STIMULANT, a SYMPATHOMIMETIC and VASOCONSTRICTOR drug incorporated into a number of proprietary cold cures taken orally, as a vasoconstrictor and DECONGESTANT both orally and by nasal spray, and in eye-drops to dilate the pupil to facilitate ophthalmic examination. In emergency situations, it can be administered by intravenous injection or infusion to increase blood pressure.
✚ Side-effects: When taken as eye-drops, there may be blurred vision, stinging, pain in the eye and photophobia. Systemic effects when taken orally (or absorbed from nasal spray or eye-drops), including hypertension and headache; changes in heart rate; vomiting, tingling and coolness of the skin.
▲ Warnings: See NORADRENALINE ACID TARTRATE. It should not be given to patients with hyperthyroidism or severe hypertension.
✪ Related entries: Anadin Cold Control Capsules; Anadin Cold Control Flu Strength Hot Lemon;Beechams All-In-One; Beechams Cold and Flu Hot Blackcurrant; Beechams Cold and Flu Hot Lemon; Beechams Flu-Plus Caplets; Beechams Flu-Plus Hot Berry Fruits; Beechams Flu-Plus Hot Lemon; Beechams Powders Capsules; Betnovate; Fenox Nasal Drops; Fenox Nasal Spray; Isopto Frin; Lemsip Cold + Flu Breathe Easy; Lemsip Cold + Flu Max Strength; Lemsip Cold + Flu Max Strength Capsules; Lemsip Cold + Flu Original Lemon; Minims Phenylephrine Hydrochloride; Paracets Plus Capsules; Phenylephrine Injection.

Phenylephrine Injection

(Sovereign) is a proprietary, prescription-only preparation of the SYMPATHOMIMETIC and VASOCONSTRICTOR drug phenylephrine hydrochloride. It can be used to treat cases of acute hypotension, particularly in emergency situations as a temporary measure. It is available in a form for injection.
✚▲ Side-effects/warnings: See PHENYLEPHRINE HYDROCHLORIDE.

phenylpropanolamine hydrochloride

is a SYMPATHOMIMETIC and VASOCONSTRICTOR drug which is used systemically as an upper airways DECONGESTANT in the symptomatic relief of allergic disorders, such as asthma and hay fever (when it is often administered with an ANTIHISTAMINE), and also for the symptomatic relief of colds and flu (often in combination with an ANALGESIC). Administration can be by several routes, including orally in various forms.
✚▲ Side-effects/warnings: See EPHEDRINE HYDROCHLORIDE. Also, phenylpropanolamine may aggravate conditions such as diabetes, glaucoma and prostatic enlargement.

P

✪ Related entries: Benylin Day and Night; Contac 400; Day Nurse Capsules; Day Nurse Liquid; Sinutab Tablets.

phenytoin

is an ANTICONVULSANT and ANTI-EPILEPTIC drug which is used to treat most forms of epilepsy (except absence seizures) and trigeminal (facial) neuralgia, and in neurosurgery. Administration (as phenytoin or phenytoin sodium) is either oral or by injection.

✚ Side-effects: These include, depending on whether taken orally or by injection, nausea, vomiting, confusion, headache, dizziness, nervousness, insomnia; rarely, movement disorders, peripheral nerve disorders, slurred speech, eye-flicker and blurred vision, rashes, acne, enlargement of the gums, growth of excess hair and blood disorders; also a number of other side-effects.

▲ Warnings: It should be administered with caution to patients with liver impairment or who are pregnant or breast-feeding; avoid its use in those with porphyria. Withdrawal of treatment should be gradual. Medical advice should be sought if there is fever, rash, sore throat, bruising or mouth ulcers. Some ANTIDEPRESSANT agents (and St John's wort) may decrease the blood concentration and effects of phenytoin. Some ulcer-healing drugs (CIMETIDINE and PROTON-PUMP INHIBITOR agents) may increase its effects.

✪ Related entries: Epanutin; Epanutin Ready Mixed Parenteral.

Phillips' Milk of Magnesia

(GSK Consumer Healthcare) is a proprietary, non-prescription preparation of the ANTACID magnesium hydroxide. It can be used to relieve stomach discomfort, indigestion, hyperacidity, heartburn, flatulence and constipation. It is available as a suspension and is not normally given to children under one, except on medical advice.

✚▲ Side-effects/warnings: See MAGNESIUM HYDROXIDE.

Phillips' Milk of Magnesia Tablets

(GSK Consumer Healthcare) is a proprietary, non-prescription preparation of the ANTACID magnesium hydroxide. It can be used to relieve indigestion, nausea, biliousness, acid stomach, heartburn and flatulence. It is available as tablets and is not normally given to children under six, except on medical advice.

✚▲ Side-effects/warnings: See MAGNESIUM HYDROXIDE.

Phimetin

(BHR) is a proprietary, prescription-only preparation of the H_2-ANTAGONIST cimetidine. It can be used as an ULCER-HEALING DRUG for benign peptic ulcers (in the stomach or duodenum), gastro-oesophageal reflux, dyspepsia and associated conditions. It is available as tablets.

✚▲ Side-effects/warnings: See CIMETIDINE.

pHiso-Med

(Sanofi-Synthelabo) is a proprietary, non-prescription preparation of the ANTISEPTIC chlorhexidine (as gluconate). It can be used as a soap or shampoo substitute in acne and seborrhoeic conditions, and also for bathing babies in maternity units to prevent cross infection. It is available as a solution.

✚▲ Side-effects/warnings: See CHLORHEXIDINE.

pholcodine

is a weak OPIOID which is used as a cough treatment as an ANTITUSSIVE constituent in many cough linctuses or syrups (in preference to stronger opioids of the NARCOTIC ANALGESIC type). Although its action resembles that of other opioids, it has no appreciable analgesic effect or addictive liability.

✚▲ Side-effects/warnings: See OPIOID; but normally has only mild adverse effects.

✪ Related entries: Benylin Children's Dry Coughs; Care Pholcodine Linctus; Galenphol Linctus; Galenphol Paediatric Linctus; Hill's Balsam Dry Cough Liquid; Pavacol-D; Tixylix Cough and Cold; Tixylix Daytime; Tixylix Night-Time SF.

Phosphate-Sandoz

(HK Pharma) is a proprietary, non-prescription compound preparation of potassium bicarbonate, sodium acid phosphate and sodium bicarbonate. It can be used as a MINERAL SUPPLEMENT to provide calcium or phosphate. It is available as tablets.

✚▲ Side-effects/warnings: See POTASSIUM BICARBONATE; SODIUM ACID PHOSPHATE; SODIUM BICARBONATE.

phosphodiesterase inhibitor 🅴

drugs are a relatively new class which work by

inhibiting certain enzymes and so affect the heart, especially the heart muscle (myocardium), in ways that are very similar to the SYMPATHOMIMETIC drugs acting at beta-adrenoceptors, and are also vasodilators (see VASODILATOR). They have so far mainly been used in short-term HEART FAILURE TREATMENT, especially where other drugs have been unsuccessful. The group includes ENOXIMONE and MILRINONE. The vasodilator action is utilized in SILDENAFIL (an impotence treatment for men).

photodynamic therapy

(photochemotherapy) is a method of drug treatment where drugs are used as photosensitizers, so that light radiation in the visible and near ultraviolet region of the spectrum is activated to produce the required pharmacological effect. In the past, this principle was used with drugs based on plant pigment (eg buttercups) combined with natural ultraviolet light to treat skin conditions such as vitiligo and psoriasis. In more recent times, intense UVB lamps or laser light of a certain wavelength (non-thermal red light) have been used to activate synthetic compounds. Where activation produced cytotoxic metabolites, this procedure has been evaluated in local ANTICANCER treatment for superficial carcinomas. Currently, the drug VERTEPORFIN is licensed for use in the photodynamic treatment of subfoveal choroidal neovascularization associated with age-related macular degeneration or with pathological myopia. This actually results in some damage to the macula (a central area of the retina), but principally it damages networks of small, recently formed blood vessels which are the cause of the problem. Eventually, these would cause scarring if allowed to grow and then contract, as usually happens in a particular form of macular degeneration called 'wet'. Also, the drug PORFIMER SODIUM has been licensed for photodynamic therapy of non-small cell lung cancer and obstructing oesophageal cancer. It accumulates in malignant tissue and is activated by laser light to produce its cytotoxic effect.

Photofrin

(Sinclair) is a newly introduced proprietary, prescription-only preparation of porfimer sodium, which is a CYTOTOXIC drug used in photodynamic therapy for ANTICANCER treatment of non-small cell lung cancer and oesophageal cancer. It is available in a form for injection.

✚▲ Side-effects/warnings: See PORFIMER SODIUM.

Phyllocontin Continus

(Napp) is a proprietary, non-prescription preparation of the BRONCHODILATOR aminophylline. It can be used as an ANTI-ASTHMATIC, and is available as tablets and modified-release tablets (*Forte tablets*) and paediatric tablets.

✚▲ Side-effects/warnings: See AMINOPHYLLINE.

Physeptone

(Martindale) is a proprietary, prescription-only preparation of the (OPIOID) NARCOTIC ANALGESIC and ANTITUSSIVE methadone hydrochloride, and is on the Controlled Drugs list. It can be used to treat severe pain, in detox therapy, and is available as tablets and in a form for injection.

✚▲ Side-effects/warnings: See METHADONE HYDROCHLORIDE.

Physiotens

(Solvay) is a proprietary, prescription-only preparation of the ANTIHYPERTENSIVE moxonidine. It can be used to treat mild to moderate essential hypertension, and is available as tablets.

✚▲ Side-effects/warnings: See MOXONIDINE.

Phytex

(Forest) is a proprietary, non-prescription compound preparation of several ANTIFUNGAL and KERATOLYTIC drugs, including salicylic acid, tannic acid and boric acid (with ethyl acetate and alcohol). It can be used to treat fungal (*Candida*) infections of the skin and nails, and is available as a paint for topical application.

✚▲ Side-effects/warnings: See SALICYLIC ACID.

phytomenadione

(vitamin K_1) is a natural form of VITAMIN K and is normally obtained from vegetables and dairy products. Phytomenadione can be used to treat vitamin K deficiency, but not a deficiency caused by malabsorption states (in such cases vitamin K_1 or MENADIOL SODIUM PHOSPHATE, the synthetic form of vitamin K_3, must be used). It is given as a single intramuscular injection, or by mouth to prevent vitamin K deficiency bleeding in newborn babies. Administration is either oral or by slow intravenous injection.

✚▲ Side-effects/warnings: See VITAMIN K.

✪ **Related entries: Konakion; Konakion MM; Konakion MM Paediatric.**

Picolax

(Nordic; Ferring) is a proprietary, non-prescription preparation of the (*stimulant*) LAXATIVE sodium picosulfate and magnesium citrate. It can be used to evacuate the bowels before surgery, radiography or endoscopy, and is available as an oral solution.

✚▲ Side-effects/warnings: See SODIUM PICOSULFATE.

pilocarpine

is a PARASYMPATHOMIMETIC drug. It can be applied to the eye to treat glaucoma by improving drainage of aqueous fluid from the eye, and to constrict the pupil of the eye after it has been dilated for ophthalmic examination (administration is as eye-drops). It can be used to alleviate the symptoms of salivary gland hypofunction with dry mouth following irradiation for head and neck cancer (administration is oral).

✚ Side-effects: When taken orally, there may be sweating; chills; diarrhoea or constipation, nausea and vomiting, abdominal pain, hypertension, abnormal vision, tears, dizziness, rhinitis, weakness, increased urinary frequency, headache, dyspepsia, vasodilatation, flushing. Other possible side-effects include effects on the heart and breathing, confusion and tremors. When used for glaucoma treatment, there may be browache and headache, which may get worse in the weeks following treatment. There may also be blurred vision, itching, burning and smarting, and other effects on the eye.

▲ Warnings: It is not used in pregnancy and breast-feeding. Systemic effects do not apply, or are rare, when application is to the eye. When used as eye-drops, blurring may affect the ability to perform skilled tasks, such as driving.

✪ **Related entries: Minims Pilocarpine Nitrate; Pilogel; Salagen.**

Pilogel

(Alcon) is a proprietary, prescription-only preparation of the PARASYMPATHOMIMETIC pilocarpine (with carbomer gel). It can be used in GLAUCOMA TREATMENT and to facilitate inspection of the eye. It is available as an eye gel.

✚▲ Side-effects/warnings: See CARBOMER; PILOCARPINE.

pimozide

is an ANTIPSYCHOTIC drug (of the *diphenylbutylpiperidines* chemical group) which is used to treat patients suffering from psychotic disorders, such as schizophrenia, hypochondriacal psychosis and paranoid psychosis. It can also be used to treat Gilles de la Tourette syndrome. Administration is oral.

✚▲ Side-effects/warnings: There are a number, see CHLORPROMAZINE HYDROCHLORIDE, but it is less sedating. It is not to be given to patients who are breast-feeding or with certain heart arrhythmias. ECGs may be taken before and during treatment.

✪ **Related entry: Orap.**

pindolol

is a BETA-BLOCKER which can be used as an ANTIHYPERTENSIVE for raised blood pressure and as an ANTI-ANGINA treatment to relieve symptoms and improve exercise tolerance. Administration is oral. It is also available, as an antihypertensive treatment, in a compound preparation with a DIURETIC.

✚▲ Side-effects/warnings: See PROPRANOLOL HYDROCHLORIDE.

✪ **Related entries: Viskaldix; Visken.**

pioglitazone

is a newly introduced drug which is used in DIABETIC TREATMENT of Type II diabetes (non-insulin-dependent diabetes mellitus; NIDDM; maturity-onset diabetes). It is one of the thiazolidinedione group which reduces peripheral insulin resistance, and this causes a reduction of blood-glucose concentration. Treatment with pioglitazone is started by a physician experienced in treating Type II diabetes and should always be used in combination with metformin (or with a SULPHONYLUREA if METFORMIN HYDROCHLORIDE is inappropriate). Authorities have recommended pioglitazone combination therapy as an alternative to insulin for certain people. Administration is oral.

✚ Side-effects: Gastrointestinal disturbances,

oedema, weight gain, anaemia, headache, visual disturbances, dizziness, pain in the joints, impotence, blood in the urine; also less commonly hypoglycaemia, fatigue, sweating, altered blood lipids, proteinuria.
▲ Warnings: Pioglitazone should not be given to people with liver impairment or heart failure, or to anyone who is pregnant or breast-feeding. Liver and cardiovascular function will be monitored during treatment. There have been rare reports of liver dysfunction; so immediate medical attention should be sought if symptoms develop that indicate liver problems, such as abdominal pain, nausea and vomiting, fatigue and dark urine; and treatment will be discontinued if jaundice occurs.
✪ **Related entry: Actos.**

piperacillin

is a broad-spectrum ANTIBACTERIAL and (PENICILLIN) ANTIBIOTIC which is used to treat many serious or compound forms of bacterial infection, particularly those caused by *Pseudomonas aeruginosa*, and in prophylaxis after surgery. Administration is by intravenous injection or infusion.
✚▲ Side-effects/warnings: See BENZYLPENICILLIN.
✪ **Related entries: Pipril; Tazocin.**

piperazine

is an ANTHELMINTIC drug (a PHENOTHIAZINE) which is used to treat infestation by roundworm or threadworm. Administration is oral.
✚ Side-effects: There may be nausea and vomiting with diarrhoea and colic, drowsiness; there may also be allergic reactions, such as urticaria. Rarely, there is dizziness and lack of muscular coordination ('worm wobble').
▲ Warnings: It should be administered with caution to patients with certain kidney or liver disorders, epilepsy, neurological disease or who are pregnant.
✪ **Related entry: Pripsen Piperazine Phosphate Powder.**

piperazine estrone sulphate

see ESTROPIPATE.

piperazine oestrone sulphate

see ESTROPIPATE.

Piportil Depot

(JHC) is a proprietary, prescription-only preparation of the ANTIPSYCHOTIC drug pipotiazine palmitate. It can be used in maintenance therapy of patients with psychotic disorders, such as chronic schizophrenia. Administration is by a long-acting depot deep intramuscular injection.
✚▲ Side-effects/warnings: See PIPOTIAZINE PALMITATE.

pipothiazine palmitate

see PIPOTIAZINE PALMITATE.

pipotiazine palmitate

(pipothiazine palmitate) is a PHENOTHIAZINE derivative, which is used as an ANTIPSYCHOTIC in maintenance therapy of patients with schizophrenia and other psychoses. Administration is by injection.
✚▲ Side-effects/warnings: See CHLORPROMAZINE HYDROCHLORIDE. There may be pain, redness and swelling at the injection site.
✪ **Related entry: Piportil Depot.**

Pipril

(Lederle; Wyeth) is a proprietary, prescription-only preparation of the broad-spectrum ANTIBACTERIAL and (PENICILLIN) ANTIBIOTIC piperacillin. It can be used to treat a range of bacterial infections, and is available in a form for intravenous injection or infusion.
✚▲ Side-effects/warnings: See PIPERACILLIN.

piracetam

is an ANTI-EPILEPTIC drug which is used in the treatment of cortical myoclonus (involuntary spasmic contractions of muscles of the body). There are also unconfirmed reports that it is a NOOTROPIC AGENT, a cognition enhancer that allegedly improves mental performance. Administration is oral.
✚ Side-effects: Diarrhoea, weight gain, sleepiness, insomnia, depression, rash and overactivity.
▲ Warnings: It should not be used in patients with severe liver or kidney impairment, or who are pregnant or breast-feeding. Withdrawal of treatment should be gradual.
✪ **Related entry: Nootropil.**

Piriton

(Stafford-Miller; GSK) is a proprietary, non-prescription preparation of the ANTIHISTAMINE chlorphenamine maleate (chlorpheniramine

maleate). It can be used to treat allergic conditions, such as hay fever and urticaria, and is available as tablets and a syrup; it is also available on a prescription-only basis in a form for injection.
✚▲ Side-effects/warnings: See CHLORPHENAMINE MALEATE.

Piriton Allergy Tablets

(Stafford-Miller; GSK) is a proprietary, non-prescription preparation of the ANTIHISTAMINE chlorphenamine maleate (chlorpheniramine maleate). It can be used for symptomatic relief of allergic conditions, such as hay fever, nettle rash, heat rash, insect bites and stings and urticaria, and is available as tablets. It is not normally given to children under six years, except on medical advice.
✚▲ Side-effects/warnings: See CHLORPHENAMINE MALEATE.

Piriton Syrup

(Stafford-Miller; GSK) is a proprietary, non-prescription preparation of the ANTIHISTAMINE chlorphenamine maleate (chlorpheniramine maleate). It can be used for symptomatic relief of allergic conditions, such as hay fever, nettle rash, heat rash, insect bites and stings and urticaria, and is available as a syrup. It is not normally given to children under one, except on medical advice.
✚▲ Side-effects/warnings: See CHLORPHENAMINE MALEATE.

piroxicam

is a (NSAID) NON-NARCOTIC ANALGESIC and ANTIRHEUMATIC drug. It has a long duration of action and is used to treat pain and inflammation in rheumatic disease and other musculoskeletal disorders, including juvenile arthritis and acute gout. Administration can be oral, topical (gel or suppositories) or by injection.
✚▲ Side-effects/warnings: See NSAID. It may cause pain at the injection site; it may cause pancreatitis or gastrointestinal disturbances, especially in the elderly. It should not be used by anyone with porphyria. There is a relatively high risk of gastric bleeding.
✪ Related entries: Brexidol; Feldene; Feldene P Gel; Flamatrol; Kentene; Pirozip.

Pirozip

(Ashbourne) is a proprietary, prescription-only preparation of the (NSAID) NON-NARCOTIC ANALGESIC and ANTIRHEUMATIC piroxicam. It can be used to treat acute gout, arthritic and rheumatic pain and other musculoskeletal disorders. It is available as capsules.
✚▲ Side-effects/warnings: See PIROXICAM.

Pitressin

(Goldshield) is a proprietary, prescription-only preparation of the HORMONE vasopressin. It can be administered as a DIABETES INSIPIDUS TREATMENT. Alternatively, it can be used to treat the bleeding of varices (varicose veins) in the oesophagus. It is available in a form for injection.
✚▲ Side-effects/warnings: See VASOPRESSIN.

pivmecillinam hydrochloride

is an ANTIBACTERIAL and ANTIBIOTIC drug, one of the extensive penicillin-like BETA-LACTAM group, but within a new class called *mecillinams* (it is converted in the body to mecillinam, the active drug). It can be used to treat infections caused by Gram-negative bacteria, including *Pseudomonas aeruginosa, Escherichia coli*, klebsiella, enterobacter and salmonellae infections. Administration is oral.
✚▲ Side-effects/warnings: See BENZYLPENICILLIN. Also: vomiting, nausea, diarrhoea, dyspepsia, blood changes. Not used in caritinine deficiency, obstruction and other gastrointestinal disorders. Caution in pregnancy, liver and kidney tests needed with prolonged use.
✪ Related entry: Selexid.

Piz Buin SPF 30 Sun Block Lotion

(Novartis Consumer Health) is a proprietary, non-prescription SUNSCREEN lotion that protects the skin from ultraviolet radiation in people who suffer from skin photosensitivity because of genetic or other conditions or after radiotherapy. It is a cream-coloured skin lotion, containing the pigment titanium dioxide (along with butylmethoxydibenzoyl methane and ethyl hexyl methoxycinnamate), which is applied prior to exposure to the sun.
✚▲ Side-effects/warnings: TITANIUM DIOXIDE.

pizotifen

is an ANTIHISTAMINE and SEROTONIN antagonist which can be used as an ANTIMIGRAINE treatment, particularly for headaches in which blood pressure inside the blood vessels plays a part, such as migraine and cluster headache. Administration is oral.

✚ Side-effects: Anticholinergic effects, drowsiness, increased appetite and weight gain, occasionally nausea and dizziness.

▲ Warnings: It should be administered with care to patients with urinary retention, kidney impairment, closed-angle glaucoma; or who are pregnant or breast-feeding. Drowsiness may impair the performance of skilled tasks, such as driving.

✪ **Related entry: Sanomigran.**

Plaquenil

(Sanofi-Synthelabo) is a proprietary, prescription-only preparation of hydroxychloroquine sulphate, which has ANTI-INFLAMMATORY and ANTIRHEUMATIC properties. It can be used to treat rheumatoid arthritis (including juvenile arthritis) and lupus and systemic discoid erythematosus. It is available as tablets.

✚▲ Side-effects/warnings: See HYDROXYCHLOROQUINE SULPHATE.

Plavix

(Bristol-Myers Squibb; Sanofi-Synthelabo) is a proprietary, prescription-only preparation of the ANTIPLATELET drug clopidogrel (as hydrogen sulphate). It can be used to prevent thrombosis, and is available as tablets.

✚▲ Side-effects/warnings: See CLOPIDOGREL.

Plendil

(AstraZeneca) is a proprietary, prescription-only preparation of the CALCIUM-CHANNEL BLOCKER felodipine. It can be used as an ANTIHYPERTENSIVE and in ANTI-ANGINA treatment, and is available as modified-release tablets.

✚▲ Side-effects/warnings: See FELODIPINE.

Plesmet

(Link) is a proprietary, non-prescription preparation of ferrous glycine sulphate. It can be used as an IRON supplement in iron deficiency ANAEMIA TREATMENT, and is available as a syrup.

✚▲ Side-effects/warnings: See FERROUS GLYCINE SULPHATE.

pneumococcal polysaccharide vaccine

see PNEUMOCOCCAL VACCINE.

pneumococcal vaccine

(pneumococcal polysaccharide vaccine) is a VACCINE used for IMMUNIZATION against pneumonia. There are two types. First, 'polyvalent unconjugated pneumococcal polysaccharide vaccine' is officially recommended for the immunization of people over the age of two years who have any of a number of conditions, including sickle-cell disease, severe spleen dysfunction, chronic kidney, liver, heart or lung disease, coeliac syndrome, diabetes mellitus, immunodeficiency syndrome or immunosuppression treatment (including HIV infection). Second, 'polyvalent pneumococcal polysaccharide conjugated vaccine' has been recently introduced for the prevention of pneumococcal disease in children between two months and two years. Administration is by subcutaneous or intramuscular injection.

✚▲ Side-effects/warnings: See VACCINE.

✪ **Related entry: Pnu-Imune; Pneumovax II; Prevenar.**

Pneumovax II

(Aventis Pasteur) is a proprietary, prescription-only vaccine preparation of PNEUMOCOCCAL VACCINE in the form 'polyvalent unconjugated pneumococcal polysaccharide vaccine'. It can be used for the prevention of pneumococcal pneumonia in people over two years for whom the risk of contracting the disease is unusually high. It is available in a form for injection.

✚▲ Side-effects/warnings: See VACCINE.

Pnu-Imune

(Wyeth) is a proprietary, prescription-only vaccine preparation of PNEUMOCOCCAL VACCINE in the form 'polyvalent unconjugated pneumococcal polysaccharide vaccine'. It can be used for the prevention of pneumococcal pneumonia in people over two years for whom the risk of contracting the disease is unusually high. It is available in a form for injection.

✚▲ Side-effects/warnings: See VACCINE.

Podophyllin Paint, Compound, BP

is a non-proprietary, prescription-only preparation the KERATOLYTIC agent podophyllum (in benzoin tincture). It can be used for men and women to treat external genital warts (applied weekly by trained nurses). It is

available as a solution for topical application.
✚▲ Side-effects/warnings: See PODOPHYLLUM.

podophyllum
is a KERATOLYTIC and caustic agent which can be used to treat and dissolve warts (including certain anogenital warts), and also to reduce the production of new skin cells. Podophyllotoxin is the main active constituent of podophyllum, and some preparations contain only this. Administration is topical.
✚ Side-effects: It may cause considerable irritation (particularly to eyes), avoid face, normal skin and open wounds.
▲ Warnings: Do not use if pregnant or breast-feeding.
✪ **Related entries: Condyline; Podophyllin Paint, Compound, BP; Posalfilin; Warticon.**

Poliomyelitis Vaccine, Inactivated
(Farillon) (Pol/Vac – Inact) is a non-proprietary, prescription-only VACCINE preparation of poliomyelitis vaccine inactivated (Salk). It can be used to provide immunity from infection by polio, and is available in a form for injection.
✚▲ Side-effects/warnings: See POLIOMYELITIS VACCINES.

Poliomyelitis Vaccine, Live (Oral)
(District Health Authorities; Farillon) (Pol/Vav – Oral) is a non-proprietary, prescription-only VACCINE preparation of poliomyelitis vaccine live, (oral) (Sabin), which contains 'live' but attenuated polio viruses. It can be used to confer immunity from infection, and is available in a form for oral administration.
✚▲ Side-effects/warnings: See POLIOMYELITIS VACCINES.

poliomyelitis vaccines
is a VACCINE used for IMMUNIZATION that is available in two types. Poliomyelitis vaccine, inactivated (Salk) is a suspension of dead viruses injected into the body so that the body produces antibodies and becomes immune. Poliomyelitis vaccine live, (oral) (Sabin) is a suspension of live but attenuated polio viruses (of polio virus types 1, 2 and 3) for oral administration. In the UK, the live oral vaccine is more commonly used and the administration is generally simultaneous with diphtheria-pertussis-tetanus (triple) vaccine during the first year of life with a booster at school-entry age, and another before leaving school. The inactivated vaccine remains available for those patients who, for some reason, cannot use the live vaccine (eg immunodeficiency disorders).
✚▲ Side-effects/warnings: See VACCINE. Strict personal hygiene is important (eg wash hands after changing nappies of recently vaccinated babies).
✪ **Related entries: Poliomyelitis Vaccine, Inactivated; Poliomyelitis Vaccine, Live (Oral).**

Pollinex
(Allergy) is a proprietary, prescription-only preparation of DESENSITIZING VACCINE. It is available in a version of grass or tree pollen extract for treatment of seasonal allergic hay fever due to grass or tree pollen and is used to hyposensitize people who have not responded to anti-allergy drugs. It is available in a form for subcutaneous injection.
✚▲ Side-effects/warnings: See: DESENSITIZING VACCINE.

poloxamer '188'
is a SURFACTANT wetting agent which used in combination with LAXATIVE dantron is an effective laxative: versions are called CO-DANTHRAMER 25/200 and CO-DANTHRAMER 75/1000. Administration is oral.
✚▲ Side-effects/warnings: Used on an occasional basis it is thought to be safe.
✪ **Related entries: Ailax; Codalax; Codalax Forte; co-danthramer 25/200; co-danthramer 75/1000; Danlax.**

Pol/Vac (Inact)
is an abbreviation for POLIOMYELITIS VACCINE, INACTIVATED.

Pol/Vac (Oral)
is an abbreviation for POLIOMYELITIS VACCINE, LIVE (ORAL).

polyacrylic acid
see CARBOMER.

Polyfax
(Dominion) is a proprietary, prescription-only compound preparation of the ANTIBACTERIAL and ANTIBIOTIC drugs, the (POLYMYXIN) polymyxin B sulphate and bacitracin zinc. It can

be used to treat infections of the skin and the eye, and is available for topical application as a skin ointment and an eye ointment.

✚▲ Side-effects/warnings: See BACITRACIN ZINC; POLYMYXIN B SULPHATE.

polymixin

see POLYMYXIN.

polymyxin

(polymixin) is the name of a chemical class of ANTIBIOTIC used for their ANTIBACTERIAL actions. They work by disrupting the bacterial cell membrane, so killing growing bacteria (they are *bactericidal*; that is, they kill bacteria rather than simply inhibit their growth). They are active against Gram-negative bacteria, including *Pseudomonas aeruginosa*, and are used to treat skin infections, burns and wounds. The antibiotics of this group can be administered by injection or topical application; although COLISTIN (polymyxin E) is not absorbed orally it can be used to sterilize the bowel. See also POLYMYXIN B SULPHATE.

polymyxin B sulphate

is an ANTIBACTERIAL and (POLYMYXIN) ANTIBIOTIC which can be used to treat several forms of bacterial infections of ear, eye and skin. Its use is restricted because it is very toxic and because of this toxicity it is mainly administered topically.

✚▲ Side-effects/warnings: Minimal on topical application.

✪ **Related entries: Gregoderm; Maxitrol; Neosporin; Otosporin; Polyfax; Polytrim.**

polysaccharide-iron complex

is a drug rich in IRON which is used in iron-deficiency ANAEMIA TREATMENT to restore iron to the body or prevent deficiency. Administration is oral.

✚▲ Side-effects/warnings: See FERROUS SULPHATE.

✪ **Related entries: Niferex.**

polystyrene sulphonate resins

are used to treat excessively high levels of potassium in the blood (hyperkalaemia), for example, in dialysis patients. Administration is either oral or by topical application in the form of a retention enema.

✚ Side-effects: Treatment by enemas may cause rectal ulcers. Also gastrointestinal effects (eg nausea, diarrhoea).

▲ Warnings: Some resins should not be given to patients with hyperparathyroidism, sarcoidosis, multiple myeloma or metastatic cancer; care is needed in those with congestive heart failure, impaired kidney function, in pregnancy or breast-feeding, and in other conditions. An adequate fluid intake must be maintained.

✪ **Related entries: Calcium Resonium; Resonium A.**

Polytar AF

(Stiefel) is a proprietary, non-prescription preparation of coal tar (with pyrithione). It can be used to treat scaly scalp disorders such as psoriasis, seborrhoeic dermatitis and dandruff, and is available as a shampoo.

✚▲ Side-effects/warnings: See COAL TAR.

Polytar Emmollient

(Stiefel) is a proprietary, non-prescription preparation of coal tar with arachis oil and liquid paraffin. It can be used to treat skin conditions such as psoriasis and eczema, and is available as a bath additive.

✚▲ Side-effects/warnings: See COAL TAR; LIQUID PARAFFIN.

Polytar Liquid

(Stiefel) is a proprietary, non-prescription preparation of coal tar. It can be used to treat scalp conditions, including psoriasis, eczema, seborrhoeic dermatitis and dandruff, and is available as a shampoo.

✚▲ Side-effects/warnings: See COAL TAR.

Polytar Plus

(Stiefel) is a proprietary, non-prescription preparation of coal tar. It can be used to treat scalp conditions such as psoriasis, eczema, seborrhoeic dermatitis and dandruff, and is available as a shampoo.

✚▲ Side-effects/warnings: See COAL TAR.

polythiazide

is one of the THIAZIDE class of DIURETIC. It can be used as an ANTIHYPERTENSIVE, either alone or in conjunction with other types of drugs, and in the treatment of oedema. Administration is oral.

✚▲ Side-effects/warnings: See BENDROFLUMETHIAZIDE.

P

✪ Related entry: Nephril.

Polytrim

(Dominion) is a proprietary, prescription-only compound preparation of the ANTIBACTERIAL and SULPHONAMIDE-like drugtrimethoprim and the ANTIBIOTIC polymyxin B sulphate. It can be used to treat bacterial infections in the eye, and is available as eye-drops and an eye ointment.
✚▲ Side-effects/warnings: See POLYMYXIN B SULPHATE; TRIMETHOPRIM.

polyvinyl alcohol

is a constituent in several preparations that are used as artificial tears to treat dryness of the eye (eg tear deficiency due to disease).
Administration is by topical application.
✚▲ Side-effects/warnings: It is regarded as safe in normal topical use.
✪ Related entries: Hypotears; Ocufen; Sno Tears.

Ponstan

(Chemidex) is a proprietary, prescription-only preparation of the (NSAID) NON-NARCOTIC ANALGESIC and ANTIRHEUMATIC mefenamic acid. It can be used to treat pain in rheumatoid arthritis, osteoarthritis and other musculoskeletal disorders and period pain. It is available as capsules, tablets (*Ponstan Forte*) and as a paediatric oral suspension.
✚▲ Side-effects/warnings: See MEFENAMIC ACID.

porfimer sodium

is an ANTICANCER drug which is used in PHOTODYNAMIC THERAPY where it accumulates in malignant tissue and is activated by laser light to produce its CYTOTOXIC effect. It can be used to treat non-small cell lung cancer and obstructing oesophageal cancer. Given by intravenous injection.
✚ Side-effects: See CYTOTOXIC; there may be photosensitivity (so avoid exposure of skin and eyes to direct sunlight or bright indoor light) and also constipation.
▲ Warnings: See CYTOTOXIC. It is a specialist drug and full patient assessment and suitability will be determined prior to treatment. It is not used in people with severely impaired liver function or those who have tracheo-oesophageal or broncho-oesophageal fistula; or porphyria.

Pork Actrapid

(Novo Nordisk) is a proprietary, prescription-only preparation of highly purified porcine SOLUBLE INSULIN. It is used in DIABETIC TREATMENT to treat and maintain diabetic patients, and is available in vials for injection. It has a relatively short duration of action.
✚▲ Side-effects/warnings: See INSULIN.

Pork Insulatard

(Novo Nordisk) is a proprietary, prescription-only preparation of (porcine) ISOPHANE INSULIN. It is used in DIABETIC TREATMENT to treat and maintain diabetic patients, and is available in vials for injection and has an intermediate duration of action.
✚▲ Side-effects/warnings: See INSULIN.

Pork Mixtard 30

(Novo Nordisk) is a proprietary, prescription-only preparation of BIPHASIC ISOPHANE INSULIN (porcine) containing both ISOPHANE INSULIN and SOLUBLE INSULIN (in a proportion of 70% to 30% respectively). It is used to treat and maintain diabetic patients, has an intermediate duration of action, and is available in vials for injection.
✚▲ Side-effects/warnings: See INSULIN.

Posalfilin

(Norgine) is a proprietary, non-prescription compound preparation of the KERATOLYTIC agents salicylic acid and podophyllum (resin). It can be used to treat and remove plantar warts (verrucas) but not anogenital warts, and is available as an ointment for topical application.
✚▲ Side-effects/warnings: See PODOPHYLLUM; SALICYLIC ACID.

Posiject

(Boehringer Ingelheim) is a proprietary, prescription-only preparation of the CARDIAC STIMULANT dobutamine hydrochloride, which has SYMPATHOMIMETIC and BETA-RECEPTOR STIMULANT properties. It can be used to treat serious heart disorders, such as cardiogenic shock, septic shock, during heart surgery and in cardiac infarction. It is available in a form for intravenous infusion.
✚▲ Side-effects/warnings: See DOBUTAMINE HYDROCHLORIDE.

Potaba

(Glenwood) is a proprietary, non-prescription preparation of potassium aminobenzoate. It can

be used to treat scleroderma and Peyronie's disease, and is available as capsules, tablets and as a powder in sachets (called *Envules*).
✚▲ Side-effects/warnings: See POTASSIUM AMINOBENZOATE.

potassium aminobenzoate

is used in the treatment of disorders associated with excess fibrous tissue, such as scleroderma and Peyronie's disease. There is uncertainty, however, about how it works and how well. Administration is oral.
✚ Side-effects: There may be nausea; anorexia (if so treatment may have to be discontinued).
▲ Warnings: It should not be administered to patients who are taking sulphonamides and with caution to those with kidney disease.
✪ **Related entry: Potaba.**

potassium bicarbonate

is used primarily as a potassium supplement to correct potassium deficiency, especially due to or following severe loss of body fluids (eg chronic diarrhoea). Administration is either oral or by injection or intravenous infusion.
✚▲ Side-effects/warnings: It is regarded as safe in normal use in antacids. Its use in electrolyte correction requires specialist monitoring.
✪ **Related entries: Algicon; Gaviscon Advance; Phosphate-Sandoz; Resolve; Sando-K.**

potassium-channel activator 🄴

drugs work by opening pores in cell membranes which allow potassium ions to pass more readily, which has the effect of making these cells electrically less excitable. In blood vessels such drugs have VASODILATOR effects, which cause a reduction of the heart's workload and generally lowers blood pressure. An example is NICORANDIL, which can be used as an ANTI-ANGINA treatment to prevent and treat attacks of angina pectoris.

potassium chloride

is used primarily as a potassium supplement to correct potassium deficiency, especially due to or following severe loss of body fluids (eg chronic diarrhoea) or during or after treatment with drugs that deplete body reserves (eg some DIURETIC drugs). It is incorporated into body fluid replacement media such as artificial saliva and Balanced Salt Solution. It may also be used as a substitute for natural salt (SODIUM CHLORIDE) in cases where sodium, for one reason or another, is inadvisable. Administration is either oral or by injection or intravenous infusion.
✚▲ Side-effects/warnings: It is considered safe at the recommended dosage.
✪ **Related entries: Burinex K; Centyl K; Dioralyte Natural; Dioralyte Relief; Dioralyte Tablets Raspberry Flavour; Diumide-K Continus; Glandosane; Lasikal; Luborant; Neo-NaClex-K; Sando-K; Slow-K Tablets.**

potassium citrate

when administered orally has the effect of making the urine alkaline instead of acid, which is an action that is useful for relieving pain in some infections of the urinary tract or the bladder. Administration is oral.
✚ Side-effects: There may be a mild diuretic effect.
▲ Warnings: It should be administered with caution to patients with heart disease or impaired kidney function.
✪ **Related entries: Care Potassium Citrate Mixture; Cystopurin; Dioralyte Natural; Dioralyte Relief; Effercitrate; Micolette Micro-enema.**

Potassium Citrate Mixture BP

see EFFERCITRATE.

potassium hydroxyquinoline sulphate

is a drug that has both ANTIBACTERIAL and ANTIFUNGAL properties. It is used mostly as a constituent in anti-inflammatory and antibiotic creams and ointments, for example, in preparations used to treat acne. It is used topically.
✚ Side-effects: Rarely, it may cause sensitivity reactions.
✪ **Related entries: Quinocort; Quinoderm Cream; Quinoderm Cream 5; Quinoderm Lotio-Gel 5%; Quinoped Cream; Valderma Cream.**

potassium permanganate

is a general ANTISEPTIC and DISINFECTANT agent which can be used in solution for cleaning burns and abrasions, and for maintaining asepsis in wounds that are suppurating or weeping.
✚▲ Side-effects/warnings: Avoid contact with mucous membranes, to which it is an irritant. It stains skin and fabric.

✪ **Related entry: Permitabs.**

povidone
is a constituent of artificial tears, which are used to treat extremely dry eyes due to certain disorders. It is available as eye-drops.
✚▲ Side-effects/warnings: It is regarded as safe in normal topical use.
✪ **Related entry: Liquifilm Tears; Oculotect.**

povidone-iodine
is a complex of iodine on an organic carrier and is used as an ANTISEPTIC. It is applied topically to the skin, especially in sensitive areas (such as the vulva), acne of the scalp and is also used as a mouthwash. It works by slowly releasing the iodine it contains and is available as a gel, an oral solution or vaginal inserts (pessaries).
✚ Side-effects: Rarely, there may be sensitivity reactions.
▲ Warnings: These depend on how and where it is applied, but it should be used with care by patients with certain kidney diseases, who are pregnant or planning to become pregnant, breast-feeding, on broken skin, and in thyroid disorders.
✪ **Related entries: Betadine Antiseptic Paint; Betadine Dry Powder Spray;Betadine Gargle and Mouthwash; Betadine Ointment; Betadine Shampoo; Betadine Vaginal Gel; Betadine Vaginal Pessaries; Betadine VC Kit; Savlon Dry Antiseptic.**

Powergel
(Menarini) is a proprietary, prescription-only preparation of the (NSAID) NON-NARCOTIC ANALGESIC and ANTIRHEUMATIC ketoprofen, which also has COUNTER-IRRITANT, or RUBEFACIENT, actions. It can be applied to the skin for symptomatic relief of underlying muscle or joint pain, and is available as a gel for topical application to the skin.
✚▲ Side-effects/warnings: See KETOPROFEN; but adverse effects on topical application are limited.

Pragmatar
(Alliance) is a proprietary, non-prescription compound preparation of coal tar (as cetyl alcohol-coal tar distillate) and salicylic acid. It can be used for scaly scalp disorders such as cradle cap, and seborrhoeic conditions such as dandruff, and is available as a cream.
✚▲ Side-effects/warnings: COAL TAR; SALICYLIC ACID.

pralidoxime mesilate
(P2S) is an ANTIDOTE which is used in conjunction with an ANTICHOLINERGIC (ANTIMUSCARINIC) drug (usually ATROPINE SULPHATE) to treat poisoning by organophosphorous compounds (eg insecticides). Administration is by injection.
✚ Side-effects: Drowsiness, dizziness, visual disturbances, muscular weakness, nausea, headache, also speeding of the heart and breathing.
▲ Warnings: It should not be used to treat poisoning by carbamates or organophosphorous compounds which don't have anticholinesterase activity. Use with caution in patients with myasthenia gravis or impaired kidney function.

pramipexole
is an ANTIPARKINSONISM drug that works by stimulating the DOPAMINE receptors in the brain (a DOPAMINE-RECEPTOR STIMULANT), and which is similar to BROMOCRIPTINE in that it is used to improve symptoms and signs of the disease, often in combination with LEVODOPA. Administration is oral.
✚ Side-effects: Constipation, nausea, drowsiness (with sudden falling asleep), visual hallucinations, uneven gait (dose may need changing).
▲ Warnings: Not used when breast-feeding. Caution in kidney impairment; psychotic disorders; severe cardiovascular disease; in pregnancy. Eye testing is recommended because there is a risk of pramipexole causing visual disorders.
✪ **Related entry: Mirapexin.**

pramocaine hydrochloride
see PRAMOXINE HYDROCHLORIDE.

pramoxine hydrochloride
(pramocaine hydrochloride) is a LOCAL ANAESTHETIC included in some proprietary preparations that are used for haemorrhoids. Administration is by topical application.
✚▲ Side-effects/warnings: It is regarded as safe in normal topical use.
✪ **Related entry: Anugesic-HC.**

pravastatin sodium
is a (*statin*) LIPID-REGULATING DRUG used in

hyperlipidaemia to reduce the levels, or change the proportions, of various lipids in the bloodstream (particularly where there is heart disease, or a risk of heart attacks or stroke). It is usually administered only to patients in whom a strict and regular dietary regime, alone, or some other therapy is not having the desired effect. Administration is oral.

✚▲ Side-effects/warnings: See SIMVASTATIN. Also, rash, fatigue and chest pain. Patients should report any muscle weakness, pain or tenderness to their doctor.

✪ **Related entry: Lipostat.**

Praxilene

(Lipha) is a proprietary, prescription-only preparation of the VASODILATOR naftidrofuryl oxalate. It can be used to help improve blood circulation to the hands and feet when this is impaired, for example, in peripheral vascular disease (Raynaud's phenomenon), and for cerebral vascular disease. Available as tablets.

✚▲ Side-effects/warnings: See NAFTIDROFURYL OXALATE.

praziquantel

is an ANTHELMINTIC drug which is the drug of choice in treating infestation caused by schistosomes, which are the worms that can colonize the blood vessels of a human host and cause bilharziasis, and is also useful in the treatment of tapeworm infestation. It has a low toxicity and is administered orally. (It is available only on a named-patient basis in the UK.)

✚▲ Side-effects/warnings: This is a specialist drug given only after full assessment.

✪ **Related entry: Cysticide.**

prazosin hydrochloride

is a selective ALPHA-ADRENOCEPTOR BLOCKER which is used as an ANTIHYPERTENSIVE, in the treatment of urinary retention (eg in benign prostatic hyperplasia; BPH) and sometimes in peripheral vascular disease (Raynaud's phenomenon) or heart failure. Administration is oral.

✚ Side-effects: See selective ALPHA-ADRENOCEPTOR BLOCKER. Drowsiness and sedation, dizziness and hypotension (particularly on standing); weakness and lack of energy, depression, headache, dry mouth, nausea, urinary frequency and incontinence, palpitations and, rarely, speeding of the heart, incontinence and prolonged erections.

▲ Warnings: Initially, it may cause marked postural hypotension, so the patient should lie down when given the drug or it should be taken on retiring to bed. It is not to be used in certain forms of congestive heart failure (eg aortic stenosis). It should be administered with care to those who are pregnant or breast-feeding or with certain kidney disorders.

✪ **Related entries: Alphavase; Hypovase.**

Precortisyl

(Hoechst Marion Roussel; Aventis Pharma) is a proprietary, prescription-only preparation of the CORTICOSTEROID and ANTI-INFLAMMATORY prednisolone. It can be used in the treatment of allergic and inflammatory conditions. It is available as tablets in several different forms and strengths (eg *Precortisyl Forte*).

✚▲ Side-effects/warnings: See PREDNISOLONE.

Predenema

(Forest) is a proprietary, prescription-only preparation of the CORTICOSTEROID prednisolone (as sodium metasulphobenzoate). It can be used as an ANTI-INFLAMMATORY treatment for rectal inflammation (eg in ulcerative colitis), and is available as a retention enema.

✚▲ Side-effects/warnings: See PREDNISOLONE.

Predfoam

(Forest) is a proprietary, prescription-only preparation of the CORTICOSTEROID prednisolone (as metasulphobenzoate sodium). It can be used as an ANTI-INFLAMMATORY treatment for inflammation of the rectum (eg in ulcerative colitis) and proctitis, and is available as a rectal foam enema.

✚▲ Side-effects/warnings: See PREDNISOLONE.

Pred Forte

(Allergan) is a proprietary, prescription-only preparation of the CORTICOSTEROID and ANTI-INFLAMMATORY prednisolone (as acetate). It can be used to treat inflammatory conditions in and around the eye, and is available as eye-drops.

✚▲ Side-effects/warnings: See PREDNISOLONE.

prednisolone

is a synthetic, *glucocorticoid* CORTICOSTEROID

P

with ANTI-INFLAMMATORY properties. It is used in the treatment of a number of rheumatic and allergic or inflammatory conditions (particularly those affecting the eye, joints or the lungs) and collagen disorders. It is also an effective treatment for ulcerative colitis, Crohn's disease, rectal or anal inflammation, haemorrhoids and as an IMMUNOSUPPRESSANT in the treatment of myasthenia gravis. It may also be used for systemic corticosteroid therapy. It is also used as an ANTICANCER drug in the treatment of the lymphatic cancer Hodgkin's disease and other forms of lymphoma, and may also be helpful in halting the progress of hormone-linked breast cancer. Administration (as prednisolone, prednisolone acetate or prednisolone sodium phosphate) can be oral, by topical application or by injection.

✚▲ Side-effects/warnings: See CORTICOSTEROID. The type and severity of any side-effects depends on the route of administration. Systemic side-effects are unlikely with topical application, but there may be local reactions.

✪ **Related entries: Deltacortril Enteric; Deltastab; Minims Prednisolone; Precortisyl; Pred Forte; Predenema; Predfoam; Predsol; Predsol-N; Scheriproct.**

Predsol

(Celltech) is a proprietary, prescription-only preparation of the CORTICOSTEROID prednisolone (as sodium phosphate). It can be used as an ANTI-INFLAMMATORY treatment for inflammation of the rectum (eg in ulcerative colitis and Crohn's disease) and for non-infected, inflammatory ear and eye conditions. It is available as a retention enema, suppositories and as ear- or eye-drops.

✚▲ Side-effects/warnings: See PREDNISOLONE.

Predsol-N

(Predsol) is a proprietary, prescription-only compound preparation of the CORTICOSTEROID prednisolone (as sodium phosphate) and the ANTIBACTERIAL and (AMINOGLYCOSIDE) ANTIBIOTIC neomycin sulphate. It can be used to treat inflammatory ear and eye conditions, and is available as ear- and eye-drops.

✚▲ Side-effects/warnings: See NEOMYCIN SULPHATE; PREDNISOLONE.

Pregaday

(Celltech) is a proprietary, non-prescription compound preparation of ferrous fumarate and folic acid. It can be used as an IRON and folic acid supplement during pregnancy, and is available as tablets.

✚▲ Side-effects/warnings: See FERROUS FUMARATE; FOLIC ACID.

Pregnyl

(Organon) is a proprietary, prescription-only preparation of the HORMONE human chorionic gonadotrophin (human chorionic gonadotropin; HCG). It can be used to treat delayed puberty in boys, and as an infertility treatment in women suffering from specific hormonal deficiency contributing to infertility. It is available in a form for injection.

✚▲ Side-effects/warnings: See CHORIONIC GONADOTROPHIN.

Premarin

(Wyeth) is a proprietary, prescription-only preparation of the OESTROGEN comprised of (equine) conjugated oestrogens. It can be used in HRT, and is available as tablets in a calendar pack and as an intravaginal cream.

✚▲ Side-effects/warnings: See CONJUGATED OESTROGENS.

Premique

(Wyeth) is a proprietary, prescription-only preparation of the OESTROGEN of conjugated oestrogens and medroxyprogesterone acetate. It can be used in HRT (including for osteoporosis prophylaxis), and is available as tablets, and tablets in a calendar pack.

✚▲ Side-effects/warnings: See OESTROGEN; MEDROXYPROGESTERONE ACETATE.

Prempak-C

(Wyeth) is a proprietary, prescription-only compound preparation of the female SEX HORMONES the OESTROGEN conjugated oestrogens and the PROGESTOGEN norgestrel. It can be used in HRT, and is available as tablets in two forms of calendar pack.

✚▲ Side-effects/warnings: See CONJUGATED OESTROGENS; NORGESTREL.

Prepadine

(Berk; APS) is a proprietary, prescription-only preparation of the (TRICYCLIC) ANTIDEPRESSANT dosulepin hydrochloride. It can be used to treat

depressive illness, especially in cases where some degree of sedation is deemed necessary, and is available as tablets and capsules.
✚▲ Side-effects/warnings: See DOSULEPIN HYDROCHLORIDE.

Prescal
(Novartis) is a proprietary, prescription-only preparation of the CALCIUM-CHANNEL BLOCKER isradipine. It can be used as an ANTIHYPERTENSIVE, and is available as tablets.
✚▲ Side-effects/warnings: See ISRADIPINE.

Preservex
(UCB Pharma) is a proprietary, prescription-only preparation of the (NSAID) NON-NARCOTIC ANALGESIC and ANTIRHEUMATIC aceclofenac. It can be used to treat pain and inflammation in rheumatoid arthritis, for ankylosing spondylitis, and for short-term treatment of osteoarthritis. It is available as tablets.
✚▲ Side-effects/warnings: See ACECLOFENAC.

Prestim
(ICN) is a proprietary, prescription-only compound preparation of the BETA-BLOCKER timolol maleate and the (THIAZIDE) DIURETIC bendroflumethiazide. It can be used as an ANTIHYPERTENSIVE for raised blood pressure, and is available as tablets.
✚▲ Side-effects/warnings: See BENDROFLUMETHIAZIDE; TIMOLOL MALEATE.

Prevenar
(Wyeth) is a proprietary, prescription-only vaccine preparation of PNEUMOCOCCAL VACCINE in the form 'polyvalent pneumococcal polysaccharide conjugated vaccine'. It can be used for the prevention of pneumococcal pneumonia in infants under six months and children from one to two years old for whom the risk of contracting the disease is unusually high. It is available in a form for intramuscular injection.
✚▲ Side-effects/warnings: See VACCINE.

PR Heat Spray
(Crookes) is a proprietary, non-prescription compound preparation of methyl salicylate and camphor which all have COUNTER-IRRITANT, or RUBEFACIENT, actions, and the VASODILATOR ethyl nicotinate. It can be applied to the skin for symptomatic relief of underlying muscle or joint pain, sprains and bruises, and is available as a spray for topical application. It is not normally given to children under five years, except on medical advice.
✚▲ Side-effects/warnings: See CAMPHOR; ETHYL NICOTINATE; METHYL SALICYLATE. Avoid inflamed, broken skin and mucous membranes.

Priadel
(Sanofi-Synthelabo; Delandale) is a proprietary, prescription-only preparation of the ANTIMANIA drug lithium. It can be used to treat acute mania, manic-depressive bouts and recurrent depression, and is available as tablets (as lithium carbonate; Sanofi-Synthelabo) or a sugar-free liquid preparation (as lithium citrate; Delandale).
✚▲ Side-effects/warnings: See LITHIUM.

prilocaine hydrochloride
is a LOCAL ANAESTHETIC which is used extensively for relatively minor surgical procedures, especially by injection in dentistry and nerve block. Administration is by injection (in several forms) or by topical application.
✚▲ Side-effects/warnings: See LIDOCAINE HYDROCHLORIDE. It may cause methaemoglobinaemia (an abnormal form of haemoglobin that does not transport oxygen) that may require correction. It is avoided in those who have anaemia or pre-existing methaemoglobinaemia.
✪ Related entries: Citanest; Citanest with Octapressin; Emla.

Primacor
(Sanofi-Synthelabo) is a proprietary, prescription-only preparation of the PHOSPHODIESTERASE INHIBITOR milrinone. It can be used, in the short term, in HEART FAILURE TREATMENT for acute heart failure, especially where other drugs have not been successful. It is available in a form for intravenous infusion or injection.
✚▲ Side-effects/warnings: See MILRINONE.

primaquine
is an (*8-aminoquinoline*) ANTIMALARIAL drug which is used to destroy parasitic forms in the liver that are not destroyed by chloroquine. Administration is oral.
✚ Side-effects: There may be nausea and vomiting, abdominal pain and blood disorders.

P

▲ Warnings: It should be administered with caution to patients who are pregnant or breast-feeding, or who have G6PD deficiency.

Primaxin

(MSD) is a proprietary, prescription-only compound preparation of the ANTIBACTERIAL and (BETA-LACTAM) ANTIBIOTIC imipenem and the ENZYME INHIBITOR cilastatin, which is a combination known as imipenem with cilastatin. It can be used to treat infections such as those of the urethra and cervix and to prevent infection during operations. It is available in a form for intravenous injection or infusion.
✚▲ Side-effects/warnings: See IMIPENEM WITH CILASTATIN.

primidone

is an ANTICONVULSANT and ANTI-EPILEPTIC drug which is used in the treatment of all forms of epilepsy (except absence seizures) and for essential tremor. It is largely converted in the body to the BARBITURATE drug phenobarbital and therefore has similar actions and effects. Administration is oral.
✚▲ Side-effects/warnings: See PHENOBARBITAL; but there may also be drowsiness, unsteady gait, nausea, rash and disturbances of vision. It often causes hypersensitivity reactions, and is given gradually over several weeks.
✪ Related entry: Mysoline.

Primolut N

(Schering Health) is a proprietary, prescription-only preparation of the PROGESTOGEN norethisterone. It can be used to treat uterine bleeding, abnormally heavy menstruation and other menstrual problems, endometriosis and premenstrual syndrome. It is available as tablets.
✚▲ Side-effects/warnings: See NORETHISTERONE.

Primperan

(Berk; APS) is a proprietary, prescription-only preparation of the ANTI-EMETIC and ANTINAUSEANT metoclopramide hydrochloride. It can be used for the treatment of nausea and vomiting, particularly when associated with gastrointestinal disorders and after treatment with radiation or cytotoxic drugs. It also has gastric MOTILITY STIMULANT actions and can be used in the treatment of non-ulcer dyspepsia, gastric stasis and for prevention of reflux oesophagitis. It is available as tablets and as an oral solution.
✚▲ Side-effects/warnings: See METOCLOPRAMIDE HYDROCHLORIDE. Note the side-effects in young people in particular.

Prioderm Cream Shampoo

(SSL) is a proprietary, non-prescription preparation of the SCABICIDAL and PEDICULICIDAL drug malathion. It can be used to treat infestations of the scalp and pubic hair by lice (pediculosis), or of the skin by the itch-mite (scabies). It is available as a shampoo. It is not normally used on children under six months, except on medical advice.
✚▲ Side-effects/warnings: See MALATHION.

Prioderm Lotion

(SSL) is a proprietary, non-prescription preparation of the SCABICIDAL and PEDICULICIDAL drug malathion. It can be used to treat lice infestations of the scalp (pediculosis), or of the skin by the itch-mite (scabies). It is available as a lotion. It is not normally used on children under six months, except on medical advice.
✚▲ Side-effects/warnings: See MALATHION.

Priorix

(SmithKline Beecham; GSK) is a proprietary, prescription-only preparation of a VACCINE (MMR vaccine) that can be used for the prevention of measles, mumps and rubella (German measles) in children. It is available in a form for injection.
✚▲ Side-effects/warnings: See MMR VACCINE.

Pripsen Mebendazole Tablets

(SSL) is a proprietary, non-prescription preparation of the ANTHELMINTIC drug mebendazole. It can be used to treat infections by threadworm (enterobiasis), and is available as tablets. It is not normally given to children under two years, except on medical advice.
✚▲ Side-effects/warnings: See MEBENDAZOLE.

Pripsen Piperazine Phosphate Powder

(SSL) is a proprietary, non-prescription compound preparation of the ANTHELMINTIC drug piperazine (as phosphate) with the

LAXATIVE senna. It can be used to treat infestation by pinworm, threadworm and roundworm, and is available as an oral powder. It is not normally given to children under one year, except on medical advice.

✚▲ Side-effects/warnings: See PIPERAZINE; SENNA.

Pro-Banthine

(Hansam) is a proprietary, prescription-only preparation of the ANTICHOLINERGIC propantheline bromide. It can be used as an ANTISPASMODIC for gastrointestinal disorders involving spasm and in the treatment of adult enuresis (urinary incontinence). It is available as tablets.

✚▲ Side-effects/warnings: See PROPANTHELINE BROMIDE.

Probecid

(IDIS) is a non-proprietary, prescription-only preparation of probenecid available on a named-patient basis only. It can be used to prevent nephrotoxicity associated with the ANTIVIRAL drug CIDOFOVIR. It is available as tablets.

✚▲ Side-effects/warnings: See PROBENECID.

probenecid

is a drug that alters the way the kidney excretes chemicals, and is used for several purposes. First, by inhibiting the excretion from the body of certain ANTIBIOTIC drugs (mainly of the PENICILLIN and CEPHALOSPORIN classes), it increases their duration of action, though it is now rarely used for this purpose. Second, it is always given with the ANTIVIRAL drug CIDOFOVIR because it helps to protect the kidney from the toxicity of the latter. Third, because it increases the excretion of uric acid from the blood into the urine, it can be used in the prevention of attacks of chronic gout which involve high levels of uric acid (hyperuricaemia; though it is now less used for this purpose). Administration is oral as tablets.

✚ Side-effects: There may be nausea and vomiting, hair loss, increased urination, headache and flushing, dizziness and rash, sore gums; rarely, hypersensitivity, liver and kidney changes and blood disorders.

▲ Warnings: It is not to be used in patients with blood disorders, certain kidney disorders, porphyria, acute gout or who are using aspirin or other salicylates. When first administering, certain concurrent treatments are required, such as colchicine and a NSAID (not aspirin), and an adequate fluid intake (two litres a day) must be maintained. Administer with caution to those with peptic ulcers, renal impairment or G6PD deficiency. (It is not for acute attacks, but if acute attack occurs during treatment, probenicid should be continued.)

✪ **Related entries: Benuryl; Probecid.**

Probeta-LA

(Trinity) is a proprietary, prescription-only preparation of the BETA-BLOCKER propranolol hydrochloride. It can be used, for example as an ANTIHYPERTENSIVE for raised blood pressure, as an ANTI-ANGINA treatment to relieve symptoms and improve exercise tolerance. It is available as modified-release capsules.

✚▲ Side-effects/warnings: See PROPRANOLOL HYDROCHLORIDE.

procainamide hydrochloride

has LOCAL ANAESTHETIC properties and is used as an ANTI-ARRHYTHMIC to treat heartbeat irregularities, especially ventricular arrhythmias after a heart attack. Administration can be either oral or by injection.

✚ Side-effects: There may be nausea, diarrhoea, high temperature, slow heart rate and rashes. There may also be heart and/or skin or blood disorders; psychosis and lupus-like symptoms especially after prolonged treatment.

▲ Warnings: It should not be administered to patients with certain cardiovascular disorders, those who have lupus erythematosus, or who are breast-feeding. Administer with caution to those with asthma, the neuromuscular disease myasthenia gravis, impaired kidney and liver function or who are pregnant.

✪ **Related entry: Pronestyl.**

procaine

is a LOCAL ANAESTHETIC which, though once popular, is now seldom used because it has been overtaken by anaesthetics that are longer-lasting and better absorbed through mucous membranes. It cannot be used as a surface anaesthetic because it is poorly absorbed. However, it is still available and can be used for regional anaesthesia or by infiltration, usually in combination with adrenaline acid tartrate

(epinephrine). Administration (as procaine hydrochloride) is by injection.
✚ Side-effects: Rarely, there are sensitivity reactions.

procarbazine

is a CYTOTOXIC drug which is used as an ANTICANCER treatment for the lymphatic cancer Hodgkin's disease. Administration is oral.
✚▲ Side-effects/warnings: See CYTOTOXIC. There may be a hypersensitivity rash. Alcohol must be avoided because there is a serious interaction (DISULFIRAM-like).

prochlorperazine

is a PHENOTHIAZINE derivative which is used as an ANTIPSYCHOTIC drug in the treatment of psychotic disorders, such as schizophrenia and mania, as an ANXIOLYTIC in the short-term treatment of anxiety; also as an ANTI-EMETIC and ANTINAUSEANT in the prevention of nausea caused by chemotherapy, radiotherapy, or by the vertigo and labyrinthine disorders.
Administration (as prochlorperazine maleate or prochlorperazine mesilate) can be oral, topical or by injection.
✚▲ Side-effects/warnings: See CHLORPROMAZINE HYDROCHLORIDE; extrapyramidal symptoms may occur, particularly in children, the elderly or debilitated.
✪ Related entries: Buccastem; Stemetil.

Proctosedyl

(Hoechst Marion Roussel; Aventis Pharma) is a proprietary, prescription-only compound preparation of the CORTICOSTEROID and ANTI-INFLAMMATORY hydrocortisone and the LOCAL ANAESTHETIC cinchocaine (dibucaine hydrochloride). It can be used to treat various painful conditions of the anus and rectum, including haemorrhoids, and is available as an ointment and suppositories.
✚▲ Side-effects/warnings: See CINCHOCAINE; HYDROCORTISONE.

procyclidine hydrochloride

is an ANTICHOLINERGIC (ANTIMUSCARINIC) drug which is used in the treatment of some types of parkinsonism (see ANTIPARKINSONISM). It increases mobility and decreases rigidity and tremor, but has only a limited effect on bradykinesia. The tendency to produce an excess of saliva is also reduced. It is thought to work by correcting the over-effectiveness of the neurotransmitter ACETYLCHOLINE (cholinergic excess), which is caused by the dopamine deficiency that occurs in parkinsonism. Administration, which may be in conjunction with other drugs used for the relief of parkinsonism, is either oral or by injection.
✚▲ Side-effects/warnings: See BENZHEXOL HYDROCHLORIDE.
✪ Related entries: Arpicolin; Kemadrin.

Pro-Epanutin

(Parke-Davis; Pfizer) is a proprietary, prescription-only preparation of the ANTICONVULSANT and ANTI-EPILEPTIC fosphenytoin sodium. It can be used in the emergency treatment of status epilepticus and convulsive seizures during neurosurgical operations. It is available in a form for injection.
✚▲ Side-effects/warnings: See FOSPHENYTOIN SODIUM.

Profasi

(Serono) is a proprietary, prescription-only preparation of the HORMONE human chorionic gonadotrophin (human chorionic gonadotropin; HCG). It can be used to treat delayed puberty in boys, and as an infertility treatment for women suffering from specific hormonal deficiency. It is available in a form for injection.
✚▲ Side-effects/warnings: See CHORIONIC GONADOTROPHIN.

Proflex Pain Relief

(Novartis Consumer Health) is a proprietary, non-prescription preparation of the (NSAID) NON-NARCOTIC ANALGESIC and ANTIRHEUMATIC ibuprofen. It can be used for the symptomatic relief of rheumatic and muscular pain, backache, sprains, strains, sports injuries, lumbago and fibrositis. It is available as a cream for massage into the effected area. It is not normally given to children, except on medical advice.
✚▲ Side-effects/warnings: See IBUPROFEN.

Proflex Sustained Relief Capsules

(Novartis Consumer Health) is a proprietary, non-prescription preparation of the (NSAID) NON-NARCOTIC ANALGESIC and ANTIRHEUMATIC ibuprofen. It can be used as a RUBEFACIENT, or counter-irritant, to relieve muscular pain,

rheumatic pain, lumbago and fibrositis. It is available as tablets and is not normally given to children, except on medical advice.
✚▲ Side-effects/warnings: See IBUPROFEN.

progesterone

is a sex hormone (see SEX HORMONES), a PROGESTOGEN, that is found predominantly in women but also in men. In women, it is produced and secreted mainly by the ovaries (and also the placenta of pregnant women) and the adrenal glands. It prepares the lining of the uterus (the endometrium) every menstrual cycle to receive a fertilized ovum. Most cycles do not result in fertilization (conception), but if a fertilized ovum does implant in the endometrium the resulting formation of a placenta ensures the continuation of the supply of progesterone and this prevents ovulation. In men, small quantities of progesterone are secreted by the testes and the adrenal glands. Therapeutically, progesterone is administered to women to treat various menstrual and gynaecological disorders (eg menopausal symptoms, certain types of infertility, premenstrual syndrome, and postnatal depression). Administration is either by topical application, as anal or vaginal suppositories (pessaries), or by injection.
✚▲ Side-effects/warnings: See PROGESTOGEN.
✪ Related entries: Crinone; Cyclogest; Gestone.

progestogen 🅱

is the name of the group of (STEROID) SEX HORMONES formed and released by the ovaries and placenta in women, the adrenal gland and in small amounts by the testes in men. Physiologically, progestogens prepare the lining of the uterus (endometrium) for pregnancy, maintain it throughout pregnancy and prevent the further release of eggs (ovulation). They include the natural progestogen PROGESTERONE and those like it (DYDROGESTERONE, HYDROXYPROGESTERONE CAPROATE and MEDROXYPROGESTERONE ACETATE) and the analogues of TESTOSTERONE (eg NORGESTREL and NORETHISTERONE; and the analogues and derivatives of norgestrel DESOGESTREL, GESTODENE, LEVONORGESTREL and NORGESTIMATE. All are synthesized for therapeutic use and have many uses, including treatment of menstrual disorders (menorrhagia and severe dysmenorrhoea), endometriosis (inflammation of the tissues normally lining the uterus), in HRT, in recurrent (habitual) abortion, to relieve the symptoms of premenstrual syndrome and sometimes in the treatment of breast, endometrial and prostate cancers. The most common use is as constituents (with or without OESTROGEN) in ORAL CONTRACEPTIVE preparations. Mainly progestogens are given orally, but there are also forms for contraception that are given by deep intramuscular injection, by implant (subdermal; under the skin), or from an intra-uterine container device that slowly releases the drug into the cavity of the uterus.
✚ Side-effects: Depending on the dose, use and the particular progestogen administered; acne, skin rash, oedema, gastrointestinal disturbances, changes in libido, breast discomfort, premenstrual syndrome, irregular periods, flushing, sleep disturbances, depression, irritability, fluid retention, nausea.
▲ Warnings: It should not be administered to patients with undiagnosed vaginal bleeding, certain cardiovascular disorders, porphyria or certain cancers. Use with care in those with diabetes, heart, liver or kidney disorders, epilepsy, depression, or who are breast-feeding.

Prograf

(Fujisawa) is a proprietary, prescription-only preparation of the IMMUNOSUPPRESSANT tacrolimus. It can be used to prevent tissue rejection in transplant patients, and is available as capsules and in a form for intravenous infusion.
✚▲ Side-effects/warnings: See TACROLIMUS.

proguanil hydrochloride

is an ANTIMALARIAL drug which is used to prevent the contraction of malaria by visitors to tropical countries (in combination with ATOVAQUONE). Administration is oral.
✚ Side-effects: There may be mild stomach disorders, diarrhoea, occasional skin reactions, mouth ulcers and hair loss.
▲ Warnings: It should be administered with caution to patients who suffer from severely impaired kidney function or who are pregnant (folate supplements are required).
✪ Related entries: Malarone; Paludrine; Paludrine/Avloclor.

Progynova

(Schering Health) is a proprietary, prescription-

only preparation of the OESTROGEN estradiol (as valerate). It can be used as HRT to treat menopausal symptoms, and is available as tablets.
✚▲ Side-effects/warnings: See ESTRADIOL.

Progynova TS

(Schering Health) is a proprietary, prescription-only preparation of the OESTROGEN estradiol (as valerate). It can be used to treat menopausal symptoms in HRT, and is available as skin patches.
✚▲ Side-effects/warnings: See ESTRADIOL.

prolactin

is a HORMONE secreted into the bloodstream by the anterior pituitary gland in both men and women. Its main role is indeed the control of milk production in women, but it also influences many aspects of body function. Its release is controlled by the hypothalamus through a factor called prolactin-release inhibiting factor (PRIF), which is probably the neurotransmitter mediator DOPAMINE. This fact is important, because it explains why the drug BROMOCRIPTINE, which stimulates dopamine RECEPTORS, can be used to suppress prolactin secretion and why a dopamine ANTAGONIST increases it. Bromocriptine, when clinically necessary, can therefore be used to prevent or suppress milk production after normal birth or in disease states where there is excessive secretion of prolactin with associated galactorrhea (excessive milk production). Over-production of prolactin can also occur when there is a pituitary tumour or, as a side-effect when patients are being treated with dopamine antagonist ANTIPSYCHOTIC drugs, METOCLOPRAMIDE HYDROCHLORIDE, DOMPERIDONE or METHYLDOPA. Prolactin itself is not used in therapeutics.

Proleukin

(Chiron) is a proprietary, prescription-only preparation of the IMMUNOMODULATOR drug aldesleukin. It can be used for ANTICANCER treatment in certain patients with metastatic renal cell carcinoma, and is available in a form for injection.
✚▲ Side-effects/warnings: See ALDESLEUKIN.

Proluton Depot

(Schering Health) is a proprietary, prescription-only preparation of the PROGESTOGEN hydroxyprogesterone caproate. It can be used to treat recurrent miscarriage, and is available in a form for long-lasting (depot) injection.
✚▲ Side-effects/warnings: See HYDROXYPROGESTERONE CAPROATE.

promazine hydrochloride

is chemically one of the PHENOTHIAZINE derivatives. It is used as an ANTIPSYCHOTIC drug to tranquillize agitated and restless patients, especially the elderly. Administration is either oral or by injection.
✚▲ Side-effects/warnings: See CHLORPROMAZINE HYDROCHLORIDE.

promethazine hydrochloride

is an ANTIHISTAMINE, chemically a PHENOTHIAZINE derivative, which also has HYPNOTIC properties. It is used to treat the symptoms of allergic conditions, such as hay fever and urticaria, for motion sickness, and can also be used in the emergency treatment of anaphylactic shock. It has a SEDATIVE action and can be administered as a preoperative medication, to treat temporary sleep disorders, and is included in some cough preparations. Administration can be either oral or by injection. See also PROMETHAZINE TEOCLATE.
✚▲ Side-effects/warnings: See ANTIHISTAMINE. Intramuscular injections may be painful. Avoid its use in patients with porphyria. Because of its sedative side-effects, the performance of skilled tasks, such as driving, may be impaired.
✪ Related entries: Medised; Medised Sugar Free Colour Free; Night Nurse Capsules; Night Nurse Liquid; Pamergan P100; Phenergan; Sominex; Tixylix Night-Time SF.

promethazine teoclate

(promethazine theoclate) is chemically a PHENOTHIAZINE derivative and is a form of the ANTIHISTAMINE promethazine hydrochloride, but with a slightly longer duration of action. It can be used as an ANTINAUSEANT to prevent nausea, vertigo and vomiting caused by motion sickness or infection of the ear. It can also be used for severe nausea in pregnancy. Administration is oral.
✚▲ Side-effects/warnings: See ANTIHISTAMINE. Because of its sedative property, the performance of skilled tasks, such as driving, may be impaired.
✪ Related entry: Avomine.

promethazine theoclate

see PROMETHAZINE TEOCLATE.

P

Pronestyl
(Squibb; Bristol-Myers Squibb) is a proprietary, prescription-only preparation of the ANTI-ARRHYTHMIC drug procainamide hydrochloride. It can be used to treat irregularities in the heartbeat, especially after a heart attack, and is available as tablets and in a form for injection.
✚▲ Side-effects/warnings: See PROCAINAMIDE HYDROCHLORIDE.

Propaderm
(GlaxoWellcome; GSK) is a proprietary, prescription-only preparation of the CORTICOSTEROID beclometasone dipropionate. It can be used to treat severe, non-infective skin inflammation, such as eczema and psoriasis, and is available as a cream and an ointment for topical application.
✚▲ Side-effects/warnings: See BECLOMETASONE DIPROPIONATE.

propafenone hydrochloride
is an ANTI-ARRHYTHMIC drug which is used to prevent and treat a number of irregularities of the heartbeat. Administration is oral.
✚ Side-effects: Nausea, vomiting, diarrhoea or constipation; fatigue, headache, dizziness; rash, postural hypotension (especially in the elderly), dry mouth, bitter taste, blurred vision and occasionally heart and blood disorders.
▲ Warnings: It should be administered with care in the elderly, those who are pregnant or with certain kidney, liver or airways disorders. Avoid in patients with severe heart conditions, myasthenia gravis.
✪ **Related entry: Arythmol.**

Propain Caplets
(Sankyo Pharma) is a proprietary, non-prescription compound preparation of the (OPIOID) NARCOTIC ANALGESIC codeine phosphate, the ANTIHISTAMINE diphenhydramine hydrochloride, the NON-NARCOTIC ANALGESIC and ANTIPYRETIC paracetamol and the STIMULANT caffeine. It can be used to relieve pain, including headache, toothache, migraine, muscular pain and period pain, and to relieve cold and flu symptoms and fever. It is available as scored tablets and is not normally given to children, except on medical advice.
✚▲ Side-effects/warnings: See CAFFEINE; CODEINE PHOSPHATE; DIPHENHYDRAMINE HYDROCHLORIDE; PARACETAMOL.

propamidine isethionate
is an ANTIBACTERIAL which is used specifically to treat infections of the eyelids or conjunctiva, including acanthamoeba keratitis (sometimes in conjunction with other drugs). Administration is by topical application in the form of eye-drops.
✪ **Related entry: Brolene Eye Drops.**

propantheline bromide
is an ANTICHOLINERGIC (ANTIMUSCARINIC) drug which is used in the treatment of gastrointestinal disorders that involve muscle spasm of the intestinal wall, of urinary frequency and adult enuresis (urinary incontinence), and gustatory sweating. Administration is oral as tablets.
✚▲ Side-effects/warnings: See ATROPINE SULPHATE.
✪ **Related entry: Pro-Banthine.**

Propecia
(MSD) is a proprietary, prescription-only preparation (not available on the NHS) of the ANTI-ANDROGEN finasteride, which is a sex hormone antagonist (see SEX HORMONES; ANTAGONIST). It can be used to treat male-pattern baldness, and is available as tablets.
✚▲ Side-effects/warnings: See FINASTERIDE.

Propess
(Ferring) is a proprietary, prescription-only preparation of the PROSTAGLANDIN dinoprostone. It can be used to promote cervical ripening and induce labour at term, and is available as pessaries.
✚▲ Side-effects/warnings: See DINOPROSTONE.

Propine
(Allergan) is a proprietary, prescription-only preparation of the SYMPATHOMIMETIC dipivefrine hydrochloride. It can be used as a GLAUCOMA TREATMENT to reduce intraocular pressure, and is available as eye-drops.
✚▲ Side-effects/warnings: See DIPIVEFRINE HYDROCHLORIDE.

propiverine hydrochloride
is an ANTICHOLINERGIC (ANTIMUSCARINIC) drug which can be used as an ANTISPASMODIC to treat urinary frequency, incontinence and bladder spasms. Administration is oral.
✚ Side-effects: These include dry mouth, blurred vision, gastrointestinal disturbances,

P

hypotension, drowsiness, tiredness, difficulty in urination, flushing of the face, irritability, restlessness, hot flushes, rash and heart speeding.
▲ Warnings: It should not be administered to patients with intestinal obstruction, severe ulcerative colitis, toxic megacolon, glaucoma, myasthenia gravis or bladder obstruction, liver or kidney impairment, or who are pregnant or breast-feeding. Administer with care to those with certain heart disorders, hyperthyroidism, prostatic hypertrophy, hiatus hernia with reflux oesophagitis.
✪ **Related entry: Detrunorm.**

Pro-plus Tablets

(Roche) is a proprietary, non-prescription preparation of the STIMULANT caffeine. It can be used to give rapid relief of temporary tiredness, and is not given to children, except on medical advice.
✚▲ Side-effects/warnings: See CAFFEINE.

propranolol hydrochloride

is a BETA-BLOCKER which can be used as an ANTIHYPERTENSIVE for raised blood pressure, as an ANTI-ANGINA treatment to relieve symptoms and improve exercise tolerance and as an ANTI-ARRHYTHMIC to regularize heartbeat and to treat and prevent myocardial infarction or after attacks. It can also be used as an ANTITHYROID drug for short-term treatment of thyrotoxicosis, with an ALPHA-ADRENOCEPTOR BLOCKER for phaeochromocytoma, as an ANTIMIGRAINE treatment to prevent attacks and as an ANXIOLYTIC, particularly for symptomatic relief of tremor and palpitations (and for some other types of tremor). Administration is either oral or by injection. It is also available, as an antihypertensive treatment, in the form of compound preparations with DIURETIC drugs.
✚ Side-effects: Slowing of the heart rate, hypotension, asthma-like symptoms and bronchospasm, gastrointestinal disturbances, poor circulation in the extremities, fatigue and sleep-disturbance; heart failure in susceptible patients. There may be rashes and dry eyes. (When beta-blockers are given as eye-drops, not all these warnings apply.)
▲ Warnings: It should not be administered to patients with asthma or obstructive disease of the airways, history of heart failure, cardiogenic shock or certain abnormal heart rhythms. It should be administered with caution to those with certain liver or kidney disorders, in late pregnancy, who are breast-feeding, diabetics or with myasthenia gravis. It may increase sensitivity to allergens.
✪ **Related entries: Angilol; Bedranol SR; Beta-Prograne; Half-Beta-Prograne; Half-Inderal LA; Inderal; Inderal-LA; Inderetic; Inderex; Lopranol-LA; Probeta-LA.**

propylthiouracil

is a drug that acts as an indirect HORMONE ANTAGONIST by inhibiting the thyroid gland's production of THYROID HORMONES, therefore treating an excess of thyroid hormones in the blood and the symptoms that it causes (thyrotoxicosis). Treatment can be on a maintenance basis over a long period (with dosage adjusted to optimum effect), or it can be used just before surgical removal of the thyroid gland. It is prescribed in particular to patients who are sensitive to the antithyroid drug carbimazole. Administration is oral.
✚▲ Side-effects/warnings: See CARBIMAZOLE. Also, rarely it may cause blood disorders, hepatitis, effects on the skin, lupus erythematous-like syndrome.

Proscar

(MSD) is a proprietary, prescription-only preparation of the ANTI-ANDROGEN finasteride, which is a sex hormone (see SEX HORMONES) ANTAGONIST. It can be used to treat benign prostatic hyperplasia in men, and is available as tablets.
✚▲ Side-effects/warnings: See FINASTERIDE.

prostacyclin

see EPOPROSTENOL.

prostaglandin 🅱

is the name given to any of a family of LOCAL HORMONE mediators (so-called because they exert their effects near to where they are formed), which are produced naturally by many organs and tissues in the body, both normally and in disease states. Naturally occurring members of the family include prostaglandin E_2 (DINOPROSTONE), prostaglandin F_2 (dinoprost; formerly used) and prostacyclin (EPOPROSTENOL). They are used therapeutically along with synthetic analogues that are similar to the natural ones (eg MISOPROSTOL; used as an ULCER-HEALING DRUG). A prostaglandin present naturally in the walls of blood vessels, EPOPROSTENOL (prostacyclin), can be given therapeutically by intravenous infusion for its ANTIPLATELET activity to help prevent formation of blood thrombi during procedures such as kidney dialysis. The uses of the prostaglandins reflect their high potency in causing such bodily actions as contraction of the uterus, softening and dilation of the cervix at the base of the uterus (they may be used as ABORTIFACIENT drugs, eg GEMEPROST) and dilation of blood vessels (eg ALPROSTADIL which is used to maintain patency of ductus arteriosus in babies). LATANOPROST and TRAVOPROST (prostaglandin analogues) are used in open-angle glaucoma and ocular hypertension. The side-effects of these agents used as drugs reflect their other powerful actions; such as stimulating the intestine causing pain, diarrhoea, actions on the brain to cause fever and prolongation of bleeding.

Prostap 3

(Wyeth) is a proprietary, prescription-only preparation of leuprorelin acetate and can be used as an ANTICANCER drug for cancer of the prostate gland. It is available in a form for subcutaneous injection.

✚▲ Side-effects/warnings: See LEUPRORELIN ACETATE.

Prostap SR

(Wyeth) is a proprietary, prescription-only preparation of leuprorelin acetate and can be used as an ANTICANCER drug for cancer of the prostate gland and to treat endometriosis. It is available in a form for injection.

✚▲ Side-effects/warnings: See LEUPRORELIN ACETATE.

Prostin E2

(Pharmacia & Upjohn; Pharmacia) is a proprietary, prescription-only form of the PROSTAGLANDIN dinoprostone. It is used mainly to induce labour. It is available as tablets, vaginal tablets (pessaries), a vaginal gel and in forms for injection.

✚▲ Side-effects/warnings: See DINOPROSTONE.

Prostin VR

(Pharmacia & Upjohn; Pharmacia) is a proprietary, prescription-only form of the PROSTAGLANDIN alprostadil (prostaglandin PGE_1). It is used to maintain newborn babies with heart defects (to maintain patent ductus arteriosus), while preparations are made for corrective surgery in intensive care. It is available in a form for intravenous infusion.

✚▲ Side-effects/warnings: See ALPROSTADIL.

Prosulf

(CP) is a proprietary, prescription-only preparation of protamine sulphate. It can be used to counteract heparin overdose, and is available in a form for injection.

✚▲ Side-effects/warnings: See PROTAMINE SULPHATE.

protamine sulfate

see PROTAMINE SULPHATE.

protamine sulphate

(protamine sulfate) can be used to treat an overdose of heparin. Administration is by slow intravenous injection.

✚▲ Side-effects/warnings: Slowing of the heart rate, hypotension and flushing, nausea, vomiting and hypersensitivity reactions.

✪ **Related entry: Prosulf.**

protamine zinc insulin

is a form of purified INSULIN, prepared as a sterile complex with protamine and zinc, which is used in DIABETIC TREATMENT to maintain diabetic patients. It is available in vials for injection and has a long duration of action.

✚▲ Side-effects/warnings: See INSULIN.

✪ **Related entry: Hypurin Bovine Protamine Zinc.**

protein C concentrate

is a vitamin K-dependent natural ANTICOAGULANT. It is prepared from blood plasma obtained from healthy human donors and used as a HAEMOSTATIC in patients with congenital protein C deficiency. It is available, only on prescription, in a form for intravenous infusion.

✚ Side-effects: Heart arrhythmias, fever, thrombosis and bleeding are possible side-effects and rarely allergic reactions.

▲ Warnings: It is used with caution in people who are known to be hypersensitive to heparin.

✪ **Related entry: Ceprotin.**

P

Prothiaden
(Knoll) is a proprietary, prescription-only preparation of the (TRICYCLIC) ANTIDEPRESSANT dosulepin hydrochloride. It can be used to treat depressive illness, especially in cases where some degree of sedation is deemed necessary, and is available as tablets and capsules.
✚▲ Side-effects/warnings: See DOSULEPIN HYDROCHLORIDE.

protirelin
is a synthetic version of *thyrotrophin-releasing hormone* (TRH), a hypothalamic HORMONE produced and secreted by the hypothalamus. TRH in turn acts on the anterior pituitary gland to produce and secrete thyrotrophin (thyroid-stimulating hormone; TSH), a hormone that then causes the production and secretion of yet other hormones in the body. Therapeutically, it is used primarily to assess thyroid function in patients who suffer from under-activity of the pituitary gland (hypopituitarism) or from over-activity of the thyroid gland (hyperthyroidism). Administration is by injection.
✚ Side-effects: There is commonly nausea. It may cause flushing, dizziness, faintness, raised blood pressure and pulse rate, a strange taste in the mouth and a desire to urinate. Occasionally, there may be bronchospasm.
▲ Warnings: Administer with caution to patients with severe under-activity of the pituitary gland, myocardial ischaemia, asthma and obstructive airways disease or who are pregnant or breast-feeding.

Protium
(Knoll) is a proprietary, prescription-only preparation of the PROTON-PUMP INHIBITOR pantoprazole. It can be used as an ULCER-HEALING DRUG and for associated conditions, and is available as tablets and in a form for injection.
✚▲ Side-effects/warnings: See PANTOPRAZOLE.

proton-pump inhibitor 🅱
drugs are a type of ULCER-HEALING DRUG. They work by inhibiting gastric acid secretion in the parietal cells (acid-producing cells) of the stomach lining by interfering with the action of the ion (proton) pump that is responsible for the secretion of acid. They can be used to treat the symptoms of dyspepsia, which is caused by over-production of acid (hyperacidity), chronic problems associated with peptic ulcers (gastric or duodenal), oesophagitis (inflammation of the oesophagus caused by regurgitation of acid and enzymes), for Zollinger-Ellison syndrome, and for the eradication of *Helicobactor pylori* infection when used in combination with antibiotics. They can also be used as an alternative to treatment with H_2-ANTAGONIST. Examples of proton-pump inhibitors are LANSOPRAZOLE, OMEPRAZOLE, PANTOPRAZOLE and RABEPRAZOLE SODIUM.
✚ Side-effects: Proton-pump inhibitors may cause headache, diarrhoea, rashes and itching, dizziness, nausea and vomiting, constipation, flatulence, abdominal pain, bronchospasm, muscle and joint pain, blurred vision, depression and dry mouth. They decrease gastric acidity so may increase the risk of gastrointestinal infections.
▲ Warnings: Proton-pump inhibitors should be used with caution in patients who have liver disease or are pregnant or breast-feeding. Before treatment, it should be confirmed that there is no gastric cancer or other disease.

Provera
(Pharmacia) is a proprietary, prescription-only preparation of the sex hormone medroxyprogesterone acetate (a synthetic PROGESTOGEN). In women it can be used as an ANTICANCER drug for cancer of the kidney or uterine endometrium, and in endometriosis or dysfunctional uterine bleeding. It is available as tablets.
✚▲ Side-effects/warnings: See MEDROXYPROGESTERONE ACETATE.

Provigil
(Cephalon) is a proprietary, prescription-only preparation of the CNS STIMULANT modafinil, and is used to treat narcolepsy. Available as tablets.
✚▲ Side-effects/warnings: See MODAFINIL.

Pro-Viron
(Schering) is a proprietary, prescription-only preparation of mesterolone, which has ANDROGEN (male sex hormone) activity. It can be used to make up hormonal deficiency, and is available as tablets.
✚▲ Side-effects/warnings: See MESTEROLONE.

proxymetacaine
is a LOCAL ANAESTHETIC which can be used (as

P

hydrochloride) by topical application in ophthalmic treatments

✚ Side-effects: There may be slight stinging on initial application.

✪ **Related entries: Minims Proxymetacaine and Fluorescein; Minims Proxymetacaine Hydrochloride.**

Prozac

(Dista; Lilly) is a proprietary, prescription-only preparation of the (SSRI) ANTIDEPRESSANT fluoxetine hydrochloride, which has less SEDATIVE effects than some other antidepressants, and has recently been used to treat bulimia nervosa. It is available as capsules and a liquid.

✚▲ Side-effects/warnings: See FLUOXETINE.

pseudoephedrine hydrochloride

is a SYMPATHOMIMETIC with BRONCHODILATOR, VASOCONSTRICTOR and DECONGESTANT properties. It is sometimes used to treat obstructive airways disease, but is most commonly included in a number of proprietary preparations for treating cold symptoms. Its actions and effects are very similar to those of the closely related drug ephedrine hydrochloride.

✚▲ Side-effects/warnings: See EPHEDRINE HYDROCHLORIDE.

✪ **Related entries: Actifed Compound Linctus; Actifed Expectorant; Actifed Syrup; Actifed Tablets; Adult Meltus Expectorant with Decongestant; Adult Meltus for Dry Tickly Coughs and Catarrh; Benylin Cough and Congestion; Benylin Four Flu Liquid; Benylin Four Flu Tablets; Bronalin Decongestant Elixir; Dimotane Co; Dimotane Co Paediatric; Dimotane Expectorant; Galpseud; Junior Meltus for Dry Tickly Coughs and Catarrh; Lemsip Pharmacy Flu Strength; Lemsip Pharmacy Powercaps; Nurofen Cold & Flu; Robitussin Chesty Cough with Congestion; Robitussin Night-Time; Sudafed Expectorant; Sudafed Linctus; Sudafed Tablets; Sudafed-Co Tablets; Tixycolds Syrup; Tixylix Cough and Cold; Vicks Medinite.**

Psoriderm

(Dermal) is a proprietary, non-prescription compound preparation of coal tar (with lecithin). It can be used for psoriasis of skin and scalp, and is available as a cream, a scalp lotion and a bath emulsion.

✚▲ Side-effects/warnings: See COAL TAR.

Psorin

(Ayrton Saunders) is a proprietary, non-prescription compound preparation of dithranol, salicylic acid and coal tar. It can be used to treat psoriasis, and is available as an ointment and scalp gel.

✚▲ Side-effects/warnings: See COAL TAR; DITHRANOL; SALICYLIC ACID.

PTH

see PARATHYROID HORMONE.

Pulmicort

(Astra) is a proprietary, prescription-only preparation of the CORTICOSTEROID budesonide. It can be used to prevent asthma attacks and is available in various forms with inhalers including *Pulmicort LS*, *Respules* solution, and a dry powder used with the *Turbohaler*.

✚▲ Side-effects/warnings: See BUDESONIDE.

Pulmo Bailly

(Roche Consumer Health) is a proprietary, non-prescription preparation of the (OPIOID) ANTITUSSIVE codeine phosphate and the EXPECTORANT guaiacol. It can be used to give symptomatic relief of coughs associated with colds, bronchial catarrh, flu and infections such as laryngitis. It is available as a liquid.

✚▲ Side-effects/warnings: See CODEINE PHOSPHATE; GUAIACOL.

Pulmozyme

(Roche) is a proprietary, prescription-only preparation of dornase alfa, a human enzyme, and can be used in cystic fibrosis to improve lung function. It is available in a form for inhalation by jet nebulizer.

✚▲ Side-effects/warnings: See DORNASE ALFA.

Puregon

(Organon) is a proprietary, prescription-only HORMONE preparation of recombinant human FOLLICLE-STIMULATING HORMONE (FSH) in the form follitropin beta. It can be used to treat infertility in women and is available in a form for injection.

✚▲ Side-effects/warnings: See FOLLITROPIN BETA.

purgative 🅸

see LAXATIVE.

P

Puri-Nethol

(GlaxoWellcome; GSK) is a proprietary, prescription-only preparation of the (CYTOTOXIC) ANTICANCER mercaptopurine. It can be used in the treatment of acute leukaemias, and is available as tablets.
✚▲ Side-effects/warnings: See MERCAPTOPURINE.

Pylorid

(GlaxoWellcome; GSK) is a proprietary, prescription-only preparation of the H_2-ANTAGONIST and ULCER-HEALING DRUG ranitidine bismuth citrate. It can be used to treat benign peptic ulcers (in the stomach or duodenum) and, in conjunction with antibiotics, duodenal ulceration associated with *Helicobacter pylori* infection. It is available as tablets.
✚▲ Side-effects/warnings: See RANITIDINE BISMUTH CITRATE.

Pyralvex

(Norgine) is a proprietary, non-prescription preparation of salicylic acid and rhubarb extract (anthraquinone glycosides), which have a COUNTER-IRRITANT, or RUBEFACIENT, action. It can be applied to the mouth for symptomatic relief of pain from mouth ulcers and denture irritation. It is available as an oral paint and is not normally used for children, except on medical advice.
✚▲ Side-effects/warnings: See SALICYLIC ACID.

pyrazinamide

is an ANTIBACTERIAL drug and is one of the major forms of ANTITUBERCULAR treatment. It is generally used in combination with other drugs, such as ISONIAZID and RIFAMPICIN for maximum effect. Because pyrazinamide is only active against dividing forms of *Mycobacterium tuberculosis*, it is most effective in the early stages of treatment (ie the first few months). Administration is oral as tablets.
✚ Side-effects: There may be symptoms of liver malfunction, including high temperature, severe weight loss and jaundice. There may be nausea and vomiting, sensitivity reactions, such as urticaria, joint pain and blood disorders.
▲ Warnings: It should not be administered to patients with serious liver damage or porphyria; it should be administered with caution to patients with impaired kidney function, diabetes or gout. Patients should be aware of, and look for signs of liver disorders (eg vomiting, jaundice, malaise) and report these to the doctor.
✪ **Related entries: Rifater; Zinamide.**

pyridostigmine

is an ANTICHOLINESTERASE drug which enhances the effects of the neurotransmitter acetylcholine (and of certain cholinergic drugs). Because of this property, it has PARASYMPATHOMIMETIC actions. It is more commonly used to treat the neuromuscular transmission disorder *myasthenia gravis*. Administration is oral.
✚▲ Side-effects/warnings: See NEOSTIGMINE; but it has generally weaker parasympathomimetic actions and has fewer side-effects.
✪ **Related entry: Mestinon.**

pyrimethamine

is an ANTIMALARIAL drug which is mainly used in combination with DAPSONE or SULFADOXINE to prevent or treat malaria. It can also sometimes be used, along with a sulphonamide, to treat the protozoal infection toxoplasmosis.
Administration is oral as tablets.
✚ Side-effects: There may be rashes, insomnia and blood disorders.
▲ Warnings: It should be administered with caution to patients with certain liver or kidney disorders, or who are pregnant of breast-feeding. A high dosage requires regular blood counts.
✪ **Related entries: Daraprim; Fansidar; Maloprim.**

Pyrogastrone

(Sanofi-Synthelabo) is a proprietary, prescription-only compound preparation of the CYTOPROTECTANT drug carbenoxolone sodium, the ANTACID agents aluminium hydroxide, magnesium trisilicate and sodium bicarbonate, and the DEMULCENT agent ALGINIC ACID. It can be used to treat oesophageal inflammation and ulceration, and is available as tablets and an oral liquid.
✚▲ Side-effects/warnings: See ALGINIC ACID; ALUMINIUM HYDROXIDE; CARBENOXOLONE SODIUM; MAGNESIUM TRISILICATE; SODIUM BICARBONATE.

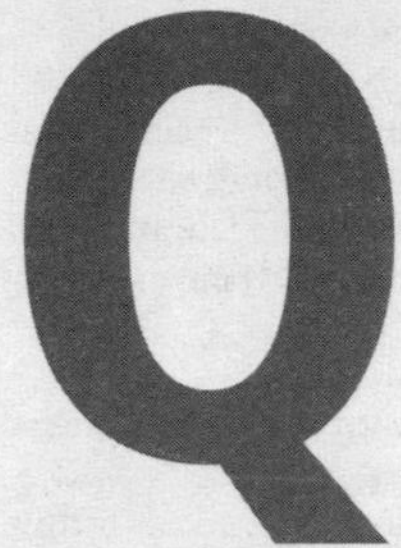

Quellada-M Cream Shampoo

(Stafford-Miller; GSK) is a proprietary, non-prescription preparation of the SCABICIDAL and PEDICULICIDAL drug malathion. It can be used to treat infestations of the scalp and pubic hair by lice (pediculosis), and is available as a shampoo. It is not normally given to children under six months, except on medical advice.

✚▲ Side-effects/warnings: See MALATHION.

Quellada-M Liquid

(Stafford-Miller; GSK) is a proprietary, non-prescription preparation of the SCABICIDAL and PEDICULICIDAL drug malathion. It can be used to treat infestations of the scalp and pubic hair by lice (pediculosis) or of the skin by the itch-mite (scabies), and is available as a liquid. It is not normally given to children under six months, except on medical advice.

✚▲ Side-effects/warnings: See MALATHION.

Questran

(Squibb; Bristol-Myers Squibb) is a proprietary, prescription-only preparation of the LIPID-REGULATING DRUG colestyramine. It can be used in hyperlipidaemia to modify the proportions, of lipids in the bloodstream. It has various other uses, including as an ANTIDIARRHOEAL and, in certain circumstances, in biliary disturbances. It is available as a powder to be taken with liquids.

✚▲ Side-effects/warnings: See COLESTYRAMINE.

Questran Light

(Squibb; Bristol-Myers Squibb) is a proprietary, prescription-only preparation of the LIPID-REGULATING DRUG colestyramine. It can be used in hyperlipidaemia to modify the proportions of various lipids in the bloodstream. It has various other uses, including as an ANTIDIARRHOEAL and in biliary disturbances. It is available as a powder (containing the sweetener aspartame) to be taken with liquids.

✚▲ Side-effects/warnings: See COLESTYRAMINE.

quetiapine

is an ANTIPSYCHOTIC drug (one of a group sometimes termed 'atypical' antipsychotics) which can be used for the treatment of schizophrenia in patients. It is taken orally.

✚ Side-effects: Atypical antipsychotics include weight gain, dizziness, postural hypotension, extrapyramidal symptoms (usually mild and transient, but occasionally tardive dyskinesia on long-term administration). Also: drowsiness, dyspepsia, constipation, dry mouth, changes in liver enzymes and blood counts, blood lipids, weakness, rhinitis, tachycardia; anxiety, fever, muscle pain, rash, effects on the heart.

▲ Warnings: Atypical antipsychotics are used with caution in patients with cardiovascular disease, history of epilepsy, and Parkinson's disease; they may affect performance of skilled tasks including driving. Quetiapine is not used in breast feeding. Care is required in its use in those who are pregnant, or who have liver or kidney impairment.

✪ **Related entry: Seroquel.**

quinagolide

is a drug with similar actions to bromocriptine as a DOPAMINE-RECEPTOR STIMULANT. It can be used to treat HORMONE disorders (hyperprolactinaemia disorders), such as prolactinoma. Administration is oral as tablets.

✚▲ Side-effects/warnings: See BROMOCRIPTINE. There may also be hypotensive actions, which may be disturbing, anorexia, abdominal pain, diarrhoea, insomnia, oedema, fainting, flushing and nasal congestion. It is not to be given to patients who are pregnant.

✪ **Related entry: Norprolac.**

quinalbarbitone sodium

see SECOBARBITAL SODIUM.

quinapril

is an ACE INHIBITOR and a powerful VASODILATOR which can be used as an ANTIHYPERTENSIVE and in congestive HEART FAILURE TREATMENT, often when other treatments are not appropriate. It is frequently used in conjunction with other classes of drug,

Q

particularly (THIAZIDE) DIURETIC drugs. Administration is oral.
✚ Side-effects: See ACE INHIBITOR. Also, muscle weakness, chest pains, oedema, flatulence, depression, nervousness, insomnia, blurred vision, impotence, back pain and muscle pains.
▲ Warnings: See ACE INHIBITOR.
✪ Related entries: Accupro; Accuretic; Acezide.

quinidine

is a CINCHONA ALKALOID and is chemically related to QUININE. It is also used as an ANTI-ARRHYTHMIC drug to treat heartbeat irregularities (supraventricular tachycardias and ventricular arrhythmias). Administration is oral.
✚▲ Side-effects/warnings: See PROCAINAMIDE HYDROCHLORIDE. There may also be effects on the heart and a number of different blood disorders. It is not to be given to patients with heart block.
✪ Related entry: Kinidin Durules.

quinine

is a CINCHONA ALKALOID and was for a long time the main treatment for malaria. Today, it has been almost completely replaced by synthetic and less toxic drugs (eg CHLOROQUINE). However, quinine is still used (as quinine sulphate or quinine hydrochloride) against falciparum malaria in cases that prove to be resistant to the newer drugs, or for emergency cases in which large doses are necessary. It can also be used to relieve nocturnal leg cramps. Administration is either oral or by intravenous infusion.
✚ Side-effects: Toxic effects (especially in overdose) – called *cinchonism* – include nausea, headache, abdominal pain, visual disturbances, tinnitus, a rash and confusion. Some patients may experience visual disturbances and temporary blindness, sensitivity reactions and blood disorders, hot flushes skin, confusion, and kidney effects.
▲ Warnings: It should not be administered to patients with certain optic nerve and heart disorders or haemoglobinurea. It should be administered with caution to those who suffer from heart block, atrial fibrillation, who have G6PD deficiency or who are pregnant. It is very toxic in overdose.

Quinocort

(Quinoderm Ltd) is a proprietary, prescription-only compound preparation of the ANTI-INFLAMMATORY and CORTICOSTEROID hydrocortisone and the ANTIFUNGAL and ANTIBACTERIAL potassium hydroxyquinoline sulphate. It can be used to treat inflammation, particularly when associated with fungal infections, and is available as a cream for topical application.
✚▲ Side-effects/warnings: See HYDROCORTISONE; POTASSIUM HYDROXYQUINOLINE SULPHATE.

Quinoderm Cream

(Quinoderm) is a proprietary, non-prescription compound preparation of the KERATOLYTIC and ANTIMICROBIAL benzoyl peroxide and the ANTIFUNGAL and ANTIBACTERIAL potassium hydroxyquinoline sulphate. It can be used to treat acne, and is available as a cream for topical application. It is not normally given to children, except on medical advice.
✚▲ Side-effects/warnings: See BENZOYL PEROXIDE; POTASSIUM HYDROXYQUINOLINE SULPHATE.

Quinoderm Cream 5

(Quinoderm) is a proprietary, non-prescription compound preparation of the KERATOLYTIC and ANTIMICROBIAL benzoyl peroxide (5%) and the ANTIFUNGAL and ANTIBACTERIAL potassium hydroxyquinoline sulphate. It can be used to treat acne, and is available as a cream for topical application. It is not normally given to children, except on medical advice.
✚▲ Side-effects/warnings: See BENZOYL PEROXIDE; POTASSIUM HYDROXYQUINOLINE SULPHATE.

Quinoderm Lotio-Gel 5%

(Quinoderm) is a proprietary, non-prescription compound preparation of the KERATOLYTIC and ANTIMICROBIAL benzoyl peroxide (5%) and the ANTIFUNGAL and ANTIBACTERIAL potassium hydroxyquinoline sulphate. It can be used to treat acne, and is available as a gel for topical application.
✚▲ Side-effects/warnings: See BENZOYL PEROXIDE; POTASSIUM HYDROXYQUINOLINE SULPHATE.

quinolone

(4-quinolone; fluoroquinolone) drugs are ANTIBACTERIAL drugs often used to treat infections in patients who are allergic to penicillin or whose strain of bacterium is resistant to standard antibiotics. They are ANTIBIOTIC-like, sharing many of their important characteristics with antibiotics – and are usually grouped with antibiotics – but actually all members of the quinolone group are purely synthetic in origin; so are not strictly antibiotics (in the sense meaning derived, at least in the case of the original members, from micro-organisms). Although the quinolones are active against a wide range of infective bacterial organisms, they are usually more effective against Gram-negative organisms and also have useful activity against some Gram-positive organisms. They are especially used for complicated urinary tract infections, bacterial prostatitis, cervicitis and gonorrhoea; and generally in circumstances where other antibiotics classes are less effective. They work by damaging the internal structure of bacteria (ie they are *bactericidal*). Side-effects are usually mild, and are not common – usually rash and gastrointestinal disorders. Chemically, they are related to NALIDIXIC ACID and the names of more recently introduced members end with *-oxacin*. See CIPROFLOXACIN; LEVOFLOXACIN; NORFLOXACIN; OFLOXACIN.

✚ Side-effects: There may be nausea, diarrhoea, vomiting, dyspepsia, abdominal pain; headache, dizziness, sleep disorders, rash, pruritus, fever, photosensitivity; joint and muscle pains, blood disorders. Less frequently, there may be anaphylaxis, anorexia, confusion, hallucinations and sensory disturbances, and others.

▲ Warnings: It should be administered with caution to children or adolescents; to patients with epilepsy, kidney or liver impairment; G6PD-deficiency, or who are pregnant or breast-feeding. There is a risk of convulsions being precipitated in those showing no previous tendencies by other drugs (eg by NSAIDS). Avoid excessive exposure to sunlight. If there is tendon pain or inflammation, the treatment should be stopped and the limb rested, and the doctor informed. Some inorganic compounds which can be taken orally for medical purposes (eg as ANTACID agents) or as nutritional supplements (eg in multivitamin preparations) can reduce the effectiveness of some quinolones. These include salts of magnesium, calcium (eg CALCIUM CARBONATE), zinc and IRON.

Quinoped Cream

(Quinoderm) is a proprietary, non-prescription compound preparation of the ANTIFUNGAL drug potassium hydroxyquinoline sulphate and the KERATOLYTIC and ANTIMICROBIAL benzoyl peroxide. It can be used to treat athlete's foot, and is available as a cream.

✚▲ Side-effects/warnings: See BENZOYL PEROXIDE; POTASSIUM HYDROXYQUINOLINE SULPHATE.

quinupristin with dalfopristin

is a combination of two ANTIBIOTIC drugs with ANTIBACTERIAL properties that belong to the unusual group, the streptogramin antibiotics. These two antibiotics are only used together, to treat infections that have failed to respond or are resistant to other antibiotics, for instance MRSA (methicillin-resistant *Staphylococcus aureus*), hospital-acquired pneumonia, soft-tissue infection with *E. faecium* and Gram-positive infections or in people who are unable to tolerate other antibiotics. They need to be given in conjunction with other antibiotics for some infections. Administration is by injection.

✚ Side-effects: This is a specialist drug, and a full explanation will be given. Nausea and vomiting, diarrhoea or constipation, abdominal pain, anxiety, insomnia, dizziness, blood and liver effects, headache, rash and itching, muscle and joint pains, tingling in the extremities, and a variety of other side-effects.

▲ Warnings: Caution in kidney and liver impairment, pregnancy or breast-feeding.

✪ **Related entry: Synercid.**

Qvar

(3M) is a proprietary, prescription-only preparation of the CORTICOSTEROID and ANTI-ASTHMATIC beclometasone dipropionate. It can be used to prevent asthmatic attacks, and is available in an aerosol for inhalation (in a variety of forms, including *Qvar 50; Qvar 100; Qvar 50 Autohaler; Qvar 100 Autohaler*).

✚▲ Side-effects/warnings: See BECLOMETASONE DIPROPIONATE.

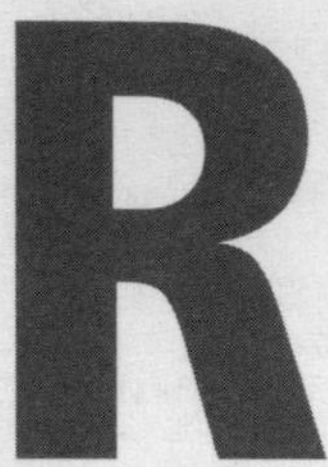

rabeprazole sodium

is an ULCER-HEALING DRUG. It works as an inhibitor of gastric acid secretion in the parietal (acid-producing) cells of the stomach lining by acting as a PROTON-PUMP INHIBITOR. It is used for the treatment of benign gastric and duodenal ulcers, gastro-oesophageal reflux disease and duodenal ulcer associated with *Helicobacter pylori*. Administration is oral.

✚▲ Side-effects/warnings: See PROTON-PUMP INHIBITOR. Also reported, inflammation of the lining of the mucous membrane of the mouth, chest pain, cough, rhinitis, sinusitis, blood changes, insomnia, nervousness, drowsiness, weakness, taste disturbance, anorexia or weight gain, flu-like syndrome, sweating, weight gain.

✪ **Related entry: Pariet.**

Rabies Immunoglobulin

(PHLS; BPL; SNBTS) (Antirabies Immunoglobulin Injection) is a non-proprietary, prescription-only preparation of a SPECIFIC IMMUNOGLOBULIN. It can be used in IMMUNIZATION to give immediate immunity against infection by rabies. It is available in a form for intramuscular injection and infiltration around the wound (eg a bite).

✚▲ Side-effects/warnings: See IMMUNIZATION.

rabies immunoglobulin

(HTIG) is a SPECIFIC IMMUNOGLOBULIN of human origin, which is used in IMMUNIZATION to give immediate *passive immunity* against infection by rabies and can be used in conjunction with RABIES VACCINE. Administration is by intramuscular injection and injection at the site of the bite.

✚▲ Side-effects/warnings: See IMMUNIZATION.

✪ **Related entry: Rabies Immunoglobulin.**

Rabies Vaccine

(Aventis Pasteur) is a proprietary, prescription-only VACCINE preparation which can be used to prevent contracting rabies. It is available in a form for injection.

✚▲ Side-effects/warnings: See RABIES VACCINE.

rabies vaccine

is a VACCINE (an inactivated virus) used for the IMMUNIZATION to prevent contracting rabies (but does not treat people already infected with rabies). It is administered to medical workers and their relatives, who may come into contact with rabid animals or with people who have been bitten by an animal that might be rabid. It can also be routinely administered to people who work with animals (eg vets) to prevent contracting rabies. The vaccine is of a type known as a *human diploid cell vaccine* and is administered by a course of injections.

✚▲ Side-effects/warnings: See VACCINE.

✪ **Related entry: Rabies Vaccine; Rabipur.**

Rabipur

(MASTA) is a proprietary, prescription-only VACCINE preparation (inactivated Flury LEP rabies virus) which can be used to prevent contracting rabies. It is available in a form for intramuscular injection.

✚▲ Side-effects/warnings: See RABIES VACCINE.

Radian B Heat Spray

(Roche Consumer Health) is a proprietary, non-prescription compound preparation of camphor, menthol, aspirin and methyl salicylate, which all have COUNTER-IRRITANT, or RUBEFACIENT, actions. It can be applied to the skin for symptomatic relief of muscle and rheumatic pain, sciatica, lumbago, fibrosis and muscle stiffness. It is available as a spray and is not normally given to children under six, except on medical advice.

✚▲ Side-effects/warnings: See ASPIRIN; CAMPHOR; MENTHOL; METHYL SALICYLATE.

Radian B Ibuprofen Gel

(Roche Consumer Health) is a proprietary, non-prescription compound preparation of the NSAID and antirheumatic agent ibuprofen, which has a COUNTER-IRRITANT, or RUBEFACIENT, action. It can be applied to the skin for symptomatic relief of muscle and rheumatic pain, sciatica, lumbago, fibrosis and muscle stiffness. It is available as a gel for application to the skin and is not normally given to children under 14, except on medical advice.

✚▲ Side-effects/warnings: See IBUPROFEN; but adverse effects are minimal on topical application.

Radian B Muscle Lotion

(Roche Consumer Health) is a proprietary, non-prescription compound preparation of camphor, menthol, salicylic acid and ammonium salicylate, which all have COUNTER-IRRITANT, or RUBEFACIENT, actions. It can be applied to the skin for symptomatic relief of backache, sprains, strains, neuralgia, muscle and rheumatic pain. It is available as a spray for application to the skin and is not normally given to children under six years, except on medical advice.
✚▲ Side-effects/warnings: See AMMONIUM SALICYLATE; CAMPHOR; MENTHOL; SALICYLIC ACID.

Radian B Muscle Rub

(Roche Consumer Health) is a proprietary, non-prescription compound preparation of camphor, menthol, methyl salicylate and capsicum oleoresin, which all have COUNTER-IRRITANT, or RUBEFACIENT, actions. It can be applied to the skin for symptomatic relief of muscle and rheumatic pain, pulled, sprained and stiff muscles, and muscle stiffness. It is available as an ointment for topical application to the skin. Not normally used for children under six, except on medical advice.
✚▲ Side-effects/warnings: See CAPSICUM OLEORESIN; CAMPHOR; MENTHOL; METHYL SALICYLATE. It should not be used on inflamed or broken skin or mucous membranes.

Ralgex Cream

(SSL) is a proprietary, non-prescription compound preparation of glycol monosalicylate and capsicum oleoresin, which act as COUNTER-IRRITANT, or RUBEFACIENT agents, and the VASODILATOR methyl nicotinate, and is used for the symptomatic relief of muscle pain and stiffness, sciatica, lumbago and fibrositis. It is available as a cream for topical application to the skin and is not normally used for children, except on medical advice.
✚▲ Side-effects/warnings: See CAPSICUM OLEORESIN; GLYCOL SALICYLATE; METHYL NICOTINATE. It should not be applied to broken skin and abrasions.

Ralgex Freeze Spray

(SSL) is a proprietary, non-prescription of glycol monosalicylate (with propellants) which acts as a COUNTER-IRRITANT, or RUBEFACIENT, for the symptomatic relief of muscle pain and stiffness, backache, sciatica and lumbago. It is available as a spray for topical application to the skin and is not normally used for children under five years, except on medical advice.
✚▲ Side-effects/warnings: See GLYCOL SALICYLATE.

Ralgex Heat Spray

(SSL) is a proprietary, non-prescription compound preparation of glycol monosalicylate which acts as COUNTER-IRRITANT, or RUBEFACIENT, and the VASODILATOR methyl nicotinate, and is used for the symptomatic relief of muscle pain and stiffness, sciatica and lumbago. It is available as a spray for topical application to the skin and is not normally used for children under five years, except on medical advice.
✚▲ Side-effects/warnings: See GLYCOL SALICYLATE; METHYL NICOTINATE.

Ralgex Stick

(SSL) is a proprietary, non-prescription compound preparation of menthol, methyl salicylate, glycol salicylate, ethyl salicylate and capsicum oleoresin, which have COUNTER-IRRITANT, or RUBEFACIENT actions, for the symptomatic relief of muscle pain and stiffness, sciatica and lumbago. It is available as an embrocation stick for topical application to the skin and is not normally used for children, except on medical advice.
✚▲ Side-effects/warnings: See CAPSICUM OLEORESIN; ETHYL SALICYLATE; GLYCOL SALICYLATE; MENTHOL; METHYL SALICYLATE.

raloxifene hydrochloride

is an agent that has weak OESTROGEN activity at some sites in the body, but anti-oestrogen actions at others. Chemically, it is not a STEROID, but like some oestrogens it can be used as a form of hormone replacement therapy (HRT), though only for postmenopausal women with increased risk of osteoporosis for the prevention of vertebral fractures. It does not, however, reduce other menopausal symptoms. Administration is oral.
✚ Side-effects: Venous blood clots (thromboembolism and thrombophlebitis), leg cramps, hot flushes, peripheral oedema.
▲ Warnings: It is not to be used in individuals with

a history of venous thromboembolism, undiagnosed uterine bleeding, breast or uterine cancer, liver disease or severe kidney impairment; impaired bile secretion in the intestine (cholestasis), or in pregnancy and breast-feeding. Used with caution where there are risk factors for venous thromboembolism, and treatment should be stopped if there is to be prolonged immobilization.
✪ **Related entry: Evista.**

raltitrexed

is an (*antimetabolite*) CYTOTOXIC drug which is used primarily as an ANTICANCER treatment of colon cancer. Administration is by injection.
✚▲ Side-effects/warnings: See CYTOTOXIC.
✪ **Related entry: Tomudex.**

ramipril

is an ACE INHIBITOR and acts as a VASODILATOR. It can be used as an ANTIHYPERTENSIVE and in congestive HEART FAILURE TREATMENT and sometimes following myocardial infarction (damage to heart muscle, usually after a heart attack). It is often used in conjunction with other classes of drug, particularly (THIAZIDE) DIURETIC drugs. Administration is oral.
✚ Side-effects: See ACE INHIBITOR. Also heart arrhythmias, angina and chest pain, fainting, cerebrovascular accident, myocardial infarction, loss of appetite, dry mouth, skin reactions; exacerbation of Raynaud's syndrome; conjunctivitis, confusion, nervousness and anxiety, depression, impotence, decreased libido, alopecia, bronchitis and muscle cramps.
▲ Warnings: See ACE INHIBITOR.
✪ **Related entries: Triapin; Tritace.**

Ranitic

(Tillomed) is a proprietary, prescription-only preparation of the H_2-ANTAGONIST and ULCER-HEALING DRUG ranitidine (as hydrochloride). It can be used to treat benign peptic ulcers (in the stomach or duodenum), gastro-oesophageal reflux, dyspepsia and associated conditions. It is available as tablets.
✚▲ Side-effects/warnings: See RANITIDINE.

ranitidine

is an effective and extensively prescribed H_2-ANTAGONIST and ULCER-HEALING DRUG. It is used in the treatment of benign peptic (gastric and duodenal) ulcers, NSAID-induced ulceration, and as prophylaxis to relieve heartburn in cases of reflux oesophagitis, Zollinger-Ellison syndrome and a variety of conditions where reduction of acidity is beneficial. It is now also available without prescription – in a limited amount and for short-term uses only – for the relief of heartburn, dyspepsia and hyperacidity. It works by reducing the secretion of gastric acid, so reducing erosion and bleeding from peptic ulcers and allowing them a chance to heal. However, treatment with ranitidine should not start before a full diagnosis of gastric bleeding or serious pain has been made, because its action in restricting gastric secretions may possibly mask the presence of stomach cancer. It can also be used to treat ulceration induced by NSAID treatment. Administration can be either oral or by injection. (Although it is a prescription-only drug when used for the treatment of ulcers and related conditions, it can be sold over-the-counter in limited quantities and dosage for occasional indigestion and heartburn for people over 16 years.)
✚▲ Side-effects/warnings: See H_2-ANTAGONIST. Also, there may be agitation, increased heart rate, skin symptoms, hair loss, visual disturbances. It should not be used by people with porphyria.
✪ **Related entries: Ranitic; Rantec; Zaedoc; Zantac; Zantac 75 Relief Tablets.**

ranitidine bismuth citrate

(ranitidine bismutrex) is a compound of the extensively prescribed H_2-ANTAGONIST and ULCER-HEALING DRUG ranitidine, together with bismuth. It can be used in the treatment of benign peptic (gastric or duodenal) ulcers. In the treatment of duodenal ulceration associated with *Helicobacter pylori* infection it is used in conjunction with an ANTIBIOTIC, CLARITHROMYCIN with either AMOXICILLIN or METRONIDAZOLE. Ranitidine works by reducing the secretion of gastric acid and (together with the antibiotic) helps to eliminate the bacterium associated with peptic ulceration. Administration is oral.
✚▲ Side-effects/warnings: See H_2-ANTAGONIST; also TRIPOTASSIUM DICITRATOBISMUTHATE. Also, it may darken tongue or blacken faeces; rarely there is a speeding of the heart, agitation, visual disturbances, hair loss, skin symptoms. It is not used in porphyria, pregnancy or breast-feeding, kidney impairment.
✪ **Related entry: Pylorid.**

ranitidine bismutrex

see RANITIDINE BISMUTH CITRATE.

Rantec

(Berk; APS) is a proprietary, prescription-only preparation of the H_2-ANTAGONIST and ULCER-HEALING DRUG ranitidine (as hydrochloride). It can be used to treat benign peptic ulcers (in the stomach or duodenum), gastro-oesophageal reflux, dyspepsia and associated conditions. It is available as tablets.

✚▲ Side-effects/warnings: See RANITIDINE.

Rapamune

(Wyeth) as a recently introduced proprietary, prescription-only preparation of the IMMUNOSUPPRESSANT sirolimus. It can be used to prevent tissue rejection in kidney transplant patients, and is available as an oral solution which is drunk after mixing with water or orange juice.

✚▲ Side-effects/warnings: See SIROLIMUS.

Rapifen

(Janssen-Cilag) is a proprietary, prescription-only preparation of the (OPIOID) NARCOTIC ANALGESIC alfentanil (as hydrochloride), and is on the Controlled Drugs list. It can be used in outpatient surgery, short operational procedures and for the enhancement of anaesthesia. It is available in a form for injection.

✚▲ Side-effects/warnings: See ALFENTANIL.

Rapilysin

(Roche) is a proprietary, prescription-only preparation of the FIBRINOLYTIC drug reteplase. It can be used to treat myocardial infarction, and is available in a form for injection.

✚▲ Side-effects/warnings: See RETEPLASE.

Rapitil

(Rhône-Poulenc Rorer; Aventis Pharma) is a proprietary, prescription-only preparation of the ANTI-ALLERGIC drug nedocromil sodium. It can be used to treat allergic conjunctivitis in the eye, and is available as eye-drops.

✚▲ Side-effects/warnings: See NEDOCROMIL SODIUM.

rasburicase

is an enzyme (see ENZYMES), urate oxidase, produced by by recombinant DNA technology, which helps to break down urea in the blood. It can be used to prevent or treat an acute rise in blood urea caused by chemotherapy for blood cancers. It is given by intravenous infusion.

✚ Side-effects: Rasburicase can cause fever, nausea and vomiting; less often it may cause headache, diarrhoea, rash, bronchospasm and other hypersensitivity reactions, and haemolytic anaemia.

▲ Warnings: It should be not be administered to patients susceptible to haemolytic anaemia, including G6PD deficiency, or who are pregnant or breast-feeding. There will be monitoring for hypersensitivity reactions and allergies.

razoxane

is a synthetic CYTOTOXIC drug which is used as in ANTICANCER therapy for some forms of cancer, including leukaemia. Administration is oral.

✚▲ Side-effects/warnings: See CYTOTOXIC.

Rebetol

(Schering-Plough) is a proprietary, prescription-only preparation of the ANTIVIRAL drug tribavirin. It can be used to treat chronic hepatitis C (in combination with interferon alfa-2b). It is available as capsules.

✚▲ Side-effects/warnings: See TRIBAVIRIN.

Rebif

(Serono) is a proprietary, prescription-only preparation of the drug interferon (in the form of beta-1a). It can be used to treat relapsing-remitting multiple sclerosis. It is available in a form for subcutaneous injection.

✚▲ Side-effects/warnings: See INTERFERON.

reboxetine

is an 'atypical' ANTIDEPRESSANT drug that can be used to treat depressive illness. As for the *selective serotonin re-uptake inhibitor* (SSRI) group of antidepressants, its mechanism of action is thought to be principally through inhibiting an amine-pump responsible for the re-uptake of a neurotransmitter in the brain, but rather than SEROTONIN uptake into nerve endings within the brain, it is believed to be a selective noradrenaline uptake inhibitor (SNRI). Administration is oral as tablets.

✚ Side-effects: Insomnia; sweating; dizziness, vertigo and postural hypotension; tingling in the extremities, impotence, pain on urination and urinary retention (mainly in men), dry mouth, constipation, speeding of the heart.

R

▲ Warnings: Care in severe kidney or liver impairment, in the elderly, pregnancy or breast-feeding, in those with a history of epilepsy, manic-depressive disorders, prostatic hypertrophy, urinary retention, glaucoma. Drowsiness may impair the performance of skilled tasks such as driving. It should not be used in pregnancy and breast-feeding.
✪ **Related entry: Edronax.**

recombinant human insulin analogue
see INSULIN LISPRO.

Recombinate
(Hyland Immuno) is a proprietary, prescription-only preparation of factor VIII fraction (octocog alfa), which acts as a HAEMOSTATIC drug to reduce or stop bleeding in the treatment of disorders in which bleeding is prolonged and potentially dangerous (mainly haemophilia A). It is available in a form for intravenous injection or infusion.
✚▲ Side-effects/warnings: See FACTOR VIII FRACTION (DRIED).

Redoxon
(Roche Consumer Health) is a proprietary, non-prescription preparation of vitamin C (ascorbic acid). It can be used to treat the symptoms of vitamin C deficiency, and is available as chewable tablets (adults and children), effervescent tablets (adults and children over six) and slow-release tablets (adults only).
✚▲ Side-effects/warnings: See ASCORBIC ACID.

Reductil
(Abbott) is a proprietary preparation of the APPETITE SUPPRESSANT sibutramine. It can be used to assist in OBESITY TREATMENT, and is available as capsules.
✚▲ Side-effects/warnings: See SIBUTRAMINE.

ReFacto
(Wyeth) is a proprietary, prescription-only preparation of factor VIII fraction (octocog alfa), which acts as a HAEMOSTATIC drug to reduce or stop bleeding in the treatment of disorders in which bleeding is prolonged and potentially dangerous (mainly haemophilia A). It is available in a form for intravenous injection or infusion.
✚▲ Side-effects/warnings: See FACTOR VIII FRACTION (DRIED).

Refludan
(Hoechst Marion Roussel; Aventis Pharma) is a proprietary, prescription-only preparation of the (parenteral) ANTICOAGULANT lepirudin. It can be used to treat thromboembolic disease in patients who show adverse reactions to heparin, and is available in a form for injection.
✚▲ Side-effects/warnings: See LEPIRUDIN.

Refolinon
(Pharmacia) is a proprietary, prescription-only preparation of calcium folinate. It can be used to counteract the folate-antagonist activity and consequent toxic effects of certain ANTICANCER drugs, especially METHOTREXATE. It is available as tablets and in a form for injection.
✚▲ Side-effects/warnings: See CALCIUM FOLINATE.

Regaine Extra Strength
(Pharmacia) is a proprietary, non-prescription preparation of the VASODILATOR minoxidil. It can be used to treat male-pattern baldness, and is available as a topical solution. It should not be used by anyone over 65 years or under 18 years.
✚▲ Side-effects/warnings: See MINOXIDIL.

Regaine Regular Strength
(Pharmacia) is a proprietary, non-prescription preparation of the VASODILATOR minoxidil. It can be used to treat male-pattern baldness (in men and women), and is available as a topical solution. It should not be used by anyone over 65 years or under 18 years.
✚▲ Side-effects/warnings: See MINOXIDIL.

Regranex
(Janssen-Cilag) is a prescription-only, proprietary preparation of becaplermin, a growth factor (see GROWTH FACTORS) that is under evaluation as an adjunct in the treatment of ulcers found in neuropathic diabetic disease. It is used in the form of a gel.
✚▲ Side-effects/warnings: see BECAPLERMIN.

Regulan Lemon & Lime
(Procter & Gamble) is a proprietary, non-prescription preparation of the (*bulking-agent*) LAXATIVE ispaghula husk. It can be used to treat a number of gastrointestinal disorders that require a high-fibre diet, including irritable bowel syndrome, diverticular disease and to relieve

constipation. It is available as a powder for solution in water. It is not normally given to children under six, except on medical advice.
✚▲ Side-effects/warnings: See ISPAGHULA HUSK.

Regulose

(Novartis) is a proprietary, non-prescription preparation of the (*osmotic*) LAXATIVE lactulose. It can be used to relieve constipation, and is available as an oral solution.
✚▲ Side-effects/warnings: See LACTULOSE.

Regurin

(Galen) is a newly introduced proprietary, prescription-only preparation of the ANTICHOLINERGIC trospium chloride. It can be used as an ANTISPASMODIC in the treatment of urinary disorders, such as incontinence. It is available as tablets.
✚▲ Side-effects/warnings: See TROSPIUM CHLORIDE.

Relaxit Micro-enema

(Crawford) is a proprietary, non-prescription preparation of sodium citrate, glycerol, the SURFACTANT sodium lauryl sulphate; with sorbic acid and sorbitol. Used as a LAXATIVE. Available as an enema.
✚▲ Side-effects/warnings: See GLYCEROL; SODIUM CITRATE; SODIUM LAURYL SULPHATE; SORBITOL.

Relaxyl Capsules

(SSL) is a proprietary, non-prescription preparation of the ANTISPASMODIC drug alverine citrate. It can be used to treat muscle spasm of the gastrointestinal tract, for example, in irritable bowel syndrome, and is available as capsules. It is not normally given to children, except on medical advice.
✚▲ Side-effects/warnings: See ALVERINE CITRATE.

Relenza

(GlaxoWellcome; GSK) is a prescription-only, proprietary preparation of the ANTIVIRAL drug zanamivir, and can be used in the treatment of influenza A or B. It may be given to shorten the duration of infection. It is available in the form of a dry powder for inhalation. At the time of writing, there are restrictions on its NHS prescription.
✚▲ Side-effects/warnings: See ZANAMIVIR.

Relifex

(SmithKline Beecham; GSK) is a proprietary, prescription-only preparation of the (NSAID) NON-NARCOTIC ANALGESIC and ANTIRHEUMATIC nabumetone. It can be used to treat and relieve pain and inflammation, particularly osteoarthritic and rheumatic pain. It is available as tablets and a sugar-free oral suspension.
✚▲ Side-effects/warnings: See NABUMETONE.

Relpax

(Pfizer) is a proprietary, prescription-only preparation of the ANTIMIGRAINE drug eletripan (as hydrobromide). It can be used to treat acute migraine attacks, and is available as tablets.
✚▲ Side-effects/warnings: See **eletripan**.

Remedeine

(Napp) is a proprietary, prescription-only compound analgesic preparation of the NON-NARCOTIC ANALGESIC paracetamol and the (OPIOID) NARCOTIC ANALGESIC dihydrocodeine tartrate, in the ratio 500:20 mg. It can be used as a painkiller, and is available as tablets, effervescent tablets (and as *Forte tablets* and *Forte effervescent tablets* in a combination of 500:30 mg).
✚▲ Side-effects/warnings: See DIHYDROCODEINE TARTRATE; PARACETAMOL. Some forms should be avoided by people with kidney impairment.

Remegel Original

(SSL) is a proprietary, non-prescription preparation of the ANTACID calcium carbonate. It can be used to relieve heartburn, acid indigestion and upset stomach. It is available as chewable tablets and is not normally given to children, except on medical advice. It is also available in *Alpine Mint with Lemon* and *Freshmint* flavours.
✚▲ Side-effects/warnings: See CALCIUM CARBONATE.

remifentanil

is an (OPIOID) NARCOTIC ANALGESIC which is used in the induction of anaesthesia and during surgery to supplement the effect of GENERAL ANAESTHETIC drugs. Administration is by intravenous infusion.
✚▲ Side-effects/warnings: See OPIOID.
✪ **Related entry: Ultiva.**

Reminyl

(Shire) is a prescription-only form of the ANTICHOLINESTERASE galantamine (as hydrobromide) which can be used in DEMENTIA

R

TREATMENT. It is available as tablets.
✚▲ Side-effects/warnings: See GALANTAMINE.

Remnos
(DDSA) is a proprietary, prescription-only preparation of the BENZODIAZEPINE nitrazepam. It can be used as a relatively long-acting HYPNOTIC for the short-term treatment of insomnia, where a degree of sedation during the daytime is acceptable. It is available as tablets.
✚▲ Side-effects/warnings: See NITRAZEPAM.

Rennie Deflatine
(Roche Consumer Health) is a proprietary, non-prescription compound preparation of the ANTACID agents calcium carbonate and magnesium carbonate, with the ANTIFOAMING AGENT dimeticone (as simeticone/simethicone). It can be used to relieve acid indigestion, heartburn, dyspepsia, bloating and flatulence. It is available as tablets and is not normally given to children under six years, except on medical advice.
✚▲ Side-effects/warnings: See CALCIUM CARBONATE; DIMETICONE; MAGNESIUM CARBONATE.

Rennie Duo
(Roche Consumer Health) is a proprietary, non-prescription compound preparation of the ANTACID agents calcium carbonate and magnesium carbonate and the DEMULCENT alginic acid (as sodium alginate). It is used to relieve the symptoms of indigestion and gastro-oesophageal reflux, and is available as an oral suspension. It is not normally given to children, except on medical advice.
✚▲ Side-effects/warnings: ALGINIC ACID; CALCIUM CARBONATE, MAGNESIUM CARBONATE.

Rennie Rap-Eze
(Roche Consumer Health) is a proprietary, non-prescription preparation of the ANTACID calcium carbonate. It can be used to relieve acid indigestion, heartburn, upset stomach, dyspepsia and biliousness. It is available as tablets and is not normally given to children, except on medical advice.
✚▲ Side-effects/warnings: See CALCIUM CARBONATE.

ReoPro
(Lilly) is a proprietary, prescription-only preparation of the ANTIPLATELET drug abciximab, which inhibits platelet aggregation and thrombus formation. It is used by specialist doctors in certain types of coronary angioplasty operations. Administration is by injection.
✚▲ Side-effects/warnings: See ABCIXIMAB.

repaglinide
is a newly introduced drug which is used in DIABETIC TREATMENT of Type II diabetes (non-insulin-dependent diabetes mellitus; NIDDM; maturity-onset diabetes), particularly in patients who are not totally dependent on additional supplies of INSULIN, in diabetes that is not controlled by diet and exercise. It works by stimulating insulin release from the pancreas, and can be used together with another diabetic drug, METFORMIN HYDROCHLORIDE. Administration is oral.
✚ Side-effects: Constipation or diarrhoea, abdominal pain, nausea and vomiting; hypersensitivity reactions including rashes; changed liver enzymes. Insulin needs to be substituted for this drug during certain illnesses and infections and for surgery.
▲ Warnings: It should not be used in pregnancy or breast-feeding, where there is severe kidney or liver impairment, or in certain diabetic states.
✪ **Related entry: NovoNorm.**

Replenate
(BPL) is a proprietary, prescription-only preparation of dried human factor VIII fraction. It acts as a HAEMOSTATIC to reduce or stop bleeding in the treatment of disorders in which bleeding is prolonged and potentially dangerous (mainly haemophilia A). It is available in a form for intravenous injection or infusion.
✚▲ Side-effects/warnings: See FACTOR VIII FRACTION (DRIED).

Replenine-VF
(BPL) is a proprietary, prescription-only (heat-treated) preparation of factor IX fraction, dried, which is prepared from human blood plasma. It can be used in treating patients with a deficiency in factor IX (haemophilia B), and is available in a form for intravenous infusion.
✚▲ Side-effects/warnings: See FACTOR IX FRACTION, DRIED.

Requip
(SmithKline Beecham; GSK) is a proprietary,

prescription-only preparation of the DOPAMINE-RECEPTOR STIMULANT a drug ropinirole (as hydrochloride). It can be used as an ANTIPARKINSONISM drug, and is available as tablets.
✚▲ Side-effects/warnings: See ROPINIROLE.

Resolve

(SSL) is a proprietary, non-prescription preparation of the NON-NARCOTIC ANALGESIC paracetamol, vitamin C (ascorbic acid) and various ANTACID salts (sodium carbonate, potassium bicarbonate, with citric acid). It can be used to treat headache with stomach upset, particularly after overindulgence. It is available as sachets to make an effervescent drink, and is not normally given to children under 16 years, except on medical advice.
✚▲ Side-effects/warnings: See ASCORBIC ACID; SODIUM CARBONATE; PARACETAMOL; POTASSIUM BICARBONATE.

Resonium A

(Sanofi-Synthelabo) is a proprietary, non-prescription preparation of sodium polystyrene sulphonate, which is a resin that can be used to treat high blood potassium levels. It is available in the form of a powdered resin to be taken by mouth or for use as a rectal enema.
✚▲ Side-effects/warnings: See POLYSTYRENE SULPHONATE RESINS.

resorcinol

is a KERATOLYTIC agent which, when applied topically, causes skin to peel and relieves itching. It is also used in ointments and lotions for the treatment of acne.
✚ Side-effects: There may be local irritation.
▲ Warnings: It is not to be used if there are local infections; avoid the eyes, mouth and mucous membranes. Prolonged use may affect the functioning of the thyroid gland.
✪ **Related entry: Eskamel.**

respiratory stimulant

(analeptic) drugs are central nervous stimulants that show some degree of selectivity for respiratory stimulation. They have little current use but DOXAPRAM HYDROCHLORIDE is sometimes used to relieve severe respiratory failure in patients who suffer from chronic obstructive airways disease, or who undergo respiratory depression following major surgery, particularly in cases where ventilatory support is not possible. A number of them were once used as ANTIDOTE agents in the event of overdose and poisoning by respiratory depressants, but have been discontinued because effective doses were close to those causing toxic effects, especially convulsions. Overdose with respiratory depressants, such as BENZODIAZEPINE and OPIOID drugs, is now treated with specific receptor ANTAGONIST agents.

Respontin

(A&H; GSK) is a proprietary, prescription-only preparation of the ANTICHOLINERGIC and BRONCHODILATOR ipratropium bromide. It can be used to treat the symptoms of chronic bronchitis, and is available as a nebulizer solution.
✚▲ Side-effects/warnings: See IPRATROPIUM BROMIDE.

Restandol

(Organon) is a proprietary, prescription-only preparation of the ANDROGEN (male sex hormone) testosterone (as undecanoate). It can be used to treat hormone deficiency in men, and is available as capsules.
✚▲ Side-effects/warnings: See TESTOSTERONE.

reteplase

has enzyme (see ENZYMES) activity and is used therapeutically as a FIBRINOLYTIC drug because it has the property of breaking up blood clots. It is used rapidly in acute myocardial infarction. Administration is by injection.
✚▲ Side-effects/warnings: See FIBRINOLYTIC.
✪ **Related entry: Rapilysin.**

Retin-A

(Janssen-Cilag) is a proprietary, prescription-only preparation of the (RETINOID) tretinoin. It can be used to treat severe acne, and is available as a cream, a gel and a lotion.
✚▲ Side-effects/warnings: See TRETINOIN.

retinoid

drugs are a group of chemical agents derived from RETINOL (another name for vitamin A). Retinol is normally concerned in regulating epithelial (surface tissues, including skin) cell growth and differentiation. Synthetic analogues of retinol used as drugs can be given to treat a number of skin

R

conditions, including acne, psoriasis and rarer conditions such as Darier's disease. One, TRETINOIN, is used to induce remission in acute promyelocytic leukaemia. However drugs with such an action are toxic, so are generally used by topical application as a gel or cream. When used orally it is under strict medical supervision; and because they influence cell division they are potentially teratogenic (affect the developing fetus) and so they are not administered to women who are or may become pregnant. See ACITRETIN; ADAPALENE; ISOTRETINOIN; TAZAROTENE; TRETINOIN.

retinol

is the chemical term for vitamin A, which is a fat-soluble vitamin found in meats, liver and milk products and is also synthesized in the body from constituents in green vegetables and carrots. Retinol is essential for growth and the maintenance of mucous membranes. It is particularly useful in supporting the part of the eye's retina that allows vision in the dark and a deficiency may cause night-blindness and dry eyes. It is administered therapeutically to make up vitamin deficiency (which is rare in Western countries). Administration is usually oral or topical as an emulsion, but it can also be by injection. Derivatives of Vitamin A (retinoids) are used by topical application to treat acne.

✚ Side-effects: Massive overdose can cause rough skin, dry hair, effects on the liver and blood.

▲ Warnings: In view of evidence suggesting that high levels of vitamin A may cause birth defects, women who are (or may become) pregnant are advised not to take vitamin A supplements (including tablets and fish-liver oil drops), except on the advice of a doctor or an antenatal clinic; nor should they eat liver or products such as liver paté.

✪ Related entries: Halycitrol; Vitamin A Palmitate; Vitamin Tablets (with Calcium and Iodine) for Nursing Mothers.

Retinova

(Janssen-Cilag) is a proprietary, prescription-only preparation of the (RETINOID) tretinoin. It can be used to treat photodamage to the skin due to chronic exposure to the sun, and is available as a cream.

✚▲ Side-effects/warnings: See TRETINOIN.

Retrovir

(GlaxoWellcome; GSK) is a proprietary, prescription-only preparation of the ANTIVIRAL drug zidovudine (azidothymidine; AZT). It can be used in the treatment of HIV infection, and is available as capsules, tablets, a syrup and in a form for intravenous infusion.

✚▲ Side-effects/warnings: See ZIDOVUDINE.

reviparin sodium

is a *low molecular weight* heparin which is used as an ANTICOAGULANT. It has some advantages over heparin when used in the long-duration prevention of venous thrombo-embolism, particularly in orthopaedic use. Administration is by injection.

✚▲ Side-effects/warnings: See HEPARIN.

✪ Related entry: Clivarine.

Rheumacin LA

(Hillcross) is a proprietary, prescription-only preparation of the (NSAID) NON-NARCOTIC ANALGESIC and ANTIRHEUMATIC drug indometacin (indomethacin). It can be used to relieve pain and inflammation, particularly rheumatic and arthritic pain and to treat other musculoskeletal disorders (including and inflammation of joints and tendons), period pain and acute gout. It is available as modified-release capsules.

✚▲ Side-effects/warnings: See INDOMETACIN.

Rheumox

(Goldshield) is a proprietary, prescription-only preparation of the (NSAID) NON-NARCOTIC ANALGESIC and ANTIRHEUMATIC azapropazone. It can be used to relieve pain and inflammation only of severe rheumatoid arthritis, ankylosing spondylitis and acute gout. It is available as capsules and tablets.

✚▲ Side-effects/warnings: See AZAPROPAZONE.

Rhinocort Aqua

(AstraZeneca) is a proprietary, prescription-only preparation of the CORTICOSTEROID budesonide. It can be used to treat nasal rhinitis and nasal polyps, and is available as a nasal aerosol. (It can be sold to the public without prescription for seasonal rhinitis subject to certain safeguards including age restriction.)

✚▲ Side-effects/warnings: See BUDESONIDE.

Rhinolast

(ASTA Medica) is proprietary, prescription-only preparation of the ANTIHISTAMINE azelastine

hydrochloride. It can be used for the symptomatic relief of allergic rhinitis, and is available as a nasal spray.
✚▲ Side-effects/warnings: See AZELASTINE HYDROCHLORIDE.

Rhinolast Allergy
(ASTA Medica) is proprietary, non-prescription preparation of the ANTIHISTAMINE azelastine hydrochloride. It can be used for the symptomatic relief of seasonal and perennial allergic rhinitis, and is available as a nasal spray. It is not normally given to children under five years.
✚▲ Side-effects/warnings: See AZELASTINE HYDROCHLORIDE.

rhubarb
in a powdered form is sometimes used as a *stimulant* LAXATIVE and is a constituent of some proprietary laxative preparations.
✚▲ Side-effects/warnings: It is regarded as safe in normal topical use, but unstandardized preparations (where the amount of rhubarb is unknown) can cause undesirably powerful actions.
✪ **Related entries: Jackson's Herbal Laxative; Pyralvex.**

Rhumalgan CR
(Lagap) is a proprietary, prescription-only version of the (NSAID) NON-NARCOTIC ANALGESIC and ANTIRHEUMATIC diclofenac sodium. It can be used to treat arthritic and rheumatic pain and other musculoskeletal disorders. It is available as modified-release tablets.
✚▲ Side-effects/warnings: See DICLOFENAC SODIUM.

ribavirin
(tribavirin) is an ANTIVIRAL drug which inhibits a wide range of DNA and RNA viruses. It can be used to treat severe bronchiolitis caused by the respiratory syncytial virus (RSV) and certain other serious diseases, including Lassa fever and chronic hepatitis C (together with one of the INTERFERON group of drugs). It is administered by injection or aerosol inhalation.
✚▲ Side-effects/warnings: It is a specialist drug, and there will be full assessment and patient monitoring throughout treatment. Possible side-effects will be explained.
✪ **Related entries: Rebetol; Virazole.**

Ridaura
(Yamanouchi) is a proprietary, prescription-only preparation of the ANTIRHEUMATIC auranofin. It can be used to treat rheumatoid arthritis, and is available as tablets.
✚▲ Side-effects/warnings: See AURANOFIN.

Rideril
(DDSA) is a proprietary, prescription-only preparation of the ANTIPSYCHOTIC thioridazine. It can be used to treat and tranquillize psychotic patients (eg schizophrenic and manic patients), and is used in the short-term treatment of anxiety. It is available as tablets.
✚▲ Side-effects/warnings: See THIORIDAZINE.

rifabutin
is an ANTIBACTERIAL, ANTITUBERCULAR and ANTIBIOTIC drug, a member of the rifamycin family. It can be used for the prevention of *Mycobacterium avium* infection in immunocompromised patients and for the treatment of pulmonary tuberculosis and other mycobacterial disease. Administration is oral.
✚▲ Side-effects/warnings: See RIFAMPICIN; there may also be blood and liver disorders, nausea, vomiting and hypersensitivity reactions, flu-like symptoms. Urine, saliva and other bodily secretions may turn orange-red.
✪ **Related entry: Mycobutin.**

Rifadin
(Aventis Pharma) is a proprietary, prescription-only preparation of the ANTIBACTERIAL and ANTIBIOTIC rifampicin. It can be used as an ANTITUBERCULAR drug to treat other serious infections. It is available as capsules, as a syrup and in a form for intravenous infusion.
✚▲ Side-effects/warnings: See RIFAMPICIN.

rifampicin
is an ANTIBACTERIAL, ANTITUBERCULAR and ANTIBIOTIC drug. It is one of the principal drugs used in the treatment of tuberculosis, mainly in combination with other antitubercular drugs, such as isoniazid or pyrazinamide, in order to cover resistance and for maximum effect. It acts against *Mycobacterium tuberculosis* and sensitive Gram-positive bacteria by inhibiting the bacterial RNA polymerase enzyme. It is also effective in the treatment of leprosy, brucellosis, legionnaires' disease and serious staphylococcal infections.

R

Additionally, it may be used to prevent meningococcal meningitis and *Haemophilus influenzae* (type b) infection. Administration can be either oral or by intravenous injection or infusion.

✚ Side-effects: There are many side-effects, including the following: gastrointestinal problems, such as nausea, vomiting, diarrhoea, anorexia and weight loss; some patients also undergo the symptoms of flu, breathlessness, collapse and shock. Rarely, there is kidney failure, liver dysfunction, jaundice, muscle weakness, alteration in the composition of the blood and/or discolouration of the urine, saliva and other body secretions. Sensitivity reactions, such as a rash or urticaria, and menstrual disturbances.

▲ Warnings: It should not be administered to patients with jaundice or porphyria; it should be administered with caution to those with impaired liver function, or who are pregnant or breast-feeding. One other effect of the drug is that soft contact lenses may become discoloured. It may reduce the reliability of the contraceptive pill.

✪ **Related entries: Rifadin; Rifater; Rifinah; Rimactane; Rimactazid.**

Rifater

(Aventis Pharma) is a proprietary, prescription-only compound preparation of the ANTIBACTERIAL drugs rifampicin, isoniazid and pyrazinamide. It can be used in the ANTITUBERCULAR treatment of pulmonary tuberculosis in the initial, intensive phase, and is available as tablets.

✚▲ Side-effects/warnings: See ISONIAZID; PYRAZINAMIDE; RIFAMPICIN.

Rifinah

(Aventis Pharma) is a proprietary, prescription-only compound preparation of the ANTIBACTERIAL drugs rifampicin and isoniazid. It can be used in ANTITUBERCULAR treatment, and is available as tablets in two strengths, *Rifinah 150* and *Rifinah 300*.

✚▲ Side-effects/warnings: See ISONIAZID; RIFAMPICIN.

Rilutek

(Rhône-Poulenc Rorer; Aventis Pharma) is a proprietary, prescription-only preparation of the specialist drug riluzole, which is used in the treatment of patients with amyotrophic lateral sclerosis. It is available as tablets.

✚▲ Side-effects/warnings: See RILUZOLE.

riluzole

is a specialist drug which is used in the treatment of patients with amyotrophic lateral sclerosis. Administration is oral.

✚ Side-effects: Nausea, vomiting, weakness, increased heart rate, sleepiness, headache, dizziness, vertigo, pain, loss of sensation.

▲ Warnings: It should be administered with care where there is a history of abnormal liver function; if there is a risk of blood disorders; dizziness or vertigo may affect performance of skilled tasks, such as driving. It is not to be given to patients who are pregnant or breast-feeding, or who have liver or kidney impairment.

✪ **Related entry: Rilutek.**

Rimacid

(Ranbaxy) is a proprietary, prescription-only preparation of the (NSAID) NON-NARCOTIC ANALGESIC and ANTIRHEUMATIC indometacin (indomethacin). It can be used to treat the pain and inflammation of rheumatic disease and other musculoskeletal disorders, period pain and acute gout, and is available as capsules.

✚▲ Side-effects/warnings: See INDOMETACIN.

Rimacillin

(Ranbaxy) is a proprietary, prescription-only preparation of the broad-spectrum ANTIBACTERIAL and (PENICILLIN) ANTIBIOTIC ampicillin. It can be used to treat systemic bacterial infections. It is available as capsules and an oral suspension.

✚▲ Side-effects/warnings: See AMPICILLIN.

Rimactane

(Swedish Orphan Int AB) is a proprietary, prescription-only preparation of the ANTIBACTERIAL and ANTIBIOTIC rifampicin. It can be used particularly in ANTITUBERCULAR treatment, but it may also be used to treat other serious infections, and is available as capsules, a syrup and in a form for intravenous infusion.

✚▲ Side-effects/warnings: See RIFAMPICIN.

Rimactazid

(Swedish Orphan Int AB) is a proprietary, prescription-only compound preparation of the ANTIBACTERIAL drugs rifampicin and isoniazid.

It can be used in ANTITUBERCULAR treatment, and is available as tablets in two strengths, *Rimactazid 150* and *Rimactazid 300*.
✚▲ Side-effects/warnings: See ISONIAZID; RIFAMPICIN.

Rimafen

(Ranbaxy) is a proprietary, prescription-only preparation of the (NSAID) NON-NARCOTIC ANALGESIC, ANTIRHEUMATIC and ANTIPYRETIC ibuprofen. It can be used to relieve pain, particularly the pain of rheumatic disease and other musculoskeletal disorders, period pain and pain following operations and fever. It is available as tablets.
✚▲ Side-effects/warnings: See IBUPROFEN.

Rimapam

(Ranbaxy) is a proprietary, prescription-only preparation of the BENZODIAZEPINE diazepam. It can be used as an ANXIOLYTIC in the short-term treatment of anxiety, as a HYPNOTIC to relieve insomnia, as an ANTICONVULSANT and ANTI-EPILEPTIC for status epilepticus and febrile convulsions in children, as a SEDATIVE in preoperative medication, as a SKELETAL MUSCLE RELAXANT and to assist in the treatment of alcohol withdrawal symptoms. It is available as tablets.
✚▲ Side-effects/warnings: See DIAZEPAM.

Rimapurinol

(Ranbaxy) is a proprietary, prescription-only preparation of the ENZYME INHIBITOR allopurinol, which is a XANTHINE-OXIDASE INHIBITOR. It can be used to treat excess uric acid in the blood and so prevent renal stones and attacks of gout. It is available as tablets.
✚▲ Side-effects/warnings: See ALLOPURINOL.

rimexolone

is a CORTICOSTEROID with ANTI-INFLAMMATORY and ANTI-ALLERGIC properties. It is used to suppress the symptoms of eye inflammation (eg uveitis, or after eye operations). Administration is topical as eye-drops.
✚▲ Side-effects/warnings: See CORTICOSTEROID. Serious systemic effects are unlikely with topical application, though there may be local reactions.
✪ Related entry: Vexol.

Rimoxallin

(Ranbaxy) is a proprietary, prescription-only preparation of the broad-spectrum ANTIBACTERIAL and (PENICILLIN) ANTIBIOTIC amoxicillin. It can be used to treat systemic bacterial infections, and is available as capsules and an oral suspension.
✚▲ Side-effects/warnings: See AMOXICILLIN.

Rinatec

(Boehringer Ingelheim) is a proprietary, prescription-only preparation of the ANTICHOLINERGIC and BRONCHODILATOR ipratropium bromide. It can be used to treat watery rhinitis, and is available as a metered spray.
✚▲ Side-effects/warnings: See IPRATROPIUM BROMIDE. Avoid spraying near the eyes.

Rinstead Adult Gel

(Schering-Plough Consumer Health) is a proprietary, non-prescription compound preparation of the LOCAL ANAESTHETIC benzocaine and the ANTISEPTIC agent CHLORO-XYLENOL. It can be used for the temporary relief of pain caused by mouth ulcers, denture spots and soreness of the gums, and is available as a gel for topical application. It is not normally given to children, except on medical advice.
✚▲ Side-effects/warnings: See BENZOCAINE; CHLOROXYLENOL.

Rinstead Sugar Free Pastilles

(Schering-Plough Consumer Health) is a proprietary, non-prescription compound preparation of the ANTISEPTIC agent CETYLPYRIDINIUM CHLORIDE and also menthol. It can be used for the temporary relief of pain caused by mouth ulcers, denture sore spots and soreness of the gums, and is available as pastilles which dissolve in the mouth. It is not normally given to children, except on medical advice.
✚▲ Side-effects/warnings: See CETYLPYRIDINIUM CHLORIDE; MENTHOL.

Rinstead Teething Gel

(Schering-Plough Consumer Health) is a proprietary, non-prescription compound preparation of the LOCAL ANAESTHETIC LIDOCAINE HYDROCHLORIDE (lignocaine) and the ANTISEPTIC agent CETYLPYRIDINIUM CHLORIDE. It can be used for the temporary relief of pain caused by teething and mouth ulcers, and is available as a gel for topical application. Rinstead Teething Gel is not normally given to babies

under three months, except on medical advice.
✚▲ Side-effects/warnings: See CETYLPYRIDINIUM CHLORIDE; LIDOCAINE HYDROCHLORIDE.

risedronate sodium

is a recently introduced drug (a BISPHOSPHONATE) that is a CALCIUM METABOLISM MODIFIER. It is used in the treatment and prevention of osteoporosis (including corticosteroid-induced osteoporosis) in postmenopausal women, and (at a different dose) for Paget's disease of the bone. Administration is oral.
✚ Side-effects: There may be gastrointestinal effects which might include dyspepsia, nausea, diarrhoea or constipation, oesophageal tightening, and inflammation of the duodenum; also headache and musculoskeletal pain; ringing in the ears (tinnitus), inflammation of the tongue, oedema, weight loss, breathing problems, bronchitis and sinusitis, rash, nocturia, and effects on the eyes such as poor sight, corneal lesion, dry eye and inflammation of the iris of the eye.
▲ Warnings: Risedronate is not suitable for people who have low blood calcium levels, and is not given to pregnant women or women who are breast-feeding. It is used with caution for people who suffer from certain conditions including oesophageal abnormalities or who have impaired kidney function. People who have certain disturbances of bone and mineral metabolism (eg vitamin-D deficiency or low blood calcium levels) will have these disturbances corrected before treatment is started. Before commencing treatment, counselling will be given to explain how and when to take the tablets, and to explain that food and drink (especially calcium-containing products such as milk) must be avoided for at least two hours before or after taking the drug and that iron and mineral supplements and antacids should also be avoided.
✪ **Related entry: Actonel.**

Risperdal

(Janssen-Cilag, Organon) is a proprietary, prescription-only preparation of the ANTIPSYCHOTIC drug risperidone. It can be used to tranquillize patients suffering from psychotic disorders, and is available as tablets and a liquid.
✚▲ Side-effects/warnings: See RISPERIDONE.

risperidone

is an ANTIPSYCHOTIC drug (one of a group sometimes termed 'atypical' antipsychotics) which is used for patients suffering from acute and chronic psychotic disorders. Administration is oral.
✚ Side-effects: Atypical antipsychotics include weight gain, dizziness, postural hypotension, extrapyramidal symptoms (usually mild and transient, but occasionally tardive dyskinesia on long-term administration). Also insomnia, agitation and anxiety, headache, drowsiness, difficulty in concentrating, fatigue, blurred vision, nausea and vomiting, constipation, dyspepsia, abdominal pain, menstrual, sexual and breast disorders, and a number of other side-effects have been reported.
▲ Warnings: Atypical antipsychotics are used with caution in patients with cardiovascular disease, history of epilepsy, and Parkinson's disease; may affect performance of skilled tasks, including driving. Caution in pregnancy; liver or kidney impairment.
✪ **Related entry: Risperdal.**

Ritalin

(Novartis) is a proprietary, prescription-only preparation of methylphenidate hydrochloride, and is on the Controlled Drugs list. Although a weak STIMULANT in adults, it can be used to treat hyperkinesis (hyperactivity) or attention-deficit hyperactivity disorder (ADHD) in children. It is available as tablets.
✚▲ Side-effects/warnings: See METHYLPHENIDATE HYDROCHLORIDE.

ritodrine hydrochloride

is a SYMPATHOMIMETIC and BETA-RECEPTOR STIMULANT drug which can be used in obstetrics to prevent or delay premature labour by relaxing the uterus. Administration is either oral or by injection.
✚▲ Side-effects/warnings: Muscle tremor, nausea, vomiting, sweating, effects of the heart and blood pressure. It is a specialist drug usually used under hospital conditions.
✪ **Related entry: Yutopar.**

ritonavir

is a (*protease inhibitor*) ANTIVIRAL drug which is often used together with (*reverse transcriptase*) antivirals, and can be used in the treatment of progressive or advanced HIV infection. Administration is oral.
✚ Side-effects: Nausea, vomiting, diarrhoea,

abdominal pain; taste disturbance, throat irritation, dyspepsia and loss of appetite; vasodilatation; headache, insomnia and sleep disturbance, dizziness, muscle weakness and paraesthesia, changes in kidney function, pancreatitis, blood changes, and a number of other reported symptoms.

▲ Warnings: It is a specialist drug, and there will be full assessment and patient monitoring throughout treatment. It is not given to patients who are breast-feeding or where there is severely impaired liver function. Administer with caution to those with certain kidney disturbances, haemophilia or who are pregnant.

✪ Related entry: Norvir.

rituximab

represents a new type of specialist drug. It is a monoclonal antibody (a form of pure antibody produced by a type of molecular engineering) which causes lysis of B lymphocytes, so effectively it can be regarded as a specific CYTOTOXIC agent with defined IMMUNOSUPPRESSANT actions. It has recently been introduced for ANTICANCER treatment in individuals who have chemotherapy-resistant advanced follicular lymphoma. Administration is by injection.

✚▲ Side-effects/warnings: see CYTOTOXIC. It has widespread toxicity, and is used only under close supervision of a hospital specialist.

✪ Related entry: MabThera.

rivastigmine

is an ANTICHOLINESTERASE drug used for the symptomatic treatment of mild to moderate dementia of Alzheimer's disease. It is thought only to slow the rate of cognitive deterioration in about half of patients treated. Authorities have identified those patients that may benefit by assessing what is known as a mini mental-state examination (MMSE) score. Diagnosis and treatment is initiated by specialists with assessment throughout treatment. It is administered orally.

✚ Side-effects: Muscle weakness, anorexia and weight loss, dizziness, nausea, vomiting and abdominal pain, dyspepsia, drowsiness, agitation and confusion, insomnia, depression, headache, sweating, feeling of being unwell, tremor; rarely angina pectoris, gastrointestinal haemorrhage, fainting, convulsions; there can be bladder outflow obstruction.

▲ Warnings: It should not be used in women who are breast-feeding. It should be used with care in kidney or liver impairment; certain heart abnormalities; in patients at risk of developing peptic ulcers; in obstructive airways disease, or those who are pregnant.

✪ Related entry: Exelon.

Rivotril

(Roche) is a proprietary, prescription-only preparation of the BENZODIAZEPINE clonazepam. It can be used as an ANTICONVULSANT and ANTI-EPILEPTIC to treat most forms of epilepsy, especially myoclonus, status epilepticus. It is available as tablets and in a form for injection.

✚▲ Side-effects/warnings: See CLONAZEPAM.

rizatriptan

is a (TRIPTAN) ANTIMIGRAINE drug, which is used to treat acute migraine attacks (but not to prevent attacks). It works as a VASOCONSTRICTOR (through acting as a serotonin receptor stimulant selective for SEROTONIN 5-HT_1 receptors), producing a rapid constriction of blood vessels surrounding the brain. Administration is oral.

✚ Side-effects: See SUMATRIPTAN for general side-effects of drugs of this class. Rizatriptan may cause drowsiness, palpitations, speeding of the heart, dry mouth, diarrhoea, dyspepsia, thirst, discomfort in the pharynx, difficulty in breathing, headache, tingling in the extremities, decreased alertness, nervousness, insomnia, muscle tremor and uneven gait, vertigo, mental confusion, muscle pains and weakness, sweating, itching and urticaria, blurred vision; rarely fainting, hypertension.

▲ Warnings: See SUMATRIPTAN for general warnings for drugs of this class. It is not used in patients with peripheral vascular disease. Drowsiness may impair the performance of skilled tasks, such as driving.

✪ Related entry: Maxalt.

Roaccutane

(Roche) is a proprietary, prescription-only preparation of isotretinoin. It can be used to treat severe acne that proves to be unresponsive to more common treatments, and is available as oral capsules.

✚▲ Side-effects/warnings: See ISOTRETINOIN.

Robaxin

(Shire) is a proprietary, prescription-only

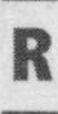

preparation of the SKELETAL MUSCLE RELAXANT methocarbamol. It can be used to relieve acute muscle spasm, and is available as tablets and in a form for injection.
✚▲ Side-effects/warnings: See METHOCARBAMOL.

Robinul

(Anpharm) is a proprietary, prescription-only preparation of the ANTICHOLINERGIC drug glycopyrronium bromide. It can be used before operations for drying up saliva and other secretions. It is available in a form for injection.
✚▲ Side-effects/warnings: See GLYCOPYRRONIUM BROMIDE.

Robinul-Neostigmine

(Anpharm) is a proprietary, prescription-only compound preparation of the ANTICHOLINERGIC drug glycopyrronium bromide and the ANTICHOLINESTERASE neostigmine (as metisulphate). It can be used at the end of operations to reverse the actions of competitive neuromuscular blocking agents. It is available in a form for injection.
✚▲ Side-effects/warnings: See GLYCOPYRRONIUM BROMIDE; NEOSTIGMINE.

Robitussin Chesty Cough Medicine

(Whitehall) is a proprietary, non-prescription preparation of the EXPECTORANT agent guaifenesin (guaiphenesin). It can be used to relieve coughs, and is available as an oral liquid. It is not to be given to children under one year, except on medical advice.
✚▲ Side-effects/warnings: See GUAIFENESIN.

Robitussin Chesty Cough with Congestion

(Whitehall) is a proprietary, non-prescription preparation of the EXPECTORANT agent guaifenesin (guaiphenesin) and the SYMPATHOMIMETIC and DECONGESTANT pseudoephedrine hydrochloride. It can be used to relieve chesty coughs and nasal congestion, and is available as an oral liquid. It is not to be given to children under two, except on medical advice.
✚▲ Side-effects/warnings: See GUAIFENESIN; PSEUDOEPHEDRINE HYDROCHLORIDE.

Robitussin Dry Cough

(Whitehall) is a proprietary, non-prescription preparation of the (OPIOID) ANTITUSSIVE dextromethorphan hydrobromide. It can be used for the symptomatic relief of persistent dry, irritant cough, and is available as an oral liquid. It is not to be given to children under six years, except on medical advice.
✚▲ Side-effects/warnings: See DEXTROMETHORPHAN HYDROBROMIDE.

Robitussin Night-Time

(Whitehall) is a proprietary, non-prescription compound preparation of the (OPIOID) ANTITUSSIVE codeine phosphate, the ANTIHISTAMINE brompheniramine maleate and the SYMPATHOMIMETIC and DECONGESTANT pseudoephedrine hydrochloride. It can be used for the symptomatic relief of coughs associated with colds and other respiratory disorders in children. It is available as a liquid and is not normally given to children under four, except on medical advice.
✚▲ Side-effects/warnings: See BROMPHENIRAMINE MALEATE; CODEINE PHOSPHATE; PSEUDOEPHEDRINE HYDROCHLORIDE.

Rocaltrol

(Roche) is a proprietary, prescription-only preparation of calcitriol, which is a VITAMIN D analogue. It can be used to treat vitamin D deficiency, and is available as capsules.
✚▲ Side-effects/warnings: See CALCITRIOL.

Rocephin

(Roche) is a proprietary, prescription-only preparation of the ANTIBACTERIAL and (CEPHALOSPORIN) ANTIBIOTIC drug ceftriaxone, which can be used to treat and prevent bacterial infections. It is available in a form for injection.
✚▲ Side-effects/warnings: See CEFTRIAXONE.

RoC Total Sunblock Cream

(Johnson & Johnson) is a proprietary, non-prescription SUNSCREEN which contains constituents that protect the skin from ultraviolet radiation. It contains several agents, including TITANIUM DIOXIDE, avobenzone and ethylhexyl *p*-methoxycinnamate. A patient whose skin condition requires this sort of protection may be prescribed it at the discretion of their doctor.
✚▲ Side-effects/warnings: TITANIUM DIOXIDE.

rocuronium bromide

is a *non-depolarizing* SKELETAL MUSCLE

RELAXANT which is used to induce muscle paralysis during surgery. Administration is by injection.

✚▲ Side-effects/warnings: It is a specialist drug used by anaesthetists in hospital.

✪ **Related entry: Esmeron.**

rofecoxib

is a (NSAID) NON-NARCOTIC ANALGESIC and ANTIRHEUMATIC drug, which is used to treat pain and inflammation in osteoarthritis. Administration is oral.

✚ Side-effects: See NSAID. Also, mouth ulcers, weight gain, chest pain, sleep disturbance, depression, eczema, and muscle cramps reported.

▲ Warnings: See NSAID. Also, rofecoxib it is not used in people with active peptic ulceration or gastrointestinal bleeding; with inflammatory bowel disease or severe congestive heart failure. Caution is required in people with a history of cardiac failure and other heart disorders, hypertension and oedema for any other reason.

✪ **Related entry: Vioxx.**

Roferon-A

(Roche) is a proprietary, prescription-only preparation of interferon (in the form of alpha-2a, rbe). It can be used as an ANTICANCER drug in the treatment of hairy cell leukaemias, myelogenous leukaemia, certain renal cell carcinoma, progressive cutaneous T-cell lymphoma, follicular non-Hodgkin's lymphoma, as an adjunct to surgery in malignant melanoma and AIDs-related Kaposi's sarcoma, and also as an ANTIVIRAL for chronic active hepatitis B and C. It is available in a form for injection.

✚▲ Side-effects/warnings: See INTERFERON.

Rogitine

(Alliance) is a proprietary, prescription-only preparation of the ALPHA-ADRENOCEPTOR BLOCKER phentolamine mesilate. It can be used as an ANTIHYPERTENSIVE and in the diagnosis of phaeochromocytoma. It is available in a form for injection.

✚▲ Side-effects/warnings: See PHENTOLAMINE MESILATE.

Rohypnol

(Roche) is a proprietary, prescription-only preparation of the BENZODIAZEPINE flunitrazepam. It can be used as a HYPNOTIC for the short-term treatment of insomnia, and is available as tablets. It is on the Controlled Drugs list.

✚▲ Side-effects/warnings: See FLUNITRAZEPAM.

Rommix

(Ashbourne) is a proprietary, prescription-only preparation of the ANTIBACTERIAL and (MACROLIDE) ANTIBIOTIC erythromycin (as ethyl succinate). It can be used to treat and prevent many forms of infection, and is available as tablets and a liquid oral mixture.

✚▲ Side-effects/warnings: See ERYTHROMYCIN.

ropinirole

is an ANTIPARKINSONISM drug that works by stimulating the DOPAMINE receptors in the brain (ie is a DOPAMINE-RECEPTOR STIMULANT), and which is similar to BROMOCRIPTINE in that it is used to improve symptoms and signs of the disease, either alone or in combination with LEVODOPA. Administration is oral.

✚ Side-effects: Nausea and vomiting; sudden falling asleep; oedema of the legs; abdominal pain; sometimes severe hypotension and slow heart rate; reports of hallucinations and confusion.

▲ Warnings: It should not be administered to patients with severe kidney and liver disease; or to those who are pregnant or breast-feeding. Administer with caution where there is severe cardiovascular disease or major psychiatric disease. It may affect the performance of skilled tasks, such as driving. Withdrawal is gradual.

✪ **Related entry: Requip.**

rose bengal

is a dye which is used for ophthalmic diagnostic procedures in the eye (eg to detect foreign bodies). Administration is by topical application in the form of eye-drops.

✚▲ Side-effects/warnings: It is regarded as safe in normal topical use.

✪ **Related entry: Minims Rose Bengal.**

rosiglitazone

is a newly introduced drug which is used in DIABETIC TREATMENT of Type II diabetes (non-insulin-dependent diabetes mellitus; NIDDM; maturity-onset diabetes). It is one of the thiazolidinedione group which reduces peripheral insulin resistance, and this causes a

R

reduction of blood-glucose concentration. Treatment with rosiglitazone is started by a physician experienced in treating Type II diabetes and should always be used in combination with metformin (or with a SULPHONYLUREA if METFORMIN HYDROCHLORIDE is inappropriate). Authorities have recommended pioglitazone combination therapy an alternative to insulin for certain people. Administration is oral.
✚ Side-effects: Gastrointestinal disturbances, oedema, weight gain, headache, anaemia, fatigue, hypoglycaemia; less commonly dizziness, paraesthesia, rash, hair loss, shortness of breath, altered blood lipids, thrombocytopenia.
▲ Warnings: Rosiglitazone should not be given to people with liver impairment or heart failure, or to anyone who is pregnant or breast-feeding, and it is used with care in people with impaired kidney function. Liver and cardiovascular function will be monitored during treatment. There have been rare reports of liver dysfunction; so immediate medical attention should be sought if symptoms develop that indicate liver problems, such as abdominal pain, nausea and vomiting, fatigue and dark urine; and treatment will be discontinued if jaundice occurs.
✪ Related entry: Avandia.

Rowachol

(Rowa) is a proprietary, prescription-only preparation of plant oils, including TERPENE (borneol, camphene, cineole, menthol and pipene in olive oil). It can be used, with other drugs, to treat biliary disorders by increasing biliary cholesterol solubility. It is available as capsules.
✚▲ Side-effects/warnings: See CINEOLE; MENTHOL; TERPENE.

Rowatinex

(Rowa) is a proprietary, prescription-only preparation of plant oils containing a number of terpene compounds (anethol, borneol, camphene, cineole, fenchone, pinene). It can be used to help expulsion of urinary tract calculi (stones), and is available as capsules.
✚▲ Side-effects/warnings: See TERPENE.

Rozex

(Stafford-Miller; GSK) is a proprietary, prescription-only preparation of the ANTIMICROBIAL metronidazole, which has ANTIBACTERIAL and ANTIPROTOZOAL actions and can be used to treat acute acne rosacea outbreaks. It is available as a topical cream and gel.
✚▲ Side-effects/warnings: See METRONIDAZOLE.

rubefacient

agents are also called COUNTER-IRRITANT. The name derives from the fact that these agents cause a reddening of the skin by causing the blood vessels of the skin to dilate, which gives a soothing feeling of warmth. The term *counter-irritant* refers to the idea that irritation of the sensory nerve endings alters or offsets pain in the underlying muscle or joints that are served by the same nerves. See CAPSAICIN; CAPSICUM OLEORESIN; CHOLINE SALICYLATE; ETHYL SALICYLATE; GLYCOL SALICYLATE; METHYL SALICYLATE; MENTHOL; SALICYLIC ACID; TURPENTINE OIL.

rubella vaccine

(Rub/Vac (live)) is a VACCINE used for IMMUNIZATION against rubella (German measles). It is medically recommended for (not previously immunized) medical staff who, as potential carriers, might put pregnant women at risk from infection and also for women of child-bearing age, because German measles during pregnancy constitutes a serious risk to the fetus. As a precaution, vaccination should not take place if the patient is pregnant or likely to become pregnant within the following three months. The vaccine is prepared as a freeze-dried suspension of live, but attenuated, viruses grown in cell cultures. Administration is by injection. The substitution of a universal vaccination programme in schools for boys and girls by the combined MR vaccine (against measles and rubella) and the MMR programme for infants has meant that the rubella vaccination treatment alone is likely to become obsolete. It is given by injection.
✚▲ Side-effects/warnings: See VACCINE. It should be avoided in early pregnancy.
✪ Related entry: Ervevax.

Rub/Vac

is an abbreviation for RUBELLA VACCINE.

Rusyde

(CP) is a proprietary, prescription-only preparation of the (*loop*) DIURETIC furosemide (frusemide). It can be used to treat oedema, particularly pulmonary (lung) oedema, in patients with chronic heart failure and low urine production due to kidney failure (oliguria). It is available as tablets.

✚▲ Side-effects/warnings: See FUROSEMIDE.

rutosides

also known as oxerutins are derivatives of rutin, which is a vegetable substance. They are thought to work by reducing the fragility and permeability of certain blood vessels and may therefore be effective in preventing small haemorrhages and swellings (though there are doubts as to their efficacy). In mixtures, called oxerutins, they are used to treat oedema associated with chronic venous insufficiency.

✚ Side-effects: Flushing, rashes, headache and gastrointestinal disturbances.

✪ Related entry: Paroven.

Rynacrom

(Pantheon) is a proprietary, non-prescription preparation of the ANTI-ALLERGIC drug sodium cromoglicate. It can be used in the prevention of allergic rhinitis, and is available as a nasal spray.

✚▲ Side-effects/warnings: See SODIUM CROMOGLICATE.

Rynacrom Allergy Nasal Spray

(Aventis Pharma) is a proprietary, non-prescription compound preparation of the ANTI-ALLERGIC drug sodium cromoglicate and the SYMPATHOMIMETIC and DECONGESTANT xylometazoline hydrochloride. It can be used in the prevention of allergic rhinitis, and is available as a nasal spray.

✚▲ Side-effects/warnings: See SODIUM CROMOGLICATE; XYLOMETAZOLINE HYDROCHLORIDE.

Rynacrom Compound

(Pantheon) is a proprietary, non-prescription compound preparation of the ANTI-ALLERGIC drug sodium cromoglicate and the SYMPATHOMIMETIC and DECONGESTANT xylometazoline hydrochloride. It can be used in the prevention of allergic rhinitis, and is available as a nasal spray.

✚▲ Side-effects/warnings: See SODIUM CROMOGLICATE; XYLOMETAZOLINE HYDROCHLORIDE.

Rythmodan

(Borg) is a proprietary, prescription-only preparation of the ANTI-ARRHYTHMIC disopyramide (as disopyramide phosphate), and is available as capsules and in a form for injection.

✚▲ Side-effects/warnings: See DISOPYRAMIDE.

Rythmodan Retard

(Borg) is a proprietary, prescription-only preparation of the ANTI-ARRHYTHMIC disopyramide (as disopyramide phosphate), and is available as modified-release tablets.

✚▲ Side-effects/warnings: See DISOPYRAMIDE.

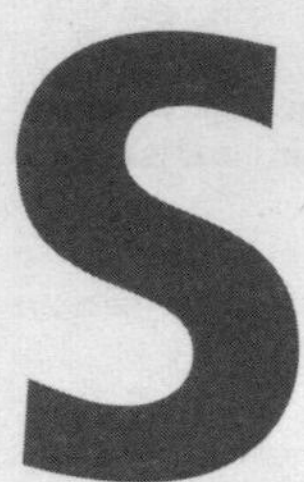

Sabril

(Hoechst Marion Roussel; Aventis Pharma) is a proprietary, prescription-only preparation of the ANTICONVULSANT and ANTI-EPILEPTIC drug vigabatrin. It is available as tablets and a powder for oral administration (taken immediately in water or a soft drink).
✚▲ Side-effects/warnings: See VIGABATRIN.

Saizen

(Serono) is a proprietary, prescription-only preparation of somatropin, which is the biosynthetic form of the pituitary HORMONE human growth hormone. It can be used to treat hormonal deficiency and associated symptoms (in particular, short stature), and is available in a form for intramuscular or subcutaneous injection, and in 'Clickeasy' and 'Easyject' forms for subcutaneous injection.
✚▲ Side-effects/warnings: See SOMATROPIN.

Salactol Wart Paint

(Dermal) is a proprietary, non-prescription preparation of the KERATOLYTIC agent salicylic acid (with lactic acid). It can be used to remove warts, verrucas, corns and calluses, and is available as a liquid paint.
✚▲ Side-effects/warnings: See SALICYLIC ACID.

Salagen

(Chiron) is a proprietary, prescription-only preparation of the PARASYMPATHOMIMETIC pilocarpine. It can be used to alleviate the symptoms of salivary gland hypofunction for dry mouth following irradiation for head and neck cancer. It is available as tablets.
✚▲ Side-effects/warnings: See PILOCARPINE.

Salamol Easi-Breathe

(IVAX) is a proprietary, prescription-only preparation of the beta-receptor stimulant salbutamol. It can be used as a BRONCHODILATOR in reversible obstructive airways disease, such as in ANTI-ASTHMATIC treatment. It is available as a CFC-free metered aerosol inhalant.
✚▲ Side-effects/warnings: See SALBUTAMOL.

Salamol Steri-Neb

(IVAX) is a proprietary, prescription-only preparation of the BETA-RECEPTOR STIMULANT salbutamol. It can be used as a BRONCHODILATOR in reversible obstructive airways disease, such as in ANTI-ASTHMATIC treatment. It is available as an inhaler solution.
✚▲ Side-effects/warnings: See SALBUTAMOL.

Salatac Wart Gel

(Dermal) is a proprietary, non-prescription preparation of the KERATOLYTIC agent salicylic acid (with lactic acid). It can be used to remove warts, verrucas, calluses and corns and is available as a gel.
✚▲ Side-effects/warnings: See SALICYLIC ACID.

Salazopyrin

(Pharmacia) is a proprietary, prescription-only preparation of the AMINOSALICYLATE sulfasalazine. It can be used to treat active rheumatoid arthritis, ulcerative colitis and Crohn's disease. It is available as tablets, enteric-coated tablets (called *EN-Tabs*), an oral suspension, suppositories and a retention enema.
✚▲ Side-effects/warnings: See SULPHASALAZINE.

Salbulin

(3M) is a proprietary, prescription-only preparation of the BETA-RECEPTOR STIMULANT salbutamol (as salbutamol sulphate). It can be used as a BRONCHODILATOR in reversible obstructive airways disease, such as in ANTI-ASTHMATIC treatment. It is available as a metered aerosol inhalant.
✚▲ Side-effects/warnings: See SALBUTAMOL.

salbutamol

is a SYMPATHOMIMETIC and BETA-RECEPTOR STIMULANT with good beta$_2$-receptor selectivity. It is mainly used as a BRONCHODILATOR in reversible obstructive airways disease and as an ANTI-ASTHMATIC treatment in severe acute asthma (including in emergency), in obstetrics as a SMOOTH MUSCLE RELAXANT to prevent or delay premature labour by relaxing the uterus.

Administration can be oral, by inhalation or by intravenous injection or infusion.

✚▲ Side-effects/warnings: There may be a fine muscle tremor, particularly of the hands; headache and nervous tension, palpitations, dilation of blood vessels in the extremities, a speeding of the heart (normally minimal with aerosol administration), sleep and behavioural problems in children, and very occasionally muscle cramps. Infusion or high doses can lead to a lowering of blood potassium levels. Some hypersensitivity reactions have been reported, including (paradoxical) bronchoconstriction, urticaria and angioedema. Administer with caution to patients with certain disorders of the thyroid gland and heart, with hypertension, diabetes (in intravenous use) and who are breast-feeding or pregnant (except when used to delay premature labour). There may be pain at the site of injection. For its use in premature labour, also see RITODRINE HYDROCHLORIDE for side-effects/warnings.

✪ **Related entries: Aerocrom; Aerolin Autohaler; Airomir; Asmasal Clickhaler; Asmaven; Combivent; Maxivent; Salamol Easi-Breathe; Salamol Steri-Neb; Salbulin; Ventide; Ventmax SR; Ventodisks; Ventolin; Volmax.**

salcatonin

(*calcitonin (salmon)*) is a synthetic form of the thyroid hormone CALCITONIN (in the same form that is found in salmon). Its function is to lower the levels of calcium and phosphate in the blood, and the overall effect is to lower calcium levels and to regulate these levels with the correspondingly opposite action of a PARATHYROID HORMONE. Therapeutically, it has the same effect and is used in the short term to lower blood levels of calcium when they are abnormally high (hypercalcaemia) and to treat Paget's disease of the bone, bone pain in neoplastic disease, postmenopausal osteoporosis. It is given by injection.

✚ Side-effects: There may be nausea, vomiting, flushing and dizziness. There may also be a tingling sensation in the hands, a peculiar taste in the mouth, diarrhoea and inflammation at the site of injection rash; allergic reactions including anaphylaxis.

▲ Warnings: Caution if there is history of allergy, kidney impairment, heart failure, pregnancy or breast-feeding. Prolonged use of calcitonin derived from animals may eventually lead to the body producing antibodies against it and consequent neutralization of its effect. Some patients may become hypersensitive to animal calcitonin.

✪ **Related entries: Calsynar; Forcaltonin; Miacalcic.**

salicylamide

is used topically as a constituent with a COUNTER-IRRITANT, or RUBEFACIENT, action. It can be applied to the skin for symptomatic relief of underlying muscle or joint pain.

✚▲ Side-effects/warnings: On topical administration there may be local irritation. It should not be used on broken skin or mucous membranes.

✪ **Related entry: Intralgin.**

salicylate 🅴

drugs are a class of drugs that include ASPIRIN and are chemically related to salicylic acid, which is a simple, single-ringed, organic molecule that occurs naturally as a component of salicin (a glycoside found in willow bark) and methyl salicylate (in oil of wintergreen). These natural products have been known for centuries to have antirheumatic actions, which derive from an inherent ANTI-INFLAMMATORY activity. Both the two natural medicines are irritant and poisonous if taken by mouth and the salt SODIUM SALICYLATE is rather irritant if administered orally. However, in 1899, the semi-synthetic drug ester acetylsalicylic acid, was introduced under the trade name *Aspirin* as an ANALGESIC, ANTIPYRETIC and ANTIRHEUMATIC drug. Today, aspirin is still widely used as a generic drug and has been joined by a number of other salicylate drugs with similar actions and uses, for example, the aspirin-paracetamol ester BENORYLATE and DIFLUNISAL.

From the use of oil of wintergreen (containing METHYL SALICYLATE) as a topically applied treatment for muscle and joint aches and pains, several similar derivatives were developed with similar actions, for example, AMMONIUM SALICYLATE, CHOLINE SALICYLATE, DIETHYLAMINE SALICYLATE, ETHYL SALICYLATE and GLYCOL SALICYLATE. Although it is not clear how these drugs act, it seems likely that they act as COUNTER-IRRITANT, also known as RUBEFACIENT, agents though there is probably also some systemic absorption.

Further uses of salicylates include the AMINOSALICYLATE drugs (containing a 5-aminosalicylic acid component) which are used to treat active Crohn's disease and to induce and maintain remission of the symptoms of ulcerative colitis, and are also sometimes used to treat rheumatoid arthritis. Drugs in this group include MESALAZINE, OLSALAZINE SODIUM and SULFASALAZINE, which combine within the one chemical both 5-aminosalicylic acid and the antibacterial SULPHONAMIDE.

In strong solution, salicylic acid is the standard, classic KERATOLYTIC agent, which can be used in the treatment of acne and to clear the skin of thickened, horny patches (hyperkeratoses) and scaly areas that occur in some forms of eczema, ichthyosis and psoriasis.

salicylic acid

is a KERATOLYTIC agent that also has some ANTIFUNGAL activity. It can be used to treat minor skin conditions and infections, such as athlete's foot, acne vulgaris and psoriasis. It is also incorporated into some topical preparations that are rubbed into the skin as a COUNTER-IRRITANT, or RUBEFACIENT, treatment to relieve pain in soft tissues, including underlying muscle and joints. It is also used to remove warts and calluses, and for fungal nail infections (such as tinea). Administration is by topical application in a variety of forms, included in many compound preparations.

✚ Side-effects: There may be excessive drying, sensitivity and local irritation. After prolonged use there may be systemic effects and toxicity, especially if large skin areas are treated.

▲ Warnings: Avoid broken or inflamed skin. Certain preparations of this drug should not be used by diabetics or those with impaired blood circulation. Some preparations are not recommended for use in pregnancy.

✪ Related entries: Acnisal; Aserbine; Bazuka Extra Strength Gel; Bazuka Gel; Benzoic Acid Ointment, Compound, BP; Capasal Therapeutic Shampoo; Carnation Callous Caps; Carnation Corn Caps; Carnation Verruca Treatment; Coal Tar and Salicylic Acid Ointment, BP; Cocois; Compound W; Cuplex; Diprosalic; Duofilm; Ionil T; Monphytol; Movelat Relief Cream; Movelat Relief Gel; Occlusal; Phytex; Posalfilin; Pragmatar; Psorin; Pyralvex; Radian B Muscle Lotion; Salatac Wart Gel; Salactol Wart Paint; Scholl Callous Removal Pads; Scholl Corn and Callous Removal Liquid; Scholl Corn Removal Pads; Scholl Corn Removal Plasters (Fabric); Scholl Corn Removal Plasters (Washproof); Scholl Polymer Gel Callous Removal Pads; Scholl Polymer Gel Corn Removers; Scholl Seal and Heal Verruca Removal Gel; Scholl Verruca Removal System; TCP Antiseptic Ointment; Verrugon; Zinc and Salicylic Acid Paste, BP.

Salivace

(Penn) is a proprietary, non-prescription compound preparation of CARMELLOSE SODIUM and various other salts and constituents. It is used as a form of ARTIFICIAL SALIVA for application to the membranes of the mouth and throat in conditions that make the mouth abnormally dry (including after radiotherapy or in Sicca syndrome). It is available as an oral spray.

Salivix

(Provalis) is a proprietary, non-prescription compound preparation of malic acid, sodium phosphate and calcium lactate. It is used as a form of ARTIFICIAL SALIVA for application to the membranes of the mouth and throat in conditions that make the mouth abnormally dry. It is available as pastilles.

✚▲ Side-effects/warnings: See MALIC ACID.

salmeterol

is a SYMPATHOMIMETIC and BETA-RECEPTOR STIMULANT with β_2-receptor selectivity. It is mainly used as a BRONCHODILATOR in reversible obstructive airways disease and as an ANTI-ASTHMATIC treatment in severe acute asthma. It is similar to salbutamol but has a much longer duration of action. Therefore it may be used to prevent asthma attacks throughout the night after inhalation before going to bed and also for long-duration prevention of exercise-induced bronchospasm. It is administered by inhalation as an aerosol or powder. It would normally be used in conjunction with long-term ANTI-INFLAMMATORY prophylactic (preventive) therapy (eg with CORTICOSTEROID drugs or SODIUM CROMOGLICATE).

✚▲ Side-effects/warnings: See SALBUTAMOL; but the effects are more prolonged. There is a significant incidence of (paradoxical) bronchospasm. (Users will be cautioned not to exceed the stated dose and if a previously effective

dose fails to relieve symptoms, they should consult their doctor.) It should not be used to relieve acute attacks.
✪ **Related entries: Seretide; Serevent.**

Salofalk

(Cortecs) is a proprietary, prescription-only preparation of the AMINOSALICYLATE mesalazine. It can be used to treat ulcerative colitis, and is available as tablets, suppositories and an enema.
✚▲ Side-effects/warnings: See MESALAZINE.

Sandimmun

(Novartis) is a proprietary, prescription-only preparation of the IMMUNOSUPPRESSANT ciclosporin. It can be used to prevent tissue rejection in transplant patients, to treat severe, active rheumatoid arthritis and certain severe, resistant skin conditions (under specialist supervision). It is available as capsules, an oral solution and in a form for injection.
✚▲ Side-effects/warnings: See CICLOSPORIN.

Sandocal

(Novartis) is a proprietary, non-prescription preparation of calcium carbonate, calcium lactate gluconate, calcium carbonate and citric acid. It can be used as a MINERAL SUPPLEMENT in cases of calcium deficiency. It is available as effervescent tablets in two strengths, *Sandocal-400* and *Sandocal-1000*.
✚▲ Side-effects/warnings: See CALCIUM CARBONATE.

Sando-K

(HK Pharma) is a proprietary, non-prescription MINERAL SUPPLEMENT that contains potassium chloride and potassium bicarbonate. It is used to make up deficient blood levels of potassium, and is available as effervescent tablets.
✚▲ Side-effects/warnings: See POTASSIUM BICARBONATE; POTASSIUM CHLORIDE.

Sandostatin

(Novartis) is a proprietary, prescription-only preparation of octreotide. It can be used as an ANTICANCER drug to treat the symptoms following the release of hormones from certain neuroendocrine tumours, and for acromegaly. It is available in forms for injection.
✚▲ Side-effects/warnings: See OCTREOTIDE.

Sandostatin LAR

(Novartis) is a proprietary, prescription-only preparation of octreotide. It can be used as an ANTICANCER drug to treat the symptoms following the release of hormones from certain neuroendocrine tumours. It is available in a form for injection.
✚▲ Side-effects/warnings: See OCTREOTIDE.

Sandrena

(Organon) is a proprietary, prescription-only preparation of the OESTROGEN estradiol. It can be used in HRT and is available in the form of a gel for topical application.
✚▲ Side-effects/warnings: See ESTRADIOL.

SangCya

(Sangstat) is a proprietary, prescription-only preparation of the IMMUNOSUPPRESSANT ciclosporin. It can be used to prevent tissue rejection in transplant patients, to treat severe, active rheumatoid arthritis and certain severe, resistant skin conditions (under specialist supervision). It is available as an oral solution.
✚▲ Side-effects/warnings: See CICLOSPORIN.

Sanomigran

(Novartis) is a proprietary, prescription-only preparation of the ANTIMIGRAINE drug pizotifen. It can be used to treat headache, particularly migraine and cluster headache, and is available as tablets and an elixir.
✚▲ Side-effects/warnings: See PIZOTIFEN.

saquinavir

is a (*protease inhibitor*) ANTIVIRAL drug, which is often used together with (*reverse transcriptase*) antivirals, and can be used in the treatment of progressive or advanced HIV infection. Administration is oral.
✚ Side-effects: Nausea, diarrhoea, abdominal pain; mouth ulceration; loss of appetite; headache, rash or skin eruptions; dizziness, muscle weakness and paraesthesia; changes in kidney function, blood changes and a number of other reported symptoms.
▲ Warnings: It is a specialist drug, and there will be full assessment and patient monitoring throughout treatment. It is not given to patients who are breast-feeding or who have severely impaired liver function. It should be adminstered with caution to those with certain kidney or liver disturbances, haemophilia, diabetes, or who are pregnant.
✪ **Related entries: Fortovase; Invirase.**

S

Saventrine IV

(Pharmax) is a proprietary, prescription-only preparation of the SYMPATHOMIMETIC isoprenaline (as isoprenaline hydrochloride). It can be used as a CARDIAC STIMULANT to treat a dangerously low heart rate or heart block. It is available in a form for intravenous infusion.
✚▲ Side-effects/warnings: See ISOPRENALINE.

Savlon Antiseptic Cream

(Novartis Consumer Health) is a proprietary, non-prescription preparation of the ANTISEPTIC chlorhexidine (as gluconate) and cetrimide. It can be used to clean lesions, ranging from minor skin disorders or blisters to minor burns and small wounds, and to prevent all types of infection from developing. It is available as a cream.
✚▲ Side-effects/warnings: See CETRIMIDE; CHLORHEXIDINE.

Savlon Antiseptic Liquid

(Novartis Consumer Health) is a proprietary, non-prescription preparation of the ANTISEPTIC agents chlorhexidine (as gluconate) and cetrimide. It can be used to clean lesions, ranging from minor skin disorders or blisters to minor burns and small wounds, and to prevent different types of infection from developing. It is available as a liquid.
✚▲ Side-effects/warnings: See CETRIMIDE; CHLORHEXIDINE.

Savlon Antiseptic Wound Wash

(Novartis Consumer Health) is a proprietary, non-prescription preparation of the ANTISEPTIC chlorhexidine (as gluconate). It can be used to clean lesions, ranging from minor skin disorders or blisters to minor burns and small wounds, and to prevent infection from developing. It is available as a liquid.
✚▲ Side-effects/warnings: See CHLORHEXIDINE.

Savlon Dry Antiseptic

(Novartis Consumer Health) is a proprietary, non-prescription preparation of the ANTISEPTIC povidone-iodine. It can be used for first aid treatment of cuts, grazes, minor burns and scalds to protect against infection, and is available as a spray. It should not be used for new burns or on low birthweight babies.
✚▲ Side-effects/warnings: See POVIDONE-IODINE.

scabicidal 🅱

agents are used to kill the mites that cause scabies, which is an infestation by the itch-mite *Sarcoptes scabiei*. The female mite tunnels into the top surface of the skin in order to lay her eggs, causing severe irritation as she does so. Newly hatched mites, also causing irritation with their secretions, then pass easily from person to person on direct contact. Every member of an infected household should be treated and clothing and bedding should be disinfected. Treatment is usually with local application of a cream containing MALATHION or PERMETHRIN, which kills the mites. BENZYL BENZOATE may also be used, but can be an irritant itself.

Scheriproct

(Schering Health) is a proprietary, prescription-only compound preparation of the CORTICOSTEROID prednisolone (as hexanoate) and the LOCAL ANAESTHETIC cinchocaine (dibucaine hydrochloride). It can be used by topical application to treat haemorrhoids, and is available as an ointment and suppositories.
✚▲ Side-effects/warnings: See CINCHOCAINE; PREDNISOLONE.

Scholl Athlete's Foot Cream

(SSL) is a proprietary, non-prescription preparation of the ANTIFUNGAL drug tolnaftate. It can be used to prevent and treat fungal infections responsible for athlete's foot, and is available as a cream.
✚▲ Side-effects/warnings: See TOLNAFTATE.

Scholl Athlete's Foot Powder

(SSL) is a proprietary, non-prescription preparation of the ANTIFUNGAL drug tolnaftate. It can be used to prevent and treat fungal infections responsible for athlete's foot, and is available as a powder.
✚▲ Side-effects/warnings: See TOLNAFTATE.

Scholl Athlete's Foot Spray Liquid

(SSL) is a proprietary, non-prescription preparation of the ANTIFUNGAL drug tolnaftate. It can be used to prevent and treat fungal infections responsible for athlete's foot. Available as a spray.
✚▲ Side-effects/warnings: See TOLNAFTATE.

Scholl Callous Removal Pads

(SSL) is a proprietary, non-prescription

preparation of the KERATOLYTIC salicylic acid. It can be used to treat callouses and is available as a medicated plaster. It is not normally used on children under 16 years, except on medical advice
✚▲ Side-effects/warnings: See SALICYLIC ACID.

Scholl Corn and Callous Removal Liquid

(SSL) is a proprietary, non-prescription preparation of the KERATOLYTIC salicylic acid and camphor, which has mild COUNTER-IRRITANT, or RUBEFACIENT, properties. It can be used to treat corns and callouses and is available as a liquid. It is not normally used on children under 16 years, except on medical advice
✚▲ Side-effects/warnings: See CAMPHOR; SALICYLIC ACID.

Scholl Corn Removal Pads

(SSL) is a proprietary, non-prescription preparation of the KERATOLYTIC salicylic acid. It can be used to treat callouses and is available as a medicated plaster. It is not normally used on children under 16 years, except on medical advice.
✚▲ Side-effects/warnings: See SALICYLIC ACID.

Scholl Corn Removal Plasters (Fabric)

(SSL) is a proprietary, non-prescription preparation of the KERATOLYTIC salicylic acid. It can be used to treat corns and is available as a medicated plaster. It is not normally used on children under 16 years, except on medical advice.
✚▲ Side-effects/warnings: See SALICYLIC ACID.

Scholl Corn Removal Plasters (Washproof)

(SSL) is a proprietary, non-prescription preparation of the KERATOLYTIC salicylic acid. It can be used to treat corns and is available as a medicated plaster. It is not normally used on children under 16, except on medical advice.
✚▲ Side-effects/warnings: See SALICYLIC ACID.

Scholl Polymer Gel Callous Removal Pads

(SSL) is a proprietary, non-prescription preparation of the KERATOLYTIC salicylic acid. It can be used to treat callouses and is available as a medicated plaster. It is not normally used on children under 16, except on medical advice.
✚▲ Side-effects/warnings: See SALICYLIC ACID.

Scholl Polymer Gel Corn Removers

(SSL) is a proprietary, non-prescription preparation of the KERATOLYTIC salicylic acid. It can be used to treat corns and is available as a medicated plaster. It is not normally used on children under 16, except on medical advice.
✚▲ Side-effects/warnings: See SALICYLIC ACID.

Scholl Seal and Heal Verruca Removal Gel

(SSL) is a proprietary, non-prescription preparation of the KERATOLYTIC salicylic acid with camphor. It can be used to treat common warts on the hands and feet and is available as a liquid gel. It is not normally used on children, except on medical advice.
✚▲ Side-effects/warnings: See CAMPHOR; SALICYLIC ACID.

Scholl Verruca Removal System

(SSL) is a proprietary, non-prescription preparation of the KERATOLYTIC salicylic acid. It can be used to treat common warts on the hands and feet and is available as a medicated plaster. It is not normally given to babies, except on medical advice
✚▲ Side-effects/warnings: See SALICYLIC ACID.

Scopoderm TTS

(Novartis) is a proprietary, prescription-only preparation of the ANTICHOLINERGIC drug hyoscine (as base). It can be used as an ANTINAUSEANT in the treatment of motion sickness. It is available as a self-adhesive patch that is placed on a hairless area of skin (usually behind an ear), the drug is then absorbed through the skin.
✚▲ Side-effects/warnings: See HYOSCINE HYDROBROMIDE.

scopolamine hydrobromide

is another name, which is standard in the USA, for HYOSCINE HYDROBROMIDE.

Sea-Legs

(SSL) is a proprietary, non-prescription preparation of the ANTIHISTAMINE and ANTINAUSEANT drug meclozine hydrochloride. It can be used to treat and prevent motion sickness,

and is available as tablets. It is not normally given to children under two years, except on medical advice.
✚▲ Side-effects/warnings: See MECLOZINE HYDROCHLORIDE.

Secadrex

(Akita) is a proprietary, prescription-only compound preparation of the BETA-BLOCKER acebutolol and the (THIAZIDE) DIURETIC hydrochlorothiazide. It can be used as an ANTIHYPERTENSIVE for raised blood pressure, and is available as tablets.
✚▲ Side-effects/warnings: See ACEBUTOLOL; HYDROCHLOROTHIAZIDE.

secobarbital sodium

(quinalbarbitone sodium) is a BARBITURATE with a rapid onset of action and is used as a HYPNOTIC to promote sleep in conditions of severe, intractable insomnia, only in patients already taking barbiturates. Administration is oral. Preparations containing secobarbital sodium are on the Controlled Drugs list.
✚▲ Side-effects/warnings: See BARBITURATE.
✪ Related entries: Seconal Sodium; Tuinal.

Seconal Sodium

(Flynn) is a proprietary, prescription-only preparation of the BARBITURATE secobarbital sodium (quinalbarbitone sodium), and is on the Controlled Drugs list. It can be used as a HYPNOTIC to treat persistent and intractable insomnia, and is available as capsules.
✚▲ Side-effects/warnings: See SECOBARBITAL SODIUM.

Sectral

(Akita) is a proprietary, prescription-only preparation of the BETA-BLOCKER acebutolol. It can be used as an ANTIHYPERTENSIVE for raised blood pressure, as an ANTI-ANGINA treatment to relieve symptoms and improve exercise tolerance and as an ANTI-ARRHYTHMIC to regularize heartbeat and to treat myocardial infarction. It is available as capsules and tablets.
✚▲ Side-effects/warnings: See ACEBUTOLOL.

Securon

(Knoll) is a proprietary, prescription-only preparation of the CALCIUM-CHANNEL BLOCKER verapamil hydrochloride. It can be used as an ANTIHYPERTENSIVE, as an ANTI-ANGINA drug in the prevention of attacks and as an ANTI-ARRHYTHMIC to correct certain heart irregularities. It is available as tablets and in a form for injection.
✚▲ Side-effects/warnings: See VERAPAMIL HYDROCHLORIDE.

Securon SR

(Knoll) is a proprietary, prescription-only preparation of the CALCIUM-CHANNEL BLOCKER verapamil hydrochloride. It can be used as an ANTIHYPERTENSIVE, as an ANTI-ANGINA drug in the prevention of attacks and after myocardial infarction. It is available as modified-release tablets.
✚▲ Side-effects/warnings: See VERAPAMIL HYDROCHLORIDE.

sedative 🅱

drugs calm and soothe, relieving anxiety and nervous tension and disposing a patient towards drowsiness. They are used particularly as a premedication prior to surgery. At higher doses, many sedatives can act as HYPNOTIC drugs (eg the BARBITURATE group), but when administered in doses lower than those used to induce sleep have mainly a sedative action but with some sleepiness. The terms *minor tranquillizer* or ANXIOLYTIC are now more commonly used to describe benzodiazepine-like sedatives that relieve anxiety without causing excessive sleepiness.
▲ Warnings: Many over-the-counter and herbal remedies (eg valerian and kava kava) may interfere with the effects of sedatives and can increase or reduce their efficacy or cause adverse reactions (eg increased sedation).

Select-A-Jet Dopamine

(Celltech) is a proprietary, prescription-only preparation of the SYMPATHOMIMETIC and CARDIAC STIMULANT dopamine (as dopamine hydrochloride). It can be used to treat cardiogenic shock following a heart attack or during heart surgery. It is available as a liquid in vials for dilution and intravenous infusion.
✚▲ Side-effects/warnings: See DOPAMINE.

selegiline

is an ENZYME INHIBITOR which is used in ANTIPARKINSONISM treatment because it inhibits one of the enzymes (monoamine-oxidase type B) that break down the neurotransmitter DOPAMINE in the brain. It is thought that dopamine deficiency in the brain causes Parkinson's disease. It is often used in combination with LEVODOPA (which is converted to dopamine in the brain) to treat the symptoms of parkinsonism. Its enzyme-inhibiting property, in effect, supplements and extends the action of levodopa and (in many but not all patients) it also minimizes some side-effects. Administration is oral.

✚ Side-effects: Constipation or diarrhoea, nausea and vomiting, dry mouth, inflammation of the lining of the mouth and sore throat, hypotension, depression, confusion, psychosis, agitation, headache, tremor, dizziness and vertigo, sleep disturbances; back pain, muscle cramps and joint pain, difficulty in urination, skin reactions.

▲ Warnings: It is not used in people with active gastric and duodenal ulceration, certain cardiovascular disorders, psychosis, pregnancy and breast-feeding. The side-effects are aggravated by the combination of selegiline and levodopa, and the dose of levodopa may have to be reduced.

✪ Related entries: Eldepryl; Zelapar.

selenium sulphide

is a substance that is used as an anti-dandruff agent in some shampoos.

✚▲ Side-effects/warnings: It is regarded as safe in normal topical use. However, undue absorption can produce systemic toxicity (although very low amounts are actually *required* in the dietary intake). Avoid abraded skin.

✪ Related entry: Selsun.

Selexid

(Leo) is a proprietary, prescription-only preparation of the ANTIBACTERIAL and ANTIBIOTIC drug pivmecillinam hydrochloride, a penicillin-like BETA-LACTAM. It can be used to treat a range of infections. It is available as tablets.

✚▲ Side-effects/warnings: See PIVMECILLINAM HYDROCHLORIDE.

Selsun

(Abbott) is a proprietary, non-prescription shampoo which contains SELENIUM SULPHIDE, and is used to treat seborrheic dermatitis and dandruff. It is available as a shampoo, and should not be used on children under five years, except on medical advice.

✚▲ Side-effects/warnings: See SELENIUM SULPHIDE.

Semi-Daonil

(Hoechst Marion Roussel; Aventis Pharma) is a proprietary, prescription-only preparation of the SULPHONYLUREA glibenclamide. It can be used in DIABETIC TREATMENT of Type II diabetes (non-insulin-dependent diabetes mellitus; NIDDM; maturity-onset diabetes), and is available as tablets (at half the strength of DAONIL).

✚▲ Side-effects/warnings: See GLIBENCLAMIDE.

Semprex

(GlaxoWellcome; GSK) is a proprietary, prescription-only preparation of the ANTIHISTAMINE acrivastine. It can be used to treat the symptoms of allergic disorders, such as hay fever and urticaria, and is available as capsules.

✚▲ Side-effects/warnings: See ACRIVASTINE.

senna

is a traditional, powerful (*stimulant*) LAXATIVE which is still in fairly widespread use. It works by increasing the muscular activity of the intestinal walls and may take from 8 to 12 hours to have any relieving effect on constipation. Senna preparations can also be administered to evacuate the bowels before an abdominal radiographic, surgery or endoscopy.

✚ Side-effects: It may cause griping, abdominal cramp and discoloured urine.

▲ Warnings: It should not be administered to patients who suffer from intestinal blockage. Care is necessary in women who are breast-feeding.

✪ Related entries: Califig California Syrup of Figs; Califig Herbal Laxative Tablets with Senna; Care Senna Laxative Tablets; Ex-Lax Senna; Jackson's Herbal Laxative; Manevac; Nylax with Senna; Pripsen Piperazine Phosphate Powder; Senokot Granules; Senokot Syrup; Senokot Tablets.

Senokot Granules

(Reckitt Benckiser Healthcare) is a proprietary, non-prescription preparation of the (*stimulant*) LAXATIVE senna. It can be used to relieve constipation, and is available as granules. It is not normally given to children, except on medical advice.

✚▲ Side-effects/warnings: See SENNA.

Senokot Syrup

(Reckitt Benckiser Healthcare) is a proprietary,

non-prescription preparation of the (*stimulant*) LAXATIVE senna. It can be used to relieve constipation, and is available as a syrup. It is not normally given to children under six years, except on medical advice.
✚▲ Side-effects/warnings: See SENNA.

Senokot Tablets

(Reckitt Benckiser Healthcare) is a proprietary, non-prescription preparation of the (*stimulant*) LAXATIVE senna. It can be used to relieve constipation, and is available as tablets. It is not normally given to children, except on medical advice.
✚▲ Side-effects/warnings: See SENNA.

Septrin

(GlaxoWellcome; GSK) is a proprietary, prescription-only compound preparation of the (SULPHONAMIDE) ANTIBACTERIAL sulfamethoxazole and the sulphonamide-like antibacterial trimethoprim, which is a combination called co-trimoxazole. It can be used to treat bacterial infections, and is available as tablets, a suspension (in adult and paediatric strengths), stronger tablets (*Forte*) and in a form for intravenous infusion.
✚▲ Side-effects/warnings: See CO-TRIMOXAZOLE.

Serc

(Solvay) is a proprietary, prescription-only preparation of betahistine hydrochloride, which has ANTINAUSEANT properties. It can be used to treat nausea associated with vertigo, tinnitus and hearing loss in Ménière's disease, and is available as tablets (in two strengths).
✚▲ Side-effects/warnings: See BETAHISTINE HYDROCHLORIDE.

Serdolect

(Lundbeck) is a proprietary, prescription-only preparation of the ANTIPSYCHOTIC drug sertindole. It can be used to tranquillize patients suffering from schizophrenia, and is available as tablets. (Currently, this product is available only on a named-patient basis for patients stabilized on sertindole in whom other antipsychotics have previously failed.)
✚▲ Side-effects/warnings: See SERTINDOLE.

Serenace

(IVAX) is a proprietary, prescription-only preparation of the ANTIPSYCHOTIC drug haloperidol. It can be used to treat psychotic disorders, such as schizophrenia. It can also be used in the short-term treatment of severe anxiety, for some involuntary motor disturbances and for intractable hiccup. It is available as a liquid, tablets, capsules and in a form for injection.
✚▲ Side-effects/warnings: See HALOPERIDOL.

Seretide

(A&H; GSK) is a proprietary, prescription-only compound preparation of the CORTICOSTEROID fluticasone propionate and the SYMPATHOMIMETIC, BRONCHODILATOR and BETA-RECEPTOR STIMULANT salmeterol (as xinafoate). It can be used as a treatment for the symptomatic relief of obstructive airways disease, as an ANTI-ASTHMATIC. It is available as an aerosol inhalant and as a dry powder for inhalation (called *Seretide Accuhaler Seretide Evohaler* for use in a special inhaler).
✚▲ Side-effects/warnings: See FLUTICASONE PROPIONATE; SALMETEROL.

Serevent

(A&H; GSK) is a proprietary, prescription-only preparation of the BETA-RECEPTOR STIMULANT salmeterol (as xinafoate; hydroxynaphthoate). It can be used as a BRONCHODILATOR in reversible obstructive airways disease and as an ANTI-ASTHMATIC treatment. It is a drug with unusual properties, in that it has a very prolonged duration of action. Therefore it is not to be used to relieve acute attacks, but instead is largely used to give overnight protection (though it should be taken in conjunction with corticosteroids or similar drugs). It is available as an aerosol and as a powder for inhalation using the *Diskhaler* or *Accuhaler* devices.
✚▲ Side-effects/warnings: See SALMETEROL. (Users will be cautioned not to exceed the stated dose and if a previously effective dose fails to relieve symptoms, they should consult their doctor.)

sermorelin

is an analogue of growth hormone-releasing hormone (somatorelin; GHRH). It is used therapeutically in a newly introduced test primarily to assess secretion of growth hormone. Administration is by injection.

✚ Side-effects: It may cause flushing of the face and pain at the injection site.
▲ Warnings: Administer with care to patients with epilepsy, hypothyroidism or who are being treated with antithyroid drugs. Do not use in pregnancy or breast-feeding. Caution must be taken when prescribing to those who are obese, hyperglycaemic or have increased fatty acids in their blood.
✪ **Related entry: Geref 50.**

Seroquel

(AstraZeneca) is a proprietary, prescription-only preparation of the ANTIPSYCHOTIC quetiapine (as fumarate). It can be used to treat schizophrenia. It is available as tablets.
✚▲ Side-effects/warnings: See QUETIAPINE.

serotonin

(5-HT; 5-hydroxytryptamine) is a natural mediator in the body with neurotransmitter and LOCAL HORMONE roles. As a neurotransmitter in the brain, it mediates chemical messages on its release to excite or inhibit other nerves. It also interacts with a range of RECEPTORS (specific types of recognition sites on cells). A number of important drug classes have been developed that work by mimicking, modifying or antagonizing serotonin's actions, including drugs that selectively modify its effect at receptors. Serotonin levels in the brain are thought to be an important determinant of mood and ANTIDEPRESSANTS modify levels of serotonin (and other monoamines, such as NORADRENALINE). One of the most recently developed classes of antidepressants, the SSRI class (eg FLUOXETINE), is named after the drugs' mechanisms of action – selective serotonin re-uptake inhibitors. The ANXIOLYTIC, BUSPIRONE HYDROCHLORIDE is thought to work by stimulating a certain type of serotonin receptor in the brain (5-HT_{1A}) and can be used for the short-term relief of anxiety. Serotonin is also involved in the process of perception and its function is thought to be disrupted in psychotic illness (eg schizophrenia); part of the evidence for this is that drugs such as LSD both induce mental states with psychotic features and are able to interact with some types of serotonin receptors.

Serotonin and its receptors also have other important roles. For example, a newly developed class of ANTINAUSEANT and ANTI-EMETIC drugs is the 5-HT_3-receptor antagonists (eg GRANISETRON, ONDANSETRON and TROPISETRON) and are of particular value in treating vomiting caused by chemotherapy by, in part, blocking the local hormone actions of serotonin in the intestine. Another recently developed group of drugs including SUMATRIPTAN, NARATRIPTAN, RIZATRIPTAN and ZOLMITRIPTAN can be used to treat acute migraine attacks, which work by mimicking certain vascular actions of 5-HT, producing a rapid constriction of blood vessels surrounding the brain through stimulating serotonin 5-HT_1 receptors. Serotonin, itself, is not used in clinical medicine.

Seroxat

(SmithKline Beecham; GSK) is a proprietary, prescription-only preparation of the (SSRI) ANTIDEPRESSANT paroxetine, which has fewer SEDATIVE effects than some other antidepressants. It is available as an oral liquid and tablets.
✚▲ Side-effects/warnings: See PAROXETINE.

sertindole

is an ANTIPSYCHOTIC drug (one of a group sometimes termed 'atypical' antipsychotics) which can be used to tranquillize patients suffering from schizophrenia. Administration is oral. (Currently, use of this drug is suspended, following reports of heart arrhythmias, and is available only on a named-patient basis for those who are already taking the drugs or for whom other antipsychotics have previously failed.)
✚ Side-effects: Of atypical antipsychotics include weight gain, dizziness, postural hypotension, extrapyramidal symptoms (usually mild and transient, but occasionally tardive dyskinesia on long-term administration). Also with sertindole, heart rhythm changes, peripheral oedema, dry mouth, difficulties in breathing, nasal congestion, dyspnoea, tingling in the extremities, decreases in the volume of ejaculate; also other side-effects.
▲ Warnings: Atypical antipsychotics are used with caution in patients with cardiovascular disease, history of epilepsy, and Parkinson's disease; may affect performance of skilled tasks, including driving. Also, caution in liver impairment; diabetes. Not used in pregnancy or breast-feeding, severe liver impairment, or with certain heart abnormalities (including those due to effects of other drugs).

✪ **Related entry: Serdolect.**

sertraline

is an ANTIDEPRESSANT drug of the recently developed SSRI group. It is used to treat depressive illness and has the advantage over some other antidepressant drugs because it has relatively fewer SEDATIVE and ANTICHOLINERGIC (ANTIMUSCARINIC) side-effects. It is also used to treat obsessive-compulsive disorders. Administration is oral.

✚▲ Side-effects/warnings: See SSRI. Also speeding of the heart, confusion and memory loss, hallucinations, aggressive behaviour, psychosis, hypersensitivity reactions (rash and other skin reactions; photosensitivity, angioedema, muscle pains), liver changes, abnormal milk secretion, menstrual irregularities, tingling in the extremities; also various other side-effects reported.

✪ **Related entry: Lustral.**

Setlers Antacid Peppermint Tablets

(Stafford-Miller; GSK) is a proprietary, non-prescription preparation of the ANTACID calcium carbonate. It can be used to relieve heartburn, indigestion, dyspepsia and nervous indigestion. It is available as tablets and is not normally given to children under 12 years, except on medical advice. Also available in *Fruit* and *Spearmint* flavours.

✚▲ Side-effects/warnings: See CALCIUM CARBONATE.

Setlers Heartburn and Indigestion Liquid

(Stafford-Miller; GSK) is a proprietary, non-prescription compound preparation of the ANTACID agents calcium carbonate and sodium bicarbonate and the DEMULCENT alginic acid (as sodium alginate). It can be used to relieve dyspepsia associated with gastric reflux, redflux oesophagitis, regurgitation and hiatus hernia. It is available as an oral suspension and is not normally given to children under six years, except on medical advice.

✚▲ Side-effects/warnings: See ALGINIC ACID; CALCIUM CARBONATE; SODIUM BICARBONATE.

Setlers Wind-eze

(Stafford-Miller; GSK) is a proprietary, non-prescription preparation of the ANTIFOAMING AGENT dimeticone (as simethicone). It can be used to relieve flatulence and bloating. It is available as chewable tablets and is not normally given to children, except on medical advice.

✚▲ Side-effects/warnings: See DIMETICONE.

Setlers Wind-eze Gel Caps

(Stafford-Miller; GSK) is a proprietary, non-prescription preparation of the ANTIFOAMING AGENT dimeticone (as simethicone). It can be used to relieve bloating and flatulence. It is available as capsules and is not normally given to children, except on medical advice.

✚▲ Side-effects/warnings: See DIMETICONE.

Sevredol

(Napp) is a proprietary, prescription-only preparation of the (OPIOID) NARCOTIC ANALGESIC morphine sulphate. It is available as tablets and oral solutions. (Some preparations are on the Controlled Drugs list.)

✚▲ Side-effects/warnings: See MORPHINE SULPHATE.

sex hormones 🅱

are endocrine (blood-borne) hormones (see HORMONE) that largely determine the development of the internal and external genitalia and secondary sexual characteristics (growth of hair, breasts and depth of voice). For convenience they are divided into male and female hormones, but both groups are produced to some extent by both sexes. They are all steroids (see STEROID) and chemically very similar. The main *male sex hormones* are called androgens (see ANDROGEN), of which TESTOSTERONE is the principal member. In men, androgens are produced primarily by the testes; in both men and women, they are also produced by the adrenal glands; and in women, small quantities are secreted by the ovaries. In medicine, there are a number of synthetic androgens that are used to make up hormonal deficiency and which can also be used in ANTICANCER treatment.

Female sex hormones are called OESTROGEN and PROGESTERONE. They are produced and secreted mainly by the ovary and the placenta during pregnancy; and to a lesser extent, in men and women, by the adrenal cortex; and, in men, by the testes.

Natural and synthetic oestrogens are used therapeutically, sometimes in combination with progestogens (see PROGESTOGEN), to treat menstrual, menopausal or other gynaecological problems, as ORAL CONTRACEPTIVE (and as parenteral contraceptives by injection or implantation) and for HRT (hormone replacement therapy). See also: ANTI-ANDROGEN; ANTI-OESTROGEN; CONTRACEPTIVE.

sibutramine

is an APPETITE SUPPRESSANT which is used, under medical supervision and on a short-term basis, to aid weight loss in OBESITY TREATMENT, maintain weight loss in the severely obese who are at risk from hypertension, diabetes mellitus, or disorders of fat metabolism. It works by inhibiting reuptake of norepinephrine, serotonin and dopamine in the central nervous system (CNS). Some antidepressants work in a similar way.

✚ Side-effects: Most commonly people taking sibutramine experience dry mouth, constipation and insomnia, though there may also be nausea and effects on the heart and cardiovascular system, such as tachycardia and palpitations, hypertension and vasodilation. There may also be light-headedness, headache, anxiety, sweating, paraesthesia, changes in taste and blurring of vision.

▲ Warnings: Sibutramine should not be used by women who are pregnant or breast-feeding. It is not suitable for people who have certain cardiovascular disorders such as coronary artery disease or congestive heart failure, tachycardia, peripheral arterial occlusive disease, arrhythmias, uncontrolled hypertension or cerebrovascular disease; or who have had major eating disorders or psychiatric illness, Gilles de la Tourette syndrome; hyperthyroidism, hypertrophy of the prostate, phaeochromocytoma, certain types of glaucoma or who have abused drugs or alcohol in the past. There will be monitoring throughout treatment. It is prescribed with caution for people with epilepsy, sleep apnoea syndrome or who have impaired liver or kidney function.

✪ Related entry: Reductil.

sildenafil

is used in IMPOTENCE TREATMENT for men with erectile dysfunction. It is a PHOSPHODIESTERASE INHIBITOR that acts as a powerful VASODILATOR in the blood vessels of the penis. It is taken orally.

✚ Side-effects: Dyspepsia (acid stomach); headache, flushing, dizziness, visual disturbances (including blue-coloured vision), nasal congestion; prolonged erection reported in some cases.

▲ Warnings: It should not be used concurrent to treatment with NITRATE drugs (eg in heart failure, angina); in conditions in which sexual activity is inadvisable; and in hereditary degenerative retinal disorders. It is used with caution in certain heart or cardiovascular disorders, where there is anatomical deformation of penis; liver impairment; or where there is predisposition to prolonged erection (eg in sickle-cell anaemia, leukaemia, multiple myeloma). Its onset of action (and effects) may be delayed if taken with food.

✪ Related entry: Viagra.

silver nitrate

is a powerful KERATOLYTIC agent which is used to treat verrucas and common warts. It also has an ANTISEPTIC action. It is used topically.

✚ Side-effects: It stains skin and fabric.

▲ Warnings: Surrounding skin and broken skin should be avoided. It is not suitable for application to large areas, or to the face and anogenital regions.

✪ Related entry: AVOCA.

silver sulfadiazine

(silver sulphadiazine) is an ANTIBACTERIAL preparation of silver combined with the SULPHONAMIDE sulphadiazine. It has a broad spectrum of antibacterial activity, as well as the ASTRINGENT and ANTISEPTIC properties of the silver. It is used primarily to inhibit infection of burns and bedsores. Administration is by topical application.

✚ Side-effects: These are rare, but there may be sensitivity reactions, such as rashes, burning, itching, effects on the blood (which may require stopping treatment).

▲ Warnings: It should not be administered to patients who are allergic to sulphonamides, who are pregnant or breast-feeding; it should be administered with caution to those with impaired function of the liver or kidneys, G6PD deficiency.

✪ Related entry: Flamazine.

simeticone

see DIMETICONE.

Simple Eye Ointment

is a non-proprietary, bland, sterile preparation of liquid paraffin and wool fat in yellow soft

paraffin. It is used as an eye treatment both as a night-time eye lubricant (in conditions that cause dry eyes) and to soften the crusts caused by infections of the eyelids (blepharitis).
✚▲ Side-effects/warnings: See LIQUID PARAFFIN; WOOL FAT; YELLOW SOFT PARAFFIN.

Simulect

(Novartis) is a proprietary, prescription-only preparation of the IMMUNOSUPPRESSANT basiliximab. It can be used to prevent rejection in kidney transplant patients (under specialist supervision). It is available in a form for injection.
✚▲ Side-effects/warnings: See BASILIXIMAB.

simvastatin

is a (*statin*) LIPID-REGULATING DRUG used in hyperlipidaemia to reduce the levels, or change the proportions, of various lipids in the bloodstream. It is usually administered only to patients in whom a strict and regular dietary regime, alone, is not having the desired effect, or who have high total blood cholesterol levels and coronary heart disease. Administration is oral.
✚ Side-effects: Rash, nausea, headache, hair loss, anaemia, dizziness, depression, tingling in the extremities, nerve disturbances, hepatitis and jaundice, pancreatitis; hypersensitivity syndrome, vomiting diarrhoea, flatulence.
▲ Warnings: It should not be administered to patients who are pregnant or breast-feeding (and avoid pregnancy for at least one month after stopping treatment), porphyria and kidney impairment. Patients should report any muscle weakness, pain or tenderness to their doctor.
✪ **Related entry: Zocor.**

Sinemet

(DuPont; Bristol-Myers Squibb) is a proprietary, prescription-only compound preparation of levodopa and carbidopa, which is a combination called co-careldopa. It can be used to treat parkinsonism, but not the parkinsonian symptoms induced by drugs (see ANTIPARKINSONISM), and is available as tablets in various strengths (called *Sinemet-62.5*, *Sinemet-110*, *Sinemet-275* and *Sinemet-Plus*).
✚▲ Side-effects/warnings: See LEVODOPA.

Sinemet CR

(DuPont; Bristol-Myers Squibb) is a proprietary, prescription-only compound preparation of levodopa and carbidopa, which is a combination called co-careldopa. It can be used to treat parkinsonism, but not the parkinsonian symptoms induced by drugs (see ANTIPARKINSONISM), and is available as modified-release tablets with a carbidopa/levodopa ratio of 1:4.
✚▲ Side-effects/warnings: See LEVODOPA.

Sinequan

(Pfizer) is a proprietary, prescription-only preparation of the (TRICYCLIC) ANTIDEPRESSANT doxepin. It can be used to treat depressive illness, especially in cases where sedation is required, and is available as capsules.
✚▲ Side-effects/warnings: See DOXEPIN.

Singulair

(MSD) is a proprietary, prescription-only preparation of the ANTI-ALLERGIC and ANTI-ASTHMATIC drug montelukast, a LEUKOTRIENE-RECEPTOR ANTAGONIST. It is used for the prevention (prophylaxis) of asthma symptoms. It is available as chewable tablets and tablets.
✚▲ Side-effects/warnings: See MONTELUKAST.

Sinthrome

(Alliance) is a proprietary, prescription-only preparation of the synthetic ANTICOAGULANT acenocoumarol (nicoumalone). It can be used to prevent the formation of clots in heart disease, after heart surgery (especially following implantation of prosthetic heart valves) and to prevent venous thrombosis and pulmonary embolism. It is available as tablets.
✚▲ Side-effects/warnings: See ACENOCOUMAROL.

Sinutab Tablets

(Warner Lambert Consumer Healthcare; Pfizer) is a proprietary, non-prescription compound preparation of the NON-NARCOTIC ANALGESIC paracetamol and the SYMPATHOMIMETIC and DECONGESTANT phenylpropanolamine hydrochloride. It can be used for the symptomatic relief of sinus pain, nasal congestion, hay fever, colds and flu. It is available as tablets and is not normally given to children under six years, except on medical advice.
✚▲ Side-effects/warnings: See PARACETAMOL; PHENYLPROPANOLAMINE HYDROCHLORIDE.

Siopel

(Bioglan) is a proprietary, non-prescription

preparation of the ANTISEPTIC cetrimide and the ANTIFOAMING AGENT dimeticone and arachis oil. It can be used as a BARRIER CREAM to treat and dress itching or infected skin, nappy rash and bedsores, and also to protect and sanitize a stoma (an outlet on the skin surface following the surgical curtailment of the intestines). It is available as a cream.

✚▲ Side-effects/warnings: See ARACHIS OIL; CETRIMIDE; DIMETICONE.

sirolimus

is a recently introduced IMMUNOSUPPRESSANT drug, actually an ANTIBIOTIC related to the macrolide family. It is used particularly to limit tissue rejection during and following kidney transplant surgery (in combination with CICLOSPORIN and a corticosteroid). Administration is oral.

✚ Side-effects: These are extensive and include abdominal pain and diarrhoea, tachycardia, effects on the blood, including anaemia and thrombocytopenia, hyperlipidaemias (raised levels of several blood lipids), enzyme changes, lowered blood potassium, pain in the joints and acne. Also, several less common symptoms such as nose bleeds and rash.

▲ Warnings: It is not to be administered to patients who are pregnant or breast-feeding. Caution is required in those with impaired liver function.

✪ Related entry: Rapamune.

skeletal muscle relaxant 🅴

drugs act to reduce tone or spasm in the voluntary (skeletal) muscles of the body. They include those drugs – called *neuromuscular blocking drugs* – that are used in surgical operations to paralyse skeletal muscles that are normally under voluntary nerve control (but because the muscles involved in respiration are also paralysed, the patient usually needs to be artificially ventilated). The use of these drugs means that lighter levels of anaesthesia are required. Drugs of this sort work by acting at *nicotinic* RECEPTORS on the muscle that recognize ACETYLCHOLINE, the neurotransmitter released from nerves to contract the muscle. There are two sorts of drug that achieve this effect, the *non-depolarizing* skeletal muscle relaxants (eg ATRACURIUM BESILATE, CISATRACURIUM, GALLAMINE TRIETHIODIDE, MIVACURIUM CHLORIDE, ROCURONIUM BROMIDE and VECURONIUM BROMIDE) and the *depolarizing* skeletal muscle relaxants (eg SUXAMETHONIUM CHLORIDE). The action of the non-depolarizing blocking agents may be reversed at the end of the operation, so that normal respiration may return, by administering an ANTICHOLINESTERASE drug (eg NEOSTIGMINE).

They work in a different way to DANTROLENE SODIUM which acts directly on skeletal muscle, and may be used when there is chronic severe spasticity of the muscles.

There are some quite different drugs (eg BACLOFEN and DIAZEPAM) that also effect muscle tone but do not work in the same way as the skeletal muscle relaxants discussed above, instead they act at some site in the central nervous system to reduce nervous activity and indirectly lower muscle tone. These drugs are used when some defect or disease causes spasm in muscle. The new drug TIZANIDINE which is used to treat spasticity caused by multiple sclerosis or due to injury or disease of the spinal cord, works in a different way again (it is an ALPHA-ADRENOCEPTOR STIMULANT acting at alpha-$_2$ receptors in the central nervous system).

All the drugs discussed in this entry are quite distinct and different from SMOOTH MUSCLE RELAXANT drugs.

Skelid

(Sanofi-Synthelabo) is a proprietary, prescription-only preparation of the CALCIUM METABOLISM MODIFIER tiludronic acid (as tiludronate disodium). It can be used to treat Paget's disease of the bone. It is available as tablets.

✚▲ Side-effects/warnings: See TILUDRONIC ACID.

Skinoren

(Schering Health) is a proprietary, prescription-only preparation of azelaic acid, which has mild ANTIBACTERIAL and KERATOLYTIC properties. It can be used to treat skin conditions, such as acne, and is available as a cream.

✚▲ Side-effects/warnings: See AZELAIC ACID.

Slofedipine

(Sterwin) is a proprietary, prescription-only preparation of the CALCIUM-CHANNEL BLOCKER nifedipine. It can be used as an ANTI-ANGINA treatment in the prevention of attacks, and as an

S

ANTIHYPERTENSIVE. It is available as modified release tablets.
✚▲ Side-effects/warnings: See NIFEDIPINE.

Slofedipine XL

(Sterwin) is a proprietary, prescription-only preparation of the CALCIUM-CHANNEL BLOCKER nifedipine. It can be used as an ANTI-ANGINA treatment in the prevention of attacks, and as an ANTIHYPERTENSIVE. It is available as modified release tablets.
✚▲ Side-effects/warnings: See NIFEDIPINE. This formulation of nifedipine is not suitable for people with certain liver or gastrointestinal conditions.

Slo-Phyllin

(Lipha) is a proprietary, non-prescription preparation of the BRONCHODILATOR theophylline. It can be used as an ANTI-ASTHMATIC and chronic bronchitis treatment, and is available as modified-release capsules for prolonged effect.
✚▲ Side-effects/warnings: See THEOPHYLLINE. To be swallowed whole with fluid or soft food.

Slow-Fe

(Novartis) is a proprietary, prescription-only preparation of ferrous sulphate. It can be used as an IRON supplement in iron deficiency ANAEMIA TREATMENT, and is available as modified-release tablets.
✚▲ Side-effects/warnings: See FERROUS SULPHATE.

Slow-Fe Folic

(Novartis) is a proprietary, prescription-only compound preparation of ferrous sulphate and folic acid. It can be used as an IRON and folic acid supplement during pregnancy, and is available as modified-release tablets.
✚▲ Side-effects/warnings: See FERROUS SULPHATE; FOLIC ACID.

Slow-K Tablets

(Alliance) is a proprietary, non-prescription preparation of potassium chloride. It can be used as a potassium supplement to prevent or treat blood deficiency of potassium, and is available as modified-release tablets. It is not given to children, except on medical advice.
✚▲ Side-effects/warnings: See POTASSIUM CHLORIDE.

Slow-Trasicor

(Novartis) is a proprietary, prescription-only preparation of the BETA-BLOCKER oxprenolol hydrochloride. It can be used as an ANTIHYPERTENSIVE for raised blood pressure and as an ANTI-ANGINA treatment. It is available as modified-release tablets.
✚▲ Side-effects/warnings: See OXPRENOLOL HYDROCHLORIDE.

Slozem

(Lipha) is a proprietary, prescription-only preparation of the CALCIUM-CHANNEL BLOCKER diltiazem hydrochloride. It can be used as an ANTIHYPERTENSIVE and ANTI-ANGINA treatment, and is available as modified-release capsules.
✚▲ Side-effects/warnings: See DILTIAZEM HYDROCHLORIDE.

smallpox vaccine

(Var/Vac) consists of a suspension of live (but attenuated) viruses and was used in IMMUNIZATION to prevent infection with smallpox. It is no longer required for public inoculation anywhere in the world because global eradication of smallpox has now been achieved. However, smallpox vaccine also works against other poxes (such as *vaccinia*) and is still used in specialist centres by researchers who work there with dangerous viruses, so need to be immunized. Also, this vaccine is now being manufactured again in quantity because of anxiety about the possible use of the smallpox virus in terrorist attacks. Technically, therefore, smallpox vaccine is still available on prescription.
✚▲ Side-effects/warnings: See VACCINE.

smooth muscle relaxant

drugs act on smooth (involuntary) muscles (such as the intestines and blood vessels) throughout the body to reduce spasm (ANTISPASMODIC), cause relaxation and to decrease motility. They can work by a variety of mechanisms, though the term is often reserved for those drugs that act directly on smooth muscle, rather than those that work indirectly through blocking or modifying the action of vasoconstrictor hormones or neurotransmitters (eg ACE INHIBITOR, ALPHA-ADRENOCEPTOR BLOCKER and BETA-BLOCKER drugs). Smooth muscle relaxants may be used for a number of purposes: drugs that dilate blood vessels may be used as ANTIHYPERTENSIVE agents to lower blood pressure (eg CALCIUM-CHANNEL BLOCKER drugs for long-term treatment and SODIUM NITROPRUSSIDE for a hypertensive crisis); in ANTI-ANGINA treatment to treat angina pectoris (eg calcium-channel blockers for long-term prevention and GLYCERYL TRINITRATE for acute attacks); to improve circulation in the extremities in the treatment of peripheral vascular disease (eg INOSITOL NICOTINATE and PENTOXIFYLLINE); in ANTI-ASTHMATIC treatment as BRONCHODILATOR drugs (eg BETA-RECEPTOR STIMULANT drugs and THEOPHYLLINE); to reduce spasm or colic of the intestine (eg MEBEVERINE HYDROCHLORIDE); and to relax the uterus in premature labour (beta-receptor stimulants). Drugs of the smooth muscle relaxant class are quite distinct from those of the SKELETAL MUSCLE RELAXANT class.

Sno Phenicol

(Chauvin) is a proprietary, prescription-only preparation of the ANTIBACTERIAL and ANTIBIOTIC chloramphenicol. It can be used to treat bacterial infections in the eye, and is available as eye-drops.
✚▲ Side-effects/warnings: See CHLORAMPHENICOL.

Sno Tears

(Chauvin) is a proprietary, non-prescription preparation of polyvinyl alcohol. It can be used as artificial tears where there is dryness of the eye due to disease, and is available as eye-drops.
✚▲ Side-effects/warnings: See POLYVINYL ALCOHOL.

Sodiofolin

(Medac) is a proprietary, prescription-only preparation of folinic acid (as disodium salt), which can be used to counteract some of the toxic effects of certain anticancer drugs, especially METHOTREXATE. It is available in a form for injection.
✚▲ Side-effects/warnings: See CALCIUM FOLINATE.

Sodium Bicarbonate, BP

is a non-proprietary, non-prescription liquid formulation of sodium bicarbonate and can be used as an ANTACID. It is available as a solution.
✚▲ Side-effects/warnings: See SODIUM BICARBONATE.

sodium acid phosphate

is a mineral salt which is mainly used in combination either with other phosphorus salts as a phosphorus supplement or a proprietary LAXATIVE enema to treat infections of the urinary tract. It is available in proprietary laxative preparations as an enema, suppositories and as tablets.
✚▲ Side-effects/warnings: It is regarded as safe in normal topical use.
✪ **Related entries: Carbalax; Fleet Phospho-soda; Fleet Ready-to-use Enema; Fletchers' Phosphate Enema; Phosphate-Sandoz.**

sodium alginate

see ALGINIC ACID.

Sodium Amytal

(Flynn) is a proprietary, prescription-only preparation of the BARBITURATE amobarbital (as sodium), and is on the Controlled Drugs list. It can be used as a HYPNOTIC to treat persistent and intractable insomnia, and as an ANTI-EPILEPTIC for severe episodes in specialist epilepsy centres. It is available as capsules.
✚▲ Side-effects/warnings: See AMOBARBITAL.

sodium aurothiomalate

is a form in which GOLD can be used as an ANTI-INFLAMMATORY and ANTIRHEUMATIC drug in the treatment of severe conditions of active rheumatoid arthritis and juvenile arthritis. It works extremely slowly and takes several months to have any beneficial effect. Administration is by injection.
✚ Side-effects: Severe reactions in a few patients and blood disorders; skin reactions, mouth ulcers; rarely, peripheral nerve disorders, fibrosis, liver toxicity and jaundice, hair loss and colitis.
▲ Warnings: It should not be administered to patients with blood disorders or bone marrow disease or porphyria, severe kidney or liver impairment; certain skin disorders, lupus erythematosus and certain other disorders; or who are pregnant or breast-feeding. Regular blood counts and monitoring of a wide range of body functions during treatment is necessary. Tell your doctor if you develop sore throat, infection, fever, unexplained bruising, bleeding or purple patches, mouth ulcers, metallic taste, rashes, cough or breathlessness.
✪ **Related entry: Myocrisin.**

S

sodium bicarbonate

is an ANTACID and is used for the rapid relief of indigestion. It is a constituent of many proprietary preparations that are used to relieve hyperacidity, dyspepsia and for the symptomatic relief of heartburn and a peptic ulcer. It is also used to provide relief from discomfort in mild infections of the urinary tract; also, it is incorporated into some ear-drops to soften wax. It is also sometimes used in infusion media to replace lost electrolytes or to relieve conditions of severe metabolic acidosis – when the acidity of body fluids is badly out of balance with the alkalinity – which may occur in kidney failure or diabetic coma. Administration is oral (except when in ear-drops).

✚ Side-effects: Belching, when used as an antacid.

▲ Warnings: It should be taken with care by patients with impaired kidney, liver or heart function or who are on a low-sodium diet. Avoid prolonged use.

✪ **Related entries: Actonorm Powder; Alka-Seltzer Original; Alka-Seltzer XS; Asilone Heartburn Liquid; Asilone Heartburn Tablets; Bisodol Extra Strong Mint; Bisodol Heartburn Relief; Bisodol Indigestion Relief Powder; Bisodol Indigestion Relief Tablets; Bisodol Wind Relief; Canesten Oasis; Cymalon; Dioralyte Tablets Raspberry Flavour; Eno; Gastrocote Liquid; Gastrocote Tablets; Gaviscon 250; Gaviscon 500 Lemon Flavour Tablets; Jaaps Health Salts; Liquid Gaviscon; Min-I-Jet Sodium Bicarbonate; Neo Gripe Mixture; Nurse Harvey's Gripe Mixture; Original Andrews Salts; Peptac Liquid; Phosphate-Sandoz; Pyrogastrone; Setlers Heartburn and Indigestion Liquid;Sodium Bicarbonate, BP; Topal; Woodward's Gripe Water.**

sodium calcium edetate

(sodium calciumedetate) is used as an ANTIDOTE to treat poisoning by heavy metals, especially lead. It acts as a CHELATING AGENT by binding to metals to form a compound that can be excreted from the body. Administration is by injection.

✚ Side-effects: There are a number, but the drug is only used under specialist care.

▲ Warnings: Caution in kidney impairment.

✪ **Related entry: Ledclair.**

sodium carbonate

is used as an ANTACID as a constituent of a proprietary effervescent preparations that are used to relieve hyperacidity, indigestion and flatulence. Also, it can be used to make the urine more alkaline in treating cystitis in adult women. Administration is oral.

✚▲ Side-effects/warnings: It should taken with care by patients with impaired kidney, liver or heart function or who are on a low-sodium diet. Avoid prolonged use.

✪ **Related entries: Canesten Oasis; Cymalon; Eno; Resolve.**

sodium carboxymethyl cellulose

see CARMELLOSE SODIUM.

sodium chloride

is an essential constituent of the human body for both blood and tissues. It is the major form in which the mineral element sodium appears. Sodium is involved in the balance of body fluids, in the nervous system and is essential for the functioning of the muscles. Sodium chloride, or salt, is contained in many foods, but too much salt can lead to oedema, dehydration and/or hypertension. Therapeutically, sodium chloride is widely used as saline solution (0.9%) or dextrose saline (to treat dehydration and shock), as a medium with which to effect bladder irrigation, as a sodium supplement in patients with low sodium levels, as an eye-wash, nose-drops, a mouthwash and by topical application in solution as a cleansing lotion.

✚ Side-effects: Overdosage can lead to hypertension, dehydration or oedema.

▲ Warnings: It should be administered with caution to patients with heart failure, hypertension, fluid retention or impaired kidney function.

✪ **Related entries: Dioralyte Natural; Dioralyte Relief; Dioralyte Tablets Raspberry Flavour; Glandosane; Minims Saline.**

sodium citrate

is an alkaline compound which is used in investigation and treatment of urinary tract procedures (eg to make the urine more alkaline in treating cystitis in women), and in electrolyte replacement preparations for treating losses in diarrhoea. It is available in several proprietary compound LAXATIVE enema preparations. Administration is oral.

✚ Side-effects: There may be dry mouth and mild diuresis.

▲ Warnings: It should be administered with

caution to patients with impaired kidney function, heart disease or who are pregnant.
✪ **Related entries: Bronalin Expectorant Linctus; Bronalin Junior Linctus; Canesten Oasis; Care Cystitis Relief; Cymalon; Dioralyte Natural; Dioralyte Relief; Micolette Micro-enema; Micralax Micro-enema; Relaxit Micro-enema.**

sodium clodronate

is a CALCIUM METABOLISM MODIFIER, a BISPHOSPHONATE that affects calcium metabolism and is used to treat high calcium levels and bone pain due to metastases associated with malignant tumours and bone lesions. Administration can be either oral or by slow intravenous infusion. Dietary counselling of patients is advised, particularly with regard to avoiding food containing calcium during oral treatment.
✚ Side-effects: There may be nausea and diarrhoea and skin reactions.
▲ Warnings: It should not be administered to patients with certain kidney disorders or who are pregnant or breast-feeding. Kidney and liver function and white blood-cell count will be monitored; an adequate fluid intake should be maintained. Food should not be taken one hour before and after treatment.
✪ **Related entries: Bonefos; Loron.**

sodium cromoglicate

(sodium cromoglycate) is an ANTI-ALLERGIC drug. It is used to prevent recurrent asthma attacks (but not to treat acute attacks) and allergic symptoms in the eye (eg allergic conjunctivitis), intestine (eg food allergy) and elsewhere. It is not clear how it works, but its ANTI-INFLAMMATORY activity appears to involve a reduction in the release of inflammatory mediators. Administration can be by inhalation, topically to the eye or nose, and by mouth.
✚ Side-effects: Depending on the route of administration, there may be coughing or transient bronchospasm. Inhalation of the dry powder preparation may cause irritation of the throat. Local irritation in the nose. Nausea, vomiting or joint pain.
✪ **Related entries: Aerocrom; Clarityn Allergy Eyedrops; Cromogen Easi-Breathe; Hay-Crom Aqueous; Hay-Crom Hay Fever Eye Drops; Intal; Nalcrom; Opticrom Allergy Eye Drops; Opticrom Aqueous; Optrex Allergy Eye Drops; Rynacrom; Rynacrom Allergy Nasal Spray; Rynacrom Compound; Vividrin.**

sodium cromoglycate

see SODIUM CROMOGLICATE.

sodium feredetate

(sodium ironedetate) is a drug rich in IRON which is used in iron-deficiency ANAEMIA TREATMENT to restore iron to the body or prevent deficiency. Administration is oral.
✚▲ Side-effects/warnings: See FERROUS SULPHATE.
✪ **Related entry: Sytron.**

sodium fluoride

see FLUORIDE.

sodium fusidate

see FUSIDIC ACID.

sodium hypochlorite

is a powerful oxidizing agent which can be used in solution as an ANTISEPTIC for cleansing abrasions, burns and ulcers. It is not commonly used today because it can be an irritant to some people, but there are a number of non-proprietary solutions available in various concentrations.
✚▲ Side-effects/warnings: It can have a marked irritant effect so is not generally recommended as an antiseptic (though is a good disinfectant), and can bleach fabrics.
✪ **Related entry: Chlorasol.**

sodium ironedetate

see SODIUM FEREDETATE.

sodium lauryl sulphate

is a salt with detergent and SURFACTANT properties. It is incorporated into the formulation of a number of proprietary skin preparations, shampoos and enemas.
✚▲ Side-effects/warnings: It is considered safe in use as directed, though hypersensitivity reactions have been reported.
✪ **Related entries: Alcoderm; Dentinox Cradle Cap Treatment Shampoo; Relaxit Micro-enema.**

sodium nitrite

is a compound that is used in the emergency treatment of cyanide poisoning and often in

combination with sodium thiosulphate. Administration is by injection. See ANTIDOTE.
✚ Side-effects: Flushing and headache.

sodium nitroprusside

is a VASODILATOR which can be used acutely as an ANTIHYPERTENSIVE to control severe hypertensive crises, in HEART FAILURE TREATMENT and as a HYPOTENSIVE for controlled low blood pressure in surgery. Administration is by intravenous infusion.
✚ Side-effects: Headache, dizziness, sweating, nausea and retching, and palpitations. Patients may also experience abdominal pain and anxiety.
▲ Warnings: It should not be administered to patients with severely impaired liver function or vitamin B_{12} deficiency; it is administered with caution to those with impaired kidney function, impaired blood circulation, hypothyroidism, hypothermia, who are elderly, pregnant or breast-feeding, or have ischaemic heart disease. Blood pressure and blood tests may be carried out during treatment.

sodium perborate

is an ANTISEPTIC which is used in solution as a mouthwash.
▲ Warnings: It should not be used for long periods of time (over seven days) or borate poisoning may occur; it should be used with care in those with renal impairment.
✪ **Related entry: Bocasan.**

sodium phenylbutyrate

is a soluble salt of the amino acid phenylbutyric acid, and is used in METABOLIC DISORDER TREATMENT for urea cycle disturbances where there is a build-up of ammonia in the body. It is given orally.
✚▲ Side-effects/warnings: It is a specialist drug and advice is necessary in assessing patients. Caution is necessary if there is kidney or liver impairment.
✪ **Related entry: Ammonaps.**

sodium picosulfate

(sodium picosulphate) is a (*stimulant*) LAXATIVE which works by stimulating motility of the intestine and can be used to relieve constipation and to prepare patients for radiological procedures, endoscopy or surgery. Administration is oral.
✚ Side-effects: Abdominal cramps.
▲ Warnings: It should not be administered to patients who suffer from intestinal blockage.
✪ **Related entries: Dulco-lax Perles; Laxoberal; Picolax.**

sodium picosulphate

see SODIUM PICOSULFATE.

sodium salicylate

is a soluble (NSAID) NON-NARCOTIC ANALGESIC and ANTIRHEUMATIC drug. It can be used to treat rheumatic disease and other musculoskeletal disorders. Administration is oral. See also SALICYLATE and SALICYLIC ACID.
✚▲ Side-effects/warnings: See NSAID.
✪ **Related entry: Jackson's Febrifuge.**

sodium stibogluconate

is an ANTIPROTOZOAL drug which can be used to treat various forms of the tropical disease leishmaniasis (or kala-azar), which is caused by parasitic protozoa transmitted in sandfly bites and leaves extensive, unsightly lesions on the skin. Administration is by slow intravenous or intramuscular injection.
✚ Side-effects: There may be vomiting, coughing and chest pain, headache, lethargy, effects on heart and liver, fever, sweating, vertigo, bleeding gums and nose, anorexia. The injection may be painful.
▲ Warnings: It should not be administered to patients who are breast-feeding, or have serious kidney impairment; it is used with caution in certain heart, liver or kidney disorders or who are pregnant.
✪ **Related entry: Pentostam.**

sodium tetradecyl sulphate

is a drug used in sclerotherapy, which is a technique to treat varicose veins by the injection of an irritant solution. Administration is by injection.
✚▲ Side-effects/warnings: See ETHANOLAMINE OLEATE.
✪ **Related entry: Fibro-Vein.**

sodium thiosulphate

is a compound that is used in the emergency treatment of cyanide poisoning and often in combination with sodium nitrite. Administration is by injection. See ANTIDOTE.

sodium valproate

is an ANTICONVULSANT and ANTI-EPILEPTIC drug. It is a valuable drug for treating all forms of epilepsy, particularly tonic-clonic seizures (grand mal) in primary generalized epilepsy. Recently, valproic acid as semisodium salt has been introduced for the treatment of the manic phase associated with manic-depressive illness. Administration can be either oral or by injection.
✚ Side-effects: These include stomach irritation and nausea, unsteady gait and muscle tremor, increased appetite and weight gain, thinning and curling hair, oedema, blood changes. It may cause pancreas and liver damage.
▲ Warnings: It should not be administered to patients with liver disease or a family history of liver dysfunction. Treatment should be stopped immediately if there is vomiting, jaundice, drowsiness, anorexia, or loss of seizure control; rashes; various signs of liver of blood disorder. Patients or their carers should be instructed how to recognize signs of blood or liver disorders, and they are advised to seek immediate medical attention if symptoms develop.
✪ Related entries: Convulex; Depakote; Epilim; Epilim Chrono; Epilim Intravenous; Orlept.

Sofradex

(Florizel) is a proprietary, prescription-only compound preparation of the (ANTIBACTERIAL) ANTIBIOTIC framycetin sulphate and gramicidin, also the ANTI-INFLAMMATORY and CORTICOSTEROID dexamethasone. It can be used to treat inflammation and infection in the eye or outer ear, and is available as drops and an ointment.
✚▲ Side-effects/warnings: See DEXAMETHASONE; FRAMYCETIN SULPHATE; GRAMICIDIN.

Soframycin

(Florizel) is a proprietary, prescription-only preparation of the broad-spectrum, ANTIBACTERIAL and (AMINOGLYCOSIDE) ANTIBIOTIC framycetin sulphate. It can be used to treat bacterial infections of the eye, and is available as eye-drops.
✚▲ Side-effects/warnings: See FRAMYCETIN SULPHATE.

Solaraze

(Bioglan) is a proprietary, prescription-only preparation of the (NSAID) NON-NARCOTIC ANALGESIC diclofenac sodium, which also has COUNTER-IRRITANT, OR RUBEFACIENT, actions. It can be used for the symptomatic relief of actinic keratosis by topical application to the skin, and is available as a gel.
✚▲ Side-effects/warnings: See DICLOFENAC SODIUM; but adverse effects on topical application are limited.

Solarcaine Cream

(Schering-Plough Consumer Health) is a proprietary, non-prescription compound preparation of the LOCAL ANAESTHETIC benzocaine and the ANTISEPTIC triclosan. It can be used to give relief from sunburn, insect bites, minor burns and skin injuries, and is available as a cream. It should not be given to children under three years, except on medical advice.
✚▲ Side-effects/warnings: See BENZOCAINE; TRICLOSAN.

Solarcaine Gel

(Schering-Plough Consumer Health) is a proprietary, non-prescription preparation of the LOCAL ANAESTHETIC lignocaine hydrochloride. It can be used to treat local pain and skin irritation, and is available as a gel. It is not used by children under three years, except on medical advice.
✚▲ Side-effects/warnings: See LIGNOCAINE HYDROCHLORIDE.

Solarcaine Lotion

(Schering-Plough Consumer Health) is a proprietary, non-prescription compound preparation of the LOCAL ANAESTHETIC benzocaine and the ANTISEPTIC triclosan. It can be used to give relief from sunburn, insect bites, minor burns and skin injuries, and is available as a lotion. It should not be given to children under three years, except on medical advice.
✚▲ Side-effects/warnings: See BENZOCAINE; TRICLOSAN.

Solarcaine Spray

(Schering-Plough Consumer Health) is a proprietary, non-prescription compound preparation of the LOCAL ANAESTHETIC benzocaine and the ANTISEPTIC triclosan. It can be used to give relief from sunburn, insect bites, minor burns and skin injuries, and is available as a spray. It should not be given to children under three years, except on medical advice.

✚▲ Side-effects/warnings: See BENZOCAINE; TRICLOSAN.

Solian
(Sanofi-Synthelabo) is a proprietary, prescription-only preparation of the ANTIPSYCHOTIC amisulpride. It can be used to treat schizophrenia. It is available as tablets.
✚▲ Side-effects/warnings: See AMISULPRIDE.

Solpadeine Capsules
(GSK Consumer Healthcare) is a proprietary, non-prescription compound preparation of the NON-NARCOTIC ANALGESIC paracetamol, the (OPIOID) NARCOTIC ANALGESIC codeine phosphate (a combination known as co-codamol 8/500) and the STIMULANT caffeine. It can be used to relieve pain, including headache, period pain and rheumatic and musculoskeletal pain. It is available as capsules and is not to be given to children, except on medical advice.
✚▲ Side-effects/warnings: See CAFFEINE; CODEINE PHOSPHATE; PARACETAMOL.

Solpadeine Max
(GSK Consumer Healthcare) is a proprietary, non-prescription compound preparation of the NON-NARCOTIC ANALGESIC paracetamol and the (OPIOID) NARCOTIC ANALGESIC codeine phosphate (a combination known as co-codamol). It can be used to relieve pain, including headache, period pain and rheumatic and musculoskeletal pain. It is available as tablets and is not to be given to children, except on medical advice.
✚▲ Side-effects/warnings: See CODEINE PHOSPHATE; PARACETAMOL.

Solpadeine Soluble Tablets
(GSK Consumer Healthcare) is a proprietary, non-prescription compound preparation of the NON-NARCOTIC ANALGESIC paracetamol, the (OPIOID) NARCOTIC ANALGESIC codeine phosphate (a combination known as co-codamol 8/500) and the STIMULANT caffeine. It can be used to relieve headache, period pain, rheumatic and musculoskeletal pain, fever, sore throat and cold and flu symptoms. It is available as soluble tablets and is not to be given to children under seven years, except on medical advice.
✚▲ Side-effects/warnings: See CAFFEINE; CODEINE PHOSPHATE; PARACETAMOL.

Solpadeine Tablets
(GSK Consumer Healthcare) is a proprietary, non-prescription compound preparation of the NON-NARCOTIC ANALGESIC paracetamol, the (OPIOID) NARCOTIC ANALGESIC codeine phosphate (a combination known as co-codamol 8/500) and the STIMULANT caffeine. It can be used to relieve headache, period pain, rheumatic and musculoskeletal pain, fever, sore throat and cold and flu symptoms. It is available as tablets and is not to be given to children, except on medical advice.
✚▲ Side-effects/warnings: See CAFFEINE; CODEINE PHOSPHATE; PARACETAMOL.

Solpadol
(Sanofi-Synthelabo) is a proprietary, prescription-only compound analgesic preparation of the (OPIOID) ANTITUSSIVE codeine phosphate and the NON-NARCOTIC ANALGESIC paracetamol (a combination known as co-codamol 30/500). It can be used as a painkiller, and is available as tablets (*Caplets*), capsules and effervescent tablets.
✚▲ Side-effects/warnings: See CODEINE PHOSPHATE; PARACETAMOL.

Solpaflex Tablets
(GSK) is a proprietary, non-prescription compound analgesic preparation of the (OPIOID) ANTITUSSIVE codeine phosphate and the NON-NARCOTIC ANALGESIC ibuprofen. It can be used as a painkiller (for example, for backache, headache and period pain), to treat fever and relieve cold and flu symptoms. It is available as tablets (*Caplets*), capsules an effervescent tablets, and is not to be given to children, except on medical advice.
✚▲ Side-effects/warnings: See CODEINE PHOSPHATE; IBUPROFEN.

soluble insulin
(insulin injection; neutral insulin) is a form of purified bovine and/or porcine insulin or human insulin, prepared as a sterile solution, which is used in DIABETIC TREATMENT to maintain diabetic patients. Administration is by injection and it has a short-acting duration of action.
✚▲ Side-effects/warnings: See INSULIN.
✪ Related entries: Human Actrapid; Human Mixtard 10; Human Mixtard 20; Human Mixtard 30; Human Mixtard 30 ge; Human Mixtard 40;

Human Mixtard 50; Human Velosulin; Humulin M2; Humulin M3; Humulin M5; Humulin S; Hypurin Porcine Biphasic Isophane 30/70 Mix; Hypurin Bovine Neutral; Hypurin Porcine Neutral; Pork Actrapid; Pork Mixtard 30.

Solu-Cortef

(Pharmacia) is a proprietary, prescription-only preparation of the CORTICOSTEROID and ANTI-INFLAMMATORY hydrocortisone (as sodium succinate). It can be used to treat inflammation, allergic symptoms and shock, and is available in a form for injection.

✚▲ Side-effects/warnings: See HYDROCORTISONE.

Solu-Medrone

(Pharmacia) is a proprietary, prescription-only preparation of the CORTICOSTEROID and ANTI-INFLAMMATORY methylprednisolone (as acetate). It can be used in the treatment of allergic disorders, shock and cerebral oedema, and is available in a form for injection.

✚▲ Side-effects/warnings: See METHYLPREDNISOLONE.

Solvazinc

(Provalis) is a proprietary, non-prescription preparation zinc sulphate. It can be used as a MINERAL SUPPLEMENT to correct zinc deficiency. It is available as effervescent tablets.

✚▲ Side-effects/warnings: See ZINC SULPHATE.

somatotrophin

see SOMATOTROPIN.

somatotropin

(somatotrophin) is a name for the pituitary HORMONE human growth hormone (HGH). It was isolated from the pituitary glands of cadavers, which when used to treat short stature (dwarfism) brought with it the risk of acquiring Creutzfeldt-Jakob disease due to contamination. It has now been replaced in the UK by SOMATROPIN, which is a biosynthetic form (produced by genetic engineering) of human growth hormone and so has no risk of contamination.

somatropin

(biosynthetic human growth hormone) is the name given to the synthetic form of the pituitary HORMONE human growth hormone. The name is used to distinguish it from the natural human product somatotropin (HGH) that it replaced in the UK. Somatotropin was isolated from the pituitary glands of cadavers and consequently brought with it the risk of acquiring Creutzfeldt-Jakob disease due to contamination. Somatropin is used to treat short stature (dwarfism) when the condition is due to growth hormone deficiency (eg in Turner syndrome); also for chronic renal insufficiency in children. It is mainly used when the bones are still forming and is administered by injection.

✚ Side-effects: Headache (which may need further investigation), visual problems, nausea and vomiting occur (may need further investigation), fluid retention and oedema, joint pain, muscle pain, tingling feeling, hypothyroidism, injection site reaction; leukaemia in children with growth hormone deficiency has also been reported.

▲ Warnings: A full specialist assessment of patient suitability will be made. It is not to be used by pregnant women. It is given with caution to those with diabetes, breast-feeding, other pituitary hormone deficiencies, or open bone epiphyses.

✪ Related entries: Genotropin; Humatrope; Norditropin; Saizen; Zomacton.

Somatuline Autogel

(Ipsen) is a proprietary, prescription-only preparation of lanreotide. It can be used as an ANTICANCER drug and to treat the symptoms following the release of hormones from certain carcinoid and non-carcinoid tumours and for acromegaly. It is available in a form for intramuscular injection.

✚▲ Side-effects/warnings: See LANREOTIDE.

Somatuline LA

(Ipsen) is a proprietary, prescription-only preparation of lanreotide. It can be used as an ANTICANCER drug and to treat the symptoms following the release of hormones from certain neuroendocrine tumours, and for acromegaly. It is available in a form for intramuscular injection.

✚▲ Side-effects/warnings: See LANREOTIDE.

Sominex

(SSL) is a proprietary, non-prescription preparation of the ANTIHISTAMINE promethazine

hydrochloride. It can be used to help induce sleep in the treatment of temporary sleep disturbances, and is available as tablets. It is not normally given to children under 16 years, except on medical advice.
✚▲ Side-effects/warnings: See PROMETHAZINE HYDROCHLORIDE.

Somnite
(Norgine) is a proprietary, prescription-only preparation of the BENZODIAZEPINE nitrazepam. It can be used as a relatively long-acting HYPNOTIC for the short-term treatment of insomnia, where a degree of sedation during the daytime is acceptable. It is available as an oral suspension.
✚▲ Side-effects/warnings: See NITRAZEPAM.

Sonata
(Lundbeck) is a proprietary, prescription-only preparation of the recently introduced HYPNOTIC drug zaleplon. It can be used for the short-term treatment of insomnia, and is available as capsules.
✚▲ Side-effects/warnings: See ZALEPLON.

Soneryl
(Concord) is a proprietary, prescription-only preparation of the BARBITURATE butobarbital (butobarbitone), and is on the Controlled Drugs list. It can be used as a HYPNOTIC to treat persistent and intractable insomnia, and is available as tablets.
✚▲ Side-effects/warnings: See BUTOBARBITAL.

Soothelip
(Bayer) is a proprietary, non-prescription preparation of the ANTIVIRAL drug aciclovir (acyclovir). It can be used to treat cold sores. It is available as a cream. It is not normally given to children, except on medical advice.
✚▲ Side-effects/warnings: See ACICLOVIR.

sorbitol
is a sweet-tasting carbohydrate which is used as a sugar-substitute (particularly by diabetics) and as the carbohydrate component in some nutritional supplements that are administered by intravenous injection or infusion. It is also used as a constituent of ARTIFICIAL SALIVA and is in some LAXATIVE preparations.
✚▲ Side-effects/warnings: It is regarded as safe in normal topical use.
✪ Related entries: Glandosane; Luborant; Micolette Micro-enema; Micralax Micro-enema; Relaxit Micro-enema.

Sotacor
(Squibb; Bristol-Myers Squibb) is a proprietary, prescription-only preparation of the BETA-BLOCKER sotalol hydrochloride. It is used as an ANTI-ARRHYTHMIC to regularize heartbeat in serious conditions, and is available as tablets and in a form for injection.
✚▲ Side-effects/warnings: See SOTALOL HYDROCHLORIDE.

sotalol hydrochloride
is a BETA-BLOCKER which can be used as an ANTI-ARRHYTHMIC to regularize heartbeat in life-threatening situations. Administration can be either oral or by injection.
✚▲ Side-effects/warnings: See PROPRANOLOL HYDROCHLORIDE. It may cause abnormal heart rhythms. It is not to be used if there are certain heart conditions or kidney failure, and should be used with care when there is severe diarrhoea.
✪ Related entries: Beta-Cardone; Sotacor.

spasmolytic
see ANTISPASMODIC.

Spasmonal
(Norgine) is a proprietary, non-prescription preparation of the ANTISPASMODIC alverine citrate. It can be used to treat muscle spasm of the gastrointestinal tract and period pain, and is available as capsules (a stronger version is called *Spasmonal Forte*).
✚▲ Side-effects/warnings: See ALVERINE CITRATE.

Spasmonal Fibre
(Norgine) is a proprietary, non-prescription compound preparation of the ANTISPASMODIC alverine citrate and the (*bulking-agent*) LAXATIVE sterculia. It can be used to treat irritable bowel syndrome, and is available as oral granules.
✚▲ Side-effects/warnings: See ALVERINE CITRATE; STERCULIA.

specific immunoglobulin
is used to give immediate *passive immunity*. Protection is achieved by administering a blood component prepared in much the same way as

NORMAL IMMUNOGLOBULIN, except that the blood plasma pooled is from donors with high levels of the particular antibody that is required (eg for hepatitis B, rabies, tetanus or varicella-zoster). Administration is by injection.

✚▲ Side-effects/warnings: See IMMUNIZATION.

✪ **Related entries: anti-D (Rh0) immunoglobulin; hepatitis B immunoglobulin (HBIG); rabies immunoglobulin; tetanus immunoglobulin; varicella-zoster immunoglobulin.**

Spectraban Lotion

(Stiefel) is a proprietary, non-prescription SUNSCREEN lotion. It contains constituents that protect the skin from ultraviolet radiation, including aminobenzoic acid and padimate-O, with UVB protection (SPF25). It can be used by people who suffer from photosensitivity because of genetic or other disorders or due to radiotherapy.

✚▲ Side-effects/warnings: See AMINOBENZOIC ACID.

Spectraban Ultra

(Stiefel) is a proprietary, non-prescription SUNSCREEN lotion. It contains constituents that protect the skin from ultraviolet radiation, including titanium dioxide, padimate-O, oxybenzone and butylmethoxydibenzoyl, with both UVB (SPF28) and UVA protection (SPF 6). It can be used by people who suffer from photosensitivity because of genetic or other disorders or due to radiotherapy.

✚▲ Side-effects/warnings: See TITANIUM DIOXIDE.

spermicidal contraceptive

drugs kill sperm and are intended to be used as an adjunct to (ie used as well as) barrier methods of contraception, such as the condom (sheath) or diaphragm (Dutch cap), but should never be regarded as a sole means of contraception. Most spermicidal preparations consist of a spermicide, which is usually chemically an alcohol ester (eg NONOXINOL), within a jelly liquid or cream base. Administration is topical.

✪ **Related entries: Delfen; Duragel; Gynol II; Ortho-Creme; Orthoforms.**

spironolactone

is a DIURETIC of the *aldosterone-antagonist* type. It is also *potassium-sparing* and so can be used in conjunction with other types of diuretic, such as the THIAZIDE, which cause loss of potassium, to obtain a more beneficial action. It can be used to treat oedema associated with aldosteronism (abnormal production of aldosterone by the adrenal gland), in HEART FAILURE TREATMENT, nephrotic syndrome and fluid retention and ascites caused by cirrhosis of the liver. Administration is oral.

✚ Side-effects: Gastrointestinal disturbances, headache, confusion, impotence and gynaecomastia (enlargements of breasts) in men; irregular menstruation in women; skin rashes, lethargy, disturbances of liver, blood and bone function.

▲ Warnings: It should not be administered to patients with severe kidney failure; raised potassium or lowered sodium levels in the blood; who are pregnant or breast-feeding; or who have Addison's disease. Administer with caution to those with certain liver or kidney disorders (blood electrolytes should be monitored).

✪ **Related entries: Aldactide 25; Aldactide 50; Aldactone; co-flumactone 25/25; co-flumactone 50/50; Lasilactone; Spirospare.**

Spirospare

(Ashbourne) is a proprietary, prescription-only preparation of the (*aldosterone-antagonist* and *potassium-sparing*) DIURETIC spironolactone, which is often used in conjunction with other types of diuretic, such as the THIAZIDE, that cause a loss of potassium. It can be used in HEART FAILURE TREATMENT, to treat oedema associated with aldosteronism, kidney disease and fluid retention and ascites caused by cirrhosis of the liver. It is available as tablets.

✚▲ Side-effects/warnings: See SPIRONOLACTONE.

Sporanox

(Janssen-Cilag) is a proprietary, prescription-only preparation of the ANTIFUNGAL drug itraconazole. It can be used to treat infections, especially candidiasis infections, and is available as an oral liquid, capsules and in a form for intravenous infusion.

✚▲ Side-effects/warnings: See ITRACONAZOLE.

Sprilon

(Smith and Nephew) is a proprietary, non-prescription compound preparation of zinc

oxide, the ANTIFOAMING AGENT dimeticone, wool fat, wool alcohol, white soft paraffin and liquid paraffin. It can be used as a BARRIER CREAM to treat leg ulcers, bedsores or applied to areas of the skin that require protection from urine or faeces (as in nappy rash or around a stoma – an outlet on the skin surface following the surgical curtailment of the intestines). Available as a spray.
✚▲ Side-effects/warnings: See DIMETICONE; LIQUID PARAFFIN; WHITE SOFT PARAFFIN; WOOL FAT; ZINC OXIDE.

SSRI

drugs are recently developed ANTIDEPRESSANT agents which are used to relieve the symptoms of depressive illness, and currently are the most widely prescribed class of antidepressant drugs. Some can also be used in anxiety disorders, obsessive-compulsive disorder and panic attacks. Like the MONOAMINE-OXIDASE INHIBITOR (MAOIs) and TRICYCLIC classes, the SSRI antidepressants are thought to work by modifying the actions of a mood-modifying amine neurotransmitter in the brain. The abbreviation SSRI stands for Selective Serotonin Re-uptake Inhibitor, because the mechanism of action is thought to be principally through inhibiting the amine-pump responsible for the re-uptake of the neurotransmitter 5-hydroxytryptamine (5-HT, SEROTONIN; chemically an amine) into nerve endings within the brain, an action that consequently increases levels of this mood-elevating amine in the brain. The SSRIs (CITALOPRAM, FLUOXETINE, FLUVOXAMINE MALEATE, PAROXETINE and SERTRALINE) seem to be effective in a good proportion of patients and have the advantage of being better tolerated than TRICYCLIC antidepressants, having fewer SEDATIVE and ANTICHOLINERGIC (ANTIMUSCARINIC) side-effects (eg dry mouth and gastrointestinal effects). Treatment often takes at least two weeks before any benefit is achieved: also, treatment should not begin immediately before or after some other types of antidepressant have been taken. Withdrawal of treatment must be gradual.

There are other drugs which are similar but have additional or slightly different actions: REBOXETINE is more active in inhibiting re-uptake of NORADRENALINE (Selective Noradrenaline Uptake Inhibitor; SNRI) and VENLAFAXINE inhibits both noradrenaline and serotonin uptake. Both have little sedative action. NEFAZODONE, like the SSRIs, inhibits serotonin reuptake, but additionally is a serotonin-receptor blocker.
✚ Side-effects: Gastrointestinal effects (related to dose); including nausea and vomiting, loss of appetite and weight (anorexia), dyspepsia, abdominal pain, diarrhoea or constipation; generally anorexia with weight loss; hypersensitivity reactions. Also, dry mouth, headache, nervousness, anxiety and insomnia; tremor, dizziness, muscle weakness, movement disorders, drowsiness, convulsions, loss of libido and failure of orgasm, sweating, purple blotches, hypomania or mania. SSRIs are generally less sedating and have fewer ANTICHOLINERGIC (antimuscarinic) and adverse heart effects than tricyclic antidepressants.
▲ Warnings: SSRIs should not be used if the person has a manic phase. An SSRI should not be started until some weeks after stopping an MAOI, and *vice versa*. Care is required in epilepsy, certain heart, liver and kidney disorders, and in pregnancy and breast-feeding. Driving may be affected. Unlike MAOIs, SSRIs do not cause food reactions. Herbal or other alternative remedies for depression, in particular St John's wort, should not be taken at the same time as SSRIs because serious adverse reactions can result.

stannous fluoride

see FLUORIDE.

Staril

(Squibb; Bristol-Myers Squibb) is a proprietary, prescription-only preparation of the ACE INHIBITOR fosinopril. It can be used as an ANTIHYPERTENSIVE and in congestive HEART FAILURE TREATMENT, and is available as tablets.
✚▲ Side-effects/warnings: See FOSINOPRIL.

Starlix

(Novartis) is a recently introduced proprietary, prescription-only preparation of nateglinide. It can be used in DIABETIC TREATMENT of Type II diabetes (non-insulin-dependent diabetes mellitus; NIDDM; maturity-onset diabetes), and is available as tablets.
✚▲ Side-effects/warnings: See NATEGLINIDE.

stavudine

(d4T) is a (*reverse transcriptase*) ANTIVIRAL drug

which can be used in the treatment of HIV infection. Administration is oral.

✚ Side-effects: There may be peripheral neuropathy (eg numbness, tingling, pain in hands and feet); pancreatitis; nausea and vomiting, diarrhoea, constipation and abdominal discomfort; chest pain and shortness of breath, muscle weakness; headache, insomnia, mood changes; muscular pain, flu symptoms; rash and other allergic symptoms; rarely, blood disturbances, pancreatitis, and others.

▲ Warnings: It is a specialist drug, and there will be full assessment and patient monitoring throughout treatment. It is not administered to patients who are breast-feeding. It should be administered with caution to those with a history of peripheral neuropathy or pancreatitis, kidney impairment or who are pregnant.

✪ Related entry: Zerit.

Stelazine

(Goldshield) is a proprietary, prescription-only preparation of the (PHENOTHIAZINE derivative) ANTIPSYCHOTIC drug trifluoperazine. It can be used to treat and tranquillize psychotic patients (such as schizophrenics), particularly those experiencing behavioural disturbances. The drug can also be used in the short-term treatment of severe anxiety and as an ANTI-EMETIC and ANTINAUSEANT for severe nausea and vomiting. It is available as tablets, syrup and capsules (*Spansules*).

✚▲ Side-effects/warnings: See TRIFLUOPERAZINE.

Stemetil

(Castlemead) is a proprietary, prescription-only preparation of the PHENOTHIAZINE derivative prochlorperazine (as maleate or mesilate), which has a range of applications. In this preparation it is used as an ANTINAUSEANT and ANTI-EMETIC to relieve the symptoms of nausea. It can also be used as an ANTIPSYCHOTIC for schizophrenia and other psychoses and for the short-term treatment of severe anxiety. It is available as tablets, effervescent granules, a syrup, suppositories and in a form for injection.

✚▲ Side-effects/warnings: See PROCHLORPERAZINE.

sterculia

is a vegetable gum that can absorb large amounts of water and is used as a (*bulking-agent*) LAXATIVE. It works by increasing the overall mass of faeces and so stimulating bowel movement, though the full effect may not be achieved for several hours. It is a useful alternative for patients who cannot tolerate bran in treating a range of bowel conditions, including diverticular disease and irritable bowel syndrome. It has been used (controversially) as an APPETITE SUPPRESSANT to treat serious obesity with the intention that small amounts of food ingested may be bulked up internally, so making the patient feel full. Administration is oral.

✚▲ Side-effects/warnings: See ISPAGHULA HUSK.

✪ Related entries: Normacol; Normacol Plus.

Steripod Chlorhexidine

(SSL) is a proprietary, non-prescription preparation of the ANTISEPTIC chlorhexidine (as gluconate). It can be used for swabbing and cleaning wounds and burns, and is available as a solution.

✚▲ Side-effects/warnings: See CHLORHEXIDINE.

Steripod Chlorhexidine/Cetrimide

(SSL) is a proprietary, non-prescription preparation of the ANTISEPTIC chlorhexidine (as gluconate) and cetrimide. It can be used for swabbing and cleaning wounds and burns, and is available as a solution.

✚▲ Side-effects/warnings: See CHLORHEXIDINE; CETRIMIDE.

steroid 🅴

is the term used to describe any of a class of naturally occurring and synthetic agents whose structure is based chemically on a steroid nucleus (a rather complex structure that consists of three six-member rings and one five-member ring). There are a number of important groups of chemicals in the body that are steroids, including all the CORTICOSTEROID hormones of the adrenal cortex (*glucocorticoids* or *mineralocorticoids*), all the SEX HORMONES (see ANDROGEN, PROGESTOGEN and ANABOLIC STEROID), all VITAMINS of the vitamin-D group (CALCIFEROL and analogues) and the bile acids (ie URSODEOXYCHOLIC ACID and analogues). Synthetic chemical analogues of the majority of these have an important part in medicine.

Ster-Zac Bath Concentrate

(SSL InternationalS) is a proprietary, non-

S

prescription preparation of the ANTISEPTIC triclosan. It can be used to prevent skin infections, and is available as a liquid for adding to a bath. It is not normally given to children, except on medical advice.
✚▲ Side-effects/warnings: See TRICLOSAN.

Ster-Zac Powder
(SSL) is a proprietary, non-prescription preparation of the ANTISEPTIC hexachlorophene. It can be used for staphylococcal skin infections in babies and also pressure sores. Available as a powder.
✚▲ Side-effects/warnings: See HEXACHLOROPHENE.

Stesolid
(Alpharma) is a proprietary, prescription-only preparation of the BENZODIAZEPINE diazepam. It can be used as an ANXIOLYTIC for the sort-term treatment of anxiety, as a HYPNOTIC to relieve insomnia, as an ANTICONVULSANT for febrile convulsions in children (when the oral route is not appropriate. It is available as a rectal solution (rectal tube).
✚▲ Side-effects/warnings: See DIAZEPAM.

Stiedex
(Stiefel) is a proprietary, prescription-only preparation of the CORTICOSTEROID and ANTI-INFLAMMATORY desoximetasone. It can be used in the treatment of severe, acute inflammation and chronic skin disorders, including psoriasis, and is available as a lotion and oily cream.
✚▲ Side-effects/warnings: See DESOXIMETASONE.

Stiemycin
(Stiefel) is a proprietary, prescription-only preparation of the ANTIBACTERIAL and (MACROLIDE) ANTIBIOTIC erythromycin. It can be used to treat acne, and is available as a solution for topical application.
✚▲ Side-effects/warnings: See ERYTHROMYCIN.

stilbestrol
see DIETHYLSTILBESTROL.

stilboestrol
see DIETHYLSTILBESTROL.

Stilnoct
(Sanofi-Synthelabo) is a proprietary, prescription-only preparation of the HYPNOTIC drug zolpidem tartrate. It can be used for the short-term treatment of insomnia, and is available as tablets.
✚▲ Side-effects/warnings: See ZOLPIDEM TARTRATE.

Stimlor
(Berk; APS) is a proprietary, prescription-only preparation of the VASODILATOR naftidrofuryl oxalate. It can be used to help improve blood circulation to the hands and feet when this is impaired, for example, in peripheral vascular disease (Raynaud's phenomenon), and for cerebral vascular disease. Available as capsules.
✚▲ Side-effects/warnings: See NAFTIDROFURYL OXALATE.

stimulant 🅱
drugs activate body systems or functions. In general, the term is used to describe drugs that stimulate the central nervous system (CNS stimulants). Therapeutically, they can be used to treat patients suffering from narcolepsy, which is an extreme tendency to fall asleep when engaged in monotonous activities or when in quiet surroundings (eg MODAFINIL). There is a tendency for those who use stimulant drugs on a regular basis to become drug dependant and show a withdrawal syndrome when they stop taking the drug. Preparations of one of the most powerful and best-known stimulants, DEXAMFETAMINE SULPHATE (dexamphetamine), are on the Controlled Drugs list. CAFFEINE and related compounds are mild stimulants and for medical purposes caffeine is incorporated into several proprietary compound analgesic preparations that are used as cold remedies.
▲ Warnings: Herbal remedies used for their stimulant properties, such as Siberian ginseng, could be dangerous if taken with stimulant drugs prescribed by your doctor or bought over-the-counter.

Strefen
(Crooks) is a proprietary, prescription-only preparation of the (NSAID) NON-NARCOTIC ANALGESIC flurbiprofen. It can be used topically for relief of sore throat, and is available as lozenges.
✚▲ Side-effects/warnings: See FLURBIPROFEN. Move the lozenge around the mouth to help prevent mouth ulcers.

Strepsils Cough Lozenges
(Crookes Healthcare) is a proprietary, non-prescription preparation of the ANTITUSSIVE dextromethorphan hydrobromide. It can be used for the relief of dry ticklish coughs and is available as lozenges. It is not normally given to children under 12 years, except on medical advice.
✚▲ Side-effects/warnings: See DEXTROMETHORPHAN HYDROBROMIDE.

Strepsils Extra
(Crookes Healthcare) is a proprietary, non-prescription preparation of the ANTISEPTIC hexylresorcinol. It can be used for symptomatic relief of severe sore throat, and is available in the form of a lozenge. It is not given to children under six years, except on medical advice.
✚▲ Side-effects/warnings: See HEXYLRESORCINOL.

Strepsils Honey and Lemon
(Crookes Healthcare) is a proprietary, non-prescription compound preparation of the ANTISEPTIC amylmetacresol with dichlorobenzyl alcohol. It can be used for the relief of minor mouth and throat infections, and is available as lozenges.
✚▲ Side-effects/warnings: See AMYLMETACRESOL.

Strepsils Menthol and Eucalyptus
(Crookes Healthcare) is a proprietary, non-prescription compound preparation of the ANTISEPTIC amylmetacresol with dichlorobenzyl alcohol and menthol (as levomenthol). It can be used for the relief of minor mouth and throat infections and nasal congestion. It is available as a lozenge.
✚▲ Side-effects/warnings: See AMYLMETACRESOL; MENTHOL.

Strepsils Original
(Crookes Healthcare) is a proprietary, non-prescription preparation of the ANTISEPTIC amylmetacresol (with dichlorobenzyl alcohol). It can be used for relief of infections associated with sore throat, and is available as a lozenge.
✚▲ Side-effects/warnings: See AMYLMETACRESOL.

Strepsils Pain Relief Plus
(Crookes Healthcare) is a proprietary, non-prescription compound preparation of the LOCAL ANAESTHETIC lidocaine hydrochloride (lignocaine) and the ANTISEPTIC amylmetacresol (with dichlorobenzyl alcohol). It can be used for symptomatic relief of infections associated with sore throat, and is available in the form of a lozenge. It should not be given to children, except on medical advice.
✚▲ Side-effects/warnings: See AMYLMETACRESOL; LIDOCAINE HYDROCHLORIDE.

Strepsils Pain Relief Spray
(Crookes Healthcare) is a proprietary, non-prescription preparation of the LOCAL ANAESTHETIC lidocaine hydrochloride (lignocaine). It can be used for relief of infections associated with sore throat, and is available as a spray. It should not be given to children, except on medical advice.
✚▲ Side-effects/warnings: See LIDOCAINE HYDROCHLORIDE.

Strepsils Sugar Free Lozenges
(Crookes Healthcare) is a proprietary, non-prescription preparation of the ANTISEPTIC amylmetacresol (with dichlorobenzyl alcohol). It can be used for symptomatic relief of infections associated with sore throat, and is available in the form of a lozenge.
✚▲ Side-effects/warnings: See AMYLMETACRESOL.

Strepsils with Vitamin C 100 mg
(Crookes Healthcare) is a proprietary, non-prescription compound preparation of the ANTISEPTIC amylmetacresol (with dichlorobenzyl alcohol) and ascorbic acid. It can be used for symptomatic relief of infections associated with sore throat, and is available in the form of a lozenge.
✚▲ Side-effects/warnings: See ASCORBIC ACID; AMYLMETACRESOL.

Streptase
(Hoechst Marion Roussel; Aventis Pharma) is a proprietary, prescription-only preparation of the FIBRINOLYTIC drug streptokinase. It can be used to treat thrombosis and embolism, and is available in a form for injection.
✚▲ Side-effects/warnings: See STREPTOKINASE.

streptokinase
is used therapeutically as an FIBRINOLYTIC drug,

because it has the property of breaking up blood clots. It is used rapidly in such serious conditions as venous thrombi, pulmonary embolism and myocardial infarction. It is also used topically as a desloughing agent in treatment of ulcers. Administration is by intravenous injection or infusion.

✚▲ Side-effects/warnings: See FIBRINOLYTIC.

✪ **Related entries: Streptase; Varidase Topical.**

streptomycin

is an ANTIBACTERIAL and ANTIBIOTIC drug which is an original member of the AMINOGLYCOSIDE family. In the UK today, it is used almost exclusively for the treatment of tuberculosis, in combination with other antibiotics. Treatment takes between 6 and 18 months. It can also be used with DOXYCYCLINE as an adjunct in brucellosis treatment. Administration is normally by injection.

✚▲ Side-effects/warnings: See GENTAMICIN; there may also be hypersensitivity reactions and tingling sensations in the mouth.

Stugeron 15 Tablets

(Johnson & Johnson • MSD) is a proprietary, non-prescription preparation of the ANTIHISTAMINE cinnarizine. It can be used as an ANTINAUSEANT to prevent and treat nausea and vomiting caused by motion sickness in travelling. It is available as tablets.

✚▲ Side-effects/warnings: See CINNARIZINE.

Stugeron Forte

(Janssen-Cilag) is a proprietary, non-prescription preparation of the ANTIHISTAMINE cinnarizine. It is used as a VASODILATOR to treat peripheral vascular disease (Raynaud's phenomenon). This stronger preparation is available as capsules.

✚▲ Side-effects/warnings: See CINNARIZINE.

Sublimaze

(Janssen-Cilag) is a proprietary, prescription-only preparation of the (OPIOID) NARCOTIC ANALGESIC fentanyl (as hydrochloride), and is on the Controlled Drugs list. It can be used to treat moderate to severe pain, including during operations. It is available in a form for injection.

✚▲ Side-effects/warnings: See FENTANYL.

Subutex

(Schering-Plough) is a proprietary, prescription-only preparation of the (OPIOID) NARCOTIC ANALGESIC buprenorphine (as hydrochloride), and is on the Controlled Drugs list. It can be used as part of therapy for those dependent (addicted to) opioids, and is available as sublingual tablets (to be retained under the tongue).

✚▲ Side-effects/warnings: See BUPRENORPHINE.

sucralfate

is a complex of aluminium hydroxide and sulphated sucrose, which can be used as a long-term treatment of gastric and duodenal ulcers. It has very little ANTACID action, but is thought to work as a CYTOPROTECTANT by forming a barrier over an ulcer, so protecting it from acid and the enzyme pepsin and allowing it to heal. Administration is oral.

✚ Side-effects: Constipation, diarrhoea, nausea, indigestion, gastric discomfort, dry mouth, skin rash and itching, insomnia, dizziness, vertigo and drowsiness.

▲ Warnings: It should be administered with caution to patients with kidney disorders or who are pregnant or breast-feeding.

✪ **Related entry: Antepsin.**

Sudafed-Co Tablets

(Warner Lambert Consumer Healthcare; Pfizer) is a proprietary, non-prescription compound preparation of the SYMPATHOMIMETIC and DECONGESTANT pseudoephedrine hydrochloride and the NON-NARCOTIC ANALGESIC paracetamol. It can be used for the symptomatic relief of conditions where upper respiratory congestion is associated with raised body temperature or pain, including colds and flu. It is available as tablets and is not normally given to children under six years, except on medical advice.

✚▲ Side-effects/warnings: See PARACETAMOL; PSEUDOEPHEDRINE HYDROCHLORIDE.

Sudafed Decongestant Nasal Spray

(Warner Lambert Consumer Healthcare; Pfizer) is a proprietary, non-prescription preparation of the SYMPATHOMIMETIC and VASOCONSTRICTOR xylometazoline hydrochloride. It can be used as a NASAL DECONGESTANT for the symptomatic relief of nasal congestion such as with the common cold and flu, perennial and allergic rhinitis (such as hay fever) and sinusitis. It is available as a (metered dose) nasal spray and is not given to children, except on medical advice.

✚▲ Side-effects/warnings: See XYLOMETAZOLINE HYDROCHLORIDE.

Sudafed Elixir

(Warner Lambert Consumer Healthcare; Pfizer) is a proprietary, non-prescription preparation of the SYMPATHOMIMETIC and DECONGESTANT pseudoephedrine hydrochloride. It can be used for the symptomatic relief of allergic and vasomotor rhinitis and colds and flu. It is available as a liquid and is not normally given to children under two years, except on medical advice.

✚▲ Side-effects/warnings: See PSEUDOEPHEDRINE HYDROCHLORIDE.

Sudafed Expectorant

(Warner Lambert Consumer Healthcare; Pfizer) is a proprietary, non-prescription compound preparation of the SYMPATHOMIMETIC and DECONGESTANT pseudoephedrine hydrochloride and the EXPECTORANT agent guaifenesin (guaiphenesin). It can be used for the symptomatic relief of upper respiratory tract disorders accompanied by productive cough. It is available as a liquid and is not normally given to children under two years, except on medical advice.

✚▲ Side-effects/warnings: See GUAIFENESIN; PSEUDOEPHEDRINE HYDROCHLORIDE.

Sudafed Linctus

(Warner Lambert Consumer Healthcare; Pfizer) is a proprietary, non-prescription compound preparation of the SYMPATHOMIMETIC and DECONGESTANT pseudoephedrine hydrochloride and the (OPIOID) ANTITUSSIVE dextromethorphan hydrobromide. It can be used for the symptomatic relief of dry coughs accompanied by congestion of the upper airways. It is available as a liquid and is not normally given to children under two years, except on medical advice.

✚▲ Side-effects/warnings: See DEXTROMETHORPHAN HYDROBROMIDE; PSEUDOEPHEDRINE HYDROCHLORIDE.

Sudafed Nasal Spray

(Warner Lambert Consumer Healthcare; Pfizer) is a proprietary, non-prescription preparation of the SYMPATHOMIMETIC and VASOCONSTRICTOR oxymetazoline hydrochloride. It can be used as a NASAL DECONGESTANT for symptomatic relief of nasal congestion associated with a wide variety of upper respiratory tract disorders. It is available as a nasal spray and is not normally given to children under six years, except on medical advice.

✚▲ Side-effects/warnings: See OXYMETAZOLINE HYDROCHLORIDE.

Sudafed Tablets

(Warner Lambert Consumer Healthcare; Pfizer) is a proprietary, non-prescription preparation of the SYMPATHOMIMETIC and VASOCONSTRICTOR pseudoephedrine hydrochloride. It can be used as a NASAL DECONGESTANT for the symptomatic relief of rhinitis, the common cold and flu. It is available as tablets and is not given to children, except on medical advice.

✚▲ Side-effects/warnings: See PSEUDOEPHEDRINE HYDROCHLORIDE.

Sudocream Antiseptic Healing Cream

(Pharmax) is a proprietary, non-prescription compound preparation of zinc oxide, lanolin, benzyl benzoate, benzyl cinnamate and benzyl alcohol. It can be used for nappy rash, bedsores, eczema, chilblains, sunburn and acne. It is available as a cream.

✚▲ Side-effects/warnings: See BENZYL BENZOATE; LANOLIN; ZINC OXIDE.

Sudocrem Antiseptic Cream

(Pharmax) is a proprietary, non-prescription compound preparation of zinc oxide, benzyl alcohol, benzyl benzoate, hypoallergenic lanolin and various other minor constituents. It can be used as an EMOLLIENT and a BARRIER CREAM for nappy rash and incontinence dermatitis, and other minor wounds and sunburn. It is applied as a topical cream.

✚▲ Side-effects/warnings: See BENZYL BENZOATE; LANOLIN; ZINC OXIDE.

Sulazine EC

(Alpharma) is a proprietary, prescription-only preparation of the AMINOSALICYLATE sulphasalazine. It can be used to treat active rheumatoid arthritis, ulcerative colitis and Crohn's disease. It is available as enteric-coated tablets.

✚▲ Side-effects/warnings: See SULPHASALAZINE.

S

sulconazole nitrate
is an (AZOLE) ANTIFUNGAL drug which is used to treat skin infections, particularly those caused by tinea; also for vaginal candidiasis. Administration is by topical application.
✚▲ Side-effects/warnings: See CLOTRIMAZOLE. Avoid contact with the eyes.
✪ **Related entry: Exelderm.**

Suleo-M Lotion
(SSL) is a proprietary, non-prescription preparation of the SCABICIDAL and PEDICULICIDAL drug malathion. It can be used to treat infestations of the scalp by lice (pediculosis). It is available as a lotion and is not normally used for children under six months, except on medical advice.
✚▲ Side-effects/warnings: See MALATHION.

sulfabenzamide
(sulphabenzamide) is a (SULPHONAMIDE) ANTIBACTERIAL drug which is combined with two similar drugs, sulfacetamide and sulfathiazole, in a proprietary preparation that can be used to treat bacterial infections of the vagina and the cervix, and to prevent infection following gynaecological surgery. Administration is by topical application.
✚▲ Side-effects/warnings: There may be sensitivity reactions, local irritation, Candidiasis.
✪ **Related entry: Sultrin.**

sulfacetamide
(sulphacetamide) is a (SULPHONAMIDE) ANTIBACTERIAL drug which is available only combined with two similar drugs, SULFABENZAMIDE and SULFATHIAZOLE, in a proprietary preparation that can be used to treat bacterial infections of the vagina and the cervix, and to prevent infection following gynaecological surgery. Administration is by topical application.
✚▲ Side-effects/warnings: There may be sensitivity reactions. It should not be used by patients who are pregnant.
✪ **Related entry: Sultrin.**

sulfadiazine
(sulphadiazine) is a (SULPHONAMIDE) ANTIBACTERIAL drug which can be used to treat serious bacterial infections, and to prevent recurrence of rheumatic fever. Administration can be either oral or by intravenous injection or infusion. It is available as two non-proprietary, prescription-only forms, tablets and in a form for injection. (See also SILVER SULFADIAZINE.)
✚▲ Side-effects/warnings: See CO-TRIMOXAZOLE.

sulfadoxine
is a long-acting (SULPHONAMIDE) ANTIBACTERIAL drug, which is used solely in combination with the ANTIMALARIAL drug PYRIMETHAMINE to prevent or treat malaria.
✚▲ Side-effects/warnings: There may be serious side-effects; it should be administered with caution to patients who are pregnant or breast-feeding.
✪ **Related entry: Fansidar.**

sulfalene
see SULFAMETOPYRAZINE.

sulfamethoxazole
(sulphamethoxazole) is a (SULPHONAMIDE) ANTIBACTERIAL drug which can be used, in combination with another sulphonamide-like antibacterial drug trimethoprim (a combination called co-trimoxazole), to treat a wide range of serious infections, especially of the urinary tract, the upper respiratory tract; also for *Pneumocystis carinii*. infection. It is given orally or by injection.
✚▲ Side-effects/warnings: See CO-TRIMOXAZOLE.
✪ **Related entries: Chemotrim; Fectrim; Septrin.**

sulfametopyrazine
(sulfalene) is a long-acting (SULPHONAMIDE) ANTIBACTERIAL drug which is used primarily in the treatment of chronic bronchitis and infections of the urinary tract. Administration is oral.
✚▲ Side-effects/warnings: See CO-TRIMOXAZOLE.
✪ **Related entry: Kelfizine W.**

sulfasalazine
(sulphasalazine) is an AMINOSALICYLATE which combines within the one chemical a SULPHONAMIDE constituent (with ANTIBACTERIAL properties) and an aminosalicylate (5-aminosalicylic acid) component. It can be used to treat active Crohn's disease and to induce and maintain remission of the symptoms of ulcerative colitis. It is also sometimes used to treat rheumatoid arthritis.

Administration can be either oral or topical as suppositories or a retention enema.
✚ Side-effects: Nausea, vomiting and discomfort in the upper abdomen; rash, headache; rarely, fever, skin, lung or eye disorders and a number of other complaints. Some preparations may stain contact lenses. Patients should tell their doctor if they have any unexplained bruising, bleeding, sore throat, fever or malaise, because of possible effects on the blood requiring treatment to be stopped.
▲ Warnings: It should not be administered to patients known to be sensitive to salicylates (aspirin-type drugs) or to sulphonamides; it should be administered with caution to those with liver or kidney disease, G6PD deficiency or who are pregnant or breast-feeding.
✪ **Related entries: Salazopyrin; Sulazine EC; Ucine.**

sulfathiazole

(sulphathiazole) is a (SULPHONAMIDE) ANTIBACTERIAL drug which is combined with two similar drugs, sulfacetamide and sulfabenzamide, in a proprietary preparation that can be used to treat bacterial infections of the vagina and the cervix, and to prevent infection following gynaecological surgery. Administration is topical.
✚ Side-effects: There may be sensitivity reactions.
▲ Warnings: It should not be used by patients with severe kidney damage, or who are pregnant.
✪ **Related entry: Sultrin.**

sulfinpyrazone

(sulphinpyrazone) is a drug that is used to prevent gout and to treat hyperucaemia. It works by promoting the excretion of uric acid in the urine. Administration is oral.
✚ Side-effects: Gastrointestinal disturbances, allergic skin reactions, salt and water retention, rarely blood disorders, ulceration and bleeding in the gastrointestinal tract, kidney failure and changes in liver function.
▲ Warnings: See PROBENECID. Regular blood counts are advisable and avoid using in patients with NSAID hypersensitivity or heart disease. (It is not for acute attacks, but if an acute attack occurs during treatment, sulfinpyrazone should be continued.)
✪ **Related entry: Anturan.**

sulindac

is a (NSAID) NON-NARCOTIC ANALGESIC and ANTIRHEUMATIC drug. It is used to treat pain and inflammation in rheumatic disease and other musculoskeletal disorders, and in acute gout. Administration is oral.
✚▲ Side-effects/warnings: see NSAID. It is prescribed with care to patients who have had kidney stones. An adequate fluid intake must be maintained. Urine may become discoloured. Skin reactions are more common than with many other NSAIDs.
✪ **Related entry: Clinoril.**

sulphadiazine

see SULFADIAZINE.

sulpha drugs

see SULPHONAMIDE.

sulphamethoxazole

see SULFAMETHOXAZOLE.

sulphasalazine

see SULFASALAZINE.

sulphathiazole

see SULFATHIAZOLE.

sulphinpyrazone

see SULFINPYRAZONE.

sulphonamide 🅱

drugs (sulpha or sulfa drugs) are derivatives of a red dye, prontosil, which was discovered in the 1930s and which is converted in the body to sulphanilamide. This class of drugs has the property of preventing the growth of bacteria. They were the first group of drugs suitable for ANTIMICROBIAL use as relatively safe (at that time) ANTIBACTERIAL agents. Today, they, along with other similar synthetic classes of chemotherapeutic drugs, are commonly referred to as ANTIBIOTIC drugs, although, strictly speaking, they are not *antibiotics* (in the literal sense of agents produced by, or obtained from, micro-organisms that inhibit the growth of, or destroy, other micro-organisms). Their antibacterial action stems from their chemical similarity to a compound required by bacteria to generate the essential growth factor, folic acid. This similarity inhibits the production of folic acid by bacteria (and therefore growth), while the human host is able to utilize folic acid in the diet.

Most sulphonamides are administered orally and are rapidly absorbed into the blood. They are short-acting and may have to be taken several times a day. Their quick progress through the body and excretion in the urine makes them particularly suited for the treatment of urinary infections (since they work within the urine-conducting tubules). One or two sulphonamides are long-acting (and may be used to treat diseases such as malaria or leprosy) and another one or two are poorly absorbed (consequently, they were, until recently, used to treat intestinal infections since they are retained within the intestines where this is the site of the infection, not being absorbed into the body). The best-known and most-used sulphonamides include SULFADIAZINE and SULFAMETOPYRAZINE. Compared to more recent antibacterial drugs, sulphonamides tend to cause more side-effects, particularly nausea, vomiting, diarrhoea and headache, some of which (especially sensitivity reactions) may become serious. For instance, bone-marrow damage may result from prolonged treatment. Such serious hypersensitivity reactions are more of a risk with the longer-acting sulphonamides, which can accumulate in the body. As a general rule, patients being treated with sulphonamides should try to avoid sunlight. The sulphonamides are largely being replaced by newer antibacterials with greater activity, fewer problems with bacterial resistance and less risk of side-effects, and are reserved for certain serious infections (eg CO-TRIMOXAZOLE is the drug of choice for *Pneumocystis carinii* pneumonia). See also: SILVER SULFADIAZINE; SULFADOXINE; SULFAMETHOXAZOLE; SULPHONE.

sulphone 🅱

drugs are closely related to the SULPHONAMIDE group. They have similar therapeutic action, and are therefore used for similar purposes. They are particularly successful in preventing the growth of the bacteria responsible for leprosy, for dermatitis herpetiformis, and also as an ANTIMALARIAL for prophylaxis. The only member of this group that is still commonly used is the valuable drug DAPSONE.

sulphonylurea 🅱

drugs were derived from a SULPHONAMIDE and have the effect of reducing blood levels of glucose, so they can be used orally in DIABETIC TREATMENT. They work by promoting the secretion of INSULIN from the pancreas and are thus useful in treating the form of hyperglycaemia that occurs in Type II diabetes (non-insulin-dependent diabetes mellitus; NIDDM; maturity-onset diabetes) where there is still some insulin production. They should be used in conjunction with a modified diet. Several drugs increase the hypoglycaemic effect of sulphonylureas (eg ETHANOL, MAOI antidepressants, PHENYLBUTAZONE), and some that depress them (eg *loop class* DIURETIC agents and CORTICOSTEROID drugs). See CHLORPROPAMIDE; GLIBENCLAMIDE; GLICLAZIDE; GLIMEPIRIDE; GLIPIZIDE; GLIQUIDONE; TOLBUTAMIDE.

sulphur

is a non-metallic element which was thought to be active against external parasites and fungal infections of the skin, but this would now appear to have little scientific basis. Consequently, sulphur now has a less common use in creams, ointments and lotions for treating skin disorders, such as acne, dermatitis and psoriasis.

✚▲ Side-effects/warnings: May cause irritation. Avoid eyes, mucous membranes and mouth.

✪ **Related entries: Clearasil Treatment Cream Regular (Colourless); Cocois; Eskamel; TCP Antiseptic Ointment.**

sulpiride

is an ANTIPSYCHOTIC drug (of the *benzamides* chemical group) which is used for schizophrenia and, quite separately from its antipsychotic uses, disorders that may cause tremor, tics, involuntary movements or involuntary utterances (such as Gilles de la Tourette syndrome). Administration is oral.

✚▲ Side-effects/warnings: See CHLORPROMAZINE HYDROCHLORIDE; but is less sedating and does not cause jaundice or skin reactions. It is not used in people with porphyria or who are breast-feeding.

✪ **Related entries: Dolmatil; Sulpor; Sulpitil.**

Sulpitil

(Pharmacia) is a proprietary, prescription-only preparation of the ANTIPSYCHOTIC drug sulpiride. It can be used to treat the symptoms of schizophrenia, and quite separately from its

antipsychotic uses, to treat other conditions that may cause tremor, tics, involuntary movements or involuntary utterances (such as Gilles de la Tourette syndrome). It is available as tablets.
✚▲ Side-effects/warnings: See SULPIRIDE.

Sulpor

(Rosemont) is a proprietary, prescription-only preparation of the ANTIPSYCHOTIC drug sulpiride. It can be used to treat the symptoms of schizophrenia, and is available as an oral solution.
✚▲ Side-effects/warnings: See SULPIRIDE.

Sultrin

(Janssen-Cilag) is a proprietary, prescription-only compound preparation of the (SULPHONAMIDE) ANTIBACTERIAL drugs sulfacetamide, sulfabenzamide and sulfathiazole. It can be used to treat bacterial infections of the vagina and cervix, and to prevent infection following gynaecological surgery. It is available as a cream. (It should not be used by people who are sensitive to peanuts since it contains arachis oil.)
✚▲ Side-effects/warnings: See SULFACETAMIDE; SULFABENZAMIDE; SULFATHIAZOLE.

sumatriptan

is a (TRIPTAN) ANTIMIGRAINE drug, which is used to treat acute migraine attacks (but not to prevent attacks). It works as a VASOCONSTRICTOR (through acting as a serotonin receptor stimulant selective for SEROTONIN 5-HT_1 receptors), producing a rapid constriction of blood vessels surrounding the brain. It is also used (by injection) for cluster headache. Administration is oral as tablets, by self-injection, or as a nasal spay (it is absorbed into the circulation from the nasal mucosa).
✚ Side-effects: These include chest pain and tightness in parts of the body including the chest or throat, which may indicate constriction of the blood vessels of the heart (or of anaphylaxis), sometimes intense, and in these cases therapy should be discontinued. There may be sensations of tingling, heaviness, pressure, heat, flushing, dizziness, a feeling of weakness, drowsiness and fatigue, changes in liver function, reports of nausea and vomiting. Sumatriptan may cause drowsiness, transient increase in blood pressure, hypotension (low blood pressure), slowing or speeding of the heart; also seizures have been reported.
▲ Warnings: Drugs of this class (ie those stimulating SEROTONIN 5-HT_1 receptors) are used only with great caution in conditions predisposing to coronary artery disease (pre-existing heart diseases including ischaemic heart disease; previous myocardial infarction; coronary vasospasm including some types of angina, or in those with uncontrolled hypertension). They should not be used at the same time, or shortly after using ERGOTAMINE TARTRATE or other migraine therapies. Ergotamine-like antimigraine drugs should not be taken until six hours after this type of antimigraine drug; and this type of antimigraine drug should not be taken until at least 24 hours after an ergotamine-like antimigraine drug. They should be used with care in patients with impaired kidney function, or by those with sensitivity to sulphonamides. The dose should not be repeated within one migraine attack.

MAOI and SSRI ANTIDEPRESSANT drugs (and the herbal remedy St John's wort) and ERGOT ALKALOID drugs should be avoided by people taking sumatriptan-like ('triptan') drugs. There can be important interactions between conventional drugs, alternative remedies or supplements where either the therapeutic effect of the drugs taken can be changed or there may be adverse reactions, some of which can be serious. Any prescription, over-the-counter medicines, supplements, herbal remedies or other alternative therapies that you are using, have recently used or plan to use should be discussed with your doctor or pharmacist before you take any drugs of this type. Important interactions will be detailed in the Patient Information Leaflet.

Sumatriptan is used with care in people who are pregnant or breast-feeding. It may cause drowsiness and so impair the performance of skilled tasks, such as driving.
✪ Related entry: Imigran.

sunscreen

creams and lotions contain chemical agents that partly block the passage of ultraviolet radiation from the sun and certain radiation therapies to the skin. Ultraviolet radiation harms the skin and exacerbates many skin conditions. It can be divided into two wavelength bands: UVB causes sunburn and contributes to skin cancer and ageing; UVA causes problems by sensitizing the skin to certain drugs and, in the long term, may

S

contribute to skin cancers. A number of substances offer protection against UVB, but are less effective against UVA. Some preparations also contain substances, such as TITANIUM DIOXIDE, which are reflective and provide some protection against UVA. The sun-protection factor, or SPF, of a preparation indicates the degree of protection against burning by UVB. For example, an SPF of 4 allows a person to stay in the sun four-times longer than an unprotected person without burning. A star-rating system is used by some sunscreens to indicate the degree of protection against UVA relative to UVB. For example, a rating of 4 stars means equal protection against UVA and UVB; lower ratings mean greater protection against UVB than UVA. Sunscreens with an SPF greater than 15 may be prescribed for patients whose skin condition require this sort of preparation (eg those abnormally sensitive to UV radiation due to genetic disorders, or to radiotherapy, or those with recurrent or chronic herpes simplex labialis). Examples of preparations (see entries) are: AMBRE SOLAIRE; E45 SUN LOTION; PIZ BUIN SPF 30 SUN BLOCK LOTION; ROC TOTAL SUNBLOCK CREAM; SPECTRABAN LOTION; SPECTRABAN ULTRA.

Sunsense Ultra

(Lagap) is a proprietary, non-prescription SUNSCREEN lotion that protects the skin from UVA and UVB ultraviolet radiation (UVB-SPF 60). It containins the pigment titanium dioxide (along with oxybenzone and ethylkexyl-*p*-cinnammimate).

✚▲ Side-effects/warnings: TITANIUM DIOXIDE.

Supralip 160

(Fournier) is a proprietary, prescription-only preparation of the LIPID-REGULATING DRUG fenofibrate. It can be used in hyperlipidaemia to change the proportions of various lipids in the bloodstream. It is available as modified-release tablets.

✚▲ Side-effects/warnings: See FENOFIBRATE.

Suprax

(Rhône-Poulenc Rorer; Aventis Pharma) is a proprietary, prescription-only preparation of the ANTIBACTERIAL and (CEPHALOSPORIN) ANTIBIOTIC cefixime. It can be used to treat a range of acute bacterial infections, and is available as tablets and a paediatric oral suspension.

✚▲ Side-effects/warnings: See CEFIXIME.

Suprecur

(Shire) is a proprietary, prescription-only preparation of the HORMONE buserelin. It can be used in women to treat endometriosis and in infertility treatment. It is available as a nasal spray (it is absorbed into the systemic circulation from the nasal mucosa) and in a form for injection.

✚▲ Side-effects/warnings: See BUSERELIN.

Suprefact

(Shire) is a proprietary, prescription-only preparation of the HORMONE buserelin. It can be used in men as an ANTICANCER treatment for cancer of the prostate gland. It is available as a nasal spray and in a form for injection.

✚▲ Side-effects/warnings: See BUSERELIN.

surfactant 🅴

agents have a detergent action that lowers surface tension so allowing wetting. Sometimes they are incorporated into medicinal formulations simply to improve the physical properties of the preparations. But some are incorporated because, in themselves, they are necessary for the actions of the drug preparation, for instance in shampoos, enemas and skin preparations. Examples include SODIUM LAURYL SULPHATE and related salts (sodium lauryl sulphoacetate; sodium lauryl ether sulphate and sodium lauryl ether sulphosuccinate), POLOXAMER '188' and DOCUSATE SODIUM.

Surgam

(Florizel) is a proprietary, prescription-only preparation of the (NSAID) NON-NARCOTIC ANALGESIC and ANTIRHEUMATIC tiaprofenic acid. It can be used to treat the pain of rheumatic disease and other musculoskeletal disorders. It is available as tablets and modified-release capsules (*Surgam SA*).

✚▲ Side-effects/warnings: See TIAPROFENIC ACID.

Surmontil

(Futuna) is a proprietary, prescription-only preparation of the (TRICYCLIC) ANTIDEPRESSANT trimipramine. It can be used to treat depressive illness, especially in cases where there is a need for sedation. It is available as tablets and as capsules

(in the form of trimipramine maleate).
✚▲ Side-effects/warnings: See TRIMIPRAMINE.

Suscard

(Forest) is a proprietary, non-prescription preparation of the VASODILATOR and ANTI-ANGINA drug glyceryl trinitrate. It can be used in HEART FAILURE TREATMENT and to treat and prevent angina pectoris. It is available as modified-release buccal tablets (which dissolve between the upper lip and gums).
✚▲ Side-effects/warnings: See GLYCERYL TRINITRATE.

Sustac

(Forest) is a proprietary, non-prescription preparation of the VASODILATOR and ANTI-ANGINA drug glyceryl trinitrate. It can be used to prevent angina pectoris, and is available as modified-release tablets.
✚▲ Side-effects/warnings: See GLYCERYL TRINITRATE.

Sustenon 100

(Organon) is a proprietary, prescription-only preparation of the ANDROGEN (male sex hormone) testosterone (as propionate, isocaproate and phenylpropionate). It can be used to treat hormone deficiency in men, and is available in a form for long-lasting (oily depot) injection.
✚▲ Side-effects/warnings: See TESTOSTERONE.

Sustenon 250

(Organon) is a proprietary, prescription-only preparation of the ANDROGEN (male sex hormone) testosterone (as isocaproate and decanoate). It can be used to treat hormone deficiency in men, and is available in a form for long-lasting (oily depot) injection.
✚▲ Side-effects/warnings: See TESTOSTERONE.

Sustiva

(DuPont; Bristol-Myers Squibb) is a proprietary, prescription-only preparation of the ANTIVIRAL drug efavirenz. It can be used in the treatment of HIV infection, and is available as capsules.
✚▲ Side-effects/warnings: See EFAVIRENZ.

suxamethonium chloride

is a (*depolarizing*) SKELETAL MUSCLE RELAXANT which is used to induce muscle paralysis during surgery. Administration is by injection.
✚▲ Side-effects/warnings: It is a specialist drug used by anaesthetists in hospital. It is not to be administered to people with a family history of malignant hyperthermia or low blood cholinesterase levels. There may be muscle pain on recovery from anaesthesia.
✪ Related entry: Anectine.

Symbicort

(AstraZeneca) is a proprietary, prescription-only compound preparation of the CORTICOSTEROID budesonide and the SYMPATHOMIMETIC, BRONCHODILATOR and BETA-RECEPTOR STIMULANT formoterol fumarate. It can be used as a treatment for the symptomatic relief of obstructive airways disease, such as an ANTI-ASTHMATIC treatment. It is available as a dry powder for inhalation in several forms and strengths.
✚▲ Side-effects/warnings: See BUDESONIDE; FORMOTEROL FUMARATE.

Symmetrel

(Alliance) is a proprietary, prescription-only preparation of the ANTIPARKINSONISM drug amantadine hydrochloride, which also has some ANTIVIRAL activity. It is used to treat parkinsonism, but not the parkinsonian symptoms induced by drugs. It can also be used to prevent certain types of influenza and to treat herpes zoster (shingles). It is available as capsules and as a syrup.
✚▲ Side-effects/warnings: See AMANTADINE HYDROCHLORIDE.

sympathomimetic

drugs have effects that mimic those of the sympathetic nervous system. There are two main types (though several sympathomimetics belong to both types): the ALPHA-ADRENOCEPTOR STIMULANT drugs (eg PHENYLEPHRINE HYDROCHLORIDE and OXYMETAZOLINE HYDROCHLORIDE) are VASOCONSTRICTOR drugs and are used particularly in NASAL DECONGESTANT preparations and preparations for relieving cold symptoms; the other type is the BETA-RECEPTOR STIMULANT class (eg SALBUTAMOL, ORCIPRENALINE SULPHATE, TERBUTALINE SULPHATE) which are widely used as BRONCHODILATOR drugs, particularly in ANTI-ASTHMATIC treatment and also as CARDIAC

STIMULANT drugs (eg ISOPRENALINE). A distinction may be made between the *direct sympathomimetics* such as those examples given above, which achieve selectivity of action within the body by only acting at one receptor type (recognition site for hormones or neurotransmitters), as compared to the *indirect sympathomimetics* (eg EPHEDRINE HYDROCHLORIDE and PSEUDOEPHEDRINE HYDROCHLORIDE) that work by releasing NORADRENALINE and ADRENALINE from nerves of the sympathetic nervous system and adrenal medulla and consequently show no selectivity of action, which therapeutically is a disadvantage. See DOBUTAMINE HYDROCHLORIDE; DOPAMINE; FENOTEROL HYDROBROMIDE; METARAMINOL; METHOXAMINE HYDROCHLORIDE.
▲ Warnings: There can be serious reactions if sympthomimetics (such as over-the-counter nasal decongestants) are taken with other drugs such as MAOIS or some herbal remedies.

Synacthen
(Alliance) is a proprietary, prescription-only preparation of tetracosactide, which can be used to test adrenal gland function. It is available in a form for injection.
✚▲ Side-effects/warnings: See TETRACOSACTIDE.

Synacthen Depot
(Alliance) is a proprietary, prescription-only preparation of tetracosactide, which can be used to test adrenal gland function. It is available in a form for injection.
✚▲ Side-effects/warnings: See TETRACOSACTIDE.

Synagis
(Abbott) is a proprietary, prescription-only preparation of the ANTIVIRAL drug palivizumab, which can be used to treat viral infection caused by respiratory syncytial virus (RSV). Available in a form for injection.
✚▲ Side-effects/warnings: See PALIVIZUMAB.

Synalar
(Bioglan) is a proprietary, prescription-only preparation of the CORTICOSTEROID and ANTI-INFLAMMATORY fluocinolone acetonide. It can be used to treat severe, acute inflammatory skin disorders, such as eczema and psoriasis. It is available as a cream, gel or ointment in different strengths: *Synalar*, *Synalar 1 in 4 Dilution* and *Synalar 1 in 10 Dilution*.
✚▲ Side-effects/warnings: See FLUOCINOLONE ACETONIDE.

Synalar C
(Bioglan) is a proprietary, prescription-only compound preparation of the CORTICOSTEROID and ANTI-INFLAMMATORY fluocinolone acetonide and the ANTIMICROBIAL clioquinol. It can be used to treat skin infections with inflammation, and is available as an ointment and a cream for topical application.
✚▲ Side-effects/warnings: See CLIOQUINOL; FLUOCINOLONE ACETONIDE.

Synalar N
(Bioglan) is a proprietary, prescription-only compound preparation of the CORTICOSTEROID and ANTI-INFLAMMATORY fluocinolone acetonide and the ANTIBACTERIAL and (AMINOGLYCOSIDE) ANTIBIOTIC neomycin sulphate. It can be used to treat skin infections with inflammation, and is available as an ointment and a cream for topical application.
✚▲ Side-effects/warnings: See FLUOCINOLONE ACETONIDE; NEOMYCIN SULPHATE.

Synarel
(Pharmacia) is a proprietary, prescription-only preparation of nafarelin, which is an analogue of the hypothalamic hormone GONADORELIN (gonadothrophin-releasing hormone; GnRH). It can be used to treat endometriosis and also infertility, and is available as a nasal spray.
✚▲ Side-effects/warnings: See NAFARELIN.

Syndol
(SSL) is a proprietary, non-prescription compound preparation of the NON-NARCOTIC ANALGESIC paracetamol, the (OPIOID) NARCOTIC ANALGESIC codeine phosphate, the ANTIHISTAMINE doxylamine succinate and the STIMULANT caffeine. It can be used to treat mild to moderate pain, including tension headache, toothache, period pain, muscle pain, neuralgia and pain following surgery. It is available as tablets and is not normally given to children, except on medical advice.
✚▲ Side-effects/warnings: See CAFFEINE; CODEINE PHOSPHATE; DOXYLAMINE; PARACETAMOL.

Synercid
(Rhône-Poulenc Rorer; Aventis Pharma) is a

proprietary, prescription-only preparation, that is a compound preparation of two ANTIBIOTIC drugs with ANTIBACTERIAL properties, quinupristin with dalfopristin, which are only used together to treat infections that have failed to respond or are resistant to other antibiotics. Administration is by injection.
✚▲ Side-effects/warnings: See QUINUPRISTIN WITH DALFOPRISTIN.

Synflex
(Roche) is a proprietary, prescription-only preparation of the (NSAID) NON-NARCOTIC ANALGESIC and ANTIRHEUMATIC naproxen (as sodium). It can be used to relieve pain and inflammation, particularly rheumatic and arthritic pain and also of acute gout and other musculoskeletal disorders, period pain and acute gout. It is available as tablets.
✚▲ Side-effects/warnings: See NAPROXEN.

Synphase
(Searle; Pharmacia) is a proprietary, prescription-only compound preparation that can be used as a (*triphasic*) ORAL CONTRACEPTIVE of the *COC* (standard strength) type that combines an OESTROGEN and a PROGESTOGEN, in this case ethinylestradiol and norethisterone. It is available as tablets in a calendar pack.
✚▲ Side-effects/warnings: See ETHINYLESTRADIOL; NORETHISTERONE.

Syntaris
(Roche) is a proprietary, prescription-only preparation of the CORTICOSTEROID flunisolide. It can be used to prevent and treat nasal rhinitis and hay fever, and is available as a nasal spray. (A form is available for sale to the public, with restrictions including age.)
✚▲ Side-effects/warnings: See FLUNISOLIDE.

Syntocinon
(Alliance) is a proprietary, prescription-only preparation of the natural pituitary HORMONE oxytocin, which can be administered therapeutically to induce or assist labour. It is available in a form for intravenous injection or infusion.
✚▲ Side-effects/warnings: See OXYTOCIN.

Syntometrine
(Alliance) is a proprietary, prescription-only compound preparation of the ALKALOID ergometrine maleate and the natural HORMONE oxytocin. It can be used to assist the third and final stage of labour (delivery of the placenta) and to control postnatal bleeding following incomplete abortion. It is available in a form for injection.
✚▲ Side-effects/warnings: See ERGOMETRINE MALEATE; OXYTOCIN.

Syscor MR
(Forest) is a proprietary, prescription-only preparation of the CALCIUM-CHANNEL BLOCKER nisoldipine. It can be used as an ANTI-ANGINA treatment in the prevention of attacks and as an ANTIHYPERTENSIVE. It is available as modified-release tablets.
✚▲ Side-effects/warnings: See NISOLDIPINE.

Sytron
(Link) is a proprietary, non-prescription preparation of sodium feredetate. It can be used as an IRON supplement in iron-deficiency ANAEMIA TREATMENT, and is available in the form of an oral elixir.
✚▲ Side-effects/warnings: See SODIUM FEREDETATE.

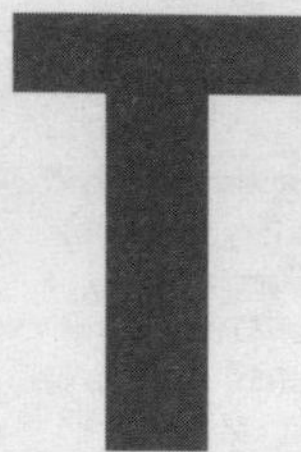

tacalcitol

is an analogue of vitamin D which is used as a skin treatment for plaque psoriasis. Administration is topical.

✚ Side-effects: There may be local irritation including itching, burning, erythema and tingling in the extremities.

▲ Warnings: It should not be used in patients with disorders of calcium metabolism. Administer with care to those who are pregnant. Avoid the scalp or contact with eyes and body areas not being treated.

✪ **Related entry: Curatoderm.**

tacrolimus

is an IMMUNOSUPPRESSANT drug, an ANTIBIOTIC related to the macrolide family. It is used particularly to limit tissue rejection during and following organ transplant surgery (particularly of liver or kidney). Administration is either oral or by intravenous infusion.

✚▲ Side-effects/warnings: See CYCLOSPORIN. Do not administer to patients who are sensitive to macrolide antibiotics, pregnant or breast-feeding. Potassium supplements should be avoided when taking tacrolimus or there is a risk of hyperkalemia (high blood potassium levels) developing. Grapefruit juice should also be avoided because it can increase the level of tacrolimus in the blood.

✪ **Related entry: Prograf.**

Tagamet

(SmithKline Beecham) is a proprietary, prescription-only preparation of the H_2-ANTAGONIST and ULCER-HEALING DRUG cimetidine. It can be used to treat benign peptic ulcers (in the stomach or duodenum), gastro-oesophageal reflux, dyspepsia and associated conditions. It is available as tablets, effervescent tablets, a syrup and in a form for intravenous injection.

✚▲ Side-effects/warnings: See CIMETIDINE.

Tagamet 100

(GSK Consumer Healthcare) is a proprietary preparation of the H_2-ANTAGONIST and ULCER-HEALING DRUG cimetidine. It is available without a prescription in a limited amount for short-term use for dyspepsia, heartburn, hyperacidity and associated conditions, and is available as tablets. It should not be given to children under 16 years, except on medical advice.

✚▲ Side-effects/warnings: See CIMETIDINE.

Tambocor

(3M) is a proprietary, prescription-only preparation of the specialist ANTI-ARRHYTHMIC flecainide acetate. It can be used to treat heartbeat irregularities, and is available as tablets and in a form for injection.

✚▲ Side-effects/warnings: See FLECAINIDE ACETATE.

Tamofen

(Pharmacia) is a proprietary, prescription-only preparation of the sex HORMONE ANTAGONIST tamoxifen. It inhibits the effect of OESTROGEN and because of this is used primarily as an ANTICANCER drug for cancers that depend on the presence of oestrogen in women, particularly breast cancer. It may also be used to treat certain conditions of infertility. It is available as tablets.

✚▲ Side-effects/warnings: See TAMOXIFEN.

tamoxifen

is a sex HORMONE ANTAGONIST, an ANTI-OESTROGEN, which antagonizes the natural oestrogen present in the body and can be useful in treating infertility in women whose condition is linked to the persistent presence of oestrogens and a consequent failure to ovulate. A second, and major, use is as an ANTICANCER drug in the treatment of existing oestrogen-dependent breast cancer (both in pre- and postmenopausal women). A related, but still experimental, use is as a prophylactic (preventive) treatment in women considered to be at risk of developing breast cancer. Administration is oral.

✚ Side-effects: Severe side-effects are not common. Hot flushes, vaginal bleeding or discharge, suppression of menstruation, itching vulva, vaginal discharge, gastrointestinal upsets, headache, light-headedness, oedema, hair loss, blood disturbances (fall in platelet count and porphyria), visual disturbances, blood and liver disturbances. Some patients with breast cancer may experience pain.

▲ Warnings: It should not be administered to patients who are pregnant or breast-feeding. There may be swelling within the ovaries. Changes in the endometrium including a small risk of endometrial cancer have been reported; for this reason abnormal vaginal bleeding or discharge, changes in menstruation, pelvic pain or pressure, should be reported to your doctor.

✪ Related entries: Emblon; Nolvadex; Tamofen.

Tampovagan

(Co-Pharma) is a proprietary, prescription-only preparation of a form of diethylstilbestrol, which is a sex hormone (see SEX HORMONES) analogue with OESTROGEN activity. It can be used in topical HRT (hormone replacement therapy) to treat conditions of the vagina caused by hormonal deficiency (generally atrophic vaginitis in the menopause). It is available as vaginal inserts (pessaries).

✚▲ Side-effects/warnings: See DIETHYLSTILBESTROL.

tamsulosin hydrochloride

is a selective ALPHA-ADRENOCEPTOR BLOCKER which can be used to treat urinary retention in benign prostatic hyperplasia. Administration is oral.

✚▲ Side-effects/warnings: See selective ALPHA-ADRENOCEPTOR BLOCKER. It is not used in people with severe liver impairment.

✪ Related entry: Flomax MR.

Tanatril

(Trinity) is a proprietary, prescription-only preparation of the ACE INHIBITOR imidapril hydrochloride. It can be used as an ANTIHYPERTENSIVE, and is available as tablets.

✚▲ Side-effects/warnings: See IMIDAPRIL HYDROCHLORIDE.

Targocid

(Hoechst Marion Roussel; Aventis Pharma) is a proprietary, prescription-only preparation of the ANTIBACTERIAL and ANTIBIOTIC teicoplanin. It can be used to treat serious infections, and is available in a form for injection or intravenous infusion.

✚▲ Side-effects/warnings: See TEICOPLANIN.

Tarivid

(Hoechst Marion Roussel; Aventis Pharma) is a proprietary, prescription-only preparation of the (QUINOLONE) ANTIBIOTIC-like ANTIBACTERIAL ofloxacin. It can be used to treat a wide range of infections. It is available as tablets and in a form for intravenous infusion.

✚▲ Side-effects/warnings: See OFLOXACIN.

Tarka

(Knoll) is a proprietary, prescription-only compound preparation of the ACE INHIBITOR trandolapril together with the CALCIUM-CHANNEL BLOCKER verapamil hydrochloride. It can be used as an ANTIHYPERTENSIVE and is available as capsules.

✚▲ Side-effects/warnings: See TRANDOLAPRIL; VERAPAMIL HYDROCHLORIDE.

Tavanic

(Hoechst Marion Roussel; Aventis Pharma) is a proprietary, prescription-only preparation of the (QUINOLONE) ANTIBIOTIC-like ANTIBACTERIAL levofloxacin. It can be used to treat a wide range of infections. It is available as tablets and in a form for intravenous infusion.

✚▲ Side-effects/warnings: See LEVOFLOXACIN.

Tavegil

(Novartis) is a proprietary, non-prescription preparation of the ANTIHISTAMINE clemastine (as hydrogen fumarate). It can be used to treat the symptoms of allergic disorders, such as hay fever and urticaria, and is available as tablets and a liquid.

✚▲ Side-effects/warnings: See CLEMASTINE.

Taxol

(Squibb; Bristol-Myers Squibb) is a proprietary, prescription-only preparation of the ANTICANCER drug paclitaxel. It can be used to treat ovarian and breast cancer, and non-small cell lung cancer. It is available in a form for intravenous infusion.

✚▲ Side-effects/warnings: See PACLITAXEL.

Taxotere

(Aventis Pharma) is a proprietary, prescription-only preparation of the ANTICANCER drug docetaxel. It can be used to treat breast cancer, and is available in a form for intravenous infusion.

✚▲ Side-effects/warnings: See DOCETAXEL.

tazarotene

is chemically a RETINOID (a derivative of RETINOL,

T

or vitamin A) and can be used to treat mild to moderate plaque psoriasis. Administration is by topical application.

✚ Side-effects: local irritation (may require discontinuation), burning, rash, redness and other skin conditions, rarely stinging and inflamed, dry or painful skin.

▲ Warnings: It should not be used in pregnancy or breast-feeding. Patients should wash hands immediately after use, and avoid contact with eyes, face, hair-covered scalp, eczematous or inflamed skin. Also avoid excessive exposure to UV light (including sunlight and solariums); do not apply cosmetics or other skin treatment within one hour of application.

✪ Related entry: Zorac.

tazobactam

is used as a PENICILLINASE INHIBITOR to combat bacterial resistance. It works as an ENZYME INHIBITOR by inhibiting the penicillinase enzymes ('beta-lactamases') that are produced by some bacteria. These enzymes can inactivate many antibiotics of the penicillin family, and it is used combined with the (PENICILLIN) ANTIBIOTIC piperacillin.

✚▲ Side-effects/warnings: It is only used combined with antibiotics.

✪ Related entry: Tazocin.

Tazocin

(Lederle; Wyeth) is a proprietary, prescription-only compound preparation of the broad-spectrum ANTIBACTERIAL and (PENICILLIN) ANTIBIOTIC piperacillin and the PENICILLINASE INHIBITOR tazobactam, which, by preventing degradation by bacterium-derived beta-lactamase enzyme, confers *penicillinase-resistance* to the antibiotic. It can be used to treat many serious or compound forms of bacterial infection, including skin infections, septicaemia and of the respiratory and urinary tracts, particularly infections caused by *Pseudomonas aeruginosa*. It is available in a form for intravenous injection or infusion.

✚▲ Side-effects/warnings: See PIPERACILLIN; TAZOBACTAM.

TCP Antiseptic Ointment

(Warner Lambert Consumer Healthcare; Pfizer) is a proprietary, non-prescription preparation of camphor, sulphur, methyl salicylate, salicylic acid and the ANTISEPTIC termed *TCP antiseptic* (based on halogenated phenols), iodine and tannic acid, and can be used to relieve piles, and for treating cuts, spots and pimples, grazes, minor burns and scalds, insect bites and stings. It is available as an ointment.

✚▲ Side-effects/warnings: See CAMPHOR, IODINE, METHYL SALICYLATE, SALICYLIC ACID; SULPHUR.

TCP First Aid Antiseptic Cream

(Warner Lambert Consumer Healthcare; Pfizer) is a proprietary, non-prescription preparation of the ANTISEPTIC agents triclosan, chloroxylenol and TCP liquid antiseptic. It can be used to cleanse spots, pimples, grazes, wounds and skin to prevent infection, and is available as a cream.

✚▲ Side-effects/warnings: See CHLOROXYLENOL; TRICLOSAN.

TCP Liquid Antiseptic

(Warner Lambert Consumer Healthcare; Pfizer) is a proprietary, non-prescription preparation of the ANTISEPTIC phenol (with halogenated phenols). It can be used for the symptomatic relief of sore throat, including those associated with colds and flu, and is available as a solution for use as a gargle. It can also be used for grazes, bites, boils and mouth ulcers when it is applied topically.

✚▲ Side-effects/warnings: See PHENOL.

TCP Sore Throat Lozenges

(Warner Lambert Consumer Healthcare; Pfizer) is a proprietary, non-prescription preparation of the ANTISEPTIC hexylresorcinol, and can be used to relieve minor sore throats. It is available as lozenges. It is not normally given to children under six years, except on medical advice.

✚▲ Side-effects/warnings: See HEXYLRESORCINOL.

Tears Naturale

(Alcon) is a proprietary, non-prescription preparation of HYPROMELLOSE (with dextran '70'). It can be used as artificial tears for tear deficiency, and is available as eye-drops.

✚▲ Side-effects/warnings: See HYPROMELLOSE.

tegafur with uracil

is a compound preparation of uracil with the (*antimetabolite*) CYTOTOXIC drug tegafur, which is

used as an ANTICANCER treatment primarily of solid tumours, particularly for metastatic colorectal cancer. It is a pro-drug (that is, it is converted in the body to) of FLUOROURACIL, which prevents the cancer cells from replicating and so prevents the growth of the cancer. It is always used combined with uracil which prevents fluorouracil breaking down once in the body, but has no direct action against the cancer. It is taken orally.
✚▲ Side-effects/warnings: See CYTOTOXIC; but serious toxicity is unusual.
✪ **Related entry: Uftoral.**

Tegretol
(Novartis) is a proprietary, prescription-only preparation of the ANTICONVULSANT and ANTI-EPILEPTIC drug carbamazepine. It can be used in the preventive treatment of most forms of epilepsy (except absence seizures), and for trigeminal neuralgia. It is available as tablets, chewable tablets, a liquid, suppositories and as modified-release tablets called *Tegretol Retard*.
✚▲ Side-effects/warnings: See CARBAMAZEPINE.

teicoplanin
is an ANTIBACTERIAL and ANTIBIOTIC drug of the glycopeptide family. It is similar to VANCOMYCIN, but with a longer duration of action so it can be taken only once a day. It has activity primarily against Gram-positive bacteria, inhibiting the synthesis of components of the bacterial cell wall. It can be used in the treatment of serious infections, including endocarditis, dialysis-associated peritonitis, in orthopaedic surgery, and for infections caused by *Staphylococcus aureus* (including MRSA). Administration is by intravenous injection or infusion.
✚ Side-effects: It is a specialist drug, and patients will be carefully evaluated for treatment. There may be diarrhoea, nausea and vomiting, headache; severe allergic reactions, bronchospasm, fever and rash; blood disorders; ringing in the ears and mild loss of hearing; local reactions at the injection site; loss of balance has been reported.
▲ Warnings: Tests on liver and kidney function are required, also blood counts and hearing tests. Administered with caution to patients who are elderly, pregnant or breast-feeding. Its use may have deleterious effects on the organs of the ear, on the kidney and liver; blood concentrations of the drug in the blood, along with liver and kidney function, should be monitored during treatment.
✪ **Related entry: Targocid.**

Telfast 120
(Hoechst Marion Roussel; Aventis Pharma) is a proprietary, prescription-only preparation of the ANTIHISTAMINE drug fexofenadine hydrochloride. It can be used to treat the symptoms of allergic disorders such as seasonal allergic rhinitis (hay fever).
✚▲ Side-effects/warnings: See FEXOFENADINE HYDROCHLORIDE.

Telfast 180
(Hoechst Marion Roussel; Aventis Pharma) is a proprietary, prescription-only preparation of the ANTIHISTAMINE fexofenadine. It can be used to treat allergic symptoms, such as chronic idiopathic urticaria (itching and rashes), and is available as tablets.
✚▲ Side-effects/warnings: See FEXOFENADINE HYDROCHLORIDE.

telmisartan
is an ANGIOTENSIN-RECEPTOR BLOCKER, which is a class of drugs that work by blocking angiotensin receptors. Angiotensin II is a circulating HORMONE that is a powerful VASOCONSTRICTOR and so blocking its effects leads to a fall in blood pressure. Therefore valsartan can be used as an ANTIHYPERTENSIVE. Administration is oral.
✚ Side-effects: Angiotensin-receptor antagonists in general cause orthostatic hypotension (particularly in those on diuretics), raised blood potassium and angioedema. Also, gastrointestinal upsets, inflamed pharynx, back pain, sometimes anaemia and raised blood changes.
▲ Warnings: Angiotensin-receptor antagonists in general should be avoided in breast-feeding. Administered with care to those who have biliary obstruction or kidney impairment.
✪ **Related entry: Micardis.**

temazepam
is a BENZODIAZEPINE which is used as a relatively short-acting HYPNOTIC for the short-term treatment of insomnia and as a preoperative medication. Administration is oral.
✚▲ Side-effects/warnings: See BENZODIAZEPINE.

Temgesic
(Schering-Plough) is a proprietary, prescription-only preparation of the (OPIOID) NARCOTIC

T

ANALGESIC buprenorphine (as hydrochloride), and is on the Controlled Drugs list. It can be used to treat pain including during operations, and is available as sublingual tablets (to be retained under the tongue) and in a form for injection.
✚▲ Side-effects/warnings: See BUPRENORPHINE.

Temodal
(Schering-Plough) is a proprietary, prescription-only preparation of the ANTICANCER drug temozolomide. It can be used in treatment of malignant glioma, and is available as capsules.
✚▲ Side-effects/warnings: See TEMOZOLOMIDE.

temozolomide
is a (CYTOTOXIC) ANTICANCER drug which can be used in second-line treatment of malignant glioma. Administration is oral.
✚▲ Side-effects/warnings: See CYTOTOXIC.
✪ **Related entry: Temodal.**

Tenben
(Galen) is a proprietary, prescription-only compound preparation of the BETA-BLOCKER atenolol and the DIURETIC bendroflumethiazide (bendrofluazide). It can be used as an ANTIHYPERTENSIVE, and is available as capsules.
✚▲ Side-effects/warnings: See ATENOLOL; BENDROFLUMETHIAZIDE.

Tenchlor
(Berk; APS) is a proprietary, prescription-only compound preparation of the BETA-BLOCKER atenolol and the DIURETIC chlortalidone (a combination called co-tenidone). It can be used as an ANTIHYPERTENSIVE for raised blood pressure, and is available as tablets.
✚▲ Side-effects/warnings: See ATENOLOL; CHLORTALIDONE.

tenecteplase
is a synthesized (recombinant DNA technology) enzyme (see ENZYMES), and is used therapeutically as a FIBRINOLYTIC, because it can break up blood clots. It is used in serious conditions such as myocardial infarction (heart attack). Administration is by injection.
✚▲ Side-effects/warnings: See FIBRINOLYTIC.
✪ **Related entry: Metalyse.**

Tenif
(AstraZeneca) is a proprietary, prescription-only compound preparation of the BETA-BLOCKER atenolol and the CALCIUM-CHANNEL BLOCKER nifedipine. It can be used as an ANTIHYPERTENSIVE for raised blood pressure and in ANTI-ANGINA treatment. Available as capsules.
✚▲ Side-effects/warnings: See ATENOLOL; NIFEDIPINE.

Tenkicin
(Kent) is a proprietary, prescription-only preparation of the ANTIBACTERIAL and (PENICILLIN) ANTIBIOTIC phenoxymethylpenicillin. It can be used to treat a range of infections, and is available as tablets and an oral solution (as the potassium salt).
✚▲ Side-effects/warnings: See PHENOXYMETHYLPENICILLIN.

Tenkorex
(Kent) is a proprietary, prescription-only preparation of the ANTIBACTERIAL and (CEPHALOSPORIN) ANTIBIOTIC cefalexin. It can be used to treat many forms of infection, including of the urogenital tract, and is available as capsules, tablets and an oral suspension.
✚▲ Side-effects/warnings: See CEFALEXIN.

Tenoret 50
(AstraZeneca) is a proprietary, prescription-only compound preparation of the BETA-BLOCKER atenolol and the DIURETIC chlortalidone. It can be used as an ANTIHYPERTENSIVE for raised blood pressure, and is available as tablets.
✚▲ Side-effects/warnings: See ATENOLOL; CHLORTALIDONE.

Tenoretic
(AstraZeneca) is a proprietary, prescription-only compound preparation of the BETA-BLOCKER atenolol and the DIURETIC chlortalidone. It can be used as an ANTIHYPERTENSIVE for raised blood pressure, and is available as tablets.
✚▲ Side-effects/warnings: See ATENOLOL; CHLORTALIDONE.

Tenormin
(AstraZeneca) is a proprietary, prescription-only preparation of the BETA-BLOCKER atenolol. It can be used as an ANTIHYPERTENSIVE for raised blood pressure, as an ANTI-ANGINA treatment to relieve symptoms and improve exercise tolerance and as an ANTI-ARRHYTHMIC to regularize heartbeat

and to treat myocardial infarction. It is available as tablets (of various strengths and forms), a syrup and in a form for injection.
✚▲ Side-effects/warnings: See ATENOLOL.

tenoxicam
is a (NSAID) NON-NARCOTIC ANALGESIC and ANTIRHEUMATIC drug. It has a long duration of action and is used to treat pain and inflammation in rheumatic disease and other musculoskeletal disorders. Administration can be either oral or by injection.
✚▲ Side-effects/warnings: See NSAID and NAPROXEN.
✪ **Related entry: Mobiflex.**

Tensipine MR
(Genus) is a proprietary, prescription-only preparation of the CALCIUM-CHANNEL BLOCKER nifedipine. It can be used as an ANTI-ANGINA treatment in the prevention of attacks, and as an ANTIHYPERTENSIVE. It is available as modified-release tablets.
✚▲ Side-effects/warnings: See NIFEDIPINE.

Tensium
(DDSA) is a proprietary, prescription-only preparation of the BENZODIAZEPINE diazepam. It can be used as an ANXIOLYTIC for the short-term treatment of anxiety, as a HYPNOTIC to relieve insomnia, as an ANTICONVULSANT and ANTI-EPILEPTIC for status epilepticus and febrile convulsions in children, as a SEDATIVE in preoperative medication, as a SKELETAL MUSCLE RELAXANT and to assist in the treatment of alcohol withdrawal symptoms. It is available as tablets.
✚▲ Side-effects/warnings: See DIAZEPAM.

Tensopril
(Norton) is a proprietary, prescription-only preparation of the ACE INHIBITOR captopril. It can be used as an ANTIHYPERTENSIVE and in HEART FAILURE TREATMENT, usually in conjunction with other classes of drug. It is available as tablets.
✚▲ Side-effects/warnings: See CAPTOPRIL.

Teoptic
(Novartis Ophthalmics) is a proprietary, prescription-only preparation of the BETA-BLOCKER carteolol hydrochloride. It can be used for GLAUCOMA TREATMENT, and is available as eye-drops.
✚▲ Side-effects/warnings: See CARTEOLOL HYDROCHLORIDE.

terazosin
is a selective ALPHA-ADRENOCEPTOR BLOCKER which is used as an ANTIHYPERTENSIVE and also in the treatment of urinary retention (eg in benign prostatic hyperplasia). Administration is oral.
✚▲ Side-effects/warnings: See selective ALPHA-ADRENOCEPTOR BLOCKER.
✪ **Related entries: Hytrin; Hytrin BPH.**

terbinafine
is an ANTIFUNGAL drug which is used to treat ringworm infections of the skin and fungal infections of the nails. Unlike most other antifungals it can be taken by mouth and so is available as tablets as well as a cream.
✚ Side-effects: When taken orally, there may be loss of appetite, abdominal discomfort, nausea and diarrhoea, headache, muscle and joint ache, rash, light sensitivity, taste disturbances and liver disorders. Used topically, there may be itching, redness, stinging, and allergic reactions (if so, treatment should be stopped).
▲ Warnings: It should be administered with care to patients with abnormal liver or kidney function, who are pregnant or breast-feeding. Avoid contact of the cream with the eyes.
✪ **Related entry: Lamisil.**

terbutaline sulphate
is a SYMPATHOMIMETIC and a BETA-RECEPTOR STIMULANT with good beta$_2$-receptor selectivity. It is mainly used as a BRONCHODILATOR in reversible obstructive airways disease, such as an ANTI-ASTHMATIC treatment. It can also be used in obstetrics to prevent or delay premature labour by relaxing the uterus. Administration is oral, by injection or inhalation.
✚▲ Side-effects/warnings: See SALBUTAMOL (and RITODRINE HYDROCHLORIDE for use in labour).
✪ **Related entries: Bricanyl; Monovent.**

terfenadine
is a recently developed ANTIHISTAMINE with fewer sedative side-effects than some older members of its class. It can be used for the symptomatic relief of allergic symptoms, such as hay fever and urticaria.

Its active metabolite is fexofenadine hydrochloride, which has largely replaced it because of concerns about safety. Only a generic preparation of terfenadine is available, and this is on a prescription-only basis. Administration is oral.
✚▲ Side-effects/warnings: See ANTIHISTAMINE. Although the incidence of sedative and anticholinergic effects is low, there may still be drowsiness which may impair the performance of skilled tasks, such as driving. There may be erythema multiforme or milk production. Certain serious disturbances of heart rhythm have been observed after excessive dose and when used in combination with certain other drugs.
▲ Warnings: Terfenadine is used with care in pregnancy and breast-feeding. It is not used in people with certain heart disorders (particularly arrhythmias) or liver impairment. Grapefruit and grapefruit juice should be avoided because they inhibit the metabolism of terfenadine, thereby causing toxic effects. Also grapefruit juice can increase the concentration of terfenadine in the blood. There are several drugs that should not be used by people taking terfenadine because of the risk of serious interactions.

Teril CR

(Taro) is a proprietary, prescription-only preparation of the ANTICONVULSANT and ANTI-EPILEPTIC carbamazepine. It can be used to treat most forms of epilepsy (except absence seizures), trigeminal neuralgia and in the management of manic-depressive illness. It is available as tablets.
✚▲ Side-effects/warnings: See CARBAMAZEPINE.

terlipressin

is a form of the pituitary HORMONE antidiuretic hormone (ADH) or vasopressin. It can be used as a VASOCONSTRICTOR to treat bleeding from varices (varicose veins) in the oesophagus. Administration is by injection.
✚▲ Side-effects/warnings: See VASOPRESSIN; but side-effects are usually milder.
✪ Related entry: Glypressin.

terpene 🄴

is the term used to describe chemically unsaturated hydrocarbons that are found in terpene plant oils and resins. Examples include CINEOLE, MENTHOL, pinene, turpineol and squalene. Examples that are chemically larger include the caratenoids and VITAMIN A. Mixtures of some terpenes are used to in the treatment of biliary disorders. Menthol, which is the most widely used of all the terpenes, is included in inhalant preparations intended to clear nasal or catarrhal congestion in conditions such as colds, rhinitis or sinusitis. It is also included in some COUNTER-IRRITANT, or RUBEFACIENT, preparations that are rubbed into the skin to relieve muscle or joint pain.
✚▲ Side-effects/warnings: There seem to be only a few adverse reactions with topical application, even though their action would appear to involve irritation of sensory nerve endings. Some that are administered orally interact with contraceptives or coagulants.

Terra-Cortril

(Pfizer) is a proprietary, prescription-only compound preparation of the ANTI-INFLAMMATORY and CORTICOSTEROID hydrocortisone and the ANTIBACTERIAL and (TETRACYCLINES) ANTIBIOTIC oxytetracycline (as hydrochloride). It can be used for local or topical application to treat skin disorders in which bacterial or other infection is also implicated. It is available as a topical ointment.
✚▲ Side-effects/warnings: See HYDROCORTISONE; OXYTETRACYCLINE.

Terra-Cortril Nystatin

(Pfizer) is a proprietary, prescription-only compound preparation of the ANTI-INFLAMMATORY and CORTICOSTEROID hydrocortisone, the ANTIFUNGAL and ANTIBIOTIC nystatin and the ANTIBACTERIAL and (TETRACYCLINES) antibiotic oxytetracycline (as hydrochloride). It can be used to treat skin disorders caused by fungal or bacterial infection, and is available as a cream.
✚▲ Side-effects/warnings: See HYDROCORTISONE; NYSTATIN; OXYTETRACYCLINE.

Terramycin

(Pfizer) is a proprietary, prescription-only preparation of the ANTIBACTERIAL and (TETRACYCLINES) ANTIBIOTIC oxytetracycline. It can be used to treat a wide range of infections, and is available as tablets.
✚▲ Side-effects/warnings: See OXYTETRACYCLINE.

Tertroxin

(Goldshield) is a proprietary, prescription-only

preparation of liothyronine sodium, which is a form of the thyroid hormone (see THYROID HORMONES) triiodothyronine. It can be used to make up hormonal deficiency (hypothyroidism) and therefore to treat the associated symptoms. It is available as tablets.
✚▲ Side-effects/warnings: See LIOTHYRONINE SODIUM.

Testosterone

(Organon) is a proprietary, prescription-only preparation of the ANDROGEN (male sex hormone) testosterone. It can be used to treat hormone deficiency in men, and sometimes in women (as part of HRT), and is available as an implant.
✚▲ Side-effects/warnings: See TESTOSTERONE.

testosterone

is an ANDROGEN and the principal male sex hormone (see SEX HORMONES). It is produced (in men) mainly in the testes with other androgens that promote the development and maintenance of the male sex organs and in the development of the secondary male sexual characteristics. It is also made in small amounts in women. Therapeutically, it can be administered in men to treat hormonal deficiency, for instance for delayed puberty, also in women for certain cancers (eg breast cancer) and sometimes as part of HRT. Administration can be oral, by injection, as implants or skin patches.
✚▲ Side-effects/warnings: See ANDROGEN. Sperm production may be suppressed. Patches may cause local irritation and allergic reactions; they should not be worn in the bath or when swimming.
✪ **Related entries: Andropatch; Restandol; Sustenon 100; Sustenon 250; Testosterone; Testosterone Enantate; Virormone.**

Testosterone Enantate

(Cambridge) is a proprietary, prescription-only preparation of the male sex hormone (see SEX HORMONES) testosterone enanthate, which is an ANDROGEN. It can be used to treat hormone deficiency in men and as an ANTICANCER treatment for hormone-related cancer in women. It is available in a form for long-acting (oily depot) injection.
✚▲ Side-effects/warnings: See TESTOSTERONE.

Tetabulin

(Hyland Immuno) (Tetanus Immunoglobulin) is a proprietary, prescription-only preparation of tetanus immunoglobulin, human (HTIG), which is a SPECIFIC IMMUNOGLOBULIN. It can be used in IMMUNIZATION to give immediate *passive immunity* against infection by the tetanus organism. Administration is by intramuscular injection.
✚▲ Side-effects/warnings: See IMMUNIZATION.

Tetanus Immunoglobulin

(BPL; SNBTS) (Antitetanus Immunoglobulin Injection) is a non-proprietary, prescription-only preparation of tetanus immunoglobulin, human (HTIG), which is a SPECIFIC IMMUNOGLOBULIN that can be used in immunization to give immediate *passive immunity* against infection by the tetanus organism. Administration is by intramuscular injection.
✚▲ Side-effects/warnings: See IMMUNIZATION.

tetanus immunoglobulin

(HTIG) is a SPECIFIC IMMUNOGLOBULIN of human origin, which is a form of immunoglobulin used for IMMUNIZATION to give immediate *passive immunity* against infection by tetanus. It is mostly used as an added precaution in treating patients with contaminated wounds, and can be used in dressing wounds. It can be considered just a precautionary measure because today almost everybody has established immunity through a VACCINE administered at an early age and vaccination is in any case readily available for those at risk. Administration is by intramuscular injection or sometimes intravenous infusion. In established cases it may be given together with the ANTIMICROBIAL drug METRONIDAZOLE.
✚▲ Side-effects/warnings: See IMMUNIZATION.
✪ **Related entries: Tetabulin; Tetanus Immunoglobulin; Tetanus Immunoglobulin for Intravenous Use.**

Tetanus Immunoglobulin for Intravenous Use

(BPL; SNBTS) is a non-proprietary, prescription-only preparation of TETANUS IMMUNOGLOBULIN, human (HTIG), which is a SPECIFIC IMMUNOGLOBULIN that can be used in IMMUNIZATION to give immediate passive immunity against infection by the tetanus organism for suspected or proven clinical tetanus. Administration is by intravenous injection. Available on a named-patient basis only.

✚▲ Side-effects/warnings: See IMMUNIZATION.

Tetanus Immunoglobulin Injection
see TETABULIN.

tetanus toxoid
see TETANUS VACCINE.

tetanus vaccine
(tetanus toxoid) is used in IMMUNIZATION to provide protection against infection by the tetanus organism. It is a *toxoid-type* VACCINE, which is a vaccine made from a toxin produced by a microbe, in this case tetanus bacteria, that is modified to make it non-infective and which then stimulates the body to form the appropriate antitoxin (antibody). In tetanus vaccine, the bacterial toxoid is adsorbed onto a mineral carrier and is usually given as one constituent of the *triple vaccine* ADSORBED DIPHTHERIA, TETANUS AND PERTUSSIS VACCINE (DTPer/Vac/Ads) or the *double vaccine* ADSORBED DIPHTHERIA AND TETANUS VACCINE (DT/Vac/Ads), which are administered during early life. However, tetanus vaccine can be administered by itself at any age for those who are at special risk from being infected. Administration is by injection, and a 'booster' injection is given after ten years.
✚▲ Side-effects/warnings: See VACCINE.
✪ **Related entries: ACT-HIB DTP dc; Adsorbed Diphtheria and Tetanus Vaccine; Adsorbed Diphtheria and Tetanus Vaccine for Adolescents and Adults; Adsorbed Diphtheria, Tetanus and Pertussis Vaccine; Adsorbed Diphtheria, Tetanus and [whole-cell] Pertussis Vaccine; Adsorbed Tetanus Vaccine; Diftavax; Infanrix; Infanrix-HIB.**

tetrabenazine
is a drug that is used to assist a patient to regain voluntary control of movement, or at least to lessen the extent of involuntary movements, in Huntingdon's chorea and related disorders. It is thought to work by reducing the amount of DOPAMINE in the nerves in the brain. Administration is oral.
✚ Side-effects: Drowsiness, gastrointestinal disturbance, depression, hypotension, extrapyramidal symptoms (muscle tremor and rigidity).
▲ Warnings: It is used with caution in people who are pregnant and its use is avoided in those who are breast-feeding. Because of its drowsiness effect, the performance of skilled tasks, such as driving, may be impaired.

tetracaine
(amethocaine) is a LOCAL ANAESTHETIC which is used particularly in ophthalmic treatments and anaesthesia prior to venepuncture or cannulation of veins. Administration is by topical application.
✚▲ Side-effects/warnings: See LIDOCAINE HYDROCHLORIDE. Also, hypersensitivity reactions have been reported. It is absorbed rapidly through mucous membranes and so should not be applied to inflamed, traumatized or highly vascular surfaces.
✪ **Related entries: Ametop; Minims Amethocaine Hydrochloride.**

tetracosactide
(tetracosactrin) is a synthetic HORMONE, an analogue of the pituitary hormone corticotropin (corticotrophin; ACTH), which acts on the adrenal glands to release corticosteroids, especially HYDROCORTISONE. It is used to test adrenal function. Administration is oral.
✚▲ Side-effects/warnings: See CORTICOSTEROID. There is a risk of anaphylaxis.
✪ **Related entries: Synacthen; Synacthen Depot.**

tetracosactrin
see TETRACOSACTIDE.

tetracycline
is a broad-spectrum ANTIBACTERIAL and ANTIBIOTIC of the TETRACYCLINES family, and gave its name to this family of similar antibiotics. It can be used to treat many forms of infection, for example, infections of the urinary and respiratory tract (eg chronic bronchitis), of the genital tract, ears, eyes, mouth ulcers and skin (acne). Administration is oral.
✚ Side-effects: There may be nausea and vomiting with diarrhoea; headache and visual disturbances. Occasionally, there is sensitivity to light or other sensitivity reactions, such as rashes (if so, discontinue treatment), pancreatitis and colitis, effects on the liver, photosensitivity.
▲ Warnings: It should not be administered to patients who are aged under 12 years, because of tooth colouration, or who are pregnant or breast-feeding, or who have systemic lupus erythematosus. Administered with caution to those

with impaired liver or kidney function.
✪ **Related entries: Achromycin; Deteclo; Economycin; Topicycline.**

tetracyclines

are a group of very broad-spectrum ANTIBACTERIAL and ANTIBIOTIC drugs. They have a very wide spectrum of activity. Apart from being effective against bacteria (they are *bacteriostatic*), they also inhibit the growth of chlamydia (a virus-like bacterium that causes genitourinary tract infections, eye infections and psittacosis *Chlamydia psittaci*), Rickettsia (a virus-like bacterium that causes, for example, Q fever); mycoplasma (a minute nonmotile organism that causes, for example, mycoplasmal pneumonia (*Mycoplasma pneumoniae*)); and spirochaetes (eg (*Borrelia burghdorferi*) that causes Lyme disease). They are valuable in brucellosis, cholera, plague and many other infections.

The tetracyclines act by inhibiting protein biosynthesis in sensitive micro-organisms and penetrate human macrophages and are therefore useful in combating micro-organisms, such as mycoplasma, that can survive and multiply within macrophages. Although they have been used to treat a very wide range of infections, the development of bacterial resistance has meant that their uses have become more specific (ie restricted to specific indications, in an effort to limit the spread of resistance). Treatment of atypical pneumonia due to chlamydia, rickettsia or mycoplasma is a notable indication for tetracyclines, while treatment of chlamydial urethritis and pelvic inflammatory disease is another. They are effective in treating exacerbations of chronic bronchitis and serious acne. Most tetracyclines are badly absorbed from a stomach that contains milk, ANTACID (calcium salts or magnesium salts) or IRON salts (eg in ANAEMIA TREATMENT); and most (except doxycycline and minicycline) may exacerbate kidney failure and so should be avoided when treating patients with kidney disease. They may be deposited in growing bone and teeth (causing staining and potential deformity), and should therefore not be administered to children under 12 years or to pregnant women. Side-effects are not generally very serious, but include gastrointestinal complaints.

The best-known and most-used tetracyclines include TETRACYCLINE (which they were all named after), DOXYCYCLINE and OXYTETRACYCLINE. The members of the tetracycline family have generic names ending *-cycline*. Administration is oral. See CHLORTETRACYCLINE; DEMECLOCYCLINE HYDROCHLORIDE; LYMECYCLINE; MINOCYCLINE.
▲ Warnings: Some inorganic compounds, such as magnesium, calcium, iron and zinc, which are taken orally for medical purposes (eg as ANTACID drugs) or as nutritional supplements (eg in multivitamin preparations) can reduce the effectiveness of certain tetracyclines if taken at the same time.

Tetralysal 300

(Galderma) is a proprietary, prescription-only preparation of the ANTIBACTERIAL and (TETRACYCLINES) ANTIBIOTIC lymecycline. It can be used to treat infections of many kinds, and is available as capsules.
✚▲ Side-effects/warnings: See LYMECYCLINE.

Tet/Vac/Ads

is an abbreviation for ADSORBED TETANUS VACCINE.

Teveten

(Solvay) is a proprietary, prescription-only preparation of the ANGIOTENSIN-RECEPTOR BLOCKER eprosartan (as mesilate). It can be used as an ANTIHYPERTENSIVE, and is available as tablets.
✚▲ Side-effects/warnings: See EPROSARTAN.

Theo-Dur

(AstraZeneca) is a proprietary, non-prescription preparation of the BRONCHODILATOR theophylline. It can be used as an ANTI-ASTHMATIC, and is available as modified-release tablets.
✚▲ Side-effects/warnings: See THEOPHYLLINE.

theophylline

is a BRONCHODILATOR drug which is mainly used as an ANTI-ASTHMATIC and for the treatment of chronic obstructive airways disease. Chemically, it is classed as a xanthine. Administration is oral as tablets and capsules (mainly modified-release forms capable of working for up to 12 hours), as a liquid and in a form for injection. It is also available in the form of chemical derivatives, eg AMINOPHYLLINE.

✚ Side-effects: There may be nausea and gastrointestinal disturbances, headache, an increase or irregularity in the heartbeat and/or insomnia; convulsions may occur when given intravenously.

▲ Warnings: Safety depends very much on the concentration in the blood, but this depends on many factors, including whether the person smokes or drinks, his or her age, health and concurrent drug therapy. For this reason a full assessment will be made, and treatment should initially be gradual and progressively increased until control of bronchospasm is achieved. It is administered with caution to patients who suffer from certain heart or liver disorders, who are pregnant or breast-feeding, and where there is a risk of low blood potassium (hypokalaemia), or who have hyperthyroidism, peptic ulcer or epilepsy. It should not be used in patients with porphyria. The herbal remedy St John's wort should be avoided because it can reduce the blood-level of theophylline.

✪ Related entries: Do-Do Chesteze; Nuelin; Nuelin SA; Slo-Phyllin; Theo-Dur; Uniphyllin Continus.

thiabendazole

see TIABENDAZOLE.

thiazide

drugs have a DIURETIC action: they inhibit sodium (and accompanying chloride) reabsorption at the beginning of the distal convoluted tubule of the kidney and may be used for prolonged periods. Their uses include as ANTIHYPERTENSIVE drugs (either alone or in conjunction with other types of diuretic or other drugs) and in the treatment of oedema associated with heart failure. There may be some depletion of potassium, but this can be treated with potassium supplements or the co-administering of *potassium-sparing* diuretics. Administration is oral. See BENDROFLUMETHIAZIDE; BENZTHIAZIDE; CHLORTALIDONE; CLOPAMIDE; CYCLOPENTHIAZIDE; HYDROCHLOROTHIAZIDE; HYDROFLUMETHIAZIDE; INDAPAMIDE; METOLAZONE; POLYTHIAZIDE; XIPAMIDE.

thioguanine

see TIOGUANINE.

thioridazine

is an ANTIPSYCHOTIC drug (a PHENOTHIAZINE) which is used to treat and tranquillize psychotic patients (such as schizophrenics), particularly those experiencing behavioural disturbances. The drug may also be used in the short-term treatment of anxiety and to calm agitated, elderly patients. Administration is oral.

✚▲ Side-effects/warnings: See CHLORPROMAZINE HYDROCHLORIDE; but has fewer sedative, hypothermia and extrapyramidal (muscle tremor and rigidity) symptoms; but is more likely to cause hypotension, effects on the heart, and there may be eye disorders and sexual dysfunction. Its use is avoided in patients with porphyria and those who suffer from any of a number of heart conditions. It is now restricted to second-line treatment of schizophrenia in adults under specialist supervision.

✪ Related entries: Melleril; Rideril.

thiotepa

is an (*alkylating agent*) CYTOTOXIC drug which is used as an ANTICANCER drug in the treatment of tumours in the bladder and sometimes for breast cancer. It works by interfering with the DNA of new-forming cells, so preventing cell replication. Administration is by injection or instillation into the bladder.

✚▲ Side-effects/warnings: See CYTOTOXIC.

thrombolytic

drugs break up or dissolve thrombi (blood clots). See FIBRINOLYTIC.

thymol

is obtained from the essential oil of the plant thyme. It can be used as a weak ANTISEPTIC, particularly to treat minor skin problems, and also in DECONGESTANT preparations for inhalation. It is sometimes used in combination with the essential oils of other plants.

✚▲ Side-effects/warnings: It is regarded as safe in normal topical use.

✪ Related entries: Compound Thymol Glycerin, BP; Karvol Decongestant Capsules.

thymoxamine

see MOXISYLYTE.

thyroid hormones

are secreted by the thyroid gland at the base of the neck. There are two major forms, both containing iodine. One form is THYROXINE (L-thyroxine; T_4 (80%), and the other is TRIIODOTHYRONINE (L-tri-iodothyronine; T_3 (20%)). They are transported in the bloodstream to control functions throughout the body. Both these hormones, in the form of their sodium salts (also known, in their therapeutic form as LEVOTHYROXINE SODIUM and LIOTHYRONINE SODIUM, respectively), are used therapeutically to make up a hormonal deficiency on a regular maintenance basis and to treat associated symptoms. They may also be used in the treatment of hypothyroidism (myxoedema), Hashimotos's thyroiditis, goitre and thyroid cancer. A third hormone, CALCITONIN, is secreted by a different cell type in the thyroid gland and has a different physiological role. It is concerned with lowering calcium levels in the blood (and a form of it, SALCATONIN (*calcitonin (salmon)*), is used therapeutically for this).

thyroid-stimulating hormone

see THYROTROPHIN.

thyrotrophin

(thyroid-stimulating hormone; TSH) is an anterior pituitary HORMONE. It controls the release of THYROID HORMONES from the thyroid gland and is itself controlled by the hypothalamic hormone TRH (thyrotrophin-releasing hormone) and by high levels of thyroid hormone in the blood. In the case of clinical defects at some stage in this system of control, diagnostic tests are necessarily a matter for specialist clinics. Nowadays, it is considered less helpful to make direct diagnosis using thyrotrophin itself in stimulation tests, because it is easier to chemically measure the concentration of thyrotrophin and thyroid hormones (T_3 and T_4) in the blood, so TSH is only occasionally used for diagnosis purposes.

thyrotrophin-releasing hormone

see PROTIRELIN.

thyroxine

is a natural blood-borne (endocrine) HORMONE released by the thyroid gland. The other major thyroid hormone is TRIIODOTHYRONINE. (In turn, the release of these hormones is regulated by the endocrine hormone THYROTROPHIN (thyroid-stimulating hormone; TSH), which is secreted by the pituitary gland.) Therapeutically, thyroxine is used in the form of LEVOTHYROXINE SODIUM (sodium L-throxine; T_4).

thyroxine sodium

see LEVOTHYROXINE SODIUM.

tiabendazole

(thiabendazole) is an (AZOLE) ANTHELMINTIC drug. It is used in the treatment of infestations by worm parasites, particularly those of the *Strongyloides* species that reside in the intestines but may migrate into the tissues. It is also used to treat other worm infestations resistant to common drugs. The usual course of treatment is intensive. Administration is oral.

✚ Side-effects: There may be nausea, vomiting, diarrhoea and anorexia; dizziness and drowsiness; and headache and itching. Possible hypersensitivity reactions include fever with chills, rashes and other skin disorders and occasionally tinnitus or liver damage, visual disorders.

▲ Warnings: It should be administered with caution to patients with impaired kidney or liver function. Treatment should be withdrawn if hypersensitivity reactions occur. It is not to be administered to pregnant or breast-feeding women. It may impair the performance of skilled tasks, such as driving.

✪ **Related entry: Triasox.**

tiagabine

is an ANTICONVULSANT and ANTI-EPILEPTIC drug. It can be used to assist in the control of partial seizures. Administration is oral.

✚ Side-effects: Diarrhoea, tiredness, nervousness, dizziness and tremor, difficulties in concentrating, emotional changes, speech impairment; rarely, confusion, depression, drowsiness, psychosis; blood changes reported.

▲ Warnings: Care in liver impairment; may impair performance of skilled tasks (eg driving).

✪ **Related entry: Gabitril.**

tiaprofenic acid

is a (NSAID) NON-NARCOTIC ANALGESIC and ANTIRHEUMATIC drug, which is used to treat pain and inflammation in rheumatic disease and other musculoskeletal disorders. Administration is oral.

✚▲ Side-effects/warnings: See NSAID. It may cause cystitis and bladder irritation and so should

not be used where there is a history of urinary tract disorders and treatment must be stopped if adverse effects occur (such as increased frequency of urination, pain or blood in the urine).
✪ **Related entry: Surgam.**

tibolone
is a drug that has both OESTROGEN and PROGESTOGEN activity. It can be used to treat menopausal problems in HRT (hormone replacement therapy). Administration is oral.
✚▲ Side-effects/warnings: See OESTROGEN; PROGESTOGEN.
✪ **Related entry: Livial.**

ticarcillin
is an ANTIBACTERIAL and (PENICILLIN) ANTIBIOTIC drug. It has improved activity against a number of important Gram-negative bacteria, including *Pseudomonas aeruginosa*. It can be used to treat serious infections, such as septicaemia and peritonitis, and also infections of the respiratory and urinary tracts. One of its proprietary forms also contains CLAVULANIC ACID. Administration is by intravenous injection or infusion.
✚▲ Side-effects/warnings: See BENZYLPENICILLIN.
✪ **Related entry: Timentin.**

Ticlid
(Sanofi-Synthelabo) is a proprietary, prescription-only preparation of the ANTIPLATELET drug ticlopidine hydrochloride. It can be used to prevent thrombosis, and is available as tablets.
✚▲ Side-effects/warnings: See TICLOPIDINE.

ticlopidine
is an ANTIPLATELET (antithrombotic) drug which is used to prevent thrombosis (blood-clot formation), but does not have an ANTICOAGULANT action. It works by stopping platelets sticking to one another or to the walls of blood vessels. It is used to reduce complications in patients with history of atherosclerotic disease (ischaemic stroke, myocardial infarction or peripheral arterial disease, ischaemic stroke, and with people with intermittent claudication). Administration is oral.
✚ Side-effects: Bleeding and a variety of blood disorders (some serious); nausea, diarrhoea (discontinue if severe / persistent); elevated liver enzymes. Rarely, hepatitis, jaundice; increased blood cholesterol; various hypersensitivity reactions including skin rashes and itching.
▲ Warnings: It should not be used when there is any recent bleeding or risk of bleeding (including acute haemorrhagic stroke and active gastroduodenal ulcer; history of bleeding associated with blood disorders, or in breast-feeding. It is avoided for some days after heart attacks or ischaemic stroke. It should be used with caution in pregnancy, liver or kidney liver impairment. It should be discontinued if there are certain changes in blood counts or before surgery or pregnancy. Patients and their carers should know how to recognize signs of blood disorders or jaundice, and be advised to seek immediate medical attention if symptoms such as fever, sore throat, mouth ulcers, bruising or bleeding develop.
✪ **Related entry: Ticlid.**

Tiger Balm White (Regular Strength)
(SSL) is a proprietary, non-prescription compound preparation of camphor and menthol, which have COUNTER-IRRITANT, or RUBEFACIENT, actions, along with clove oil and cajuput. It can be applied to the skin to relieve temporarily minor muscular aches and pains. It is available as an ointment for topical application to the skin, and is not normally given to children under two years, except on medical advice.
✚▲ Side-effects/warnings: See CAMPHOR; MENTHOL.

Tilade
(Pantheon) is a proprietary, prescription-only preparation of the ANTI-ASTHMATIC drug nedocromil sodium. It can be used to prevent recurrent attacks of asthma, and is available in a form for inhalation.
✚▲ Side-effects/warnings: See NEDOCROMIL SODIUM.

Tildiem
(Sanofi-Synthelabo) is a proprietary, prescription-only preparation of the CALCIUM-CHANNEL BLOCKER diltiazem hydrochloride. It can be used as an ANTIHYPERTENSIVE and as an ANTI-ANGINA drug. It is available as modified-release tablets.
✚▲ Side-effects/warnings: See DILTIAZEM HYDROCHLORIDE.

Tildiem LA

(Sanofi-Synthelabo) is a proprietary, prescription-only preparation of the CALCIUM-CHANNEL BLOCKER diltiazem hydrochloride. It can be used as an ANTIHYPERTENSIVE and as an ANTI-ANGINA drug. It is available as modified-release capsules.

✚▲ Side-effects/warnings: See DILTIAZEM HYDROCHLORIDE.

Tildiem Retard

(Sanofi-Synthelabo) is a proprietary, prescription-only preparation of the CALCIUM-CHANNEL BLOCKER diltiazem hydrochloride. It can be used as an ANTIHYPERTENSIVE and as an ANTI-ANGINA drug. It is available as modified-release tablets.

✚▲ Side-effects/warnings: See DILTIAZEM HYDROCHLORIDE. The tablet membrane is porous so the drug comes out, but the tablet may pass through the whole gastrointestinal system intact.

Tiloryth

(Tillomed) is a proprietary, prescription-only preparation of the ANTIBACTERIAL and (MACROLIDE) ANTIBIOTIC erythromycin. It can be used to treat and prevent many forms of infection, and is available as capsules.

✚▲ Side-effects/warnings: See ERYTHROMYCIN.

tiludronate disodium

see TILUDRONIC ACID.

tiludronic acid

is a CALCIUM METABOLISM MODIFIER, a BISPHOSPHONATE used (as tiludronate disodium) to treat Paget's disease of the bone. Administration is oral.

✚ Side-effects: Stomach pain and nausea, diarrhoea; rarely, dizziness, headache and skin reactions.

▲ Warnings: It is administered with caution to patients with certain kidney disorders. It is not for use in pregnancy or breast-feeding.

✪ **Related entry: Skelid**

Timentin

(SmithKline Beecham; GSK) is a proprietary, prescription-only compound preparation of the ANTIBACTERIAL and (PENICILLIN) ANTIBIOTIC ticarcillin and the PENICILLINASE INHIBITOR clavulanic acid, which inhibits enzymes produced by some bacteria and thereby imparting *penicillinase-resistance* on ticarcillin. This combination can be used to treat serious infections that occur in patients whose immune systems are undermined by disease or drugs, and where the responsible micro-organism is resistant to ticarcillin alone. (Patients with such conditions are generally in hospital.) It is available in a form for intravenous injection or infusion.

✚▲ Side-effects/warnings: See CLAVULANIC ACID; TICARCILLIN.

Timodine

(R&C; Reckitt Benckiser) is a proprietary, prescription-only compound preparation of the CORTICOSTEROID hydrocortisone, the ANTIFUNGAL and ANTIBIOTIC nystatin and the ANTISEPTIC benzalkonium chloride together with the ANTIFOAMING AGENT dimethicone. It can be used to treat fungal infections and mild skin inflammation, and is available as a cream for topical application.

✚▲ Side-effects/warnings: See BENZALKONIUM CHLORIDE; DIMETICONE; HYDROCORTISONE; NYSTATIN.

timolol maleate

is a BETA-BLOCKER which can be used as an ANTIHYPERTENSIVE for raised blood pressure, as an ANTI-ANGINA treatment to relieve symptoms and improve exercise tolerance, and for prophylaxis after myocardial infarction. It can also be used as an ANTIMIGRAINE treatment to prevent attacks. Administration is oral. It is also available, as an antihypertensive, in the form of a compound preparation with a DIURETIC. Additionally, it can be used as a GLAUCOMA TREATMENT and is administered topically as eye-drops.

✚▲ Side-effects/warnings: See PROPRANOLOL HYDROCHLORIDE. There may be some systemic absorption after using eye-drops, so some of the side-effects listed under PROPRANOLOL HYDROCHLORIDE may be seen. Dry eyes, stinging, redness, pain and some local allergic reactions, including conjunctivitis may also occur. It is not used in uncontrolled heart failure, bradycardia or other heart problems.

✪ **Related entries: Betim; Cosopt; Glau-opt; Moducren; Prestim; Timoptol; Xalacom.**

Timonil Retard

(CP) is a proprietary, prescription-only

T

preparation of the ANTICONVULSANT and ANTI-EPILEPTIC carbamazepine. It can be used to treat most forms of epilepsy (except absence seizures), trigeminal neuralgia and in the management of manic-depressive illness. It is available as tablets.
✚▲ Side-effects/warnings: See CARBAMAZEPINE.

Timoptol

(MSD) is a proprietary, prescription-only preparation of the BETA-BLOCKER timolol maleate. It can be used for GLAUCOMA TREATMENT, and is available as eye-drops (in *Ocumeter* units). Another eye-drop preparation, *Timoptol- LA*, is also available.
✚▲ Side-effects/warnings: See TIMOLOL MALEATE.

Timpron

(Berk; APS) is a proprietary, prescription-only preparation of the (NSAID) NON-NARCOTIC ANALGESIC and ANTIRHEUMATIC naproxen. It can be used to relieve pain of musculoskeletal disorders, particularly rheumatic and arthritic pain, period pain and acute gout. It is available as tablets and modified-release tablets (*Timpron EC*).
✚▲ Side-effects/warnings: See NAPROXEN.

Tinaderm Cream

(Schering-Plough Consumer Health) is a proprietary, non-prescription preparation of the ANTIFUNGAL drug tolnaftate. It can be used to treat athlete's foot, and is available as a cream.
✚▲ Side-effects/warnings: See TOLNAFTATE.

Tinaderm-M

(Schering-Plough Consumer Health) is a proprietary, prescription-only compound preparation of the ANTIFUNGAL and ANTIBIOTIC nystatin and the antifungal tolnaftate. It can be used to treat *Candida* fungal infections of the skin and nails. Available as a cream.
✚▲ Side-effects/warnings: See NYSTATIN; TOLNAFTATE.

Tinaderm Plus Powder

(Schering-Plough Consumer Health) is a proprietary, non-prescription preparation of the ANTIFUNGAL drug tolnaftate. It can be used to treat athlete's foot, and is available as a powder.
✚▲ Side-effects/warnings: See TOLNAFTATE.

tinidazole

is an (AZOLE) AMOEBICIDAL drug with ANTIBACTERIAL and ANTIPROTOZOAL properties. It can be used to treat anaerobic infections, such as bacterial vaginitis, and protozoal infections, such as giardiasis, trichomoniasis and amoebiasis. It can also be used to treat acute ulcerative gingivitis, to prevent infection following abdominal surgery, and for *Helicobacter pylori* eradication. Administration is oral.
✚▲ Side-effects/warnings: See METRONIDAZOLE.
✪ **Related entry: Fasigyn.**

tinzaparin sodium

is a low molecular weight version of heparin. It has some advantages as an ANTICOAGULANT when used for long-term prevention of venous thrombo-embolism, particularly in orthopaedic use. Administration is by injection.
✚▲ Side-effects/warnings: See HEPARIN.
✪ **Related entry: Innohep.**

tioconazole

is an (AZOLE) ANTIFUNGAL drug which is used to treat fungal infections of the nails. It is available as a lotion and a cream, which are applied to the nails and surrounding area.
✚ Side-effects: There may be local irritation, most commonly during the first week (discontinue if it persists).
✪ **Related entry: Trosyl.**

tioguanine

(thioguanine) is an (*antimetabolite*) CYTOTOXIC drug and is used as an ANTICANCER treatment of acute leukaemias. Administration is oral.
✚▲ Side-effects/warnings: See CYTOTOXIC.
✪ **Related entry: Lanvis.**

tirofiban

is an ANTIPLATELET (antithrombotic) drug which is used to prevent thrombosis (blood-clot formation). It works by stopping platelets sticking to one another or to the walls of blood vessels. It can be used (together with heparin and aspirin) to prevent thrombosis in myocardial infarction, as part of ANTI-ANGINA treatment. Administration is by intravenous infusion.
✚▲ Side-effects/warnings: Used only under hospital specialist supervision.
✪ **Related entry: Aggrastat.**

Tisept

(SSL) is a proprietary, non-prescription

compound preparation of the ANTISEPTIC chlorhexidine (as gluconate) and cetrimide. It can be used as a general skin disinfectant and as an antiseptic for cleaning wounds. It is available as a solution.

✚▲ Side-effects/warnings: See CETRIMIDE; CHLORHEXIDINE.

titanium dioxide

is a white pigment incorporated into several SUNSCREEN preparations. It provides some degree of protection from ultraviolet UVA and UVB radiation.

✚▲ Side-effects/warnings: It is regarded as safe in normal topical use.

✪ Related entries: Ambre Solaire; Delph; E45 Sun Lotion; Metanium; Piz Buin SPF 30 Sun Block Lotion; RoC Total Sunblock Cream; Sunsense Ultra; Spectraban Ultra.

Titralac

(3M) is a proprietary, non-prescription preparation of calcium carbonate. It can be used as a phosphate-binding agent (for hyper-phosphataemia, eg in renal failure). Available as tablets.

✚▲ Side-effects/warnings: See CALCIUM CARBONATE.

Tixycolds Cold and Allergy Nasal Drops

(Novartis Consumer Health) is a proprietary, non-prescription preparation of the SYMPATHOMIMETIC and VASOCONSTRICTOR xylometazoline hydrochloride. It can be used as a NASAL DECONGESTANT for the symptomatic relief of nasal congestion, perennial and allergic rhinitis (such as hay fever) and sinusitis. It is available as nasal drops and is not given to children under three months, except on medical advice.

✚▲ Side-effects/warnings: See XYLOMETAZOLINE HYDROCHLORIDE.

Tixycolds Cold and Hayfever Inhalant Capsules

(Novartis Consumer Health) is a proprietary, non-prescription preparation of turpentine oil, camphor, eucalyptus oil and menthol. It can be used for the relief of nasal congestion associated with head colds, catarrh, flu and hay fever. It is available as capsules and the oil is sprinked on, for example, bedlinen at night, and is not given to children under three months, except on medical advice.

✚▲ Side-effects/warnings: See CAMPHOR; MENTHOL; TURPENTINE OIL.

Tixycolds Syrup

(Novartis Consumer Health) is a proprietary, non-prescription preparation of the SYMPATHOMIMETIC and DECONGESTANT pseudoephedrine hydrochloride and the ANTIHISTAMINE diphenhydramine hydrochloride. It can be used for relieving the symptoms of colds and flu, for the symptomatic relief of nasal congestion and blocked sinuses and aid restful sleep. It is available as a linctus and is not given to children under one year, except on medical advice.

✚▲ Side-effects/warnings: See PSEUDOEPHEDRINE HYDROCHLORIDE; DIPHENHYDRAMINE HYDROCHLORIDE.

Tixylix Baby Syrup

(Novartis Consumer Health) is a proprietary, non-prescription preparation of glycerol which can be used to relieve dry, tickly coughs. It is available as a syrup and is not normally given to infants under three months, except on medical advice.

✚▲ Side-effects/warnings: See GLYCEROL.

Tixylix Chesty Cough

(Novartis Consumer Health) is a proprietary, non-prescription preparation of the EXPECTORANT agent guaifenesin (guaiphenesin). It can be used to relieve chesty coughs, sore throats and hoarseness. It is available as a linctus. It is not normally given to children under one year, except on medical advice.

✚▲ Side-effects/warnings: See GUAIFENESIN.

Tixylix Cough and Cold

(Novartis Consumer Health) is a proprietary, non-prescription compound preparation of the (OPIOID) ANTITUSSIVE pholcodine, the ANTIHISTAMINE chlorphenamine maleate (chlorpheniramine maleate) and the SYMPATHOMIMETIC and DECONGESTANT pseudoephedrine hydrochloride. It can be used to relieve dry, tickly coughs, runny nose and congestion. It is available as a linctus and is not normally given to children under one year, except on medical advice.

✚▲ Side-effects/warnings: See CHLORPHENAMINE MALEATE; PHOLCODINE; PSEUDOEPHEDRINE HYDROCHLORIDE.

T

Tixylix Daytime
(Novartis Consumer Health) is a proprietary, non-prescription preparation of the (OPIOID) ANTITUSSIVE pholcodine. It can be used for the symptomatic relief of tickly coughs. It is available as a linctus and is not normally given to children under one year, except on medical advice.
✚▲ Side-effects/warnings: See PHOLCODINE.

Tixylix Night-Time SF
(Novartis Consumer Health) is a proprietary, non-prescription compound preparation of the (OPIOID) ANTITUSSIVE pholcodine and the ANTIHISTAMINE promethazine hydrochloride. It can be used for the symptomatic relief of tickly coughs, especially for irritating coughs at night. It is available as a linctus and is specifically formulated for children aged between one year and ten years (it is not recommended for children under one year or over ten years, or for adults).
✚▲ Side-effects/warnings: See PHOLCODINE; PROMETHAZINE HYDROCHLORIDE.

Tixymol
(Novartis Consumer Health) is a proprietary, non-prescription preparation of the NON-NARCOTIC ANALGESIC and ANTIPYRETIC paracetamol. It can be used to treat mild to moderate pain. such as teething pain, and to reduce fever in children. However, it is not normally given to children under three months, except on medical advice (it can be used for post vaccination fever in infants under three months). It is available as a liquid suspension.
✚▲ Side-effects/warnings: See PARACETAMOL.

tizanidine
is a SKELETAL MUSCLE RELAXANT which can be used for relieving severe muscle spasticity associated with multiple sclerosis or spinal cord injury or disease. Administration is oral.
✚ Side-effects: Drowsiness and fatigue, dizziness, nausea and gastrointestinal disturbances, dry mouth, hypotension; also, insomnia, hallucinations, bradycardia, and effects on the liver.
▲ Warnings: It is administered with caution to the elderly or those with kidney impairment, in pregnancy and breast-feeding: liver function should be monitored at first and in those who develop unexplained nausea, anorexia or fatigue, or those with impaired heart and liver function. Drowsiness may impair the performance of skilled tasks, such as driving. Alcohol's effects are enhanced.
✪ **Related entry: Zanaflex.**

Tobi
(PathoGenesis) is a proprietary, prescription-only preparation of the ANTIBACTERIAL and (AMINOGLYCOSIDE) ANTIBIOTIC tobramycin. It can be used to treat serious bacterial infections, particularly *Pseudomonas aeruginosa* infection in cystic fibrosis patients (over six years), and is available in a form for inhalation.
✚▲ Side-effects/warnings: See TOBRAMYCIN.

Tobradex
(Alcon) is a proprietary, prescription-only compound preparation of the ANTI-INFLAMMATORY and CORTICOSTEROID dexamethasone, the ANTIBACTERIAL and (AMINOGLYCOSIDE) ANTIBIOTIC tobramycin. It can be used to treat inflammation of the eye when infection is also present, and is available as eye-drops.
✚▲ Side-effects/warnings: See DEXAMETHASONE; TOBRAMYCIN.

tobramycin
is an ANTIBACTERIAL and ANTIBIOTIC drug of the AMINOGLYCOSIDE group. It is effective against some Gram-positive and Gram-negative bacteria and is used primarily for the treatment of serious Gram-negative infections caused by *Pseudomonas aeruginosa*, because it is significantly more active against this organism than gentamicin (the most commonly used of this class of antibiotic). Like other aminoglycosides, it is not absorbed from the intestine (except in the case of local infection or liver failure) and so is administered by injection or intravenous infusion (eg for urinary tract infections). It is also available as eye-drops to treat bacterial infections of the eye.
✚▲ Side-effects/warnings: See GENTAMICIN.
✪ **Related entries: Nebcin; Tobi; Tobradex.**

tocopherol
see ALPHA TOCOPHERYL ACETATE; VITAMIN E.

tocopheryl acetate
see ALPHA TOCOPHERYL ACETATE; VITAMIN E.

Tofranil
(Novartis) is a proprietary, prescription-only preparation of the (TRICYCLIC) ANTIDEPRESSANT

imipramine hydrochloride. It can be used to treat depressive illness, particularly in patients who are withdrawn and apathetic, and may also be used to treat bed-wetting at night by children. It is available as tablets and a syrup.
✚▲ Side-effects/warnings: See IMIPRAMINE HYDROCHLORIDE.

tolbutamide
is a SULPHONYLUREA which is used in DIABETIC TREATMENT for Type II diabetes (non-insulin-dependent diabetes mellitus; NIDDM; maturity-onset diabetes). Administration is oral.
✚▲ Side-effects/warnings: See GLIBENCLAMIDE; however, it may be chosen for patients with renal impairment and in the elderly because it is shorter-acting.

tolfenamic acid
is a (NSAID) NON-NARCOTIC ANALGESIC. It can be used to relieve pain in acute migraine attacks. Administration is oral.
✚▲ Side-effects/warnings: See NSAID.
✪ **Related entry: Clotam.**

tolnaftate
is a mild ANTIFUNGAL drug which is used primarily in the topical treatment of infections caused by the tinea species (eg athlete's foot). Administration is by topical application
✚▲ Side-effects/warnings: Rarely, sensitivity reactions.
✪ **Related entries: Mycil Athlete's Foot Spray; Mycil Ointment; Mycil Powder; Scholl Athlete's Foot Cream; Scholl Athlete's Foot Powder; Scholl Athlete's Foot Spray Liquid; Tinaderm Cream; Tinaderm Plus Powder; Tinaderm-M.**

tolterodine tartrate
is an ANTICHOLINERGIC (ANTIMUSCARINIC) drug which can be used as an ANTISPASMODIC to treat urinary frequency, incontinence and urgency. Administration is oral.
✚ Side-effects: These include dry mouth, blurred vision, constipation, nausea, dyspepsia and abdominal pain, flatulence, vomiting, headache, drowsiness, nervousness, tingling in the extremities, dry eyes, dry skin; less commonly blurred vision, chest pain, confusion, difficulty in urination.
▲ Warnings: It should not be administered to patients with angle-closure glaucoma; urinary retention; myasthenia gravis; certain gastrointestinal disorders. Administered with care to those with bladder or gastrointestinal obstruction; hiatus hernia; neuropathy; liver or kidney impairment.
✪ **Related entries: Detrusitol; Detrusitol XL.**

Tomudex
(AstraZeneca) is a proprietary, prescription-only preparation of the ANTICANCER drug raltitrexed which can be used as a treatment for cancer of the colon, and is available in a form for injection.
✚▲ Side-effects/warnings: See RALTITREXED.

Topal
(Ceuta) is a proprietary, non-prescription compound preparation of the ANTACID agents aluminium hydroxide; magnesium carbonate; sodium bicarbonate and the DEMULCENT alginic acid (with lactose and sucrose). It can be used for the symptomatic relief of heartburn, reflux oesophagitis and hiatus hernia, and is available as tablets.
✚▲ Side-effects/warnings: See ALGINIC ACID; ALUMINIUM HYDROXIDE; MAGNESIUM CARBONATE; SODIUM BICARBONATE.

Topamax
(Janssen-Cilag) is a proprietary, prescription-only preparation of the ANTI-EPILEPTIC drug topiramate. It is available as tablets and sprinkle capsules (swallowed whole or sprinkled over food).
✚▲ Side-effects/warnings: See TOPIRAMATE.

Topicycline
(Shire) is a proprietary, prescription-only preparation of the ANTIBACTERIAL and (TETRACYCLINES) ANTIBIOTIC tetracycline (as hydrochloride). It can be used to treat acne, and is available as a solution for topical application.
✚▲ Side-effects/warnings: See TETRACYCLINE.

topiramate
is an ANTI-EPILEPTIC drug. Administration is oral.
✚ Side-effects: Abdominal pains, nausea, anorexia and weight loss; confusion; impaired speech, memory and concentration, depression, emotional, behaviour, and mood changes; unsteady and abnormal gait, tingling in the extremities, dizziness, drowsiness and fatigue, muscle weakness, various visual disturbances;

taste changes, also psychotic symptoms, aggression, cognitive problems, blood changes.
▲ Warnings: It should not be administered to patients who are breast-feeding. Used with care in those who are pregnant or have liver or kidney impairment. Withdrawal of treatment should be gradual. Plenty of liquid should be drunk.
✪ **Related entry: Topamax.**

topotecan
is a CYTOTOXIC drug, one of a new group of drugs termed the *topoisomerase I inhibitors*, used as an ANTICANCER drug in the treatment of ovarian cancer. Administration is by intravenous infusion.
✚▲ Side-effects/warnings: See CYTOTOXIC.
✪ **Related entry: Hycamtin**

Toradol
(Roche) is a proprietary, prescription-only preparation of the (NSAID) NON-NARCOTIC ANALGESIC ketorolac trometamol. It can be used in the short-term management of moderate to severe acute postoperative pain, and is available as tablets and in a form for injection.
✚▲ Side-effects/warnings: See KETOROLAC TROMETAMOL.

torasemide
is a powerful (*loop*) DIURETIC which can be used to treat oedema and as an ANTIHYPERTENSIVE. Administration is oral.
✚▲ Side-effects/warnings: See FRUSEMIDE. It should be avoided in people who are pregnant or breast-feeding.
✪ **Related entry: Torem.**

Torem
(Roche) is a proprietary, prescription-only preparation of the (*loop*) DIURETIC torasemide. It can be used to treat oedema and as an ANTIHYPERTENSIVE. It is available as tablets.
✚▲ Side-effects/warnings: See TORASEMIDE.

toremifene
is a sex HORMONE ANTAGONIST, an ANTI-OESTROGEN. It antagonizes the natural oestrogen present in the body and is used in treating hormone-dependent metastatic breast cancer in postmenopausal women. Administration is oral.
✚▲ Side-effects/warnings: See TAMOXIFEN. It is not to be administered to patients with severe liver impairment, endometrial hyperplasia or a history of thromboembolic disease. Any abnormal vaginal bleeding or discharge, pelvic pain or pressure, or menstrual disturbances should be reported to the doctor.
✪ **Related entry: Fareston.**

Totaretic
(CP) is a proprietary, prescription-only compound preparation of the BETA-BLOCKER atenolol and the DIURETIC chlortalidone (a combination called co-tenidone). It can be used as an ANTIHYPERTENSIVE for raised blood pressure, and is available as tablets.
✚▲ Side-effects/warnings: See ATENOLOL; CHLORTALIDONE.

Tracrium
(GlaxoWellcome; GSK) is a proprietary, prescription-only preparation of the (*non-depolarizing*) SKELETAL MUSCLE RELAXANT atracurium besilate. It can be used to induce muscle paralysis during surgery, and is available in a form for injection.
✚▲ Side-effects/warnings: See ATRACURIUM BESILATE.

Tractocile
(Ferring) is a recently introduced proprietary, prescription-only preparation of the OXYTOCIN-RECEPTOR ANTAGONIST drug atosiban (as acetate). It is used to prevent premature labour, and is available in a form for intravenous infusion.
✚▲ Side-effects/warnings: See ATOSIBAN.

tramadol hydrochloride
is a NARCOTIC ANALGESIC which is similar to morphine in relieving pain, but probably with fewer side-effects. However, there seem to be some differences in the mechanisms by which it produces analgesia (additional effects on serotonin- and noradrenaline-utilizing nerve pathways within the CNS) so it does not represent a typical OPIOID. It has less constipating action, addictive liability or respiratory depression compared to typical opioids. Administration can be either oral or by injection.
✚▲ Side-effects/warnings: See OPIOID. Effects on blood pressure, psychiatric reactions (hallucinations and confusion) and anaphylactic reactions have been reported. Administered with

care to epileptics. It should not be given to those who are pregnant or breast-feeding.
✪ **Related entries: Dromadol SR; Dromadol XL; Tramake; Zamadol; Zydol; Zydol SR; Zydol XL.**

Tramake

(Galen) is a proprietary, prescription-only preparation of the (OPIOID) NARCOTIC ANALGESIC tramadol hydrochloride. It can be used to relieve pain, but seems to differ from typical opioids in its mode of action, and is available as capsules and effervescent powder (called *Tramake Insts*).
✚▲ Side-effects/warnings: See TRAMADOL HYDROCHLORIDE.

tramazoline hydrochloride

is an ALPHA-ADRENOCEPTOR STIMULANT, a SYMPATHOMIMETIC and VASOCONSTRICTOR drug which can be used as a NASAL DECONGESTANT to treat allergic rhinitis. Administration is topical as an aerosol.
✚▲ Side-effects/warnings: See EPHEDRINE HYDROCHLORIDE.
✪ **Related entry: Dexa-Rhinaspray Duo.**

Trandate

(Celltech) is a proprietary, prescription-only preparation of the mixed BETA-BLOCKER and ALPHA-ADRENOCEPTOR BLOCKER labetalol hydrochloride. It can be used as an ANTIHYPERTENSIVE to reduce blood pressure, including in pregnancy, after myocardial infarction, in angina and during surgery. It is available as tablets and in a form for injection.
✚▲ Side-effects/warnings: See LABETALOL HYDROCHLORIDE.

trandolapril

is an ACE INHIBITOR and acts as a VASODILATOR. It can be used as an ANTIHYPERTENSIVE and often in conjunction with other classes of drug, particularly (THIAZIDE) DIURETIC drugs; also after myocardial infarction and ventricular malfunction. Administration is oral.
✚ Side-effects: See ACE INHIBITOR. Also speeding of the heart and irregular rhythms and other effects on the cardiovascular system, intestinal obstruction, dry mouth, skin reactions, muscle weakness, hair loss, breathing difficulties.
▲ Warnings: See ACE INHIBITOR.
✪ **Related entries: Gopten; Odrik; Tarka.**

tranexamic acid

is an antifibrinolytic drug which is used to stem bleeding in circumstances such as dental extraction, prostatectomy, and in a haemophiliac patient or menorrhagia (excessive menstrual bleeding). It may also be used in hereditary angioedema and in thrombolytic drug overdose. It works by inhibiting activation of plasminogen, an enzyme in the blood that dissolves blood clots. Administration can be either oral or by injection.
✚ Side-effects: There may be nausea and vomiting with diarrhoea; an injection may cause temporary giddiness.
▲ Warnings: It is administered with caution to those with impaired kidney function or who are pregnant. Prolonged treatment requires regular eye checks and liver function tests. It is not used in people with thromboembolic disease.
✪ **Related entry: Cyklokapron.**

tranquillizer 🅱

is a term sometimes used to describe any of a group of drugs that calm, soothe and relieve anxiety, and many also cause some degree of sedation. Although it is somewhat misleading, tranquillizers are often classified in two groups *major tranquillizers* and *minor tranquillizers*. The major tranquillizers, which are also called NEUROLEPTIC or ANTIPSYCHOTIC drugs, are used primarily to treat severe mental disorders, such as psychoses (including schizophrenia and mania). They are extremely effective in restoring a patient to a calmer, less-disturbed state of mind. The hallucinations, both auditory and visual, the gross disturbance of logical thinking and to some extent the delusions typical of psychotic states are generally well controlled by these drugs. Violent, aggressive behaviour that presents a danger to the patients themselves, and to those that look after them, is also effectively treated by major tranquillizers. For this reason they are often used in the *management* of difficult, aggressive, antisocial individuals. But the tranquillizing effect is of secondary importance in the treatment of, for example, schizophrenics; and in some patients it is a debilitating side-effect. Major tranquillizers that are commonly administered include the PHENOTHIAZINE derivatives (eg CHLORPROMAZINE HYDROCHLORIDE, PROCHLORPERAZINE and THIORIDAZINE) and such drugs as FLUPENTIXOL and HALOPERIDOL. Minor tranquillizers are also *calming drugs*, but

T

they are ineffective in the treatment of psychotic states. Their principal applications are as ANXIOLYTIC, HYPNOTIC and SEDATIVE drugs. The best-known and most-used minor tranquillizers are undoubtedly the BENZODIAZEPINE drugs (eg DIAZEPAM). However, prolonged treatment with minor tranquillizers can lead to dependence (addiction).

Transiderm-Nitro

(Novartis) is a proprietary, non-prescription preparation of the VASODILATOR drug glyceryl trinitrate, which can be used as an ANTI-ANGINA drug and to prevent phlebitis and extravasation. It is available as a self-adhesive dressing (patch), which, when placed on the chest, allows the drug to be absorbed through the skin (transdermally) to give lasting relief.

✚▲ Side-effects/warnings: See GLYCERYL TRINITRATE.

Transvasin Heat Rub

(SSL) is a proprietary, non-prescription compound preparation of the COUNTER-IRRITANT, or RUBEFACIENT, tetrahydrofurfuryl salicylate, and the VASODILATOR ethyl nicotinate and hexyl nicotinate. It can be used for the symptomatic relief of muscular aches and pains, and is available as a cream for topical application to the skin.

✚▲ Side-effects/warnings: See ETHYL NICOTINATE.

Transvasin Heat Spray

(SSL) is a proprietary, non-prescription preparation of diethylamine salicylate (and hydroxyethyl salicylate) which have COUNTER-IRRITANT, or RUBEFACIENT, actions, and the VASODILATOR methyl nicotinate. It can be applied to the skin for the symptomatic relief of musculoskeletal rheumatic conditions, and is available as a spray. It is not normally given to children under five, except on medical advice.

✚▲ Side-effects/warnings: See DIETHYLAMINE SALICYLATE; METHYL NICOTINATE.

Tranxene

(Boehringer Ingelheim) is a proprietary, prescription-only preparation of the ANXIOLYTIC clorazepate dipotassium. It can be used principally for the short-term treatment of anxiety, and is available as capsules.

✚▲ Side-effects/warnings: See CLORAZEPATE DIPOTASSIUM.

tranylcypromine

is an ANTIDEPRESSANT of the MONOAMINE-OXIDASE INHIBITOR (MAOI) class. It has, however, some STIMULANT effect and so is not as frequently used as some other antidepressants. Administration is oral.

✚▲ Side-effects/warnings: See PHENELZINE; but do not use in patients with overactive thyroid secretion. It can cause hypertensive crisis with a throbbing headache (treatment may need to be discontinued).

✪ Related entry: Parnate.

Trasicor

(Novartis) is a proprietary, prescription-only preparation of the BETA-BLOCKER oxprenolol hydrochloride. It can be used as an ANTIHYPERTENSIVE for raised blood pressure, as an ANTI-ANGINA treatment to relieve symptoms and improve exercise tolerance and as an ANTI-ARRHYTHMIC to regularize heartbeat. It can also be used as an ANXIOLYTIC, particularly for symptomatic relief of tremor and palpitations. It is available as tablets.

✚▲ Side-effects/warnings: See OXPRENOLOL HYDROCHLORIDE.

Trasidrex

(Novartis) is a proprietary, prescription-only compound preparation of the BETA-BLOCKER oxprenolol hydrochloride and the (THIAZIDE) DIURETIC cyclopenthiazide (called *co-prenozide 160/0.25*. It can be used as an ANTIHYPERTENSIVE for raised blood pressure, and is available as tablets.

✚▲ Side-effects/warnings: See CYCLOPENTHIAZIDE; OXPRENOLOL HYDROCHLORIDE.

trastuzumab

is one of a relatively new class of drug, a monoclonal antibody (a form of pure antibody produced by a type of molecular engineering). In this case the cloned antibody is one that causes lysis (destruction) of B lymphocytes, so effectively it can be regarded as a specific CYTOTOXIC agent with defined IMMUNOSUPPRESSANT actions. It has been recently introduced as an ANTICANCER drug for the treatment of metastatic breast cancer in patients whose tumours overexpress the human epidermal growth factor receptor 2 (HER2). Authorities have indicated that trastuzumab treatment should be reserved for patients who have previously received appropriate chemotherapy or for whom chemotherapy is not appropriate.

✚ Side-effects: This is a specialist drug and possible side-effects will be explained prior to its use and there will be constant monitoring. There may be reactions because the drug is infused, including chills, fever, hypersensitivity reactions, such as anaphylaxis, urticaria and angioedema, effects on the airways and heart; gastrointestinal symptoms, asthenia, headache, chest pains, arthralgia, myalgia, lowered blood pressure.

▲ Warnings: Trastuzumab should not be used if breast-feeding or where there is severe shortness of breath at rest. It is used with caution in people with certain cardiovascular conditions such as heart failure, hypertension, or coronary artery disease; or who are pregnant.

✪ **Related entry: Herceptin.**

Trasylol

(Bayer) is a proprietary, prescription-only preparation of aprotinin, which is a HAEMOSTATIC drug used to prevent life-threatening clot-formation, for instance, in open-heart surgery, removal of tumours and in surgical procedures in patients with certain blood disorders (hyperplasminaemias). It is available in a form for injection.

✚▲ Side-effects/warnings: See APROTININ.

Travasept 100

(Baxter) is a proprietary, non-prescription compound preparation of the ANTISEPTIC cetrimide and chlorhexidine (as acetate). It can be used for cleaning wounds and obstetrics, and is available as a solution.

✚▲ Side-effects/warnings: See CETRIMIDE; CHLORHEXIDINE.

Travatan

(Alcon) is proprietary prescription-only preparation of the PROSTAGLANDIN analogue travoprost. It can be used as a GLAUCOMA TREATMENT in open-angle glaucoma and ocular hypertension, and is available as eye-drops.

✚▲ Side-effects/warnings: See TRAVOPROST.

travoprost

is a PROSTAGLANDIN, a synthetic prostaglandin $F_{2\alpha}$ analogue, which has been recently introduced as a novel GLAUCOMA TREATMENT to reduce intraocular pressure in open-angle glaucoma and ocular hypertension in patients for whom other drugs are not suitable. Administration is topical in the form of eye-drops.

✚ Side-effects: See under LATANOPROST; also, headache, itching of the eyes, inflammation of the cornea of the eyes, discomfort in bright light. Rarely, its use may result in slowing of the heart and low blood pressure, aching brow, conjunctivitis and swollen eyelids.

▲ Warnings: See under LATANOPROST.

✪ **Related entry: Travatan.**

Traxam

(Goldshield) is a proprietary, prescription-only preparation of felbinac (an active metabolite of fenbufen), which has (NSAID) NON-NARCOTIC ANALGESIC and COUNTER-IRRITANT, or RUBEFACIENT, actions. It can be used for the symptomatic relief of underlying muscle or joint pain, and is available as a foam or gel for topical application to the skin.

✚▲ Side-effects/warnings: See FELBINAC; but adverse effects on topical application are limited.

Traxam Pain Relief Gel

(Whitehall) is a proprietary, non-prescription preparation of felbinac (an active metabolite of fenbufen), which has (NSAID) NON-NARCOTIC ANALGESIC and COUNTER-IRRITANT, or RUBEFACIENT, actions. It can be used for the symptomatic relief of underlying muscle or joint pain, and is available as a gel for topical application to the skin. It is not normally given to children, except on medical advice.

✚▲ Side-effects/warnings: See FELBINAC; but adverse effects on topical application are limited.

trazodone hydrochloride

is an ANTIDEPRESSANT drug that, though chemically is TRICYCLIC-related, has additional actions that make it 'atypical' in its spectrum of action and has fewer ANTICHOLINERGIC effects than most tricyclics. It is used to treat depressive illness, particularly in cases where some degree of sedation (see SEDATIVE) is required. Administration is oral.

✚▲ Side-effects/warnings: see AMITRIPTYLINE HYDROCHLORIDE; but fewer anticholinergic (antimuscarinic) and cardiovascular effects. In rare

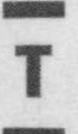

cases there may be priapism (prolonged erection), when it should be discontinued immediately.
✪ Related entry: Molipaxin.

Trental
(Borg) is a proprietary, prescription-only preparation of the VASODILATOR pentoxifylline (oxpentifylline). It can be used to help improve blood circulation to the hands and feet when this is impaired, for example, in peripheral vascular disease (Raynaud's phenomenon). It is available as modified-release tablets.
✚▲ Side-effects/warnings: See PENTOXIFYLLINE.

treosulfan
is an (*alkylating agent*) CYTOTOXIC drug which is used as an ANTICANCER treatment specifically of ovarian cancer. It works by interfering with the DNA of new-forming cells and so preventing cell replication. Administration can be either oral or by injection.
✚▲ Side-effects/warnings: See CYTOTOXIC. There may be skin pigmentation.

tretinoin
is chemically a RETINOID (a derivative of RETINOL, or vitamin A) and can be used to treat acne, also to treat photodamaged skin. Recently, it has been introduced for the induction of remission in acute promyelocytic leukaemia. Administration is oral or by topical application.
✚ Side-effects: When used topically, there may be irritation or skin peeling, redness, changes in skin pigmentation and sensitivity to light. It is used orally under specialist hospital conditions: there are extensive side-effects.
▲ Warnings: Tretinoin should not be applied to broken skin. It should be kept away from the eyes, mouth and mucous membranes. It is not to be used in combination with other keratolytics, or with sun-ray lamps. Do not use if pregnant, or where there is eczema or sunburned skin. Given orally, it is a specialist hospital treatment. Vitamin A, for example, as a nutritional supplement, should be avoided by people taking tretinoin since there is an increased risk of hypervitaminosis A. There can be important interactions between conventional drugs, alternative remedies or supplements where either the therapeutic effect of the drugs taken can be changed or there may be adverse reactions, some of which can be serious. Any prescription, over-the-counter medicines, supplements, herbal remedies or other alternative therapies that you are using, have recently used or plan to use should be discussed with your doctor or pharmacist before you take drugs of this type. Important interactions will be detailed in the Patient Information Leaflet.
✪ Related entries: Acticin; Aknemycin Plus; Retin-A; Vesanoid.

TRH
see PROTIRELIN.

Tri-Adcortyl
(Squibb; Bristol-Myers Squibb) is a proprietary, prescription-only compound preparation of the ANTI-INFLAMMATORY and CORTICOSTEROID triamcinolone (in the form of acetonide), the ANTIBACTERIAL and ANTIBIOTIC drugs gramicidin and neomycin sulphate and the ANTIFUNGAL and antibiotic nystatin. It can be used for the treatment of severe infective skin inflammation, such as eczema and psoriasis, especially in cases that have not responded to less-powerful therapies. It is available as a cream and an ointment for topical application.
✚▲ Side-effects/warnings: See GRAMICIDIN; NEOMYCIN SULPHATE; NYSTATIN; TRIAMCINOLONE.

Tri-Adcortyl Otic
(Squibb; Bristol-Myers Squibb) is a proprietary, prescription-only compound preparation of the ANTI-INFLAMMATORY and CORTICOSTEROID triamcinolone (in the form of acetonide), the ANTIBACTERIAL and ANTIBIOTIC drugs gramicidin and neomycin sulphate and the ANTIFUNGAL and antibiotic nystatin. It can be used for the treatment of severe eczematous infective inflammation of the outer ear, and is available as an ear ointment.
✚▲ Side-effects/warnings: See GRAMICIDIN; NEOMYCIN SULPHATE; NYSTATIN; TRIAMCINOLONE.

Triadene
(Schering Health) is a proprietary, prescription-only compound preparation which can be used as a (*triphasic*) ORAL CONTRACEPTIVE of the *COC* (standard strength) type that combines an OESTROGEN and a PROGESTOGEN, in this case ethinylestradiol and gestodene. It is available as

tablets in a calendar pack.
✚▲ Side-effects/warnings: See ETHINYLESTRADIOL; GESTODENE.

TriamaxCo

(Ashbourne) is a proprietary, prescription-only compound preparation of the (*potassium-sparing*) DIURETIC triamterene and the (THIAZIDE) diuretic hydrochlorothiazide (a combination also called co-triamterzide 50/25). It can be used in the treatment of oedema and as an ANTIHYPERTENSIVE. It is available as tablets.
✚▲ Side-effects/warnings: See HYDROCHLOROTHIAZIDE; TRIAMTERENE. Urine may appear blue.

triamcinolone

is a synthetic CORTICOSTEROID with ANTI-INFLAMMATORY and ANTI-ALLERGIC properties. It is used to suppress the symptoms of inflammation, especially when it is caused by allergic disorders. It is sometimes used to prevent and treat conditions such as allergic rhinitis and severe inflammatory skin disorders such as eczema (where weaker corticosteroids are ineffective) and psoriasis, but it is usually given by direct injection to treat inflammatory conditions of the joints to release pain and increase mobility and reduce deformity. It can be given orally, also there are several proprietary topical preparations available that are mainly used to treat severe, non-infective skin inflammation, such as eczema, or inflammation in the mouth. (It is used in the form of triamcinolone; triamcinolone acetonide and triamcinolone hexacetonide.)
✚▲ Side-effects/warnings: See CORTICOSTEROID. These depend on route of administration and dose, but serious systemic effects are unlikely with topical application, though there may be local sensitivity reactions.
✪ Related entries: Adcortyl in Orabase; Adcortyl Intra-articular/ Intradermal; Audicort; Aureocort; Kenalog; Kenalog Intra-articular/ Intramuscular; Nasacort; Tri-Adcortyl; Tri-Adcortyl Otic.

Triam-Co

(IVAX) is a proprietary, prescription-only compound preparation of the (THIAZIDE) DIURETIC hydrochlorothiazide and the (*potassium-sparing*) diuretic triamterene (a combination called co-triamterzide 50/25). It can be used in the treatment of oedema and as an ANTIHYPERTENSIVE. It is available as tablets.
✚▲ Side-effects/warnings: See HYDROCHLOROTHIAZIDE; TRIAMTERENE. Urine may appear blue.

triamterene

is a mild DIURETIC of the *potassium-sparing* type and so causes the retention of potassium. It is therefore used as an alternative to or, more commonly, in combination with other diuretics that normally cause a loss of potassium from the body (such as the THIAZIDE and *loop* diuretics). It can be used to treat oedema, as an ANTIHYPERTENSIVE (in combination with other drugs). Administration is oral.
✚ Side-effects: Gastrointestinal upsets, skin rashes, dry mouth, fall in blood pressure on standing and raised blood potassium. There are also reports of blood disorders and light-sensitivity.
▲ Warnings: See AMILORIDE HYDROCHLORIDE. Urine may be coloured blue.
✪ Related entries: Dyazide; Dytac; Dytide; Frusene; Kalspare; Triam-Co.

Triapin

(Hoechst Marion Roussel; Aventis Pharma) is a proprietary, prescription-only compound preparation of the ACE INHIBITOR ramipril, together with the CALCIUM-CHANNEL BLOCKER felodipine. It can be used as an ANTIHYPERTENSIVE. It is available as tablets in two strengths (one called *Triapin mite*).
✚▲ Side-effects/warnings: See FELODIPINE; RAMIPRIL.

Triasox

(IDIS) is a proprietary, prescription-only preparation of the ANTHELMINTIC drug tiabendazole. It can be used to treat intestinal infestations, especially by the *Strongyloides* species, and to assist in the treatment of resistant infections by hookworm, whipworm and roundworm. It is available as tablets on a named-patient basis only.
✚▲ Side-effects/warnings: See TIABENDAZOLE.

triazole 🅱

see AZOLE.

tribavirin

see RIBAVIRIN.

T

Triclofos Oral Solution, BP

(triclofos elixir) is a non-proprietary, prescription-only preparation of the HYPNOTIC triclofos sodium. It is used to treat insomnia in children and the elderly, and is available as an elixir.

✚▲ Side-effects/warnings: See TRICLOFOS SODIUM.

triclofos elixir

see TRICLOFOS ORAL SOLUTION, BP.

triclofos sodium

is used as a HYPNOTIC to treat insomnia. Administration is oral.

✚▲ Side-effects/warnings: See CHLORAL HYDRATE; but with less stomach irritation.

✪ **Related entry: Triclofos Oral Solution, BP**

triclosan

is an ANTISEPTIC agent which is used to prevent the spread of an infection on the skin. It is available as a hand rub and a powder to be added to a bath.

✚▲ Side-effects/warnings: Avoid contact with the eyes.

✪ **Related entries: Aquasept Skin Cleanser; Clearasil Treatment Cream Regular (Colourless); Dettol Antiseptic Cream; Oilatum Junior Flare-Up; Solarcaine Cream; Solarcaine Lotion; Solarcaine Spray; Ster-Zac Bath Concentrate; TCP First Aid Antiseptic Cream.**

tricyclic 🅱

drugs are one of the three main, original classes of ANTIDEPRESSANT drugs that are used to relieve the symptoms of depressive illness, especially effective in *endogenous depression*. They constitute a well-established class of drugs, having been used for many years, but they do have SEDATIVE actions which can cause drowsiness and difficulties in concentrating, and many other troublesome side-effects such as dry mouth, blurred vision, constipation, postural hypotension and urinary retention. Since depression is commonly associated with loss of appetite and sleep disorders, an early benefit of tricyclic treatment may be an improvement of these symptoms. Some are also useful in the management of panic attacks and bed-wetting in children. Chemically, they are mainly dibenzazepine or dibenzcycloheptene derivatives and notable examples include AMITRIPTYLINE HYDROCHLORIDE, DOSULEPIN HYDROCHLORIDE, DOXEPIN and IMIPRAMINE HYDROCHLORIDE. Some examples are chemically not tricyclics because they do not have the characteristic three-ringed structure, but are pharmacologically similar and so are often classed under this heading (eg MIANSERIN HYDROCHLORIDE). They are believed to work by blocking the uptake of neurotransmitter amines (SEROTONIN and NORADRENALINE) by nerve terminals in the brain (though their side-effects are partly due to their largely unwanted ANTICHOLINERGIC actions). Treatment often takes some weeks to show maximal beneficial effects. Anxious or agitated patients respond better to those tricyclics which have more pronounced sedative properties (eg amitriptyline and doxepin), whereas withdrawn patients are prescribed less-sedative tricyclics (eg imipramine). See AMITRIPTYLINE HYDROCHLORIDE for principal uses, side-effects and warnings.

▲ Warnings: There are important, potentially dangerous interactions with a number of other drugs, including alcohol. Other types of antidepressant, including herbal or other alternative remedies for depression, in particular St John's wort, should not be taken at the same time as tricyclics since serious adverse reactions can occur.

Tridestra

(Orion) is a proprietary, prescription-only compound preparation of the OESTROGEN estradiol (as valerate) and the PROGESTOGEN medroxyprogesterone acetate. It can be used to treat menopausal problems in HRT and osteoporosis prevention, and is available as tablets.

✚▲ Side-effects/warnings: See MEDROXYPROGESTERONE ACETATE; ESTRADIOL.

trientine dihydrochloride

is a CHELATING AGENT which is used as a METABOLIC DISORDER TREATMENT to reduce the abnormally high levels of copper in the body that occur in Wilson's disease. It is given to patients who cannot tolerate the more commonly used PENICILLAMINE. Administration is oral.

✚ Side-effects: Nausea.

▲ Warnings: It should be administered with care to patients who are pregnant.

✪ **Related entry: Trientine Dihydrochloride Capsules.**

Trientine Dihydrochloride Capsules
(Anstead) is a proprietary, prescription-only preparation of the CHELATING AGENT trientine dihydrochloride. It can be used as a METABOLIC DISORDER TREATMENT to reduce the abnormally high levels of copper in the body that occur in Wilson's disease. It is given to patients who cannot tolerate the more commonly used PENICILLAMINE, and is available as capsules.
✚▲ Side-effects/warnings: See TRIENTINE DIHYDROCHLORIDE.

trifluoperazine
is chemically a PHENOTHIAZINE derivative. It is used as a powerful ANTIPSYCHOTIC drug to treat and tranquillize psychotic patients (such as schizophrenics), particularly those experiencing some form of behavioural disturbance. It can also be used for the short-term treatment of severe anxiety and as an ANTI-EMETIC and ANTINAUSEANT for severe nausea and vomiting caused by underlying disease or drug therapies. Administration is oral.
✚▲ Side-effects/warnings: See CHLORPROMAZINE HYDROCHLORIDE; but it causes less sedation, hypotension, hypothermia and anticholinergic effects; though there is a greater frequency of various movement disturbances, including extrapyramidal symptoms (muscle tremor and rigidity).
✪ **Related entry: Stelazine.**

Trifyba
(Sanofi-Synthelabo) is a proprietary, non-prescription preparation of the natural (*bulking-agent*) LAXATIVE bran (wheat fibre), and is available as a powder.
✚▲ Side-effects/warnings: See BRAN.

trihexyphenidyl hydrochloride
see BENZHEXOL HYDROCHLORIDE.

Triiodothyronine
(Goldshield) is a proprietary, prescription-only preparation of liothyronine sodium, which is a form of the thyroid hormone (see THYROID HORMONES) triiodothyronine. It can be used to make up hormonal deficiency (hypothyroidism) in emergency situations (eg hypothyroid coma). It is available in a form for injection.
✚▲ Side-effects/warnings: See LIOTHYRONINE SODIUM.

triiodothyronine
is a natural blood-borne (endocrine) HORMONE released by the thyroid gland. The other major thyroid hormone is THYROXINE. (In turn, the release of these two hormones is regulated by the endocrine hormone THYROTROPHIN (thyroid-stimulating hormone; TSH), which is secreted by the pituitary gland.) Therapeutically, triiodothyronine is administered in the form known as LIOTHYRONINE SODIUM (actually it is L-tri-iodothyronine; T_3).

Trileptal
(Novartis) is a newly introduced proprietary, prescription-only preparation of the ANTICONVULSANT and ANTI-EPILEPTIC oxcarbazepine. It can be used to treat some forms of epilepsy (partial seizures with or without secondary generalized tonic-clonic seizures absence seizures). It is available as tablets.
✚▲ Side-effects/warnings: See OXCARBAZEPINE.

trilostane
is an ENZYME INHIBITOR which inhibits the production of both *glucocorticoid* and *mineralocorticoid* CORTICOSTEROID by the adrenal glands. It can therefore be used to treat conditions that result from the excessive secretion of corticosteroids into the bloodstream (such as Cushing's syndrome and primary hyper-aldosteronism). It can also be used to treat post-menopausal breast cancer. Administration is oral.
✚ Side-effects: There may be flushing, swelling and tingling of the mouth, watery nose, nausea, vomiting, diarrhoea; rarely, rashes and blood changes.
▲ Warnings: It is a specialist drug, and a full assessment of patient suitability will be carried out. It is not given to patients who are pregnant, breast-feeding or have impaired liver or kidney function.
✪ **Related entry: Modrenal.**

trimeprazine tartrate
see ALIMEMAZINE TARTRATE.

trimetaphan camsilate
(trimetaphan camsylate) is a GANGLION-BLOCKER drug which lowers blood pressure by reducing vascular tone normally induced by the sympathetic nervous system. It is short-acting and can be used as a HYPOTENSIVE for controlled

blood pressure during surgery. Administration is by injection or intravenous infusion.
✚ Side-effects: There may be an increase in the heart rate and depression of respiration, increased intraocular pressure, dilated pupils and constipation.
▲ Warnings: Trimetaphan camsilate should be administered with caution to patients with certain heart or kidney disorders, diabetes, Addison's disease, degenerative disease of the brain and in the elderly. It is not to be given to patients who are pregnant or with severe arteriosclerosis.

trimetaphan camsylate

see TRIMETAPHAN CAMSILATE.

trimethoprim

is an ANTIBACTERIAL drug which is similar to drugs of the SULPHONAMIDE group. It is used to treat and prevent the spread of many forms of bacterial infection, but particularly infections of the urinary and respiratory tracts. It has been used in combination with the sulphonamide SULFAMETHOXAZOLE, because the combined effect is considered to be greater than twice the individual effect of either drug. This is the basis of the medicinal compound CO-TRIMOXAZOLE. More recently there has been a move away from the compound preparation to the use of trimethoprim alone. It is effective in many situations (eg urinary tract infections and bronchitis) and lacks many of the side-effects of sulfamethoxazole. Administration can be either oral or by injection. (It is also available for topical use with POLYMYXIN B SULPHATE for eye infections.)
✚ Side-effects: There may be nausea, vomiting and gastrointestinal disturbances; rashes may break out with pruritus (itching) and there may be effects on blood.
▲ Warnings: It should not be administered to patients who have severe kidney impairment or certain blood disorders; it is administered with care to those who are pregnant or breast-feeding, or have impaired kidney function. Prolonged treatment requires frequent blood counts. Patients should look out for signs of blood disorders (eg bruising, fever, sore throat, mouth ulcers, bleeding) and report them to their doctor.
✪ **Related entries: Chemotrim; Fectrim; Monotrim; Polytrim; Septrin; Trimopan.**

trimetrexate

is an ANTIPROTOZOAL drug. It is used to treat pneumonia caused by the protozoan micro-organism *Pneumocystis carinii* in patients whose immune system has been suppressed as in HIV infection (normally where standard treatment is not appropriate). Administration is by injection.
✚ Side-effects: Diarrhoea, vomiting, mouth and gastrointestinal ulceration; blood disorders; fever; confusion, rarely seizures, disturbed liver enzymes and blood electrolytes, rash and very rarely anaphylactic shock.
▲ Warnings: This is a specialist drug given with careful supervision. It is not used in patients who are pregnant or breast-feeding, and (for men and women) avoid conception for at least six months after treatment. Administration requires concurrent use of calcium folinate and specialist monitoring.
✪ **Related entry: Neutrexin.**

Tri-Minulet

(Wyeth) is a proprietary, prescription-only compound preparation which can be used as a (*triphasic*) ORAL CONTRACEPTIVE of the *COC* (standard strength) type that combines an OESTROGEN and a PROGESTOGEN, in this case ethinylestradiol and gestodene. It is available as tablets in a calendar pack.
✚▲ Side-effects/warnings: See ETHINYLESTRADIOL; GESTODENE.

trimipramine

is an ANTIDEPRESSANT of the TRICYCLIC class. It is used to treat depressive illness, especially in cases where sedation (see SEDATIVE) is required. Administration is oral.
✚▲ Side-effects/warnings: See AMITRIPTYLINE HYDROCHLORIDE.
✪ **Related entry: Surmontil.**

Trimopan

(Berk; APS) is a proprietary, prescription-only preparation of the SULPHONAMIDE-like ANTIBACTERIAL drug trimethoprim. It can be used to treat infections (eg of the urinary tract). It is available as a sugar-free suspension.
✚▲ Side-effects/warnings: See TRIMETHOPRIM.

Trimovate

(GlaxoWellcome; GSK) is a proprietary, prescription-only compound preparation of the

CORTICOSTEROID clobetasone butyrate, the ANTIBACTERIAL and (TETRACYCLINE) ANTI-BIOTIC oxytetracycline and the ANTIFUNGAL and antibiotic nystatin. It can be used to treat skin infections, and is available as a cream for topical application.
✚▲ Side-effects/warnings: See CLOBETASONE BUTYRATE; NYSTATIN; OXYTETRACYCLINE. It stains clothing.

Trinordiol

(Wyeth) is a proprietary, prescription-only compound preparation which can be used as a (*triphasic*) ORAL CONTRACEPTIVE of the *COC* (standard strength) type that combines an OESTROGEN and a PROGESTOGEN, in this case ethinylestradiol and levonorgestrel. It is available as tablets in a calendar pack.
✚▲ Side-effects/warnings: See ETHINYLESTRADIOL; LEVONORGESTREL.

TriNovum

(Janssen-Cilag) is a proprietary, prescription-only compound preparation which can be used as a (*triphasic*) ORAL CONTRACEPTIVE of the *COC* (standard strength) type that combines an OESTROGEN and a PROGESTOGEN, in this case ethinylestradiol and norethisterone. It is available as tablets in a calendar pack.
✚▲ Side-effects/warnings: See ETHINYLESTRADIOL; NORETHISTERONE.

tripotassium dicitratobismuthate

(bismuth chelate) is a CYTOPROTECTANT drug. It coats the mucosa of the stomach and can be used as an ULCER-HEALING DRUG for benign peptic ulcers in the stomach and duodenum. It may also have a specific action on the bacterial organism *Helicobacter pylori*, which is associated with peptic ulcers. Administration is oral.
✚ Side-effects: The compound may darken the tongue and the faeces and cause nausea and vomiting.
▲ Warnings: It should not be given to patients with kidney impairment or who are pregnant. It is important to follow the instructions on how and when to take this drug, and to avoid drinking milk (on its own) during treatment.
✪ Related entry: De-Noltab.

triprolidine hydrochloride

is an ANTIHISTAMINE which can be used for the symptomatic relief of allergic symptoms, such as hay fever and urticaria. It is also used in some cough and decongestant preparations. Administration is oral.
✚▲ Side-effects/warnings: See ANTIHISTAMINE. Because of its sedative property, the performance of skilled tasks, such as driving, may be impaired.
✪ Related entries: Actifed Compound Linctus; Actifed Expectorant; Actifed Syrup; Actifed Tablets.

Triptafen

(Goldshield) is a proprietary, prescription-only compound preparation of the (TRICYCLIC) ANTIDEPRESSANT amitriptyline hydrochloride and the ANTIPSYCHOTIC perphenazine, in the ratio of 12.5:1. It can be used to treat depressive illness, particularly in association with anxiety, and is available as tablets. *Triptafen-M* is a similar preparation but with a lower proportion of amitriptyline hydrochloride (5:1).
✚▲ Side-effects/warnings: See AMITRIPTYLINE HYDROCHLORIDE; PERPHENAZINE.

triptan

drugs, also called $5HT_1$ agonists, are a chemical class of agents with potent VASOCONSTRICTOR actions, acting as serotonin-receptor stimulant drugs selective for serotonin $5\text{-}HT_1$ receptors, producing a rapid constriction of blood vessels surrounding the brain. They have fairly recently been introduced in ANTIMIGRAINE treatment for acute migraine attacks rather than prevention. Sumatriptan, given by subcutaneous injection, can also be used for cluster headache. Administration is oral, by self-injection or by a nasal spray. Because they are used after the onset of an attack, quick absorption into the blood circulation is essential, so although they can be taken orally they work much more quickly when self-injected or taken by nasal spray (where they are absorbed across the nasal mucosa). See: ALMOTRIPTAN; NARATRIPTAN; RIZATRIPTAN; SUMATRIPTAN; ZOLMITRIPTAN.

triptorelin

is an analogue of GONADORELIN (gonadothrophin-releasing hormone; GnRH), which is a hypothalamic HORMONE. On prolonged administration it acts as an indirect HORMONE ANTAGONIST in that it reduces the pituitary gland's secretion of gonadotrophin (after an initial surge), which results in reduced secretion of SEX HORMONES by the ovaries or testes. It can be used to treat endometriosis (a growth of the lining of the uterus at inappropriate sites) and is also used as an ANTICANCER drug for cancer of the prostate gland. Administration is by injection.

✚▲ Side-effects/warnings: See BUSERELIN. There may also be transient hypertension, dry mouth, muscle ache and weakness, increase in painful urination. There may be irritation at the injection site.

✪ **Related entry: De-capeptyl sr.**

Trisequens

(Novo Nordisk) is a proprietary, prescription-only compound preparation of the OESTROGEN estradiol and the PROGESTOGEN norethisterone (as acetate). It can be used to treat menopausal problems and osteoporosis prevention, including in HRT. It is available as tablets in a calendar pack and also in a higher strength form, *Trisequens Forte*.

✚▲ Side-effects/warnings: See NORETHISTERONE; ESTRADIOL.

trisodium edetate

is a CHELATING AGENT that binds to calcium and forms an inactive complex. It can therefore be used as an ANTIDOTE to treat conditions in which there is excessive calcium in the bloodstream (hypercalcaemia), and can also be used in the form of a solution to treat calcification of the cornea, or lime burns, of the eye. Administration for treating hypercalcaemia is by intravenous infusion and for the eye it is by topical application as a solution.

✚ Side-effects: Nausea, diarrhoea and cramps; pain in the limb where it is injected. An overdose may lead to kidney damage.

▲ Warnings: It is not given to patients with impaired kidney function.

✪ **Related entry: Limclair.**

Tritace

(Aventis Pharma) is a proprietary, prescription-only preparation of the ACE INHIBITOR ramipril. It can be used as an ANTIHYPERTENSIVE and in HEART FAILURE TREATMENT, often in conjunction with other classes of drug, and is available as capsules.

✚▲ Side-effects/warnings: See RAMIPRIL.

Trizivir

(GlaxoWellcome; GSK) is a proprietary, prescription-only compound preparation of the ANTIVIRAL agents abacavir, lamivudine and zidovudine. It can be used in the treatment of HIV infection, and is available as tablets.

✚▲ Side-effects/warnings: See ABACAVIR; LAMIVUDINE; ZIDOVUDINE.

Tropergen

(Goldshield) is a proprietary, prescription-only compound preparation of the (OPIOID) ANTIDIARRHOEAL diphenoxylate hydrochloride and the ANTICHOLINERGIC atropine sulphate (a combination called co-phenotrope). It can be used to treat chronic diarrhoea, for example, in mild chronic ulcerative colitis. Dependence may occur with prolonged use. It is available as tablets.

✚▲ Side-effects/warnings: See ATROPINE SULPHATE; DIPHENOXYLATE HYDROCHLORIDE.

tropicamide

is a short-acting ANTICHOLINERGIC (ANTIMUSCARINIC) drug, which can be used to dilate the pupil and paralyse the focusing of the eye for ophthalmic examination. Administration is topical as eye-drops.

✚▲ Side-effects/warnings: See ATROPINE SULPHATE; but there should be few side-effects because of topical administration, apart from initial stinging and blurred vision. It should not be used in patients with raised intraocular pressure (pressure in the eyeball). Patients should not drive for two hours after treatment.

✪ **Related entries: Minims Tropicamide; Mydriacyl.**

tropisetron

is an ANTI-EMETIC and ANTINAUSEANT drug. It gives relief from nausea and vomiting, especially in patients receiving chemotherapy to prevent nausea and vomiting. It acts as a serotonin receptor antagonist, blocking the action of the naturally occurring mediator SEROTONIN. Administration can be either oral or by injection.

✚ Side-effects: Constipation, diarrhoea, abdominal pain, headache, hypersensitivity reactions, fatigue, drowsiness, and dizziness (which may impair the performance of skilled tasks, such as driving).

▲ Warnings: It should be administered with care to patients with certain cardiovascular disorders, or who are pregnant or breast-feeding.

✪ **Related entry: Navoban.**

Tropium

(DDSA) is a proprietary, prescription-only preparation of the BENZODIAZEPINE chlordiazepoxide. It can be used as an ANXIOLYTIC for the short-term treatment of anxiety and (used with other drugs) to alleviate acute alcohol withdrawal symptoms. Available as capsules.

✚▲ Side-effects/warnings: See CHLORDIAZEPOXIDE.

trospium chloride

is an ANTICHOLINERGIC (ANTIMUSCARINIC) drug which can be used as an ANTISPASMODIC to treat urinary frequency, incontinence and urgency. Administration is oral.

✚▲ Side-effects/warnings: See ATROPINE SULPHATE; also flatulence, chest pain and breathing difficulties, rash and weakness.

✪ **Related entry: Regurin.**

Trosyl

(Pfizer) is a proprietary, prescription-only preparation of the ANTIFUNGAL drug tioconazole. It can be used to treat fungal infections of the nails, and is available as a nail solution.

✚▲ Side-effects/warnings: See TIOCONAZOLE.

Trusopt

(MSD) is a proprietary, prescription-only preparation of the CARBONIC-ANHYDRASE INHIBITOR dorzolamide. It is used in GLAUCOMA TREATMENT, and is available as eye-drops.

✚▲ Side-effects/warnings: See DORZOLAMIDE.

tryptophan

is an amino acid present in an ordinary, well-balanced diet and from which the natural body substance serotonin (5-hydroxytryptamine; 5-HT) is derived. Dysfunction of serotonin, in its neurotransmitter role in nerve-tracts in the brain, is thought to contribute to depression. Therapeutic administration of tryptophan has been used in ANTIDEPRESSANT treatment, but was withdrawn from general use because of an association with a dangerous side-effect called eosinophilia-myalgia syndrome. It can be used by hospital specialists in patients only where no alternative treatment is suitable and with registration and constant monitoring. Administration is oral.

✚▲ Side-effects/warnings: It is a specialist drug used under hospital conditions. Light-headedness, drowsiness, headache, nausea, eosinophilia-myalgia syndrome. It should not be administered to patients known to have defective metabolism of tryptophan in the diet, or who have a history of eosinophilia-myalgia syndrome. It is administered with extra caution to those who are pregnant or breast-feeding.

✪ **Related entry: Optimax.**

TSH

see THYROTROPHIN.

tuberculin

(in the form *tuberculin purified protein derivative; PPD*) is a diagnostic agent prepared from the heat-treated products of species of mycobacterium. It is used to test whether or not a person has antibodies to tuberculosis, to see if they have been in contact with the infection or whether a vaccination has 'taken'. It is used either in the *Mantoux test* (where tuberculin is injected intradermally) or the *Heaf test* (multiple puncture of the skin), where a positive result (for the antibody) is indicated by the skin of the site on the forearm becoming red, raised and hard.

✚▲ Side-effects/warnings: This is a specialist diagnostic agent.

✪ **Related entry: Tuberculin PPD.**

Tuberculin PPD

(District Health Authorities; Farillon) is a preparation of tuberculin (in the form *tuberculin purified protein derivative; PPD*) and is a diagnostic agent used in the *tuberculin test* to see whether or not a person has antibodies to tuberculosis. It is applied intradermally to the skin of the forearm.

✚▲ Side-effects/warnings: see TUBERCULIN.

Tub/Vac/BCG (Perc)

is an abbreviation for a VACCINE, the live version of BCG VACCINE (against tuberculosis) for *percutaneous* administration by multiple puncture of the skin.

Tuinal

(Flynn) is a proprietary, prescription-only compound preparation of the BARBITURATE amobarbital (amylobarbitone, as sodium) and secobarbital sodium (quinalbarbitone sodium), and is on the Controlled Drugs list. It can be used as a HYPNOTIC to treat persistent and intractable

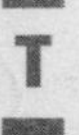

insomnia, and is available as capsules.
✚▲ Side-effects/warnings: See AMOBARBITAL; SECOBARBITAL SODIUM.

Tums Assorted Fruit Flavours

(GSK Consumer Healthcare) is a proprietary, non-prescription preparation of calcium carbonate. It can be used to relieve heartburn and indigestion, and is available as tablets. It is not normally given to children, except on medical advice.
✚▲ Side-effects/warnings: See CALCIUM CARBONATE.

turpentine oil

is a COUNTER-IRRITANT, or RUBEFACIENT, agent. It is included in certain compound preparations that are used by topical application for the symptomatic relief of pain associated with rheumatism, neuralgia, fibrosis and sprains and stiffness of the joints. It is also used, along with other constituents, as an inhalant in DECONGESTANT preparations to relieve cold symptoms.
✚▲ Side-effects/warnings: It is regarded as safe when used topically at correct dosage, though it does have a mild irritant action – and should not be applied to broken skin.
✪ Related entries: Deep Heat Rub; Ellimans Universal Embrocation; Goddard's Embrocation; Tixycolds Cold and Hayfever Inhalant Capsules; Vicks Vaporub; Wax Wane Ear Drops; Woodward's Baby Chest Rub.

Twinrix

(SmithKline Beecham; GSK) is a proprietary, prescription-only double VACCINE preparation of hepatitis B vaccine (rby), prepared from yeast cells by recombinant DNA technique, together with inactivated hepatitis A virus. It can be used to protect people at risk from infection with both hepatitis A and B, and is available in a form for intramuscular injection. There are different *Adult* and *Paediatric* forms.
✚▲ Side-effects/warnings: see HEPATITIS A VACCINE; HEPATITIS B VACCINE.

Tylex

(Schwarz) is a proprietary, prescription-only compound analgesic preparation of the (OPIOID) ANTITUSSIVE codeine phosphate and the NON-NARCOTIC ANALGESIC paracetamol (a combination known as co-codamol 30/500). It can be used as a painkiller, and is available as capsules and effervescent tablets.
✚▲ Side-effects/warnings: See CODEINE PHOSPHATE; PARACETAMOL.

Typherix

(SmithKline Beecham; GSK) is a proprietary, prescription-only VACCINE preparation of the typhoid vaccine, and is available in a form for injection.
✚▲ Side-effects/warnings: See TYPHOID VACCINE.

Typhim Vi

(Aventis Pasteur) is a proprietary, prescription-only VACCINE preparation of the typhoid vaccine (Vi capsular polysaccharide typhoid vaccine), and is available in a form for injection.
✚▲ Side-effects/warnings: See TYPHOID VACCINE.

typhoid vaccine

is a suspension of polysaccharide (or live attenuated for oral use) typhoid bacteria *Salmonella typhi*). However, full protection is not guaranteed and travellers at risk are advised not to eat uncooked food or to drink untreated water. Administration can be either oral or by deep subcutaneous or intramuscular injection or orally.
✚▲ Side-effects/warnings: See VACCINE.
✪ Related entries: Hepatyrix; Typherix; Typhim Vi; Vivotif.

tyrothricin

is a weak ANTISEPTIC agent which is incorporated in some lozenges for sore throats.
✚▲ Side-effects/warnings: Considered safe in normal topical use at recommended concentrations.
✪ Related entry: Tyrozets.

Tyrozets

(Johnson & Johnson · MSD) is a proprietary, non-prescription compound preparation of the ANTISEPTIC agent TYROTHRICIN and the LOCAL ANAESTHETIC benzocaine. It can be used to relieve minor mouth and throat irritations, and is available as lozenges. It is not normally given to children under three years, except on medical advice.
✚▲ Side-effects/warnings: See BENZOCAINE; TYROTHRICIN.

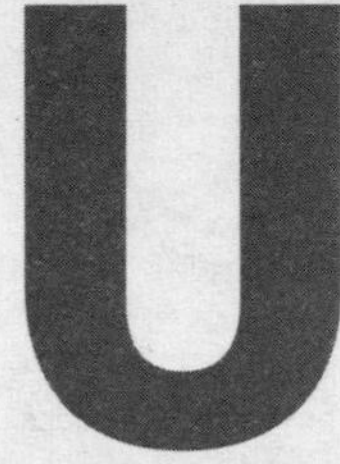

Ubretid

(Rhône-Poulenc Rorer; Aventis Pharma) is a proprietary, prescription-only preparation of the ANTICHOLINESTERASE and PARASYMPATHOMIMETIC distigmine bromide. It can be used to stimulate the bladder and to treat myasthenia gravis. It is available as tablets.

✚▲ Side-effects/warnings: See DISTIGMINE BROMIDE.

Ucerax

(UCB Pharma) is a proprietary, prescription-only preparation of the ANTIHISTAMINE hydroxyzine hydrochloride, which has some additional ANXIOLYTIC properties. It can be used to relieve allergic symptoms, such as pruritus (itching and rashes), and also for short-term treatment of anxiety. It is available as tablets and a syrup.

✚▲ Side-effects/warnings: See HYDROXYZINE HYDROCHLORIDE.

Ucine

(Ashbourne) is a proprietary, prescription-only preparation of the AMINOSALICYLATE sulphasalazine. It can be used to treat active rheumatoid arthritis, ulcerative colitis and Crohn's disease. It is available as enteric-coated tablets.

✚▲ Side-effects/warnings: See SULPHASALAZINE.

Uftoral

(Squibb; Bristol-Myers Squibb) is a recently inroduced proprietary, prescription-only compound preparation of the ANTICANCER drug combination tegafur with uracil. Available as capsules.

✚▲ Side-effects/warnings: See TEGAFUR WITH URACIL.

ulcer-healing drug 🅱

refers to any of a group of drugs used to promote healing of ulceration of the gastric (stomach) and duodenal (first part of small intestine) linings and so are used in the treatment of peptic ulcers. A number of classes of drugs may be used, including H_2-ANTAGONIST drugs (eg CIMETIDINE and RANITIDINE), PROTON-PUMP INHIBITOR drugs (eg OMEPRAZOLE), PROSTAGLANDIN analogues (eg MISOPROSTOL), BISMUTH CHELATE compounds (eg TRIPOTASSIUM DICITRATOBISMUTHATE). The drug CARBENOXOLONE SODIUM, which has a poorly understood mode of action, is no longer used for peptic ulceration, instead being used for oesophageal ulceration and inflammation. The first two classes act principally by reducing the secretion of peptic acid by the stomach's mucosal lining. The other drugs have complex actions that include a beneficial increase in blood flow to the mucosa, alterations in natural protective secretions (CYTOPROTECTANT actions), or antimicrobial actions against an infection by the bacterial organism *Helicobacter pylori*, which is associated with peptic ulcers. These classes may be combined in treatment, and RANITIDINE BISMUTH CITRATE combines two actions in one chemical compound. Other types of drug may reduce the discomfort of some peptic ulcers without necessarily being ulcer-healing drugs (eg ANTACID agents and ANTICHOLINERGIC drugs).

Ultec

(Berk; APS) is a proprietary, prescription-only of the H_2-ANTAGONIST and ULCER-HEALING DRUG cimetidine. It can be used to treat benign peptic ulcers (in the stomach or duodenum), gastro-oesophageal reflux, dyspepsia and associated conditions. It is available as tablets.

✚▲ Side-effects/warnings: See CIMETIDINE.

Ultiva

(Elan) is a proprietary, prescription-only preparation of the (OPIOID) NARCOTIC ANALGESIC remifentanil (as hydrochloride). It can be used for the induction of anaesthesia and during surgery to supplement the effect of GENERAL ANAESTHETIC drugs. It is available in a form for intravenous infusion.

✚▲ Side-effects/warnings: See REMIFENTANIL.

Ultra Chloraseptic

(Prestige Brands) is a proprietary, non-prescription compound preparation of the LOCAL

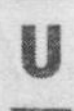

ANAESTHETIC benzocaine. It can be used to relieve the pain of a sore throat, and is available as a throat spray. It is not normally given to children under six years, except on medical advice.
✚▲ Side-effects/warnings: See BENZOCAINE.

Ultralanum Plain
(Schering Health) is a proprietary, prescription-only preparation of the CORTICOSTEROID and ANTI-INFLAMMATORY fluocortolone (as fluocortolone hexanoate and fluocortolone pivalate). It can be used to treat severe, inflammatory skin disorders, such as eczema and psoriasis, and is available as a cream and an ointment for topical application.
✚▲ Side-effects/warnings: See FLUOCORTOLONE.

Ultraproct
(Schering Health) is a proprietary, prescription-only compound preparation of the CORTICOSTEROID and ANTI-INFLAMMATORY fluocortolone (as hexanoate) and the LOCAL ANAESTHETIC cinchocaine (dibucaine hydrochloride). It can be used to treat haemorrhoids, and is available as an ointment and suppositories for topical application.
✚▲ Side-effects/warnings: See CINCHOCAINE; FLUOCORTOLONE.

undecenoate
see UNDECENOIC ACID.

undecenoic acid
and its salts (eg zinc undecenoate) have ANTIFUNGAL activity and are incorporated into a number of topical preparations for the treatment of fungal infections of the skin, particularly athlete's foot. Administration is by topical application.
✚▲ Side-effects/warnings: It is regarded as safe in normal topical use.
✪ **Related entries: Ceanel Concentrate; Mycota Cream; Mycota Powder; Mycota Spray.**

Unguentum M
(Crooks Healthcare) is a proprietary, non-prescription compound preparation of LIQUID PARAFFIN, WHITE SOFT PARAFFIN and several other constituents. It can be used as an EMOLLIENT for dry skin and related disorders such as nappy rash, pruritis and dermatitis, and is available as a cream.
✚▲ Side-effects/warnings: See LIQUID PARAFFIN; WHITE SOFT PARAFFIN.

Uniphyllin Continus
(Napp) is a proprietary, non-prescription preparation of the BRONCHODILATOR theophylline. It can be used as an ANTI-ASTHMATIC and to treat bronchitis. It is available as modified-release tablets for prolonged effect.
✚▲ Side-effects/warnings: See THEOPHYLLINE.

Uniroid-HC
(Chemidex) is a proprietary, prescription-only compound preparation of the CORTICOSTEROID hydrocortisone and the LOCAL ANAESTHETIC cinchocaine. It can be used by topical application to treat haemorrhoids, and is available as an ointment and as suppositories.
✚▲ Side-effects/warnings: See CINCHOCAINE; HYDROCORTISONE.

Unisept
(SSL) is a proprietary, non-prescription preparation of the ANTISEPTIC chlorhexidine (as gluconate). It can be used to clean wounds and burns, and is available in sachets for making up into a solution.
✚▲ Side-effects/warnings: See CHLORHEXIDINE.

Univer
(Elan) is a proprietary, prescription-only preparation of the CALCIUM-CHANNEL BLOCKER verapamil hydrochloride. It can be used as an ANTIHYPERTENSIVE and in ANTI-ANGINA treatment. It is available as modified-release capsules.
✚▲ Side-effects/warnings: See VERAPAMIL HYDROCHLORIDE.

Uprima
(Abbott) is a prescription-only preparation of apomorphine hydrochloride in a recently introduced form used in IMPOTENCE TREATMENT for erectile dysfunction. It is available as sublingual (under the tongue) tablets.
✚▲ Side-effects/warnings: See APOMORPHINE HYDROCHLORIDE.

Urdox
(CP) is a proprietary, prescription-only preparation of ursodeoxycholic acid. It is used to dissolve gallstones, and is available as tablets.

✚▲ Side-effects/warnings: See URSODEOXYCHOLIC ACID.

urea

is a chemical incorporated as a HYDRATING AGENT into a number of skin preparations; for example, creams that are used to treat eczema and psoriasis. It is also included in ear-drop preparations used for dissolving and washing out earwax.

✚▲ Side-effects/warnings: It is regarded as safe in normal topical use.

✪ **Related entries: Alphaderm; Aquadrate; Calmurid; Calmurid HC; E45 Itch Relief Cream; Eucerin; Exterol Ear Drops; Nutraplus; Otex Ear Drops.**

Uriben

(Rosemont) is a proprietary, prescription-only preparation of the (QUINOLONE) ANTIBIOTIC-like ANTIBACTERIAL nalidixic acid. It can be used to treat infections, particularly those of the urinary tract, and is available as an oral suspension.

✚▲ Side-effects/warnings: See NALIDIXIC ACID.

Urispas 200

(Shire) is a proprietary, prescription-only preparation of the ANTICHOLINERGIC drug flavoxate hydrochloride. It can be used as an ANTISPASMODIC in the treatment of urinary frequency and incontinence, and is available as tablets.

✚▲ Side-effects/warnings: See FLAVOXATE HYDROCHLORIDE.

urofollitrophin

see UROFOLLITROPIN.

urofollitropin

(urofollitrophin) is a form of the sex hormone, FOLLICLE-STIMULATING HORMONE (FSH), which is also found in an extract that can be prepared from urine from menopausal women. Urofollitropin is used as an infertility treatment in women whose infertility is due to abnormal pituitary gland function, or who do not respond to the commonly used fertility drug CLOMIPHENE CITRATE. It is also used in superovulation treatment for assisted conception, such as in IVF. It is used by injection.

✚▲ Side-effects/warnings: See HUMAN MENOPAUSAL GONADOTROPHINS.

✪ **Related entry: Metrodin High Purity.**

Uromitexan

(ASTA Medica) is a proprietary, prescription-only preparation of mesna. It is used to combat haemorrhagic cystitis, which is a serious complication caused by certain CYTOTOXIC drugs. It is available as tablets and in a form for injection.

✚▲ Side-effects/warnings: See MESNA.

ursodeoxycholic acid

is a drug which can dissolve some gallstones *in situ*. It is also used in primary biliary cirrhosis. Administration is oral.

✚ Side-effects: Vomiting, nausea, diarrhoea, skin itching.

▲ Warnings: Not for use in pregnant women or in certain conditions such as chronic liver disease, peptic ulceration, some gastrointestinal conditions, or non-functioning gall bladder.

✪ **Related entries: Destolit; Urdox; Ursofalk; Ursogal.**

Ursofalk

(Provalis) is a proprietary, prescription-only preparation of ursodeoxycholic acid. It can be used to dissolve gallstones and biliary cirrhosis. Available as capsules and an oral suspension.

✚▲ Side-effects/warnings: See URSODEOXYCHOLIC ACID.

Ursogal

(Galen) is a proprietary, prescription-only preparation of ursodeoxycholic acid. It is used to dissolve gall-stones, and is available as tablets and capsules.

✚▲ Side-effects/warnings: See URSODEOXYCHOLIC ACID.

Utinor

(MSD) is a proprietary, prescription-only preparation of the (QUINOLONE) ANTIBIOTIC-like ANTIBACTERIAL norfloxacin. It can be used to treat infections, particularly of the urinary tract, and is available as tablets.

✚▲ Side-effects/warnings: See NORFLOXACIN.

Utovlan

(Pharmacia) is a proprietary, prescription-only preparation of the PROGESTOGEN norethisterone. It can be used to treat uterine bleeding, abnormally heavy menstruation, endometriosis, premenstrual syndrome and other menstrual problems. It is available as tablets.

✚▲ Side-effects/warnings: See NORETHISTERONE.

V

vaccine ⊠

preparations are used for IMMUNIZATION to confer what is known as *active immunity* against specific infections: that is, they cause a patient's own body to create a defence, in the form of antibodies (immunoglobulins), against the microbe or its toxic products. Vaccines can be one of three types. The first type of vaccines are those administered in the form of a suspension of *dead* (inactivated) viruses (eg INFLUENZA VACCINE) or bacteria (eg TYPHOID VACCINE). The second type may be *live* but weakened, or 'attenuated', viruses (eg RUBELLA VACCINE) or bacteria (eg BCG VACCINE). The third and final type of vaccines are *toxoids* (extracts of detoxified exotoxins), which are suspensions containing extracts of the toxins released by the invading organism, which then stimulate the formation of antibodies against the toxin of the disease, rather than the organism itself. Vaccines that incorporate dead micro-organisms or toxoids generally require a series of administrations (usually three) to build up a sufficient supply of antibodies in the body. 'Booster' shots may thereafter be necessary at regular intervals to reinforce immunity, for example, after ten years in the case of the tetanus vaccine. Vaccines that incorporate live micro-organisms may confer immunity with a single dose, because the organisms multiply within the body, although some live vaccines still require three administrations, for example, oral *poliomyelitis vaccine*. They are used in the general population, also special ones for high-risk groups of people (such as those travelling abroad). Administration is either by injection or mouth.

✚ Side-effects: These range from little or no reactions to severe discomfort, high temperature and pain; a mild form of the disease (eg rubella and measles) and these vary accordingly (eg with typhoid vaccination; diarrhoea, abdominal cramps, nausea and vomiting). There may be redness and swelling at the site of injection; some vaccines (including meningococcal group C vaccine) can cause dizziness, headache, nausea and vomiting, and irritability. Rarely, there may be anaphylactic shock.

▲ Warnings: A full assessment will be made of patient suitability. Vaccination should not be administered to patients who have a febrile (feverish) illness or any form of infection. Vaccines containing live material should not be administered routinely to patients who are pregnant, or who are known to have an immunodeficiency disorder. Many should not be administered to breast-feeding women (eg botuinum toxin). After vaccination, patients will be required to wait for some time (to ensure that there is no serious reaction, such as anaphylaxis).

Vagifem

(Novo Nordisk) is a proprietary, prescription-only preparation of the OESTROGEN estradiol. It can be used to treat conditions of the vagina caused by hormonal deficiency (generally, atrophic vaginitis in the menopause). It is available as vaginal tablets (pessaries) that come with disposable applicators.

✚▲ Side-effects/warnings: See ESTRADIOL.

Vaginyl

(DDSA) is a proprietary, prescription-only preparation of the ANTIMICROBIAL metronidazole, with both ANTIPROTOZOAL and ANTIBACTERIAL properties. It is used to treat a range of infections, and is available as tablets.

✚▲ Side-effects/warnings: See METRONIDAZOLE.

Vagisil Medicated Creme

(Combe International) is a proprietary, non-prescription preparation of the LOCAL ANAESTHETIC lidocaine hydrochloride. It can be used for the temporary relief of pain and itches and irritation around the female genitalia, and is available as a cream. It is not normally given to children, except on medical advice.

✚▲ Side-effects/warnings: See LIDOCAINE HYDROCHLORIDE.

valaciclovir

is a prodrug of aciclovir, an ANTIVIRAL drug. It can be used to treat herpes zoster and herpes simplex infections of the skin and mucous membranes (including initial and recurrent genital herpes). Administration is oral.

✚▲ Side-effects/warnings: See ACICLOVIR; nausea and headache have been reported.

✪ **Related entry: Valtrex.**

Valclair

(Sinclair) is a proprietary, prescription-only preparation of the BENZODIAZEPINE diazepam. It can be used as an ANXIOLYTIC for the short-term treatment of anxiety, as an ANTICONVULSANT for febrile conditions in children, especially when the oral route is inappropriate. It is available as suppositories.

✚▲ Side-effects/warnings: See DIAZEPAM.

Valderma Cream

(Roche Consumer Health) is a proprietary, non-prescription preparation of the ANTISEPTIC, ANTIBACTERIAL and ANTIFUNGAL agents POTASSIUM HYDROXYQUINOLINE SULPHATE and chlorocresol. It can be used to treat minor skin problems such as spots, and is available as a cream.

✚▲ Side-effects/warnings: See POTASSIUM HYDROXYQUINOLINE SULPHATE.

Valium

(Roche) is a proprietary, prescription-only preparation of the BENZODIAZEPINE diazepam. It can be used as an ANXIOLYTIC for the short-term treatment of anxiety, as a HYPNOTIC to relieve insomnia, as an ANTICONVULSANT and ANTI-EPILEPTIC for status epilepticus, in febrile convulsions in children, as a SEDATIVE in preoperative medication, as a SKELETAL MUSCLE RELAXANT and to help alleviate alcohol withdrawal symptoms. It is available as tablets, an oral solution and a form for injection.

✚▲ Side-effects/warnings: See DIAZEPAM.

Vallergan

(Castlemead) is a proprietary, prescription-only preparation of the ANTIHISTAMINE alimemazine tartrate (trimeprazine tartrate). It can be used to treat the symptoms of allergic disorders, particularly urticaria and pruritus. It also has SEDATIVE properties. It can be used for premedication prior to surgery. It is available as tablets and a syrup (in two strengths).

✚▲ Side-effects/warnings: See ALIMEMAZINE TARTRATE.

Valoid

(CeNeS) is a proprietary, preparation of the ANTIHISTAMINE and ANTINAUSEANT cyclizine (as hydrochloride (tablets), or lactate (for injection)). It can be used to treat nausea, vomiting, vertigo, motion sickness and disorders of the balance function of the inner ear. It is available without prescription as tablets and in a form for injection only on prescription.

✚▲ Side-effects/warnings: See CYCLIZINE.

Valpeda Foot Cream

(Roche Consumer Health) is a proprietary, non-prescription preparation of halquinol, which has ANTIFUNGAL and ANTIBACTERIAL properties. It can be used to treat common bacterial and fungal infections of the feet, including athlete's foot. It is available as a cream for topical application.

✚▲ Side-effects/warnings: See HALQUINOL.

valproic acid

see SODIUM VALPROATE.

valsartan

is an ANGIOTENSIN-RECEPTOR BLOCKER, which is a class of drugs that work by blocking angiotensin receptors. Angiotensin II is a circulating HORMONE that is a powerful VASOCONSTRICTOR and so blocking its effects leads to a fall in blood pressure. Therefore valsartan can be used as an ANTIHYPERTENSIVE. Administration is oral.

✚▲ Side-effects/warnings: See LOSARTAN POTASSIUM. Also, fatigue and, rarely, disturbances of the blood count. Should not be used in severe liver impairment, biliary obstruction, or breast-feeding; and used with care in kidney impairment.

✪ **Related entry: Diovan.**

Valtrex

(GSK) is a proprietary, prescription-only preparation of the ANTIVIRAL drug valaciclovir. It can be used to treat herpes zoster and herpes simplex infections of skin and mucous membranes (including initial and recurrent genital herpes). Administration is oral.

✚▲ Side-effects/warnings: See VALACICLOVIR.

Vancocin

(Lilly) is a proprietary, prescription-only preparation of the ANTIBACTERIAL and ANTIBIOTIC vancomycin (as hydrochloride). It

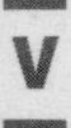

can be used to treat certain infections, such as pseudomembranous colitis and certain types of endocarditis. It is available as capsules (*Matrigel capsules*) and in a form for injection.
✚▲ Side-effects/warnings: See VANCOMYCIN.

vancomycin

is an ANTIBACTERIAL and ANTIBIOTIC drug which is primarily active against Gram-positive bacteria and works by inhibiting the synthesis of components of the bacterial cell wall. It is only used in special situations, for example, in the treatment of pseudomembranous colitis (a superinfection of the gastrointestinal tract), which can occur after treatment with broad-spectrum antibiotics. Another use is in the treatment of multiple-drug-resistant staphylococcal infections (such as MRSA), particularly endocarditis. Administration is oral to treat colitis and by intravenous infusion for systemic infections.
✚ Side-effects: These include kidney damage and tinnitus. There may be blood disorders, chills, fever, rashes and other complications.
▲ Warnings: It is a specialist drug and patients will be carefully evaluated for suitability for treatment. It should not be administered to patients with impaired kidney function, or who are deaf. It should be administered with caution to patients who are pregnant or breast-feeding. Blood counts, kidney function tests and hearing tests are required.
✪ **Related entry: Vancocin.**

Varicella-Zoster Immunoglobulin

(PHLS; BPL; SNBTS) (Antivaricella-Zoster Immunoglobulin) is a non-proprietary, prescription-only preparation of a SPECIFIC IMMUNOGLOBULIN and is used to give immediate immunity against infection by varicella-zoster (chickenpox) virus. Administration is by intramuscular injection.
✚▲ Side-effects/warnings: See IMMUNIZATION.

varicella-zoster immunoglobulin

(VZIG) is a SPECIFIC IMMUNOGLOBULIN, which is a form of immunoglobulin that is used in IMMUNIZATION to give immediate *passive immunity* against infection by the varicella-zoster virus (chickenpox or herpes zosta), but is used only in immunosuppressed patients at risk, neonates whose mothers develop chickenpox seven days before, or 28 days after delivery, and pregnant women. (Varicella VACCINE is also available, but only on a named-patient basis.) Administration is by intramuscular injection.
✚▲ Side-effects/warnings: See IMMUNIZATION.
✪ **Related entry: Varicella-Zoster Immunoglobulin.**

Varidase Topical

(Lederle; Wyeth) is a proprietary, prescription-only preparation of the powdered enzymes streptokinase and streptodornase. It can be used, with a desloughing agent, to cleanse and soothe skin ulcers. It can also be administered through a catheter to dissolve clots in the urinary bladder. It is available as a powder.
✚▲ Side-effects/warnings: See STREPTOKINASE.

Var/Vac

is an abbreviation for variola vaccine (in fact made from *vaccinia* virus). See SMALLPOX VACCINE.

Vascace

(Roche) is a proprietary, prescription-only preparation of the ACE INHIBITOR cilazapril. It can be used as an ANTIHYPERTENSIVE in conjunction with other classes of drug, particularly (THIAZIDE) DIURETIC drugs, and is available as tablets.
✚▲ Side-effects/warnings: See CILAZAPRIL.

Vaseline Dermacare

(Elida Faberge) is a proprietary, non-prescription compound preparation of WHITE SOFT PARAFFIN and dimeticone. It can be used as an EMOLLIENT for dry skin, eczema, scaly or itchy skin and related disorders. It is available as a cream and a lotion.
✚▲ Side-effects/warnings: DIMETICONE; WHITE SOFT PARAFFIN.

vasoconstrictor 🅱

drugs cause a narrowing (constricting) of the blood vessels and therefore a reduction in blood flow and an increase in blood pressure. They are used to increase blood pressure in circulatory disorders, in cases of shock or where pressure has fallen during lengthy or complex surgery. Different vasoconstrictors work in different ways, but many are sympathomimetics (see SYMPATHOMIMETIC) with ALPHA-ADRENOCEPTOR STIMULANT properties. Most vasoconstrictors have an effect on mucous membranes and therefore may be used to relieve nasal congestion (eg OXYMETAZOLINE HYDROCHLORIDE and XYLOMETAZOLINE HYDROCHLORIDE). Some are used to prolong the effects of local anaesthetics (eg ADRENALINE ACID TARTRATE; epinephrine). Vasoconstrictors used in circulatory shock include METHOXAMINE HYDROCHLORIDE, NORADRENALINE (norepinephrine) and PHENYLEPHRINE HYDROCHLORIDE.

vasodilator

drugs dilate blood vessels and thereby increase blood flow. Drugs of this class work in a number of different ways: some have SMOOTH MUSCLE RELAXANT activity and act directly on the blood vessels (eg NITRATE compounds and CALCIUM-CHANNEL BLOCKER drugs); whereas others act indirectly by blocking or modifying the action of hormones (see HORMONE) or neurotransmitters (eg ALPHA-ADRENOCEPTOR BLOCKER and ACE INHIBITOR drugs). Vasodilator drugs are used for a number of purposes when blood flow needs to be increased, including as ANTI-ANGINA drugs (eg GLYCERYL TRINITRATE), in acute hypertensive crisis (eg SODIUM NITROPRUSSIDE), as ANTIHYPERTENSIVE drugs to treat chronic raised blood pressure (eg HYDRALAZINE HYDROCHLORIDE and NIFEDIPINE) and to treat poor circulation in the extremities (peripheral vascular disease, or Raynaud's Phenomenon, eg INOSITOL NICOTINATE).

Vasogen Cream

(Pharmax) is a proprietary, non-prescription compound preparation of zinc oxide, dimeticone and calamine. It can be used for nappy rash, bedsores and the skin around a stoma (an outlet on the skin surface following surgical curtailment of the intestines). It is available as a cream.

✚▲ Side-effects/warnings: See CALAMINE; DIMETICONE; ZINC OXIDE.

vasopressin

is one of the pituitary hormones (see HORMONE) secreted by the posterior lobe of the pituitary gland. It is also known as *antidiuretic hormone*, or ADH. Naturally, it occurs in two forms called argipressin and lypressin, but only the former is currently used therapeutically. It is used mainly to treat pituitary-originated diabetes insipidus, but it is a powerful VASOCONSTRICTOR and can also be used to treat bleeding from varices (varicose veins) of the oesophagus. There are alternative synthetic forms of vasopressin (DESMOPRESSIN and TERLIPRESSIN), which all differ in their duration of action and uses. Administration is by intravenous injection or infusion.

✚ Side-effects: Peripheral vasoconstriction with pallor of skin; nausea, vomiting, belching, abdominal cramps and an urge to defecate, headache, fluid retention, tremor, vertigo; hypersensitivity reactions, constriction of coronary arteries (possibly leading to angina and heart pain).

▲ Warnings: Dosage will be adjusted to individual response in order to balance water levels in the body. Great care is necessary in patients with asthma, epilepsy, certain kidney disorders, migraine, heart failure, who are pregnant or have certain vascular disorders. Treatment must not be prolonged and should be carefully and regularly monitored; intermittent treatment is needed to avoid water overloading.

✪ **Related entry: Pitressin.**

Vasoxine

(GSK) is a proprietary, prescription-only preparation of the SYMPATHOMIMETIC and VASOCONSTRICTOR methoxamine hydrochloride. It can be used to treat cases of acute hypotension, such as where blood pressure has dropped because of induction of general anaesthesia, and is available in a form for intravenous injection or infusion.

✚▲ Side-effects/warnings: See METHOXAMINE HYDROCHLORIDE.

Vectavir

(Novartis) is a proprietary, prescription-only preparation of the ANTIVIRAL drug penciclovir. It can be used to treat herpes labialis, and is available in a cream for topical application.

✚▲ Side-effects/warnings: See PENCICLOVIR.

vecuronium bromide

is a (*non-depolarizing*) SKELETAL MUSCLE RELAXANT which is used to induce muscle paralysis during surgery. Administration is by injection.

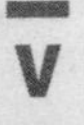

✚▲ Side-effects/warnings: It is a specialist drug used by anaesthetists in hospital.
✪ **Related entry: Norcuron.**

Veganin Tablets

(Warner Lambert Consumer Healthcare; Pfizer) is a proprietary, non-prescription compound analgesic preparation of the NON-NARCOTIC ANALGESIC and ANTIRHEUMATIC aspirin, the non-narcotic analgesic and ANTIPYRETIC paracetamol and the (OPIOID) ANTITUSSIVE codeine phosphate. It can be used to treat the symptoms of flu, headache, rheumatism, toothache and period pain. It is available as tablets and is not to be given to children, except on medical advice.
✚▲ Side-effects/warnings: See ASPIRIN; CODEINE PHOSPHATE; PARACETAMOL.

Velbe

(Lilly) is a proprietary, prescription-only preparation of the ANTICANCER drug vinblastine sulphate. It can be used in the treatment of a range of cancers. It is available in a form for injection.
✚▲ Side-effects/warnings: See VINBLASTINE SULPHATE.

Velosef

(Squibb; Bristol-Myers Squibb) is a proprietary, prescription-only preparation of the ANTIBACTERIAL and (CEPHALOSPORIN) ANTIBIOTIC cefradine. It can be used to treat a range of bacterial infections, and is available as capsules, a syrup and in a form for injection.
✚▲ Side-effects/warnings: See CEFRADINE.

venlafaxine

is an ANTIDEPRESSANT that has similarities to the SSRI group, but can be referred to as a *selective serotonin and noradrenaline uptake inhibitor* (SNRI) in that it seems to work by inhibiting uptake of both these NEUROTRANSMITTER, and so has less sedative and ANTICHOLINERGIC (ANTIMUSCARINIC) side-effects than the *tricyclics*. It can be used to treat depressive illness and administration is oral.
✚ Side-effects: Nausea, dry mouth, headache, sleep disturbances, dizziness; constipation, weakness, sweating, nervousness, convulsions (when it should be discontinued); gastrointestinal and various other side-effects have also been reported.
▲ Warnings: Should not be used in patients with liver or kidney impairment, pregnancy or breast-feeding. Should be used with caution if there is a history of myocardial infarction or certain heart diseases, epilepsy, blood pressure monitoring may be required. Caution if there is epilepsy. It may affect driving.
✪ **Related entry: Efexor.**

Venofer

(Syner-Med) is a proprietary, prescription-only preparation of a complex of IRON (as sucrose) which can be used as an iron supplement in iron-deficiency ANAEMIA TREATMENT, and is available in a form for injection.
✚▲ Side-effects/warnings: See IRON SUCROSE.

Ventide

(A&H; GSK) is a proprietary, prescription-only compound preparation of the CORTICOSTEROID beclometasone dipropionate and the SYMPATHOMIMETIC, BRONCHODILATOR and BETA-RECEPTOR STIMULANT salbutamol. It can be used as a treatment for the symptomatic relief of obstructive airways disease, such as in ANTI-ASTHMATIC treatment. It is available as an aerosol inhalant and as a dry powder for inhalation (called *Rotacaps* and *Paediatric Rotacaps*; used in a special inhaler *Ventide Rotahaler*).
✚▲ Side-effects/warnings: See BECLOMETASONE DIPROPIONATE; SALBUTAMOL.

Ventmax SR

(Trinity) is a proprietary, prescription-only preparation of the BETA-RECEPTOR STIMULANT salbutamol (as salbutamol sulphate). It can be used as a BRONCHODILATOR in reversible obstructive airways disease, such as in ANTI-ASTHMATIC treatment. It is available as capsules.
✚▲ Side-effects/warnings: See SALBUTAMOL.

Ventodisks

(A&H; GSK) is a proprietary, prescription-only preparation of the BETA-RECEPTOR STIMULANT salbutamol (as salbutamol sulphate). It can be used as a BRONCHODILATOR in reversible obstructive airways disease, such as in ANTI-ASTHMATIC treatment in severe acute asthma. It is available in the form of disks of dry powder for use with the *Diskhaler* device.
✚▲ Side-effects/warnings: See SALBUTAMOL.

Ventolin

(A&H; GSK) is a proprietary, prescription-only preparation of the BETA-RECEPTOR STIMULANT salbutamol (as salbutamol sulphate). It can be used as a BRONCHODILATOR in reversible obstructive airways disease, such as in ANTI-ASTHMATIC treatment. It is available in many forms: as a sugar-free syrup, ampoules for injection, an infusion fluid, an aerosol-metered inhalant (*Evohaler*), as ampoules for nebulization spray (under the name *Nebules*), as a respirator solution and as a powder for inhalation (under the name *Accuhaler* and *Rotacaps*).

✚▲ Side-effects/warnings: See SALBUTAMOL.

Vepesid

(Bristol-Myers Squibb) is a proprietary, prescription-only preparation of the (CYTOTOXIC) ANTICANCER drug etoposide. It can be used in the treatment of cancers, particularly lymphoma or small cell carcinoma of the bronchus, or cancer of the testicle. It is available as capsules and in a form for injection.

✚▲ Side-effects/warnings: See ETOPOSIDE.

Veracur

(Typharm) is a proprietary, non-prescription preparation of the KERATOLYTIC agent formaldehyde. It can be used to treat warts, especially verrucas (plantar warts), and is available as a gel.

✚▲ Side-effects/warnings: See FORMALDEHYDE.

verapamil hydrochloride

is a CALCIUM-CHANNEL BLOCKER which is used as an ANTI-ANGINA drug in the prevention and treatment of attacks, as an ANTI-ARRHYTHMIC to correct heart irregularities and as an ANTIHYPERTENSIVE and after myocardial infarction as prophylaxis. Administration can be either oral or by intravenous injection or infusion.

✚ Side-effects: There may be constipation, nausea and vomiting; headache, dizziness, muscle and joint pain, tingling in the extremities, flushing, fatigue; swollen ankles; rarely, there may be impairment of liver function; allergic skin reactions; gynaecomastia (enlargement of breasts in males); abnormal growth of the gums, and heart and cardiovascular problems on prolonged treatment.

▲ Warnings: It should not be taken by patients with certain heart disorders or porphyria. Administered with caution in patients with certain liver or heart disorders, or who are pregnant or breast-feeding. Grapefruit juice should be avoided since it affects the metabolism of the drug.

✪ Related entries: Cordilox; Cordilox MR; Ethimil MR; Half Securon SR; Securon; Tarka; Univer; Verapress MR; Vertab SR 240.

Verapress MR

(Dexcel) is a proprietary, prescription-only preparation of the CALCIUM-CHANNEL BLOCKER verapamil hydrochloride. It can be used as an ANTIHYPERTENSIVE. It is available as modified-release tablets.

✚▲ Side-effects/warnings: See VERAPAMIL HYDROCHLORIDE.

Vermox

(Janssen-Cilag) is a proprietary, prescription-only preparation of the ANTHELMINTIC drug mebendazole. It can be used to treat infections by roundworm, threadworm, whipworm and hookworm and similar intestinal parasites. It is available as chewable tablets and a liquid oral suspension.

✚▲ Side-effects/warnings: See MEBENDAZOLE.

Verrugon

(Pickles) is a proprietary, non-prescription preparation of the KERATOLYTIC agent salicylic acid. It can be used to remove plantar warts (verrucas), and is available as an ointment.

✚▲ Side-effects/warnings: See SALICYLIC ACID.

Vertab SR 240

(Trinity) is a proprietary, prescription-only preparation of the CALCIUM-CHANNEL BLOCKER verapamil hydrochloride. It can be used as an ANTIHYPERTENSIVE and in ANTI-ANGINA treatment. It is available as modified-release tablets.

✚▲ Side-effects/warnings: See VERAPAMIL HYDROCHLORIDE.

verteporfin

is a newly introduced drug for specialist use only for photodynamic treatment of subfoveal choroidal neovascularization associated with age-related macular degeneration or with pathological myopia (see PHOTODYNAMIC THERAPY). Following intravenous infusion, verteporfin is activated by local irradiation using non-thermal red light to produce CYTOTOXIC derivatives. Treatment with verteporfin is always carried out by specialists.

✚ Side-effects: Visual disturbances, which might include blurred vision, flashing lights and visual-field defects. There may also be nausea, back pain, weakness, pruritus, hypercholesterolaemia, hypertension, chest pain, fainting and fever. Rarely, there may be other eye problems such as tear disorders or subretinal or vitreous haemorrhage. At the site of the injection there may also be reactions.

▲ Warnings: People with porphyria or who are breast-feeding should not have this treatment and it is suitable only with care for people who have liver impairment, biliary obstruction or who are pregnant. Exposure of unprotected skin and eyes to bright light should be avoided during infusion and for 48 hours afterwards because of possible photosensitivity.

✪ **Related entry: Visudyne.**

Vesanoid

(Roche) is a proprietary, prescription-only preparation of the (RETINOID) tretinoin. It can be used as an ANTICANCER drug to treat acute promyelocytic leukaemia, and is available as capsules.

✚▲ Side-effects/warnings: See TRETINOIN.

Vexol

(Alcon) is a proprietary, prescription-only preparation of the CORTICOSTEROID and ANTI-INFLAMMATORY rimexolone. It can be used to treat inflammatory eye disorders. It is available as eye-drops.

✚▲ Side-effects/warnings: See RIMEXOLONE.

Viagra

(Pfizer) is a prescription-only preparation of the VASODILATOR sildenafil (as citrate), and is used in IMPOTENCE TREATMENT for men to manage penile erectile dysfunction. At the time of writing, there are certain NHS restrictions on patients for whom it may be prescribed. It is available as tablets.

✚▲ Side-effects/warnings: See SILDENAFIL.

ViATIM

(Aventis Pasteur) is a proprietary, prescription-only VACCINE preparation of hepatitis A vaccine. It can be used to for immunization against hepatitis A infection in people aged over 16 years. It is available in a form for injection.

✚▲ Side-effects/warnings: See HEPATITIS A VACCINE.

Viazem XL

(Genus) is a proprietary, prescription-only preparation of the CALCIUM-CHANNEL BLOCKER diltiazem hydrochloride. It can be used as an ANTIHYPERTENSIVE and as an ANTI-ANGINA drug. It is available as modified-release capsules.

✚▲ Side-effects/warnings: See DILTIAZEM HYDROCHLORIDE.

Vibramycin

(Pfizer) is a proprietary, prescription-only preparation of the ANTIBACTERIAL and (TETRACYCLINES) ANTIBIOTIC doxycycline. It can be used to treat a wide range of infections, and is available as capsules.

✚▲ Side-effects/warnings: See DOXYCYCLINE.

Vibramycin D

(Pfizer) is a proprietary, prescription-only preparation of the ANTIBACTERIAL and (TETRACYCLINES) ANTIBIOTIC doxycycline. It can be used to treat a wide range of infections, and is available as soluble tablets.

✚▲ Side-effects/warnings: See DOXYCYCLINE.

Vicks Inhaler

(Proctor & Gamble) is a proprietary, non-prescription preparation of camphor and menthol with pine needle oil. It can be used as a NASAL DECONGESTANT for the relief of nasal congestion. It is available as a nasal stick and is not given to children under six years, except on medical advice.

✚▲ Side-effects/warnings: See CAMPHOR; MENTHOL.

Vicks Medinite

(Procter & Gamble) is a proprietary, non-prescription compound preparation of the NON-NARCOTIC ANALGESIC and ANTIPYRETIC paracetamol, the (OPIOID) ANTITUSSIVE dextromethorphan hydrobromide, the ANTIHISTAMINE doxylamine (as succinate), and the SYMPATHOMIMETIC and DECONGESTANT pseudoephedrine hydrochloride. It can be used for the symptomatic relief of colds and flu, and is

available as a syrup. It is not normally given to children under ten years, except on medical advice.
✚▲ Side-effects/warnings: See DEXTROMETHORPHAN HYDROBROMIDE; DOXYLAMINE; PARACETAMOL; PSEUDOEPHEDRINE HYDROCHLORIDE.

Vicks Sinex Decongestant Nasal Spray

(Procter & Gamble) is a proprietary, non-prescription preparation of the SYMPATHOMIMETIC and VASOCONSTRICTOR oxymetazoline hydrochloride. It can be used as a NASAL DECONGESTANT for the symptomatic relief of nasal congestion associated with a wide variety of upper respiratory tract disorders, such as hay fever and colds. It is available as a nasal spray and is not normally given to children under six years, except on medical advice.
✚▲ Side-effects/warnings: See OXYMETAZOLINE HYDROCHLORIDE.

Vicks Vaporub

(Proctor & Gamble) is a proprietary, non-prescription preparation of turpentine oil, eucalyptus oil, camphor and menthol. It can be used to relieve nasal congestion, cough caused by colds and sore throat. It is available as an ointment that is rubbed onto the chest and back and the vapours inhaled. It is not given to children under six months, except on medical advice.
✚▲ Side-effects/warnings: See CAMPHOR; MENTHOL; TURPENTINE OIL.

Vicks Vaposyrup for Chesty Coughs

(Procter & Gamble) is a proprietary, non-prescription preparation of the EXPECTORANT guaifenesin (guaiphenesin). It can be used to relieve coughs and loosen the throat. It is available as a syrup. It is not normally given to children under two, except on medical advice.
✚▲ Side-effects/warnings: See GUAIFENESIN.

Vicks Vaposyrup for Dry Coughs

(Procter & Gamble) is a proprietary, non-prescription preparation of the (OPIOID) ANTITUSSIVE dextromethorphan hydrobromide. It can be used for relieving and calming coughs, and is available as a syrup. It is not normally given to children under two years, except on medical advice.
✚▲ Side-effects/warnings: See DEXTROMETHORPHAN HYDROBROMIDE.

Vicks Vaposyrup for Tickly Coughs

(Proctor & Gamble) is a proprietary, non-prescription preparation of menthol (as levomenthol). It can be used to relieve dry, irritating cough associated with the common cold. It is not given to children under six years, except on medical advice.
✚▲ Side-effects/warnings: See MENTHOL.

Videx

(Bristol-Myers Squibb) is a proprietary, prescription-only preparation of the ANTIVIRAL drug didanosine. It can be used in the treatment of HIV infection, and is available as tablets.
✚▲ Side-effects/warnings: See DIDANOSINE.

Videx EC

(Squibb; Bristol-Myers Squibb) is a proprietary, prescription-only preparation of the ANTIVIRAL drug didanosine. It can be used in the treatment of HIV infection, and is available as modified-release capsules.
✚▲ Side-effects/warnings: See DIDANOSINE.

vigabatrin

is an ANTI-EPILEPTIC drug which is used to treat epilepsy, especially in cases where other anti-epileptic drugs have not been effective (including infant spasms in West's syndrome). Administration is oral.
✚ Side-effects: These include; fatigue, dizziness, drowsiness, depression, headache, mood changes, nervousness and irritability, confusion, aggression, memory, visual and gastrointestinal disturbances; weight gain; psychotic episodes and excitation and agitation in children, and others.
▲ Warnings: It is administered with caution to patients with kidney impairment, who are pregnant or breast-feeding, or where there is a history of psychosis, depression or behavioural problems. Any problems with vision should be reported to the doctor, and vision is best checked regularly. Withdrawal should be gradual.
✪ **Related entry: Sabril.**

vinblastine sulphate

is a CYTOTOXIC drug and one of the VINCA ALKALOIDS. It can be used as an ANTICANCER treatment of acute leukaemias, lymphomas and

V

some solid tumours. Administration is by injection.
✚▲ Side-effects/warnings: See CYTOTOXIC.
✪ **Related entry: Velbe.**

Vinca alkaloids

are a type of CYTOTOXIC drug derived from the periwinkle *Vinca rosea*. They work by halting the process of cell replication and are therefore used as ANTICANCER drugs, particularly for acute leukaemias, lymphomas and some solid tumours. Their toxicity inevitably causes some serious side-effects, in particular, some loss of nerve function at the extremities, muscle weakness, constipation and bloating, all of which may be severe. There may be suppression of blood cells by the bone marrow. See VINBLASTINE SULPHATE; VINCRISTINE SULPHATE; VINDESINE SULPHATE; VINORELBINE.

vincristine sulphate

is a CYTOTOXIC drug and one of the VINCA ALKALOIDS. It is used as an ANTICANCER drug, particularly in the treatment of acute leukaemias, lymphomas and some solid tumours. Administration is by injection.
✚▲ Side-effects/warnings: See CYTOTOXIC. It causes little myelosuppression.
✪ **Related entry: Oncovin.**

vindesine sulphate

is a CYTOTOXIC drug and one of the VINCA ALKALOIDS. It is used as an ANTICANCER drug, particularly in the treatment of leukaemias, lymphomas and some solid tumours. Administration is by injection.
✚▲ Side-effects/warnings: See CYTOTOXIC.
✪ **Related entry: Eldisine.**

vinorelbine

is a CYTOTOXIC drug and one of the (semisynthetic) VINCA ALKALOIDS. It has been introduced as an ANTICANCER drug, for advanced breast cancer and for advanced non-small cell lung cancer. Administration is by injection.
✚▲ Side-effects/warnings: See CYTOTOXIC.
✪ **Related entry: Navelbine.**

Vioform-Hydrocortisone

(Novartis Consumer Health) is a proprietary, prescription-only compound preparation of the CORTICOSTEROID hydrocortisone and the ANTIMICROBIAL clioquinol. It can be used to treat inflammatory skin disorders, and is available as a water-based cream and an ointment.
✚▲ Side-effects/warnings: See CLIOQUINOL; HYDROCORTISONE.

Vioxx

(MSD) is a proprietary, prescription-only preparation of the (NSAID) NON-NARCOTIC ANALGESIC and ANTIRHEUMATIC rofecoxib. It can be used to relieve pain, particularly for symptomatic relief in osteoarthritis. It is available as tablets, *Vioxx Acute tablets* and an oral suspension.
✚▲ Side-effects/warnings: See ROFECOXIB.

Viracept

(Roche) is a proprietary, prescription-only preparation of the ANTIVIRAL nelfinavir (as mesilate). It can be used in the treatment of HIV infection, and is available as tablets and an oral powder.
✚▲ Side-effects/warnings: See NELFINAVIR.

Viraferon

(Schering-Plough) is a proprietary, prescription-only preparation of interferon (in the form alpha-2b, rbe). It can be used in the treatment of chronic active hepatitis B and chronic hepatitis C, and is available in a form for subcutaneous injection.
✚▲ Side-effects/warnings: See INTERFERON.

ViraferonPeg

(Schering-Plough) is a recently introduced proprietary, prescription-only preparation of the IMMUNOMODULATOR interferon (in the form peginterferon alpha-2b, rbe). It can be used combined with ribavirin to treat chronic hepatitis C or alone if treatment with ribavirin is not tolerated or is not suitable. It is available in a form for subcutaneous injection.
✚▲ Side-effects/warnings: See INTERFERON.

Viramune

(Boehringer Ingelheim) is a proprietary, prescription-only preparation of the ANTIVIRAL drug nevirapine. It can be used in the treatment of HIV infection, and is available as tablets and a suspension.
✚▲ Side-effects/warnings: See NEVIRAPINE.

Virasorb Cold Sore Cream

(SSL) is a proprietary, non-prescription preparation of the ANTIVIRAL drug aciclovir (acyclovir). It can be used to treat recurrent cold sores. It is available as a cream.

✚▲ Side-effects/warnings: See ACICLOVIR.

Virazole

(ICN) is a proprietary, prescription-only preparation of the ANTIVIRAL drug tribavirin. It can be used to treat serious respiratory infections. It is available in a form for inhalation.
✚▲ Side-effects/warnings: See TRIBAVIRIN.

Virgan

(Chauvin) is a recently introduced proprietary, prescription-only preparation of the ANTIVIRAL ganciclovir. It can be used to treat viral infections of the eye, including acute herpetic keratitis. It is available in the form of gel eye-drops.
✚▲ Side-effects/warnings: See GANCICLOVIR.

Viridal

(Schwarz) is a PROSTAGLANDIN, alprostadil (PGE_1). It is a prescription-only IMPOTENCE TREATMENT for men to manage penile erectile dysfunction. It is used by intracavernosal injection into the penis, and is available in a form for injection in packs called *Duo* and *Continuation Pack*.
✚▲ Side-effects/warnings: See ALPROSTADIL.

Virormone

(Ferring) is a proprietary, prescription-only preparation of the male sex hormone (see SEX HORMONES) testosterone (as testosterone propionate). In men, it can be used in hormone replacement therapy and for delayed puberty in boys; in women, as an ANTICANCER drug for breast cancer. It is available in a form for injection and as skin patches.
✚▲ Side-effects/warnings: See TESTOSTERONE.

Visclair

(Sinclair) is a proprietary, non-prescription preparation of the MUCOLYTIC and EXPECTORANT mecysteine hydrochloride (methyl cysteine hydrochloride). It can be used to reduce the viscosity of sputum and thus facilitate expectoration in patients with chronic asthma or bronchitis. It is available as tablets.
✚▲ Side-effects/warnings: See MECYSTEINE HYDROCHLORIDE.

Viscotears

(Novartis Ophthalmics) is a proprietary, non-prescription preparation of CARBOMER. It can be used as artificial tears where there is dryness of the eye due to disease (eg ketanoconjunctivitis). It is available as a liquid gel for application to the eye.
✚▲ Side-effects/warnings: See CARBOMER.

Viskaldix

(Novartis) is a proprietary, prescription-only compound preparation of the BETA-BLOCKER pindolol and the DIURETIC clopamide. It can be used as an ANTIHYPERTENSIVE for raised blood pressure, and is available as tablets.
✚▲ Side-effects/warnings: See CLOPAMIDE; PINDOLOL.

Visken

(Novartis) is a proprietary, prescription-only preparation of the BETA-BLOCKER pindolol. It can be used as an ANTIHYPERTENSIVE for raised blood pressure and as an ANTI-ANGINA treatment to relieve symptoms and improve exercise tolerance. It is available as modified-release tablets.
✚▲ Side-effects/warnings: See PINDOLOL.

Vista-Methasone

(Martindale) is a proprietary, prescription-only preparation of the CORTICOSTEROID and ANTI-INFLAMMATORY betamethasone (as sodium phosphate). It can be used to treat non-infective inflammation in the ear (eg in eczema), eye or nose, and is available as drops.
✚▲ Side-effects/warnings: See BETAMETHASONE.

Vista-Methasone-N

(Martindale) is a proprietary, prescription-only compound preparation of the ANTI-INFLAMMATORY and CORTICOSTEROID betamethasone (as sodium phosphate) and the ANTIBACTERIAL and (AMINOGLYCOSIDE) ANTI-BIOTIC neomycin sulphate. It can be used to treat inflammation in the ear, eye, or nose, and is available as drops.
✚▲ Side-effects/warnings: See BETAMETHASONE; NEOMYCIN SULPHATE.

Vistide

(Pharmacia) is a proprietary, prescription-only preparation of the ANTIVIRAL cidofovir. It can be used to treat viral infections in AIDS patients, and is available in a form for intravenous infusion.
✚▲ Side-effects/warnings: See CIDOFOVIR.

Visudyne

(Novartis Ophthalmics) is a newly introduced

proprietary, prescription-only preparation of the drug verteporfin. It can be used for photodynamic treatment of subfoveal choroidal neovascularization associated with age-related macular degeneration or with pathological myopia. It is available in a form for intravenous infusion.
✚▲ Side-effects/warnings: See VERTEPORFIN.

vitamin

is the term used to describe a substance that is required in small quantities for growth, development and proper functioning of the body. Because many of the vitamins cannot be synthesized by the body, they must be obtained from a normal, well-balanced diet. The lack of any one vitamin causes a specific deficiency disorder, which may be treated by the use of vitamin supplements.

vitamin A

is another term for RETINOL.

Vitamin A Palmitate

(Cambridge) is a proprietary, prescription-only preparation of retinol, or VITAMIN A, and can be used in vitamin A deficiency. It is available in a form for injection.
✚▲ Side-effects/warnings: See RETINOL.

vitamin B

is the collective term for a number of water-soluble vitamins, which are found particularly in dairy products, cereals and liver. See CYANOCOBALAMIN; FOLIC ACID; NICOTINAMIDE; NICOTINIC ACID.

vitamin C

see ASCORBIC ACID.

vitamin D

occurs in four main forms, D_1, D_2, D_3 and D_4, which are produced in plants or in human skin by the action of sunlight. Vitamin D facilitates the absorption of calcium and, to a lesser extent, phosphorus from the intestine and so promotes good deposition into the bones. A deficiency of vitamin D therefore results in bone deficiency disorders, such as rickets in children. It is readily available in a normal, well-balanced diet and particularly good sources include eggs, milk, cheese and fish-liver oil, which can be used as a dietary supplement. Vitamin D deficiency is most commonly found in communities eating unleavened bread, in the elderly and where certain diseases prevent proper absorption from food. The preferred therapeutic method (despite the cost) of replacing vitamin D in cases of severe deficiency is by using quantities of one of the synthetic vitamin D analogues, such as ALFACALCIDOL, CALCITRIOL, DIHYDROTACHYSTEROL and ERGOCALCIFEROL. However, as with most vitamins, prolonged administration of large doses can produce adverse effects (hypervitaminosis).
✚ Side-effects: There may be nausea, vomiting, anorexia, lassitude, diarrhoea, weight loss, sweating, headache, thirst, polyuria, dizziness and vertigo.
▲ Warnings: An overdose may cause kidney damage. Calcium levels should be monitored and use with care in those who are breast-feeding (high levels of calcium may reach the baby).
✪ Related entries: Halycitrol; Vitamin Tablets (with Calcium and Iodine) for Nursing Mothers.

vitamin E

(tocopherols) is a group of related substances that occur in foodstuffs, especially vegetable oils, nuts, leafy vegetables, cereals, wheat germ, meat and egg yolk. As a vitamin it has essential roles as a natural antioxidant and free-radical scavenger, protecting particularly fats from oxidation. The main important natural form is alpha tocopherol, and that used in medicine is ALPHA TOCOPHERYL ACETATE). In therapeutics, it is used to treat deficiency due to malabsorption, such as in abetalipoproteinaemia in young children with congenital cholestasis or cystic fibrosis and as a vitamin supplement. Some people take it in higher doses as a free-radical scavenger in the belief of protection against a number of disease states. Administration is oral.

vitamin K

is a fat-soluble vitamin that occurs naturally in two forms, vitamin K_1 (also called PHYTOMENADIONE) and vitamin K_2, and is an essential requirement for a healthy body. Vitamin K_1 is found in food and particularly good sources include fresh root vegetables, fruit, seeds, dairy products and meat. Vitamin K_2 is synthesized in the intestine by bacteria and this source supplements the dietary form. Vitamin K is necessary for blood-clotting factors (the name derives from the German name, *Koagulation* vitamin), and is also important for the proper calcification of bone.

Both forms of the vitamin require the secretion of bile salts by the liver and fat absorption from the intestine in order to be taken up into the body. For this reason, when treating vitamin K deficiency due to malabsorption disorders (eg due to obstruction of the bile ducts or in liver disease) a synthetic form, vitamin K_3 (usually called MENADIOL SODIUM PHOSPHATE) is administered, because it is water-soluble and therefore effective when taken orally in such disease states. However, in adults, deficiency of vitamin K is rare because it is so readily available in a normal, balanced diet, but medical administration may be required in fat malabsorption states, where the intestinal flora is disturbed by ANTIBIOTIC or certain ANTICOAGULANT (eg acenocoumarol) drugs. Vitamin K is given routinely to newborn babies to prevent vitamin-K-deficiency bleeding. Chronic overdose due to vitamin supplements (hypervitaminosis) can be dangerous.

✚ Side-effects: There may be liver damage if high doses are taken for a long period. Skin and allergic reactions have been reported.

▲ Warnings: It should be administered with caution to patients who are pregnant or susceptible to red-blood-cell haemolysis due to G6PD enzyme deficiency or vitamin E deficiency. See also MENADIOL SODIUM PHOSPHATE; PHYTOMENADIONE.

✪ Related entries: Konakion; Konakion MM; Konakion MM Paediatric; Konkion Neonatal Injection.

Vitamin Tablets (with Calcium and Iodine) for Nursing Mothers

(Sussex) is a non-proprietary, non-prescription MULTIVITAMIN preparation of vitamins A, C and D together with calcium (calcium hydrogen phosphate) and iodine (as potassium iodide). It is recommended by the Department of Health for routine supplementation to the diet of nursing mothers. It is available direct to families under the Welfare Food Scheme or direct to the public from maternity and child health clinics. It is available as tablets.

✚▲ Side-effects/warnings: See ASCORBIC ACID; RETINOL; VITAMIN D. Women who are (or may become) pregnant are advised not to take this supplement except on the advice of a doctor or antenatal clinic.

Vitrasert

(Bausch & Lomb) is a proprietary, prescription-only preparation of the ANTIVIRAL ganciclovir. It can be used to treat for sight-threatening viral infections and in immunocompromised patients. It is available in a form specifically for eye-infection as slow-release ocular implants.

✚▲ Side-effects/warnings: See GANCICLOVIR.

Vitravene

(Novartis Ophthalmics) is prescription-only preparation of the ANTIVIRAL fomivirsen sodium. It is used specifically for the local treatment of cytomegalovirus retinitis in patients with AIDS when other therapies have not worked or are not suitable. It is given by injection into the posterior chamber of the eye (intravitreal).

✚▲ Side-effects/warnings: See FOMIVIRSEN SODIUM.

Vividrin

(Pharma-Global) is a proprietary, preparation of the ANTI-ALLERGIC drug sodium cromoglicate. It can be used to prevent or treat allergic conditions of the eye such as conjunctivitis and is available (on prescription) as eye-drops, and as a nasal spray (non-prescription) for allergic conditions of the nose such as allergic rhinitis.

✚▲ Side-effects/warnings: See SODIUM CROMOGLICATE.

Vivotif

(MASTA) is a proprietary, prescription-only VACCINE preparation of typhoid vaccine as a *live* (attenuated) oral vaccine. It is available as capsules (which should be stored in the fridge).

✚▲ Side-effects/warnings: See TYPHOID VACCINE.

Volmax

(A&H) is a proprietary, prescription-only preparation of the BETA-RECEPTOR STIMULANT salbutamol (as salbutamol sulphate). It can be used as a BRONCHODILATOR in reversible obstructive airways disease, such as in ANTI-ASTHMATIC treatment. It is available as tablets.

✚▲ Side-effects/warnings: See SALBUTAMOL.

Volraman

(Eastern) is a proprietary, prescription-only

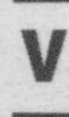

preparation of the (NSAID) NON-NARCOTIC ANALGESIC and ANTIRHEUMATIC diclofenac sodium. It can be used to treat arthritic and rheumatic pain, other musculoskeletal disorders and acute gout. Available as tablets.

✚▲ Side-effects/warnings: See DICLOFENAC SODIUM.

Voltarol

(Novartis) is a proprietary, prescription-only preparation of the (NSAID) NON-NARCOTIC ANALGESIC and ANTIRHEUMATIC diclofenac sodium. It can be used to treat arthritic and rheumatic pain and other musculoskeletal disorders. It is available as tablets, dispersible tablets, modified-release tablets (*Voltarol 75 mg SR*, *Voltarol Retard*), a form for migraine called *Voltarol Rapid*, suppositories, and in a form for injection.

✚▲ Side-effects/warnings: See DICLOFENAC SODIUM.

Voltarol Emulgel

(Novartis) is a proprietary, prescription-only preparation of the (NSAID) NON-NARCOTIC ANALGESIC diclofenac sodium (as diethylammonium), which also has COUNTER-IRRITANT, or RUBEFACIENT, actions. It can be used for the symptomatic relief of underlying muscle or joint pain and is available as a gel for topical application to the skin.

✚▲ Side-effects/warnings: See DICLOFENAC SODIUM; but adverse effects on topical application are limited.

Voltarol Ophtha

(Novartis Ophthalmics) is a proprietary, prescription-only preparation of the (NSAID) NON-NARCOTIC ANALGESIC diclofenac sodium. It can be used by topical application to inhibit contraction of the pupil of the eye, for other ophthalmic procedures, and is available as eye-drops.

✚▲ Side-effects/warnings: See DICLOFENAC SODIUM.

VZIG

see VARICELLA-ZOSTER IMMUNOGLOBULIN

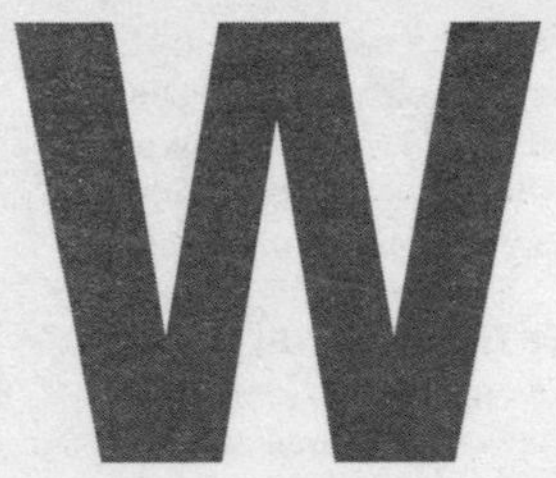

warfarin sodium

is an ANTICOAGULANT which can be used to prevent the formation of clots in heart disease, after heart surgery (especially following implantation of prosthetic heart valves) and venous thrombosis and pulmonary embolism for transient ischaemic attacks. Administration is oral.
✚ Side-effects: Haemorrhaging. There may be hypersensitivity reactions, rashes, hair loss, diarrhoea, skin problems ('purple toes'), kidney problems, nausea and vomiting.
▲ Warnings: Warfarin sodium should be administered with care to patients with certain kidney or liver disorders and after recent operations. It should not be used by patients with severe hypertension, bacterial endocarditis, peptic ulcer or who are pregnant. Aspirin taken concurrently may increase bleeding, some antidepressants (and St John's wort), alcohol (in large amounts), and vitamin K (and some dietary supplements) may increase the effects of warfarin, with a risk of bleeding.
✪ Related entry: Marevan.

Warticon

(Stiefel) is a proprietary, prescription-only preparation of the KERATOLYTIC agent podophyllotoxin, the main active constituent of podophyllum. It can be used to treat and remove warts on the external genitalia of men (*Warticon*), also from women (*Warticon Fem*), and is available as a solution (with applicator) and a cream for topical application.
✚▲ Side-effects/warnings: See PODOPHYLLUM.

Wasp-Eze Ointment

(SSL) is a proprietary, non-prescription preparation of the ANTIHISTAMINE antazoline hydrochloride. It can be used to relieve wasp and other insect stings and bites, and is available as an ointment. It is not used for children under one year, except on medical advice.
✚▲ Side-effects/warnings: See ANTAZOLINE.

Wasp-Eze Spray

(SSL) is a proprietary, non-prescription compound preparation of the ANTIHISTAMINE mepyramine maleate and the LOCAL ANAESTHETIC benzocaine. It can be used to relieve wasp and other insect stings and bites, nettle stings and jellyfish stings, and is available as a spray.
✚▲ Side-effects/warnings: See BENZOCAINE; DIPHENHYDRAMINE HYDROCHLORIDE.

Waxsol Ear Drops

(Norgine) is a proprietary, non-prescription preparation of docusate sodium. It can be used for the dissolution and removal of ear wax, and is available as ear-drops.
✚▲ Side-effects/warnings: See DOCUSATE SODIUM.

Wax Wane Ear Drops

(Thornton & Ross) is a proprietary, non-prescription preparation of turpentine oil, terpineol and chloroxylenol. It can be used to dissolve hard ear wax prior to its removal by syringing, and is available as ear-drops.
✚▲ Side-effects/warnings: See CHLOROXYLENOL; TURPENTINE OIL.

Welldorm

(S&N Hlth.) is a proprietary, prescription-only preparation of the HYPNOTIC drug chloral hydrate (in the form of cloral betaine (chloral betaine)). It can be used to treat short-term insomnia, and is available as tablets and an elixir.
✚▲ Side-effects/warnings: See CHLORAL HYDRATE.

Wellvone

(GlaxoWellcome; GSK) is a proprietary, prescription-only preparation of the ANTIPROTOZOAL drug atovaquone. It can be used to treat pneumonia caused by the protozoan micro-organism *Pneumocystis carinii* in patients with suppressed immune systems. It is available as tablets.
✚▲ Side-effects/warnings: See ATOVAQUONE.

white soft paraffin

is used as a base for ointments and is also

incorporated into EMOLLIENT preparations.
✚▲ Side-effects/warnings: It is regarded as safe in normal topical use. See also LIQUID PARAFFIN.
✪ **Related entries: Cetraben Emollient Cream; E45; Emulsifying Ointment, BP; Lacri-Lube; Lubri-Tears; Sprilon; Unguentum M; Vaseline Dermacare; Zinc and Salicylic Acid Paste, BP.**

Whitfield's Ointment

see BENZOIC ACID OINTMENT, COMPOUND, BP.

WinRho SDF

(Octapharma) is a proprietary, prescription-only preparation of anti-D Rh_0 immunoglobulin. It can be used to prevent rhesus-negative mothers from making antibodies against fetal rhesus-positive cells that may pass into the mother's circulation during childbirth. The result of this is to protect a future child from haemolytic disease of the newborn. It is available in a form for injection.
✚▲ Side-effects/warnings: See ANTI-D (RHO) IMMUNOGLOBULIN.

Woodward's Baby Chest Rub

(SSL) is a proprietary, non-prescription preparation of turpentine oil, eucalyptus oil and menthol. It can be used to relieve nasal congestion due to colds. It is available as an ointment that is rubbed onto the chest and back and the vapours inhaled. It is not given to children under three months, except on medical advice.
✚▲ Side-effects/warnings: See CAMPHOR; MENTHOL; TURPENTINE OIL.

Woodward's Colic Drops

(SSL) is a proprietary, non-prescription preparation of the ANTIFOAMING AGENT dimeticone (as simethicone). It can be used to relieve wind and griping pain in infants (under two years), and is available as a oral drops.
✚▲ Side-effects/warnings: See DIMETICONE.

Woodward's Gripe Water

(SSL) is a proprietary, non-prescription preparation of the ANTACID sodium bicarbonate (with dill seed oil). It can be used to relieve wind and griping pain in infants (under one years), and is available as an oral suspension.
✚▲ Side-effects/warnings: See SODIUM BICARBONATE.

Woodward's Teething Gel

(SSL) is a proprietary, non-prescription compound preparation of the LOCAL ANAESTHETIC lidocaine hydrochloride and the ANTISEPTIC cetylpyridinium chloride. It can be used for the temporary relief of pain caused by teething in babies over three months, and is available as a gel for topical application.
✚▲ Side-effects/warnings: See CETYLPYRIDINIUM CHLORIDE; LIDOCAINE HYDROCHLORIDE.

wool fat

which contains lanolin, is a greasy preparation of hydrous wool fat in a yellow soft paraffin base. It is used as a protective BARRIER CREAM on cracked, dry or scaling skin and encourages hydration.
✚▲ Side-effects/warnings: Local reactions may occur in sensitive people. See also LANOLIN.
✪ **Related entries: Decubal Clinic; E45; Hewletts Cream; Kamillosan; Lubri-Tears; Simple Eye Ointment; Sprilon.**

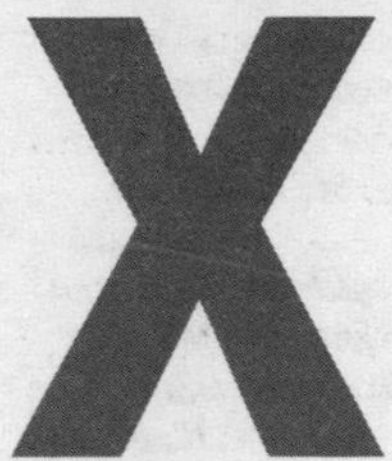

Xalacom

(Pharmacia) is proprietary prescription-only preparation of the PROSTAGLANDIN analogue latanoprost with the BETA-BLOCKER timolol. It can be used as a GLAUCOMA TREATMENT in open-angle glaucoma and ocular hypertension. It is available as eye-drops.
✚▲ Side-effects/warnings: See LATANOPROST; TIMOLOL MALEATE.

Xalatan

(Pharmacia) is proprietary, prescription-only preparation of the PROSTAGLANDIN analogue latanoprost. It can be used as a GLAUCOMA TREATMENT in open-angle glaucoma and ocular hypertension, and is available as eye-drops.
✚▲ Side-effects/warnings: See LATANOPROST.

Xanax

(Pharmacia) is a proprietary, prescription-only preparation of the BENZODIAZEPINE alprazolam. It can be used as an ANXIOLYTIC for the short-term treatment of anxiety, and is available as tablets.
✚▲ Side-effects/warnings: See ALPRAZOLAM.

xanthine-oxidase inhibitor

agents are ENZYME INHIBITOR drugs which work by inhibiting the enzyme (xanthine-oxidase) in the body that synthesizes uric acid and so can be used in the treatment of gout (because gout is caused by the deposition of uric acid crystal in the synovial tissue of joints). The most widely used xanthine-oxidase inhibitor is ALLOPURINOL, which is administered for the long-term treatment of gout (but not acute attacks which would be made worse).

Xanthomax

(Ashbourne) is a proprietary, prescription-only preparation of the ENZYME INHIBITOR allopurinol, which is a XANTHINE-OXIDASE INHIBITOR. It can be used to treat excess uric acid in the blood and so prevent renal stones and attacks of gout. It is available as tablets.
✚▲ Side-effects/warnings: See ALLOPURINOL.

Xatral

(Sanofi-Synthelabo) is a proprietary, prescription-only preparation of the ALPHA-ADRENOCEPTOR BLOCKER alfuzosin. It can be used to treat urinary retention (eg in benign prostatic hyperplasia), and is available as tablets.
✚▲ Side-effects/warnings: See ALFUZOSIN.

Xatral XL

(Sanofi-Synthelabo), is a proprietary, prescription-only preparation of the ALPHA-ADRENOCEPTOR BLOCKER alfuzosin. It can be used to treat urinary retention (eg in benign prostatic hyperplasia), and is available as modified-release tablets.
✚▲ Side-effects/warnings: See ALFUZOSIN.

Xefo

(CeNeS) is a proprietary, prescription-only preparation of the (NSAID) NON-NARCOTIC ANALGESIC and ANTIRHEUMATIC drug lornoxicam. It can be used to relieve the pain and inflammation in osteoarthritis and rheumatoid arthritis, with acute lumbo-sciatica, and in the short-term treatment of moderate post-operative pain. It is available as modified-release capsules and in a form for injection.
✚▲ Side-effects/warnings: See LORNOXICAM.

Xeloda

(Roche) is a proprietary, prescription-only preparation of the ANTICANCER drug capecitabine. It is available as tablets.
✚▲ Side-effects/warnings: See CAPECITABINE.

Xenical

(Roche) is a proprietary, prescription-only preparation of orlistat. It can be used adjunct in OBESITY TREATMENT, working by reducing the absorption of dietary fat. It is available as capsules.
✚▲ Side-effects/warnings: See ORLISTAT.

Xepin

(Bioglan) is a proprietary, prescription-only preparation of doxepin, commonly used as a (TRICYCLIC) ANTIDEPRESSANT but which in this

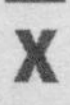

preparation acts as a topical ANTIHISTAMINE to treat pruritus (itching) associated with eczema. It is available as a cream.
✚▲ Side-effects/warnings: See DOXEPIN.

xipamide
is a DIURETIC of the THIAZIDE-related class. It can be used as an ANTIHYPERTENSIVE (either alone or in conjunction with other drugs) and also in HEART FAILURE TREATMENT and associated oedema. Administration is oral.
✚▲ Side-effects/warnings: See BENDROFLUMETHIAZIDE. Also, there may be mild dizziness and gastrointestinal upsets.
✪ **Related entry: Diurexan.**

Xylocaine
(AstraZeneca) is a series of proprietary, mainly prescription-only preparations of the LOCAL ANAESTHETIC lidocaine hydrochloride (lignocaine hydrochloride). They can be used for inducing anaesthesia or relieving pain by a variety of methods of application and at a number of sites. Solutions and forms for injection are available only on prescription (including dental cartridges); but ointment, gel and spray preparations are available without prescription.
✚▲ Side-effects/warnings: See LIDOCAINE HYDROCHLORIDE.

xylometazoline hydrochloride
is an ALPHA-ADRENOCEPTOR STIMULANT and SYMPATHOMIMETIC drug with VASOCONSTRICTOR properties, which is why it is mainly used as a NASAL DECONGESTANT. It is available as nose-drops and as a nasal spray, and is also a constituent of some eye-drop preparations that are used to treat allergic conjunctivitis.
✚▲ Side-effects/warnings: See EPHEDRINE HYDROCHLORIDE.
✪ **Related entries: Otradrops Adult; Otradrops Paediatric; Otraspray; Otrivine Adult Menthol Nasal Spray; Otrivine Adult Nasal Drops; Otrivine Adult Nasal Spray; Otrivine Children's Nasal Drops; Otrivine Measured Dose Sinusitis Spray; Otrivine-Antistin; Rynacrom Allergy Nasal Spray; Rynacrom Compound; Sudafed Decongestant Nasal Spray; Tixycolds Cold and Allergy Nasal Drops.**

Xyloproct
(Astra) is a proprietary, prescription-only compound preparation of the CORTICOSTEROID hydrocortisone (as acetate), the LOCAL ANAESTHETIC lidocaine hydrochloride (with aluminium acetate) and the ASTRINGENT zinc oxide. It can be used by topical application to treat haemorrhoids, and is available as an ointment.
✚▲ Side-effects/warnings: See ALUMINIUM ACETATE; HYDROCORTISONE; LIDOCAINE HYDROCHLORIDE; ZINC OXIDE.

Xyzal
(UCB Pharma) is a proprietary, prescription-only preparation of the ANTIHISTAMINE levocetirizine dihydrochloride. It can be used to treat the symptoms of allergic disorders, such as hay fever and urticaria, and is available as tablets.
✚▲ Side-effects/warnings: See LEVOCETIRIZINE HYDROCHLORIDE.

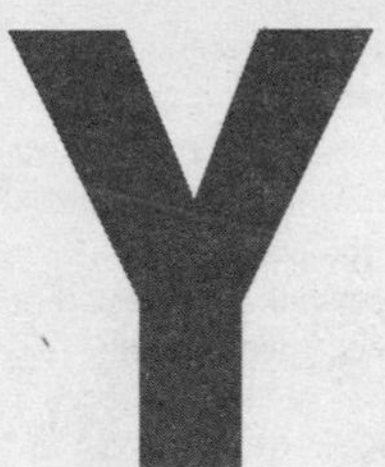

Yeast-vite

(SSL) is a proprietary, non-prescription preparation of the STIMULANT caffeine along with B vitamins. It can be used to give relief of fatigue and drowsiness. It is not given to children, except on medical advice.
✚▲ Side-effects/warnings: See CAFFEINE.

yellow fever vaccine

(Yel/Vac) is a VACCINE used for IMMUNIZATION that consists of a protein suspension containing *live*, but weakened (attenuated), yellow fever viruses that are cultured in chick embryos. Immunity lasts for at least ten years. The disease is still prevalent in many parts of Africa and South America. Administration is by subcutaneous injection.
✚▲ Side-effects/warnings: See VACCINE. It should not be administered to those who are pregnant, allergic to egg or have impaired immune systems.
✪ **Related entry: Arilvax.**

yellow soft paraffin

is used as a base for ointments and is also incorporated into EMOLLIENT preparations that are used for skin treatments.
✚▲ Side-effects/warnings: It is regarded as safe in normal topical use. See also LIQUID PARAFFIN.
✪ **Related entries: Epaderm; Simple Eye Ointment; Zinc and Coal Tar Paste, BP.**

Yel/Vac

is an abbreviation for YELLOW FEVER VACCINE.

Yutopar

(Solvay) is a proprietary, prescription-only preparation of the BETA-ADRENOCEPTOR STIMULANT ritodrine hydrochloride. It can be used to prevent or delay premature labour, and is available as tablets or in a form for intravenous infusion.
✚▲ Side-effects/warnings: See RITODRINE HYDROCHLORIDE.

Z

Zacin

(Elan) is a proprietary, prescription-only preparation of capsaicin, the main active principle of capsicum oleoresin, and has COUNTER-IRRITANT, or RUBEFACIENT, actions. It can be applied to the skin for symptomatic relief of pain in osteoarthritis.

✚▲ Side-effects/warnings: See CAPSICUM OLEORESIN.

Zaditen

(Novartis) is a proprietary, prescription-only preparation of ketotifen (as hydrogen fumarate). It can be used as an ANTI-ASTHMATIC treatment, and is available as capsules, tablets and an elixir.

✚▲ Side-effects/warnings: See KETOTIFEN.

Zaedoc

(Ashbourne) is a proprietary, prescription-only preparation of the H_2-ANTAGONIST and ULCER-HEALING DRUG ranitidine (as hydrochloride). It can be used to treat benign peptic ulcers (in the stomach or duodenum), gastro-oesophageal reflux, dyspepsia and associated conditions. It is available as tablets.

✚▲ Side-effects/warnings: See RANITIDINE.

zafirlukast

is an ANTI-ASTHMATIC drug. It can be used in the treatment of asthma to prevent mild to moderate attacks, but not to treat acute attacks. It represents a new drug class called LEUKOTRIENE-RECEPTOR ANTAGONIST drugs which work as ANTI-ALLERGIC agents by blocking the actions of leukotrienes, which are natural inflammatory mediators released in the lungs. Administration is oral.

✚ Side-effects: May cause gastrointestinal disturbances; headaches; bleeding disorders; some skin reactions and other hypersensitivity reactions, and very rarely may cause blood disorders. It is not used in breast-feeding women or those with impaired liver function.

▲ Warnings: It should be used with caution in pregnancy, the elderly, and where there is kidney impairment. Unusual symptoms need to be reported to the doctor because of current concern about development of the so-called Churg-Strauss syndrome.

✪ **Related entry: Accolate.**

zalcitabine

(ddC; DDC) is a (*reverse transcriptase inhibitor*) ANTIVIRAL drug which can be used in the treatment of HIV infection, in combination with other antiviral drugs. Administration is oral.

✚ Side-effects: It is a specialist drug, and there will be full assessment and patient monitoring throughout treatment. There are extensive side-effects, including peripheral neuropathy, nausea, vomiting, mouth ulcers, anorexia and weight loss; diarrhoea or constipation, abdominal pain; headache, dizziness and rash; mood changes and hearing and visual disorders, and other disorders.

▲ Warnings: It should not be used in patients with peripheral neuropathy or who are breast-feeding. It should be administered with care where there is a history of pancreatitis, certain heart disorders or impaired liver or kidney function, or who are pregnant.

✪ **Related entry: Hivid.**

zaleplon

is a newly introduced HYPNOTIC drug which works in the same way as the BENZODIAZEPINE group of drugs (though it is not chemically a benzodiazepine). It can be used for the short-term treatment of insomnia. Administration is oral.

✚ Side-effects: Headache, asthenia, drowsiness, dependence, dizziness, amnesia, some paradoxical effects (hostility, aggression, talkativeness, excitement).

▲ Warnings: Zaleplon should not be used by anyone who suffers from sleep apnoea syndrome, myasthenia gravis or who are breast-feeding. It should be given with care to anyone who is pregnant. It is prescribed with caution for those people with respiratory insufficiency, impaired liver function and for those who have a history of drug or alcohol abuse. It should not be used for any prolonged periods of time and withdrawal of treatment

should be gradual.
✪ **Related entry: Sonata.**

Zamadol
(ASTA Medica) is a proprietary, prescription-only preparation of the (OPIOID) NARCOTIC ANALGESIC tramadol hydrochloride. It can be used to relieve pain, but seems to differ from typical opioids in the way it works. It is available as capsules, modified-release capsules (*Zamadol SR*), and in a form for injection.
✚▲ Side-effects/warnings: See TRAMADOL HYDROCHLORIDE.

Zanaflex
(Elan) is a proprietary, prescription-only preparation of the SKELETAL MUSCLE RELAXANT tizanidine (as hydrochloride). It can be used for relieving severe spasticity of muscles in spasm (eg multiple sclerosis), and is available as tablets.
✚▲ Side-effects/warnings: See TIZANIDINE.

zanamivir
is an ANTIVIRAL drug which works as an ENZYME INHIBITOR (a neuraminidase inhibitor) that inhibits influenza virus replication. It can be used in the treatment of influenza A or B. It may be given to shorten the duration of infection. At the time of writing, there are restrictions on its NHS prescription. It is used to treat at-risk adults when influenza is circulating in the community if it is possible to commence treatment within 48 hours after the onset of symptoms. Administration is oral.
✚ Side-effects: Gastrointestinal disturbances; rarely, respiratory impairment or bronchospasm, rash.
▲ Warnings: It should not be used in breast-feeding. Administer with caution in the elderly, those with respiratory disease, immunocompromised people, or those who have chronic illnesses.
✪ **Related entry: Relenza.**

Zanidip
(Napp) is a proprietary, prescription-only preparation of the CALCIUM-CHANNEL BLOCKER lercanidipine hydrochloride. It can be used as an ANTIHYPERTENSIVE for mild to moderate essential hypertension. It is available as tablets.
✚▲ Side-effects/warnings: See LERCANIDIPINE HYDROCHLORIDE.

Zantac
(GSK) is a proprietary, prescription-only preparation of the H_2-ANTAGONIST and ULCER-HEALING DRUG ranitidine (as hydrochloride). It can be used to treat benign peptic ulcers (in the stomach or duodenum), gastro-oesophageal reflux, dyspepsia and associated conditions. It is available as tablets, effervescent tablets, a syrup and in a form for intravenous injection or infusion.
✚▲ Side-effects/warnings: See RANITIDINE.

Zantac 75 Relief Tablets
(GSK Consumer Healthcare) is a proprietary, non-prescription preparation of the H_2-ANTAGONIST and ULCER-HEALING DRUG ranitidine (as hydrochloride). It is available without a prescription only in a limited amount for indigestion, heartburn and hyperacidity, and is available as tablets. It is not normally given to children under 16 years, except on medical advice.
✚▲ Side-effects/warnings: See RANITIDINE.

Zarontin
(Parke-Davis; Pfizer) is a proprietary, prescription-only preparation of the ANTICONVULSANT and ANTI-EPILEPTIC drug ethosuximide. It can be used to treat absence (petit mal), myoclonic and some other types of seizure. It is available as capsules and a syrup.
✚▲ Side-effects/warnings: See ETHOSUXIMIDE.

Zavedos
(Pharmacia) is a proprietary, prescription-only preparation of the ANTICANCER drug idarubicin hydrochloride. It can be used to treat various cancers, and is available as capsules and in a form for injection.
✚▲ Side-effects/warnings: See IDARUBICIN HYDROCHLORIDE.

Zeffix
(GSK) is a proprietary, prescription-only preparation of the ANTIVIRAL lamivudine. It can be used in the treatment of HIV infection and chronic hepatitis B infection, and is available as tablets and as an oral solution.
✚▲ Side-effects/warnings: See LAMIVUDINE.

Zelapar
(Athena; Elan) is a proprietary, prescription-only

preparation of the ANTIPARKINSONISM drug selegiline. It can be used in the treatment of the symptoms of parkinsonism, and is available as a form of freeze-dried tablets (oral lyophilisates) that are placed on the tongue and allowed to dissolve.
✚▲ Side-effects/warnings: See SELEGILINE.

Zenapax

(Roche) is a proprietary, prescription-only preparation of the IMMUNOSUPPRESSANT daclizumab. It can be used to prevent rejection in kidney transplant patients (under specialist supervision). It is available in a form for intravenous infusion.
✚▲ Side-effects/warnings: See DACLIZUMAB.

Zentel

(SmithKline Beecham) is a proprietary, prescription-only preparation of the ANTHELMINTIC drug albendazole. It can be used for tapeworm cysts and to treat strongyloidiasis. Available as tablets (named-patient basis only).
✚▲ Side-effects/warnings: See ALBENDAZOLE.

Zerit

(Bristol-Myers Squibb) is a proprietary, prescription-only preparation of the ANTIVIRAL drug stavudine. It can be used in the treatment of HIV infection, and is available as capsules and an oral solution.
✚▲ Side-effects/warnings: See STAVUDINE.

Zestoretic

(AstraZeneca) is a proprietary, prescription-only compound preparation of the ACE INHIBITOR lisinopril and the (THIAZIDE) DIURETIC hydrochlorothiazide. It can be used as an ANTIHYPERTENSIVE and is available as tablets in two strengths, *Zestoretic 10* and *Zestoretic 20*.
✚▲ Side-effects/warnings: See HYDROCHLOROTHIAZIDE; LISINOPRIL.

Zestril

(AstraZeneca) is a proprietary, prescription-only preparation of the ACE INHIBITOR lisinopril (as dihydrate). It can be used as an ANTIHYPERTENSIVE and in HEART FAILURE TREATMENT, and is available as tablets.
✚▲ Side-effects/warnings: See LISINOPRIL.

Ziagen

(GlaxoWellcome; GSK) is a proprietary, prescription-only preparation of the ANTIVIRAL agent abacavir. It can be used in the treatment of HIV infection in combination with other drugs, and is available as tablets and an oral solution.
✚▲ Side-effects/warnings: See ABACAVIR.

Zidoval

(3M) is a proprietary, prescription-only preparation of the ANTIMICROBIAL metronidazole, which has both ANTIPROTOZOAL and ANTIBACTERIAL properties. It can be used to treat bacterial vaginosis and other infections, and is available as a gel for local vaginal application.
✚▲ Side-effects/warnings: See METRONIDAZOLE.

zidovudine

(azidothymidine; AZT) is a (*reverse transcriptase inhibitor*) ANTIVIRAL drug which is used in the treatment of HIV infection. Formerly, it was used for the treatment of advanced AIDS, but is now considered useful, by some, for the early forms of HIV virus infections before the full AIDS syndrome develops, including HIV-positive individuals who do not show symptoms of AIDS; also for pregnant women and their infants. Administration can be either oral or by intravenous infusion.
✚ Side-effects: There are many and may include disturbances in various blood cells, often to a degree requiring blood transfusions; nausea and vomiting, gastrointestinal disturbances, loss of appetite, headache, rashes, fever and sleep disturbances; abdominal pain, malaise, convulsions, pigmentation of the nails, skin and mouth, and many others.
▲ Warnings: It is a specialist drug, and there will be full assessment and patient monitoring throughout treatment. It should not be used where there are certain blood disorders or when breast-feeding. It should be administered with care to those who are pregnant, have kidney or liver impairment, or are elderly. Avoid alcohol as its effects may be enhanced. Blood tests should be carried out.
✪ Related entries: Combivir; Retrovir; Trizivir.

Zileze

(Opus; Trinity) is a proprietary, prescription-only preparation of the HYPNOTIC drug zopiclone. It can be used for the short-term treatment of insomnia, and is available as tablets.
✚▲ Side-effects/warnings: See ZOPICLONE.

Zimovane

(Rhône-Poulenc Rorer; Aventis Pharma) is a proprietary, prescription-only preparation of the HYPNOTIC drug zopiclone. It can be used for the short-term treatment of insomnia, and is available as tablets.

✚▲ Side-effects/warnings: See ZOPICLONE.

Zinacef

(GlaxoWellcome; GSK) is a proprietary, prescription-only preparation of the ANTIBACTERIAL and (CEPHALOSPORIN) ANTIBIOTIC cefuroxime. It can be used to treat a range of bacterial infections and to prevent infection following surgery. It is available in a form for injection.

✚▲ Side-effects/warnings: See CEFUROXIME.

Zinamide

(MSD) is a proprietary, prescription-only preparation of the ANTIBACTERIAL pyrazinamide. It can be used as an ANTITUBERCULAR drug, usually in combination with other antitubercular drugs, and is available as tablets.

✚▲ Side-effects/warnings: See PYRAZINAMIDE.

Zinc and Coal Tar Paste, BP

is a non-proprietary, non-prescription compound preparation of zinc oxide, yellow soft paraffin and coal tar. It can be used by topical application to treat chronic eczema and psoriasis and to relieve itching. It is available as an ointment.

✚▲ Side-effects/warnings: See COAL TAR; YELLOW SOFT PARAFFIN; ZINC OXIDE.

Zinc and Salicylic Acid Paste, BP

(Lassar's paste) is a non-proprietary, non-prescription preparation of the ASTRINGENT agent zinc oxide and the KERATOLYTIC agent salicylic acid, along with starch in white soft paraffin. It can be used in the treatment of hyperkeratotic skin disorders.

✚▲ Side-effects/warnings: See SALICYLIC ACID; ZINC OXIDE; WHITE SOFT PARAFFIN.

zinc

is a metallic element necessary to the body and is ingested as a trace element in a well-balanced diet (good sources include lean meat, seafood, vegetables and wholemeal bread). It is essential for the proper functioning in the body of over 100 enzymes essential to health, especially those building proteins and nucleic acids. Deficiency does not normally occur in individuals with a balanced diet. However, burns, liver disease and certain intestinal diseases where there is reduced absorption, may cause deficiency. Zinc deficiency may be treated with an oral MINERAL SUPPLEMENT or injection of zinc salts. Apart from its dietary importance, zinc salts such as zinc oxide or (basic) zinc carbonate (in calamine) have ASTRINGENT properties and are used to treat skin disorders.

✪ Related entries: zinc oxide; zinc sulphate

zinc oxide

is a mild ASTRINGENT agent which is used primarily to treat skin disorders, such as nappy rash, urinary rash and eczema. It is available (without prescription) in any of a number of compound forms: as a cream with arachis oil, oleic acid and wool fat, or with ichthammol and wool fat; as an ointment and as an ointment with castor oil; as a dusting powder with starch and talc; as a paste with starch and white soft paraffin, or with starch and zinc and salicylic acid paste.

✚▲ Side-effects/warnings: It is regarded as safe in normal topical use.

✪ Related entries: Anugesic-HC; Anusol Cream; Anusol Ointment; Anusol Plus HC Ointment; Anusol Plus HC Suppositories; Anusol Suppositories; Benadryl Skin Allergy Relief Cream; Benadryl Skin Allergy Relief Lotion; Calamine and Coal Tar Ointment, BP; Care Calamine Lotion; E45 Emollient Wash Cream; E45 Sun Lotion; Germolene Ointment; Germoloids Cream; Germoloids Ointment; Germoloids Suppositories; Hewletts Cream; Lacto-Calamine Lotion; Morhulin Ointment; Sprilon; Sudocrem Antiseptic Cream; Sudocream Antiseptic Healing Cream; Vasogen Cream; Zinc and Coal Tar Paste, BP; Xyloproct; Zinc and Salicylic Acid Paste, BP.

Zinc Paste

is a non-proprietary, ASTRINGENT compound made up of ZINC OXIDE and WHITE SOFT PARAFFIN (and starch). It is used as a base to which other active constituents can be added, especially within impregnated bandages. Of all such pastes that are compounded to treat and protect the lesions of skin diseases, such as eczema and psoriasis, zinc paste is the standard type. There are also pastes combining other active substances, including *zinc and ichthammol cream* and ZINC AND SALICYLIC ACID PASTE, BP.

zinc sulphate

is one form in which zinc supplements can be administered in order to make up a zinc deficiency in the body. There are several proprietary preparations administered orally. In solution, zinc sulphate is also used as an ASTRINGENT and wound cleanser, as an ANTISEBORRHOEIC against seborrhoeic dermatitis in topical preparations, and also in eye-drops.
✚ Side-effects: There may be abdominal pain or mild gastrointestinal upsets.
✪ **Related entries: Efalith; Lypsyl Cold Sore Gel; Solvazinc.**

zinc undecenoate

see UNDECENOIC ACID.

Zindaclin

(Strakan) is a proprietary, prescription-only preparation of the ANTIBACTERIAL and ANTIBIOTIC clindamycin. It can be used to treat acne, and is available as a gel for topical application.
✚▲ Side-effects/warnings: See CLINDAMYCIN.

Zineryt

(Yamanouchi) is a proprietary, prescription-only preparation of the ANTIBACTERIAL and (MACROLIDE) ANTIBIOTIC erythromycin. It can be used to treat acne, and is available as a solution for topical application.
✚▲ Side-effects/warnings: See ERYTHROMYCIN.

Zinga

(Ashbourne) is a proprietary, prescription-only preparation of the H_2-ANTAGONIST nizatidine. It can be used as an ULCER-HEALING DRUG for benign peptic ulcers (in the stomach or duodenum), gastro-oesophageal reflux, dyspepsia and associated conditions. It is available as capsules and in a form for injection.
✚▲ Side-effects/warnings: See NIZATIDINE.

Zinnat

(GlaxoWellcome; GSK) is a proprietary, prescription-only preparation of the ANTIBACTERIAL and (CEPHALOSPORIN) ANTIBIOTIC cefuroxime. It can be used to treat a range of bacterial infections and to prevent infection following surgery. It is available as tablets, sachets and an oral suspension.
✚▲ Side-effects/warnings: See CEFUROXIME.

Zirtek Allergy

(UCB Pharma) is a proprietary, non-prescription preparation of the ANTIHISTAMINE cetirizine hydrochloride. It can be used to treat the symptoms of allergic disorders, such as hay fever and allergic skin conditions, and is available as tablets. It is not normally given to children under the age of six years, except on medical advice.
✚▲ Side-effects/warnings: See CETIRIZINE HYDROCHLORIDE.

Zispin

(Organon) is a proprietary, prescription-only preparation of the 'atypical' ANTIDEPRESSANT mirtazapine. It can be used to treat depressive illness, and is available as tablets.
✚▲ Side-effects/warnings: See MIRTAZAPINE.

Zita

(Eastern) is a proprietary preparation of the H_2-ANTAGONIST and ULCER-HEALING DRUG cimetidine. It is available on prescription or without a prescription (in a limited amount and for short-term uses only in those over 16 years). It can be used to treat benign peptic ulcers (in the stomach or duodenum), gastro-oesophageal reflux, dyspepsia and associated conditions. It is available as tablets.
✚▲ Side-effects/warnings: See CIMETIDINE.

Zithromax

(Pfizer) is a proprietary, prescription-only preparation of the ANTIBACTERIAL and (MACROLIDE) ANTIBIOTIC azithromycin. It can be used to treat many forms of infection and is available as capsules, tablets and an oral suspension.
✚▲ Side-effects/warnings: See AZITHROMYCIN.

Zocor

(MSD) is a proprietary, prescription-only preparation of the LIPID-REGULATING DRUG simvastatin. It can be used in hyperlipidaemia to modify the proportions of various lipids in the bloodstream. It is available as tablets.
✚▲ Side-effects/warnings: See SIMVASTATIN.

Zofran

(GlaxoWellcome; GSK) is a proprietary,

prescription-only preparation of the ANTI-EMETIC and ANTINAUSEANT ondansetron. It can be used to give relief from nausea and vomiting, especially in patients receiving chemotherapy or after operations. It is available as tablets, as tablets dissolving on the tongue (oral lyophilisates, called *Zofran Melt*), a syrup, as suppositories or in a form for intravenous injection or infusion.
✚▲ Side-effects/warnings: See ONDANSETRON.

Zoladex

(AstraZeneca) is a proprietary, prescription-only preparation of goserelin. It can be used as an ANTICANCER drug for cancer of the prostate gland, breast and for uterine endometriosis. It is available in a form for implantation into the abdominal wall (with a syringe supplied).
✚▲ Side-effects/warnings: See GOSERELIN.

Zoladex LA

(AstraZeneca) is a proprietary, prescription-only preparation of goserelin, which is an analogue of the pituitary HORMONE gonadortelin. It can be used as an ANTICANCER drug for cancer of the prostate gland. It is available in a form for implantation into the abdominal wall (with a syringe supplied).
✚▲ Side-effects/warnings: See GOSERELIN.

zoledronic acid

is a recently introduced CALCIUM METABOLISM MODIFIER drug (a BISPHOSPHONATE) which affects calcium metabolism and is used to treat high calcium levels and bone pain due to metastases associated with malignant tumours and bone lesions. Administration is by intravenous infusion.
✚ Side-effects: Flu-like symptoms such as fever and bone and joint pain, fatigue, confusion, changes in taste, increased thirst, nausea, bradycardia, effects on blood cells, headache, vomiting, rash, pruritus, conjunctivitis, chest pain; kidney failure. There may be reactions at the site of injection.
▲ Warnings: It should not be administered to anyone who is pregnant or breast-feeding. Kidney and liver function and white cell count should be monitored and patients will be advised to maintain an adequate fluid intake. There may be monitoring thoughout treatment of certain blood levels and of kidney function. It is used with caution in those with heart disease or liver impairment.
✪ **Related entry: Zometa.**

Zoleptil

(Orion) is a proprietary, prescription-only preparation of the ANTIPSYCHOTIC zotepine. It can be used to treat schizophrenics. It is available as tablets.
✚▲ Side-effects/warnings: See ZOTEPINE.

zolmitriptan

is a (TRIPTAN) ANTIMIGRAINE drug which is used to treat acute migraine attacks (but not to prevent attacks). It works as a VASOCONSTRICTOR (through acting as a serotonin receptor stimulant selective for SEROTONIN 5-HT_1 receptors), producing a rapid constriction of blood vessels surrounding the brain. Administration is oral.
✚ Side-effects: See SUMATRIPTAN for general side-effects of drugs of this class. Zolmitriptan may cause drowsiness, short-lived increase in blood pressure; dry mouth, muscle pain and weakness; reports of impaired perception of peripheral sensations.
▲ Warnings: See SUMATRIPTAN for general warnings of drugs of this class. Zolmitriptan should not be taken within 12 hours of any other drug of this type; it should not be used in patients with certain heart defects or arrhythmias.
✪ **Related entry: Zomig.**

zolpidem tartrate

is a newly introduced HYPNOTIC drug which works in the same way as a BENZODIAZEPINE. It can be used for the short-term treatment of insomnia. Administration is oral.
✚ Side-effects: Diarrhoea, nausea, vomiting, dizziness, vertigo, headache, drowsiness during the day, memory disturbances, night-time restlessness, nightmares, confusion, depression, double vision and other visual disturbances, tremor, unsteady gait and falls.
▲ Warnings: It should not be administered to patients with certain lung conditions, psychotic illness, obstructive sleep apnoea, severe liver impairment, myasthenia gravis or who are pregnant or breast-feeding. Administer with care to those with depression, a history of alcohol or drug abuse, or liver or kidney disorders. Drowsiness may impair the performance of skilled tasks, such as driving. The effects of alcohol may be enhanced.
✪ **Related entry: Stilnoct.**

Z

Zomacton

(Ferring) is a proprietary, prescription-only preparation of somatropin, which is the biosynthetic form of the pituitary HORMONE human growth hormone. It can be used to treat hormonal deficiency and associated symptoms (in particular, short stature). It is available in forms for injection.

✚▲ Side-effects/warnings: See SOMATROPIN.

Zometa

(Novartis) is a recently introduced, proprietary, prescription-only preparation of the CALCIUM METABOLISM MODIFIER sodium zoledronic acid. It is used to treat high calcium levels associated with malignant tumours and bone lesions. It is available in a form for intravenous infusion.

✚▲ Side-effects/warnings: See ZOLEDRONIC ACID.

Zomig

(AstraZeneca) is a proprietary, prescription-only preparation of the ANTIMIGRAINE drug zolmitriptan. It can be used to treat acute migraine attacks. It is available as ordinary tablets and tablets for dissolving in the mouth after placing on the tongue (*Zomig Rapimelt*).

✚▲ Side-effects/warnings: See ZOLMITRIPTAN

Zomorph

(Link) is a proprietary, prescription-only preparation of the (OPIOID) NARCOTIC ANALGESIC morphine sulphate. It can be used primarily to relieve pain following surgery, or the pain experienced during the final stages of terminal malignant disease. It is available as modified-release capsules.

✚▲ Side-effects/warnings: See MORPHINE SULPHATE.

zopiclone

is a newly introduced HYPNOTIC drug which works in the same way as a BENZODIAZEPINE (though chemically it is not of this class). It can be used for the short-term treatment of insomnia. Administration is oral.

✚ Side-effects: Nausea, vomiting, confusion, a bitter or metallic taste in the mouth, drowsiness, headache, light-headedness; can affect coordination the next day, dizziness, depression, sensitivity reactions, including rashes; hallucinations, irritability and behavioural disturbances, including aggression, memory loss, night terrors.

▲ Warnings: It should be administered with care to patients with kidney and liver impairment, myasthenia gravis, respiratory failure or sleep apnoea syndrome, psychiatric disorders, who have a history of drug abuse or who are pregnant or breast-feeding. Avoid prolonged use. It may cause drowsiness and impair the performance of skilled tasks, such as driving. The effects of alcohol are enhanced.

✪ **Related entries: Zimovane; Zileze.**

Zorac

(Bioglan) is a is a proprietary, prescription-only preparation of tazarotene (a RETINOID). It can be used to treat mild to moderate plaque psoriasis. Administration is by topical application as a gel that is applied to the skin.

✚▲ Side-effects/warnings: See TAZAROTENE.

zotepine

is an ANTIPSYCHOTIC drug (one of a group sometimes termed 'atypical' antipsychotics) which can be used for the treatment of schizophrenia. It is taken orally.

✚ Side-effects: Those for atypical antipsychotics include weight gain, dizziness, postural hypotension, extrapyramidal symptoms (usually mild and transient, but occasionally tardive dyskinesia on long-term administration). Also for zotepine, constipation, dyspepsia, dry mouth, effects on the liver, heart rate, rhinitis, agitation and anxiety, depression, weakness, headache, insomnia, drowsiness, raised or lowered body temperature, increased salivation, blood changes, blurred vision, sweating. A number of other possible side-effects have been reported. The EEG will be taken.

▲ Warnings: Atypical antipsychotics are used with caution in patients with cardiovascular disease, history of epilepsy and Parkinson's disease; may affect performance of skilled tasks (including driving). Also, used with caution in pregnancy, if there is a personal family history of epilepsy; in certain heart defects, in liver or kidney impairment; prostatic hypertrophy, urinary retention, angle-closure glaucoma, paralytic ileus. It should not be used in breast-feeding, where there is intoxication with CNS depressants; along with high doses of concomitantly prescribed antipsychotics; in acute

gout, or a history of certain kidney disorders.
✪ **Related entry: Zoleptil**

Zoton

(Lederle; Wyeth) is a proprietary, prescription-only preparation of the PROTON-PUMP INHIBITOR lansoprazole. It can be used as an ULCER-HEALING DRUG and for associated conditions, such as gastro-oesophageal reflux, and is available as capsules and a suspension.
✚▲ Side-effects/warnings: See LANSOPRAZOLE.

Zovirax

(GSK) is a proprietary, prescription-only preparation of the ANTIVIRAL drug aciclovir (acyclovir). It can be used to treat infection by herpes simplex and herpes zoster viruses. It is available as tablets, an oral suspension, an eye ointment, a cream and in a form for intravenous infusion. (A non-prescription ointment preparation for the treatment of cold sores is also available (*Zovirax Cold Sore Cream*).)
✚▲ Side-effects/warnings: See ACICLOVIR.

Zovirax Cold Sore Cream

(GSK Consumer Healthcare) is a proprietary, non-prescription preparation of the ANTIVIRAL drug aciclovir (acyclovir). It can be used to treat infection of the lips and face by herpes simplex viruses. It is available as a cream.
✚▲ Side-effects/warnings: See ACICLOVIR.

zuclopenthixol

is an ANTIPSYCHOTIC drug that is chemically one of the *thioxanthenes*, which have similar general actions to the PHENOTHIAZINE derivatives. It can be used to treat patients with psychotic disorders, such as schizophrenia, and is particularly effective for agitated and aggressive behaviour. Administration can be either oral or by injection. It is used in the form of the dihydrochloride or acetate; also the decanoate form by deep intramuscular injection for the *long-term* maintenance of schizophrenia.
✚▲ Side-effects/warnings: See CHLORPROMAZINE HYDROCHLORIDE. It should not be used in patients with porphyria.
✪ **Related entries: Clopixol; Clopixol Acuphase; Clopixol Conc.**

Zumenon

(Solvay) is a proprietary, prescription-only preparation of the OESTROGEN of estradiol. It can be used in HRT, and is available as tablets.
✚▲ Side-effects/warnings: See ESTRADIOL.

Zyban

(GlaxoWellcome; GSK) is a proprietary, non-prescription preparation of the newly introduced drug bupropion (amfebutamone), and can be used to alleviate the withdrawal symptoms experienced when giving up smoking tobacco products (in combination with motivational support). It is available as tablets.
✚▲ Side-effects/warnings: See BUPROPION.

Zydol

(Searle; Pharmacia) is a proprietary, prescription-only preparation of the (OPIOID) NARCOTIC ANALGESIC tramadol hydrochloride. It can be used to relieve pain, but seems to differ from typical opioids in its mode of action. It is available as capsules, soluble tablets and in a form for injection.
✚▲ Side-effects/warnings: See TRAMADOL HYDROCHLORIDE.

Zydol SR

(Searle; Pharmacia) is a proprietary, prescription-only preparation of the (OPIOID) NARCOTIC ANALGESIC tramadol hydrochloride. It can be used to relieve pain, but seems to differ from typical opioids in its mode of action. It is available as modified-release tablets.
✚▲ Side-effects/warnings: See TRAMADOL HYDROCHLORIDE.

Zydol XL

(Searle; Pharmacia) is a proprietary, prescription-only preparation of the (OPIOID) NARCOTIC ANALGESIC tramadol hydrochloride. It can be used to relieve pain, but seems to differ from typical opioids in its mode of action. It is available as modified-release tablets.
✚▲ Side-effects/warnings: See TRAMADOL HYDROCHLORIDE.

Zyloric

(GlaxoWellcome; GSK) is a proprietary, prescription-only preparation of the ENZYME INHIBITOR allopurinol, which is a XANTHINE-OXIDASE INHIBITOR. It can be used to treat excess uric acid in the blood and to prevent renal stones and attacks of gout. It is available as tablets.

✚▲ Side-effects/warnings: See ALLOPURINOL.

Zyomet

(Goldshield) is a proprietary, prescription-only preparation of the ANTIMICROBIAL metronidazole, which has ANTIBACTERIAL and ANTIPROTOZOAL actions. It can be applied topically as a gel to treat acute acne rosacea outbreaks.

✚▲ Side-effects/warnings: See METRONIDAZOLE.

Zyprexa

(Lilly) is a proprietary, prescription-only preparation of the ANTIPSYCHOTIC drug olanzapine. It can be used to tranquillize patients suffering from schizophrenia, and is available as ordinary tablets and tablets for dissolving in the mouth.

✚▲ Side-effects/warnings: See OLANZAPINE.

Zyvox

(Pharmacia) is a recently introduced proprietary, prescription-only compound preparation of the ANTIBIOTIC-like (oxazolidinone) ANTIBACTERIAL agent linezolid. It can be used in the treatment of pneumonia, and skin and soft tissue infections, and is available as tablets or is given by intravenous infusion.

✚▲ Side-effects/warnings: See **linezolid.**

abuse liability of drugs
concerns the propensity to lead to drug-seeking behaviour. In the case of some drugs (especially OPIOID, such as heroin), there is a strong progression into drug **dependence** (addiction) with an associated **withdrawal syndrome**.

abuse of drugs
denotes the non-medical use of drugs – without intent to prevent, treat or cure disease – ie recreational use. The term is commonly pejorative, reflecting the extent that drugs can seriously interfere with the physical and mental health of the individual.

acute
means short-term – in contrast to **chronic** (long-term) – and can be used to describe a disease of relatively sudden onset and short duration, or for how long a drug is taken.

addiction
see **dependence**.

ADHD
see **attention-deficit hyperactivity disorder**.

adjunct
is a drug or treatment that is not essential, but aids or assists another therapy, often improving the overall efficacy of treatment (eg DISULFIRAM in the treatment of chronic alcohol dependence; BETA-BLOCKER in thyrotoxicosis treatment; a DOPAMINE-RECEPTOR STIMULANT as adjunctive to LEVODOPA in the control of Parkinson's disease).

adjuvants
are drugs not necessarily effective on their own, but which may be used in addition to other drugs to increase the latter's effectiveness (eg TAMOXIFEN with CYTOTOXIC **chemotherapy** or radiotherapy for breast cancer). In immunology it has a special meaning applied to substances such as aluminium hydroxide that are not themselves antigenic, but that markedly enhance the immune response to antigens when administered with them (eg in vaccination).

adrenal
means pertaining to the adrenal gland, which is an endocrine gland close to the kidney. It secretes hormones into the bloodstream from two main layers. Adrenocortical hormones – from the cortex, or outer layer – are usually called corticosteroids (see CORTICOSTEROID) and are classified into two types, glucocorticoids and mineralocorticoids; eg CORTISONE ACETATE, HYDROCORTISONE and aldosterone. Adrenomedullary hormones – from the medulla, or central core – include ADRENALINE and NORADRENALINE. See also **aldosteronism**.

adverse drug reactions
are seriously unpleasant or harmful effects of drugs caused by doses used for normal therapeutic use. Relatively trivial side-effects, such as a dry mouth, are not normally referred to as adverse drug reactions. These reactions are divided into groups, including type A, dose-related and expected (often inevitable given the mode of action of the drug), and type B, rare and occurring only in some patients (sometimes called idiosyncratic reactions; often an allergic reaction).

aerosols
are a means of administering drugs as fine droplets in a spray, often from a nebulizer (eg a BETA-RECEPTOR STIMULANT in asthma treatment).

aetiology
is the cause of a disease, and the study of the factors involved in causing it.

aldosteronism
is a disease caused by excessive production of aldosterone, a **hormone** produced by the cortex of the **adrenal** gland due to a **tumour** of the gland known as Conn's syndrome or sometimes as part of **heart failure**, liver damage, or a low-sodium diet. Symptoms include **hypertension**, **oedema**, thirst and tiredness. Treatment includes the use of aldosterone antagonists (eg SPIRONOLACTONE).

allergens
are foreign chemicals to which the body has become sensitive, and can cause an allergy in hypersensitive persons and thus an allergic reaction (see **allergic reactions**).

allergic reactions
are caused by the reaction of **allergens** (often foreign proteins) with antibodies (formed by the body's protective immune system: see **antibody**). These reactions may be local or generalized (as in **anaphylactic shock**). Treatment of allergic disease is with anti-allergic drugs, including the CORTICOSTEROID and ANTIHISTAMINE classes. Also, there may be allergic reactions (type B **adverse drug reactions**) to some drugs, such as PENICILLIN and/or a LOCAL ANAESTHETIC.

amenorrhoea
is a stopping or absence of menstrual periods.

anaemia
is a collection of conditions where there is a reduced capacity of the blood to carry oxygen, due to a reduction in haemoglobin levels or impaired oxygen-carrying capacity. Symptoms include tiredness and breathlessness. There may be many causes. See **iron-deficient anaemia; megaloblastic anaemia; sickle-cell disease.**

analogues
are chemicals or drugs that are closely related in chemical structure.

anaphylactic shock
see **anaphylaxis.**

anaphylaxis
is an extreme local reaction to drugs or **allergens** in hypersensitive people. An extreme generalized reaction (eg to bee stings), called **anaphylactic shock**, is treated as a medical emergency. Treatment is by injection of ANTI-ALLERGIC drugs, including CORTICOSTEROID and ANTIHISTAMINE drugs, and also ADRENALINE.

angina pectoris
is a pain felt in the centre of the chest and sometimes spreading to the arm, shoulder or jaw. It often occurs with exercise, and is due to the demand for oxygen by the heart muscle exceeding the supply, for instance, when there is an obstruction of the cardiac arteries (**atheroma**). It may be treated with ANTI-ANGINA drugs (eg BETA-BLOCKER and VASODILATOR drugs).

angioedema (angioneurotic oedema)
is caused by allergy resulting in the rapid development of swellings similar to **urticaria** of the skin, but also other sites in the body (including the larynx). The most common causes are food allergy, insect stings, infections and drug allergy (eg PENICILLIN). Treatment is with CORTICOSTEROID and ANTIHISTAMINE drugs.

anorexia
is loss of appetite, and can be induced by APPETITE SUPPRESSANT or anorectic agents. The eating disorder anorexia nervosa is characterized by an unwillingness to eat, extreme weight loss and fear of becoming fat.

anoxia
is a state where the tissues receive an inadequate oxygen supply. This may result from many causes, including anaemia, inadequate oxygen in the atmosphere (eg with high altitude), in respiratory diseases (eg **asthma** and **bronchitis**), inadequate perfusion of the tissues (eg in **angina pectoris** where there is **atheroma** of the cardiac arteries). Treatment depends on the specific cause.

antibody
is a molecule produced in humans and higher animals in response to an **antigen** which has the particular property of binding to the antigen which induced its formation and makes it harmless. Antibodies are mainly found in the immunoglobulin (gamma globulin) component of blood plasma. The production of antibodies with antigens underlies both **allergic reactions** and **immunity**.

antigen
is a term used to describe proteins that are treated by the body as foreign; antibodies (see **antibody**) in the blood react with them, making them harmless.

aplasia
means failure of development of an organ or tissue (eg aplastic anaemia).

arrhythmias (dysrhythmias)
are abnormalities of heart rhythm or rate of heartbeat. They are usually caused by disturbances of the electrical impulses and their conduction within the heart. There are a number of types of disturbance: ectopic beats are isolated irregular beats; tachycardias are where the heartbeat is too fast; and bradycardias where it is too slow; atrial flutter is a rapid beat originating within the atrium; and ventricular fibrillation is a form of cardiac arrest where the ventricles of the heart twitch in a disorganized manner. Treatment of each type of disorder is usually under specialist supervision and includes the use of drugs such as the ANTI-ARRHYTHMIC, BETA-BLOCKER, CALCIUM-CHANNEL BLOCKER and CARDIAC GLYCOSIDE groups.

asthenia
is weakness or loss of strength.

asthma
is an **obstructive airways disease** characterized by acute attacks of shortness of breath (caused by difficulty in exhalation), often with increased secretions in the airways. Bronchial asthma may be precipitated by **allergens**, noxious gases, cold, exercise and certain drugs (eg ASPIRIN). It is treated with ANTI-ALLERGIC, ANTI-INFLAMMATORY and ANTI-ASTHMATIC drugs.

ataxia
is clumsiness and a lack of co-ordination, with an

unsteady gait, impaired eye and limb movements, and speech problems. There can be many causes, but mostly involving neurological damage. Several drugs may cause ataxia as a side-effect (eg BARBITURATE, HYPNOTIC and some ANTI-EPILEPTIC drugs). ETHANOL also has similar actions.

atheroma

is a degeneration of the walls of blood vessels, causing atherosclerosis, characteristically by fatty deposits and scar tissue, and predisposes to tissue **anoxia** (eg in **angina pectoris**) and **thrombosis** (causing stroke, heart attacks, gangrene). Causal factors are thought to include smoking and a diet high in saturated animal fats. Therapy includes a low-fat diet, bypass surgery and the taking of LIPID-REGULATING DRUGS and VASODILATORS.

atherosclerosis

see **atheroma.**

attention-deficit hyperactivity disorder

(ADHD) is a condition in children characterized by hyperkinesis (hyperactivity). As part of a comprehensive treatment programme, certain drugs, such as Ritalin, may be administered.

autoimmune diseases

are conditions where the immune system attacks the body's own tissues. An increasing number of diseases are now thought to involve such auto-antibodies, including **rheumatoid arthritis**, rheumatic fever, certain types of **anaemia** (pernicious anaemia, haemolytic anaemia), **lupus erythematosus** and Hashimoto's disease of the thyroid gland.

autonomic nervous system

control of bodily function involves involuntary functions such as blood pressure, heart rate and the activity of muscles of internal organs (eg blood vessels, intestines and secretions). The sympathetic nervous system (utilizing the neurotransmitter NORADRENALINE and the hormone ADRENALINE) is primarily involved in excitation of these functions, often described as 'fight, fright and flight'. The parasympathetic nervous system (utilizing the neurotransmitter ACETYLCHOLINE) is more involved in functions such as digestive processes. See also ANTICHOLINERGIC; ANTISYMPATHETIC.

BAN

see British Approved Name.

benign

means, in general, harmless conditions within the body. In relation to a **tumour**, it is used where the growth does not invade and destroy other cells or tissue, ie it is not **malignant** (cancerous).

bioavailability

of a pharmaceutical formulation is the amount that is biologically available, after administration and subsequent absorption etc., pharmacologically to act. See **formulation.**

biotechnology

is a term that denotes application of biological techniques to chemical manufacture and is used in a variety of ways, eg **recombinant DNA technology** (**genetic engineering**).

block/blocker

refers to the process where an antagonist prevents an agonist drug exerting its effect, usually by preventing the action of the latter at a receptor (eg BETA-BLOCKER, ALPHA-ADRENOCEPTOR BLOCKER and ANGIOTENSIN-RECEPTOR BLOCKER dugs).

blood-brain barrier

is the means by which the nerves within the brain are normally kept separate from the blood cells and large molecules within the blood. In relation to drug therapy, in some instances this barrier may be a disadvantage (eg certain ANTIBIOTIC drugs may not reach central nervous system cells when treating infections). However, sometimes unwanted side-effects of drugs caused by their effects on the brain can be avoided by deliberately designing new drugs that do not cross the blood-brain barrier; eg second-generation ANTIHISTAMINES do not cause drowsiness.

BNF

is the abbreviation for *British National Formulary*, which is an impartial and critical compendium of drug types and names sponsored by the British Medical Association and the Royal Pharmaceutical Society of Great Britain. It is issued every six months to prescribing doctors.

BP

is the abbreviation for **British Pharmacopoeia.**

bradycardia

is a slowed rate of heartbeat (below 60 beats per minute). See **arrhythmias.**

bradykinesia

is slow and poor movement, as seen in Parkinson's disease and as **extrapyramidal symptoms** caused by several groups of drugs as a side-effect (eg

PHENOTHIAZINE). See also **tardive dyskinesia.**

British Approved Name (BAN)
is the official name of a generic (non-proprietary) drug that has been chosen by the Nomenclature Committee of the British Pharmacopoeia. See also **generic drug name; recommended International Non-proprietary Name.**

British Pharmacopoeia (BP)
is a formulary of official preparation as used in the UK. It may differ in the drugs included, their names and further details from equivalent formulary of other countries or areas (eg **European Pharmacopoeia**).

bronchitis
is an **obstructive airways disease** characterized by a chronic shortness of breath (caused by difficulty in exhalation) and coughing, with inflammation and increased secretions and blockage of the airways (often associated with infection by micro-organisms). Chronic bronchitis is associated with a history of smoking and air pollution. It is treated with ANTIBIOTIC, ANTI-INFLAMMATORY and ANTI-ASTHMATIC drugs.

bronchoconstriction
(or bronchospasm) is a narrowing of the bronchioles of the lungs, caused by a contraction of the **smooth muscle** surrounding the airways and often exacerbated by excessive secretions within the airways. It is very characteristic of **obstructive airways diseases**, such as **asthma**, and in **allergic reactions** to **antigen** (of which an extreme example is **anaphylactic shock**). It may also be caused by drugs acting directly on the airways (eg PARASYMPATHOMIMETIC or ANTICHOLINESTERASE drugs), in drug allergy (eg PENICILLIN) or other types of **hypersensitivity** (eg to NSAIDS). Treatment is with BRONCHODILATOR drugs and, where allergy is involved, with CORTICOSTEROID and ANTIHISTAMINE drugs.

bronchospasm
see bronchoconstriction.

brucellosis
is a rare bacterial infection, normally caught from dairy products and farm animals. It is treated with ANTIBIOTIC drugs.

buccal
is a mode of administration where tablets are held between the lip and tongue, from where the active constituents (eg NITRATE drugs) are absorbed into the blood circulation in that region of the mouth, and thence into the **systemic** circulation.

cancer
is where disease is due to unrestrained cell growth and tumours. They are described as **malignant**, as such cells or growths invade and destroy other cells or tissues. There are various types of cancers, such as **carcinoma, sarcoma, lymphoma** and **leukaemia.** If untreated, cancerous growths may be life-threatening.

capsules
are gelatine or similar containers for liquid or solid (eg powder) forms of drugs that are to be taken by mouth. They allow complex formulation of the constituent drug(s), including **modified-release preparations**, especially sustained-release versions, where release is over a period of time and so reduces the frequency of dosing.

carcinoid tumours
are cancerous growths of neuroendocrine glandular tissue leading to large and often dramatic release of potent autacoids. Argentaffinoma tumours of the gut, which release SEROTONIN (5-HT) and other mediators causing asthma-like attacks, flushing and diarrhoea, where recognized early; but phaeochromocytomas, VIPomas and other neuroendocrine tumours are similar. Treatment is usually surgical.

carcinoma
is a **malignant** type of neoplasm, a cancerous growth, which arises in the epithelium which lines the internal organs and skin. See **sarcoma.**

cardiac muscle
is the type of striated muscle that makes up the contractile muscle of the heart (but not of the **smooth muscle** of the blood vessels within the heart). The muscle is controlled by the **autonomic nervous system.**

CD
see **Controlled Drugs.**

central nervous system (CNS)
is the division of the nervous system comprising the brain within the skull and spinal cord within the vertebrae. The remainder of the nervous system is the peripheral nervous system.

chemical drug names
are not normally used outside technical circles because, although they are precise and

unambiguous, they can be very large and unwieldy. In its place is substituted an official trivial or shortened name, a generic drug name, though this may unfortunately vary between countries. For instance, N-(4-hydroxyphenyl) acetamide is a chemical name for the analgesic drug given the generic name paracetamol (UK) or acetaminophen (USA). See also **generic drug name; names of drugs.**

chemotherapy
is the treatment or prevention of disease by means of chemical substances. The term is often restricted to the treatment of disease by drugs (eg an ANTIBIOTIC) or to the treatment of cancer (ie ANTICANCER drugs) in contrast to radiotherapy.

chlamydial infection
is caused by a group of small micro-organisms called chlamydia, which physically are larger than viruses but smaller than bacteria (though, like bacteria, their infection can be treated with antibiotics). They cause a wide range of infections in humans and animals, and may spread between the two (eg psittacosis from birds). The commonest infection is by strains of Chlamydia trachomatis, causing various eye, lymph node and (sexually transmitted) genital infections.

cholestasis
is a failure of the normal bile flow to the intestine causing liver disease and jaundice. Causes include a physical obstructive jaundice due to a stone (extrahepatic biliary obstruction), liver disease (eg viral **hepatitis**) or drug-induced toxic reaction (intrahepatic cholestasis), for instance, in individuals with abnormal sensitivity to CHLORPROMAZINE HYDROCHLORIDE. The symptoms are jaundice with dark urine, pale faeces and skin itching. Treatment depends on the cause, and when due to adverse drug reaction normally reverses on discontinuing drug administration.

chronic
describes a disease of long duration, usually of slow onset and slowly reversing (if at all). It does not mean severe. See **acute.**

cirrhosis
of the liver is caused by **chronic** damage to its cells, leading to scarring and loss of function. One result is a loss of ability to metabolize toxic substances and drugs, and it may cause portal hypertension (increased blood pressure in the portal vein conveying blood from the intestine and spleen to the liver). The causes include **hepatitis** (an inflammation of the liver commonly caused by microbial infection) or heavy consumption of alcohol.

clinical pharmacology
encompasses all aspects of the scientific study of drugs in humans.

clinical trial
is a systematic study of medically active agents in humans. Such trials advance through early phases in normal volunteers (to determine duration of action and metabolism), to eventual studies in patients with disease. Commonly, new active agents are compared to existing standard treatments and to dummy treatments (placebos). To avoid bias, assessment of the efficacy of treatment may be single-blind (where either the patient or the doctor does not know the identity of treatments) or double-blind (where neither knows until the trial is finished).

colitis
is inflammation of the colon of the gut. Symptoms include pain, diarrhoea, sometimes blood or mucus, and fever. It may be due to parasitic or bacterial infections or to ulcerative colitis and Crohn's disease. Treatment of ulcerative colitis is with AMINOSALICYLATE.

colorectal
pertaining to the lower gut; the colon and rectum.

Committee on Safety of Medicines
(CSM) is an independent group set up to give advice via the **Medicines Control Agency** (MCA), which administers the Medicines Act, to the licensing authorities under the Ministry of Health.

complementary medicine (alternative medicine)
is a general term sometimes applied to non-orthodox, traditional or alternative systems of medicine and healing, including **herbal medicines, homeopathy**, faith healing, hypnosis, acupuncture and aromatherapy. These alternative treatments vary in their credibility, as many are not administered by qualified practitioners and they are not, in general, subject to objective proof of efficacy through **clinical trials.**

compliance
is the extent to which patient behaviour accords with medical advice, and in relation to drugs relates to the accuracy and frequency of taking prescribed medicines (which can be surprisingly low).

compound analgesics

are drug preparations that combine two or more ANALGESIC agents in one preparation. There are a number of proprietary preparations with some combination of the NON-NARCOTIC ANALGESIC drug PARACETAMOL, the NSAID analgesics ASPIRIN and IBUPROFEN and the (OPIOID) NARCOTIC ANALGESIC drugs CODEINE PHOSPHATE, DEXTROPROPOXYPHENE HYDROCHLORIDE and DIHYDROCODEINE TARTRATE. There are also several 'official', non-proprietary compound analgesics that contain specified amounts of various analgesics: see CO-CODAMOL, CO-CODAPRIN, CO-DYDRAMOL and CO-PROXAMOL.

compound preparation

are drug formulations that are a combination of two or more pharmacologically active constituents in a single preparation. There are many possible examples. There might be two or more drugs with similar effects (eg combinations of the ANALGESIC drugs paracetamol and aspirin), with different distinct effects (eg combinations of an analgesic with a DECONGESTANT in a cough-and-cold preparation), or one main drug combined with a supplementary drug that maintains its level in the body (eg the ANTIPARKINSONISM drug LEVODOPA can be given combined with the ENZYME INHIBITOR drug BENSERAZIDE HYDROCHLORIDE to protect the former from being broken down too rapidly in the body).

Although many proprietary preparations contain a number of active constituents, each with different pharmacological effect, medical attitudes to compound preparations are mixed. The main criticism is that in certain circumstances it may be necessary to adjust the dose of one or all of the constituents independently, in order to achieve a reliable and safe response, but this is impossible in a compound preparation. For instance, POTASSIUM CHLORIDE is now much less commonly included in preparations containing a DIURETIC that cause potassium loss from the body, because the amount of potassium required is very variable and best controlled independently of the (critical) dose of the diuretic. On the other hand, certain combinations of drugs (in a standard ratio of doses) have gained an established place in both prescription-only and non-prescription applications. Most examples of these compound preparations have a *co-* prefix, which means compound. Examples include, co-codamol 8/500 which is a compound preparation of CODEINE PHOSPHATE and PARACETAMOL, in a ratio of 8mg of codeine phosphate to 500mg of paracetamol; and CO-BENELDOPA for a combination of levodopa and benserazide hydrochloride (as described above).

constriction

is a narrowing or obstruction of a hollow organ, commonly applied to blood vessels (vasoconstriction). See VASOCONSTRICTOR.

contraindication

is where a treatment must not be used because it might be hazardous to a patient under the specified conditions (common examples being those who have liver or kidney impairments, heart conditions or who are pregnant).

Controlled Drugs (CD)

are those designated under the (UK) Misuse of Drugs Act, 1971 and Regulations (1985) and are believed most likely to cause dependence and lead to misuse. There are three classes, given in order of seriousness. Class A includes synthetic and natural OPIATE drugs (eg diamorphine (heroin), morphine, opium, methadone, pethidine, cocaine, lysergide (LSD), and class B substances when prepared for injection. Class B includes oral amphetamines, barbiturates, cannabis (though its classification is under review), codeine and pholcodine. Class C includes some drugs related to amphetamine, most benzodiazepines, androgenic and anabolic steroids, and various hormones including growth hormone. The Misuse of Drugs Regulations (1985) also define who is authorized to possess and supply Controlled Drugs, which are also divided into schedules that specify details to do with manufacture, record keeping and prescription (which must be in the prescriber's handwriting).

Crohn's disease

see colitis.

Cushing's syndrome

is caused by raised levels of the hormones called CORTICOSTEROID in the bloodstream. It can be due to excess production by the adrenal gland due to a **tumour** of that gland, tumours in the lungs and elsewhere in the periphery, to a tumour of the pituitary gland leading to excess stimulation of the **adrenal** gland, or to prolonged medical administration of corticosteroid drugs (eg in **rheumatoid arthritis, asthma** or inflammatory bowel disease). Characteristics of the syndrome include a moon-faced, rounded and red-faced appearance, obesity and humped shoulders, wasted limbs, thin and easily bruised skin, osteoporosis, hairiness in females, and a variety of other adverse effects including **diabetes**. The course of chosen treatment requires expert evaluation by an endocrinologist.

cycloplegic agents

cause cycloplegia, which is paralysis of the **smooth muscle** of the eye that accommodates the lens (that allow the eye to focus on near objects), so leaving the eye focused for distant objects. ANTICHOLINERGIC drugs may be used for this purpose in the diagnosis and treatment of disease states, or alternatively cycloplegia may be an unavoidable **side-effect** of these drugs when used for other reasons. Often cycloplegia is accompanied by mydriasis.

dependence

on a drug (addiction) is a state where regular, repeated and probably excessive taking of an agent causes the individual to become accustomed to it, resulting in detrimental effects. Stopping dosing precipitates a **withdrawal syndrome** which may have marked psychological and/or physical symptoms. See **habituation.**

diabetes

is a disease characterized by the symptom of the production of large volumes of urine. There are two different diseases, diabetes mellitus and diabetes insipidus, each with a different **aetiology**. Diabetes mellitus (itself of two main types) is caused by a defect in the pancreas leading to impaired blood glucose control, and is treated with INSULIN or ORAL HYPOGLYCAEMIC drugs (see also DIABETIC TREATMENT). Diabetes insipidus is caused by under-production of, or decreased kidney response to ANTIDIURETIC HORMONE (ADH; VASOPRESSIN) which is secreted by the pituitary gland, (see DIABETES INSIPIDUS TREATMENT).

dilatation

is a widening of a hollow organ, commonly applied to blood vessels (vasodilatation). See VASODILATOR.

diverticular disease

is the presence of small pouches or sacs protruding into the intestine, commonly the colon. Diverticulitis is when inflammation is present, and if this becomes severe it can lead to perforation of the bowel wall. Treatment is surgical, with ANTIBIOTIC drugs (when there is infection) and high-fibre diets and additives (eg BRAN, ISPAGHULA HUSK).

dose

is the amount of a drug administered, and is critical in order to achieve the desired therapeutic effect without unnecessary adverse effects or side-effects. An initial (loading) dose may be administered, followed by a smaller maintenance dose given at regular intervals appropriate to that particular drug and the metabolism and excretion (**pharmacokinetics**) in a particular patient.

drug interactions

occur when one drug changes the magnitude of effect, or duration of action or some other property (eg adverse reactions or side-effects), of the other.

drugs and medicines

are terms that are often used interchangeably. However, sometimes they are used in somewhat different senses. A drug can be defined as the active principle(s) in a medication as defined by the **generic drug name** (non-proprietary names) of the constituents; essentially what is prescribed by the medical practitioner. A medicine is the appropriate **formulation** (tablets, liquid etc.) supplied by the pharmacist to the patient (which may bear a **proprietary name**, or a generic name of the product manufactured according to a product **licence**, or may have been formulated by the pharmacist from the basic constituents (as with some BP medicines).

drug screening

is the process of testing chemical agents for given types of pharmacological activity and possible therapeutic uses.

dys-

as a prefix means abnormal or disturbed body function.

dysfunctional

means abnormal or disturbed body function.

dyskinesia

is abnormal muscle movements, such as jerking and twitching; eg in **tardive dyskinesia**.

dysmenorrhoea

is the term used for the pain or discomfort just before or during menstrual periods, probably due to hormonal effects. In general, there are few effective drugs to treat it, though ANALGESIC drugs may be used to ease the discomfort. Sometimes, in older women, it can be caused by pelvic inflammatory disease, fibroids and other disorders, which are treated with appropriate drugs. See also **amenorrhoea.**

dyspepsia (indigestion)

is disturbed digestion, characterized by discomfort or pain in the region of the stomach or lower chest after eating.

dysphoria
is a feeling or discomfort or lack of wellbeing (as opposed to euphoria).

dysrhythmia
see ARRHYTHMIAS.

dystonia
is a disorder of **skeletal muscle** tone (either increased or decreased), causing abnormal positions and movements. It is sometimes caused by disorders of the basal ganglia of the brain due to adverse drug reaction (eg PHENOTHIAZINE and ANTIPSYCHOTIC drugs). See **extrapyramidal symptoms; tardive dyskinesia.**

eclampsia
is a condition of late pregnancy, or during or directly after delivery, characterized by convulsions (and preceded in pre-eclampsia by **hypertension, oedema** and **proteinurea**). It is treated by ANTICONVULSANT drugs and in pre-eclampsia by a low-sodium diet and ANTIHYPERTENSIVE drugs.

ectopic
means not in its right or normal position.

efficacy
in therapeutics is the capacity of a drug to produce the desired effect or result.

elixir
is a medicated liquid preparation for taking by mouth, which is intended to disguise a potentially unpleasant taste by including a sweetening substance, such as GLYCEROL or ALCOHOL, and often with aromatic agents.

embolism
is a condition where an embolus (eg blood clot (thrombus), bubble of gas, fat, fragment of tissue or other material) lodges in an artery to obstruct blood flow. There are various types according to the area obstructed (eg pulmonary embolism in the case of the lung). Treatment can be by surgery, the use of drugs that can dissolve blood clots (FIBRINOLYTIC or thrombolytic drugs) or by drugs that prevent formation of further clots (ANTICOAGULANT drugs). See also **thrombosis.**

emphysema
is a component of chronic **obstructive airways disease** of the lung, where there is damage to the alveoli of the lungs (which are tiny air sacs in which oxygen exchange between air and the blood takes place), resulting in shortness of breath. It is often accompanied by chronic **bronchitis,** and can in turn lead to **heart failure** and respiratory failure. It is generally due to smoking, but is exacerbated by air pollution (and a genetic predisposition in some individuals). The damage to the alveoli cannot be repaired, but symptomatic relief may be given by BRONCHODILATOR, CORTICOSTEROID and DIURETIC drugs.

encephalopathy
is any of a group of disorders that affect the functioning of the brain.

endocarditis
is inflammation of the endocardium (the lining of the heart), and occurs usually where there has been damage due to congenital heart disease or rheumatic fever, and where the immune system is damaged (as in AIDS). Endocarditis may be caused by a number of micro-organisms, including bacteria and fungi, particularly after dental extractions and heart surgery. ANTIBIOTIC drugs may be used both prophylactically and in treatment.

endogenous
means produced within the body; in contrast to exogenous agents that are administered to the body. Some agents (eg hormones, local hormones and neurotransmitters), though released endogenously, may be administered exogenously, as drugs, in medicine.

endometriosis
is the abnormal presence of tissue similar to the endometrial lining of the uterus in various sites within the pelvis. The abnormal tissue may undergo similar responses to hormones as the endometrium, causing pain and **dysmenorrhoea.** Treatment is with HORMONE ANTAGONIST drugs or by surgery.

endometrium
is the mucous membrane layer lining the uterus within the muscle layer (myometrium).

endothelium
is the tissue that lines the blood vessels, heart and lymphatic ducts. See **epithelium.**

endotoxin
is a **toxin** that is part of the structure of a micro-organism, and which may be responsible for part of the pathogenic symptoms of (notably bacterial) infection. Endotoxins are released when the pathogenic organism binds to phagocyctic cells in

the body, or are otherwise disrupted. Usually toxicity is manifested in most body tissues. It is the counterpart of **exotoxin**. See **toxin**.

enema

is an infusion of liquid into the rectum, via the anus, as a method of administering laxatives, diagnostic agents (eg radio-opaque agents) or therapeutic drugs to act locally (eg STEROID drugs in **colitis**) or sometimes agents for absorption for systemic effects (eg PARALDEHYDE as an ANTI-EPILEPTIC).

enteral

is pertaining to the intestinal tract.

enteric-coated tablets

are covered with a layer (originally shellac varnish was used) that dissolves slowly. They are intended to prevent release until the tablet has left the stomach and enters the intestine for absorption, because the active drug is gastro-irritant (eg ASPIRIN) or is broken down by gastric juices.

epilepsy

is a group of **central nervous system** diseases characterized by a tendency to recurrent seizures (fits), usually of sudden onset. There are various schemes of classification: Grand Mal is a generalized seizure in which the patient falls down unconscious; Petit Mal (absence seizure) is a generalized seizure characterized by momentary loss of consciousness without abnormal movements; Simple Partial Seizure is where consciousness is maintained during a partial physical seizure, including Jacksonian epilepsy where twitching occurs and spreads across the body in a pattern; Complex Partial Seizure (temporal lobe epilepsy) is where conscious contact with surroundings are lost and there may be stereotyped abnormal behaviour. Status epilepticus is an extension of one of these conditions to prolonged or repeated epileptic seizures without periods for recovery, and is a medical emergency. Treatment of some of these is with ANTI-EPILEPTIC drugs (ANTICONVULSANT) appropriate to each type.

epithelium

is the tissue that covers the entire external surface of the body and lines the hollow organs of the body (except blood vessels). See **endothelium**.

erythrocytes

are red blood cells.

euphoria

is a feeling of confident wellbeing, the opposite of **dysphoria**. It can be induced by some OPIOID drugs, such as MORPHINE SULPHATE, and prolonged use of CORTICOSTEROID drugs.

European Medicines Evaluation Agency

see Medicines Control Agency.

European Pharmacopoeia (Eur. P)

like the **British Pharmacopoeia** (BP) lists official preparations of drugs. The BP and EP are gradually becoming integrated in their coverage and naming of drugs.

exocrine

glands secrete substances through a duct (for example, of the salivary glands), usually under the control of HORMONES or **neurotransmitters**.

exogenous

means from outside the body; in contrast to **endogenous** agents or influences that are from within the body.

exotoxin

is a (generally highly toxic) **toxin** secreted by micro-organisms into their surroundings, so it can work at a distance. Exotoxins may cause the symptoms of ingestion such as in food poisoning (eg botulinum toxin, cholera toxin), or symptoms of infection such as inflammation (eg diphtheria toxin) or neurological and other pathogenic symptoms (eg tetanus toxin). Exotoxins chemically are composed of two parts, one (A) comprising the toxic molecule, the other (B) comprising the protein that binds to those particular cells in body tissues where the toxicity is manifested. See **endotoxin**.

extrapyramidal disorders

see **extrapyramidal symptoms**.

extrapyramidal symptoms

of movement are caused by several groups of drugs as an adverse reaction (see **adverse drug reactions**) that is commonly a foreseeable side-effect (which may be difficult to avoid with higher dose schedules). The syndrome is due to effects of drugs on the basal ganglia and associated structures within the brain (corpus striatum and substantia nigra), and is most commonly incurred with ANTIPSYCHOTIC drugs, such as PHENOTHIAZINE agents working as DOPAMINE-RECEPTOR ANTAGONIST drugs. See also **tardive dyskinesia**.

familial diseases

are those found in some families, but not others,

and are largely genetically determined.

favism

is a disorder in some individuals characterized by a food intolerance to broad beans (*Vicia faba*), which contain a chemical that in the affected person causes rapid destruction of red blood cells (haemolytic **anaemia**). It is a genetically inherited condition and is relatively common in African, Indian and some Mediterranean peoples (in some areas it may affect up to 10% of the population). It is caused by an enzyme deficiency disorder (**G6PD-deficiency**; glucose 6-phosphate dehydrogenase deficiency) which also predisposes to serious adverse drug reactions (eg to the ANTIMALARIAL drug PRIMAQUINE).

FDA (Food and Drug Authority)

is the US authority that is concerned in evaluating evidence of a drug's safety and efficacy, clinical trials and the general process of drug registration. Its regulations have an international impact.

formulary

is a book (or increasingly a computer database) that details formulations or doses of drugs. See **British Pharmacopoeia; European Pharmacopoeia; International Pharmacopoeia.**

formulation

is the pharmaceutical term for the mode of presentation of a medicine: ie capsule, tablet, pill, cream, lotion, emulsion, solution, pessary, suppository, form for injection, etc. Modern medicines are often quite complex and sophisticated products that are stable, have reliable bioavailability, and acceptability (taste etc).

G6PD-deficiency (glucose 6-phosphate dehydrogenase enzyme deficiency)

is a genetically inherited condition and is relatively common among African, Indian and some Mediterranean peoples. Serious adverse reactions occur in affected people when they take certain drugs; for instance, the ANTIMALARIAL drug PRIMAQUINE causes red blood cell haemolysis in 5-10% of black men, leading to severe anaemia. Adverse reactions also occur to certain foodstuffs; see **favism.**

gastro-oesophageal reflux

(acid reflux) is regurgitation of acid and enzymes into the oesophagus from the stomach, of which heartburn is a symptom, and is associated with oesophagitis (inflammation of the oesophagus). It is caused by a weakness in the sphincter muscle at the bottom of the oesophagus, by hiatus hernia and is common in pregnancy. Treatment is with ANTACID and ULCER-HEALING DRUGS which reduce acid secretion.

gels

are a colloidal formulation of a medicine as a jelly-like mass, and is convenient for topical application.

generations of drugs

are 'created' when, in the development of a class of drugs, a significant advance occurs (in potency, duration of action, absorption, spectrum of action, fewer side-effects etc). Thus in a number of ANTIBIOTIC families there are first, second and third generations (eg the CEPHALOSPORIN drugs).

generic drug name

is the official non-proprietary (standard) name for the active chemical(s) in a medicine, in contrast to the proprietary name (trade or brand name) for a medicine. (Originally the term generic was applied to a class of drugs, (eg BARBITURATE, SULPHONAMIDE), though this exact usage is less common nowadays.) In the UK, doctors in general and hospital practice are encouraged to refer to, and prescribe, drugs by the generic non-proprietary name (correctly written without initial capital letters). Until recently, the name that has been used was that chosen by the Nomenclature Committee of the British Pharmacopoeia and is referred to as the **British Approved Name** (BAN). This is in most cases the same as the **recommended International Non-proprietary Name** (rINN). However, for some drugs these two official names differ, and in the UK there is a changeover in progress towards use of the rINN, either exclusively, or double-labelled with both forms. (This book uses the rINN form, with a cross-index from the BAN name.) Generally, when a prescription is written by a doctor for a proprietary drug (always written with initial capital letters: see **proprietary name**), and if it is paid for by the NHS, the pharmacist may make a generic substitution in the form of a (cheaper) equivalent non-proprietary (generic) drug. However, in some instances this is not appropriate where non-proprietary forms differ in some important respect (eg **modified-release preparations** that differ in their time-courses of release), and here the exact proprietary form is generally supplied. In any case, during the period of the patent that is granted to the inventor (commonly 16-20 years for a new chemical entity or formulation, but depending on the country concerned), only a proprietary form of the drug may be available. In this case a generic prescription will be filled with a proprietary drug (complete with packaging, etc, in the latter name). Although the generic form contains the same chemical entity as the active constituent as in the proprietary form of the drug, concern has been expressed about the bioequivalence of preparations (ie whether in actual use they have an equivalent effect), and regulatory authorities normally require proof that, at a given dose, the generic drugs substituted for their parent proprietary drug have a bioavailability that ensures equivalent pharmacological effect. See also **names of drugs.**

genes
that determine the genetic make-up of living organisms are contained in 23 pairs of chromosomes in humans. The Human Genome Project is concerned with identifying the entire gene sequence (more than 50,000 genes made up of a total of about three billion DNA base pairs). See **genome; genotype.**

genetic engineering
is a modern term meaning the use of techniques (**recombinant DNA technology**) to modify the structure of **genes**, or to create or delete genes. Potentially, these techniques may be used to correct diseases in humans due to genetic defects (eg cystic fibrosis). Use in animal husbandry is now quite advanced.

genitourinary tract (also called the urogenital or urinogenital tract)
comprises the sexual organs and bladder, and related structures.

genome
is the total genetic material of an organism, which in humans is the **genes** that are contained in 23 pairs of chromosomes.

genotype
is the total genetic complement of a set of **genes** that an individual possesses (containing contributions from both parents). Not all this information is expressed. See also **phenotype.**

glaucoma
is an eye condition characterized by a raised intraocular pressure in the eye, which if left untreated can damage the optic nerve and result in blindness. There are various forms, but the two common ones are: simple (open-angle) glaucoma, which is chronic, seen more commonly in middle-age and is often familial; and acute (closed-angle) glaucoma. The former is treated with BETA-BLOCKER drugs and certain other drugs or surgery. See also GLAUCOMA TREATMENT.

goitre
is a collection of disease states characterized by an enlarged thyroid gland. Goitre has a number of causes: a shortage of iodine in the diet – endemic goitre; **hyperplasia** (**tumour**) of the gland – sporadic goitre; swelling due to overactivity in Grave's disease – exothalmic goitre; or autoimmune thyroiditis – Hashimoto's disease. Additionally, some chemicals and drugs may cause goitre as a side-effect.

gynaecomastia
is enlargement of breasts in the male. It can be caused by elevated levels of female sex hormones (oestrogen) in the blood. Some drugs may cause it as a **side-effect** (eg CIMETIDINE, DIGOXIN, SPIRONOLACTONE).

habituation
to a drug is a state where regular (possibly excessive) taking of an agent causes the individual to become accustomed to it, but not to the extreme psychological or physical stage of dependence (addiction).

haemoglobin (hemoglobin in USA)
is the oxygen-carrying pigment of the red blood cells (erythrocytes) of the blood. Some familial abnormal forms cause **anaemia** (eg **sickle-cell disease**). Other abnormal forms that carry oxygen poorly and cause **anoxia** are caused by acute reaction with chemicals, for instance **methaemoglobin** by NITRATE drugs and a number of other drugs and chemicals, and carboxyhaemoglobin by carbon monoxide.

haemolysis
is the destruction of red blood cells (erythrocytes). It may occur within the body through infection, poisoning, the action of antibodies (see **antibody**) or as **adverse drug reactions.** Individuals with (normally familial) low levels of the enzyme glucose 6-phosphate (**G6PD-deficiency**) are particularly at risk from many drugs, including PRIMAQUINE and SULPHONAMIDE and SULPHONE drugs.

haemorrhoids (piles)
are an enlargement of the wall of the anus, sometimes caused as a consequence of prolonged constipation, and often following childbirth. There may be pain and bleeding. Treatment of first-degree haemorrhoids is normally through adjustment of diet, but second- and third-degree severity may

require surgical or similar intervention.

heart failure

is a term used for the condition in which the amount of blood pumped by the heart is not sufficient to meet the oxygen and metabolic needs of the body either during work or at rest. The causes of heart failure include disease within the heart (mainly ischaemia – an inadequate supply of blood to the muscle that can also cause angina pain) or an excessive load imposed on the heart by arterial and other forms of **hypertension**. See HEART FAILURE TREATMENT.

hepatitis

is inflammation of the liver, accompanied by damage or death of liver cells. It may be due to infection (eg viral hepatitis), toxic substances or immunological abnormalities. Infectious hepatitis is of several types: hepatitis A (infectious hepatitis) is mainly transmitted by faecal-contaminated food; hepatitis B (serum hepatitis) is transmitted by infected blood, needles and sexually. Further forms are hepatitis C (non-A, non-B hepatitis), hepatitis D and hepatitis E. Prevention by vaccination or immunization is recommended for those at risk, and treatments include avoidance of alcohol and occasionally use of interferons (see INTERFERON).

herbal medicines

are those derived from plants. The science of plant drugs is part of pharmacognosy, a traditional subject taught as part of normal training-courses for pharmacists. Today, terms such as phytopharmacy, phytopharmacology and phytotherapy are commonly used instead. Many conventional medicines with defined pharmacology and therapeutic uses are herbal in origin (or are semisynthetic derivatives of plant ALKALOID drugs), and generally use of pure principles isolated from plant material are preferred. Examples include the VINCA ALKALOIDS, OPIATE (eg MORPHINE SULPHATE), BELLADONNA ALKALOID (eg ATROPINE SULPHATE), ERGOT ALKALOID, ANTICANCER drugs and the taxanes (eg PACLITAXEL). Additionally, there are many herbal remedies of less defined properties that are used in their impure form in preference, as part of **complementary medicine** (alternative medicine). The British Herbal Medicine Association (BHMA) documents herbal medicines and makes licensed remedies in a number of therapeutic categories, and these preparations have been reviewed by the **Medicines Control Agency** (MCA).

herpes

is an inflammation with blistering of the skin or mucous membranes, caused by the herpes virus. Herpes simplex virus (HSV) is of two sorts: type I causes the common cold sore around the lips (which is contagious by contact); and type II is associated with genital herpes (which is sexually transmitted). Herpes zoster (shingles), which is caused by the varicella-zoster virus, remains in a dormant form in sensory nerves following chickenpox, and can later be activated to affect the eye (ophthalmic zoster) or skin (dermatoses). Treatment of all forms of herpes is mainly with ACICLOVIR.

Hodgkin's disease

is a **lymphoma**, a **malignant** disease, a **cancer** arising in lymphoid tissue, including lymph nodes and the spleen.

homeopathy

is a system of **complementary medicine** (alternative medicine) founded by Hahnemann in Germany around 1811. It generally uses homeopathetic substances that produce the same symptoms as the disease, and proposes that medicines become more potent according to their degree of dilution. Homeopathic medicines are labelled using a system indicating the (normally very high) degree of dilution. In the UK, most OTC homeopathic medicines do not have a **licence** from the **Medicines Control Agency** (because there is no proof of efficacy), so are not allowed to be labelled with their potential use(s). However, most carry an HR (Homeopathic Registration Scheme 1997) number certifying their safety and quality (but not their efficacy). Also, there are several homeopathic specialist NHS hospitals, and certain homeopathic medicines can be prescribed under the NHS.

homeostasis

is the physiological system that maintains the internal state of the body.

hyper-

as a prefix in medical terms denotes above normal.

hyperhidrosis

is excessive sweating and may be localized to the armpits, feet, palms or face. It may be due to hormone imbalance, anxiety, nervous system disorders or as a **side-effect** of some drugs (eg PARASYMPATHOMIMETIC drugs, ANTICHOLINESTERASE drugs, LEVODOPA, BUSERELIN, AMITRIPTYLINE HYDROCHLORIDE, THYROXINE). It is treated with topical application of ALUMINIUM CHLORIDE.

hyperlipidaemia

is a clinical condition where the blood plasma contains

very high levels of the lipids (fats) cholesterol and/or triglycerides (natural fats of the body). Deposition of lipids onto the lining of blood vessels leads to diseases such as coronary atherosclerosis (see **atheroma**) where plaques of lipid material narrow blood vessels, which contributes to **angina pectoris** attacks, and the formation of abnormal clots that go on to cause heart attacks (**myocardial infarction**) and strokes. The proportions of different lipids in the blood may be altered by appropriate modifications of diet, but LIPID-REGULATING DRUGS may also be used (generally where there is a family history of hyperlipidaemia or clinical signs indicating the need for intervention).

hyperplasia
is an increase in the production and growth of normal cells in a tissue, where the organ becomes bigger but retains its form (eg the breasts or uterus in pregnancy). See also **hypertrophy; neoplasm.**

hyperreactivity
see **hypersensitivity reaction.**

hypersensitivity
is when a pharmacological response occurs at lower than normal doses.

hypersensitivity reaction
is where the individual is prone to respond abnormally or exaggeratedly to a drug. Generally this is due to an allergic reaction where the drug (eg a PENICILLIN) is acting as an **antigen**, triggering a variety of tissue reactions such as bronchospasm (marked **bronchoconstriction** of the airways), and skin reactions (eg **urticaria**), and **anaphylactic shock.** See also **adverse drug reactions; allergic reactions.**

hypertension
is a higher than normal blood pressure for a person of that age. The World Health Organization defines hypertension as a blood pressure consistently exceeding 160/95 mm Hg (systolic/diastolic). However, because there is a considerable range of blood pressures for a population group, high blood pressure in itself may not denote hypertension, but a rising pressure with secondary pathology usually is an indication for treatment. Clinically, hypertension is divided into a number of disease states each with different **aetiology**. Essential hypertension is the most common, and here the determinants of the disease are not well understood. Renal hypertension has its origins in kidney disease (eg a narrowing of the renal arteries). The condition **phaeochromocytoma** is characterized by episodes of extreme hypertension due to release of adrenaline and noradrenaline from a tumour of adrenal gland tissue. Other specific causes of hypertension include CUSHING'S SYNDROME and pre-eclampsia. Treatment depends on cause and may involve ANTIHYPERTENSIVE drugs.

hyperthyroidism
is over-activity of the thyroid gland, with elevated levels of thyroid hormones (THYROXINE) in the bloodstream. See **goitre.**

hypertrophy
is an increase in the size of an organ or tissue brought about by an increase in the size of its cells, as in muscles with exercise (rather than of number of cells, as in a **tumour** or **hyperplasia**).

hypo-
as a prefix in medical terms denotes below normal.

hypotension
is a lower than normal blood pressure. However, since there is a considerable range of blood pressures for a population group, low blood pressure in itself may not denote any pathology. It is more normally seen as an acute medical condition due to excess loss of body fluids (eg in burns, vomiting and diarrhoea) or blood (eg haemorrhage). There are a number of other causes, including **myocardial infarction, pancreatitis,** Addison's disease and pulmonary **embolism.** Postural hypotension (orthostatic hypotension) is a temporary fall in blood pressure when the subject rises from a supine position, and is due to impaired physiological compensatory reflexes. Many drugs can cause hypotension either as part of serious **adverse drug reactions** or as a minor side-effect. Many ANTIHYPERTENSIVE drugs cause postural hypotension or periods of hypotension.

idiosyncratic responses
see **adverse drug reactions.**

immunity
is a state of protection against infection and disease through the activity of the immune system, comprising circulating antibodies (see **antibody**) and white blood cells. Therapeutically, immunization can be used to boost the immunity; active immunity can be stimulated by inoculation with VACCINES, and passive immunity by administration of IMMUNOGLOBULIN agents.

immunocompromised
is a term that refers to a person whose immune defences are very much lower than normal due to

either a congenital (present at birth) or acquired condition. The commonest deficiencies are: of the white cells (neutrophils) which are the first line of defence in acute infections; of the white cells, macrophages, and T-lymphocytes, which are involved in cell-mediated killing of foreign or 'parasitized' host cells; and of the antibodies, which neutralize and bind to foreign antigens. Examples of immunocompromised hosts include: patients receiving IMMUNOSUPPRESSANT drugs to prevent rejection of transplanted organs; patients suffering from leukaemia, or being treated with high doses of CYTOTOXIC drugs to treat cancer; and individuals with AIDS. In any of these circumstances 'opportunistic' infections are apt to occur where microbes which normally pose little threat to the healthy become highly invasive and pose a serious threat. Prophylaxis with antibacterial drugs may be required, and once infections are established they are much more difficult to eradicate, even with vigorous ANTIBIOTIC treatment.

implant
is a form of drug depot administration where a solid formulation of the drug is given at intramuscular or subcutaneous sites. The commonest used is for CONTRACEPTIVE hormone drugs.

indication
see licence.

inflammation
is an acute or chronic bodily reaction to a chemical or physical injury, or to infection. It is characterized by the 'cardinal signs': calor (heat); rubor (redness); dolor (pain); and **tumor** (swelling). Although inflammation is initially protective, chronic inflammatory diseases can be incapacitating. See ANTI-INFLAMMATORY, ANTIRHEUMATIC and CORTICOSTEROID.

infusion
is the continuous administration (by injection, most commonly intravenously) of a drug or fluid over a period of minutes, hours or days. See also **routes of administration of drugs.**

injection
of a drug or fluid is administration by means of a needle and syringe. See also **routes of administration of drugs.**

INN
see **recommended International Non-proprietary Name.**

interaction
see **drug interactions.**

International Pharmacopoeia
(Int. P) is the pharmacopoeia of the World Health Organization and is a formulary intended to meet international needs.

intolerance
is when there is a greater than expected reaction to a drug. See **hypersensitivity.**

intra-
as a prefix means within.

intradermal
injections are made into the skin. See **routes of administration of drugs.**

intraocular pressure
is the pressure within the eyeball that helps maintain its shape, and which is determined by the balance between the production and removal of aqueous humour. A build-up of pressure, **glaucoma**, is damaging to the eye (and in susceptible people may be caused by certain drugs, eg CORTICOSTEROID and ANTICHOLINERGIC drugs). The main treatment of glaucoma is with drugs; see GLAUCOMA TREATMENT.

intrathecal
injections are made into the subarachnoid space of the spinal cord. This route is used to localize the actions of LOCAL ANAESTHETIC and ANALGESIC drugs to certain segments of the body supplied by sensory nerves originating from the area of injection.

iron-deficient anaemia
is a reduced capacity of the blood to carry oxygen, due to a reduction in levels of the iron-containing pigment of the red blood cells, **haemoglobin**, which transports oxygen within the body. It can be caused by insufficient intake of iron (eg in gastrointestinal disease or in dietary insufficiency), particularly when this is required after excessive loss of blood. See ANAEMIA TREATMENT.

leucopenia
is a condition when there is a low level of leucocytes (white blood cells) in the bloodstream. It may be caused by an adverse drug reaction.

leukaemia
is a malignant growth, a cancer where abnormal white blood cells proliferate in the bone marrow.

There are several types, and treatment for some forms is available.

licence

for a medicine is obtained in the UK from the **Medicines Control Agency** (MCA) after application from a pharmaceutical company to manufacture it. The licence (product licence) is granted only for certain defined **indications**, uses for which it is deemed efficacious and safe. Medical practitioners normally conform to these indications in their prescribing, and not to do so opens the way to legal consequences. But there are certain uses that are technically 'unlicensed indications' (sometimes because there is not enough data to establish efficacy in relatively uncommon conditions and circumstances), but hospital specialists may sometimes use them for such purposes. If a drug is to be licensed for use in all member states of the European Union (EU) as a whole (as is increasingly the case), applications for a licence are made to the European Medicines Evaluation Agency (which is based in London).

linctuses

are medicated syrups that are thick and soothing enough to relieve sore throats or loosen a cough.

liniments

are medicated lotions for rubbing into the skin. Many of them contain alcohol and/or camphor, and are intended to relieve minor muscle aches and pains.

liposomes

are a drug-delivery system, and are comprised of small vesicles of phospholipid-protein membrane with an aqueous drug-containing interior. They may allow absorption from the intestine of substances, such as the peptide INSULIN, that would otherwise be digested; also, liposomes may reduce toxicity of substances given intravenously.

local

action of drugs is where application or injection is such that drug action is limited to a certain area of the body; in contrast to systemic action where the drug passes into the blood circulation and thus has a general action.

lotions

are medicated liquids used to bathe or wash skin, hair or eyes.

lozenges

contain medicaments in a hard, often sweetened and flavoured, base. They are intended to be slowly dissolved in the mouth to treat local irritation or infection.

lupus erythematosus

is a chronic inflammatory condition of the connective tissue and is an autoimmune disease (see **autoimmune diseases**); it is also caused by **adverse drug reactions** to a number of types of drugs, such as HYDRALAZINE HYDROCHLORIDE, PROCAINAMIDE HYDROCHLORIDE, ISONIAZID and SULPHASALAZINE. Treatment is with ANTI-INFLAMMATORY and IMMUNOSUPPRESSANT drugs.

Lyme disease

is caused by a bacterium (spirochaete, *Borrelia burgdorferi*), which is transmitted by the bite of a tick that lives on deer and can also infest dogs. It causes acute inflammation at the site of the bite, and after a period, headache, lethargy, fever and muscle pain develop. There can be serious chronic symptoms. Treatment is with ANTIBIOTIC drugs.

lymphoma

is a malignant disease, a cancer arising in lymphoid tissue (mainly of the nodes and spleen), such as **Hodgkin's disease**.

malignant

in general, describes any condition in the body which if untreated may be a threat to health (eg malignant **hypertension**). Specifically, it describes a **tumour** that invades and destroys other cells or tissues, ie is cancerous (see **cancer**).

MCA

see **Medicines Control Agency**.

medicines

see **drugs and medicines**.

Medicines Control Agency (MCA)

is part of the UK drugs regulatory system that administers the Medicines Act and issues the product **licence** for a drug, acting on evidence received and advice from the **Committee on Safety of Medicines** (CSM). If a drug is to be licensed for use in all member states of the European Union (EU) as a whole (as is increasingly the case), applications for a licence are made to the European Medicines Evaluation Agency (situated in London).

megaloblastic anaemia

is a group of conditions that are caused by a reduction in synthesis of **haemoglobin**, or production of abnormal red blood cells, due a deficiency of vitamin B_{12} (HYDROXOCOBALAMIN and CYANOCOBALAMIN), or FOLIC ACID, or both. There may be a number of causes. In pernicious anaemia there is a shortage in the body (it is an autoimmune disease) of a substance called intrinsic factor necessary for absorption of vitamin B_{12} from the intestine. Dietary vitamin deficiency in groups at risk is a common cause. See ANAEMIA TREATMENT.

meningitis
is inflammation of the membranes covering the brain and spinal cord (meninges), commonly through infection by bacteria or viruses. Symptoms include severe headache, fever, stiff neck, nausea and vomiting, **photophobia** and other characteristic signs. In bacterial meningitis, there may also be a red blotchy skin rash. Infections by the viral form are usually mild, but those due to bacterial forms (meningococcal infection or *Haemophilus influenza*) can be serious. Vaccination against *Haemophilus influenza* is now in routine use in babies and increasingly used for travellers to areas of risk and for local UK outbreaks (especially in young people). Also, ANTIBIOTIC drugs are used against the bacterial forms.

metabolism of drugs
is the process whereby the body detoxifies chemicals and excretes them as metabolites. It can be divided into two phases of conversion.

methaemoglobin
(methemoglobin in USA) is an oxidized form of haemoglobin that is not able to carry oxygen, so production of it can lead to toxic **anoxia**. Blood can be converted (normally reversibly) into this form by drugs and chemicals (eg NITRATE drugs and NITROFURANTOIN).

-mimetic
as a suffix means to imitate or mimic. For example, SYMPATHOMIMETICS are agents that mimic the actions of the sympathetic nervous system.

MIMS
(Monthly Index of Medical Specialities) is a comprehensive compendium of the drugs that are available to general practitioners, **pharmacists** and other healthcare professionals.

modified-release preparations
(sustained-release preparations; continuous-release preparations)
are normally **tablets** or **capsules** which are designed to release their active constituents over a period of time, either for convenience or to minimize adverse effects (A **proprietary name** often contains the term Continus, CR, LA, MA, MR, Retard, SR, XL.)

molecular biology
literally, is the study of biology at the molecular level. Recently, it has taken on special meanings and is used particularly to denote the study of **genes**, gene products and sometimes pharmaceuticals produced by processes using genetic methods.

monoclonal antibody
is a type of pure **antibody** of homogeneous and selective properties (manufactured by the techniques of **molecular biology**). Such antibodies have recently been introduced into medicine for a number of specialist treatments (see ABCIXIMAB, BASILIXIMAB, DACLIZUMAB, PALIVIZUMAB, RITUXIMAB), and show promise for the future for a range of purposes including for IMMUNIZATION and as ANTICANCER drugs. See also **antibody**.

MRSA
see **multi-drug resistance**.

multi-drug resistance
is where there is resistance to the actions of a number of different drugs of different classes. It may be, for example, in **chemotherapy** for infection where pathogenic organisms have acquired resistance to antibiotic or other antibacterial agents, each with a differing mechanism of action. An important example is MRSA (methoxycillin-resistant *Staphylococcus aureus*), a staphylococcal infection found in hospitals that has become resistant to a wide range of ANTIBIOTIC drugs. Also in the chemotherapy of **cancer**, the cancerous cells may become resistant to a number of unrelated drugs through developing a specialized mechanism that excretes the drugs from the affected cells making them ineffective.

multi-drug therapy
is when a number of drugs are used together in a concerted manner to resolve a medical problem. The term is most commonly applied to the concurrent use of drugs in **chemotherapy** for infection, especially ANTIVIRAL drugs from two or three different classes in the treatment of AIDS (eg protease inhibitors together with reverse transcriptase inhibitors), or the two or more ANTIBACTERIAL drugs with different mechanisms used in tuberculosis treatment.

myasthenia gravis
is a disorder characterized by **skeletal muscle**

weakness, particularly drooping eyelids and weak speech. It is an autoimmune disease (see **autoimmune diseases**) which causes impaired neurotransmission by acetylcholine at the neuromuscular junction, and can be treated with ANTICHOLINESTERASE drugs.

myelosuppression
is a reduction in the production of blood cells by the bone marrow. It often occurs after **chemotherapy** for cancer and may cause **anaemia**, abnormal bleeding or infection.

myocardial infarction (heart attack)
is the sudden death of part of the heart muscle, characterized by severe unremitting pain. It is usually caused by coronary **thrombosis**, obstruction of the coronary arteries. Treatment, which should be immediate, is complex. Arrhythmias of the heart are treated with ANTI-ARRHYTHMIC drugs and electrical defibrillation. Associated formation of clots can be treated by FIBRINOLYTIC drugs, as well as ANALGESIC, DIURETIC and BETA-BLOCKER drugs.

names of drugs
are of three main types. The chemical drug name (see **chemical drug names**) is the full name of the chemical that is the active component, but has the disadvantage in medical use that it is often very long and complex. The **generic drug name** (non-proprietary name) is the official 'trivial' name (eg paracetamol), and is used in normal medical prescribing and use. The **proprietary name**, the trade or brand name, is always capitalized (eg Panadol), and is used for marketing purposes and in drug packaging. See also **British Approved Name; recommended International Non-proprietary Name.**

narcolepsy
is an extreme tendency to fall asleep in a quiet environment. Although such individuals can be easily roused, stimulant drugs, such as DEXAMFETAMINE SULPHATE, may be used in its treatment.

National Institute for Clinical Excellence (NICE)
is a recently founded (April 1999) independent national body for the appraisal of new and existing therapies to assess their efficacy and cost-effectiveness, and to issue guidance around their use, especially with respect to their prescription or otherwise within the NHS. Recently, it has disallowed Relenza (ZANAMIVIR) for NHS prescription for flu prophylaxis during the 1999-2000 influenza season, but has approved (expensive) taxane ANTICANCER drug therapy for ovarian and breast cancer, and has moved on to examine conditions that warrant the use of new-generation NSAID generics and other drugs of more moderate expense.

natriuretic
means causing a sodium excretion into the urine (which is a property of DIURETIC).

nebulizer
see **aerosols**.

neoplasm
is any abnormal or new growth. Correctly, the term can be applied to relatively harmless swellings (**benign**) or cancerous (**malignant**) growths. Nevertheless, the term neoplastic disease is often loosely taken as synonymous with cancerous growth.

nephrosis (nephrotic syndrome)
are the symptoms of damage to the glomeruli (the filtering units) of the kidney. There is often **proteinurea** and **oedema**. It may be caused by diabetes mellitus, **hypertension**, poisons (eg lead and carbon tetrachloride) or as an adverse reaction to some drugs.

neuropathy
see **peripheral neuropathy**.

neurotransmitter
is the term used to describe chemical messengers which on release from a nerve-ending act nearby to excite (stimulate) or inhibit either other nerves or the cells within organs innervated by the nerves (such as the heart, intestine, skeletal muscle and glands) near to where they have been released from the nerve terminals. Neurotransmitters are therefore rather like hormones (see HORMONE), but unlike the latter they act locally rather than reaching their target tissue via the blood. Such mediators work by interacting with specific recognition sites on cells, called RECEPTORS, that 'recognize' only that mediator (or chemically similar analogues). These receptors may be blocked by drugs called receptor antagonists (see BETA-BLOCKER and ALPHA-ADRENOCEPTOR BLOCKER). Examples of neurotransmitters include ACETYLCHOLINE, DOPAMINE, NORADRENALINE and SEROTONIN (5-HT). Many drugs work by either mimicking or preventing the actions of neurotransmitters (eg most ANTIPSYCHOTIC drugs

work by blocking certain actions of dopamine in the brain).

neutropenia (granulocytopenia)
is a decrease in the number of neutrophils (one of the types of white blood cells). It may be caused by a number of diseases or as an adverse drugs reaction, and increases susceptibility to infection.

NICE
see National Institute for Clinical Excellence.

non-proprietary name
see names of drugs.

obstructive airways disease
describes conditions where there is a resistance to exhalation from the lungs due to a narrowing or obstruction to the passage of air in the bronchioles and bronchi. In medical circles these conditions are now often referred to as COPD (chronic obstructive pulmonary disease). Chronic conditions include **bronchitis** and **emphysema**, whereas **asthma** is often acute in onset (and may have an allergic component). Treatment may be with BRONCHODILATOR, ANTI-ALLERGIC (eg CORTICOSTEROID drugs), ANTI-ASTHMATIC or ANTIBIOTIC drugs, alone or in combination, according to diagnosis.

oedema
is an abnormal accumulation of fluid in the body tissues, and may be localized (eg as a swelling) or generalized (eg after **heart failure**). It can be caused by injury as a component of inflammation, or as a symptom of various diseases (heart failure, cirrhosis of the liver or nephrotic syndrome). It may also be caused by a number of drugs (eg ORAL CONTRACEPTIVE, CORTICOSTEROID and ANDROGEN drugs). Treatment of oedema depends on the cause, but DIURETIC drugs are commonly used.

oesophageal varices
are widenings in the veins supplying the oesophagus (sometimes extending down to the stomach). They can develop as a result of portal hypertension (increased blood supply to the portal vein due to liver disease, including **cirrhosis**). The varices are thin-walled and may rupture causing life-threatening haemorrhage. Treatment is with VASOPRESSIN as a VASOCONSTRICTOR drug, together with a sclerosing agent to seal the veins, followed by surgery.

ointment
is a general term that is used to describe a group of essentially greasy preparations which are insoluble in water and so do not wash off. They are used as bases for many therapeutic preparations for topical application (particularly in the treatment of dry lesions or ophthalmic complaints). Most ointments have a form of PARAFFIN as their base, but a few contain LANOLIN which may cause sensitivity reactions in some people.

oliguria
is the production of abnormally small amounts of urine. It can be due to a number of causes including kidney failure, excess sweating, blood loss, fluid retention (**oedema**) and diarrhoea. In some cases it is treated with DIURETIC drugs.

osteoarthritis
is a type of arthritis (joint inflammation) in which there is degeneration of the cartilage that lines the joints. It is exacerbated by stress and characterized by painful and stiff joints. Treatment of symptoms is by NSAIDS, CORTICOSTEROID drugs or surgery. Osteoarthritis is different from rheumatoid arthritis.

osteoporosis
is a loss of the bone tissue, leading to a tendency to become brittle and fracture. The cause can be infection, injury, hormonal, as part of **Cushing's syndrome**, in long-term CORTICOSTEROID therapy, or in the elderly and women following the menopause. HRT may be used to minimize osteoporosis in postmenopausal women.

OTC
See **over-the-counter**.

ototoxicity
is toxic damage to the inner ear, including drug-induced damage to the nerve serving the inner ear (eighth cranial nerve) the cochlea and semicircular canals, so causing some degree of deafness or loss of the sense of balance. This is a common adverse effect seen with the use of ANTIBIOTIC drugs of the AMINOGLYCOSIDE class (eg NEOMYCIN SULPHATE).

over-the-counter (OTC)
medicines are non-prescription medicines that can be bought by members of the public without a doctor's **prescription**. They are of two types; either 'P' medicines (featuring a 'P' on their packaging) that may only be dispensed by qualified pharmacists, normally in a **pharmacy**; or alternatively they may be 'GSL' (General Sales List) medicines that can be sold in any shop or outlet.

pancreatitis
is inflammation of the pancreas, and is commonly due to gallstones or alcohol abuse, though it can be caused by viral infection, **hyperlipidaemia** or a physical injury. A number of drugs may precipitate (normally acute) pancreatitis, including NSAIDS and ANTIBIOTIC drugs, and also chronic use of PARACETAMOL.

paraesthesia
means spontaneous feelings of abnormal sensations such as tingling ('pins and needles'), prickling, burning, tightness, or the feeling of a band tight around a limb or the trunk. It can be caused by pressure, peripheral nerve disease, spinal cord disease, or as a side-effect of many drugs of a number of different classes (usually reversible on stopping treatment). See also **peripheral neuropathy**.

parallel imports
is the system whereby drugs are imported for sale from a country where the drugs are sold at a cheaper price.

parasympathetic nervous system
see **autonomic nervous system**.

parenteral
means administration by any route other than the mouth (eg orally). See also **routes of administration of drugs**.

passive immunity
see IMMUNIZATION.

pastille
is a soft lozenge (see **lozenges**).

patents for drugs
may be granted to the inventor of a drug as a new chemical entity or new formulation of it. During the period of the patent (commonly 16-20 years for a new chemical entity or formulation, but depending on the circumstances, and the country concerned), only a proprietary form of the drug (with a registered **proprietary name** or brand name) may be available for prescription and clinical use. See also **generic drug name**.

pathogens
are agents that cause disease, and are normally micro-organisms (including bacteria, viruses, protozoa and fungi).

pathological
means relating to disease, or to pathology, the study of disease.

-pathy
as a suffix denotes disease (eg neuropathy, encephalopathy, retinopathy).

Patient Information Leaflet (PIL; or Product Information Leaflet)
is the technical literature placed by the drug manufacturer in the packaging of medicines, and is intended to be read by the patient or carer. In the case of **over-the-counter** (OTC) drugs (medicines that can be bought without a prescription), these safety warnings are of particular importance.

peripheral neuropathy
is disease of or damage to the peripheral nerves, and is characterized by numbness, tingling ('pins and needles'), pain or sometimes muscle weakness, particularly in the extremities. There are a number of possible causes (eg diabetic or alcoholic neuropathies). Poisoning with a number of chemicals (eg lead) may cause the syndrome and a number of drugs cause it as a side-effect (which is normally reversible on withdrawal of treatment).

peripheral vascular disease
is a narrowing of the blood vessels in the legs and sometimes arms, causing pain and coldness in the extremities. There can be a number of causes, including **atheroma**, inadequately controlled **diabetes** mellitus, deep vein **thrombosis** and varicose veins. Smokers are particularly at risk. Sometimes peripheral vascular disease occurs without evident occlusion, eg Reynaud's disease and Bueger's disease.

peristalsis
is the co-ordinated and rhythmic (involuntary) waves of muscular activity that move the contents of the intestines in the appropriate direction. The term also applies to propulsive movement in the ureter that helps move urine from the kidneys to the bladder. Peristalsis depends largely on intrinsic activity of the **smooth muscle** and the nerves within the wall of the gut, but is modulated from within the **central nervous system** via nerves of the **autonomic nervous system**. A wide variety of drugs affect peristalsis activity in the treatment of disease or as side-effects.

pernicious anaemia
see **megaloblastic anaemia**.

pessary
is a formulation of a drug inserted into the vagina. See also **suppository**.

phaeochromocytoma
is a type of growth of neuroendocrine glandular tissue of the type normally found in the **adrenal** medulla, leading to large and often dramatic release of adrenaline and noradrenaline. Treatment is with ALPHA-ADRENOCEPTOR ANTAGONIST and BETA-BLOCKER drugs, prior to surgery. See also **carcinoid tumours.**

pharmaceutical industry
is the drugs industry, concerned with the development, manufacture and marketing of drugs as medicines.

pharmacist
is a practitioner of pharmacy, whether in the pharmaceutical industry, universities, hospital pharmacies or shops and high-street pharmacies.

pharmacodynamics
is a term for the effects of drugs on the body, including mechanisms ('what the drug does to the body'). See also **pharmacokinetics.**

pharmacognosy
is the study of botanical and other sources of drugs, and the properties of crude drugs.

pharmacokinetics
is a term for the processes of absorption, distribution and metabolism of drugs ('what the body does to the drug'). See **pharmacodynamics.**

pharmacologist
is a practitioner of **pharmacology**, particularly concerned with the discovery and development of drugs, and the understanding of how drugs work. Pharmacologists are mainly employed in the pharmaceutical industry, or in research and teaching in universities and institutes.

pharmacology
is the science of drugs, the effect of chemical substances have on living processes. It can be divided into **pharmacodynamics** ('what the drug does to the body') and **pharmacokinetics** ('what the body does to the drug'). It is much concerned with the development of novel drugs.

pharmacopoeias
lists official preparation of drugs. See also **British Pharmacopoeia, International Pharmacopoeia** and **European Pharmacopoeia.**

pharmacy
is the preparation (formulation) and supply of medicines (and the place where it is done). See **pharmacist.**

phenotype
is the expression of characteristics (visual, biochemical or otherwise measurable) determined by the individual's **genes** (see **genotype**) and their interaction with the environment.

phenylketonuria
is an inherited condition due to a deficiency of the enzyme that metabolizes the natural amino acid phenylalanine (to tyrosine), which is a constituent of the protein in many foodstuffs. The condition is characterized by severe mental handicap unless the diet of affected infants is switched to special foods free of this amino acid.

photophobia
is an intolerance to light to the extent that normal levels are uncomfortable. It occurs in some eye disorders (eg acute iritis, corneal damage and chronic **glaucoma**), in some systemic infections (eg **meningitis**) or can be induced by drugs that dilate the pupil.

photosensitivity
is abnormal reaction to sunlight (eg rash). Phototoxicity is where drug treatment lowers sensitivity of the skin to ultraviolet light, so that there is burning. One form is photoallergy where the drug combines with skin protein to form an allergen (see **allergens**), to which the body reacts with an allergic reaction (see **allergic reactions**). Undesirable photosensitization is caused by a wide variety of drugs in standard usage (eg TETRACYCLINES, HYPOGLYCAEMIC, ORAL CONTRACEPTIVE, PHENOTHIAZINE, SULPHONAMIDE or SULPHONYLUREA drugs). For protection SUNSCREEN agents applied to the skin can help.

pills
are solid spherical or ovoid drug dose forms (originally made by a rolling process), which are now largely superseded by **tablets.** 'The Pill' is slang for ORAL CONTRACEPTIVES, which actually are in tablet form.

placebos
are dummy treatments, having only psychological effects, used in clinical trials.

poisons
'All things are poisonous and there is nothing that is harmless, the dose alone decides that something is no poison.' Paracelsus (1493-1541). This

statement still applies, indeed, many compounds previously regarded as poisons are today used as medicines (eg COLCHICINE from the autumn crocus (*Colchicum autumnale*) and VINCA ALKALOIDS from the periwinkle (*Vinca rosea*)).

PoM
see **Prescription-only Medicine.**

porphyria
is one of a group of several relatively uncommon disease states characterized by disturbed metabolism of the pigment haem (which occurs in the blood pigment **haemoglobin**), leading to the accumulation in the body of porphyrins, causing red, brown or bluish urine. Aside from a number of porphyric disease states, some drug-induced porphyrias are known (eg that caused by TAMOXIFEN), and many drugs should not be used in individuals who suffer from porphyria.

postural hypotension
see **hypotension.**

potency of a drug
is how strong it is, either in terms of the dose required to achieve a given effect, or the maximum effect that is achievable.

pre-eclampsia
see **eclampsia.**

prescription
is the document detailing to the **pharmacist**, the name of the patient, the drug to be prescribed, the dose and other details. Drugs of **Prescription-only Medicine** (PoM) status can only be prescribed by a qualified medical practitioner (though dentists may prescribe from the Dental Practitioners' Formulary, and nurses from a limited Nurse Prescribers' Formulary). Medical practitioners may also prescribe certain **over-the-counter** (OTC) medicines, but cannot prescribe for payment by the NHS drugs on a NHS black-list of unaccepted drugs and preparations. Drugs on the **Controlled Drugs** list are subject to special restrictions.

Prescription-only Medicine (PoM)
is one that must be prescribed by an appropriately qualified doctor on a proper **prescription** form, and can not be bought **over-the-counter** (OTC). Some drugs are subject to special restrictions, for instance, drugs on the **Controlled Drugs** list (eg OPIATE drugs) or those used only in certain hospitals or clinics and on a 'named-patient-only' basis.

priapism
is prolonged erection of the penis and is a painful condition requiring immediate treatment. It is caused by a failure of blood to drain from the spongy tissue of the penis. It can occur due to nerve damage, infection, as part of a variety of other disease states and with blood clots. It can also occur as a side-effect incurred through the use of certain drugs, such as the PROSTAGLANDIN analogue ALPROSTADIL, or SILDENAFIL (Viagra) for the treatment of impotence.

pro-drug
is a chemical form of a drug that is not in itself pharmacologically active, but is converted in the body to the active drug (eg ENALAPRIL MALEATE to enalaprilat; phenacetin to PARACETAMOL). The pro-drugs may be chemically more stable or better absorbed than the active drugs.

product licence
see **licence.**

prophylaxis
means any measure taken in disease prevention. Examples include use of VACCINE drugs and IMMUNIZATION to prevent infection, CONTRACEPTIVE products (prophylactics) to prevent conception, BETA-BLOCKER drugs in ANTI-ANGINA treatment to delay the occurrence of anginal pain on exercise, and FLUORIDE in tap-water or specific preparations to reduce dental caries.

proprietary name
is the trade name or brand name of a medicine, the name given to it by the manufacturer – in contrast to the official non-proprietary (**generic drug name**) name for the active chemical(s) in a medicine. For example, Nurofen is a proprietary name for ibuprofen. At the time of its introduction, a drug is usually protected by a patent (see **patents for drugs**) granted to the company that invented it, and for the duration of that patent (commonly 16-20 years from the date of patent a new chemical entity or formulation, but often less than ten years by the time the drug is on the market), the drug will be available only as the brand-name product. After expiry of the patent, other manufacturers can market the drug under their own proprietary names or simply under the generic name; however, they will still need to obtain a **licence** from the MCA. The later generic forms (whether with a new brand name or not) are generally cheaper, and under NHS prescribing directives will normally be substituted where the original form is more

expensive. See also **names of drugs**.

proteinurea

is the passage of increased amounts of protein in the urine. It can result from a bacterial infection of the urinary tract, and a number of other disorders including pre-eclampsia (see **eclampsia**).

pruritus

is itching, which, as well as occurring in several disease states, is a very common **side-effect** of certain drugs, especially those that release histamine in the body.

psoriasis

is a chronic skin complaint characterized by thickened patches of scaling skin. Treatment is problematical, but includes PHOTODYNAMIC THERAPY, photodynamic therapy and drug therapy, including KERATOLYTIC, RETINOID, CORTICOSTEROID and METHOTREXATE drugs.

pulmonary embolism

is an obstruction of the pulmonary (lung) circulation by a clot (thrombus; often from a site in the leg) becoming lodged in the pulmonary artery or one of its branches. It can result in **heart failure** or sudden death. Treatment is with FIBRINOLYTIC and ANTICOAGULANT drugs. See **embolism**; **thrombosis**.

pyelonephritis

is an inflammation of the kidney, usually due to bacterial infection, and can occur in acute or chronic forms. Treatment of the acute form is usually with ANTIBIOTIC drugs.

pyrexia (fever)

is a body temperature raised above normal, and is usually taken as indicating an infection. It is treated with ANTIPYRETIC drugs, such as PARACETAMOL and NSAIDS.

pyrogens

are substances that cause fever. They normally are produced as a result of microbial or other infection, with the result that the body's 'thermostat' in the brain is set too high. PROSTAGLANDIN agents are pyrogens, and NSAIDS, such as ASPIRIN, that prevent their production are commonly used ANTIPYRETIC drugs.

Raynaud's disease/syndrome

see **peripheral vascular disease**.

receptors

are proteins through which many drugs and natural mediators act to exert their effects. Receptors *recognize* and are stimulated not only by their own ('endogenous') mediators – including neurotransmitters (eg endorphins), hormones (eg insulin) and local hormones (eg histamine) – but by drugs that have been designed to mimic these mediators. They are usually situated on the surface membrane of cells and require only tiny amounts of a mediator or other chemical (called 'agonists') to trigger a reaction that can produce rapid and profound changes in that cell (for instance, biochemical changes or electrical effects). The eventual end result of many such triggered effects may be some physical effect (eg an increased rate of beating due to the action of adrenaline on the heart) or may be a psychological effect (eg a mood change due to the actions of serotonin or dopamine in the brain).

Another class of drug, the ANTAGONIST, have a different type of action; they can *occupy* (in effect, physically block) the receptor without producing changes in the cell and prevent the agonist type of drug from acting. Examples of receptor types are alpha- and beta-adrenoceptors for ADRENALINE and NORADRENALINE; muscarinic and nicotinic cholinergic receptors for acetylcholine; H_1 and H_2 for histamine; and ANDROGEN or OESTROGEN receptors for these sex hormone (see SEX HORMONES) mediators. In all cases, synthetic drugs have been produced that act, either as agonists or antagonists, at these receptors.

recombinant DNA technology

introduces new genetic material (eg that of another species) or reorganized genetic material into host cells. When done by artificial techniques, it is a form of **genetic engineering**, and is used particularly in **biotechnology** to produce biopharmaceuticals, normally proteins (eg insulins, growth hormone).

recommended International Non-proprietary Name (rINN)

is the official name of a generic (non-proprietary) drug chosen by an international commission. In most cases it is the same as the **British Approved Name** (BAN), but the UK is moving towards the universal use of entirely rINN names. Other names including the American (United States Adopted Name; USAN) and Japanese (Japanese Accepted Name; JAN) are often similar, but in some instances differ completely. See also **generic drug name**.

reflux oesophagitis

see **gastro-oesophageal reflux**.

regimen
is a systematic course of treatment.

Reye's syndrome
is seen in children and may be caused by ingestion of ASPIRIN (though it may certainly have other causes). It is rare but serious, and is characterized by a fatty liver and brain damage. The link with aspirin is not entirely clear, but since 1986 aspirin bottles have been labelled as contraindicated in children under 12 years old, unless specifically indicated (as in juvenile arthritis), and is now not recommended for adolescents or young adults except on medical advice.

rheumatoid arthritis
is a type of arthritis (joint inflammation) in which the joints of the body, particularly of the fingers, wrists and toes, become stiff, swollen, painful and eventually deformed. It is progressive, but periodic and quite different from **osteoarthritis**. Treatment is by NSAIDS, CORTICOSTEROID drugs, IMMUNOSUPPRESSANT drugs and a number of other drugs.

rhinitis
is an inflammation of the mucous membrane that lines the nose, resulting in nasal congestion and a running nose. Allergic rhinitis is associated with an allergic reaction, commonly to inhaled pollens (eg hay fever), and this can be treated with ANTIHISTAMINE, ANTI-ALLERGIC and NASAL DECONGESTANT drugs, often in the form of nasal sprays or drops. There are a number of other forms of rhinitis characterized by a hypersensitivity (vasomotor rhinitis), and some of these may be precipitated by cold, foodstuffs, pregnancy and some drugs (eg NSAIDS).

rINN
see **recommended International Non-proprietary Name**.

routes of administration of drugs
is how drugs are taken. Some common routes include: intravascular injection or infusion (into the blood vessels) mainly intravenous (into veins) but sometimes intra-arterial (into arteries), intramuscular (injection into muscles), subcutaneous (injection beneath the dermis of the skin), intradermal (injection into the skin), transdermal (across the skin; eg from skin patches), topical (application to skin or mucous membranes), per rectum (by an ointment or suppository into the rectum), intravaginally (by an ointment or pessary into the vagina), intrathecal (by injection into the subarachnoid space of the spinal cord), intranasally (often as a spray or drops), orally (by mouth), by inhalation and many other routes.

salt
means, chemically, a compound formed from a chemical reaction between an acid and a base (eg sodium chloride). Many drugs, including all ALKALOID drugs, are bases, and in this form are sometimes oils or crystals that are relatively insoluble in water; so they are used in medicine largely after being chemically changed to salts that are water-soluble (eg hydrochloride, sulphate, tartrate, phosphate). Other drugs (eg the BARBITURATE drugs, HEPARIN, NSAIDS) are acids, so are used in the form of sodium (or potassium) salts. Also, most ANTACID agents are alkaline salts that work by neutralizing excess acid.

sarcoma
is a malignant type of **neoplasm**, a cancerous growth, which arises in the connective tissue in virtually any organ of the body. See also **carcinoma**.

selectivity
of drug action is where at a given concentration a given drug acts preferentially on one receptor (see **receptors**) or tissue, and this helps minimize side-effects.

self-medication
is the use of a medicine without the intervention of a doctor, though commonly with the advice of a pharmacist, normally with OTC (available 'over-the-counter') medicines.

sickle-cell disease (or sickle-cell anaemia)
is a hereditary blood disease that occurs mostly in black people and some people of Mediterranean and Indian origin, and is caused in the child when both parents carry the defective gene. In this disease the red blood cells (erythrocytes) are abnormal, containing an abnormal form of **haemoglobin**, and cause a serious form of **anaemia**, where sickle-shaped erythrocytes are formed (sickling) when the blood is deprived of oxygen, and these cells are removed from the circulation causing jaundice and anaemia. Treatment is supportive, with supplements of FOLIC ACID, ANTIBIOTIC drugs and oxygen therapy.

side-effect
of a drug is an unwanted effect, but is dose-related and normally predictable (sometimes unavoidable). The term normally is used for relatively trivial

unwanted actions of drugs (eg dry mouth) rather than potentially serious **adverse drug reactions.**

skeletal muscle
is the type of striated muscle that makes up the majority of the musculature of the body. It is attached to the skeleton and is responsible for the movement of limbs, for breathing, etc. Nerve supply is by cholinergic fibres of the somatic (voluntary) nervous system, so the muscle is caused to contract by acetylcholine and blocked by one class of ANTICHOLINERGIC drugs.

slow acetylators
are individuals with an inherited condition where an enzyme that breaks down drugs within the body has low activity, so it is important that lower doses of such drugs (eg ISONIAZID) are taken by people with this disorder.

smooth muscle (involuntary muscle; plain muscle) unlike striated muscle has no cross-striations under the microscope, indicating an organization characteristic of muscle controlled by the autonomic nervous system, and reacting more slowly to neurotransmitters than the striated muscle controlled by the voluntary nervous system.

spasm
is an involuntary strong contraction of a muscle. In the **skeletal muscle** of the body the cause may be local (eg certain cramps) or from within the **central nervous system** (eg hiccups, tics, tetany). In **smooth muscle**, the cause may be an imbalance within the **autonomic nervous system** or the release of local hormones (eg colic, **asthma, Raynaud's disease/ syndrome**). Treatment depends on its cause.

specificity
of a drug's action is the goal of **pharmacology** (not yet been achieved), where a given drug acts on only one receptor (see **receptors**) or tissue. In practice some drugs do achieve a high selectivity.

status asthmaticus
means a prolonged asthmatic attack lasting days without any recovery period. It is regarded as a medical emergency, often treated with oxygen, intravenous BRONCHODILATOR, STEROID or RESPIRATORY STIMULANT drugs (eg DOXAPRAM HYDROCHLORIDE).

status epilepticus
see **epilepsy.**

striated muscle
is any muscle type showing cross-striations under the microscope, and includes **skeletal muscle** and **cardiac muscle**, but not **smooth muscle.**

sublingual
is a mode of administration where **tablets** are held under the tongue, from where the active constituents (eg NITRATE drugs) are absorbed into the blood circulation in that region of the mouth, and thence into the **systemic** circulation.

superinfection
is a second infection that occurs when the first is being treated. The second may be a drug-resistant strain of the first, a new pathogenic organism, or a proliferation of an existing organism that is non-pathogenic under normal circumstances. A common instance is development of candidiasis (thrush) yeast infection of mouth, anus or vagina after treatment with oral TETRACYCLINES (ANTIBIOTIC drugs).

suppository
is a drug preparation formulated into a bullet-shaped plug for insertion into the rectum. (The form used for the vagina is specifically termed **pessary.**) The active drugs may have a local action (eg LOCAL ANAESTHETIC or CORTICOSTEROID drugs) when used to treat **haemorrhoids**, or be designed for a systemic action (eg ANTI-ASTHMATIC and ANALGESIC drugs) after absorption into the bloodstream (when oral administration is not suitable).

sustained-release preparations
see **modified-release preparations.**

sympathetic nervous system
see **autonomic nervous system.**

syncope
means fainting, a temporary loss of consciousness due to decreased blood supply to the brain. It can have a number of causes including as a **side-effect** of drugs (especially ANTIHYPERTENSIVE drugs).

syndrome
is a collection of signs and symptoms that, in occurring together, constitute a given disease.

synergism
is where the combined effects of two drugs is more than simply additive.

syrup
is a concentrated or aqueous solution sweetened

with sugar or some other substance. It may be used for a local soothing effect on the throat, or to disguise the taste of drugs.

systemic
means affecting the whole body rather than a specific part of it. In the case of systemic administration of a drug (in contrast to **local** administration) it means that the drug gains access to the general or systemic circulation (which includes administration by injection, and the oral route for those drugs that are absorbed). Systemic side-effects are usually taken to mean those affecting structures outside the **central nervous system**. See **routes of administration of drugs**.

tablets
are solid drug dose forms made of compressed powder, usually in a rounded disc form, though sometimes in a longer shape similar to **capsules**. They have now largely superseded **pills**. Tablets may be soluble, effervescent, dispersible, coated or uncoated, enteric-coated (to survive through the stomach) or modified-release (see **modified-release preparations**).

tachycardia
is an increase in the rate of heartbeat above normal. See also **arrhythmias**.

tardive dyskinesia
is a syndrome with abnormality of movement (particularly of the face, tongue, jaws and limbs) characteristic of long-term use of antipsychotic drugs, such as PHENOTHIAZINE agents, working as DOPAMINE-RECEPTOR ANTAGONIST drugs. See **extrapyramidal symptoms**.

thalassaemia
is a group of inherited blood disorders that occur mostly in people of Mediterranean, Middle Eastern and Southeast Asian origin, and is caused (in two different forms) in the child when one or both parents carry the defective gene. In thalassaemia, many of the red blood cells (erythrocytes) are fragile, and are broken up resulting in haemolytic **anaemia** and iron overload in internal organs (haemosiderosis). Treatment is by whole blood transfusion and bone-marrow transplant. The iron overload can be helped with iron CHELATING AGENT drugs which promote excretion.

therapeutics
is the branch of medicine concerned with the treatment of disease. Intervention may be curative (eg use of ANTIBIOTIC drugs against infections), suppressive (eg use of INSULIN to maintain diabetics) or prophylactic (eg CHLOROQUINE for malaria).

therapeutic trial
see **clinical trial**.

thrombocytopenia
is a reduction in the number of blood platelets in the body. Because of the important role of these cells in the formation of blood clots, there may be abnormal bleeding in thrombocytopenia. There are a number of causes, including as an adverse reaction to treatment with certain drugs (eg PHENYLBUTAZONE, SULPHONAMIDE drugs, TETRACYCLINES, OESTROGEN drugs and (thiazide) DIURETIC drugs).

thrombosis
is formation of a blood thrombus (clot) within an intact vessel. A number of factors can increase clot formation, including obstruction or damage to blood vessels, and contact of blood with certain surfaces. Thrombosis in blood vessels leads to impaired blood supply and resultant **anoxia**, causing in arteries of the heart coronary thrombosis (see **myocardial infarction**) or, in the brain, stroke. Thrombosis in veins is associated with the inflammation of phlebitis and phlebothrombosis. When the thrombus becomes dislodged it may become lodged elsewhere. Drugs of both the ANTICOAGULANT and ANTIPLATELET types can be used to prevent clot formation in those at risk. See also **embolism**.

thyrotoxicosis
see **goitre**.

tinctures
are alcoholic extracts from plants, or solutions of drugs.

tinnitus
means an abnormal noise in the ear (commonly a ringing or buzzing). It may be caused by inner-ear disease, various neurological disturbances, or as a side-effect of a variety of drugs (notably including QUININE).

tolerance
is a diminished response to a drug due to prior (normally **chronic**) exposure.

topical
application of a drug means that the drug is applied to the body's surface, usually the skin, as an

ointment, lotion, spray etc. See also **routes of administration of drugs**.

toxicity

in general is a poisonous or toxic property in a chemical. In relation to drugs, the term applies particularly to **adverse drug reactions**.

toxin

means a toxic product (usually a protein or polypeptide) produced by pathogenic micro-organisms, particularly bacteria, and responsible for some of the pathological symptoms of infection. The term is sometimes extended to toxic products of higher organisms, for instance ALKALOID agents produced by plants (eg VINCA ALKALOIDS). See **exotoxin**; **endotoxin**; **toxoids**. See also ANTITOXIN.

toxoids

are extracts of detoxified exotoxins (suspensions containing extracts of the toxins released by the invading organism), which can be used to manufacture vaccines for use in IMMUNIZATION, and they work by stimulating the formation of antibodies against the toxin of the disease, rather than the organism itself (DIPHTHERIA VACCINE, TETANUS VACCINE).

tumor

is swelling, and is one of the classical signs of inflammation in a tissue. The other signs are calor (heat), rubor (redness) and dolor (pain). The swelling is due not to a growth of cell numbers or size (as is usual for tumours: see **tumour**), but to the collection of fluid between the cells.

tumour

is any abnormal swelling in any part of the body, usually with a rapid increase in the number of cells. The term can be applied to fairly harmless swelling (benign) or cancerous (**malignant**) growths. See also **cancer**.

ulcerative colitis

see **colitis**.

unlicensed use

see **licence**.

urinogenital tract

see **genitourinary tract**.

urogenital tract

see **genitourinary tract**.

urticaria

is a common skin condition (also known as nettle rash or hives) characterized by raised usually itchy wheals. It usually occurs only for a few hours, but may reoccur. It is seen in some disease states, including **angioedema**. Commonly it is caused by an allergic reaction to foodstuffs (eg shellfish, eggs or nuts), food additives (eg tartrazine) or drugs (eg PENICILLIN OR ASPIRIN). Treatment is with ANTIHISTAMINE drugs or, if severe, a CORTICOSTEROID.

vagovagal attacks

are a marked slowing of the heartbeat due to overactivity of the vagal nerve. They are often associated with anxiety.

vasoconstriction

is a narrowing of blood vessels; see VASOCONSTRICTOR.

vasodilatation

is a widening of blood vessels; see VASODILATOR.

withdrawal syndrome

is where abrupt withdrawal of a drug causes a characteristic syndrome, often with both physical and psychological discomfort or illness. Often the withdrawal effects are the opposite of those of initial use of the drug, and may be incurred both by medical and nonmedical use of drugs. Drugs especially noted for serious withdrawal syndromes include OPIOID drugs, BARBITURATE drugs, BENZODIAZEPINE drugs, amphetamine, COCAINE and NICOTINE. Treatment may consist of adoption of a gradual, rather than abrupt, withdrawal; or substitution of another or weaker drug (eg METHADONE HYDROCHLORIDE for MORPHINE SULPHATE).